Comprehensive
Dental Hygiene Care

Comprehensive
Dental Hygiene
Care

THIRD EDITION

Irene R. Woodall
R.D.H., M.A., Ph.D.

Clinical Associate Professor, Department of Dental Hygiene, University of Colorado School of Dentistry, Denver, CO; and Director, Clinical Studies, Vipont Pharmaceutical, Inc., Fort Collins, CO

Bonnie R. Dafoe
R.D.H., B.S.

Formerly Clinical Instructor, School of Dental Hygiene, University of Michigan, Ann Arbor, Michigan

Nancy Stutsman Young
R.D.H., M.Ed.

Assistant Professor, Dental Hygiene Program, Indiana University School of Dentistry, Indianapolis, Indiana

Leslie Weed-Fonner
R.D.H., M.Ed., M.S.W.

Coordinator, Community Services of Bangkok, Bangkok, Thailand

Samuel L. Yankell
Ph.D., R.D.H.

Research Professor, Department of Periodontics, University of Pennsylvania School of Dental Medicine, Philadelphia, Pennsylvania

with **781** illustrations and **4** color plates

THE C. V. MOSBY COMPANY

ST. LOUIS • BALTIMORE • PHILADELPHIA • TORONTO • 1989

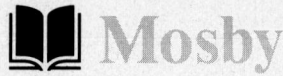 Mosby

Editor: Robert W. Reinhardt
Assistant editor: Maureen Slaten
Project manager: Patricia Gayle May
Editing/Production: Editing, Design & Production, Inc.
Designer: Liz Fett

THIRD EDITION

The C.V. Mosby Company
11830 Westline Industrial Drive, St. Louis, Missouri 63146

Library of Congress Cataloging in Publication Data

Comprehensive dental hygiene care / Irene R. Woodall . . . [et al.]—
   3rd ed.
      p. cm.
   Includes bibliographies and index.
   ISBN 0-8016-5661-3
   1. Dental hygiene.   I. Woodall, Irene R. (Irene Rita)
II. Title: Dental hygiene care.
   [DNLM: 1. Dental Prophylaxis.   WU 113 C737]
RK60.7.C65 1989
617.6′01—dc19
DNLM/DLC
for Library of Congress   88-29132
                                                         CIP

C/RRD/RRD   9   8   7   6   5   4   3   2

The chapter on restorative procedures is a revised, condensed version of Operative Dentistry Procedures for Dental Auxiliaries, The C.V. Mosby Company, 1981, and was written by:

Eric E. Spohn, D.D.S.
Professor, Department of Oral Health Science and Director, Dental Auxiliary Training Programs, University of Kentucky, College of Dentistry

Thomas G. Berry, D.D.S., M.A.
Chairman, Department of Restorative Dentistry, University of Texas Dental School at San Antonio, San Antonio, TX

Wendy A. Halowski, DIP.D.H., B.S., M.S.
Clinical Instructor, University of British Columbia, Vancouver, B.C. Canada

Other chapters were contributed by:

Donna J. Stach, R.D.H., M.Ed.
Acting Chairman, Department of Dental Hygiene School of Dentistry, University of Colorado, Denver, CO

R. Hunter Rackley, R.D.H, M.H.E.
Assistant Professor, Department of Dental Hygiene, Indiana University School of Dentistry, Indianapolis, IN

Donna Karras, R.D.H., M.A., E.M.T.
Formerly, Clinical Assistant Professor, Department of Dental Hygiene, School of Dentistry, University of Colorado, Denver, CO

Jill Ann Jaroski, R.D.H., B.S.D.H.
Research Dental Hygienist, Vipont Pharmaceutical, Inc., Fort Collins, CO

Judith A. Brown, R.D.H., B.S.
Monitor, Clinical Research, Vipont Pharmaceutical, Inc., Fort Collins, CO

Carol Janz, R.D.H., B.S.
Shawn O'Neill-Hoffman, R.D.H., M.S.
Marcia Collins, M.S.
Kathleen Ross, R.D.H., B.S.
Water-Pik, Inc., Fort Collins, CO

BIOGRAPHICAL DATA

Irene R. Woodall was awarded a certificate in dental hygiene from the University of Detroit, a bachelor of science degree in social sciences and philosophy from Grand Valley State College, and a master of arts degree in communications from Western Michigan University. She holds a doctorate in organizational development from Temple University.

During the first 12 years of her career in dental hygiene, she practiced in general and periodontics practices, held a variety of offices in the Michigan and American Dental Hygienists' Associations, taught in both university and community and junior college programs, and directed the dental hygiene program at Kalamazoo Valley Community College from 1971 to 1976. She developed and chaired the program for the Third International Symposium on Dental Hygiene in 1973.

In 1976 she was appointed Assistant Professor and Chairperson of the Department of Dental Hygiene at the University of Pennsylvania and in 1977 authored her first book, *Leadership, Management, and Role Delineation: Issues for the Dental Team.* She is the author of many articles and learning packages and has taught a variety of continuing education courses and workshops, ranging from clinical instrumentation to communications skills and peer review mechanisms.

Irene is currently Director of Clinical Studies at Vipont Pharmaceutical, Inc. and holds a faculty appointment at the University of Colorado. She received the 1988 ADHA/Warner-Lambert Award for excellence in dental hygiene for her role as a change agent. Irene is Senior Editor of *RDH* magazine. She is married and has two daughters.

Bonnie R. Dafoe received her diploma in dental hygiene from the Madison Area Technical College, Madison, Wisconsin, in 1970. She was employed for 5 years as a clinical practitioner for a general dentist and for 1 year as a clinical practitioner for a pedodontist.

In 1974 she spent the summer as a clinical instructor with the Dental Hygiene Department of Guy's Hospital in London, England. In 1975, as a clinical instructor at the University of Pennsylvania, she acquired expanded function skills in periodontics, anesthesia, restorative procedures, and intraoral photography. After taking her bachelor of science degree as a summa cum laude graduate of West Chester State College in 1976, she joined the University of Pennsylvania faculty to teach local anesthesia, dental health education, preclinic, periodontics, and intraoral photography in addition to clinical instruction.

Bonnie has given continuing education courses for the University of Pennsylvania and the Philadelphia component of the American Dental Hygienists' Association.

Bonnie has recently been employed in private practice and is a member of the editorial board of *RDH* magazine. She worked as a clinical instructor at the University of Michigan, School of Dental Hygiene.

She currently resides in Pennsylvania and is pursuing a graduate degree. She is married and has two children.

Nancy Stutsman Young earned an associate degree in dental hygiene and a bachelor of science degree in dental public health from Indiana University. She received her master of education degree from Temple University.

As a full-time faculty member of the Department of Dental Hygiene at the University of Pennsylvania from 1974 to 1979, she directed a wide variety of courses and prepared numerous learning packages and related audiovisual software. She served as clinic supervisor for 2 years. She is acknowledged among the faculty members as an outstanding teacher and one who is able to integrate inquiry learning into both didactic and clinical teaching.

Nancy has also taught in a community college program and has participated in research projects at the Oral Health Research Institute, Indianapolis, Indiana. She has practiced dental hygiene in the states of Indiana, Pennsylvania, and North Carolina. Nancy has also been active in professional associations and held office in the Philadelphia component of the Americal Dental Hygienists' Association. Nancy has given a number of continuing education courses.

Nancy is currently associated with the Dental Hygiene Program at the Indiana University School of Dentistry. In addition to teaching she is actively pursuing a doctorate in Higher Education Administration at Indiana University.

Leslie Weed-Fonner graduated from Temple University's dental hygiene program and earned her bachelor of science degree from Columbia University and her master of education degree from Temple University.

She has had a variety of clinical experiences in pedodontic, general, and periodontic practices, performing both traditional dental hygiene procedures and restorative, periodontal, and local anesthesia expanded functions. As a faculty member of the Department of Dental Hygiene at the University of Pennsylvania, she taught this wide range of skills to dental hygiene students for 4 years. In 1979 Leslie coordinated the Penn-EFDA Faculty Institute I: Periodontics/Anesthesia and taught dental hygiene faculty members from a variety of institutions how to perform and teach expanded functions to their students.

She has been able to combine her interests in clinical practice and teaching with her interest (and graduate degree) in group process by team teaching courses in practice management, communications, and community dentistry externships.

After participating in a Peace Corps program in the Philippines, Leslie taught in the Department of Dental Hygiene at Fairleigh Dickinson University. She pursued her interests in group process, developed in the Philippines, by earning a master of social work degree with a major in group process from Hunter College in New York City.

Leslie is married to Michael Fonner; they have two children, Zachary and Jennifer. They currently reside in Bangkok, Thailand, where Michael is teaching and Leslie is employed as a social worker in community services.

Samuel L. Yankell received his bachelor of science degree in biology from Ursinus College and attended Rutgers University to obtain a master of science degree in physiology and a doctorate in biochemistry. He received his certificate in dental hygiene from the University of Pennsylvania. Most of his career has been in industry, beginning with a position as a senior biochemist at Colgate Palmolive. He then went to Smith, Miller and Patch as Department Head of Pharmacology and Biochemistry and then to Menley & James Laboratories, a division of SmithKline Beckman Corp., as Department Head of Biological Sciences. Since 1974 he has been at the University of Pennsylvania in the Department of Periodontics. Although his primary efforts have been in research, he has lectured in biochemistry and nutrition in the dental hygiene program and was responsible for the graduate dental education course on new advances in cariology.

He is a member of many scientific organizations, including the American Association for the Advancement of Science, the American Chemical Society, the American Society for Pharmacology and Experimental Therapeutics, the European Organization for Caries Research, the International Association for Dental Research, the Society of Toxicology, and Sigma Xi. He has authored more than 200 publications in the scientific literature.

He is married to Kuna Yankell; they have two sons and a daughter and two granddaughters.

TO

My brothers, *Richard D.* and *William R. Zimmerman,* who taught me about competition and to have high expectations of myself; my mother, *Augusta V. Doktor,* who taught me how to respect my womanhood in a man's world; and my father, *William W. Zimmerman,* who taught me how to throw a ball and how to care.

IRW

My parents, *Howard and Florence Brown,* my family, *Don, Erin,* and *Andy,* and in memory of a dedicated community dentist and friend, *Dr. Jack Voll.*

BRD

Phil, with all my love, for his patience, endurance, support, and love.

NSY

Michael, Zachary, and *Jessica.*

LWF

Kuna for her continued patience, understanding, and help; to *Sandra Scott* and the general office staff; and to *Irene Woodall* for her patience.

SLY

PREFACE

We originally prepared this text to bring together our collective experiences and philosophies with regard to teaching and learning clinical dental hygiene in the hope that dental hygiene can continue to grow in degree of responsibility and participation among the health care professions. The scope of the text; the emphasis on goal orientation, mastery learning, and the use of a variety of learning strategies; the sequence of skill development; the integration of behavioral and basic science principles with clinical skill development; the overlay of a program of care for individual patients using the theme of assessment-planning-implementation-evaluation; and the focus on the patient as a partner in care are the unique elements of the text and represent our collective teaching experiences over the past two decades.

This third edition is enhanced by our collective growth and diversity over the past ten years—as practitioners, educators, writers, researchers, social scientists, and as people. We also have included several other educators for selected chapters to ensure that the most up-to-date expertise was brought together to prepare this text. We have, of course, updated the content and philosophy to reflect new research findings and trends and dental hygiene practice. We have added to or expanded most chapters and have added to the color plates to provide better visualization of changes in hard and soft tissues. You will find an increased emphasis upon antimicrobial and irrigation adjunctive therapy for periodontal care as these trends continue to be studied and included in routine practice. The chapter on fluorides is expanded and updated to reflect the wide range of fluoride therapies available, the increased emphasis upon safety, and the trend toward frequent, low doses of fluoride, rather than infrequent high concentrations. While we always placed great emphasis on infection control, this edition goes even further in recommending impeccable control procedures to protect you and your patients. We hope these changes will help you learn together

and stimulate you to read the literature as research findings add to what is written in this text.

A review of the table of contents should reveal that some elements of clinical practice either not typically included or not extensively developed in other texts receive considerable attention in *Comprehensive Dental Hygiene Care*. Examples are the chapters relating to comprehensive periodontal assessment, involving the patient in learning self-assessment of oral health, planning for care, ultrasonic scaling devices, intraoral photography, pain control in dental hygiene care, case documentation, and integrating dental hygiene principles in dental practice. The content of this text reflects a substantial reliance on basic and behavioral science research as it relates to dentistry in particular and health care in general.

In addition to the content, which should support both the needs of preclinical courses and the various stages of advanced clinical learning, the *sequence* of material can be readily adapted to preclinical and subsequent courses. This sequence was developed to facilitate the use of goal orientation—for the students to begin to feel participation in and ownership of the goals of the course. The constant theme or goal of the early chapters is preparation for competent and confident clinical practice. The target or goal is the "first day" of clinic when a trusting patient appears for care. The faculty member's function is to present that day as the reason for preclinical learning and to present each chapter as one means, in tandem with classroom and clinical activities, for mastering each step along the way toward *providing the care appropriate for the patient*. Thus the first chapters are devoted to "preparing the site" so that students can operate and maintain the equipment that supports the delivery of care. The student is also prepared with the introduction to sterilization and to the prevention of cross-contamination. Later chapters introduce the student to the care of the patient, beginning with the health history and including identifying and responding to medical emergencies. Time is set aside to learn positioning at the chair and basic principles of instrumentation to facilitate sit-down, four-handed procedures and to enable students to perform the subsequent assessment steps of intraoral and extraoral examinations and chartings. Rather than teach instrumentation skills as a separate, parallel laboratory experience, we recommend teaching these techniques as a part of the material in each chapter. Once the students have gained basic competence in position, grasp, stroke, and wrist motion, they can refine and develop those skills while actually observing and recording clinical data for student partners (or patients of more advanced students). The purposeful, goal-directed use of probes and explorers seems to hasten the development of basic skills. The significance of acquiring good instrumentation skills cannot easily escape the awareness of a student who is learning to use instruments to prepare a pocket depth or caries charting.

As basic skills develop, instruments with contraangles, blades, and other features requiring greater skill development in line angle adaptation, insertion, angulation, and working stroke are introduced for continued practice. Student partners can serve an important role in developing these skills in instrumentation but cannot in many instances satisfy the need for students to find a deep pocket; observe varieties of calculus; compare tissue color, texture, shape, and consistency; and remove deposits. For those students whose partners exhibit high levels of oral health, it is particularly helpful to be paired with an advanced student who is providing care for patients with evidence of disease. An important phase of development is to see the range of cases, from health through subtle change to advanced disease.

Depending on the philosophy of the dental hygiene program, the teaching of some chapters may be delayed until the student is further along in training. Examples are ultrasonic instrumentation, curettage, and periodontal dressings.

Thus one important theme is the preparation for the "first day" of clinic as a confident and competent clinician. As each chapter is concluded, the students should ask themselves if they are ready to perform the newly acquired skills as an entry-level clinician. While some anxiousness may be felt by the students, they should begin to feel that they *can* perform basic skills safely, particularly as they practice and use each skill during preclinical education and later during "in clinic" sessions where basic skills can be developed into varying degrees of refined expertise.

A second goal orientation of preclinical learning integrated in the text that tends to increase the interest of students in their learning is that many chapters prepare the student not only for clinic, but also for additional course work in the program. The chapter on emergencies, for example, serves as an introduction to complete courses in cardiopulmonary resuscitation, first aid, and pharmacology. The chapter on health histories is a prelude to pathology and many of the basic sciences. The sequences on examination and periodontal care prepare the student for periodontics, pathology, and chemistry courses. Pointing out their relevance can facilitate positive anticipation of later course work.

The structure of each chapter makes it possible to develop shorter-range goal achievement as well. A list of suggested objectives is provided, which should be discussed with the students. They may be altered, deleted, or expanded on as a result of the discussion. In inquiry learning, the faculty member may ask the students to develop their own objectives. Comparing their objectives with the chapters' may stimulate discussion and problem-solving sessions. Content in a narrative format follows the objectives. Suggested activities and review questions follow the content. It should not be necessary to conduct formal lectures or presentations for each chapter if the students have sound reading comprehension skills. Other than a few points of clarification being offered or a piece of recent research being explained, the lecture can be replaced by class activities that tend to develop a higher level of cognitive and affective learning. Search and discovery, problem solving, case analysis, values clarification, small-group tasks, role play, inquiry, and guided discussion should be useful techniques for maximizing the opportunity for growth that is available when a class of students is together. Active involvement of the students with each other as they *use* the content of the chapters enhances their acceptance of the basic principles of dental hygiene as their own and stimulates their ability to think, create, and investigate.

In addition to its broad scope of content and its goal orientation approach, *Comprehensive Dental Hygiene Care* is organized around the program development model of assessment-planning-implementation-evaluation. Although this model has been employed in community program development for years, its usefulness in clinical, one-to-one health care designs is not widely reflected in clinical dental hygiene references. We believe this model has great relevance in providing individual patient care and that its application in clinical care ensures a well-informed, logical approach to improving health status and to preserving the challenge and stimulation, as well as the gratification, of being a practicing dental hygienist.

One additional theme that is constant in the text is that of the patient as a partner in care—as a person involved in care. We believe that care is not done *to* the patient or *on* the patient but rather *for* and *with* the patient. This stance is based on a wealth of behavioral science research and on personal humanistic philosophies that identify the need for active, rewarding involvement as a corequisite for positive, long-term change. The current emphasis on prevention and self-care models in health care draws on these principles of human behavior. In addition, we believe that a major source of satisfaction in health care delivery is the warmth and caring that emanates from an accepting, egalitarian relationship between the helper and the helped.

Our best wishes are yours as you teach and learn together as the helper and the helped. We welcome your responses and your suggestions.

IRENE R. WOODALL
BONNIE R. DAFOE
NANCY STUTSMAN YOUNG
LESLIE WEED-FONNER
SAMUEL L. YANKELL

Acknowledgments for first edition

Many people contributed their efforts to make the final preparation of the manuscript possible. Conrad Woodall, Phil Young, and Kuna Yankell were invaluable in our times of greatest need, not only with their support, but also with their willingness to type, duplicate, collate, proofread, and visit the post office and the office supply and photographic stores. Don Dafoe was especially helpful in his review of the chapters on health history and emergency procedures. Sally Verity's review of the chapters on comprehensive charting was also particularly helpful. Jan Griffin and Susan Muhler deserve a thank you for finding rare equipment items for our use.

The word processing staff, Catherine Redden, Delores DiCocco, Patricia DeVuono, and Julia Marguilles, were invaluable in their preparation of the final manuscript, especially in May and June, 1979. Emily Mintz deserves a thank you for her contribution in typing tables and letters for us.

We also wish to thank Michael Schwager for his advice and efforts in meeting our most critical photographic needs. We wish to acknowledge the case documentation prepared by Deborah Drazek while she was a student at the University of Pennsylvania and the role she, Diana Mumma, and Sharon Herr played in photograph preparation. Rosemarie Valentine's leadership and efforts in developing learning materials for the department are also gratefully acknowledged. Slides prepared by Mary Robb Gross and Catherine Schifter were especially helpful in showing the use of Gracey instruments, and we thank our colleagues for sharing them with us.

Elissa Berardi, our medical illustrator, worked long and hard to prepare the many detailed drawings for the text. Her work is beautifully done and reflects a great deal of caring for the quality of the project.

We also owe thanks to all the participants in the Penn-EFDA Faculty Institute I: Periodontics/Anesthesia for their continuous support and for sharing in the excitement during the final weeks of our efforts. We shall never forget Sue Agostini, Regina Byrne, Sue Colangelo, Sue Daniel, Kandie Dautel, Mary Ann Haag, Gwen Hlava, Joyce Jenzano, JoAnne Karr, Jane Emerson Knight, Joan Madden, Pat Mulford, Lin Nassar, Joan Gluch-Scranton, Maureen Pratt Smith, and Debbie Vlanis.

Acknowledgments for second edition

Once again, many people helped us in preparing the manuscript and in ensuring that the time and moral support were there when we needed them most. We offer our heartfelt thanks and appreciation.

For their reviews of the first edition—Phyllis Beemsterboer, Debbie Brown, Sherry Castle Harfst, Ralph Lobene, Hunter Rackley, Patricia Randolph, Karen Ridley, Ellen Rogo, and Joan Gluch Scranton.

For his review of the intraoral photography chapter—Clifford L. Freehe; and for his review of the medical history and emergencies chapters—Donald C. Dafoe.

For their assistance in locating references—Sue Seeger and Ruth Cressman at the University of Michigan dental library and Kathy Marousek, Helen Itkin, and Dorothea Colburn at the Fairleigh Dickinson dental library.

For their outstanding photographic assistance—Bonnie Dafoe, William Prior, Catherine Schifter, David Sullivan, and Robert Benedon; and for the beautiful new illustrations—Elissa Berardi.

For giving permission to use the Fairleigh Dickinson School of Dentistry facilities—Richard Oglesby.

For the index preparation and service as a photographic model—Conrad Woodall.

For the much needed time to write—Michael Fonner and Dani Kazista.

For continuing support during the project—the dental hygiene faculty at the Fairleigh Dickinson University (especially Ellen Rogo and Cheryl Westphal) and at the University of Pennsylvania (Catherine Schifter, Kate Fitzgerald, Jean Byrnes, Charlotte Hangorsky, Roberta Throne, Joyce Levy, and Joanne Prifti, and Janet Yellowitz).

For their consistent, helpful presence and support in every way during this project—Conrad Woodall, Kuna Yankell, and Phil Young.

Acknowledgments for third edition

The authors wish to thank:

For outstanding photographic assistance: *Mike Halloran, Tom Berry,* and *Dennis Thompson.*

For their patient assistance as photographic models: *Philip Young, Janet Mulherin,* and *Jennifer* and *Jonathan Tilliss.*

For assistance in reviewing and revising chapters: *Michael Sabat, Lynda Sabat, Joan Gluch Scranton, Jaclyn Gleber, Pauline Spencer, Donna Stach,* and *Sherry Harfst.*

For use of beautiful clinical facilities: the Thomas Jefferson University School of Allied Health Services, Philadelphia, PA and the University of Colorado School of Dentistry, Denver, CO.

For the latest computer skills in locating references and other research assistance: *Sherry Montgomery,* Librarian, University of Pennsylvania, School of Dental Medicine, Philadelphia, PA.

For library search services: *Conrad Woodall.*

For her wonderful talents in illustration (and music): *Elissa Berardi.*

For her assistance in manuscript preparations: *Catherine Reddon.*

For moral support and assistance with a perpetual series of details: *Diane Ware, Barb Jones,* and *Lynn Brown.*

To the authors of selected chapters for their efforts, quality work, and timeliness: *Eric Spohn, Tom Berry, Wendy Halowski, Jill Jaroski, Jan Brown, Donna Karras, Donna Stach, Hunter Rackley, Carol Janz, Shawn O'Neill-Hoffman, Marcia Collins,* and *Kathleen Ross.*

CONTENTS

Comprehensive
Dental Hygiene Care

PART ONE

PREPARATION AND ASSESSMENT

Imagine that you are anticipating the arrival of your first dental hygiene patient. What would you need to have learned to provide meaningful, helpful care to the person looking to you with trust? This text is designed to help you, the new clinician, be ready when that day arrives. This portion of the text covers the fundamental skills you must master before you see a patient. It is important to know how to operate the equipment you will have at your fingertips. You need to know how to keep from cross-infecting your patients with microorganisms brought to your operatory and how to protect yourself from infection. You also need to know how to find your way through the preparation of a dental record, how to position yourself and the patient for maximum comfort and efficiency, how to hold and use instruments, and how to prepare for a medical emergency.

The first chapter introduces dental hygiene: what it has been, is, and could be. The following chapters provide the rationale, the procedures, and related information for each of the skills mentioned above and others. Once this information has been mastered, the beginning clinician should be ready to greet a patient and begin assessing the patient's health needs.

In the development of any program or project, it is wise to take time to *assess* the situation. Moving directly to implementation without taking time to determine the reasons for the project or the unique needs of the persons for whom the project is being developed can cause considerable difficulty, delay progress, or cause ultimate failure of the project. Even the best efforts in implementation can be fraught with difficulty if these efforts are aimed at nonexistent needs or at needs that the subjects of the project do not wish to have modified. A more scientific approach to project development is to set aside assumptions and personal beliefs about needs and reasons for a project and investigate objective data from which reasons can be inferred.

Assessment includes not only objective data, but also the more subjective responses and feelings of the people for whom or with whom the project will be carried out. Even though objective signs are clear indicators of the need for change, subjective responses may override those indicators. People may not want change, or they may want change to be gradual.

In providing clinical care for patients, the principle of assessment is particularly important. Assessment data provide the baseline information for determining the general and oral health status of each patient and provide the dental professional with the opportunity to evalutate the patient's perceptions of the need or desire for change. Assessment can prevent, or help the provider anticipate, emergency situations; it can allow for the individualization of care; it provides baseline data for comparing progress and outcomes with the entering status of the patient; and it allows for rational planning.

The following chapters help clinicians prepare the clinical site and practice assessment skills with patients.

1 DENTAL HYGIENE PRACTICE

OBJECTIVES: *The reader will be able to*

1. Define a philosophy of patient-centered care.
2. Identify examples of patient-hygienist interactions that reflect the philosophy of patient-centered care.
3. Identify his or her own reasons for selecting dental hygiene as a profession.
4. Define his or her own entering expectations of dental hygiene education and of dental hygiene practice.
5. Explain why the perceptions and expectations of faculty members may differ from those of students.
6. Identify changes that occurred in the 1960s and 1970s that had a major effect on the scope of dental hygiene practice.
7. Describe the effect of state dental practice acts on the scope of practice and educational programs.
8. Identify all the procedures in each of the four phases of program development—assessment, planning, implementation, and evaluation—that a dental hygienist may perform in helping meet patient needs.
9. Define *professional culture*.
10. List at least 10 key components of dental hygiene's professional culture.

This text was written to prepare dental hygiene students for clinical practice. Its primary goal is to help students feel confident and competent on their first day of clinical practice and gain personal satisfaction from understanding how dental hygiene care contributes to the well-being of the people they serve.

The early chapters introduce the student, step by step, to the sequence of procedures typically followed in the comprehensive dental hygiene appointment plan. Later chapters address more advanced clinical skills and provide guidelines for integrating ideal principles of care into a realistic practice environment.

The philosophy of patient-centered care is integrated into each phase of care. The patient is viewed as the partner in care, involved extensively in decision making and in the self-care components necessary for restoring and maintaining the patient's oral health. The mastery of technical procedures is emphasized in the individual chapters to ensure safe and effective therapy. But in each instance the *need* for the procedure and the *way* in which the *patient* is involved in the procedure are critical components of developing the relative role of technical skill in dental hygiene care.

Many beginning students see the profession of dental hygiene as being founded on this service orientation, which is the philosophic basis for patient-centered care. For those students, the text should enhance that approach to learning dental hygiene care. Other new students, whose exposure to the profession has been somewhat limited, may focus largely on the technical components of dental hygiene practice. For those, the text should help develop a more comprehensive approach to dental hygiene care.

Additionally, this book was written to help prepare students for future roles in health care delivery by introducing a flexible approach to patient care and by introducing controversies regarding the efficacy of time-honored practice procedures.

MOTIVATIONS FOR SELECTING DENTAL HYGIENE

Persons select dental hygiene as a career for many different reasons. The initial interest of some students is derived from their own encounters with dentistry and and dental hygiene. They may have learned as patients to respect and enjoy the people in the dental office. Some students may see the traditional white garb as a sign of status and achievement. In selecting a career, students may consider the clean, reasonably relaxed atmosphere to be an attractive working environment. Students who were visited by the school dental hygienist each year may identify with the relative independence of the person who travels from school to school helping young people improve their oral health. As with most professions, a family tradition in dentistry or dental hygiene may be a major determining factor. Growing up around a dental office can have a significant effect on career awareness and interest. For some students, careful career counseling and information programs may be the reason for selecting dental hygiene.

EXPECTATIONS FOR PRACTICE

When considering a career in dental hygiene, most applicants have a few common needs or expectations. When asked what special characteristics a dental hygienist should have to function well, most students identify the ability to work well with people and the ability to use their hands. They expect to earn a reasonable income, to work in pleasant surroundings, to have flexibility in scheduling, to have the respect of the patient, and to help people. When the functional role of the dental hygienist is addressed, most see the primary duties to be "cleaning teeth" and "teaching people how to care for their teeth." Most applicants expect to work with a dentist in private practice.

There are, of course, some students whose expectations are quite different from these. Varying perceptions may result from a quite different exposure to the profession or, perhaps, to misinformation.

However, it is critical that any incoming student have clear, specific expectations and perceptions of the profession and of his or her expected performance in the educational program. Sharing these perceptions with each other and exchanging perceptions with the faculty members can be an enlightening experience and one that can prevent or at least reduce conflict. A student who expects to learn one thing but is constantly expected to learn another can experience anxiety. The knowledge that different persons can have widely varying expectations can help reduce the frustrations for a student.

Usually the more extensive exposure of dental hygiene faculty members to the profession has altered their initial perceptions of dental hygiene. A faculty member has had an opportunity to compare expectations with reality and to develop an educational approach that blends the ideal with the real. Faculty members may vary greatly with regard to their respective perceptions. Whereas one faculty member may relate primarily to practical applications of skill, another may strive to preserve ideal, conceptual approaches to patient care with a strong basic and behavioral science foundation. Still other faculty members may see their role as one of preparing hygienists for the future—dental hygiene as it "ought" to be rather than as it is.

CHANGES IN THE PROFESSION
Legal and educational changes

Many of these varying perceptions, whether among faculty or students, are due to the rapid changes that have taken place in the profession since the early 1960s. After several decades of slow—at times imperceptible—change, the profession encountered the era of "expanded functions" and the challenge of defining how its members could maintain or alter their role.

Before the flurry of debate of the 1960s, dental hygiene was for the most part practiced in solo dental practices. The role of the dental hygienist was largely defined as oral prophylaxis, patient education, and the exposing of radiographs. Particularly in the east, hygienists were employed in school systems providing dental health education, prophylaxis, and eventually fluoride treatments. (See Fig. 1-1 for a view of a school-based clinic in the early days of dental hygiene.)

The events of the 1960s and 1970s helped revise that relatively narrow scope of practice. In *Survey of Dentistry*, Hollinshead (1961) describes

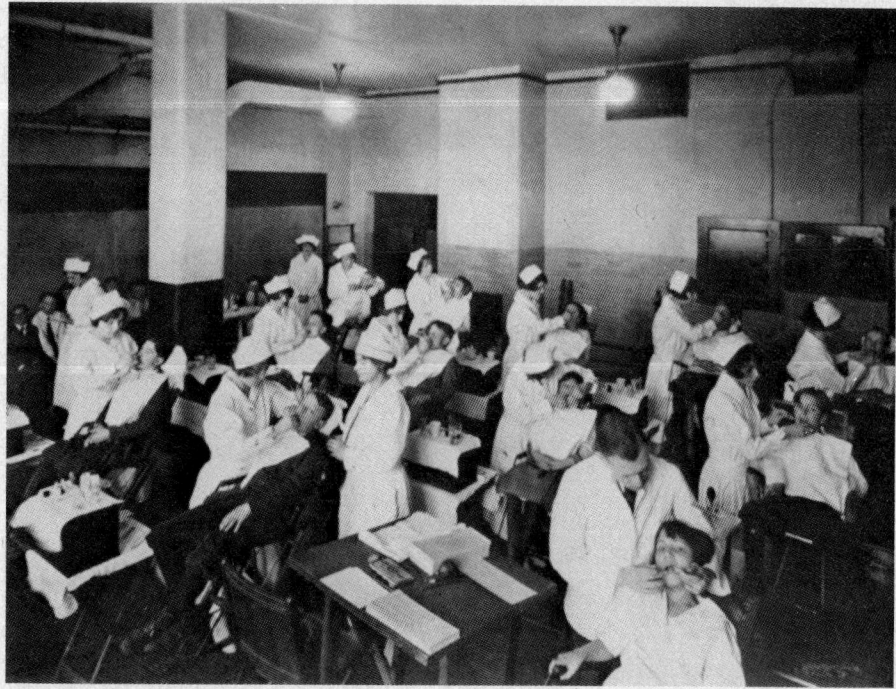

Fig. 1-1. Students in early 1900s of the Department of Oral Hygiene, University of Pennsylvania Holding Clinic in the S. Weir Mitchell School, 50th and Kingsessing Ave., Philadelphia.

the deplorable state of our nation's oral health. Many wondered how a country that was a world leader and was investing in a major space program and providing millions of dollars in aid to foreign countries could allow its own people to have such limited access to quality dental care. President Lyndon Johnson launched his War on Poverty in the mid-1960s with a call for legislation to provide comprehensive federally funded medical care for the elderly and other needy persons. Under Medicaid, states would provide dental benefits to qualified, financially handicapped persons. In addition, numerous proposals for federally supported health care for all persons were introduced in the federal legislature, some of which included dental benefits. It seemed imminent that persons previously denied medical and dental care because of financial barriers would soon be flooding the health care delivery system.

The 1970 Carnegie Commission report stated that there would soon be a great shortage of physicians and dentists: "With the advent of national health insurance, the shortcomings in our methods of health care delivery and the critical shortages of our health manpower and facilities will become even more glaringly apparent." The Carnegie Commission's recommendation for dentistry was that "progress could be achieved through more extensive use of dentist's assistants and dental hygienists and through greater emphasis on preventive programs."

Several plans developed from this recommendation, including the allocation of federal funds to increase the number of dentists, dental hygienists, physicians, nurses, and other health care providers being prepared in educational programs. Experiments to evaluate the delegation of functions to dental assistants and dental hygienists were conducted to determine whether the dentist could be relieved of some of the clinical functions he or she typically provided. In many states, as the results of the research proved to be positive, laws were debated and changed to permit auxiliary personnel to perform additional services. Curricula in dental assisting and dental hygiene programs were altered to include the new skills and knowledge required to provide these additional services.

Although dental and medical programs expanded and support personnel for dentistry and medicine increased in number and variety, national health insurance was not enacted. In 1976 the Carnegie Council (formerly the Carnegie Commission) revised its recommendations to state that increased numbers of physicians and dentists were not needed but that the number of support personnel should continue to grow and be used to provide greater varieties of health care service.

Along with deciding which skills should be added to practice, there was considerable discussion among dental hygienists about increasing the variety of settings and the range of responsibility and decision making a hygienist might assume. In the early 1970s the American Dental Hygienists' Association defined practice sites including hospitals, geriatric centers, penal institutions, and centers for the physically and mentally handicapped as appropriate and desirable locations for serving the public. Programs of care, whether for individuals or for groups, were identifed as the function of the hygienist; these were programs in which a great deal more expertise and responsibility would be required of the hygienist (ADHA Resolutions 1971, 1973, 1975, and 1976).

The number of programs rose from 70 in 1967 (ADA annual report, 1969) to 187 in 1978. The number of graduates increased from 1739 to 4847 per year between 1967 and 1977 (ADA annual report, 1978). The functions taught in various programs ranged from the most limited scope to a full array of procedures.

Bachelor's and master's degree programs available to dental hygienists increased in number and variety. In addition to the several long-standing bachelor of science programs in which clinical dental hygiene training followed previous college education in the sciences and liberal arts, newer programs offered the dental hygienist with a certificate or associate (2-year) degree the opportunity to add new skills and knowledge and earn a bachelor of science degree. Just as the 2-year basic preparation in dental hygiene varies greatly from state to state and from program to program, the content and emphasis of the bachelor's and master's degree programs vary greatly. These degree programs may focus on teacher education, public health, oral medicine, expanded functions, research, administration, biocommunications, or any combination of these elements.

A survey reported in 1986 revealed the diversity in degree programs. Some programs focus on preparation for specific alternative career settings, others provide a curriculum that encourages students to explore a variety of settings while providing a wide array of educational opportunities in management and issues analysis, and still others provide liberal arts education (Rubinstein and Brand).

The 1960s and 1970s marked a period when the definition of legally allowable clinical skills for dental hygienists changed in a variety of ways, depending on the state. It was also a time when sites and roles were reevaluated and new emphases on comprehensive care were developed that decreased the dichotomy between the interests of the "clinical hygienist" and the "community dentistry hygienist." Conceptually, at least, dental hygiene grew in scope and responsibility, but also in complexity.

The scope of practice of dental hygienists did not expand greatly during the early 1980s. The increase in the number of dentists and hygienists was not matched by the demand in the number of persons seeking care. With no national health insurance program, the cost barrier remained for many people. This was worsened by a recession that resulted in high unemployment rates, particularly in heavily industrialized regions. Suddenly dentists and hygienists working in communities where union benefits included dental insurance had barren appointment books. Workers postponed their dental care until they were back to work and benefits were reinstated. Why discuss delegating components of care to dental auxiliaries during a slow period?

The late 1980s also provided little incentive for expanded functions. Although the economy improved in the United States, dental caries was in a state of decline, particularly among young people. The emphasis turned to periodontal disease, but not with the idea of delegating its identification and treatment to dental hygienists. Rather, dentists became interested in developing their skills to include periodontal treatment. Major strides were made to change the day-to-day practice of dental hygiene during the 1970s, but there has been no continuing effort to increase the number of functions a dental hygienist can perform. Rather, the focus of the late 1980s and the agenda for the early 1990s is to secure dental hygiene as a profession that serves a vital function in identifying, treating, and preventing disease.

Issues of professionalism include defining the appropriate minimum entry criterion for licensure. Should the baccalaureate degree represent the minimum number of years of preparation? Pressure is mounting to make the 4-year degree mandatory in order for dental hygiene to make its case as a profession (Kraemer, 1985). Even if the dual entry system is retained, it is likely that there will be an effort to redefine the skills expected of graduates of the two levels, with greater expectations of the baccalaureate hygienist (Gluch-Scranton and Rigolizzo Gurenlian, 1985) and with changes in the curriculum necessary to prepare hygienists for today's and tomorrow's employment responsibilities (Cohen et al, 1985).

Other key issues are: Must dental hygienists work under dental supervision? Should dental hygienists have their own licensing and regulatory boards? Should dental hygienists accredit their own programs? Should continuing education be mandatory? What is the scope of interest for dental hygiene research? How can dental hygienists become interested in and be supported in dental hygiene research?

Practice roles

Dental hygiene is not what it was in 1960, or so it would seem from all this discussion of changed laws, functions, education, responsibilities, and practice sites. Yet, entering students often describe the dental hygienist in terms reminiscent of the pre-1960s evolution.

After 30 years of debate and attempts at regional and national planning, each state still has its own definition of dental hygiene and assisting practice, with some duties disallowed and others permitted under varying degrees of supervision. The practice of dental hygiene differs from state to state (Table 1-1).

Educational programs differ with regard to what the students learn according to the legal definition of practice in the state in which the program is located. Therefore a program located in a state where no change in the law has occurred or where the expansion of duties is limited may include only the traditional functions of scaling, polishing, fluoride treatments, exposing radiographs, and recording the medical history and intraoral findings. In another state students may learn local anesthesia, curettage, placement of restorations, and physical evaluation.

Dental hygiene enrollment has declined steadily since its peak in 1978. The 1986 Annual Report of the American Dental Association's Council on Dental Education shows that, in 1985, enrollment equalled 82% of the 11,055 students who enrolled in 1978.

Many graduates who learned expanded functions have found that they cannot use those skills even in states where they are legally allowed. Respondents to surveys of dental hygienists show that there is a gap between the functions they learned in dental hygiene school and those they perform routinely (Heine et al, 1983; Minervini et al, 1981).

It is quite possible that one factor contributing to this occurrence is the degree to which the graduate feels competent to perform such procedures, which correlates to the number of experiences the student has had in performing the service (Boyer and Nielsen, 1985). Employers need to provide opportunities for hygienists to deliver a full range of services, but dental hygiene programs need to ensure that their graduates feel capable of performing those skills by providing sufficient clinical experiences.

Even in the 1980s approximately 90% of dental hygienists are employed in private practice (ADHA, 1982; Richards, 1984; Boyer, 1986; Cohen et al, 1987).

Forty-eight states and the District of Columbia have dental hygiene representation in varying forms (Grady, 1988), ranging from full representation with one or more voting members to a committee that "advises" the board. This is a vast improvement from 20 years ago, when few states even consulted dental hygienists regarding their regulation. However, the power of dental hygiene to influence decisions is hampered by the disproportionate number of dentists on the boards and certain limitations in voting rights and privileges.

Future changes

Some people believe that the laws will continue to be revised to expand the scope of practice but

Table 1-1. Number of states with expanded function training and examination requirements for delegating specific expanded functions to dental assistants (DA) and/or hygienists (DH) as of July 1985

	Formal training in expanded function*		State board examination required (DA)*
	DA	DH	
Make radiographs	22/46	NA	10/46
Take impressions for study casts	11/40	10/45	5/40
Place periodontal dressings	7/24	7/40	5/24
Remove periodontal and surgical dressings	9/35	7/45	5/35
Remove sutures	8/38	7/44	4/38
Apply topical anesthetic agents	6/36	NA	4/36
Inspect oral cavity	4/15	NA	2/15
Polish coronal surfaces of teeth	7/18	NA	5/18
Apply anticariogenic agents topically	9/34	8/47	3/34
Administer local anesthetic agents	0/0	9/15	0/0
Place rubber dam	11/45	5/46	6/45
Remove rubber dam	11/45	6/46	4/45
Place matrix	7/34	5/38	3/34
Remove matrix	6/31	5/34	3/31
Place temporary restorations	6/26	5/35	3/26
Remove temporary restorations	5/18	4/27	3/18
Place amalgam restorations	1/6	2/11	1/6
Carve amalgam restorations	1/7	2/10	1/7
Polish amalgam restorations	4/14	10/43	4/14
Place and finish composite, resin, or silicate cement restorations	1/6	2/9	1/6
Remove excess cement from coronal surfaces of teeth	10/39	NA	5/39
Apply pit and fissure sealants	6/13	9/42	3/13
Apply cavity liners and bases	2/8	1/17	2/8
Root plane	NA	10/41	NA
Do closed soft tissue curettage	NA	8/30	NA
Administer nitrous oxide	2/5†	3/9	1/5

From American Dental Association, Division of Educational Measurements, Council on Dental Education: Legal provisions for delegating expanded functions to dental hygienists and dental assistants, Chicago, 1985.
*The number on the right of the / is the number of jurisdictions that permit delegation of the functions. NA, Not applicable as an expanded function.
†Monitoring.

at a slower pace than in the 1960s and 1970s. They see changes tied in part to nationwide economic growth and to the resulting increased demand for care (and thus, busy dentists interested in maximizing output through delegation). Employment opportunities in a variety of settings are projected by others as being a critical source of change in responsibilities. Yet others project that research findings for the control or elimination of dental disease (such as a vaccine or rinse) will drastically change the profession.

Change will probably be focused more upon practice settings in the 1990s. Hygienists graduating from baccalaureate programs report a wider array of career placement choices than was typically listed in earlier surveys (Rubinstein and Brand, 1986). A small but growing percentage of hygienists is located in nontraditional settings and finds such employment personally satisfying, flexible, challenging, and more likely to provide good benefits (Cohen et al, 1987).

Perhaps the most crucial area of change for dental hygiene surrounds the opportunity for *unsupervised* or *independent practice*. Until the mid-1980s, the idea was rarely addressed. However, Colorado legalized unsupervised practice in 1986 (Colorado, 1986) and other states have tested the legislative waters to see if a version of unsupervised practice could be allowed. Such changes open opportunities for entrepreneurial hygienists to open their own practices and for community dental hygienists to function more freely in assessing, treating, and referring patients who live in or frequently visit institutional settings.

While there has been a decrease in dental hygiene enrollment since the peak of the late 1970s, the demand for dental hygienists should increase and the scope of practice for the profession should broaden as the focus on periodontal disease sharpens and as the need for prevention and continuing oral health maintenance is accepted by the public and by dentists (Ley et al, 1984).

Thus it is important for the beginning dental hygiene student to learn the ideal, the conceptual, and the futuristic models as well as the realistic, immediately applicable models of dental hygiene. Graduates may need to be able to function within delivery systems of the past, present, and future. For this reason, the scope of practice is broadly defined as *dental hygiene care*.

Dental hygiene research

What would dental hygienists research? The simplest and easiest answer is "Every step of every dental hygiene procedure." Much of what dental hygienists (and dentists) do is based upon assumptions or conclusions drawn from individual experiences that have become a part of clinical practice. Hygienists need to know why they perform certain functions and the results of performing or not performing certain procedures. An example of an area of dental hygiene recently scrutinized by research is the simple act of polishing the teeth with an abrasive. This is a time-honored procedure taught in dental hygiene since the beginning of the profession. Yet its effect on oral health was not examined in controlled research studies until the past few years. There is some evidence that it is an ill-advised procedure; there is virtually no research evidence that it is helpful. Hygienists should be challenging every procedure and identifying procedures that could or should be added to improve the value of care. Hygienists should be going beyond what dentists and other researchers have evaluated, specifying those aspects of care that are unique to dental hygiene.

It is rumored that the dental hygiene "body of knowledge" resides in an office at the University of Iowa, where the term first received acclaim and notoriety among students of Pauline Brine. However, the dental hygiene body of knowledge can and should reside among all dental hygienists, whether in school or in the work force. Dental hygienists have, first, the obligation to know what has been discovered through research and to evaluate and apply those findings. Second, hygienists have the obligation to pose new questions and to help answer those questions so that our scope of understanding—the body of knowledge—grows. This is followed by sharing findings and stimulating others to answer new questions or to challenge findings.

Demonstrating a research mentality is critical to earning professional status. It will continue to be a key theme in the coming decade.

Professional culture

Narrowing the research scope of focus to dental hygiene from the wide array of topics that are common to many areas of dentistry is not a simple matter. There is much overlap. Dentists and hygienists share research interests in periodontal initial therapy, in fluorides, in public health education, in sealants, and in many other topics. Is there an area that is of particular interest to dental hygiene?

A key to answering that question was discovered at the 1987 dental hygiene research conference. The key may be to define dental hygiene's professional culture. *Professional culture* comprises those characteristics that are unique to the profession. It is defined by specifying the terms and conditions that describe and differentiate a profession from all other professions and from closely related vocations. While dentistry and dental hygiene share many cultural elements, there must be characteristics that differentiate dental hygienists from dentists as a group.

This new way of defining dental hygiene becomes the "germ cell" of our profession, a reference point that helps us realize who we are, even as we diversify and grow within the profession (Dickoff and James, 1988).

Three workshops with hygienists from Colorado, Mississippi, and Pennsylvania identified these common cultural characteristics: caring, gentle, meticulous, listening, communicating, detail-conscious, dedicated, prevention-oriented, service-oriented, motivated less by monetary gain than by service, female, and competent. This does not completely define dental hygiene's culture. It is a first effort.

In looking for and defining the characteristics of professional culture the following questions elicit responses that are necessary to define the culture:

1. Are there times when a person should see a dental hygienist rather than a dentist for certain aspects of care? What are they?
2. What characteristics make dental hygienists more like each other than like dentists?
3. What functions do dental hygienists attend to that dentists tend to disregard or treat perfunctorily?
4. What makes dental hygienists different from nurses and other health professionals?
5. When you envision a dental hygienist, what characteristics do you attribute to that person?
6. How are graduating dental hygienists different from entering dental hygiene students?
7. When a dental hygienist lists several characteristics, which ones trigger immediate group agreement among other hygienists?

As dental hygienists continue to define dental hygiene culture, the core of the profession should become apparent, and from that core can emerge a research focus that will identify questions, hypotheses, and projects to improve our understanding of giving care.

THE DENTAL HYGIENE APPOINTMENT

One way to define dental hygiene clinical practice is to review the procedures of the dental hygiene appointment that are implemented by providers of care who are involved in all four phases of a program of care: assessment, planning, implementation, and evaluation.

I. Assessment
  A. Comprehensive health history
  B. General physical evaluation
    1. Vital signs
    2. Extraoral examination
    3. Intraoral examination
  C. Comprehensive charting of hard and soft tissues
    1. Comprehensive caries, restorative, and tooth characteristic charting, including radiographic findings
    2. Plaque and gingival indices
    3. Calculus charting
    4. Periodontal charting
  D. Occlusal assessment
II. Planning
  A. Planning for control of disease
  B. Formulating a treatment plan
  C. Case presentation
  D. Appointment planning
III. Implementation
  A. Patient self-assessment of needs
  B. Periodontal care
    1. Scaling
    2. Root planing
    3. Curettage
  C. Topical and systemic agents for control of caries and tooth hypersensitivity
  D. Local anesthesia and nitrous oxide-oxygen conscious sedation
  E. Restorative procedures
IV. Evaluation
  A. Case documentation
  B. Success of therapy and control
  C. Cost-effectivness

Associated with these procedures are the support functions of preparing the clinical site, maintaining contamination control, anticipating and responding to emergencies, meeting legal and ethical responsibilities, developing a practice philosophy, and adapting all phases of care to patients with special needs.

This text is designed to prepare students for entry into a clinical practice that will require the performance of these functions and the acceptance of these responsibilities.

ACTIVITIES

1. Divide the class into groups of three, and appoint a recorder for each small group. Have each person share his or her definitions and expected functions of the dental hygienist with the other two members of the group. The recorder lists all the definitions and functions given by the group and presents these to the entire class. Finally, the faculty member identifies his or her definitions and list of functions. Center group discussion on differences of expectations among students and between students and faculty and the possible problems and/or benefits in the educational process that may result from the differences and similarities. The faculty member collects and retains the reports for redistribution to the students during their final week in the program so that students may identify the changes in their perceptions.
2. Have each student ask a dentist what he or she believes are the functions of a hygienist. Compare replies in class and see how accurately they reflect the skills the student will learn.
3. Discuss each of the phases of the dental hygiene appointment, using the program model of assessment, planning, implementation, and evaluation.
4. Review functions that are legally allowable in a variety of states. Summarize the variety of ways in which *supervision* is defined in a number of states. Students should select those states in which they plan to seek licensure. This information can be found in the American Dental Association's most recent edition of *Legal Provisions for Delegating Expanded Functions to Dental Hygienists and Dental Assistants*.
5. Review publications written by hygienists about their practice sites, particularly those that differ from traditional solo and group practices. Discuss the advantages and disadvantages of each and what special skills or interests a hygienist would need to fulfill each role.
6. Complete group activity 4 (p. 5) in Woodall IR: Legal, ethical, and management aspects of the dental care system, ed 3, St Louis, 1987, The CV Mosby Co.
7. Read one or more "alternative employment" profiles in Dreyer R: Career directions for dental hygienists, Holmdel, NJ, 1985, Career Directions Press. Discuss how the hygienists built upon their basic education in dental hygiene to qualify for other career opportunities.
8. Read and discuss Darby's "Collaborative Practice Model."
9. Review the current literature to locate other articles on the future of dental hygiene. Conduct a panel discussion on one of the major issues receiving current attention.

REVIEW QUESTIONS

1. Briefly define a philosophy of patient-centered care.
2. Why may faculty members' perceptions of dental hygiene education and practice differ from students' perceptions?
3. What effect do dental practice acts have
   a. On the scope of practice?
   b. On educational programs?
4. What impact might the legalization of independent practice have on dental hygiene?
5. Define *professional culture*.

REFERENCES

American Dental Hygienists Association: Who we are: a report on the "Survey of Dental Hygiene Issues: Attitudes, Perceptions, and Preferences." Dent Hyg 56(12):13, 1982.

American Dental Hygienists' Association Resolutions SR-45-71; R-17-Am-73-H; SR-18-73-H; R-30-73-H; R-10-Am-75; SR-36-Am-76; and R-56-1976-H.

Annual report on dental auxiliary education, 1968-1969. Chicago, 1969, American Dental Association, Division of Educational Measurements, Council on Dental Education.

Annual report on dental auxiliary education, 1976-1977 (suppl. 2): Employment of 1976 graduates of auxiliary programs. Chicago, 1977, American Dental Association, Division of Educational Measurements, Council on Dental Education.

Annual report on dental auxiliary education, 1977-1978. Chicago, 1978, American Dental Association, Division of Educational Measurements, Council on Dental Education.

Annual report on dental auxiliary education, 1985-86. Chicago, 1986, American Dental Association, Division of Educational Measurements, Council on Dental Education.

Boyer EM: New dental hygiene graduates: demographic and employment profile, Dent Hyg 60:204, 1986.

Boyer EM, and Nielsen NJ: The effect of student experience on dental hygienists' perceived competency, Educ Direct 10(4):4, 1985.

Boyer EM, and Nielsen-Thompson NJ: Legality and dental hygienists' performance of expanded functions, Dent Hyg 60:104, 1986.

The Carnegie Commission on Higher Education. Higher education and the nation's health: policies for medical and dental education. New York, 1970, McGraw-Hill Book Co.

The Carnegie Council on Policy Studies in Higher Education. Progress and problems in medical and dental education: federal support versus federal control. San Francisco, 1976, Jossey-Bass, Inc, Publishers.

Cohen L, LaBelle A, and Singer J: Educational preparation of hygienists working with special populations in nontraditional settings, J Dent Educ 49:592, 1985

Cohen L, Singer J, and LaBelle A: Characteristics of employment and job satisfaction in nontraditional dental hygiene practice settings, J Public Health Dent 47:88, 1987.

Colorado passes unsupervised practice. ADA News, American Dental Assoc 17(10):5, 1986.

Darby ML: Collaborative practice model: the future of dental hygiene, J Dent Educ 47:589, 1983.

Dickoff J, and James P: Organization and expansion of knowledge toward a constructive assault on the imperious distinction of pure from applied knowledge, of knowledge from technique, Dent Hyg 62:15, 1988.

Douglass CW, et al: Dental hygienists' services: a study of group and solo dental practices, Dent Hyg 56(10):17, 1982.

Gluch-Scranton J, and Rigolizzo Gurenlian J: A model for two-year and baccalaureate clinical dental hygiene education, J Dent Educ 49:95, 1985.

Grady A: Dental hygienists and state boards of dentistry: an overview of the legislative action packet, Dent Hyg 62:87, 1988.

Heine CS, et al: Dimensions of career satisfaction for the dental hygienist, Dent Hyg 57(3):22, 1983.

Hollinshead BS: Survey of dentistry, Washington, DC, 1961, American Council on Education.

Kraemer LG: The dental hygiene entry dilemma: an issue of prestige, image and professional credibility, Dent Hyg 59:117, 1985.

Legal provisions for delegating expanded functions to dental hygienists and dental assistants. Chicago, 1985, American Dental Association, Division of Educational Measurements, Council on Dental Education.

Ley E, Aker D, and Mounts C: Maintenance of an adequate dental hygiene education system, J Dent Educ 48:556, 1984.

Minervini R, et al: Assessing expanded functions performed by hygienists in Missouri, Dent Hyg 55(5):36, 1981.

Richards C: Who are we? An update based on 1984 data, Dent Hyg 59:121, 1985.

Rubinstein L, and Brand MK: A description of postcertificate dental hygiene programs, J Dent Educ 50:608, 1986.

2 PREPARING THE SITE: OPERATION AND MAINTENANCE OF EQUIPMENT

OBJECTIVES: *The reader will be able to*

1. Identify and operate and/or adjust the following operatory equipment:
   a. Dental chair, including lowering, raising, tilting, and lowering back; rotating chair; and positioning headrest, if adjustable
   b. Dental unit, including operating air-water syringe, handpiece, prophylaxis angle, saliva ejector, high-volume suction, and cuspidor (if applicable)
   c. Overhead light
   d. Clinician's and assistant's stools
   e. Sink and soap dispenser
2. Given any of the common components of the dental operatory, identify basic maintenance procedures to improve its longevity and ensure its cleanliness and satisfactory appearance.
3. Given a series of mechanical or cleanliness problems associated with equipment, identify how the problems could have been prevented.

The provision of most dental services is more easily accomplished with dental equipment specifically designed for patient, clinician, and assistant comfort and for housing special electrically powered or air-powered equipment. This includes a dental chair; a dental unit with overhead intraoral illumination, air, water, high- and slow-speed rotary engines, and high-volume evacuation equipment to remove fluids from the patient's mouth; and stools for the clinician and the assistant (Richardson and Barton, 1978; Snyder and Domer, 1983).

It is helpful to be completely familiar with the dental equipment and its function prior to seating a patient. This section presents the operation and control of various pieces of equipment. Although every operatory is different, many principles of operation and maintenance are common to most models. In addition to the generally applicable guidelines presented, a maxim to follow is to *read the directions* provided by the manufacturer. Once the directions have been reviewed, it is wise to follow suggestions for cleaning, lubricating, and securing periodic maintenance evaluations

and to retain the brochures, warranties, and instructions for future reference.

Properly maintained equipment will break down less often and require replacement less frequently. Considering the cost of dental equipment and the importance of productive hours of "chair time," care in using and maintaining equipment results in less frustration and is an important cost-effective measure (Richardson and Barton, 1978).

THE DENTAL CHAIR

Most modern dental chairs are the contour or lounge type that allow flexible patient positioning with relative ease. There are usually two or three controls located on the side of the chair back that provide a range of adjustments. One button or switch will *raise* or *lower the back* of the chair, and a second will *tilt* the entire chair back so that the footrest rises and the headrest is lowered without changing the angle between the back of the chair and the seat of the chair. An optional third button will automatically place the patient in a standard working position or return the patient to an upright seated position. The control to raise or

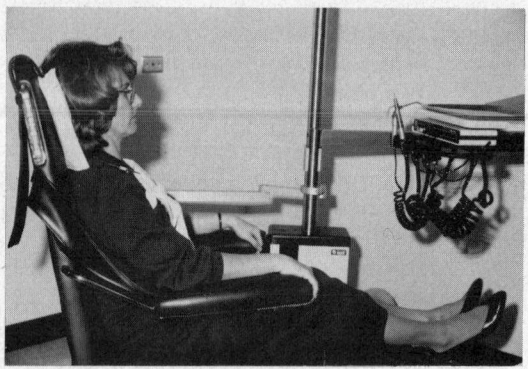

Fig. 2-1. Dental lounge chair positioned with back upright. Patient should be seated with the chair in this position as the first step in attaining the supine position.

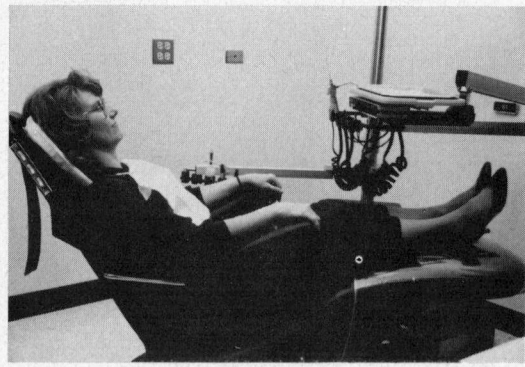

Fig. 2-2. Second step in placing patient in supine position. Chair is tilted backward so that patient's hips are well seated in angle of chair.

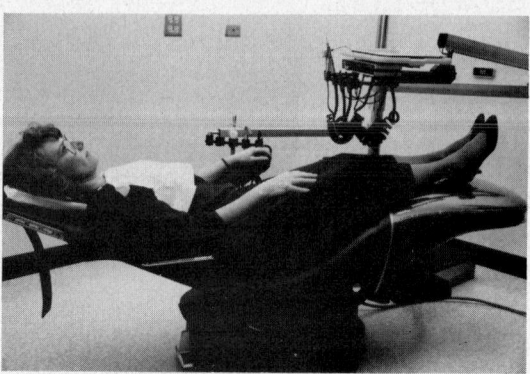

Fig. 2-3. Third step in placing patient in supine position. Back of chair is lowered until patient is in full supine position with toes and chin at approximately the same height. Overall height of chair can then be adjusted to position of seated clinician.

lower the entire chair is located at the base of the chair and is operated by foot.

With these basic controls it is possible to (1) seat the patient in an upright position, (2) tilt the chair back so that the patient's hips are well seated at the angle of the chair, (3) lower the back of the chair so that the patient is in the supine position, and (4) raise or lower the entire chair to the correct height for the clinician (Figs. 2-1 to 2-3). The patient's back should receive full support from the chair.

Most models allow for *rotating* the chair on its axis. This control is usually located at the base of the chair and allows the clinician to seat the patient with maximum space available for the patient's maneuvering and then (5) rotate the chair

to approximate other stationary equipment and to best facilitate the seating of the clinician and assistant. This is particularly useful for left-handed clinicians.

Although some chairs are secured to the floor, many others can be moved with a few hefty pushes. A few models allow for easy movement by literally floating on a cushion of air when the appropriate control is activated.

It is helpful to identify the full range of adjustment for each chair. This is helpful in obtaining optimal patient positioning and saves the clinician the embarrassment of running the chair up and down when it is obvious that it is supposed to tilt back. Some chairs have locking devices in which one press of a button will move the patient to a full reclining position. The clinician who intends only a minor chair adjustment may find this runaway chair quite unexpected (Weinert, 1971).

Headrest adjustments also vary from chair to chair. Most modern equipment uses a ring- or horseshoe-shaped pillow-style headrest that is easily adjusted and attached with adhesive material to the underside of the chair back. It can be removed entirely with the chair back, providing support for very tall patients or small children (Weinert, 1971).

For those chairs with the multijointed headrest, the best rule to follow in positioning the headrest is to seat the patient in the fully supine position and then adjust the headrest so that the pads or

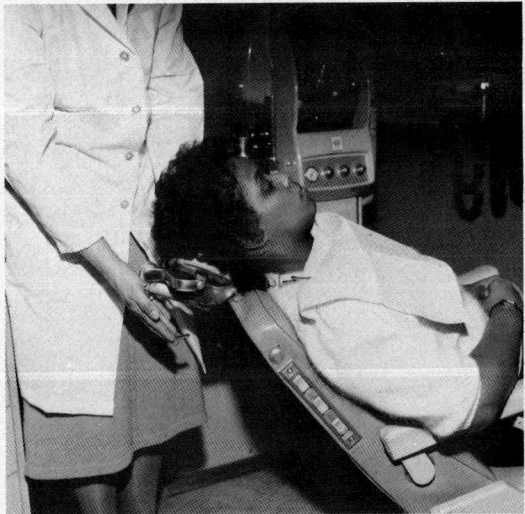

Fig. 2-4. Adjust hinged headrest so that occipital bone at base of skull is resting on padding and neck is in same plane as patient's back. When these criteria are met and patient is comfortable, lock headrest in place by pushing up on lever.

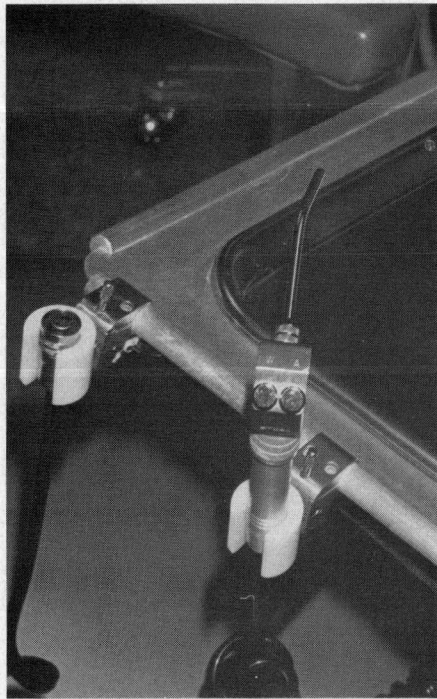

Fig. 2-5. Air-water syringe includes a button for water and a button for air; activating both buttons results in air-water spray that is ideal for flushing oral cavity. Routine use of this device eliminates the need for frequent rinsing with a cup of water.

bowl of the headrest is located behind the occipital bone. With the patient's head resting in the headrest, the clinician can raise or lower the whole unit (head and headrest) until the patient's neck is in the same plane with the spine (Fig. 2-4).

THE DENTAL UNIT

The electrical circuitry for many chairs is connected to the master switches for the dental unit. On some models the master switch is marked clearly, but on other models the switches are located in obscure, unmarked places. Again, it is wise to locate this switch before the arrival of the patient. If a modular cart is connected to the main circuitry for air and water flow, high-volume suction, and other systems, there may be a second master switch on the cart itself.

Once the master switches are activated, the following pieces of equipment should be tested for their proper function:

Air-water syringe

Sometimes referred to as a *trisyringe* or *triplex syringe* (Fig. 2-5), the air-water syringe enables the clinician or assistant to direct a stream of water, air, or an air-water spray onto the operative site

(Richardson and Barton, 1978). Usually there is one button for air and one for water, with spray resulting when both buttons are pushed simultaneously. Most quality syringes contain a heater to ensure that air and water temperatures are comfortable for the patient. The tip of the air-water syringe is usually removable and should be sterilized between patients.

The syringe has outdated the cup of water that for decades was the primary means available for rinsing. Current practices include irrigating the oral cavity with an air-water spray, with the resultant fluid and debris being evacuated by high-volume suction or an efficient saliva ejector. "Cuspidor calisthenics" throughout the appointment are no longer necessary.

Many units no longer include the flushing bowl of water. If the opportunity to swish and empty is still desired, a funnel with a paper liner (Fig. 2-6) can be connected to the high-speed suction system.

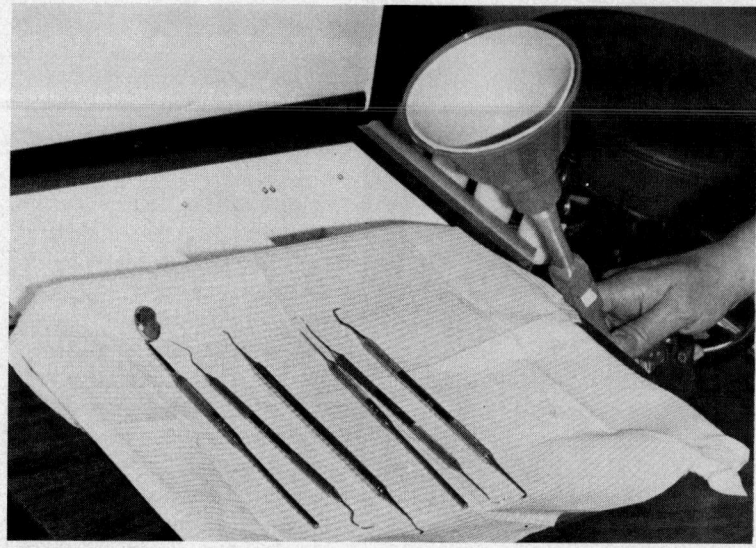

Fig. 2-6. Funnel attachment with disposable paper liner is used as a "cuspidor" and is inserted into hosing of high-volume evacuation system.

If a cuspidor is included with the unit and is used by the patients, it is important to locate the controls for the volume of water. It is possible to overflow a cuspidor if the volume of water flow is too great. Conversely, a mere trickle is inadequate to clear away debris. Usually the spout from which the water emerges swivels. The spout should be positioned so that water flows around the bowl. The trap in the cuspidor should be removed at the completion of each appointment and freed of debris to ensure proper drainage (Richardson and Barton, 1978). This task may be another reason for the growing popularity of high-volume suction. The system should be flushed with a warm solution of bleach (one part bleach to six parts water) weekly. Some other disinfectant solution should be used if the piping is of cast aluminum (Williams and Williams, 1982).

Older models provide a place for a cup of water to rest and to be refilled. On most, a single control fills the cup; some have temperature controls as well. A few models have a weight-sensitive cup rest that senses when the cup should be refilled. When the cup is replaced by the patient, the water automatically fills the cup until it reaches the predetermined optimal weight. Generally, the convenience of the cup of water adds considerably to chair time because of the time it takes to reach for the cup, swish, empty into the cuspidor, replace the cup, fill it, and resettle in the chair. Most clinicians ignore the gadget on the unit entirely, opting for the water syringe and suction instead.

Many modern units have more than one trisyringe for use by the clinician and assistant.

Oral evacuation attachments

The passively gurgling saliva ejector of yesteryear has been replaced by *high-speed suction* and an efficient *saliva ejector*. High-speed or high-volume suction was introduced to dental practice to enable rapid removal of the coolant water that accompanies the high-speed drill (Richardson and Barton, 1978). It is also useful in removing the water used with the ultrasonic scaler and in evacuating the mouth with frequent use of an air-water spray. In dental hygiene procedures in which loosened deposits, polishing pastes, and necrotic tissue need to be flushed from the sulcus surrounding each tooth, the air-water spray and the oral evacuation are close companions. Evacuation is, of course, useful for restorative procedures as well and for helping remove saliva during fluoride and sealant applications.

Saliva ejector tips traditionally have been, and still may be, bent into shapes that sit comfortably in the floor of the patient's mouth during the treatment. However, modern equipment will quickly remove a greater quantity of fluid. Saliva ejectors are often used like a reverse straw, with the patient closing his lips around the tip and letting the fluids be drawn out of his mouth.

High-speed suction will evacuate the mouth more quickly but tends to grasp cheeks or tongue.

After each patient, the line should be flushed by sucking a pint of clean water through the hosing. Tips used intraorally should be autoclaved or discarded if disposable. Many mobile carts and individual saliva ejectors contain traps to catch large particulate matter. These must be cleaned daily.

Rotary engine equipment

A complete dental operatory includes slow- and high-speed rotary equipment powered by electricity (electrotorque) or compressed air (air torque, air rotor). A slow-speed handpiece is used for finishing and polishing restorations, for some steps in cavity preparation, and for polishing teeth. It operates at approximately 6000 revolutions per minute (rpm) and offers sufficient torque power to facilitate removal of stains when an abrasive agent is applied to the tooth with a rubber cup or brush attachment. High-speed handpieces operate at over 100,000 rpm (Sockwell, 1971).

The handpieces are activated by a foot pedal, called a *rheostat*. Depending on the design, the pedal can be activated by pressing down, by moving a lever to the side, or by rotating a disk. Pushing the lever or disk in one direction causes the handpiece to move forward; moving it in the opposite direction runs it backward. Fig 2-7 shows one type of rheostat, which is activated by downward foot pressure.

It is important to know which hoses are for high speed, which hoses are for low speed, and which handpieces are intended for each. Hoses should be wiped clean with disinfectant; those covered with cloth usually require regular wiping with a dressing to keep them flexible. Hoses on retractable reels should be gently withdrawn from storage and carefully replaced. They should not be stuffed back into their compartments.

Older equipment may still rely on the belt-

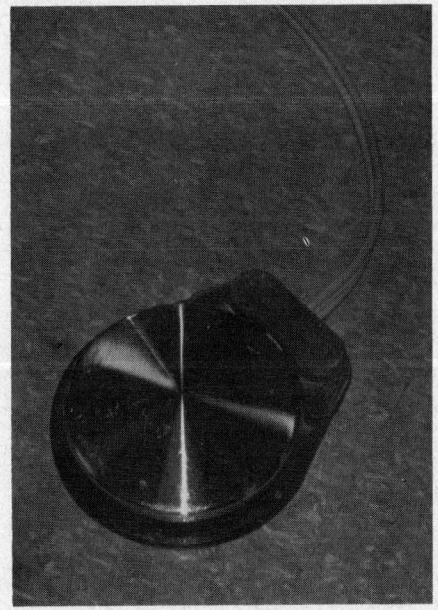

Fig. 2-7. Foot pedal adjusts speed of operation of handpiece. This style requires downward foot pressure. Other styles have a pedal that rotates with a push of the foot.

driven engine for slow-speed needs. Because an occasion to use this equipment may arise, a few precautions should be kept in mind:

1. Be certain that the belt is not frayed; change it if there is any possibility of its breaking during use.
2. Position the arm of the belt-driven engine so that it will not entangle hair (a knot of hair becoming firmly attached to the belt-driven engine is embarrassing and painful).
3. Ensure that the handpiece will reach to all areas of the dentition when the patient is in the supine position. This may require moving the entire dental chair closer to the engine, since relative positions for equipment were at one time defined by the limits of stand-up dentistry rather than those of sit-down dentistry.

Handpieces, whether for electric, air, or belt-driven engines, require regular cleaning. It is imperative to follow manufacturer's directions for each handpiece, since some require disassembling and thorough cleaning and lubricating and others are *not* to be dismantled and require only a blast of a canned cleaning/lubricating fluid especially developed for this purpose. Some handpieces should be autoclaved; others would rust and should be disinfected or dry heat sterilized (Sockwell, 1971).

The prophylaxis angle is attached to the slow-speed handpiece. This angle adapts the torque power of the handpiece to the specific purpose of polishing teeth or restorations. In almost all instances the angle needs complete disassembling and cleaning after each polishing procedure, since the abrasive polishing paste easily enters the gears of the device, wearing the gears away and usually clogging the mechanism so that it freezes shut. A few brands are sealed so that entry of contaminants is reduced or eliminated. These brands are accompanied by specific maintenance directions that must be followed carefully to ensure longevity of the angle.

There are a variety of methods for attaching rubber cups or brushes to prophylaxis angles to hold the polishing paste against the tooth. (For discussion of these methods, see Chapter 26.)

The prophylaxis angle typically presents the greatest mechanical problems for the dental hygienist. It tends to freeze when not carefully cleaned and lubricated, and it is a weak link in the control of cross-contamination. Its working parts can easily harbor debris and microorganisms; yet few are designed for the autoclave. In the best interests of controlling the spread of disease, only angles that can be cleaned and autoclaved or are disposable should be used. They are more expensive than others, but some carry guarantees and offer replacement kits for worn parts. Fortunately, they are becoming increasingly common.

Overhead light

Once all the unit controls are identified and found to be functional, it is appropriate to locate and turn on the overhead, intraoral light. Usually there is a single switch on the light itself. A special high-intensity lamp shines out onto a highly reflective concave surface that focuses the light rays so that they may be directed to illuminate the oral cavity. The reflective surface should be polished at least daily to ensure brightness. This should be done at the start of the day when the lamp is cool (Williams and Williams, 1982a).

The lamp should be allowed to cool before a burned-out bulb is replaced. Because lights often fail when they are first switched on, the lamp may still be cool to the touch and not cause a schedule delay. If the dental light has a quartz halogen bulb, only the sleeve should be handled, as fingerprints can cause the bulb to explode or to burn out more quickly. Sealed-beam bulbs require that the entire unit containing the bulb be replaced. A spare bulb or unit should be kept available for replacement and reordered according to specifications on the package as soon as a bulb is used. In some units a fuse in the dental lamp will blow at the same time that the bulb fails. Extra fuses should be kept for this purpose (Williams and Williams, 1982a).

Many overhead lights are covered by a plastic shield as a safety precaution against an exploding lamp or shattering reflector. A piece of metal flung from rotary equipment could easily trigger such an accident.

To diminish wear on the switch and the lamp, the overhead light should be turned on at the beginning of the appointment and left on for the duration of the visit. When not in use, it can be directed down from the patient's face. Turning the lamp on and off causes it to burn out more rapidly than when it is left on. As with any mechanical switch, each use causes wear. Many clinicians leave the overhead light on all day if a succession of patients is to receive care, turning it off only during extended periods of nonuse, such as during the lunch period. It should, of course, be turned off at the end of the day, as should all switches on the unit. Leaving a dental unit on for extended periods of nonuse will burn out its electrical components.

Another precaution is to shut off the water supply so that pressure is not exerted against the tubing in the unit. Rises in water pressure occur most often at night; thus so do floods in operatories where water pressure is left on overnight (Williams and Williams, 1982b).

CLINICIAN'S AND ASSISTANT'S STOOLS

When all main equipment appears to be functional and the hygienist has familiarized himself or herself with its operation, the clinician's and assistant's stools should be adjusted for their intended occupants. The height of the operator's stool should be adjusted so that the feet are flat on the floor and the thighs are parallel to the floor. The back support should be adjusted both vertically and horizontally to support the lumbar region of the back.

The height of the assistant's stool should allow an eye level approximately 4 to 6 inches above that of the clinician. This will require a ring on the stool on which the feet can rest. Because the assistant often leans forward during treatment, an abdominal rest is customary on the assistant's stool. This should be adjusted to fit below the rib cage to provide optimal body support. Neither the clinician nor the assistant should feel the pressure of the stool against the back of the thighs, because that position inhibits blood circulation to the legs (Cooper, 1974; Harris and Crabb, 1978; Richardson and Barton, 1978).

Stool adjustments should be customized for each person. Because of the wide variety of adjustment mechanisms, read equipment instructions and experiment in advance of patient arrival.

THE SINK

The sink is another essential item of equipment. It should be used for thorough scrubbing at the beginning of a clinical period and for thorough handwashing before seeing each patient and whenever an item is touched that may have microorganisms other than those specific to the patient's oral flora (cross-contaminants).

Ideally, the sink and the soap dispenser will be controlled by a foot pedal. This obviously decreases the possibility of the sink being a fomite for transferring bacteria from patient to patient.

Towel dispensers should allow the person to grasp and remove a single paper towel without touching the dispenser itself.

STORAGE CABINETRY AND TRAY SYSTEMS

Most operatories allow for some storage of supplies and instruments. The most flexible, of course, is modular or totally movable cabinetry, which can be brought to the operative site. A timesaving and safe (in terms of preventing cross-contamination) method of storing instruments and supplies is the tray system. All needed instruments and disposables for a given procedure are stored on a covered tray, which can be pulled for

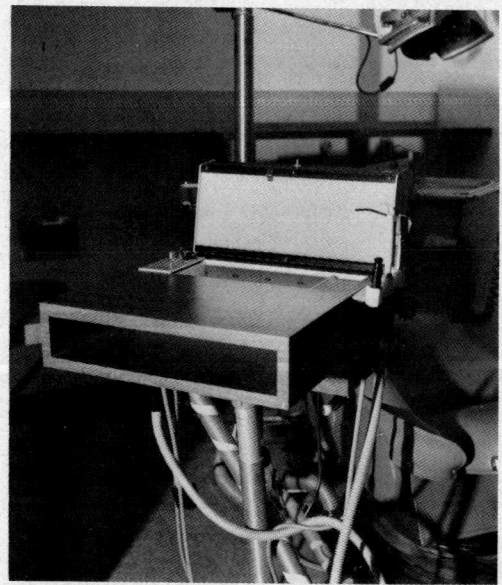

Fig. 2-8. Cart outfitted with trisyringe, evacuation system, and handpiece for slow- or high-speed use may be all that is needed as a "dental unit" for many intraoral procedures.

use when that procedure is indicated (Hillborn et al, 1974).

The mobile cart provides an alternative to the traditional over-the-patient instrument tray. The tray of instruments may be placed behind the patient's head for ready access by both the clinician and the assistant. It can hold the tri-syringe, handpiece, and suction equipment also (Hillborn, Campbell, and Hall, 1974). For traditional dental hygiene care the mobile cart may be the only "dental unit" needed (Fig. 2-8).

OTHER DENTAL OPERATORY EQUIPMENT

Other essential dental equipment includes the viewbox for mounting and interpreting radiographic film. It should be located at the chairside so that the exposed films can be readily available throughout a procedure. Likewise, it is convenient to have x-ray equipment in the operatory (Fig. 2-9) to expose films when such diagnostic aids are indicated. The room must, of course, be lead lined and provide complete protection for the clinician. Because of the cost of lead lining and the amount of room needed to manipulate radio-

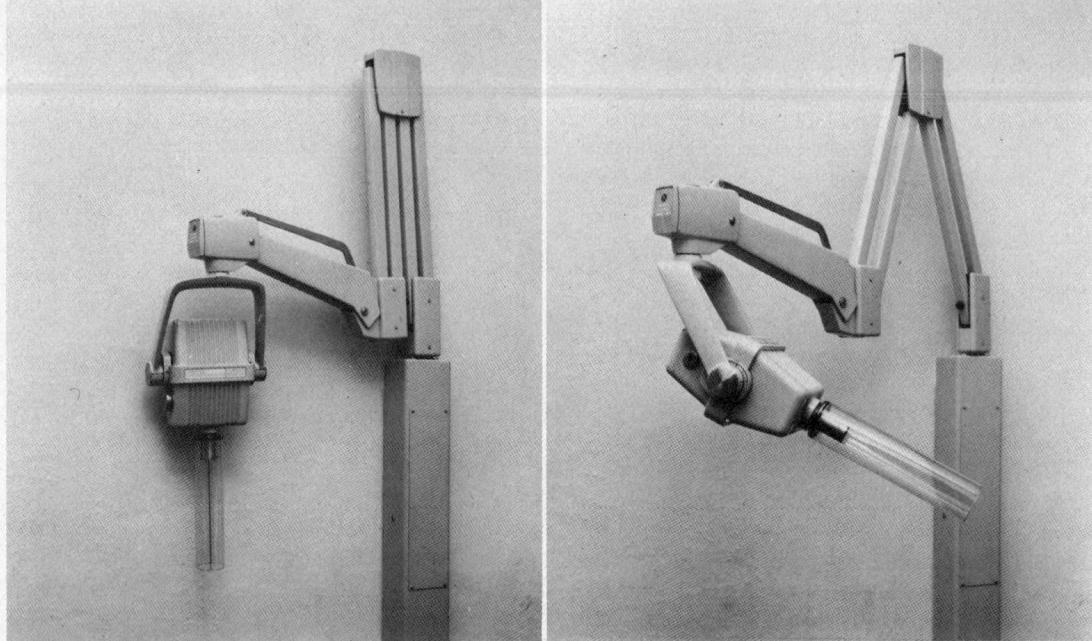

A   **B**

Fig. 2-9. **A,** X-ray unit should be stored so that all hinges are closed. This places less stress on hinges and helps prevent eventual "drifting" of head away from patient's face during its use. **B,** Improperly stored x-ray unit.

graphic equipment, such equipment is usually located in a separate operatory for a number of clinicians to use as needed.

Ultrasonic equipment for removing large calcareous deposits from teeth may be included in the operatory. Generally, there is also an amalgamator for triturating metal alloys for amalgam restorations.

Sterilizing or cleaning equipment may be located in the operatory or in an adjacent central laboratory area. Standard equipment includes an autoclave (Fig. 2-10). Ultrasonic cleaning tanks may be used to remove debris from instruments (Fig. 2-11). Dry heat sterilizing equipment may be available to sterilize items that could be dulled by steam under pressure. Maintenance of the autoclave includes using distilled water, periodically running a cycle with a cleaning agent added to the water, and testing the machine for effectiveness. Rubber seals around the door should be replaced as they show wear. (See Chapter 3 for further discussion of the use of sterilizing equipment.)

The ultrasonic cleaner should be drained when

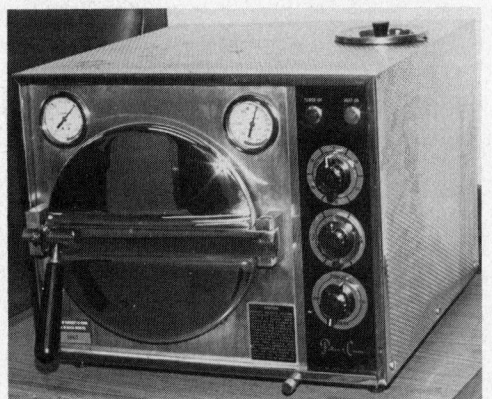

Fig. 2-10. Autoclave provides complete sterilization of instruments and other materials that are able to withstand steam under pressure.

it becomes cloudy (at least once a week). The tank should be washed and fresh solution mixed and added. Proper proportions of solution must be used, and the level of solution must be maintained to ensure proper cavitation and cleaning.

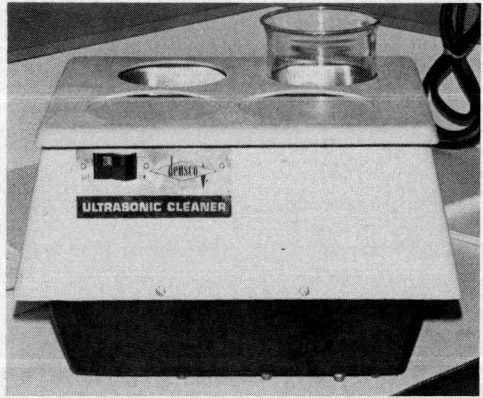

Fig. 2-11. Ultrasonic cleaner removes debris from instruments prior to their being packaged for sterilization.

Hand instruments should be handled carefully. If an instrument is dropped, the working end may bend or break. The ends of instruments should be wrapped for protection during sterilization and storage.

Cutting instruments should be routinely sharpened following autoclaving and during procedures that dull them. An autoclaved stone prevents cross-contamination. As discussed in later chapters, sharpening should maintain the intended shape rather than alter it. Instruments sharpened over a long period of time should be discarded or retipped before structural weakness predisposes them to fracture during use.

GENERAL CARE OF EQUIPMENT

It is essential that every patient be treated in a clean, safe environment. The bulk of effort will be directed toward presenting the patient with chemically disinfected or covered surfaces and sterilized instruments and equipment whenever feasible. The details of this process are discussed in Chapter 3.

Beyond sanitization, dental equipment also needs maintenance to ensure longevity and good service. The dental environment also must appear clean and tidy. For example, leather and vinyl products should be cleaned regularly with an oil soap that will prevent drying and cracking. The crease where the chair back and seat meet should be cleaned by placing the back of the chair all the way down, and the chair base should be wiped daily to remove dust and debris. The enameled portions of the unit and plastic-laminate counter tops can be cleaned and polished with glass wax or automobile polish; there are special cleaners for brushed stainless steel. The entire unit should be dusted daily.

The best check of a clean unit is to take the role of a patient yourself and enter the operatory, sit in the dental chair, and look around both from an upright and reclining position. Looking at the equipment from those perspectives provides the patient's-eye view of the otherwise hidden spot of blood, the bespeckled light reflector, the cobweb in the corner, and the red disclosing solution under the lip of the infamous cuspidor.

The benefits of this attention to detail include positive patient responses to the general environment; more dependable, functional equipment; improved safety for the patient, clinician, and assistant; and longer-lasting, newer-looking equipment.

• • •

This chapter has addressed some general points concerning cleanliness and prevention of cross-contamination. Chapter 3 focuses on aseptic techniques and control of microorganisms in the dental operatory.

ACTIVITIES

1. In groups of three, use a search and discovery technique to explore a dental operatory in the dental hygiene clinic and elsewhere. (Students should rotate from clinician to patient to assistant roles.) Locate and operate the following items:
   a. Dental chair
      (1) Raise and lower
      (2) Tilt chair back
      (3) Lower back of chair
      (4) Adjust headrest
      (5) Rotate
   b. Dental unit
      (1) Master switch(es)
      (2) Air-water syringe
         (a) Air
         (b) Water
         (c) Air-water spray
      (3) Handpiece
         (a) Mount to hose
         (b) Operate forward and reverse
         (c) Clean and store
         (d) Differentiate high and low speeds

(4) Prophylaxis angle
   (a) Mount on handpiece
   (b) Attach cup and brush
   (c) Run forward and backward
   (d) Clean and store
(5) Suction
   (a) Insert high-speed suction tip and funnel
   (b) Attach saliva ejector tip
   (c) Activate
   (d) Clean and store
c. Adjust stool to proper height
   (1) Assistant's stool
   (2) Operator's stool
d. Turn on overhead light
   (1) Change lamp in overhead light
   (2) Clean reflector and shield
e. Identify presence of
   (1) Ultrasonic scaling equipment
   (2) Amalgamator
   (3) Radiographic equipment
f. Clean the dental chair
g. Clean the dental unit
h. Operate sink and soap dispenser

2. Inspect dental equipment for proper function. Discuss how breakage or wear could be prevented.
3. Visit dental offices with modern equipment and offices with older equipment to determine how different models function and how they are maintained.
4. Attend a professional meeting where equipment is displayed. Learn about and report the differences and similarities regarding function and recommended maintenance. Calculate what an operatory of equipment costs, itemizing each essential component.
5. Change a belt on a belt-driven engine.

REVIEW QUESTIONS

1. The overhead light (should/should not) be left on throughout a treatment sequence.
2. The proper sequence for adjusting the dental chair when seating a patient is (five steps).
3. The three functions of the air-water syringe are _____ .
4. Running the prophylaxis angle backward often causes the face of the angle head or the cup/brush to _____ .
5. It is important to know the difference between high- and low-speed hoses and switches because _____ .
6. If a prophylaxis angle "freezes" or will not move, even though the handpiece itself is functional, the probable cause is _____ .
7. The clinician's stool should be adjusted so that _____ .
8. The assistant's stool should be adjusted so that _____ .
9. Leather and vinyl should be cleaned with _____ .
10. Typical equipment used for cleaning and sterilizing instruments includes _____ .

REFERENCES

Carter LM, and Yaman P: Dental instruments. St Louis, 1981, The CV Mosby Co.

Chasteen JE: Essentials of clinical dental assisting. St Louis, 1984, The CV Mosby Co.

Cooper TM: Four-handed dentistry in the team practice of dentistry, Dent Clin North Am 18:739, 1974.

Harris NO, and Crabb, LJ: Ergonomics: reducing mental and physical fatigue in the dental operatory, Dent Clin North Am 22:331, 1978.

Hillborn LB, Campbell EM, and Hall WR: Facility design and equipment considerations for the team practice of dentistry, Dent Clin North Am 18:873, 1974.

New dentist buying guide. Chicago, 1988, American Dental Association.

Richardson RE, and Barton RE: The dental assistant, ed 5, New York, 1978, McGraw-Hill Book Co.

Snyder TL, and Domer LR: Personalized guide to practice evaluation, vol 1. In Snyder TL, and Felmeister CJ, editors: Mosby's dental practice series, St Louis, 1983, The CV Mosby Co.

Sockwell CL: Dental handpieces and rotary cutting instruments, Dent Clin North Am 15:219, 1971.

Weinert AM: An evaluation of the dental lounge chair, Dent Clin North Am 15:129, 1971.

Williams KV, and Williams FT: The maintenance of dental equipment. II. Chairs and lights, Br Dent J 153(2):71 (a), 1982.

Williams KV, and Williams FT: The maintenance of dental equipment. III. Delivery and disposal systems, Br Dent J 153(3):113 (b), 1982.

3 DISEASE TRANSMISSION THEORY AND CONTROL OF CONTAMINATION

OBJECTIVES: *The reader will be able to*

1. Explain the theory of disease transmission and the necessity for asepsis in dentistry.
2. Identify common pathogenic organisms that may be found in the oral cavity and the disease entities they produce.
3. Define direct and indirect contamination and give examples that illustrate understanding of these terms.
4. Identify precautionary measures that must be taken by dental personnel to prevent disease transfer from patient to patient, patient to clinician, and clinician to patient.
5. Differentiate among the terms sanitization, disinfection, and sterilization.
6. Identify the major sources of contamination in the dental office and describe an effective method of controlling contamination or eliminating it from each source.
7. Discuss five accepted methods of instrument sterilization and identify the advantages and disadvantages of each method.
8. Discuss the choice and use of chemical disinfectants.
9. Describe an effective method of hand washing.
10. Describe the preparation of instruments for sterilization/disinfection.
11. Discuss the operation of the autoclave and the dry heat oven.
12. Discuss indications for the use of gloves, safety glasses, and face masks.
13. Describe infection control procedures for the laboratory.
14. Discuss the legal implications of following recommended infection control guidelines.

With each educational component of professional preparation, the student hygienist gains a new dimension of respect for the oral environment. This respect should center on the nature of the relationship of the hygienist to the pathogenic (disease-producing) organisms of the oral cavity. Direct and indirect exposure to these organisms occurs practically every minute of the working day.

Dentists and hygienists are in constant contact with blood, saliva, mucous membranes, and other body fluids which may be infectious. It has been estimated that a single drop of saliva may contain up to 600,000 bacteria and a spoon excavator full of dental plaque may contain an average of 200 million bacteria (Palenik and Miller, 1984a). The potential for infection of the clinician, co-workers, and patients is extremely high. Manag-ing disease transmission or, more positively, preserving the health status of patients and dental care providers depends on high standards of asepsis (freedom from pathogenic material) being rigidly applied. In this chapter, oral pathogens and modes of microbial transfer are identified. Controlling levels of contamination and procedures for maintaining asepsis are also discussed.

Some professionals may be skeptical about the need for strict standards of infection control for dental professionals and office environments. Dental treatment may seem benign in comparison with the aseptic and postinfection concerns of the medical-surgical arena. After all, patients are seen for relatively short periods of time, and the treatment in general is superficial. Right?

On the contrary, because the oral cavity supports one of the most concentrated microbial populations of the body, length of time has little significance when procedures (periodontal instrumentation, injection, extraction, endodontics) are performed that expose the underlying tissues to external agents. These procedures cannot be classified as superficial. The main routes for disease transmission occur through contact with the bloodstream and through respiratory nasal/oral secretions. Except for the surgeon, few health professionals come in closer patient contact for longer periods of treatment than the dental team.

An awareness of the infectious nature of oral organisms and their potential for transfer is important for the student to master. Beyond developing this conscience about asepsis, maintaining aseptic practices is unquestionably the hygienist's professional responsibility.

MICROFLORA OF THE ORAL CAVITY

The oral cavity provides an excellent environment for supporting a variety of organisms, including many types of bacteria, yeasts, certain fungi, mycoplasms, protozoa, and viruses. The indigenous resident flora of the oral cavity are listed in Table 3-1. The nature of the oral structures—the mucosa, tongue, and gingival crevice—and the variation in dental anatomy promote the adherence and growth of diverse microbial populations. Salivary components, exudates, and epithelial cells are an abundant intrinsic nutritional source for oral flora. In addition, the foods we ingest are extrinsic nutritional sources. These nutritional sources, ample surfaces to cling to, warmth, and moisture create a comfortable environment for an active microbial community. In fact, the concentration about the gingival sulcus and in plaque ap-

Table 3-1. Microorganisms indigenous to man

Pathogenic staphylococci	Skin, human milk, nasal passages, vagina (during pregnancy), throat, gastrointestinal tract, oral cavity, feces
Micrococci and nonpathogenic staphylococci	Skin, mucous membranes, nose, throat, vagina, postpartum uterus, oral cavity
Anaerobic micrococci	Tonsils, uterus, vagina, respiratory tract
Streptococci	Mucous surfaces, mouth, pharynx, lower intestine, genital tract, vagina
Anaerobic streptococci	Mucous surfaces, vagina, postpartum uterus, oral cavity, human feces
Enterococci	Lower intestine, feces, genitourinary tract, oral cavity, tonsils
Common neisseriae	Oral cavity, nasopharynx, nasal cavity, urethra, vagina
Veillonellae	Oral cavity
Lactobacilli	Oral cavity, gastrointestinal tract, vagina
Actinomyces	Oral cavity, throat
Corynebacteria	Mucous membranes, vagina, skin, conjunctiva, oral cavity, feces
Mycobacteria	Preputial and clitoral secretions, feces, tonsils
Clostridia	Gastrointestinal tract, feces
Enterobacteria	Feces, gastrointestinal tract, vagina, oral cavity, throat
Moraxella, Mima (Herellea) species	Conjunctiva, nose, genitourinary mucous membranes, respiratory tract
Pseudomonas species	Feces, skin, hands, external ear, axilla, perineum
Alcaligenes faecalis	Feces
Haemophilus	Conjunctiva, nose, pharynx, oral cavity, vagina
Bacteroides	Predominant in feces, lower intestine, oral cavity
Fusobacteria	Oral cavity, intestine, throat, genitalia
Anaerobic spirilla and vibrios	Oral cavity
Spirochetes	Oral cavity, genitalia, throat, tonsils, feces, gastrointestinal tract, genitourinary tract
Candida species	Oral cavity, body surfaces, throat, feces, vagina
Pityrosporon ovale	Skin
Torulopsis glabrata	Skin, mucous membranes
Dermatophytes	Skin
Trichomonads	Oral cavity, intestine, genitourinary tract
Amebas	Oral cavity, intestinal tract, vagina, genitourinary tract
Pleuropneumonia-like organisms, L forms, spheroplasts, protoplasts	Vagina, male urethra, oral cavity, throat

From Burnett GW, and Schuster GS: Pathogenic microbiology, St Louis, 1978, The CV Mosby Co.

proximates 200 billion cells per gram of sample (Burnett and Schuster, 1978).

The normal resident flora and the host generally have a cooperative relationship. Innate bacterial antagonism, salivary lysozyme and peroxidase, and immunoglobulins act to regulate the oral flora and protect the host against visiting pathogens. It is important that the reader understand the body's protective mechanisms before potential pathogens are described. Intact skin and mucous membranes offer a physical barrier against microbial invasion of the bloodstream and deeper tissues. It is interesting to note that the secretions of sweat glands maintain an average dermal pH of 5.2 to 5.8, which is bactericidal and fungicidal (Burnett and Schuster, 1978). To a large extent, once foreign particles enter the oral cavity, they are trapped in the mucus or saliva and are swallowed; gastric acid in the stomach destroys them. In a similar fashion, the respiratory tract has a mucous coat to trap large particles (10 to 50 μg) and a specialized ciliated epithelium that constantly moves the mucus down from the nasopharynx or away from the bronchi of the lungs in order to be swallowed. Smaller particles (0.5 to 5 μg) have the greatest potential for penetration and retention in the lung (Miller and Micik, 1978). Thus a number of important factors, including the individual's innate or acquired immunity and the protective physical and chemical factors mentioned above, work in concert to protect against infection.

Tables 3-2 and 3-3 summarize the bacterial and viral pathogens that may be active in the oral cavity or are significant in that they provide a means for transmission by way of the respiratory tract. Hepatitis, tuberculosis, syphilis, herpes simplex infections, and acquired immune deficiency syndrome (AIDS) are discussed in this chapter as contagious diseases that are transmitted via contact with the oral cavity.

PATHWAYS OF DISEASE TRANSMISSION

Diseases are transmitted by inanimate or human sources in a variety of ways.

Direct transmission occurs when organisms are transferred from one host to another, usually by way of the bloodstream, saliva, or respiratory secretions. Entrance to the bloodstream usually occurs when the skin is penetrated by a contaminated instrument or needle or when organisms seep into an open wound, such as a cut or torn cuticle on the clinician's hand.

The proximity of the patient and clinician make respiratory sources important. As Tables 3-2 and 3-3 indicate, most of the pathogens inhabit the nasopharynx area (Nolte, 1982). During breathing, conversation, coughing, or sneezing, organisms are sprayed into the environment, producing an aerosol (Johnson and Johnson, 1969; Miller and Micik, 1978). This collection of particles suspended in the air is capable of transmitting pathogens. The organisms may stay suspended for a period of time or may fall rapidly to contaminate the environment and the people in the operatory. Aerosol production is more significant when one considers the equipment and procedures performed by dental clinicians. Handpieces, trisyringes (air-water syringes), ultrasonic scalers, instrumentation, and even instruction of a patient in toothbrushing are responsible for creating serious aerosols (Williams, 1970). One investigator collected and cultured a sample of air from a carrier that yielded 41 viable colonies of *Mycobacterium tuberculosis*. The highest concentration of microorganisms was found within 2 feet in front of the patient where the clinician is usually positioned (Johnson and Johnson, 1969).

Aerosols and organisms carried in the dust make up airborne sources of disease transfer. Patients and workers moving in and out of the treatment area are carriers of pathogens and constantly stir up the airborne dust contaminating the environment. Some organisms (Tables 3-2 and 3-3) are able to survive on inanimate objects—counter tops, sinks, operatory equipment—for extended periods and provide a source of cross-infection. When a pathogen is transferred from one person to another by way of an inanimate source or a source other than the original carrier, *indirect transmission* has occurred.

As well as being the primary contact between the environment and the patient or between one patient and another, the clinician can be the source of disease. A clinician with an upper respiratory tract infection or, more seriously, a communicable disease such as hepatitis B, is placing the patient in jeopardy. Wearing a mask and gloves provides protection for both the clinician and the patient. Methods for maintaining asepsis are discussed later in the chapter.

Table 3-2. Summary of bacterial pathogens that may be transmitted by way of the oral cavity during dental treatment

Organism	Bacterial disease	Mode of transmission	Other
Mycobacterium tuberculosis	Tuberculosis of lungs, lymph nodes, meninges, kidneys, bone, skin, oronasopharynx tissues	Organism found in sputum; transmitted by respiratory droplet or contact with contaminated inanimate objects	Microorganisms resist chemicals and survive well on dry surfaces for weeks
Treponema pallidum	Syphilis Primary: chancre of skin, lips, tongue, oral mucosa Secondary: recurrent patch of mucosa Tertiary: gummas of oral cavity, larynx, vocal cords	Contact with oral lesions harboring organism; transmitted by contact with contaminated blood or by penetration of epithelium	Disease is highly contagious in primary and secondary stages; because of nature of symptoms women may be unaware of the disease in early stages; lesions of secondary syphilis may persist or recur for 2 to 3 years
Staphylococcus aureus	Wound infection, abscesses, cellulitis, meningitis, osteomyelitis, toxic shock syndrome	Organism found in nose, mouth, skin; transmitted by contact with contaminated blood or inanimate objects	Organism survives well on dry surfaces; 30% of population are asymptomatic nasopharyngeal carriers
Streptococcus pyogenes viridans pneumoniae	"Strep" throat, peritonsillar abscesses, pharyngitis, scarlet fever, rheumatic fever, glomerulonephritis, subacute bacterial endocarditis, pneumonia with secondary septicemia, empyema, pericarditis, and meningitis	Found in saliva, nasopharynx; transmitted by contact with contaminated blood or inanimate objects	Organism survives well on dry surfaces; approximately 10% of general population are asymptomatic nasopharyngeal carriers
Pseudomonas aeruginosa	May cause infection in almost all organs, especially in patients with lowered resistance	Lives in water supplies; transmitted through bloodstream by contaminated water supplies	Regular monitoring of water filtering system and maintenance of germ-free lines necessary to prevent transmission of organism
Candida albicans	Adult: candidiasis Child: thrush infection of skin or mucous membrane	Mouth, nails, lungs, skin, gastrointestinal tract, vagina; transmitted by contact with contaminated source	Lesion of the labial commissures occurs similar to lesion of riboflavin deficiency
Actinomyces israelii	Actinomycosis of oral cavity, face, neck, abdominal cavity, lungs	Organism inhabits tonsils, carious teeth, calculus, open wounds, extraction sites, pulp exposures; transmitted through bloodstream and tissue inoculation	Tissue infection usually occurs after repeated exposure to organism following surgery, injury, or chronic irritation
Chlamydia trachomatis	Lymphogranuloma venereum	Oral lesion (primarily tongue) can infect hands of dental personnel	A type of venereal disease seen most often in tropics
Haemophilus influenzae	Pharyngitis, sinusitis, respiratory tract infection, meningitis	Inhabitant of nasopharynx, mucus, sputum; transmitted by respiratory droplet and by contaminated objects	Organism incapsulated and may resist chemicals; organism survives longer on inanimate objects than do other organisms; 33% to 66% of normal adults are nasopharyngeal carriers
Bordetella pertussis	Whooping cough	Transmitted by respiratory droplet	Affects 90% of nonimmunized population; vaccine greatly reduces morbidity; incubation 1 to 2 weeks; course of disease runs to 6 weeks
Clostridium tetani	Tetanus	Inhabits soil and intestinal tract; dust-borne spore transmission by spores entering wound site	Spores are highly resistant to physical/chemical agents Protection: DPT vaccine

Table 3-3. Summary of viral pathogens that may be transmitted by way of the oral cavity during dental treatment

Organism	Viral disease	Mode of transmission	Other characteristics
Respiratory virus: adenovirus, coxsackievirus A, echovirus, respiratory syncytial, rhinovirus, polio virus	Upper respiratory tract infection (sore throat, cough, nasal discharge, fever, chills, muscle aches, fatigue); lower respiratory tract infection; conjunctiva; lesions of oral cavity; meningitis	Organism inhabits nose, mouth, eye; transmitted by respiratory droplet, aerosols, contaminated surfaces	Viruses occur worldwide; peak incidence in fall and winter; asymptomatic carriers and variety of strains make control difficult; all factors of transmission may not be identified as yet
Herpes virus	Simplex: "cold sores," dermatitis, keratitis (eye infection), whitlow (lesion of fingers); varicella-zoster: chicken pox (child), shingles (adult)	Saliva, direct contact with lesions, respiratory tract transmission	Repeated active phases of herpes simplex may result in chronic problem; chickenpox immunity after childhood episode; only 0.5% to 2% of population may acquire zoster varicellosus
Epstein-Barr (EB) virus	Infectious mononucleosis	Throat-oral respiratory transmission	Incubation period 4 to 49 days; possibility of treating patient in early stages
Hepatitis viruses: A B Other, as yet unidentified viruses Delta virus	Infectious hepatitis Serum hepatitis Non-A, non-B hepatitis Delta hepatitis	Saliva, feces, blood, tears, semen, sweat; transmitted by means of respiratory droplet or contact with contaminated blood	Disease on rise in general population; patient may be a carrier with or without acute episode; incubation period makes treating patient in undiagnosed or carrier state possible
Papilloma virus	Warts	Direct contact or contact with contaminated surface	Patient protection necessary if dental personnel are affected
Mumps virus Rubeola virus Rubella virus	Mumps Measles German measles	Respiratory secretions, saliva, blood, urine, contaminated surfaces	Transfer may occur during incubation phase (18 to 21 days) Vaccine available Rubella is of special concern for pregnant women, since disease may cause congenital defects or death of fetus

It is also a fact that a patient may harbor organisms naturally in the oral cavity that are capable of producing disease if they enter his or her own bloodstream. This resultant condition is referred to as an *autogenous* infection, meaning that the patient is the source of the pathogen. Some of the most prevalent organisms in the oral cavity capable of producing autogenous infection are the various types of streptococci. If during an injection organisms are "seeded" (i.e., carried) into deep tissues, or if as a result of instrumentation a bacteremia (flood of viable organisms into the bloodstream) occurs, these organisms may cause soft tissue or bone infection. In some patients a serious disease called subacute bacterial endocarditis may result (see Chapter 5).

An awareness of the variety of pathways by which microorganisms, particularly pathogenic ones, may be transmitted in the course of dental treatment is important because all human beings have the potential to contaminate themselves, each other, and the environment by direct or indirect transmission. In most cases the exact source of a resulting infection is difficult to identify. This only emphasizes the need for clinics and offices to establish and follow a strict program of infection control.

Hepatitis

The viral illnesses known as hepatitis are of special concern to the dental clinician because they can be transmitted in operatory conditions and because infected carriers are often unaware of their condition. There are at least four different types of viral hepatitis, called A; B; non-A, non-B; and delta. Common signs and symptoms include malaise, fever, loss of appetite, nausea, abdominal discomfort, and vomiting. Jaundice may or may not occur.

Hepatitis A has an incubation period of 2 to 6 weeks after being transmitted predominantly by the oral-fecal route. Children and young people are most often infected. It appears to be acute (having rapid onset), but no residual postrecovery effects result. There are no carriers of this disease. A successful vaccine for hepatitis A has not yet been developed.

In contrast, *hepatitis B* is transmitted by intimate contact with body secretions (Table 3-4). This virus is found most commonly in the blood, but can also be present in saliva, sputum, crevicular fluid, and other body fluids. Only minute quantities of contaminated blood or saliva are required to cause infection. Intraorally, the greatest concentration of hepatitis B infection is at the gingival sulcus, a location of prime concern to the hygienist as well as the dentist (Sampson, 1982).

Table 3-4. Comparison of the traditional two types of viral hepatitis

	Infectious hepatitis (A)	*Serum hepatitis (B)*
Virus transmission	Fecal-oral route; also parenteral	From blood and blood products; primarily parenteral; can be by means of oral route and contact with carrier
Incubation period	About 30 days (15 to 50)	30 to 180 days
Age preference	Children, young adults	All ages
Duration of infectious period	Virus in feces and blood 1 to 2 weeks before disease; remains 3 to 4 weeks longer	Virus in blood 3 months before disease; occasional asymptomatic carrier for as long as 5 years
Virus present	Saliva, feces, blood	Blood, feces, saliva
Clinical features*		
Onset	Acute	Slow, usually insidious
Fever	Common before jaundice	Less common
Jaundice	Rare in children, more frequent in adults	Rare in children, more frequent in adults
Severity of disease	Less severe	More severe
Prognosis	Good	Less favorable
Laboratory evaluation		
Thymol turbidity†	Increased	Normal
Abnormal SGOT‡	Transient, 1 to 3 weeks	Prolonged, 1 to 8 months
HAA (Australia antigen) in blood	Not present	Present during incubation period and acute phase; occasionally persists
Prevention and control		
Prophylactic effect of gamma globulin	Good	Possibly beneficial
Dental precautions and control	1. Emergency care during acute phase 2. Mask, gloves, and safety glasses worn 3. Sterilization of contaminated items 4. Disposables used if sterilization is impossible 5. Care with anesthetics (amides) metabolized by liver	1. Emergency care during initial phase 2. Mask, gloves, and safety glasses worn 3. Sterilization of contaminated items 4. Disposables used if sterilization is impossible 5. Care with anesthetics (amides) metabolized by liver 6. Update history at every recall visit for carrier status

Modified from Smith AL: Principles of microbiology, ed 9, St Louis, 1982, The CV Mosby Co.
*Many clinical features are the same.
†Test of liver function.
‡The enzyme serum glutamic-oxaloacetic transaminase level is elevated with liver disease.

In the dental operatory, hepatitis B may be transmitted percutaneously through wounds from sharp instruments or contaminated needles. A second mode of transmission can occur nonpercutaneously from the transfer of infected saliva or blood into breaks in the skin or mucous membranes. Transmission can also occur from contact with surfaces, such as equipment or clothing, that have been contaminated by dental aerosols.

Hepatitis B has a long incubation period of 2 to 6 months. Symptoms of hepatitis are often mild. They may mimic other common conditions such as influenza or stress-related illnesses and may include fatigue, loss of appetite, nausea, and abdominal and joint pain. Jaundice does not always occur. Conditions which result from hepatitis B include chronic hepatitis, cirrhosis, and liver cancer. There is no known cure or effective treatment for hepatitis B.

A number of population groups have been cited as belonging to high-risk groups for contact with the hepatitis B virus (Cottone, 1985). These include persons who receive frequent large volume transfusions (hemophiliacs); persons in renal dialysis units; persons in institutions for the mentally handicapped; persons who are immunosuppressed or immunodeficient; persons with a recent history of jaundice; intravenous drug abusers; promiscuous homosexual males; female prostitutes; and immigrants from Third World countries (Haiti, Indochina). This list is extensive, yet it only identifies those with a high risk of being infected with hepatitis B. Obviously, the safest recommendation is that of the National Centers for Disease Control (CDC) which states that an effective infection control program must operate under the assumption that *all* dental patients have the potential for transmitting this disease.

Hepatitis B is a major occupational hazard for dental care providers. The general practitioner and hygienist may have a risk of becoming infected with hepatitis B that is three times greater than that of the general population, and specialists such as oral surgeons and periodontists may have an even higher risk (Cottone, 1985).

In an estimated 80% of all cases of hepatitis B, the infected individual is asymptomatic or suffers only subclinical symptoms and is therefore unaware of the infection. Approximately 10% of those infected with the disease will become chronic carriers who are capable of infecting others, perhaps for years. Therefore, medical histories and examinations cannot be relied upon to identify those who are capable of transmitting the disease within the dental environment. Dental practitioners may be lulled into a false sense of security if they gauge their potential for contracting this disease solely on medical history information. An office that treats 20 patients per day might expect to encounter an active carrier of hepatitis B once in every 7 working days (Crawford, 1985). Although a few cases have documented the transmission of hepatitis from dental professionals to patients, it is far more likely that the flow of transmission is from patient to dental professional. Therefore, if proper precautions are not observed, dental professionals may not only find themselves infected, but also may unwittingly infect their family members or others with whom they have intimate contact.

The best prevention against HBV is for all dental personnel to be vaccinated with one of the hepatitis vaccines (Heptavax-B or Recombivax-HB, Merck, Sharp & Dohme). These vaccines have been proven to be safe and effective methods for prevention of this disease. Vaccination requires a series of three injections that produce antibodies in 85% to 96% of recipients. A posttest to determine seroconversion is recommended within 1 to 3 months following the last injection of the vaccine. Individuals who have not formed antibodies after the initial series should receive additional injections. Immunity is expected to last at least 5 years in most individuals who have received all three doses of the vaccine and have seroconverted (Cottone and Baker, 1985). Table 3-5 recommends procedures that should be followed following percutaneous exposure in both vaccinated and unvaccinated individuals.

The second part of this chapter discusses appropriate infection control measures that should be incorporated into dental practice to provide further protection against transmission of HBV and other infectious diseases. These recommendations should be instituted for *all* dental patients and not just those who are known to be infectious or from high-risk population groups.

The less common so-called *non-A, non-B hepatitis* has been diagnosed. In general, this form appears similar to hepatitis B and follows a simi-

Table 3-5. Recommendations for hepatitis B prophylaxis following percutaneous exposure*

Terminology:

HBsAg—Hepatitis B surface antigen

Anti-HB—antibody to HBsAg; indicates past infection and immunity to HBV, passive immunity to HBIG, or immunity due to HBV vaccine

HBIG—Hepatitis B immune globulin; made from plasma pools containing high titers of anti-HB; used for postexposure prophylaxis

	Recommended Procedure	
Source	Exposed person is vaccinated	Exposed person is not vaccinated
HBsAG positive	1. Give HBIG immediately 2. Begin HB vaccine series	1. Test exposed person anti-HBs 2. If inadequate antibody, give HBIG (x1) immediately plus HB vaccine booster
Known high risk	1. Begin HB vaccine series 2. Request that source be tested for HBsAg; if positive, give HBIG (x1)	1. Test source for HBsAg only if exposed person has inadequate antibody protection; if source is HBsAg-positive, give HBIG immediately plus HB booster dose
Low risk or unknown	Initiate HB vaccine series	No treatment required

*(Adapted from MMWR 34:331, 1985; Cottone JA, and Baker BR: Hepatitis B: recent advances and 1986 preview, CDA Journal 13:36, 1985.)

lar clinical course after an incubation period of approximately 7 weeks (Smith, 1982).

Delta hepatitis is a newly recognized form of viral hepatitis and has been shown to be a coinfection with hepatitis B (Cottone, 1986). It contains limited genetic material and requires the hepatitis B virus to act as a helper in its replication. Infection with the delta virus may occur concurrently with HBV infection, in which case the symptoms and course of the infection are similar to those of hepatitis B. Infection of delta hepatitis can also occur in an individual who is already a chronic HBV carrier. These persons are more likely to have a serious and acute fulminant form of hepatitis that can progress rapidly, resulting in severe liver damage and ultimately death. Delta hepatitis, like hepatitis B, is usually transmitted by percutaneous or permucosal exposure and can be controlled by the infection control measures recommended for hepatitis B. Fortunately, the hepatitis B vaccine will also protect against delta hepatitis, which is dependent on the former for survival.

Acquired immune deficiency syndrome (AIDS)

Since its official recognition by the Centers for Disease Control (CDC) in 1981, acquired immune deficiency syndrome (AIDS), for which there is no cure, has become a worldwide epidemic of frightening proportions. It has achieved unprecedented publicity, sometimes leading to panic, and is challenging established social, ethical, moral, legal, and medical beliefs and principles. The dental clinician is inevitably involved in these developments due to the deadly syndrome's tendency toward transmission through the exchange of body fluids.

It has been established that AIDS is caused by infection from a human immunodeficiency virus (HIV), which is transmitted through exposure to blood or other body fluids of an infected individual. The retrovirus enters the bloodstream and attacks the immune system, eventually causing its breakdown. This makes the victim vulnerable to bacteria, viruses, and fungi that would normally be harmless. The HIV incubation period varies widely among individuals, with the result that many carriers who can transmit HIV are unaware of their own infection. Clinical signs of HIV infection begin with mononucleosis-like illness symptoms and progress as opportunistic infections, such as pneumonia, tuberculosis, viral infections, meningitis, and cancers, invade the body, eventually resulting in death. Individuals at highest risk for AIDS are sexually active homo-sexual and bisexual males and intravenous drug abusers. AIDS is also transmitted through the use of contaminated needles and from mothers to un-born and nursing children, with the result that its spread into the community at large is well under way.

The number of AIDS cases increases each year. It is predicted that by 1991 there will be 270,000 cases of AIDS in the United States. The cumula-tive number of AIDS-related deaths is estimated to reach 179,000 by the end of 1991 (USPHS, 1986). Approximately 1.5 to 2 million persons are carriers of the HIV who may be infectious, and the number of carriers is constantly increas-ing. The period from the time of initial infection to the appearance of overt symptoms and diagno-sis may be as long as 7 years in some individuals (CDC, 1986; USPHS, 1986; Landesman et al, 1985).

HIV infection occurs in three stages. The first stage is an asymptomatic carrier phase in which the person may be infectious without exhibiting symptoms. An estimated 80% of infected individ-uals may be infectious to others. The second stage of infection is known as AIDS-related com-plex (ARC) and occurs in an estimated 25% of those infected with the HIV. Clinical signs in-clude long-term fever, weight loss, lymphadenop-athy, chronic diarrhea, fatigue, and night sweats. Oral findings may include candidiasis, hairy leu-koplakia, herpes simplex, xerostomia, acute gin-gival infections resembling ANUG, and acceler-ated periodontal destruction. The third stage of in-fection is AIDS. Patients live an average of 56 weeks after the diagnosis of this stage. These pa-tients frequently manifest a malignant skin cancer known as Kaposi's sarcoma, which may appear intraorally, especially on the hard palate, as single or multiple painless, reddish-blue, flat or elevated areas that are highly vascular. Other clinical find-ings are similar to those described for ARC (Neu-pert, 1987).

The primary means of transmission of HIV is through sexual contact or through contact with contaminated blood. The blood-borne route is the primary route for transmission of the virus to health care workers. Although HIV has been found in saliva, saliva has not been shown to transmit the virus. Although health care workers are at risk for contracting AIDS during contact with patients and contaminated materials, the risk is fortunately quite low. Klein and others (1988) studied the occupational risk of dental profession-als for infection with HIV and found that in spite of infrequent compliance with recommended in-fection control precautions, frequent exposure to persons at increased risk for HIV infection, and frequent accidents in which the skin was punc-tured with sharp instruments, dental professionals are at low occupational risk for HIV infection. In fact, studies indicate that this risk is less than the previously accepted risks for other infectious dis-eases such as hepatitis B or herpes.

The best means of protection for dental profes-sionals against HIV infection are barrier protec-tive techniques and compliance with the infection control procedures recommended by the CDC and the ADA and discussed later in this chapter. ADA and CDC guidelines agree that transmission con-trol is best achieved through the constant use of gloves, masks, and eye protection; the effective sterilization of dental instruments; cleanup of in-struments and surfaces in the operatory; and proper disposal of contaminated materials. Spe-cial care should always be taken when handling sharp instruments. Clothes exposed to HIV can be safely used after a normal laundry cycle or dry-cleaning. The clinician must remember that it is impossible to recognize someone with HIV with-out clinical manifestations, and the only method of protection is to assume that *every* patient has HIV and use proper barrier mechanisms accord-ingly.

The dental professional has a responsibility to treat AIDS patients just as those suffering from other diseases. Although the right of a dentist to refuse or refer treatment of a prospective new pa-tient who has AIDS has not yet been tested in the courts, refusal to treat a suspected or known AIDS carrier may be considered illegal on the grounds that such action constitutes discrimina-tion against a handicapped individual (Logan, 1987). When appropriate barrier precautions are implemented, dental professionals can safely treat these individuals. Dental clinicians are especially important because their oral findings of certain in-fections play a significant role in the diagnosis and treatment of symptoms. The dental profes-sional also has a responsibility to keep informed by keeping abreast of the rapidly proliferating literature about AIDS so that the latest breakthroughs in diagnosis and treatment can be implemented.

Tuberculosis

Tuberculosis is of special concern for dental personnel, because the oral cavity is one of the chief pathways of transmission. Sputum laden with tubercle bacilli presents the greatest danger for persons contacting the patient. *Mycobacterium tuberculosis* is resistant to many chemical disinfectants and survives well on dry surfaces, making it a matter of concern in maintaining asepsis in the dental environment.

Tuberculosis most often affects the lungs, but other sites of the disease include the mouth (especially a lesion of the tongue), skin, gastrointestinal tract, bone, and salivary glands (Burnett and Schuster, 1978; Rowe and Brooks, 1978).

Urban areas characterized by poor socioeconomic conditions have higher rates of tuberculosis than do areas with high incomes and low population densities (Nolte, 1982).

Effective therapy with medication has significantly reduced the number of deaths due to tuberculosis. Treatment consists of excision of the tubercular lesion and a regimen of medications used in various combinations. Choice of medication is dependent on the antimicrobial sensitivities of the particular strain of organisms involved. Common medications include isoniazid, rifampin, ethambutol, and streptomycin. For those frequently exposed to tuberculosis, such as family members of a tubercular patient or medical personnel working in urban areas or developing countries, a vaccine of attenuated strain is available. Protection may be only temporary with the BCG (bacille Calmette Guérin) vaccine.

Because of the increased opportunity dental personnel have for contracting tuberculosis, periodic skin testing is recommended (Rowe and Brooks, 1978).

Once tuberculosis patients are treated and cleared, they are generally followed for a yearly sputum culture and chest x-ray examination to determine any recurrence. A patient who reports a history of tuberculosis but has current medical clearance may be treated as a routine patient.

Syphilis

The incidence of venereal disease is increasing in the United States. The number of cases of gonorrhea is rising more sharply than that of syphilis, but contagious oral lesions associated with the latter disease make it of particular interest to the dental profession.

The organism that causes syphilis is *Treponema pallidum,* a spirochete that enters the body through a break—which need not be obvious—in the skin.

Syphilis has three stages. Each may be characterized by oral manifestations. From 10 days to 3 months after initial contact, a primary stage lesion may occur. This is a *chancre* and most often occurs on the genitalia, but between 5% and 12% of patients develop extragenital lesions. Greater than 50% of these extragenital chancres occur on the lips, with the tongue and tonsils being other common oral sites. Dental personnel contracting syphilis may develop a chancre of the finger(s). Transmission may occur through mishandling of contaminated dental instruments or inanimate objects such as drinking cups.

After the primary lesion heals, the secondary stage presents. The oral manifestation of this phase is a moist patch on the mucous membrane, occasionally covered by a grey membrane. These lesions are teeming with organisms and are highly infectious. This stage may last as long as 6 weeks and is followed by a nonspecific latent period. Only about one third of persons with untreated syphilis develop destructive lesions of the tertiary stage (Nolte, 1982). Although the occasion for observing a tertiary lesion is rare, tumors of granulomatous tissue, called *gummas,* may appear in the oral cavity. The most common site is the palate.

Treatment with antibiotics is indicated for syphilis. If possible, treatment should begin before the primary lesion occurs. The further along the disease is, the longer antibiotic therapy is necessary.

The dental professional should approach the examination and treatment of each patient carefully. The health history may be helpful in revealing a past episode of syphilis, in which case precautions should be taken by wearing gloves and following strict asepsis. However, some patients may be unaware of having syphilis. Primary stage lesions of the genitalia may go unnoticed, especially in women, and oral lesions may not occur at all. The primary and secondary stages pose the greatest risk for transmitting infection. At any stage, misdiagnosis of oral lesions may occur unless serologic studies are performed. For the added protection of dental personnel, some large clinics, such as those in dental schools, require a blood test as part of the admissions/screening procedure.

Herpes simplex virus infections

Infections caused by the herpes simplex virus are of particular concern to the dental professional. Transmission of these infections can occur via direct contact with oral herpetic lesions or oral secretions containing the virus, via aerosols, or via fomites such as dental instruments, handpieces, or impressions (Merchant, 1982). It has been shown that these viruses, as well as bacteria, can be transmitted by dental charts touched with contaminated gloves (Thomas et al, 1985). Four diseases caused by herpes simplex viruses are presented here. These are acute gingivostomatitis, recurrent herpes labialis, ocular keratitis, and herpetic whitlow.

Primary herpetic gingivostomatitis is commonly acquired in small children (2 to 3 years of age). Initial symptoms may mimic many acute infections, with generalized malaise, fever, regional lymphadenopathy, headache, pain on swallowing, fretfulness, sleeplessness, and refusal to eat. Within a few days the mouth and gingiva become intensely painful and inflamed. The lips, tongue, buccal mucosa, palate, pharynx, and tonsils may become involved. Scattered aphthouslike lesions appear as crops of small ulcers that coalesce to produce large, shallow, irregular ulcers with surrounding inflammation (Gross, 1981). Merchant (1982) reports that only about 10% of oral infections are clinically apparent, indicating that some children especially may be infectious without usual symptoms or complaints. Within 7 to 14 days the vesicles and ulcers heal spontaneously with no scar formation.

Recurrent oral herpes may appear as herpes labialis or oral herpes simplex. A prodromal itching, tingling, or tenderness may be present in the area 6 to 28 hours before the lesion occurs. The "cold sores" on the lip or at the mucocutaneous junction generally progress from vesicle stage to crusted stage within 2 to 4 days. Discomfort is most severe during the first 24 hours, with the course of the disease running 7 to 10 days. Generally, no scar formation occurs.

The herpes virus may remain latent at the site in the regional nerve ganglia for years. Activation of the virus may be caused by trauma, febrile illness, exposure to sunlight, fatigue, menstruation, pregnancy, allergies, or emotional stress with shedding of the virus as the result. The virus shedding may or may not produce a lesion but may put at risk susceptible individuals who are in contact.

The proof of an antibody titer to herpes simplex virus (HSV-1) does not necessarily protect against reinfection (Merchant, 1982).

The typical features of ocular keratitis include foreign body sensation in the affected eye, followed several hours later by redness, tearing, light sensitivity, and pain. Only one eye is usually involved. Complete recovery occurs within about 3 weeks (Rowe et al 1982). Ulcers may develop on the cornea, producing ocular damage. The possible debilitation and its effect on employment make recurrent ocular keratitis a serious condition for the clinician.

Herpetic whitlow is a herpes simplex virus of the fingers. Usually the infection follows a puncture wound or a passage of the virus through broken skin around fingernails. The site becomes extremely painful within 3 to 5 days. The digit frequently swells, and one or more vesicles containing clear to turbid, but never purulent, fluid develop. Typically these lesions develop in the areas around the fingernail, although other areas of the finger can be involved as well. The lesion usually resolves within 14 to 21 days, but the clinical course may be prolonged (Merchant, 1982). Rowe and others (1982) state that the risk of contracting herpes simplex virus infection of the finger or hand for the practicing dental clinician is approximately twice what it would be if he or she were a member of the control population employed in some other field. There is no effective drug treatment for herpetic whitlow and because any clinician with this problem is a risk to patients and associates, a 10- to 14-day leave from practice may be indicated (Palenik and Miller, 1982).

Unlike hepatitis B, no vaccine is available to prevent herpes simplex virus infections. As stated above, the proof of an HSV-1 antibody titer does not protect against reinfection. Treatment of herpes simplex is basically supportive in nature, with an emphasis on the prevention of secondary infection.

Topical anesthetics and compounds placed on the lesion to maintain moisture and prevent discomfort have been tried. Gross (1981) reports that topical applications of steroids have been used but have been shown to attenuate the attack and disperse the infection over a larger area. Therefore topical applications of corticosteroid creams should not be used. Compounds such as lysine (Tankersley, 1964) and bioflavonoid ascorbic acid (Terezhalmy et al 1978) have been cited to accelerate healing time. Currently, acycloguanosine (Acyclovir) has shown promise as a therapeutic agent, and research continues to find other agents to prevent, treat, and diminish recurrences of herpes simplex infections.

Protection and prevention are best obtained by taking a history to identify patients with frequent episodes of herpes. Patients with active oral lesions should not be treated when elective care can be postponed. Standard infection control measures, including barrier protection, will reduce the risk of exposure to virus-containing aerosols and saliva.

CONTROL OF MICROORGANISMS

We live in an environment that is filled with microorganisms, including the air we breathe and every surface we touch. In addition, we carry immense communities of bacteria, viruses, and other microorganisms within our own bodies. The richest reservoir of these is the mouth. Many of these microorganisms are harmless to our health, and some are necessary to assist normal functioning of the human body. Others, such as the bacteria and viruses already discussed, cause serious communicable diseases. Many pathogens, including the tubercle bacillus, hepatitis viruses, and other durable viruses and infectious bacteria, can survive for a week or more within dried body fluids on surfaces and clothing, where they can be transmitted to dental personnel, other patients, and family members.

All health professionals are concerned about preventing disease transmission and maintaining an environment where patients can be treated without the risk of contracting infection or debilitating disease. Total asepsis of the dental office is both impractical and impossible, but all attempts toward asepsis improve the likelihood that cross-contamination of pathogens from objects in the dental environment to a person or from one person to another can be prevented. An absolutely sterile office is impossible, but a safe environment is achievable. It is crucial that dental professionals be aware of the presence of pathogenic microorganisms and their potential for causing and transmitting disease. Furthermore, they must exercise all possible measures to reduce the numbers of pathogens in order to minimize the threat to patients and themselves.

The National Centers for Disease Control (CDC) has warned dental practitioners that medical histories and examinations cannot be relied upon to identify all patients who are infected with the viruses that cause hepatitis, AIDS, and other blood-borne pathogens. Therefore, "universal" precautions which are designed to prevent transmission of these diseases should be followed for all patients (CDC, 1987). The recommendations in this chapter describe the precautions that are considered at this time to be acceptable standards of care by the CDC and the American Dental Association. It is the responsibility of every dental professional and student to seek all current information regarding future additions and changes in these important guidelines to protect the health of themselves, their families, their coworkers, and those whom they serve. This chapter will discuss six important steps necessary to prevent disease transmission within the dental environment: (1) identification of contaminated surfaces; (2) sanitization of the dental environment; (3) disinfection procedures; (4) sterilization procedures; (5) use of effective barriers; and (6) personal hygiene and vaccinations.

The following definitions may be helpful in understanding contamination control terminology and recommendations:

Antiseptic. A substance that inhibits the growth and reproduction of microorganisms; usually applied to living tissues as opposed to inanimate objects.

Asepsis/aseptic. The absence of infection or infectious materials or pathogens.

-cidal. A suffix meaning "to kill" (*e.g.,* virucidal, bacteriocidal, fungicidal, sporicidal, germicidal, tuberculocidal).

Cross-contamination. The transmission of a pathogen from one person to another or from an inanimate surface to an individual.

Disinfectant. A liquid chemical agent that destroys most but not all microorganisms.

Disinfection. A process that destroys most but not all microorganisms.

HBV. Hepatitis B virus.

HIV. Human immunodeficiency virus.

Sanitization. A process of mechanical removal or reduction of the number of microorganisms, dirt, or debris (e.g., cleaning).

-static. A suffix meaning "to restrain the development of" (e.g., bacteriostatic).

Sterilant. An agent capable of resulting in sterilization.

Sterilization. A process that results in the complete destruction of *all* microorganisms.

Identification of contaminated surfaces

Surfaces in the dental environment can be contaminated by direct contact with blood, saliva, mucous membranes, or other body fluids, aerosols, splatter droplets that are generated during dental treatment, or by contact with other contaminated surfaces or contaminated hands. Contamination control of environmental surfaces involves covering them with disposable drapes or wraps, avoiding unnecessary contact with surfaces during dental treatment, and treatment by recommended disinfection and sterilization procedures. In order to select the appropriate level of contamination control for each surface in the dental environment, one must first consider the level of contamination to which it is exposed and its potential as a source of cross-contamination. When considering the level and type of contamination, the prudent dental professional will remember that the recommended standards for infection control are based on the assumption that all patients are potential carriers of infectious diseases, including the hepatitis B virus and HIV. Although complete contamination control is the ideal goal, some items cannot be sterilized because of their size or

their inability to withstand sterilization procedures. All surfaces and items in the dental environment may be classified in one of three ways:

1. *Critical surfaces* are those that actually enter the mouth and have direct contact with blood, saliva, mucous membrane, or other body fluids (e.g., all dental instruments, dental handpiece and prophy angle, air-water syringe tip, saliva ejector or high-speed evacuation tip, x-ray film holders).

2. *Semicritical surfaces* are those that may have frequent contact with aerosols generated during dental treatment or are touched by the patient or the contaminated hands of the clinician or assistant during patient treatment (*e.g.,* chair and unit controls, lamp handle and switch, bases of the air-water syringe, saliva ejector, high speed suction and handpiece, chair armrests, drawer pulls, supply container lids, bracket table rims or handles, and countertops, x-ray head and controls, water faucet handles).

3. *Noncritical surfaces* are those that are present in the dental environment but are unlikely to be contaminated by oral pathogens or touched during patient treatment (*e.g.,* floors, walls, furniture, chairs, blinds, surfaces outside the dental operatory).

All critical surfaces must be sterilized before reuse or discarded after one use (disposable). Most of the items that are listed in the semicritical category cannot be moved or are too large or incompatible with accepted sterilization methods. Therefore, they must be kept covered and/or treated with accepted chemical solutions after each patient contact. Most noncritical surfaces require routine cleaning and disinfection, but they do not require treatment after each patient unless obvious contamination is observed.

In order to establish an infection control routine that is effectively and efficiently carried out in the short amount of time between patient appointments, efforts should be made to define exactly which surfaces can and cannot be contacted during patient treatment and to restrict all contact of contaminated hands and instruments to those surfaces or areas only. This disciplined behavior will ensure that prescribed contamination control procedures will consistently treat all contaminated areas in the most effective manner and that time need not be wasted trying to clean and disinfect surfaces that should never have been contaminated. Contamination control procedures are most effective if all office staff agree to follow predetermined guidelines specifying what surfaces can and cannot be touched during patient treatment. By restricting the number of surfaces that fall within the semicritical category and by following recommended guidelines that specify optimal treatment of all surfaces according to their categories, maximal infection control can be ensured. Following identification and categorization of contaminated surfaces in the operatory, the first step in the infection control process, sanitization, can be instituted.

Sanitization

Sanitization (cleaning) involves the physical removal of germ-laden dust and dirt from floors, walls, furniture, equipment, and surfaces. The elimination of visible soil is the first step in creating a safe environment and must precede all recommended disinfection and sterilization procedures. Sanitization reduces the numbers of microorganisms on surfaces and equipment, thus increasing the effectiveness of disinfection or sterilization procedures that follow. The presence of excessive numbers of microorganisms, soil, and organic matter (such as blood or saliva) can inhibit or even prevent methods of disinfection or sterilization from destroying the target pathogens. For this reason, routine cleaning and scrubbing of all surfaces in the dental office, especially those surfaces in the dental operatory that are contacted by patients, clinicians, or dental aerosols, is mandatory as the first step in the process to prevent disease transmission.

The general working environment of the dental office should be kept meticulously clean and free of dust. This requirement includes walls, floors, furniture, curtains, cabinets, and countertops. Daily sanitization of all horizontal surfaces is necessary to remove bacteria-laden soil and dust that has entered from the outside environment. Other surfaces including walls, furniture, drapes, and blinds should be cleaned whenever they become visibly soiled. Cleaning and dusting is best accomplished with a vacuum system that removes the particles rather than a method that pushes

them around the room and back into the air. Vacuum cleaning should be followed by use of a detergent solution. The detergents or soaps used for cleaning not only enhance the ability of water to remove surface dirt and films but also have mild destructive capabilities against some less resistant pathogens. In addition, a chemical disinfectant that has been registered by the Environmental Protection Agency (EPA) as a "hospital" disinfectant should be used on contaminated surfaces to destroy pathogenic bacteria and viruses that remain after mechanical cleaning.

An especially critical area for contamination control is the lavatory, where pathogens that are spread by means of the oral-fecal route are frequently encountered. Sanitization of lavatories should include not only daily cleaning of all surfaces but also the use of strong and effective hospital disinfectants that will destroy the large numbers of bacteria found there. In addition, all bathroom supplies such as towels or cups should be disposable.

Sanitization of the dental operatory is especially important because its surfaces are constantly exposed to oral pathogens during patient treatment. Operatory sinks should be kept clean, and any standing water should be removed from sink counters following hand washing. Foot-operated faucets are the best way to reduce contamination during washing. Hand faucets should be kept cleaned and disinfected. Because these surfaces may be difficult to disinfect thoroughly, contamination can be reduced by covering them with disposable plastic film, which is replaced after each patient, or by handling them with disposable paper towels rather than with contaminated hands. All disposable refuse should be kept out of sight in trash receptacles that have been lined with disposable bags. Appropriate puncture-resistant containers should be available for disposal of contaminated needles or other sharp items. Trash containers should be emptied promptly when full. Methods of disposal for all contaminated waste materials should be in compliance with local and state ordinances. Items that pose a health hazard to others, such as disposable needles, syringes, blood-soaked materials, or hazardous chemicals, require special handling and disposal.

All surfaces in the dental operatory that would be at or above the eye level of the supine patient should be kept especially clean. Not only will these surfaces be contaminated by aerosols produced during dental procedures, but also they are frequently touched during treatment and are within the viewing range of the patient. All surfaces on the semicritical list must be routinely cleaned before being disinfected and/or covered. To check the effectiveness of operatory sanitization, it is a good idea to recline in the dental chair and take a close look at the dental operatory from where the patient sits. Cobwebs near the ceiling, a spot of blood on the dental unit, or fingerprints on the light shield that may have been undetected from the clinician's vantage point may now be visible. These areas not only indicate inconsistencies or omissions in the cleaning routine, but also affect the patient's opinion of office cleanliness. Patients may view these lapses in sanitization as a reflection of a general lack of concern not only for asepsis but also for their own health and well-being. Areas that need special spot cleaning and dusting should be attended to whenever necessary so that visible soil and dust accumulations on surfaces are promptly removed.

Disinfection

Methods of disinfection include the use of chemicals or heat to destroy microorganisms or to suppress the growth of those that remain after sanitization procedures. Disinfection methods that employ heat as the destructive agent include boiling water and hot oils. These methods are used to treat instruments or other items that are both heat-resistant and small enough to be immersed in containers of the hot liquid. Because all instruments used in dentistry are categorized as critical surfaces, they must be treated by sterilization methods. Therefore, disinfection by boiling water or hot oil is not an acceptable substitute. Disinfection methods should be used only to control contamination on surfaces or items within the dental environment that cannot be sterilized; that is, surfaces or items too large or too fragile to undergo accepted methods of sterilization.

Chemical disinfection. Chemical disinfectants may be used for immersion of small items or for disinfection of surfaces within the dental environment. Disinfectants should be chosen according to the range of bacteriostasis or bactericidal activity that is needed. Although some agents can effec-

tively destroy microorganisms, others have only the ability to suppress their growth and multiplication. Those agents that are lethal for bacteria are called *bactericides*. Others, called *viricides,* are effective only against viruses. Similar results are obtained by *fungicides* and *sporicides*. The term *germicide* is used to describe an agent that is effective against vegetative bacterial cells but not the more resistant bacteria such as *Mycobacterium tuberculosis* or HBV. Even less effective are disinfectants that are described as *bacteriostatic,* which inhibit or suppress future bacterial growth but do not actually destroy all bacteria present on the affected surface.

A variety of chemical agents have been recommended for use in dentistry as disinfectants. Only those disinfectants that have been registered by the Environmental Protection Agency (EPA) as "hospital" disinfectants and that are tuberculocidal and viricidal for both lipid and nonlipid viruses have been accepted for use in dentistry (Council on Dental Materials, Instruments, and Equipment [hereafter CDMIE], 1988). Table 3-6 provides a list of specific disinfectants that are accepted by the ADA for immersion and surface disinfection (CDMIE, 1988). Chemical disinfectants may be classified as high-, intermediate-, or low-level disinfectants depending on their range of effectiveness against pathogenic microorganisms. Table 3-7 shows the microbes that are destroyed by each level category and identifies examples of chemicals in each category.

Chemical disinfectants are effective only if the following critical factors are controlled: (1) all surfaces or items to be disinfected must first be precleaned; (2) optimal concentration of the chemical must be maintained; (3) surfaces to be treated must be in contact with the chemical for the recommended exposure time; (4) chemicals must not be used beyond their expected shelf life or period of stability; and (5) solutions must be used at the recommended temperature. Specific manufacturer's recommendations must be followed carefully for each type of chemical disinfectant to maximize control of each of these factors.

Even under ideal conditions, however, chemical solutions cannot guarantee complete and consistent decontamination of all surfaces or instruments. Chemical solutions cannot penetrate into

Table 3-6. Guide to chemical agents for disinfection and/or sterilization

Chemical[1] classification / Accepted products	Disinfectant[2,3]			Sterilant[2]
	Dilution	Time	Temperature (20 C=68 F) (25 C=77 F)	
Surface/immersion				
Chlorine compounds				
Alcide	10:1:1	3 minutes	20 C	NA[5]
Exspore	4:1:1	2 minutes	20 C	4:1:1, 6 hours, 20 C
Bleach (5.25% sodium hypochlorite)	1:10	10 minutes	20 C	NA
Iodophors				
Biocide				
Surf-A-Cide	1:213	10 minutes	-[4]	NA
ProMedyne-D				
Combination synthetic phenolics				
Dentaseptic				
Multicide	1:32	10 minutes	20 C	NA
Omni II				
Immersion				
2% Glutaraldehyde with phenolic buffer				
Sporicidin	1:16	10 minutes	20 C	Full strength, 6¾ hours, 20 C
2% Glutaraldehyde[6] acidic				
Banicide concentrate	1:40	30 minutes	20 C	1:10, 10 hours, 25 C
Banicide				
Sterall	1:4	30 minutes	20 C	Full strength, 10 hours, 25 C
Wavicide-01				
2% Glutaraldehyde[6] neutral				
Glutarex	Full strength	-	-[4]	Full strength, 10 hours, 20 C
2% Glutaraldehyde alkaline[6]				
Cidex activated dialdehyde	Full strength	45 minutes	25 C	Full strength, 10 hours, 25 C
Cidex 7	Full strength	90 minutes	25 C	Full strength, 10 hours, 25 C
CoeCide				
Germ-X	Full strength	-	-[4]	Full strength, 10 hours, 20 C
Glutall				
Omnicide				
Orthicide				
Sporex	Full strength	45 minutes	20 C	Full strength, 10 hours, 20 C
Vitacide				
Steril-Ize	Full strength	45 minutes	25 C	Full strength, 10 hours, 20 C
Centra 28				
K-Cide 10				
Maxicide				
Procide 14	Full strength	10 minutes	25 C	Full strength, 10 hours, 20 C
Procide 30				
Protec-top				
Saslow solution				

1. ADA Accepted Products as of 9/1/87; a list of currently accepted products may be obtained by contacting the office of the Council on Dental Therapeutics.
2. Always use disinfectant/sterilant products according to the instructions specified on the product label.
3. The conditions listed reflect the time required for tuberculocidal activity for reused solution, if such use is possible, at the minimum temperature and maximal dilution specified on the Environmental Protection Agency (EPA) approved product label. Tuberculocidal test methodologies may vary; consult label or manufacturer for specifics.
4. Data not available at time of publication.
5. Not approved for use as sterilants.
6. Alternate conditions, such as increased temperature or fresh solution as opposed to reused solution, may decrease disinfection time; consult label instructions for alternate uses.
(From Council on Dental Materials, Instruments, and Equipment; and Council on Dental Practice; and Council on Dental Therapeutics: Infection control recommendations for the dental office and the dental laboratory, JADA 116:241, 1988.)

Table 3-7. Level of activity of chemical disinfectants and sterilants

Level of Disinfection	Organisms destroyed						Disinfectants or Sterilants
	Vegetative bacteria	Tubercle bacillus	Spores	Fungi	Lipid Virus	Nonlipid Virus	
High	Yes	Yes	Yes	Yes	Yes	Yes	2% glutaraldehyde-phenate 2% glutaraldehydes
Intermediate	Yes	Yes	No	Yes	Yes	Yes	Iodophors Sodium hypochlorite Phenolic compounds
Low	Yes	No	No	Yes	Yes	No	Quaternary ammonium compounds*

*Quaternary ammonium compounds are not acceptable for use as disinfectants of critical or semicritical surfaces in dentistry according to CDC and ADA guidelines.
(Adapted from Terezhalmy GT et al: A rational approach to the selection of disinfectants and sterilants, Compend Contin Educ Dent 9:114, 1987.)

small recesses and destroy pathogens that may lie protected in jointed, hinged, or serrated instruments, or within the cracks and tears in the edge of a previously used rubber polishing cup. Even after recommended exposure to chemical solution, these surfaces may remain contaminated and serve as sources of cross-contamination if reused. Chemicals are most effective on smooth nonporous surfaces that can be adequately precleaned and can provide intimate contact between the pathogen and the solution. Any semicritical surface in the dental office which cannot be effectively cleaned and/or disinfected between patients must be kept covered to prevent contamination. An additional limitation of chemical disinfectants is that there are no standard, reliable methods for monitoring their effectiveness; thus there can be no guarantee that safe levels of protection have actually been achieved. This problem alone should make dental professionals wary of depending on chemical solutions for treatment of instruments or other critical items that could undergo accepted methods of sterilization.

Surface disinfection. All surfaces or items that are contaminated during patient treatment by either direct or indirect contact with oral pathogens are sources for cross-contamination for patients and dental personnel. After identifying the critical, semicritical, and noncritical items or surfaces in the dental office, one can determine which disinfectant(s) will provide effective and safe levels of contamination control.

All critical items, especially dental instruments, handpieces, and air-water syringe tips, must be sterilized after each use. Any critical item that cannot undergo sterilization must be treated by a high-level disinfectant under recommended conditions. High-level disinfectants are those that are effective against all vegetative bacteria and viruses, including the tubercle bacillus, bacterial spores, and viruses similar to the hepatitis virus. Handpieces which cannot be heat sterilized should be scrubbed with a disinfectant, rinsed, dried, and then immersed in 2% glutaraldehyde for 30 minutes if they are immersible. If not, they must be thoroughly scrubbed with a glutaraldehyde or iodophor solution, then rinsed thoroughly and flushed before patient use.

Many semicritical surfaces in the dental operatory can be protected from contamination by covering them with plastic-backed paper, plastic film, aluminum foil, or custom-designed disposable materials. Barrier covers are especially useful for surfaces that are difficult to clean and disinfect adequately in the time available between patient appointments. These disposable covers are replaced after each patient and discarded. Gloves should always be worn when removing contaminated covers. Clean hands or clean gloves should be used when replacing clean barrier covers. All surfaces in the semicritical category should be treated by an intermediate-level disinfectant unless there is reason to suspect that they might have been contaminated by the hepatitis virus, in which case high levels of disinfection are required. Intermediate-level disinfectants are effective against all microorganisms except for bacterial spores. Both the ADA and the CDC recommend the use of iodophors for surface disinfection. Iodophors are highly recommended due to their many advantages (see Table 3-8). Those items that cannot be sterilized, disposed of, or covered must be precleaned and treated with an effective disinfecting solution for the prescribed length of time following each patient contact. Noncritical items or surfaces can be safely treated with low-level disinfectants. These disinfectants are only effective against vegetative bacteria and some viruses.

The importance of adequate precleaning of all contaminated surfaces should not be underesti-mated. The process of physically removing microorganisms from surfaces through the cleaning process is as effective as directly killing them by chemicals or other methods. The term *scrubbing,* rather than *wiping,* is appropriate to describe the cleaning process to emphasize the need to use pressure and repeated strokes over the contaminated surface while applying enough disinfectant solution to wet the surface thoroughly. Large surfaces such as chairs or countertops should be sprayed with disinfectant and then wiped thoroughly with a disinfectant-soaked, absorbent paper towel (Fig. 3-1). Final cleaning is accomplished by turning the clean side of the towel over and repeating the process. Smaller items such as handles and cords for air-water syringes and saliva ejectors should be wiped twice with two sep-

Table 3-8. Advantages and disadvantages of accepted chemical agents

Chemical Agent	Advantages	Disadvantages
Chlorine compounds	Fast acting Effective against a wide variety of microbes, including HBV and tubercle bacillus Economical Recommended for hard surface disinfection	Unstable; prepare fresh solution daily Effectiveness reduced by presence of organic matter or altered pH Unpleasant odor Can corrode metals Irritates skin, eyes Can damage plastic and rubber materials Bleaching effect on clothing and other materials
Iodophors (highly recommended as a hard surface disinfectant)	EPA licensed surface disinfectant; broad spectrum effectiveness Economical Few physical side effects Color change from amber to clear indicates loss of effectiveness Residual activity on hard surfaces continues after solution has dried 3 to 30 minute contact time required for effective disinfection	Not classified as a sterilant Somewhat unstable with age at high temperature May stain light-colored surfaces after prolonged use Corrosive to some metals Inactivated by hard water Solution loses effectiveness with age Must be prepared fresh daily
Phenolic Compounds	Active in presence of detergents Broad-spectrum effectiveness; some are tuberculocidal Primary use for floors, walls, etc.	Not recommended for disinfection of critical or semicritical surfaces Not sporicidal Irregular viricidal activity; ineffective against hydrophilic viruses (e.g., HBV) Inactivated by organic matter and hard water Can damage plastics and vinyl Potentially irritating to hands
Glutaraldehydes	Used primarily for immersion of heat and/or pressure-sensitive instruments that require high-level disinfection or sterilization	Irritating to skin, mucous membrane, eyes; wearing gloves and eyeglasses recommended Odor and fumes may be offensive; use in well-ventilated room Thorough rinsing of all treated materials is required Overnight immersion can corrode some metals

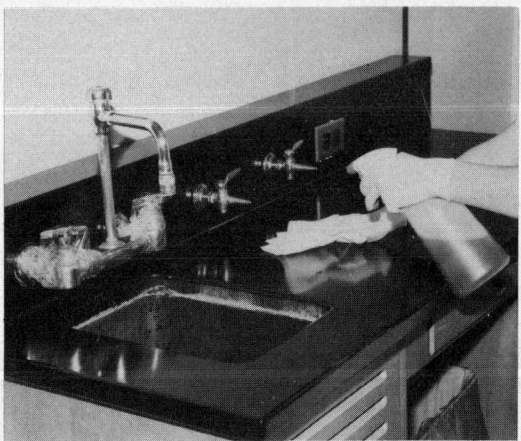

Fig. 3-1. Cleaning and disinfecting large surfaces can be accomplished efficiently with a spray bottle of the solution and a paper towel or large gauze sponges.

arate gauze squares. Removal of the majority of organic debris on these surfaces reduces the demand on the disinfecting solution and allows more intimate contact of remaining pathogens and the disinfectant. The final step in surface disinfection is to spray or wipe all surfaces to be treated with the disinfectant solution and allow those surfaces to air dry.

Practitioners should be aware of the misnomer of the term *cold sterilization* when it is used to describe a chemical method of treating instruments. This term has been traditionally used to describe the immersion of instruments in a disinfectant between patients. As sterilization is the only accepted means of treating instruments and as all chemical sterilants require immersion of instruments for a *minimum* of 6¾ to 10 hours, it is clear that the use of chemical disinfecting solutions to treat contaminated dental instruments is not an acceptable procedure by modern standards of safety. Many of the chemicals still being used in dental offices do not provide an acceptable level of safety against resistant bacteria, bacterial spores, or the hepatitis virus. Knowing this, dental professionals must consider their legal and ethical responsibilities to the patient before using chemical disinfecting solutions for treatment of instruments and other critical items when more effective and proven methods of sterilization are readily available.

Boiling water and hot oils. Both boiling water and hot oil solutions use heat as the destructive agent. Most vegetative cells are destroyed after being immersed in vigorously boiling water (100°C, 212°F) for 10 minutes. However, because many spores and certain viruses may survive this treatment, boiling cannot be considered a sterilization process. An additional problem with boiling is the corrosive effect of the water on metal. The addition of trisodium phosphate or sodium carbonate to the water will help reduce the corrosion as well as aid in removing debris from the instruments. These additives should not be used for aluminum instruments which can be corroded by the chemicals (ADA-CDT, 1984).

Immersion of instruments in hot oils or silicone fluids will produce the following effects:

Disinfection: 150°C (300°F) for 15 minutes
125°C (260°F) for 20 to 30 minutes

Sterilization: 160°C (320°F) for 60 minutes minimum

Almost any instrument that can withstand the heat of this process may be treated by this method. A special word of caution: *Hypodermic needles and syringes should never be treated with hot oil because of the danger of retained oil being injected into the bloodstream and causing an embolus.* Other disadvantages of the immersion method include the need to clean excess oil off items after sterilization or disinfection, difficulty in safely handling the hot oil solutions, and the possibility of unpleasant vapors and fumes from some heated solutions (ADA-CDT, 1984).

Antiseptics. Antiseptics are used in dentistry to reduce the number of microorganisms on living tissues, such as within the mouth or on the clinician's hands. Antiseptics are usually chemical disinfecting solutions that have been diluted so that they will not have a toxic or irritating effect when applied to human tissues. The result of this dilution is that antiseptics have a more limited ability to destroy bacterial cells than do disinfectants used on inanimate objects. Nonetheless, antiseptics can significantly reduce the chances of introducing pathogenic bacteria into the bloodstream during certain procedures. Antiseptics are commonly used before dental injections to cleanse the area so that the needle will not carry a large number of microorganisms deep into the tissue and blood supply. Antiseptics may also be used to clean an area of the mouth before a surgical procedure. The use of antiseptic mouthwashes can reduce the numbers of bacteria in the mouth before dental treatment. Many clinicians also use an antiseptic hand scrub to enhance the degerming effect of the handwashing procedure. The antiseptic may be contained in the soap or detergent that is used to cleanse the hands, or it may be a sepa-

rate solution that is applied to the hands after scrubbing. Handwashing is discussed in more detail on page 56.

Sterilization

The highest level of contamination control is *sterilization*. Sterilization results in the total destruction of all forms of microbial life. There are several methods of sterilization approved for use by

Table 3-9. Methods of sterilization

Method	Standard Conditions*	Uses	Advantages	Disadvantages	Packaging Materials
Steam under pressure (autoclave)	Temperature: 121°C (250°F) Pressure: 15 psi Time: 20 minutes	All materials except oils, greases, powders, and items that cannot withstand the required temperatures and pressure	Most reliable method Quick and efficient Wide variety of materials can be sterilized	Cannot be used for oils, greases, powders, and heat-sensitive materials May dull cutting edges of carbon steel instruments May corrode metal instruments if precautions not taken Metal and glass containers must be open to penetration by steam	(steam permeable) paper muslin nylon open containers
Dry heat (dry heat oven)	Temperature: 160° to 170°C (320° to 340°F) Time: 60 min. (170°C) or 120 min. (160°C)	Metal and glass equipment Oils, waxes, greases, powders Needles and other small instruments enclosed in glass or metal	Large capacity Low cost of equipment Does not dull cutting edges of carbon steel Only method for oils, greases, powders Does not erode ground glass surfaces Does not corrode metals Simple to operate Can penetrate closed glass and metal containers Items are dry after cycle	Requires longer time to sterilize than moist heat or chemical vapor Cannot be used on some heat-sensitive materials; temperatures above 170°C (340°F) will disjoin soldered instruments Instruments must be dry before sterilization to prevent rusting Cannot be used on liquids	(heat permeable) aluminum paper some cloth open or closed containers
Ethylene oxide gas	Temperature: 49°C (120°F) Time: 2 to 3 hours or Temperature: room temperature Time: 12 hours	Sterilization of commercial products and items in hospital environments Most dental supplies and instruments	Useful for sterilization of handpieces that cannot be autoclaved Useful for heat-sensitive items	Causes irritation to eyes and nose Inhalation must be avoided; adequate ventilation required Toxic odor may be absorbed by some plastic or rubber items; requires aeration for 1 day or more prior to use Impractical for routine sterilization between patients Equipment may be more expensive than other methods	(gas permeable) paper nylon open containers

Table 3-9. Methods of sterilization—cont'd

Method	Standard Conditions*	Uses	Advantages	Disadvantages	Packaging Materials
Chemical Vapor	Temperature: 132°C (270°F) Pressure: 20 to 40 psi Time: 20 minutes	Any item tested for vapor penetration	Does not require high temperatures of dry heat Relatively short cycle useful for handpieces Will not corrode metals (metal instruments should be predried) Items are dry after cycle	Cannot be used for materials that are sensitive to the necessary temperature or pressure Vapor must penetrate through all materials Some materials may be incompatible with the chemicals used Exposure to fumes requires ventilation	(gas permeable) paper open containers
Chemical solutions (glutaraldehyde)	Temperature: room temperature Time: 6¾ to 10 hours Requires optimal concentration of chemical solution	Plastics and other heat-sensitive materials that cannot withstand heat sterilization	Does not require heat to achieve sterilization Plastics, rubber, and other heat-sensitive materials can be sterilized Good for instruments containing bonded parts (*e.g.,* lenses, mirrors, handpieces) Chemical not affected by soaps and detergents	Requires immersion of objects for minimum of 6¾ to 10 hours to achieve sterilization Destruction of hepatitis virus is probable but not proven Irritates skin and mucous membranes; should be rinsed off instruments before their use May corrode carbon steel after 24 hours of immersion	

*Recommended conditions may vary depending on model, wrapping, size of load. Follow manufacturer's instructions and monitor with spore tests.

the American Dental Association: steam under pressure (autoclaving), dry heat, ethylene oxide gas, chemical vapor sterilizers, and chemical solutions (see Table 3-9). Of these methods, the first two, involving heat as the destructive agent, are the preferred methods, with moist heat under pressure considered the most efficient and reliable of all methods (ADA-CDT, 1984). Current recommendations regarding the preferred method(s) for sterilization of critical items in dentistry are listed in Table 3-10.

Autoclaving. Sterilization is accomplished by the action of steam under pressure in a metal chamber called an *autoclave* (Fig. 3-2). The pressure enables the temperature to reach a level high enough to ensure destruction of even the most heat-resistant bacteria. Water at normal atmospheric pressures cannot be heated to a temperature higher than boiling (100°C, 212°F), but this is not high enough to ensure complete microbial destruction. When water is heated under pressur-

ized conditions, however, its temperature can be elevated beyond the boiling point to produce a superheated effect that is capable of sterilization. No living thing can survive 10 minutes of direct exposure to saturated steam at 121°C (250°F), a temperature that is attained under ideal conditions with 15 pounds of pressure per square inch (psi) in an autoclave.

Operation of the autoclave. Preparation of the autoclave should begin by checking the water supply contained in the unit. Steam for sterilization is provided by a supply of distilled or deionized water. The water level may be viewed by lifting the cover at the top of the chamber. During the operating cycle there must be enough water available to produce a quantity of steam capable of filling the entire chamber. Therefore, the tank always should be kept filled to the indicator line.

Any package, instrument, or container to be autoclaved is loaded onto a metal tray that will be inserted into the chamber. Materials to be steril-

Table 3-10. Sterilization and disinfection of dental instruments, materials, and some commonly used items*

	Steam autoclave	Dry heat oven	Chemical vapor	Ethylene oxide	Chemical disinfection/ sterilization	Other methods/ comments
Angle attachments*	+	+	+	++	+	
Burs						
Carbon steel	−	++	++	++	−	
Steel	+	++	++	++	+	
Tungsten-carbide	+	++	+	++	+	
Condensers	++	++	++	++	+	
Dapen dishes	++	+	+	++	+	
Endodontic instruments (broaches, files, reamers)						Hot salt/glass bead sterilizer 10 to 15 seconds, 218°C (425°F)
Stainless steel handles	+	++	++	++	+	
Stainless with plastic handles	++	++	−	++	−	
Fluoride gel trays						
Heat-resistant plastic	++	− −	−	++		
Nonheat-resistant plastic	− −	− −	−	++	−	Discard (++)
Glass slabs	++	++	++	++	+	
Hand instruments						
Carbon steel	−	++	++	++	−	
	[Steam autoclave with chemical protection (1% sodium nitrite)]					
Stainless steel	++	++	++	++	+	
Handpieces*						Sterilizable preferably
Sterilizable*	(++)*	−	(+)*	++	− −	
Contra-angles*	−	−	−	++	+	Combination synthetic phenolics or iodophors (−)
Nonsterilizable*	−	−	−	++	+	
Prophylaxis angles*	+	+	+	+	+	
Impression materials						Table 2
Impression trays						
Aluminum metal	++	+	++	++	−	
Chrome-plated	++	++	++	++	+	
Custom acrylic resin	− −	− −	− −	++	+	
Plastic	− −	− −	− −	++	+	Discard (++); preferred
Instruments in packs	++	+ Small packs	++	++ Small packs	− −	
Instrument tray setups						
Restorative or surgical	+ Size limit	+	+ Size limit	++ Size limit	− −	
Mirrors	−	++	++	++	+	
Needles						
Disposable	− −	− −	− −	− −	− −	Discard (++) Do not reuse
Nitrous oxide						
Nose piece	(++)*	− −	(++)*	++	(+)*	
Hoses	(++)*	− −	(++)*	++	(+)*	
Orthodontic pliers						
High-quality stainless	++	++	++	++	+	
Low-quality stainless	−	++	++	++	−	
With plastic parts	− −	− −	− −	++	+	
Pluggers	++	++	++	++	+	
Polishing wheels and disks						
Garnet and cuttle	− −	−	−	++	− −	
Rag	++	−	+	++	− −	
Rubber	+	−	−	++	+	
Prostheses, removable	−	−	−	+	+	

Table 3-10. Sterilization and disinfection of dental instruments, materials, and some commonly used items*—cont'd

	Steam autoclave	Dry heat oven	Chemical vapor	Ethylene oxide	Chemical disinfection/ sterilization	Other methods/ comments
Rubber dam equipment						
Carbon steel clamps	−	++	++	++	−	
Metal frames	++	++	++	++	+	
Plastic frames	−	−	−	++	+	
Punches	−	++	++	++	+	
Stainless steel clamps	++	++	++	++	+	
Rubber items						
Prophylaxis cups	−	−	−	++	−	Discard (++)
Saliva evacuators, ejectors						
Low-melting plastic	−	−	−	++	+	Discard (++)
High-melting plastic	++	+	+	++	+	
Stones						
Diamond	+	++	++	++	+	
Polishing	++	+	++	++	−	
Sharpening	++	++	++	−		
Surgical instruments						
Stainless steel	++	++	++	++	+	
Ultrasonic scaling tips	+	−−	−−	++	+	
Water-air syringe tips	++	++	++	++	+	
X-ray equipment						
Plastic film holders	(++)*	−−	(+)*	++	+	
Collimating devices	−	−−	−−	++	+	

The table is adapted from *Accepted Dental Therapeutics and Dentists' Desk Reference: Materials, Instruments, and Equipment.*
*As manufacturers use a variety of alloys and materials in these products, confirmation with the equipment manufacturers is recommended, especially for handpieces and the attachments.
++Effective and preferred method.
+Effective and acceptable method.
−Effective method, but risk of damage to materials.
−−Ineffective method with risk of damage to materials.
(From Council on Dental Materials, Instruments, and Equipment; Council on Dental Practice; and Council on Dental Therapeutics: Infection control recommendations for the dental office and the dental laboratory, JADA 116:241, 1988.)

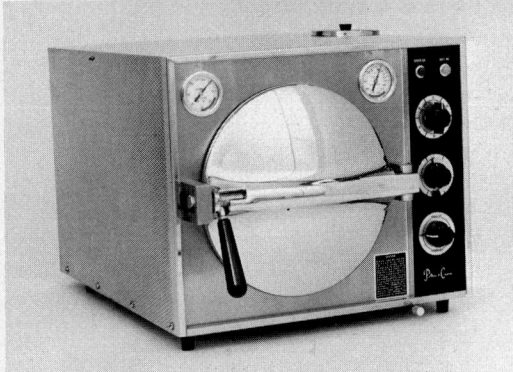

Fig. 3-2. Autoclave unit.
(Courtesy of Pelton and Crane, Charlotte, North Carolina).

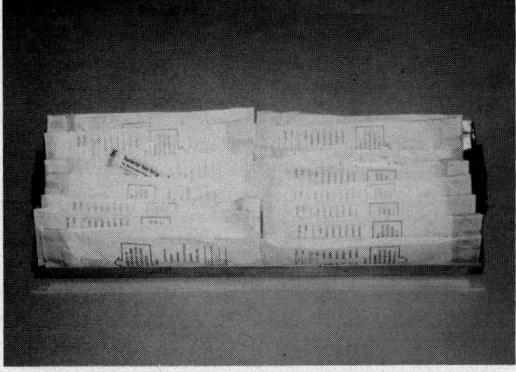

Fig. 3-3. Properly loaded trays will allow flow of steam through and around all surfaces.

ized in the autoclave should be wrapped in muslin, paper, or steam-permeable plastic bags or be held in open glass or metal containers. Do not package materials to be autoclaved in sealed or closed jars or in aluminum foil. When loading trays, place wrapped packages uniformly on edge, with no more than two layers on each tray; place open jars or containers on their sides. Packages or containers should not touch the chamber walls. The success of the sterilization procedure is dependent on the ability of the superheated steam to come in contact with all items; thus, they should be packed loosely on the tray to permit an easy flow of steam in and around all materials (Fig. 3-3). If the bags or instruments are jammed tightly against each other, it will be much more difficult for the steam to penetrate through to the innermost layers (Fig. 3-4). When trays are improperly loaded, those microorganisms that are insulated or protected from the effects of the moist heat may not be killed during the usual sterilization cycle.

After the trays are placed in the sterilization chamber, the control knob should be turned to the "fill" position, allowing the water that will later be converted to steam to enter the chamber. To ensure that there is a sufficient amount, the metal cover plate at the front of the chamber floor must be completely covered before the knob is turned to the "sterilize" position. At this time, the chamber door should be closed and locked into place. All packages should be completely sealed inside the chamber and should not be caught in the chamber door, preventing a complete seal within the chamber. In such a case, the temperature inside the chamber would not rise high enough to achieve sterilization.

When the knob is turned to the "sterilize" position, water will stop entering the chamber, and the inside temperature of the autoclave will begin to rise. The thermostatic controls on the front of the unit should be set so that when the desired temperature is reached, along with its corresponding pressure, the heat will be maintained at that level for the remainder of the sterilization cycle. Every autoclave should be equipped with a safety valve to prevent the inner chamber from reaching an unnecessarily high temperature or pressure. Once the chamber has reached the appropriate conditions for sterilization (usually 121°C at 15 psi), the timer on the unit should be set for the

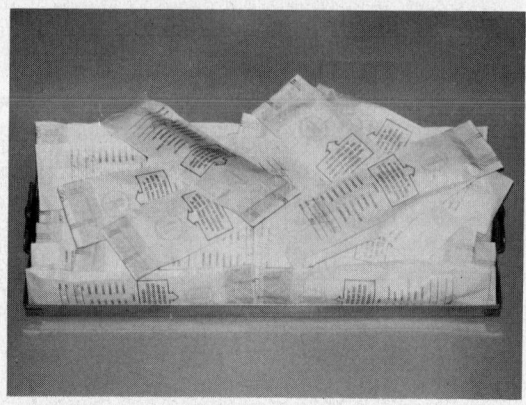

Fig. 3-4. Improperly loaded tray. Instruments are packed tightly together and tray is overloaded.

desired length of time. In most instances this will be 15 to 20 minutes. *It is important to remember that the timing of the sterilization cycle should not begin until the recommended conditions have been reached and the temperature of the contents has reached 121°C.* These conditions must then be maintained for the entire length of the cycle. At the end of this period, as indicated by the timer, the control knob can be turned to the "vent" position. The steam will escape from the chamber so that the pressure is released, and the chamber will begin to cool. These changes should be indicated by the temperature and pressure gauges as they move slowly toward zero. When both levels have been reduced to zero, the chamber door can be opened. No attempt to open the door should be made until the pressure has been eliminated within the chamber. The door should be left ajar for several minutes before trays are removed so that the bags and other materials have a chance to dry before they are stored. Even after a few minutes of cooling, however, the metal trays and their contents will still be hot and should be handled with care.

Monitoring sterilization. The effectiveness of any sterilization procedure cannot be guaranteed unless it is certain that the desired conditions such as temperature, pressure, time, and/or chemical exposure are consistently being met. Even the best gauges are not foolproof, and periodic maintenance and tests should be performed to ensure the effectiveness of all equipment. Studies of the effectiveness of dental office sterilizers have indicated that up to one third of all office sterilizers may fail testing procedures (Simonsen et al, 1979; Skaug, 1983; Palenik et al, 1986; Palenik and Miller, 1986a). Any number of factors can contribute to sterilization failure including: improper packaging or wrapping, overloading, disregard for manufacturer's instructions, or mechanical malfunction. Proper maintenance of the sterilization equipment, observation of units as they are operating, and the use of external and internal chemical monitors and biological monitors are all important steps toward ensuring that sterilization occurs.

Use of *biological spore tests* (Fig. 3-5) are the most reliable way of ensuring the effectiveness of sterilization procedures. Biological monitoring methods are available for testing the effectiveness of autoclaves, dry heat ovens, chemical vapor sterilizers, and ethylene oxide gas sterilizers. There are currently no standard procedures for biological monitoring of chemical sterilant solutions that are used for immersion of instruments. Biological monitoring utilizes special bacterial spore test strips or vials that are placed at the center of a normal load in the sterilization unit and then submitted to the usual sterilization cycle. Spore strips consist of filter paper which has been impregnated with spores and enclosed in an envelope. After sterilization, the spores are placed in a sterile growth medium and incubated for 7 days. If spores grow they turn the solution cloudy, indicating that sterilization has failed. Spore test vials contain a spore strip and an ampule which contains growth media. After processing, the vial is squeezed to crush the ampule and then incubated for 24 to 48 hours. An inexpensive incubator can be purchased to perform this test in the dental office, or test materials can be mailed to one of a number of sterilization monitoring services (Farah and Powers, 1986).

Autoclaves and chemical vapor sterilizers are tested using the organism *Bacillus stearothermophilus,* a bacterial spore that can withstand all but the most stringent sterilization conditions. The organism *B. subtilis var niger* is used to test dry heat ovens and ethylene oxide sterilizing equipment. Evidence of bacterial growth following incubation indicates that some of the bacterial

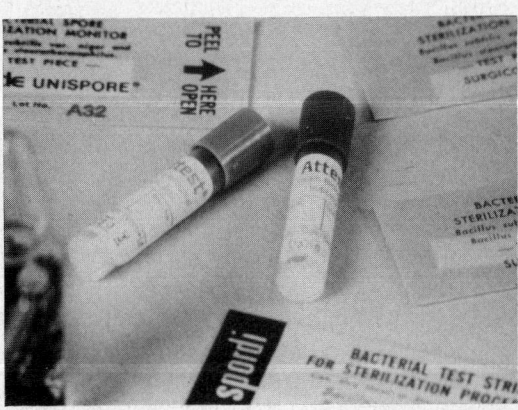

Fig. 3-5. Spore strips and test ampules are placed inside packages or containers during sterilization procedures to test whether or not sterilization has occurred.
(Courtesy of 3M Co, Minnesota.)

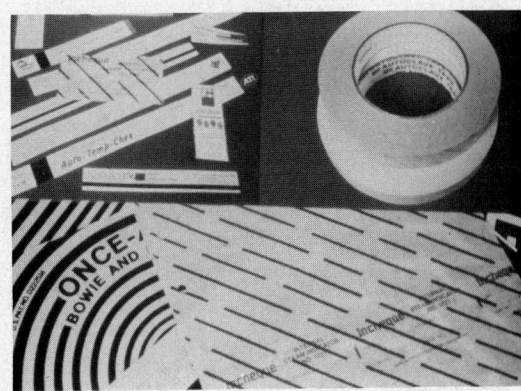

Fig. 3-6. Examples of internal *(top left)* and external chemical indicators.
(Courtesy of 3M Co, Minnesota.)

spores survived the sterilization process and that equipment malfunction or other errors have been made during the sterilization procedure. Sterilization equipment should be tested weekly by this method (CDMIE, 1988; CDC, 1986).

A second step towards ensuring sterilization is the use of *chemical indicators* (Fig. 3-6) that undergo a color change on materials that have been subjected to sterilization conditions. External chemical indicators include labels on autoclave bags and special heat-sensitive tape used to seal bags. These indicators change color when they have been exposed to sterilization temperatures and provide an easy way of discriminating between processed and nonprocessed items. Internal chemical indicators are placed inside wrapped packages to ensure that the internal contents of packages were exposed to appropriate conditions. Although chemical indicators provide a quick means of identifying a failure in sterilization procedures, they cannot be relied upon to guarantee that sterilization has actually occurred. They indicate only that the materials were exposed to the appropriate temperature or chemicals, but do not prove that the exact conditions and time required for sterilization have been met. The only method that provides conclusive evidence that sterilization has occurred is biological monitoring with spore tests. In instances where the actual results from spore test monitoring are not immediately available, however, these types of indicators can assist in the detection of improper sterilization procedures or gross equipment malfunction.

Maintenance of the autoclave should follow manufacturer's instructions and should include checking the temperature, pressure, and timer gauges daily. The door gasket should be checked regularly for signs of wear or damage. The inner surface of the chamber should be washed periodically with a mild detergent and rinsed well. Dental offices should keep written *records* to document sterilization monitoring procedures. Runnells (1985) recommended that these records be kept and stored for at least 3 years. Records should include the type of monitoring performed, sterilization conditions, dates on which tests were performed, results of biological monitoring tests, and maintenance procedures (Miller, 1987).

Dry heat. Dry heat may be used for materials that cannot withstand steam under pressure, such as oils, powders, greases, and some dental instruments and handpieces. Dry heat is the method of choice for fine endodontic instruments that need to be sterilized. The dry heat oven is much like a regular oven (Fig. 3-7). The same conditions for loading the oven apply as for loading the autoclave to ensure that all contents reach sterilization temperatures within the prescribed length of time. Instruments should be packaged in a manner that will allow the heated air to circulate freely around

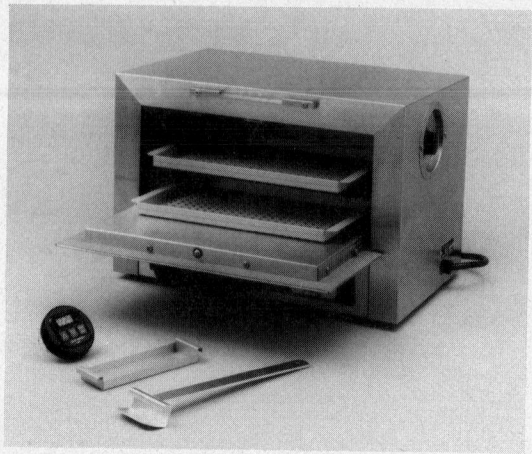

Fig. 3-7. Dry heat oven (Dri-Clave®).
(Courtesy of Columbus Dental, St Louis, Missouri.)

the contents of the oven. Appropriate wrapping materials include foil or closed glass or metal containers or trays. Cloth and paper materials may char or scorch due to the high temperatures, and some plastics may produce toxic fumes when heated to required temperatures.

Because some microorganisms are extremely resistant to dry heat, it is necessary to maintain high temperatures for a prolonged period of time until all spores have been killed. An internal temperature of 160° to 170°C (320° to 340°F) must be achieved and maintained for a minimum of 1 hour. More specific instructions as to the recommended temperatures and time required for certain materials are given in Tables 3-6 and 3-9. The length of time required to achieve the proper internal temperature depends on the size of the load, the materials being heated, and the wrapping materials used. For example, a few unwrapped metal instruments could be heated to sterilization temperatures much faster than a large number of heavily wrapped bundles. Since a certain amount of time is required to heat the entire contents of the oven to this temperature, a total sterilization period of 2 hours is often recommended. Avoid overloading the oven. Separate items by at least ½ inch and load packages no more than two layers deep with the top layer at right angles to the bottom layer. The temperature should be checked by means of a thermometer that indicates the internal temperature of the oven.

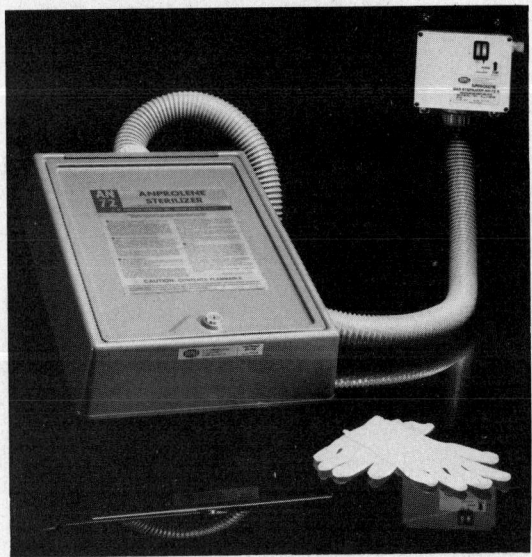

Fig. 3-8. Ethylene oxide sterilizer (Anprolene® model). (Courtesy of HW Anderson Products, Inc, Chapel Hill, North Carolina.)

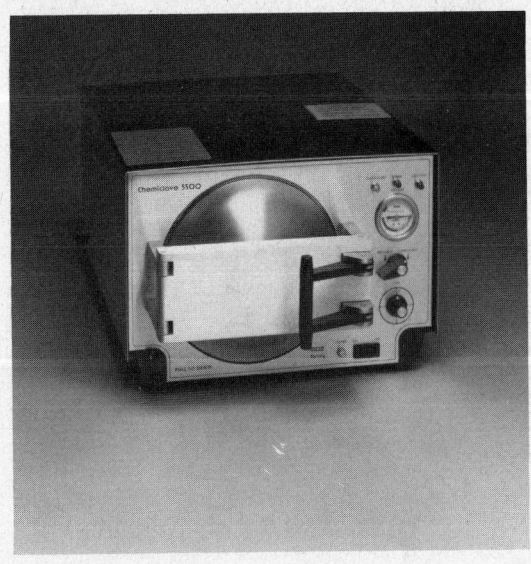

Fig. 3-9. Chemical vapor sterilizer (Chem-Clave®). (Courtesy of MDT Corp, Torrance, California.)

Bacterial spore tests are recommended to monitor the effectiveness of this equipment in achieving sterilization.

Ethylene oxide gas. A third method of sterilization is ethylene oxide gas. This method is used mainly by hospitals where large quantities of materials and instruments must be sterilized. It is also used for sterilization of some commercial products. Recently, smaller sterilizing units that are more suitable in size and expense for the dental office have been made available (Fig. 3-8). The main advantage of ethylene oxide gas sterilization is that it does not require the high temperatures of either the autoclave or the dry heat oven, which means that heat-sensitive materials, including plastic items and all handpieces, can be safely sterilized. Some units operate with cycles that require no additional moisture or pressure, and sharp items and fragile pressure-sensitive items can be safely sterilized by this method. A major disadvantage of the ethylene oxide method is its long sterilization cycle (3 to 12 hours) and the additional time required for aeration of some items; these facts render it impractical for routine sterilization of all dental instruments or supplies. In addition, ethylene oxide gas does have some

toxic properties that make it irritating to the eyes and nose. These toxic fumes can be retained by plastics or rubber materials. Rubber and plastic materials that can absorb the gas should be aerated for 24 hours or longer before being used. Prolonged inhalation of the gas in even low concentrations should be avoided, and these units should be used only in properly ventilated areas (ADA-CDT, 1984).

Chemical vapor. Chemical vapor sterilization is another method available for use in dental practices. The chemical vapor sterilizer is an autoclavelike device (Fig. 3-9) that uses a mixture of chemical vapors, including alcohol, ketone, acetone, and formaldehyde, which are heated together with water to a temperature of 270°F, under 20 psi, for 20 minutes. It is effective for materials that are heat-sensitive and cannot withstand autoclaving or dry heat temperatures. The risk of damage by rust or corrosion is also diminished by this method of sterilization because of the low water content. The chemical vapor sterilizer should not be used for any material that cannot withstand the necessary temperatures or one that is incompatible with the chemical agents. An additional disadvantage of this method is the production of chemical fumes. Therefore, these units should be operated only in well-ventilated areas. Fumes can be minimized by opening the chamber door slightly at the end of the cycle so that vapor condenses on the inside of the chamber or by venting the unit to the outside.

Wrapping materials or containers must be permeable to the chemical vapors to ensure effective exposure of chemicals to all surfaces. Do not use sealed glass jars, closed containers, or aluminum foil to hold or wrap items that will be sterilized using this method, as these materials do not permit penetration of the chemical vapor. Packages should be wrapped so as to prevent air pockets but not so tightly that air flow is obstructed. Chemical vapor sterilization should be monitored with spore test organisms to ascertain that all conditions for sterilization are being met. Maintenance should follow manufacturer's instructions and should include regular checking of all fittings and seals and weekly cleaning.

Chemical solutions. Table 3-6 lists chemical solutions that are approved for use in dentistry as sterilants (ADA, 1988). The only chemical solution that has been shown to achieve true sterilization is 2% glutaraldehyde. This chemical has been shown to destroy fungi, viruses, and bacteria including *Mycobacterium tuberculosis* after immersion for 10 minutes (disinfection). It is also capable of killing resistant bacterial spores after an immersion period of 6¾ to 10 hours (sterilization). Exposure times vary depending on the product used and the amount of biocidal activity desired (CDMIE, 1988). The manufacturer's directions for use of these chemicals should be followed carefully to ensure optimal results.

Glutaraldehyde's ability to destroy HBV is probable under recommended conditions, but it cannot be guaranteed as the etiological agent for HBV cannot be cultured. Bond and others (1983) tested the effectiveness of a number of intermediate- and high-level disinfectants, including iodophore, sodium hypochlorite, and two types of 2% glutaraldehyde, against the HBV by treating HBV-infected human plasma for 10 minutes with each disinfectant and then injecting the neutralized plasma into chimpanzees. After a 9-month observation period, none of the animals had developed hepatitis B. Although these preliminary tests indicate that glutaraldehyde and certain intermediate level disinfectants may destroy the HBV,

further studies are needed before it can be considered safe to treat critical surfaces which have been exposed to the hepatitis B virus by anything other than approved sterilization methods.

Chemical sterilant solutions should not be depended upon as a substitute for other approved measures such as the autoclave, dry heat oven, or chemical vapor sterilizer because the effectiveness of solutions is difficult to verify. Although individual manufacturers provide tests for monitoring the concentration of active glutaraldehyde remaining in solution for reuse, there is no accepted standard for biological monitoring of this method as there is for the other accepted methods. In addition, the 6¾ to 10 hours required for sterilization by 2% glutaraldehyde preparations makes them impractical for routine treatment of instruments and other critical items between patients. Glutaraldehyde solutions should be considered, however, for obtaining a high degree of disinfection or sterilization for any immersible items that cannot be sterilized by heat, such as plastics or rubber items.

Gloves and glasses should be worn when using these solutions, as they are irritating to skin and eyes. Holding containers should be kept closed and the solutions should be used in well-ventilated areas (Fig. 3-10). Instruments treated in these solutions should be rinsed thoroughly with sterile water or 70% alcohol before use. Because some rubber and plastic materials can retain the

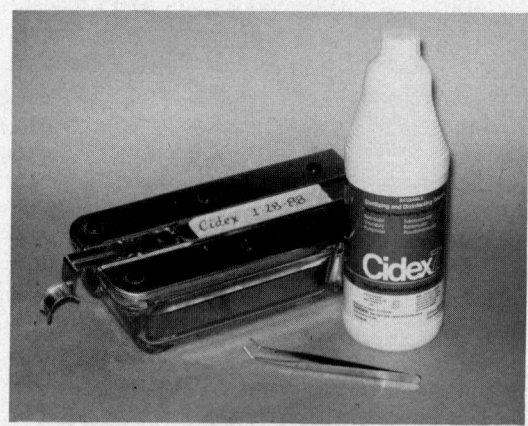

Fig. 3-10. Chemical sterilants should be used according to manufacturer's directions. Note date that solution was prepared to avoid using it beyond recommended periods of effectiveness.

chemical after repeated exposure, rinsing of these items must be particularly thorough so that the glutaraldehyde is not carried to the patient's skin, mouth, or bloodstream (Palenik and Miller, 1984).

Several other methods of sterilization including ultraviolet light, microwaves, and other forms of radiation have been used as methods of sterilization. At the present time, none of these methods is a practical alternative for use in dental offices (Runnells, 1985).

Disposable supplies and instruments

The American Dental Association states that the proper handling and preparation of instruments in the dental office should provide the practitioner with instruments that are completely free of viable bacteria, viruses, and spores while maintaining their usefulness. This can be accomplished by sterilizing reusable instruments by one of the methods discussed previously or by using disposable items that are discarded after one use. Many dental supplies, such as tongue blades, cotton-tipped applicators, aspirator tips, saliva ejectors, radiograph holders, rubber polishing cups, fluoride trays, syringes, and needles are available in disposable form. Disposable prophylaxis angles are also available. All disposable supplies are intended to be used only once and then discarded. They are not meant to be cleaned and reused under any circumstances. Disposable supplies should be stored in sterile, dry containers. Transfer of supplies into storage containers or from containers to the operating area should be accomplished using clean, gloved hands and/or sterile forceps or cotton-pliers.

There are a number of advantages to using disposable supplies. The most important advantage is the prevention of cross-contamination, because these items are used only once and then discarded. The use of disposable needles is especially valuable in the prevention of hepatitis B, because contaminated needles are known to be one of the chief causes of transmission of this serious disease. The use of disposable supplies saves considerable time and money that would otherwise be expended to clean and sterilize the supplies if they were to be reused. Disposable tray covers, patients' napkins, and headrest covers not only protect the patient and the working environment from contamination by bacterial aerosols and splatter, but also reduce significantly the time and effort needed to disinfect surfaces between patients. Use of disposable hand towels is a necessity in the dental office. Cloth towels become contaminated after only one use and cannot be safely reused until they have been cleaned and sterilized. The advantages of using disposable supplies should be weighed against the cost of purchasing them. Whenever possible, dental professionals should consider the use of disposable items for purposes of convenience and as a means of preventing cross-contamination.

Preparing instruments for sterilization

Cleaning instruments. Any instrument or other item that is to be sterilized or disinfected must be prepared by thorough cleaning, rinsing, and drying before it undergoes the chemical or heat process that will destroy the microorganisms it harbors. The presence of blood, saliva, soap films, and other organic debris not only increases the numbers of microorganisms that must be killed but also protects them against the destructive agent. The more a microorganism is protected by insulating debris, soap residue, or other microorganisms, the longer it will take for it to be destroyed. Recommended sterilization and disinfection conditions (time, concentration, temperature) depend on the intimate contact of the chemical or heating agent with the microorganism. Therefore, thorough washing, rinsing, and drying of all instruments must precede the disinfecting or sterilization process.

Instruments should be cleaned as soon as possible after they have been used to expedite the removal of blood and debris before they dry. If immediate cleaning is not possible, instruments should be soaked in a cool detergent or disinfectant solution. Ultrasonic cleaning is preferred for instrument preparation over hand scrubbing because the ultrasonic cleaner can dislodge contaminated material from grooves, hinges, and other surfaces that are not easily reached with a brush. Ultrasonic cleaning is also safer because it reduces the need to handle contaminated instruments. Protective rubber gloves should always be worn when handling contaminated instruments to prevent accidental injury and infection.

When an ultrasonic cleaner is not available, it is necessary to scrub instruments with a brush. A sterilized brush should be reserved for scrubbing

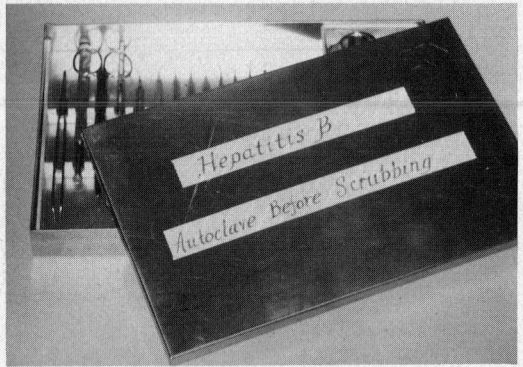

Fig. 3-11. Mark instrument trays that should be sterilized before cleaning so that they are handled with care until after they are decontaminated and safe to handle.

instruments. A detergent (not soap) is necessary for loosening blood and debris from the instrument surfaces and for reducing surface tension. During and after scrubbing, all loosened soil and blood should be rinsed off by running the instruments under cool water. All removable parts must be disassembled, and hinged instruments such as scissors must be opened to ensure that all residual detergent is completely removed. Instruments should be towel-dried prior to being sterilized by any method. Excess moisture may dilute the effects of chemicals, interfere with the achievement of sterilization in the prescribed cycle time, or contribute to rust or corrosion of certain metal instruments. A NOTE OF CAUTION: Contaminated instruments used in the treatment of a known or suspected carrier of HBV or HIV should not be scrubbed or ultrasonically cleaned before sterilization. After use, these instruments should be placed in a tray and sterilized before they are handled (Fig. 3-11). Following sterilization, the instruments should be cleaned and resterilized.

Use of the ultrasonic cleaner. Gross debris may be rinsed from contaminated instruments prior to cleaning. They are then placed into the cleaning solution, which can be either a nonfoaming commercial detergent (see manufacturer's instructions) or a solution of one part iodine surgical scrub to 19 parts detergent (Crawford, 1986). The instruments should be treated for 5 minutes in the ultrasonic bath with the cover in place to avoid splattering of the solution onto adjacent sur-

faces. Following cleaning, the instruments should be removed with forceps or heavily gloved hands, rinsed, inspected for debris, and then either rinsed in alcohol to enhance drying or dried with paper towels. Carbon steel instruments or low-quality stainless steel instruments that are likely to rust as a result of autoclaving should be dipped in protective solutions such as 1% sodium nitrite (Crawford, 1986) or amine compounds to prevent corrosion. The cleaned instruments can then be wrapped or placed in trays for sterilization. At the end of the day, the cleaning solution in the ultrasonic cleaner should be discarded, and the reservoir and tray should be disinfected with 0.5% sodium hypochlorite (Crawford, 1986).

Wrapping instruments. Unless an instrument or item will be used immediately after it is sterilized, it should be wrapped or contained in a material which is compatible with the sterilization method to be used (see Table 3-9). Follow recommendations of sterilizer manufacturers regarding the best types of packaging materials to use for each method. Sterilization bags are constructed so that, once they are sealed, they maintain the sterility of their contents unless the bag is torn or punctured. Damage to sterilization bags can be prevented by wrapping sharp instruments in a paper towel or shielding sharp edges with cotton rolls or gauze sponges before inserting them into the bag. Instruments that can be damaged by contact with other instruments, such as the head of the mouth mirror, should be wrapped separately so that they are protected from damage. The most common type of sterilization bag is made of paper and is disposable. These bags come in a variety of shapes and sizes, depending on the number and type of instruments that are being sterilized. To increase practice efficiency, it is advisable to wrap instruments together as a "tray" specific to a designated procedure. By wrapping instruments according to their intended use, only one or two sterile packages need to be opened to furnish the entire tray set-up. This fact is important because whenever a bag is opened, its entire contents are exposed to environmental contaminants and can no longer be considered sterile. By wrapping instruments with this in mind, bags need not be opened unless all instruments are to be used. Instruments used infrequently should be packaged individually. Each bag should be labeled so that instruments for any given tray set-up can be identified easily. As an added convenience, some sterilization bags are made of transparent materials so that the contents can be identified without the need for labelling or opening the bag. These bags are especially useful for singly wrapped instruments. Following are examples of instruments that may be packaged together:

Treatment procedure	Tray set-up (package together)
Initial examination	Mirror, explorer, probe, gauze sponge, tongue blade
Scaling	Assorted scalers and/or curettes
Root planing/curettage	Gracey curettes, explorer, mirror
Polishing	Mirror, prophylaxis angle, rubber cup, occlusal brush, dappen dish

Once the wrapped instruments and supplies are inserted into the labeled bag, the open end of the bag should be closed with a double fold and sealed with a piece of specially designed sterilization tape. The tape should be long enough to seal the entire fold and to lap around to the opposite side on both ends. Sealing and taping in this way will help ensure that the bag is properly sealed against recontamination during storage. Plastic bags may also be heat-sealed. Muslin or paper-wrapped packs should be resterilized if not used within 30 days. Tape-sealed paper and plastic packs should be resterilized after 4 months, and heat-sealed plastic packs can last up to 6 months before requiring resterilization (Crawford, 1986).

Instrument transfer. Clean gloves should always be worn when handling clean or sterile supplies in preparation for the next patient or when transferring supplies from one location to another. Sterile supplies should be transferred by means of sterile forceps rather than with the fingers. This precaution will help ensure that pathogens that may be transmitted by the hands are not introduced into an otherwise aseptic environment. Sterile cotton pliers may be included on each tray set-up for this purpose. When supplies are being transferred from a covered container, it is best to hold the lid top up with one hand while removing the supplies with the forceps in the other hand

(Fig. 3-5). This prevents airborne bacteria from settling onto the inside of the lid, which is then replaced on the sterile container. If it is necessary to lay the lid down, however, it should be put down with the inside surface up so that the rims of the lid are not contaminated by the countertop.

An aseptic technique should be used when removing sterile instruments from an autoclave bag for positioning on the tray. Because the bag has contacted the storage drawer and has been handled since it left the autoclave, the outside is no longer sterile. Therefore, placing the bag on the tray contaminates that surface. Instead, tear off the end of the bag and slide the wrapped instruments onto the tray without permitting contact of the bag with the contents of the tray. The contents of the tray should be kept covered until they are needed.

Reducing airborne contamination

Dental aerosols and splatter. Dental *aerosols* are tiny, invisible particles of contaminated water, blood, and saliva that are generated from the patient's mouth during dental procedures. Significantly large numbers of aerosols are produced during use of the high-speed handpiece, the air-water syringe, the ultrasonic scaler, the air polishing unit, engine polishing, and tooth brushing. The small size of these particles permits them to enter the body through the nose, mouth, and eyes. After they have entered the respiratory tract, they can penetrate deeply into its linings. Aerosols can remain suspended in the air for as long as 24 hours (Micik et al, 1969), where they continue to be sources of contamination long after the patient has left.

In addition to aerosols, the air can be contaminated by larger droplets of saliva-borne microorganisms and debris known as *splatter*. Splatter droplets are usually large enough to be visible. Their larger diameter and weight cause these particles to fall out of the air more quickly than aerosols so that they are most likely to accumulate on surfaces in the immediate treatment area, contaminating them with microorganisms from the patient's oral flora as well as other pathogens.

Miller and others (1971) compared the aerosol and splatter production of specific dental procedures with those of common nasal-oral activities. They found that using the high-speed handpiece or washing the teeth with a combined air-water spray produced contamination equal to sneezing, hissing, or tooth brushing. A prophylaxis produced the same amount of aerosol contamination as gargling, and using the ultrasonic scaler produced the same amount of contamination as a cough. Certainly, anyone would dislike having another person sneeze, hiss, gargle, or cough directly at him or her within a distance of only 8 to 12 inches, and yet most dental clinicians have to contend with these same levels of aerosol and splatter contamination continuously.

Both aerosols and splatter can contaminate the mucous membranes of the oral cavity, nose, or eyes and can lead to disease in a susceptible host. Aerosols can be the source of transmission for serious diseases, including hepatitis, tuberculosis, herpes simplex, other viral infections, and respiratory tract infections. Treatment of patients known to be infectious should be postponed until they are no longer contagious. Clinicians should avoid procedures that produce high amounts of aerosols on patients who are in high risk categories, such as carriers of HBV or HIV.

Reducing aerosol production. There are a number of ways in which the dental professional can control and reduce the amount of dental aerosols and splatter generated during treatment. The use of the rubber dam during operative procedures or at other times when this type of isolation is practical reduces aerosol production. High-speed evacuation during procedures involving the ultrasonic scaler or high-speed handpiece or when rinsing the mouth is also helpful. When the air-water syringe is used, the clinician should apply water to the area, followed by air, rather than dispensing both at the same time to produce a forced spray of water. Because bristle brushes generate more splatter during polishing procedures than do rubber cups or polishing points, use of brushes should be limited.

The number of microorganisms within the patient's mouth can be significantly reduced through the use of an antiseptic mouthwash before dental treatment (Litsky et al, 1976). Wyler and others (1971) demonstrated that the use of a pretreatment rinse with a commercially available antiseptic mouthwash reduced bacterial counts by 10 to 100 times. Although the main effect of mouth rinsing is one of mechanical removal, the antiseptic prop-

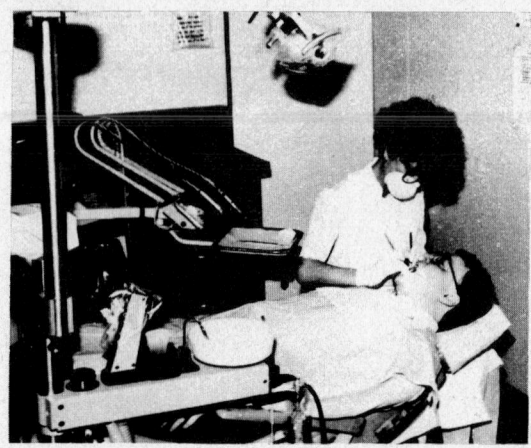

Fig. 3-12. Note the number of barrier techniques shown in this photo. How many do you see?

erties of some mouthwashes could enhance the overall reduction of microorganisms.

The direction of airflow within the dental operatory will also affect aerosols. Installation of a ceiling-to-floor laminar airflow system to direct the circulation of air in the operatory has been shown to reduce aerosols in the treatment area. The use of laminar airflow will also reduce the amount of surface contamination resulting from airborne particles (Pollock et al, 1970).

Cross-contamination due to aerosols and splatter should be controlled by using disposable paper covers on all countertops, keeping all clean and sterile supplies in closed containers, drawers, or cabinets, and disinfecting all contaminated surfaces thoroughly between patients. Dental personnel should protect themselves from aerosols and splatter through the use of barrier techniques including masks, safety glasses or face shields, gloves, and full coverage uniforms, lab coats or gowns. Disposable paper or plastic aprons, jackets, and bibs provide additional protection in reducing the amount of contamination to which uniforms are exposed, thereby reducing the potential of soiled uniforms to serve as cross-contaminants to the wearer and to other patients (Fig. 3-12). Disposable head covers and gowns provide effective barriers for dental personnel involved in the treatment of high risk patients. Dental practitioners also can reduce their exposure to aerosols and splatter by observing proper patient-operator positioning and through effective tissue retraction. Maintaining a safe operating distance from the patient's mouth, retracting soft tissues in ways that reflect liquid aerosols and splatter away from the operator, and operating from behind the patient rather than in front will all reduce exposure to airborne contaminants.

Personal hygiene and protection

Personal hygiene of all dental staff is an important step in the control of transmissible diseases. Important considerations include choice and care of uniforms or disposable coverings, hand washing and care of nails, avoiding direct contact with infected persons or lesions, wearing disposable masks, gloves, and glasses, and other practices to prevent transmission of pathogens from the office environment to the home environment.

All operating *personnel*—the dentist, the hygienist, and the assistant—participate in patient treatment and are potential sources of contamination. Dental personnel, by means of their occupation, are exposed to more disease-producing microorganisms than are most other people. If a member of the dental team contracts any sort of contagious disease, all efforts should be made to avoid transmission to other people in the office and to patients. A responsible health care provider will not risk transmitting active disease. When known disease is present in either the clinician or the patient, elective procedures should be postponed.

Uniforms. Even a healthy individual, patient or professional, carries potentially harmful bacteria on clothing, skin, and hair and in the mouth and nose. Carriers may be unaffected by these microbes, but other more susceptible individuals can contract disease if they encounter these pathogens. Health care providers can control contamination by wearing freshly laundered clothing in the dental environment. Clean clothing should be worn daily and changed if it becomes visibly soiled with blood or other contaminants. Many persons prefer to wear uniforms or full-length clinic coats because they are easily cleaned and are usually constructed of materials that do not readily give off bacteria-laden lint and threads. Styles should be selected that provide maximum protection from splatter and dental aerosols. To prevent contamination of others, they should be worn only in the dental environment and then changed before leaving that environment. Soiled garb can be commercially cleaned or placed in a plastic bag and taken home to be laundered. Contaminated clothing should be kept separate from other clothing before and during laundering. Clinic clothing should be made of materials that can be safely washed in hot water, regular laundry detergent, and bleach. Shoes worn during patient treatment also should be left at the dental office and not worn home, where small children might handle or play with them.

Unprotected street clothing is not appropriate for operating personnel for several reasons. Clothing that has been worn outside the dental office may introduce microorganisms from the outside environment into the treatment environment. At the end of the day, these personnel then carry potential pathogens that were contacted during patient treatment to their cars and homes, where they can be picked up by family members and friends. An additional problem is encountered when clothing contaminated in the dental office is combined with other family members' clothing prior to laundering, especially if laundering is not accomplished in hot water and bleach. Dental personnel must ask themselves if health risks such as these are worthwhile for the sake of fashion. Additional clothing protection is provided through the use of disposable paper or plastic bibs, aprons, or jackets which can be worn over work clothing and then discarded.

Personal hygiene is mandatory for all health care workers. Because it is known that bacteria are shed along with skin cells, dandruff, and dust from the hair and body, all exposed skin and hair must be as clean as possible. In addition, the longer the hair, the more likely it is that dandruff and bacteria may be shed because of its movement and contact with the shoulders and face. The clinician's head and face are kept close to the patient during treatment, and cross-contamination between oral pathogens and the clinician's hair (including a beard or mustache) can pose a health problem. Longer hair may also be a problem for the clinician in terms of maintaining a clear field of vision. For these reasons it is advisable that hair be kept short, pinned, or tied close to the head and out of the field of operation. Individuals who provide dental treatment for infectious or high-risk patients may consider wearing a disposable covering over their hair to protect it from contamination. At the end of the day, showering and shampooing hair will prevent transmission of pathogens to other family members.

Jewelry may be another source of contamination and should be kept to a minimum, if worn at all. Because hands and wrists cannot be adequately cleaned unless they are bare, jewelry, including all rings, bracelets, and watches, should not be worn on the hands while treating patients. Contrary to popular belief, wedding rings and watches are no less hazardous as sources of contamination than are other types of jewelry. All exposed jewelry, including earrings and necklaces, can trap and hold contaminants that are difficult, if not impossible, to remove, and they become potential reservoirs of contamination to the wearer and to other surfaces they contact.

Care of nails and hand washing. Ideally, any object that enters the patient's mouth should be sterilized or disposable to minimize the potential for cross-contamination. The most obvious and unavoidable failure of this rule is the clinician's hands. There is no acceptable way to sterilize human hands. For the protection of both the clinician and the patient, all direct care providers should wear disposable gloves during all intraoral dental procedures. As an additional measure of protection it is imperative that dental care providers give close attention to the washing and care of the hands both before putting on a new pair of gloves and after removing them. For the clinician's own protection, a close inspection of the hands should be conducted to ensure that there are no potential portals of entry for bacteria. Hangnails or small cuts or irritated areas are potential gates for infectious bacteria to enter the bloodstream. Clinicians with oozing dermatitis or exudative lesions should avoid direct patient contact until the condition has subsided (CDMIE, 1988). All breaks in the skin should be protected by keeping them covered during patient treatment procedures.

Hands and nails should be thoroughly cleaned before donning gloves and after gloves are removed. Nails should be kept short so that they will not interfere with patient comfort and effective instrument handling during intraoral procedures, and because long nails may cause tears in

disposable gloves (Parker and Williams, 1987). The protected area beneath the nail has been found to harbor residual blood and bacteria for up to 5 days in clinicians who did not routinely wear gloves (Allen et al, 1982). These studies demonstrated that the area under the nails is a potential source of cross-contamination for other patients, for the individual, and for family members. Therefore, the hand washing procedure should begin with a thorough cleaning around and under nails with an orangewood stick combined with lathering with a liquid soap or hand detergent and copious rinsing with cool water.

There are two levels of bacterial residents on the hands. A superficial layer of microorganisms, or *transient bacteria,* is found on the outer layers of the skin, under the fingernails, and around the nails. These bacteria include all the microorganisms that are picked up in the environment. A deeper level, called *resident bacteria,* forms part of the normal flora of the skin and lies deep in the crevices and folds of the skin. A quick, superficial washing will not dislodge these bacteria. This fact is significant, as many of these types are potential pathogens. Any technique of washing must be thorough enough to remove most transient bacteria and as many of the resident microorganisms as possible.

The goals of hand washing are to remove all surface dirt and contamination and to remove as much of the deeper (resident) bacteria as possible. An effective hand washing procedure should start with an initial scrub that includes a thorough lathering and scrubbing of all surfaces of the nails, fingers, hands, and lower arms. This is possible only if the hands and arms are bared of all jewelry and clothing at least to the elbow. The most important aspect of hand washing is the mechanical rubbing of all surfaces to remove soil and microorganisms, which are then rinsed away by the running water. This initial scrub should be a series of three latherings, each followed by a thorough rinsing with cool to lukewarm water, and may last for 2 to 3 minutes (Palenik and Miller, 1984b; Crawford, 1986). The initial scrub can be performed by repeated rubbing of one hand with another or with the aid of a soft, sterile brush or disposable sponge. Overzealous use of a stiff bristle brush, however, can abrade and lacerate the skin, increasing the risk of infection by oral pathogens. Scrubbing should include all surfaces of the hands and fingers and should emphasize the dominant hand, which is likely to be the more contaminated and less scrubbed hand (Maloney and Kohut, 1987).

Soap or detergent is helpful in loosening dirt, oils, and bacteria from the skin. The use of a liquid soap dispenser rather than a bar of soap will reduce cross-contamination during hand washing, as a cake or bar of soap can serve as a nutrient source and reservoir for bacteria growth after it has been used. Use of antiseptic handscrubs will enhance the destruction of bacteria in the deeper recesses of the skin. The professional should be aware of the claims made by different manufacturers regarding the bactericidal and bacteriostatic effects of antiseptic handscrubs. Whatever product is chosen should be nonirritating and gentle to the skin. The constant use of a harsh product can lead to excessive drying and skin irritation, reducing the ability of the skin to form an effective barrier against infection. A listing of accepted antimicrobial hand cleaners is available from the ADA Council on Dental Therapeutics (CDT, 1986).

When the hands are being rinsed, the water should flow from the fingertips down toward the elbow. The water should not be allowed to run back over an area that has been previously rinsed. Contaminated rinse water should not contact already clean areas. The hands should be dried with a paper towel, moving from the fingers to the hands and finally to the surfaces of the arms. A separate paper towel should be used for each hand. The faucet should be turned off either by means of foot controls or with a paper towel if hand controls are used. The paper towels should then be discarded. Care should be taken not to touch the sink, paper towel dispenser, or waste receptacle after the hands have been washed.

In addition to the initial scrubbing procedures which have been described, those individuals involved in direct patient contact must wash their hands thoroughly between each patient immediately after removing gloves and before donning clean gloves. This routine of hand washing should include two or three series of lathering followed by cool water rinses. Hands should be dried thoroughly before donning gloves. Use of hand creams should be restricted to after-work hours

since these preparations can become microbially contaminated (Palenik and Miller, 1987).

Wearing disposable gloves. The use of sterile gloves by dental clinicians will afford the highest degree of hand hygiene and protection against cross-contamination. Disposable gloves can permit the achievement and maintenance of a safer level of contamination control than can be achieved with bare hands alone. Most important, they provide an effective barrier against the entry of serious pathogens, including those responsible for syphilis, hepatitis, and other diseases transmitted by the blood or saliva of infected patients. Since it is not always possible to detect which patients may be carriers of infectious diseases, *the dental professional must wear gloves for all intraoral procedures,* especially for those procedures in which bleeding is likely to occur. The Centers for Disease Control and the ADA have recommended that gloves be worn for all procedures involving contact with blood, saliva, mucous membranes, or surfaces contaminated with body fluids or secretions. This includes all intraoral procedures and examination of oral lesions (CDC, 1986; CDMIE, 1988). Gloves should also be worn when handling soiled or contaminated instruments, surfaces, or supplies and when handling contaminated materials such as impressions or prostheses in the laboratory (Palenik and Miller, 1987).

Four types of gloves may be used in dental practice (Fig. 3-13). Sterile surgical gloves are

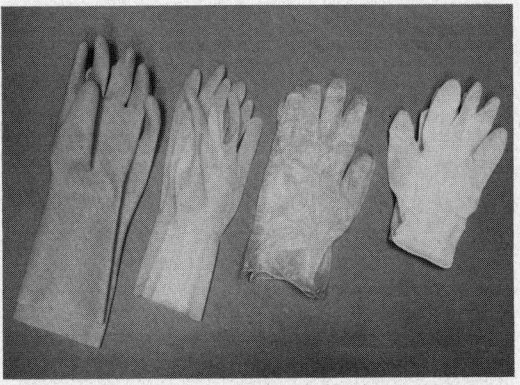

Fig. 3-13. Types of gloves. *From left to right:* puncture-resistant utility gloves, regular surgical gloves, vinyl exam gloves, latex exam gloves.

the highest quality, most expensive, and best-fitting disposable gloves. They are used most commonly for surgical or invasive procedures where maximum protection against infection must be provided for the patient and the clinician. Non-sterile, latex examination gloves are the most commonly selected gloves for use in routine dental procedures. They are available in a variety of hand sizes and may come with or without a cornstarch lubricant for ease in getting them on and off. Because there is a wide variation in sizing (palm width, finger width and length) among different manufacturers, clinicians should sample several different brands and choose the one which provides them the best fit. Some individuals may develop hypersensitive reactions either to the latex material or to the cornstarch lubricant in disposable gloves. This problem is usually alleviated through the use of nonpowdered surgical gloves or latex-free (neoprene or vinyl) examination gloves. Heavy-duty utility gloves that are puncture-resistant should be worn when handling and cleaning contaminated instruments or supplies, when using chemical sterilant solutions, and for general operatory cleaning. These gloves can be washed, disinfected or sterilized, powdered with cornstarch, and reused (Palenik and Miller, 1987).

All disposable gloves should be considered as single-use items because their present composition does not permit them to be safely washed and reused on other patients (CDC, 1986; CDMIE, 1988). Contact with hot water, soaps, detergents, and other chemicals can negatively affect glove materials by making them "tacky" and more prone to tearing. Clinicians should always inspect gloves carefully before putting them on and during treatment for signs of tears, punctures, or tackiness and should replace damaged gloves immediately before proceeding. Rings and watches and long fingernails should not be worn under gloves because of their potential for causing holes in gloves. Even new gloves may already have minute holes or tears in them and should be carefully inspected (Skaug, 1976; Clin Res Assoc, 1985). A good test is to inflate gloves with air and then hold them closed to see if there is significant leakage, which would indicate the presence of a defect in the material. Gloves should not be worn for periods of more than 1 hour on a single patient procedure. If gloves must be washed, they should be rinsed thoroughly under cool running water and then dried. New gloves should be rinsed before entering the patient's mouth to remove cornstarch residue that might have an unpleasant taste (Palenik and Miller, 1987). Dental personnel must be careful during patient treatment not to touch any part of their clothing or bodies or any other surfaces that are not protected by barrier covers, disinfection, or sterilization. If they must leave the operatory or touch surfaces which are not routinely treated or covered between patients, gloves should be removed and hands must be washed prior to contact with other surfaces. Hands must then be rewashed and new gloves put on before returning to patient treatment.

Double-gloving provides additional protection when treating patients with infectious diseases or those who are in high-risk categories as potential carriers of infections such as hepatitis B or AIDS. Inexpensive vinyl gloves, such as those used by food handlers or cafeteria workers, may also be placed over existing examination or surgical gloves which have been rinsed in cool water and dried when dental personnel have to examine a second patient briefly. The second pair of gloves should then be removed before returning to the first patient (CDMIE, 1988). This procedure should not be used when treating known infectious or high-risk patients (American Health Consultants, 1987a & b).

Use of face masks. Current guidelines from the CDC and the ADA recommend that surgical masks or chin-length plastic shields be worn for all dental procedures in which splashing or spattering of blood or other body fluids is likely (CDMIE, 1988; CDC, 1986 and 1987). A well-fitting face mask is an effective means of protection in two ways. First, it protects the patient from contamination by a clinician who has a cold or other condition that is transmittable by respiratory droplets. Since the clinician's face is in such proximity to the patient, this kind of transfer could easily occur. It may also be a source of protection for the clinician from bacteria- or virus-containing aerosols which may be generated during dental treatment.

An effective mask is one that will not only mechanically block larger particles of blood, saliva, and oral debris, but also will filter out aerosols.

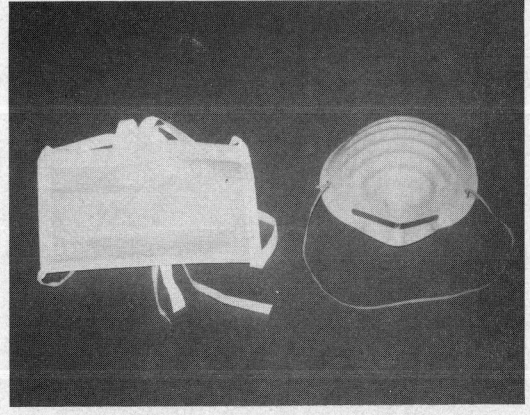

Fig. 3-14. Two popular styles of masks used in dentistry.

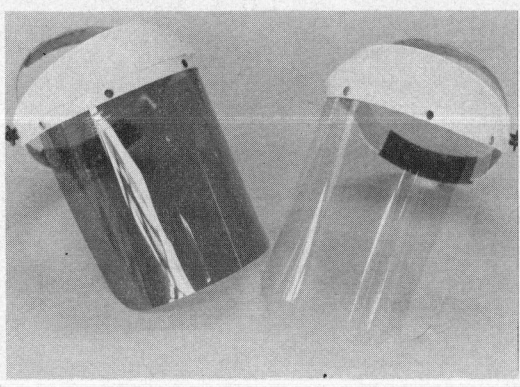

Fig. 3-15. Examples of protective shields
(Courtesy of American Shield Co, Orlando, Florida.)

Face masks should also be comfortable, fit well, and have minimal marginal leakage. Face masks are available in a wide variety of styles and materials, including paper, cloth, foam, fiberglass, and other synthetic materials. Of these, the paper, cloth, and foam masks have shown the least effectiveness, whereas the masks made of glass or synthetic fiber have been most effective in filtering aerosols, making them the best masks for dental procedures (Micik et al, 1971; Underhill et al, 1986) (Fig. 3-14).

Most face masks available to dental personnel are disposable and should be discarded after each patient or when they become visibly contaminated or wetted (Craig and Quayle, 1985). Plastic face shields are preferred by some practitioners because they provide protection to eyes, nose and mouth without some of the discomfort of close-fitting masks and because they do not interfere with communication (Fig. 3-15). Disadvantages of these shields are that they do not provide the same level of protection against aerosol contamination because they are not closely adapted to the face and they must be completely disinfected after each patient. Although disposable face masks have been shown to be effective in reducing contamination, they do not totally prevent the passage of potentially dangerous microorganisms. Additional measures for controlling airborne contaminants are discussed later in this chapter.

Use of protective eyeglasses. Protective eyeglasses or a face shield should be worn by all

dental personnel involved in chairside treatment (CDC, 1986; CDMIE, 1988). This important safety measure can prevent damage caused by bacteria-laden aerosols, accidental trauma, or flying debris. The use of ultrasonic scalers and high-speed handpieces increases the presence of aerosols containing large numbers of infectious bacteria that pose a risk to clinician and patient alike. The herpes virus is one example of a pathogen that could be transmitted from saliva or an active lesion into the eye by means of aerosols or splatter droplets. The resulting infection, recurrent herpetic keratitis, leads to impaired vision and, in some cases, blindness (Brooks et al, 1981). Safety glasses prevent damage to the eyes that could result from a particle of calculus being snapped from the tooth and propelled out of the mouth or from a slurry of abrasive and saliva that might splatter against the clinician's face during polishing procedures. Those clinicians who wear glasses can see the evidence of splatter and debris on their safety lenses following patient treatment. As both the patient's eyes and those of the dental team are in such close proximity to the working area, the risk of eye injury is high. In a survey of dental hygienists, 44% had suffered the following foreign bodies in their eyes as a result of treatment procedures: pumice/prophylaxis paste, calculus, dental materials, and contaminated water spray (Gravois and Stringer, 1980).

Patients who already wear glasses should be advised to wear them during treatment. The patient's eyes are extremely vulnerable to damage from oral debris and aerosols and from falling or mishandled instruments and dental materials. This observation is especially true for patients in the supine position (Cooley et al, 1978). Incorrect instrument or supply transfer over the patient's face could result in trauma to the eye or impaction of a foreign body. Safety glasses should be provided for patients who do not normally wear glasses. They may be of a disposable design, or they should be sterilized or disinfected between patients. Most patients will appreciate this precaution if the dental professional explains that it is recommended out of concern for their health and safety. Tinted lenses in the glasses provided for patient use will also provide shielding from overhead lighting.

Most eyeglasses fitted by prescription are now made of shatter-resistant materials, and lenses can be coated to make them scratch and fog-resistant. The clinician's glasses can be treated with antifogging cloths or cleaners that are commercially available to prevent the problem of fogging. Plastic safety glasses can be safely treated by immersion in 2% glutaraldehyde between patients (Gleason and Molinari, 1987). Those professionals who decide not to protect themselves and their patients with safety glasses should consider the economic and ethical implications of that choice.

ESTABLISHING AN EFFECTIVE ROUTINE FOR CONTAMINATION CONTROL BETWEEN PATIENTS

Now that methods of contamination control for dental personnel and the dental environment have been discussed in general, consider some of the important factors that should be considered in establishing an effective and efficient routine for treating contaminated surfaces between patient appointments. As time is limited, the person responsible for performing these tasks should already have identified the critical, semicritical, and noncritical items in the dental environment and should know which methods of treatment are appropriate for each item. In addition, care must be taken during treatment of patients not to enlarge the list of critical surfaces by touching and contaminating additional surfaces. After they have been contaminated by the patient's oral flora and

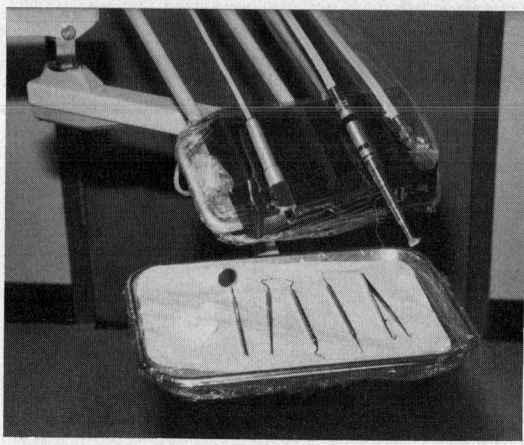

Fig. 3-16. Surface on unit and bracket table, including hoses, can be covered with clear plastic film.

saliva, the dental professional's hands should not touch any surface that is not routinely sterilized or disinfected until the hands have been washed.

Following is a discussion of specific surfaces or items that require infection control treatment both before and after patient treatment, along with recommendations for treatment.

Before cleaning and disinfecting the dental operatory at the beginning of the day, wash hands and put on gloves. All semicritical surfaces should be cleaned and disinfected with an intermediate level surface disinfectant. Whenever possible, cover semicritical surfaces with clean, disposable barrier covers to prevent them from becoming recontaminated during treatment. In most cases it takes far less time to cover these items than it does to clean and disinfect them between patients. Use of barrier coverings is especially important for surfaces or items that cannot be easily cleaned. Surfaces that may be covered include the dental chair (especially headrest and armrests), chair and unit control buttons, lamp handles and switch, the bracket table and handles, equipment cords, counter and cart surfaces, sink faucets, and any equipment or supply containers that are exposed to dental aerosols (e.g., ultrasonic and air polishing units, storage containers, patient education materials) (Figs. 3-16, 3-17, 3-18, and 3-19). In general, all clean or sterile supplies should be kept in covered containers or in draw-

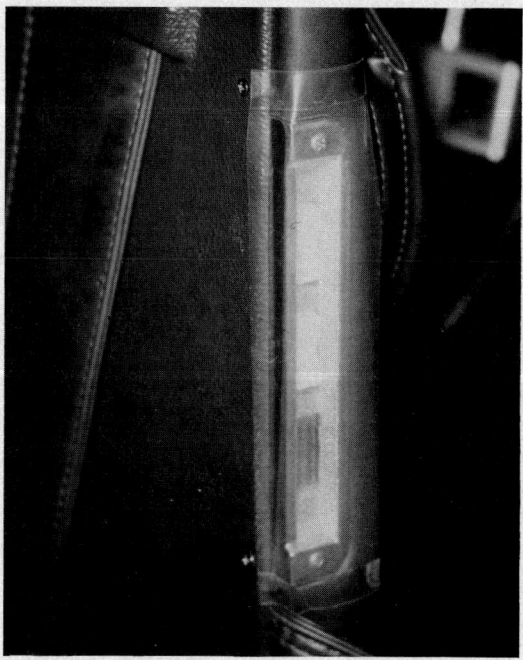

Fig. 3-17. Chair controls are easily contaminated and difficult to disinfect. Plastic covers with self-adhesive ends are a convenient way to protect these surfaces.

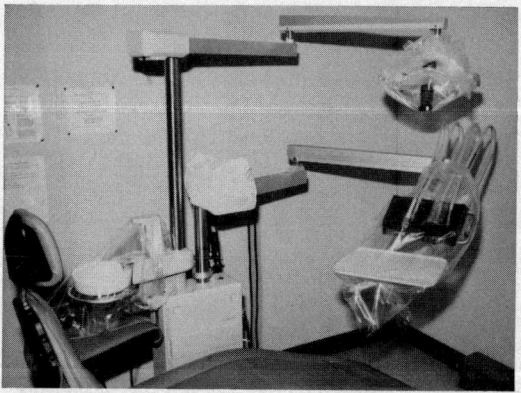

Fig. 3-19. At the end of the day, cleaned and disinfected surfaces can be kept covered overnight to protect them from aerosol particles and dust that settle out of the air.

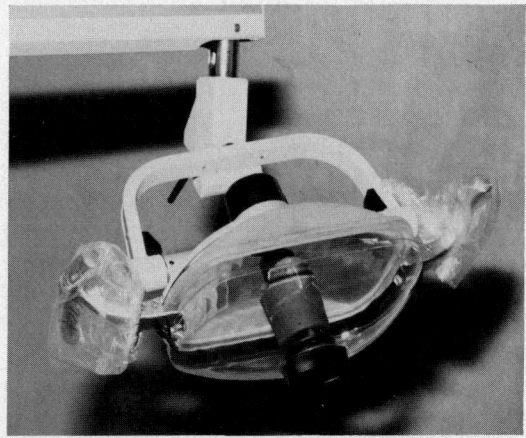

Fig. 3-18. Light handles are frequently touched during treatment. Covering them with plastic covers or film is an effective way to prevent cross-contamination.

ers where they are protected from dental aerosols and should be brought into the dental environment in quantities sufficient for each patient. Surfaces should be disinfected as needed and clean barrier coverings should then be replaced after hands have been washed and clean gloves put on.

All semicritical surfaces that cannot be covered, including saliva ejector, high speed suction, hand-held cuspidor, and handpiece bases, must be scrubbed and disinfected before and after each patient contact. Disinfection should be accomplished only with approved chemical solutions and should follow manufacturers' recommendations for use.

In many instances the *water supplies* within dental units can become contaminated with bacterial concentrations higher than those levels considered acceptable for public consumption. When water supplies are allowed to sit for long periods without being used, the effectiveness of chlorine to control bacterial growth begins to decrease. The subsequent growth of microorganisms provides a source of contamination when the water lines are again used and delivered directly into the patient's mouth by way of the drinking cup, the air-water syringe, the ultrasonic scaler, the air polisher, and the water-cooled handpiece. In addition, many modern handpieces and syringes are equipped with retraction devices that are designed to prevent water from dripping out of the ends of these items after they have been used. When this excess water is retracted back into the handpiece or syringe, it is often accompanied by contaminated water and saliva, which then contaminate the water line and the next patient treated with this equipment. The best way to prevent this contamination is to remove the retraction devices from syringes and handpieces or to install check valves (Bagga et al, 1984). In addition, all hoses that deliver water from the dental unit should be flushed for several minutes at the beginning of the day. After use, water-cooled handpieces, ultrasonic and air polishing units, and air-water syringes should have water flushed through them for 20 to 30 seconds prior to cleaning and disinfection or sterilization (CDC, 1986; CDMIE, 1988).

Equipment used for delivering nitrous oxide analgesia should be disinfected after each use. The *nitrous oxide nosepiece* should be disinfected after each use to prevent transmission of viral and upper respiratory tract infections from one patient to another. This equipment cannot be routinely sterilized because it is composed of rubber or plastic materials that cannot withstand the high temperatures of the autoclave or dry heat oven. Yagiela and others (1979) compared the effectiveness of a number of different methods for disinfecting this equipment and concluded that the most effective procedure was to wash the nosepiece thoroughly after each use with soap and water and then immerse it in a 2% alkaline glutaraldehyde solution for 10 minutes to achieve disinfection, followed by thorough rinsing in tap water. Sterilization of this equipment should be accomplished nightly, when immersion for the full 6¾- to 10-hour period, followed by a 1-hour rinse, can be accomplished.

The *x-ray supplies and equipment,* including the cone, head, and controls, should be protected from contamination with disposable barrier covers. If this is not done, these items must be scrubbed and disinfected after each use. Because the clinician is constantly going back and forth between the intraoral placement of radiographic films and the x-ray equipment, they are prime sources of cross-contamination. Whenever possible, disposable paper towels should be used to handle the head and the cone to avoid excessive contamination. Contaminated film packets should be placed on disposable paper towels until film is

removed. Film should be ejected from packets without being touched and contaminated by fingers (CDMIE, 1982). Intraoral radiographic film holders are critical surfaces and should be made of materials that are disposable or that can be sterilized between patients. X-ray viewboxes should be left on and should not be touched unless hands are clean.

The *pens and pencils* used for recording patient data, *patients' charts,* and *patient education materials* are often overlooked as sources of contamination. Pens and pencils should be wiped thoroughly with a high-level disinfectant after each patient appointment. Another safeguard is to delegate all recording and chart handling to an assistant, so that the clinician's contaminated hands never touch them. If an assistant is not available, the clinician's hands must be washed before handling these items and then washed again before resuming intraoral procedures. An alternative is to use one hand for intraoral examination and the other hand to record all data on the chart forms. Chart folders and contents should be handled only with clean hands. Pens and pencils that are used in the treatment room should remain there and not be carried to other areas where they could transfer pathogens to other patients or family members. Mirrors, demonstration models, and instructional booklets that are used during patient education should never be handled when hands are contaminated following patient treatment. Mirrors and models should be cleaned and disinfected after being handled by patients. These materials should not be left exposed on countertops during treatment when aerosols are being generated.

The *high-speed suction* and *saliva ejector tubes* should be cleaned out at the end of each day to remove residual saliva, blood, and debris. To accomplish this, the entire system should be flushed at the end of each operating day with a detergent and water followed by use of a disinfectant solution such as 1:10 sodium hypochlorite (Maloney and Kohut, 1987). Suction traps and switches should be scrubbed and disinfected. Exact instructions as to how this should be accomplished should be obtained from the manufacturer of the equipment.

After all surfaces have been cleaned, disinfected, and sterilized, sterile supplies and instruments should be placed on the bracket tray aseptically, using sterile forceps and clean, gloved hands. These items should then be kept covered until they are needed.

Laboratory asepsis

Principles of contamination control apply to all areas in the dental office, not just to the dental operatory. Another area in which stringent infection control guidelines must be applied is the dental laboratory. The following recommendations should be followed for procedures that deal with this part of the dental office. All laboratory materials, impressions, and intraoral appliances should be cleaned and disinfected before being handled, adjusted, or sent to a commercial dental laboratory (CDT, 1985; CDC, 1986).

Handling of intraoral prosthetic appliances. Dentures should be rinsed thoroughly to remove blood, saliva, and oral debris. They should then be placed in a disposable plastic cup or in a disposable zip-lock plastic bag. If dentures are to be cleaned, the appropriate solution should be added to the bag, which is then sealed and placed in the ultrasonic cleaner for the prescribed length of time. After cleaning, the denture should be removed from solution, and rinsed thoroughly. The bag should be emptied and rinsed thoroughly, and the denture can be replaced in the bag and returned to the dental operatory.

When adjustments or polishing of dentures using laboratory equipment is required or when dentures are to be returned to a commercial laboratory, they should be disinfected before being handled and treated. Dentures can be disinfected by immersing them in 1:10 sodium hypochlorite solutions for 10 to 30 minutes (CDT, 1985). Prolonged immersion of dentures with metal parts can lead to corrosion and caution is advised. Another method for disinfection of dentures has been described by Henderson and others (1987), in which dentures were scrubbed with a denture brush for one minute with 4% chlorhexidine gluconate (Hibiclens), placed in a zip-lock bag with either undiluted or diluted (1:16) buffered, alkaline glutaraldehyde, and ultrasonically treated for 10 minutes. The denture and bag were then rinsed thoroughly and the denture was again ultrasonically treated for 3 minutes in sterile water.

Impression materials should be handled with gloves, rinsed gently under water to remove blood and saliva, and disinfected prior to pouring stone casts. Manufacturer's recommendations should be followed regarding appropriate choice of disinfectants that will not distort impression material (CDC, 1986). Alginate and reversible hydrocolloid impressions may be distorted by prolonged submersion in disinfectant. At the very least, these impressions should be rinsed sequentially with water and an iodophore or be soaked in iodophore disinfectant for 10 minutes (Crawford, 1986). Herrera and Merchant (1986) reported that short-term (30-minute) immersion of impression materials in 1% sodium hypochlorite did not significantly affect the dimensional accuracy of the resultant casts and that glutaraldehydes, povidone-iodine solution, and halogenated phenol disinfectants had no apparent effect on the dimensional stability of rubber impression materials. Minagi and others (1986 and 1987) recommended immersion of silicone rubber impression materials in sodium hypochlorite solution for 60 minutes and immersion of irreversible colloid and hydrophilic impression material in 2% glutaraldehyde for 60 minutes as a means of preventing cross-contamination of viral diseases. An alternative to disinfecting impression materials is to handle the impression with gloves, pour the stone model, discard contaminated impression and gloves, and wrap the stone cast and sterilize it using ethylene oxide gas.

If impressions are sent to a *commercial laboratory,* both parties should understand the disinfection procedures that have been used. If impressions are disinfected at the dental office before transfer to the laboratory there is no need for additional disinfection treatment at the laboratory which might distort or harm the materials. All materials from high-risk patients must be clearly marked on the outside of the delivery packages for the protection of dental lab personnel. Dentures that are returned from a commercial laboratory should be disinfected and rinsed thoroughly before being handled and returned to the patient. Packaging materials in which appliances are received from dental laboratories should be discarded and not reused.

Aerosols and flying debris generated by machine grinding and rag wheel polishing can also be a potential problem. Pumice should be replaced daily and should be mixed with a 5:100 sodium hypochlorite solution to which 3 parts of green soap has been added to keep the pumice suspended (CDT, 1985). Pumice pans can be easily cleaned if they are covered with a large disposable plastic bag at the beginning of the day. At the end of the day, the bag can be turned inside out, and carefully removed so that the contaminated pumice is neatly discarded. Rag wheels should be sterilized. In offices where wheel polishing occurs only infrequently, a sterilized rag wheel can be held ready for use and only a small amount of pumice dispensed into a covered or disposable pan as needed. Pumice pans should be cleaned out daily or after use with an iodophore disinfectant. Preferred methods of disinfection and sterilization for other items used in the laboratory are listed in Table 3-9.

Barrier covers are recommended for *laboratory equipment* whenever possible. All contaminated surfaces should be cleaned and disinfected after each use with a spray bottle of an approved surface disinfectant and absorbent disposable towels or gauze sponges. For obvious reasons, dental employees should be discouraged from using dental laboratories as eating or smoking areas.

LEGAL ASPECTS OF INFECTION CONTROL

The alarming spread of lethal diseases such as hepatitis B and AIDS in recent years has not only led to major changes in standards for infection control in dentistry but has also caused dental professionals to reassess the legal implications of potential infection transfer in their practices. Failure to act in accordance with the current standard of care may be viewed by the courts as a breach of required duty and result in liability for negligence (Baker and Hawkins, 1985). Employer dentists who do not implement current infection control guidelines as set forth by the CDC and ADA may be held liable by employees or patients who contract infectious diseases as a result of dental treatment (Logan, 1987). Dental hygienists must assume a similar legal responsibility in utilizing all recommended precautions in the treatment of dental patients.

The Occupational Safety and Health Administration (OSHA) of the federal government has issued standards to ensure a safe and healthy dental workplace. These regulations require that all dentist employers must provide appropriate infection control barriers to all employees in quantities that allow for gloves, masks, and glasses to be changed with each new patient or in accordance with current infection control principles (e.g., current CDC and ADA guidelines). OSHA also requires that employees use the infection control barriers provided. Employers must inform their employees about OSHA regulations and keep them updated regarding changes in health and safety requirements. Employees must also be informed that failure to comply with these regulations is grounds for dismissal.

If a dental employer is not in compliance with these regulations, the employee should first discuss the problem with the employer to make sure that he or she is aware of the regulations. If compliance is still not implemented, the employee has the right to file a complaint with the local branch of OSHA. When filing a written and signed complaint, the employee may request that his or her name be withheld from the employer and that he or she desires notification of OSHA actions regarding the complaint. Enforcement of regulations will be implemented through inspections of dental offices as necessary and the imposition of fines against dentist employers who are found to be in violation of these rules (ADA 1987a and 1987b; ADHA, 1987; Yokom, 1988).

Employers should also inform all employees of the risk of contracting hepatitis B as an occupational hazard and of the availability of an effective vaccine. Baker and Hawkins (1985) further recommended that employers should pay for the vaccine for those high-risk dental employees who choose to receive it as a part of their duty to free the work place of the hepatitis hazard. Many states have laws and regulations describing conditions under which dental and other professionals may practice their professions that could serve as a basis for restricting the practice or revoking the license of individuals who are either infectious or carriers of infectious diseases. Professionals should consult the laws in their state for further information.

In light of these new legal implications concerning safety in the dental practice, several recommendations could prevent clinicians from encountering legal problems (Palenik and Miller, 1986b). These recommendations include (1) be aware of state-of-the-art infection control techniques as well as those peers are using; (2) be sure all staff in the office are educated as to procedures for minimizing cross-infection; (3) if there is any indication of an infection problem, cease patient contact immediately and seek medical advice; (4) do not discriminate against any patient, but if a decision not to treat a person with a serious disease has to be made, help find appropriate dental care elsewhere; and (5) consult an attorney if the issues become too complex.

CONCLUSION

It should be apparent that control of contamination when preparing the site for the patient is a very important step in patient care. Such control makes possible a comfortable, efficient, and safe environment for the patient and affords the dental personnel those same considerations.

Although the time needed for this preparatory phase may diminish with experience, its importance in providing quality care should remain a primary consideration in all phases of care.

ACTIVITIES

1. Purchase or prepare Petri dishes that contain an agar medium that will support the growth of several types of organisms. Using sterile cotton swabs, collect microbial samples from different parts of the clinic (such as counter tops, sinks, trisyringes, dental chair) or from yourself (such as skin, clothing, shoes). Wipe the contaminated swab over the agar medium and incubate for 24 to 48 hours. Observe the growth on the plates for a visual representation of the organisms present in the clinical area. As an extension of the activity, compare culture samples from both before and after sterilization and disinfection procedures. Evaluate the success of contamination control practices in the clinic.
2. View the 16 mm film, *Oral Sepsis: The Unseen Problem*. (DTB-294, 20 minutes, produced by the American Dental Association, Bureau of Audio Visual Service. Available for rental.)
3. With a lab partner, role play performing an intraoral procedure. Identify the possible sources of contamination in the area. Demonstrate how direct and indirect transmission occur.
4. Observe and report on aseptic practices in other parts of the school or other clinics.
5. Observe asepsis control in a hospital operating room.
6. Review the literature for statistics relating to the incidence of hepatitis among dental professionals and patients.
7. Discuss the implications of contracting serum hepatitis for the career of a dental professional.
8. Discuss the legal ramifications of endangering safety of practice through ineffective contamination control. Determine if there have been any malpractice suits related to this issue brought against health professionals in your state or others. Consult a lawyer about the legalities of such an issue.
9. Make a specific list of each item in the student's instrument kit, and determine how it would best be sterilized/disinfected.
10. Ask students to inspect their safety glasses after a patient appointment for signs of splatter droplets of blood and saliva or other debris.
11. Compare the germicidal effects of all disinfectants, soaps, and antiseptics available in the clinic from manufacturers' descriptions and descriptions in *Accepted Dental Therapeutics*.
12. Wipe red tempera paint on a surface normally contaminated during dental treatment to simulate saliva contamination. Have students attempt to remove it with disinfectant-soaked gauze squares. Discuss how much scrubbing was necessary to remove all traces of the paint. Draw comparisons with the amount of wiping students may normally use.

REVIEW QUESTIONS

1. Discuss the susceptibility of the dental clinician to sources of infection.
2. State the bacterial or viral disease caused by the following organisms (give the mode of transmission for each):
   a. *Mycobacterium tuberculosis*
   b. *Treponema pallidum*
   c. *Clostridium tetani*
   d. Respiratory virus (e.g., adenovirus)
   e. Hepatitis B virus
   f. Rubeola virus
3. True or false:
   a. Hepatitis A usually has no residual effects after recovery.
   b. Jaundice occurs in all cases of hepatitis.
   c. Hepatitis B virus may be transmitted by means of the saliva.

d. *Mycobacterium tuberculosis* is routinely destroyed by surface disinfection.
e. Because of an increased opportunity for contracting tuberculosis, dental personnel should have periodic skin testing performed.
f. When the patient's saliva enters the clinician's blood by way of a break in the skin, direct transmission has occurred.
g. When the hygienist punctures his/her hand while cleaning instruments, indirect transmission has occurred.
h. Aerosol production is responsible for contaminating a major portion of the dental operatory.
i. Syphilis is only contagious in the primary stage.
j. A chancre is a primary stage syphilitic lesion.
4. Define the terms sanitization, disinfection, and sterilization.
5. Describe an effective hand washing procedure.
6. List five accepted methods for instrument sterilization.
7. Describe the conditions required for sterilization when using each of the methods listed in 6.
8. Describe the recommended procedure for decontaminating the tri-syringe and the handpiece between patients.

REFERENCES

Allen AL, and Organ RJ: Occult blood accumulation under fingernails: a mechanism for the spread of blood-borne infections, JADA 105:455, 1982.

American Dental Association News 18(3):1, 1987a.

American Dental Association News 18(16):1, 1987b.

American Dental Hygienists Association: OSHA mandates protective wear, Access, November 1987, p. 1.

American Health Consultants: Companies, hospitals, scientists debate safety of disposable gloves, AIDS Alert 2:207, 1987a.

American Health Consultants: Latex vinyl gloves offer same protection against HIV. AIDS Alert 2:210, 1987b.

Bagga BS, et al: Contamination of dental units cooling water with oral microorganisms and its prevention, JADA 109:712, 1984.

Baker CH, and Hawkins VI: Law in the dental workplace: legal implications of hepatitis B for the dental profession, JADA 110:637, 1985.

Bond, WW et al: Inactivation of Hepatitis B virus by intermediate-to-high level disinfectant chemicals, J Clin Microbiol 18:535, 1983.

Brooks SL, et al: Prevalence of herpes simplex virus disease in a professional population, J Am Dent Assoc 102:31, 1981.

Burnett GW, and Schuster GS: Oral microbiology and infectious disease, Baltimore, 1978, Williams & Wilkins.

Centers for Disease Control: Recommendations for protection against viral hepatitis, MMWR 34:313, 1985.

Centers for Disease Control: Recommended infection control practice for dentistry, MMWR 35(15):237, 1986a.

Centers for Disease Control: Update: Acquired immunodeficiency syndrome—United States, MMWR 35:141, 1986b.

Centers for Disease Control: Update on hepatitis B prevention, MMWR 36:353, 1987.

Clinical Research Associates: Subject: Gloves, disposable operating, Clin Res Assoc Newsletter 9(9):2, 1985.

Cottone JA: Hepatitis B virus infection in the dental profession, J Am Dent Assoc 110:617, 1985.

Cottone JA: Delta hepatitis: another concern for dentistry, JADA 112:47, 1986.

Cottone JA, and Baker BR: Hepatitis B: recent advances and 1986 preview, CDA Journal 13:36, 1985.

Council on Dental Materials, Instruments, and Equipment: Recommendations for radiographic darkroom practices, JADA 104:886, 1982.

Council on Dental Materials, Instruments, and Equipment; Council on Dental Practice; and Council on Dental Therapeutics: Infection control recommendations for the dental office and the dental laboratory, JADA 116:241, 1988.

Council on Dental Therapeutics: ADA Council recommends hepatitis vaccine for dentist, students, and auxiliary personnel, ADA News 13(17):4, 1982.

Council on Dental Therapeutics: Accepted dental therapeutics, ed 40, Chicago, 1984, Am Dent Assoc.

Council on Dental Therapeutics: Council clarifies disinfectant use: questions on glutaraldehyde answered, ADA News 15(1):9, 1984b.

Council on Dental Therapeutics: Accepted therapeutic products, JADA 113:1018, 1986.

Council on Dental Therapeutics, and Council on Prosthetic Services and Dental Laboratory Relations: Guidelines for infection control in the dental office and the commercial dental laboratory, JADA 110:969, 1985.

Crawford JJ: Clinical Asepsis in Dentistry, ed 3, Mesquite, Tex, 1986, RA Kolstad.

Crawford JJ: State of the art practical infection control in dentistry, JADA 110:629, 1985.

Craig DC, and Quayle AA: The efficiency of face masks, Br Dent J 158:87, 1985.

Crow S: Chemical indicators, Infection Cont 4:8, 1983.

Farah JW, and Powers JM, editors: Infection control, Dental Advisor, Materials, Instruments and Equipment Quarterly 3(3):4, 1986.

Gleason MJ, and Molinari JA: Stability of safety glasses during sterilization and disinfection, JADA 115:60, 1987.

Gobette JP, et al: Hand asepsis: the efficacy of different soaps in the removal of bacteria from sterile, gloved hands, JADA 113:291, 1986.

Gravois SL, and Stringer RB: Survey of occupational health hazards in dental hygiene, Dent Hyg 54:518, 1980.

Gross ML: Herpes: an overview on diagnosis and treatment, J Ky Dent Assoc 33(3):26, 1981.

Henderson CW, et al: Evaluation of the barrier system, an infection control system for the dental laboratory, J Prosth Dent 58:517, 1987.

Herrera SP, and Merchant VA: Dimensional stability of dental impressions after immersion disinfection, JADA 113:419, 1986.

Horowitz AM, et al: Knowledge and reported use of hepatitis B vaccine by dental hygienists, J Dent Res 66:163, 1987.

Hume WR, and Matkinson, OF: Sterilizing dental instruments: evaluation of lubricating oils and microwave radiation, Oper Dent 3:93, 1978.

Johnson & Johnson: Handbook of Dental Practice Asepsis. East Windsor, NJ, 1969, Dental Products Co.

Kane MA, and Lettau LA: Transmission of HBV from dental personnel to patients, JADA 110:634, 1985.

Klein RS, et al: Low occupational risk of human immunodeficiency virus infection among dental professionals, N Engl J Med 318:86, 1988.

Kroop D: Chemical indicators, J Hosp Dent (March-April) 2:46, 1984.

Landesman S, et al: The AIDS epidemic, N Engl J Med 312:521, 1985.

Litsky BY, et al: Use of antimicrobial mouthwash to minimize the bacterial aerosol contamination generated by a high speed drill, Oral Surg 29:25, 1976.

Logan MK: Legal implications of infectious disease in the dental office, JADA 115:850, 1987.

Maloney JM, and Kohut RD: Infection control: barrier protection and the treatment environment, Dent Hyg 61:310, 1987.

Manzella JP, et al: An outbreak of herpes simplex virus type I gingivostomatitis in a dental hygiene practice, JAMA 252:2019, 1984.

Merchant VA: Herpes simplex virus infection: an occupational hazard in dental practice, J Mich Dent Assoc 64:199, 1982.

Micik RE, et al: Studies on dental aerobiology. I. Bacterial aerosols generated during dental procedures, J Dent Res 48:51, 1969.

Micik RE, et al: Studies on dental aerobiology. III. Efficiency of surgical masks in protecting dental personnel from airborne bacterial particles, J Dent Res 50:626, 1971.

Miller CH: Heat sterilization assures microbe-free instruments, Dentist (Nov-Dec) 1987.

Miller RL, et al: Studies on dental aerobiology. II. Microbial splatter discharges from the oral cavity of dental patients, J Dent Res 50:621, 1971.

Miller RL, and Micik RE: Air pollution and its control in the dental office, Dent Clin North Am 22:453, 1978.

Minagi S, et al: Disinfection method for impression materials: Freedom from fear of hepatitis B and acquired immunodeficiency syndrome, J Prosth Dent 57:451, 1986.

Minagi S, et al: Prevention of acquired immunodeficiency syndrome and hepatitis B. II: Disinfection method for hydrophilic impression materials, J Prosth Dent 58:462, 1987.

Mitchell EW: Chemical disinfecting sterilizing agents, CDA J 13:64, 1985.

Molinari JA: Surface disinfection and disinfectants, CDA J 13:73, 1985.

Molinari JA, et al: Comparison of dental surface disinfectants, Gen Dent 35:171, 1987.

Neupert AH: AIDS and the dental team, Dent Hyg 61:314, 1987.

Nolte WA: Oral microbiology, ed 4, St Louis, 1982, The CV Mosby Co.

Palenik CJ, and Miller CH: Occupational Herpetic whitlow, J Indiana Dent Assoc 61:25, 1982.

Palenik CJ, and Miller CH: Approaches to preventing disease transmission in the dental office. Part I, Dent Asepsis Rev 5(9), 1984a.

Palenik CJ, and Miller CH: Handwashing review, Dent Asepsis Rev 5(7), 1984b.

Palenik CJ, and Miller CH: The need to properly monitor the office sterilizer, Dent Asepsis Rev 7(11), 1986a.

Palenik CJ, and Miller CH: Infection control telecast. Part II. Procedures and legalities, Dent Asepsis Rev 7(4), 1986b.

Palenik CJ, and Miller CH: Use of gloves in the dental operatory, Dent Asepsis Rev 8(6):1, 1987.

Palenik, CJ, et al: A survey of sterilization practices in selected endodontic offices, J Endodontics 12:206, 1986.

Parker ME, and Williams H: Cross-infection and cross-contamination: the relationship between subgingival bacteria and fingernail length, Dent Hyg 61:68, 1987.

Pollock NL, et al: Laminar air purge of microorganisms in dental aerosols, J Am Dent Assoc 81:1131, 1970.

Price PB: Bacteriology of normal skin: a new quantitative test applied to a study of the bacterial flora and the disinfectant action of mechanical cleansing, J Infect Dis 63:301, 1983.

Rohrer M, and Boulard R: Microwave sterilization, JADA 110:194, 1985.

Rowe NH, et al: Herpetic whitlow: an occupational disease of practicing dentists, JADA 105:471, 1982.

Rowe NH, and Brooks SL: Contagion in the dental office, Dent Clin North Am 22:491, 1978.

Runnells RR: Heat and heat/pressure sterilization, CDA J 13:46, 1985.

Sampson E: Hepatitis B-protection of patient, dentist, and staff. In Proceedings of a symposium on hepatitis B: risk, prevention and the vaccine. 123rd Annual Session of American Dental Association, Las Vegas, 1982.

Schaefer ME: Infection control in dental laboratory procedures, CDA J 13:81, 1985.

Simonsen RJ, et al: An evaluation of sterilization by autoclaving in dental offices, J Dent Res 58:400, 1979 (abstract).

Skaug N: Micropunctures of rubber gloves used in oral surgery, Int J Oral Surg 5:220, 1976.

Skaug N: Proper monitoring of sterilization procedures used in oral surgery, Int J Oral Surg 12:153, 1983.

Smith AL: Principles of microbiology, ed 9, St Louis, 1982, The CV Mosby Co.

Tankersley RW: Amino acid requirements of herpes simplex virus in human cell, J Bacteriol 87:609, 1964.

Terezhalmy GP, et al: The use of water-soluble bioflavonoid-ascorbic acid complex in the treatment of recurrent herpes labialis, Oral Surg 45:56, 1978.

Thomas LE, et al: Survival of herpes simplex virus and other selected microorganisms on patient charts: potential source of infection, JADA 111:461, 1985.

Underhill TE, et al: Prevention of cross-infections in the dental environment, Comp Cont Ed Dent 7:260, 1986.

United States Public Health Service: Coolfont report: a PHS

plan for prevention and control of AIDS and the AIDS virus, Public Health Rep 101:341, 1986.

Williams GH, et al: Laminar air purge of microorganisms in dental aerosols: prophylactic procedures with the ultrasonic scaler, J Dent Res 49:1498, 1970.

Wyler D, et al: Efficacy of self-administered preoperative oral hygiene procedures in reducing the concentration of bacteria in aerosols generated during dental procedures, J Dent Res 50:509, 1971.

Yagiela JA, et al: Disinfection of nitrous oxide inhalation equipment, J Am Dent Assoc 98:191, 1979.

Yokom NG: Infection control, the government, and you, IDHA Newsletter, January 1988.

4 THE COMPLETE DENTAL RECORD

OBJECTIVES: *The reader will be able to*

1. Explain the purposes of a complete dental record.
2. List the components of a complete dental record and justify the inclusion of each component.
3. Describe and follow the guidelines for making chart entries, especially progress notes.
4. Compare and contrast treatment-oriented and problem-oriented approaches to records.
5. Define the *chart audit* and explain the purposes of a chart audit.
6. Discuss the uses of computers for maintaining dental records.

In all likelihood, you have at one time or another been treated by a physician, nurse practitioner, nurse, dentist, or dental hygienist. Think about your treatment and the records of your treatment that the health care providers have used to assist them. What would you expect to see in the record? What would you want to be excluded from the record? Have you ever read (or peeked at) the record? If so, what was your impression of its contents and of the health care providers who had written in the record?

Undoubtedly, you have come to expect that the health care provider will have an accurate, legible recording of each of your conditions or problems, visits, treatments, tests, and test results, as well as of the progress of your condition. In a nutshell, you expect that the provider will be able to glean from the record all the pertinent information needed to treat your present condition knowledgeably and adequately. In addition, you probably expect that entries will be written objectively and that the entire record will be treated with respect and confidentiality.

Patients will have these expectations of you as a dental health care provider, regarding their dental record. Patients rightfully expect health care providers to maintain accurate, adequate records about their past and present conditions, treatments, and the progress of treatment. The purpose of this chapter is to familiarize you with the functions of the dental record, its inclusions, and the approaches to maintaining a complete dental

record. In addition, confidentiality, legal responsibility, chart audits, and the use of computers are discussed.

A MEDICOLEGAL DOCUMENT

A complete dental record should include all of the information necessary to treat a patient safely and knowledgeably. The record must contain a data base that includes the patient's past and present medical and dental histories, present dental status, diagnosis of present conditions, treatment plan, treatment rendered, and financial records. The complete dental record and associated materials, such as study models, radiographs, laboratory test results, and photographs, are medicolegal documents. The records are related to medicine because they concern the general health of a patient and the ensuing treatment. They are related to the law because the records are admissible in a court of law as evidence either for or against the health care provider or the patient (Miller, 1979). As a legal document, the chart protects both the patient and the clinician, so the chart should be complete, thorough, accurate, and legible.

Miller (1979) states, "A cautious dentist (dental hygienist) will never rely on memory. He (she) will record *all* facts pertinent to a patient's history, examination, diagnosis, visits, treatments, fees, and observations, and will identify each fact by specific date. . . . Everything pertinent to a dentist's (dental hygienist's) treatment should be included in the record file. . . ." Any treatment, diagnostic aid, or diagnosis performed with the patient must be noted in the permanent record. It is important to document every interaction and treatment to ensure continuity of care for the patient and legal protection for the patient and dental personnel.

The dental record is important not only for the provision of quality care for the patient, but also as legal protection. The dental health care provider is legally responsible for protecting and respecting the personal and property rights of the patient, for providing only necessary and agreed-on care, for completing care within a reasonable amount of time, for achieving reasonably satisfactory results, for exercising "reasonable care" in performing services, and for charging reasonable fees (Miller, 1979; Morris, 1971; Woodall, 1987). In turn, the patient is responsible for paying the fee and cooperating in treatment (Miller, 1979; Morris, 1971; Woodall, 1987). If either the health care provider or the patient does not fulfill any of the responsibilities, the other party can take legal action. In most such legal cases the dental record would be used as evidence; therefore it is crucial that the record be accurate and legible. For a further discussion of patient and health care provider responsibilities, as well as malpractice, consult Woodall (1987).

Two elements of the health care provider's responsibility for protecting and respecting the personal and property rights of the patient— confidentiality and informed consent—must be emphasized. Protecting the patient's confidentiality involves respecting communications among the health care providers and the patient. It does not mean that everything between the patient and the health care provider is secret; if that were so, continuity of care would be impossible. Rather, protecting a patient's confidentiality involves ensuring that the records are not visible to other patients and that the patient's name or identifying information is removed from records being used in a professional presentation. Another example of protecting this confidentiality is not releasing a patient's records without his or her permission. Perhaps the most important way to respect a patient's confidentiality is by writing objective, truthful, and respectful chart entries. Such chart entries are discussed later in the chapter.

Informed consent, discussed in Chapter 18,

means that the patient has enough information about his or her condition to be able to accept or reject the recommended treatment. The patient's informed consent should be recorded in the dental record.

NECESSARY INCLUSIONS AND RECORD ORGANIZATION

Considering the importance of the dental record, dentally and legally, it becomes apparent that a health care provider should know the inclusions of a complete dental record. The necessary inclusions for a dental record are the patient's name on all pages; the patient's residence and employment addresses and phone numbers; the patient's date of birth, sex, and occupation; the physician's name, address, and phone number; the name of the person to contact in an emergency; medical and dental histories; examination findings and diagnosis; treatment goals; the treatment plan; the treatment provided, with dates and signatures; results of treatment, especially unexpected results; radiographs; fees charged and paid; and copies of all correspondence (Miller, 1979).

The chart should be logically organized so that it is easily read and understood. Records can be organized in many different ways. The most common format is to have a folder or envelope that contains all the forms and radiographs. It is helpful if chart folders have an envelope or pocket attached to hold the radiographs and intraoral photographs. Forms should be fastened in the sequence in which they will be prepared or reviewed at the time of the appointment.

The usual sequence of forms is as follows: basic demographic data, the patient's past and present medical and dental histories, examination findings and diagnosis, treatment goals, the treatment plan, the treatment provided with dates and signatures, results of treatment, and fees charged and paid. Radiographs, intraoral photographs, and copies of correspondence follow or are stored in the folder pocket (Miller, 1979).

Medical alerts notifying the clinician of patient conditions such as penicillin allergy, rheumatic heart disease, hepatitis, or a heart condition should be plainly visible on the front of the chart (Kilpatrick, 1974). Some charts have a symbol, colored tape, or the words "medical alert" in a prominent position on the front of the chart to alert the clinician to a medical condition that must be considered *before* treatment is begun. On seeing such an alert, the health care provider can then open the chart, refer to the medical history, and become familiar with the patient's condition. This system of symbols, tape, or "medical alert" is preferable to the system of writing the condition (*e.g.,* hepatitis) on the front of the chart, because it is more respectful of the patient's right to confidentiality.

The chart should also have an area for notation of special needs of the patient. Such needs may include special provisions to accommodate a wheelchair or referral to a specialist.

Some charts provide an area for notation of nicknames, hobbies, or special interests of the patient (Kilpatrick, 1974); these may provide the dental professional with information to put the patient at ease. It is also helpful to note emotional traumas a patient may mention to the provider, such as the death of a spouse or a recent separation; these emotional traumas may affect the patient's overall and dental health. The health care provider should remember to write these statements objectively and descriptively without violating the patient's privacy.

GUIDELINES FOR CHART ENTRIES

Considering the importance of the complete dental record, some general guidelines to help a student complete a chart are helpful. The following should be considered whenever making an entry in a patient's record.

All entries should be made *clearly, legibly,* and *in ink* or some other *permanent form* (Woodall, 1987). To be admissible as evidence in court, the data must be discernible, and it must be obvious that entries were made during the course of treatment and not after a suit was filed. Ink and computer entries can be evaluated for the length of time since they were made; thus they are valid as evidence if they reflect legitimate records of the progress of care. Pencil entries are easily changed and are difficult to evaluate concerning the time of entry; therefore pencil records in some instances may not be admissible as evidence. It should be obvious from these facts that entries should be made at each visit and that, in the face of a suit, *no attempt should be made to alter records* to try to prove a point. Such an attempt is

foolish and is an obstruction of justice (Stetler, 1962; Woodall, 1987).

Records should be retained for at least 10 years past the time a file becomes inactive (Miller, 1979). Depending on the state, a patient may file suit against a health care provider up to 6 to 10 years *after* the encounter that triggered the dissatisfaction (Stetler, 1962). The record may be the only evidence in support of the health care provider. Therefore, even if the only treatment rendered for that patient was an extraction, the record must be kept for the duration of the state's statute of limitations.

Documentation of all services rendered, data collection as well as procedures performed, should be entered in the record when they are performed. The progress notes should reflect the patient's needs identified during data collection, the diagnosis, and treatment planning. For example, a progress note stating that an amalgam was placed in tooth No. 30 should only be present if a carious lesion was charted for tooth No. 30 during data collection and subsequently included in the treatment plan.

The progress note should contain descriptive, objective statements dated and signed by the health care provider. It is always wise to compose the progress notes in a specific order so that the necessary information is always present. One such order is to report the patient's subjective findings, if any; the clinicians' objective findings; any medication administered, such as a local anesthetic; the procedure performed; complications and/or results observed; the patient's reactions; whether the treatment is complete or incomplete; the treatment to be performed at the next appointment; and the amount of time required before the next appointment. Following is a sample progress note:

6/11/88: Patient reports bleeding gums whenever she brushes. Tissues are swollen, tender, and bleed on probing; moderate to heavy subgingival calculus. Plaque and bleeding indices recorded; demonstrated Bass brushing technique. Patient performed technique and agreed to brush twice daily. Flossing reviewed; patient was not carrying floss subgingivally and was corrected. Lidocaine 2% with 1:200,000 epinephrine (72 mg lidocaine/0.038 mg epinephrine) administered in upper right quadrant: posterior superior alveolar, middle superior alveolar, anterior superior alveolar, greater palatine, nasopalatine. Ultrasonic scaler and hand instruments used to scale, root plane, and perform soft tissue curettage. Area should be evaluated at next visit and upper left quadrant treated. No adverse reactions to local anesthetic or to treatment reported or observed. Next appointment: 1 week.

LWF

By using commonly accepted abbreviations, this chart entry could be shortened as follows:

6/11/88: Pt. reports bleeding on brushing. Ging. edem., tender, BOP; mod. to heavy sub. calculus. PI & BI recorded. Bass brushing demon. & pt. performance acceptable. Pt. agreed to brush 2 ×'s daily. Flossing reviewed; not carrying sub., was corrected. Lido. 2% with Epi. 1:200,000 (72 mg lido.; 0.038 mg Epi.) admin. UR quad.: PSA, MSA, ASA, GP, NP. Scaled with ultra. & hand; RP & STC performed UR quad. Eval. next visit & scale, RP, STC UL quad. No adverse reactions to LA or tx. reported or observed. Next visit: 1 wk.

LWF

It is important to enter progress notes using accepted dental terminology or abbreviations and descriptive, objective sentences for two reasons. First, other health care providers must be able to understand the terminology used in the entry to continue care; second, the patient can gain access to the record, so no derogatory or subjective comment should be entered in the record (Howard, 1975). For example, it is highly inappropriate to enter, "Ms. Jones is a real complainer—ignore her for her own good." The following sample entry may be more appropriate: "Ms. Jones said that she hates the scraping noise of the instruments on her teeth and that she does not want me to make that noise. I explained why the noise was necessary and reassured her that the scaling was being done properly. At the end of the appointment, Ms. Jones said, that she still didn't like that sound, but her teeth feel smooth. The second entry describes the situation more completely, and if the patient ever read the entry, it is not likely that she would be offended or feel discredited. Abbreviations could be used to shorten the length of this entry.

An entry should be supported with data whenever possible so that the next health care provider can better understand the situation. If an entry stated, "Patient has poor home care procedures," the next health care provider would not have much concrete information to evaluate. However, the entry "Patient has consistently high plaque and bleeding indices; patient reports that she brushes once a day when she remembers to brush" gives the next health care provider more information about the patient's dental status without subjective judgments.

APPROACHES TO RECORD STYLE

The necessary inclusions in a dental record have been discussed, but the styles of record keeping have not. At the present time two approaches are popular. The first is the *treatment-oriented approach,* and the second is the *problem-oriented approach* (Sanger, 1973; Weed, 1969). The treatment-oriented approach has three major components: data base, treatment plan, and progress notes. The problem-oriented approach has four components: data base, problem list, treatment plan, and progress notes (Sanger, 1973; Weed, 1969). The major difference between the two approaches is the formulation of the problem list. Weed (1969) maintains that an essential element, the problem list, is missing in the traditional treatment-oriented approach.

In the treatment-oriented approach, after the data are collected, the clinician analyzes the data and formulates a treatment plan that should meet all the needs of the patient that were identified by the data collection. If the patient has complex needs, such as systemic problems as well as multiple carious lesions and areas of mobility, pocketing, and bleeding, the treatment plan may become complex and difficult to complete properly.

In the problem-oriented approach, the clinician compiles a problem list from all of the data collected. Each sign and/or symptom is identified as a problem, and each problem has an individual treatment plan with a priority number so that the most threatening problems are treated first (Weed, 1969). For example, if a patient being treated complained of bleeding gums, had gingivitis, and had one carious lesion, the problems, in order of priority, would be (1) bleeding gums, (2) gingivitis, and (3) carious lesion. In the problem-oriented approach, there is a specific step, formulating the problem list, for analysis of the data and then logical assignment of priorities. In the treatment-oriented approach, this step is not present; rather, the clinician analyzes the data as part of the treatment plan (Fig. 4-1).

Comparison of record approaches

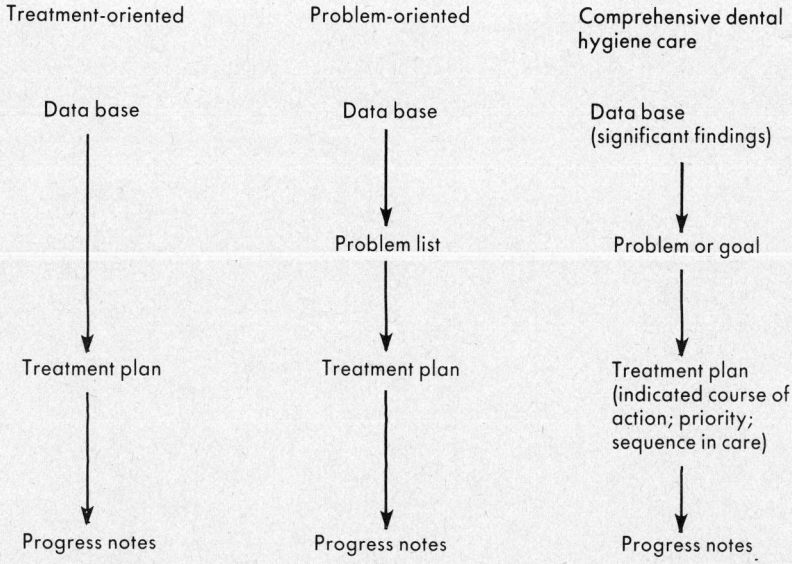

Fig. 4-1. Treatment-oriented and problem-oriented approaches are compared in the first and second columns: note that the treatment-oriented approach does not include a problem list. The approach presented in this book, a problem-oriented approach, is in the third column. Consult Chapter 18 for further explanation of terms in parentheses.

After the problem list has been formulated, a treatment plan addressing each of the problems is designed. Since the problems have already been assigned priorities, the treatment plan for the above example would be (1) bleeding gums—take baseline indices; teach modified Bass brushing and flossing; monitor patient's progress via indices; (2) gingivitis—scaling and prophylaxis; and (3) carious lesions—amalgam restoration No. 30. As can be seen, the treatment plan flows from the problem list. The problem-oriented approach is particularly helpful when a patient presents complex systemic and/or dental problems leading to an involved treatment plan. This approach is also helpful during the case presentation to the patient, as the treatments are geared to the patient's problems. Once the clinician has explained the problems to the patient in an organized fashion, the treatments are more likely to be understood by the patient.

Weed (1969) has an excellent description of the problem-oriented approach to records and a sample case, which can be studied to understand the problem-oriented approach in greater detail. The approach to records and treatment planning presented in this book (Fig. 4-1) is a problem-oriented one. The approach is described more fully in Chapter 18.

COMPUTERIZED DENTAL RECORDS

The computer is essentially a sophisticated electronic filing system that has the capability for storing all necessary patient data (Forest et al, 1986). Any information that can be stored in written form can be kept in a computer file. A tremendous advantage of the computer is its ability to sort and reference all available data across all patient records with minimal time and effort from the office staff. The second big advantage of a computer record system is the completion of several functions from one or two entries.

The computer has the capacity to integrate aspects of record keeping, financial management, patient management, clinical functions, and some miscellaneous functions (Chasteen, 1988). For a new patient, database information, such as patient identification, insurance and billing, and medical/dental status, is entered into the computer. Medical alerts can be programmed to appear not only in the patient's record but also each time he or she has an appointment scheduled.

After the clinical examination, the treatment plan is entered so that the computer can monitor status and progress whenever it is requested. Given the desired appointment length and the task to be performed, the computer can seek and schedule appropriate appointments. A series of specific instructions can customize the scheduling function; for example, extensive root planing may only be scheduled at 8:00, 11:00, and 1:00, or no more than two initial patient visits may be scheduled in a row.

The computer is excellent for financial management. It can complete insurance forms and generate monthly billings automatically. The computer can generate correspondence through its word-processing function. This can be a customized version of a form letter or a short note like "Happy Holidays" on a monthly statement. Lastly, the patient recall interval can be monitored by the computer and reminder postcards printed and addressed automatically (Chasteen, 1988). This is not an exhaustive list of the uses of a computer in dental practice, but touches on the dental record aspects only.

Computer terminals are starting to become part of the dental operatory equipment. Advances in graphics packages are making them more useful for clinical data gathering and recording. Computer-generated dental charts that utilize multiple colors and anatomically accurate restorations and pathology are now possible. Periodontal probes with electronic sensors can feed data directly to the computer regarding pocket depth. The resulting periodontal chart shows the level of the gingival margin and epithelial attachment and the difference between the two, the pocket, is shaded (Agudio et al, 1985). The resulting printout is more diagrammatic and understandable in its portrayal of the gingival status. Future projections for electronic probe/computer systems include sulcular fluid volume readings and tissue antibody measurements. The combination of this information in the computer format will make it an integral tool in disease status diagnosis.

Computers are not problem solvers; necessary information must be entered and appropriate questions asked. Computers are data management systems, and this makes them valuable tools in today's dental practice.

RECORD AUDITS

With the increasing emphasis among health care providers on thorough, complete, and accurate records and with the increasing interest of third-party carriers, such as insurance companies, in the prevention of fraud in filing claims, many health care practices have instituted record audits among the dental personnel to ensure that the charts are being completed accurately and that the necessary inclusions are present (Woodall, 1987). Fig. 4-2 is a sample chart audit form that has been used in a health care practice to audit dental records.

The audit form is completed at the conclusion of a patient's course of treatment by a clinician other than the one responsible for the patient's treatment. When performing an audit, the clinician checks the record to ensure that each of the items listed in the left column is present. If the item is present and satisfactory, an "S" is placed in the appropriate space; if the item is missing or unacceptable, a "U" is placed in the space. Once the audit is completed, the person doing the audit initials and dates the form at the top of the column. If any items are missing or unsatisfactory, the clinician responsible for the patient's care is asked to rectify the situation. Because there are several columns, the same audit form can be used after each course of a patient's treatment.

It is a wise practice to review all patient records regularly using an audit form to identify missing or inaccurate entries and to be certain that the care being delivered is appropriate for the patient's needs. By maintaining thorough, complete, and accurate charts, the health care provider will be better able to provide continuous high-quality care and provide protection for both the dental personnel and the patient.

ACTIVITIES
1. Secure sample charts from several dental care practices and:
   a. Review the charts for organization.
   b. Review the charts for the necessary inclusions.

Patient_____ Date_____

Chart number_____ Reviewer_____

Note in each box whether the item is Satisfactory (S), Unsatisfactory (U), or

Not Applicable (NA). Note the reason of each NA on the back of this form.

Place your initials and the date of the review in the appropriate boxes.

Initials

Date

1. Medical history complete, updated, signed

2. Physician's letter present, if needed

3. Oral exam complete, updated, signed

4. Chartings complete, updated, signed

5. Satisfactory radiographs taken/present

6. Satisfactory study models present, if taken

7. Satisfactory photographs present, if taken

8. Additional records present, if taken

9. Home care procedures assessed

10. Treatment plan recorded

11. Home care planned, implemented, evaluated

12. Treatment plan followed/revised

13. Progress notes complete, dated, signed

14. Recall date recorded

15. Financial records complete

16. Demographic data complete

Additional comments:

Fig. 4-2. Sample dental record audit form. See text for explanation of how to use this form.

c. Review the progress notes for thoroughness and completeness.

d. Rewrite some of the progress notes in a format that meets the criteria described in the chapter.

2. Invite a speaker from one of the companies that print dental records or market computer software packages for dental records and have him or her explain the company's record form.

3. Take a hypothetical patient, Mrs. Jones, from first contact with office through data gathering, treatment planning, appointment scheduling, multiple appointment scaling and root planing, insurance/billing,

and 3-month recall maintenance using the computer whenever possible.

3. Develop a chart audit system that could be used in a dental practice.
4. Read Chapter 19, "Problem-oriented dental record system—an alternative" and Chapter 20, "Problem-oriented record system—case example," in *Treatment Planning: A Pragmatic Approach* (Wood, 1978).

REVIEW QUESTIONS

1. Explain the purposes of dental records.
2. List the inclusions that should be part of a dental record and justify each item.
3. Name one major difference between the treatment-oriented and the problem-oriented approaches to record keeping.
4. What is the purpose of a chart audit?
5. Describe a format for writing progress notes.

REFERENCES

Agudio G, Prato GP, and Bartolucci EG: Computerized charting of probing depths, J Perio 56:766, 1985.

Chasteen JE: Personal communication, 1988.

Conger SX: The law and dental hygiene practice, Dent Hyg 57:14, 1983.

Corby CS: Are you ready for a computer? Dent Econ 68:35, 1978.

Council on Dental Practice: Computer technology in dental practice, JADA 101:938, 1980.

Crandell CE: Use of computers in dental office management, Int Dent J 30:226, 1980.

Ehrlich A, et al: Selecting a computerized account receivable system, Dent Clin North Am 25:731, 1981.

Forrest JL, Williams C, and Gurenlian JR: Improved communication through computer technology, Dent Hyg 60:558, 1986.

Gairola G, and Skaff K: Ethical reasoning in dental hygiene practice, Dent Hyg 57:16, 1983.

Granger B: Legal aspects of dental hygiene practice, Dent Hyg 54:43, 1980.

Howard WW: Dental practice planning, St Louis, 1975, The CV Mosby Co.

Johnson D: Structured case presentations: cornerstone to informed patients, Gen Dent 27:62, 1979.

Kilpatrick HC: Work simplification in dental practice: applied time and motion studies. Philadelphia, 1974, WB Saunders Co.

Kramer, IRH: Computers in clinical and laboratory diagnosis, Int Dent J 30:214, 1980.

Mahler TM, et al: Computers in preventive dentistry, Int Dent J 30:201, 1980.

Miller SL: Legal aspects of dentistry, New York, 1979, GP Putnam's Sons.

Morris WO: Some thoughts on dental malpractice, Int Dent J 26:175, 1976.

Sanger RG, and Boone ME: Problem-oriented dental record system—an alternative. In Wood NK, editor: Treatment planning: a pragmatic approach, St Louis, 1978, The CV Mosby Co.

Sloan RF: Computer application in orthodontics, Int Dent J 30:189, 1980.

Snyder, Felmeister, & Co: Computer management for dental practice ADA Council on Dental Practice Seminar Manual, 1982.

Stetler CJ, and Moritz AR: Doctor and patient and the law, St Louis, 1962, The CV Mosby Co.

Warner R and Segal H: Ethical issues of informed consent in dentistry, Chicago, 1980, Quintessence Publishing Co, Inc.

Weed LL: Medical records, medical education, and patient care, Cleveland, 1969, Case Western Reserve University, Year Book Medical Publishers, Inc.

Wood NK, editor: Treatment planning: a pragmatic approach, St Louis, 1978, The CV Mosby Co.

Woodall IR: Legal, ethical, and management aspects of the dental care system, ed 3, St Louis, 1987, The CV Mosby Co.

5 THE COMPREHENSIVE HEALTH HISTORY

OBJECTIVES: *The reader will be able to*

1. Explain the reasons for a comprehensive health history to a skeptical patient.
2. State the rationale for combining questionnaire and interview techniques to obtain the necessary patient information.
3. Identify and use the communication skills that help ensure a thorough health history.
4. List the components of a comprehensive health history and explain the relevance of each.
5. Identify responses that necessitate consultation with the dentist and/or physician.
6. Identify specific conditions and/or responses that indicate the need for antibiotic premedication, sedation, alteration of medication, special appointment planning, additional laboratory studies, and special precautions to prevent disease transmission and allergic reactions.
7. List history update questions to be asked at recall appointments.
8. Given various responses to questions, identify appropriate follow-up questions or procedures to ensure gathering of complete data.
9. Given a patient with a variety of medical problems, conduct a complete health history and prepare a review of systems.
10. Explain the rationale for a medical classification system.
11. Explain the rationale for a medical release letter.
12. Explain the need for use of the *Physicians' Desk Reference*.

Observing necessary precautions that may relate to specific medical problems or medications is a professional responsibility. Before dental services are offered to any patient, an assessment of the overall health status is necessary. Providing safe treatment is the prime objective in planning dental care consistent with a patient's health status. Advances in medical diagnosis and therapeutic agents enable many people with serious medical conditions to function at a near normal level of activity. For this reason, completing a comprehensive health history is essential to familiarize the health care provider with each patient's unique health profile.

RATIONALE FOR COMPLETING A HEALTH HISTORY

There are a number of reasons for completing a health history.

First, the information *provides continuity be-*tween medical and dental care. Establishing communication and cooperation between the physician and the dental professional ensures that all aspects of the patient's health needs can be addressed. Oral conditions and other physical conditions are often closely related. Measles, for instance, may be diagnosed by the recognition of Koplik's spots (white or bluish spots surrounded by an inflamed red zone) found on the buccal mucosa 24 hours before the general skin rash appears (Kerr and Ash, 1978). Conditions such as a red, swollen tongue and cracking skin at the corners of the mouth may be observed, which may indicate a nutritional deficiency in riboflavin. In chronic medical conditions such as diabetes mellitus, the patient's resistance to infection may be lowered, making him or her prone to periodontal disease.

Informing the patient about areas where medicine and dentistry are related is important in providing total patient care. For example, medications prescribed by the physician may affect oral conditions. Phenytoin (Dilantin) is an anticonvulsant medication often prescribed for the treatment of epilepsy. This medication has the potential to increase the gingiva's response to irritation (plaque, calculus) (Angelopoulous, 1975; Braham, 1977; Israel, 1974). For many patients the result of taking this medication is gingival enlargement, or hyperplasia.

A number of patients still find routine visits to the dentist anxiety producing. Patients with medical conditions such as angina pectoris or hypertension may be adversely affected by stress. Identifying patients who have medical or emotional conditions that may be aggravated by the stress of a visit to the dentist can be crucial for providing appropriate and successful treatment.

A complete health history may help the dental care provider *avoid medical emergencies and identify precautions the clinician and patient should observe*. It is not difficult to imagine what could happen if a medically compromised patient were treated without proper assessment of health status. Administering a local anesthetic agent to a patient who is sensitized or allergic to one of its constituents could produce a severe and possibly fatal anaphylactic reaction.

Patients who have heart valve disease due to rheumatic fever or congenital heart defects and patients with heart valves that have been surgically replaced with artificial prostheses must be medicated with an antibiotic before and after dental treatment. Patients with a history of surgical procedures in which foreign matter or prostheses have been implanted may require antibiotic protection, which should be determined by consultation with their physician. Examples of such implants are cardiac pacemaker implants and Dacron patches used to repair congenital heart defects. Patients with kidney disease who have hemodialysis shunts require antibiotic protection to prevent infection at the site of the prosthesis. Patients who have received prosthetic joints, and those who have organ transplants (e.g., kidney) also require antibiotic premedication. These patients are susceptible to subacute bacterial endocarditis following the inevitable bacteremia that occurs during procedures such as prophylaxis, curettage, endodontic therapy, tooth extraction, or more extensive periodontal surgery (Kaye, 1983; Weinstein

and Schlesinger, 1974; Prevention, 1985). Bacteremia refers to the presence of viable bacteria in the circulating blood. Antibiotic protection is recommended with all dental procedures that are likely to cause trauma to the tissue and allow oral bacteria to enter the bloodstream in these susceptible individuals.

A study by Baltch and others (1982) describes 56 patients with moderate to severe periodontal disease. Twenty-eight with valvular heart disease received intravenous penicillin before a dental cleaning procedure was performed, and 28 without known disease did not receive the drug. None of the subjects had bacteremia before cleaning, but 5 minutes after the procedure, 61% of the group that had not received penicillin were bacteremic versus 11% of the treated group. From these patients 71 microorganisms were isolated, including 53 anaerobes and 18 aerobes. Only 11 of the isolates were found in the patients receiving prophylaxis with the antibiotic.

As subacute bacterial endocarditis is of particular concern in dental care, the disease process is described in some detail. Following the bacteremia caused by a gingival procedure, the bacteria attaches to the susceptible person's affected cardiac valve endothelium or artificial prosthesis. *Streptococcus viridans* is the bacteria most commonly found as the cause of subacute bacterial endocarditis, although other bacteria, including *Staphylococcus aureus,* have been implicated as the cause of the infection (Durack, Kaplan, and Bisno, 1983; Kaye, 1983). The organisms proliferate, forming bacterial masses and clumps. With the growth of these bacteria and the consequent infection and destruction of the cardiac tissue, the valve is unable to maintain its function. In other patients the surgical graft becomes infected and incompetent. Clinically, the patient exhibits a low-grade fever, slowly developing anemia, loss of appetite, and fatigue. With undiagnosed and untreated subacute bacterial endocarditis, the patient's life expectancy seldom exceeds 3 to 6 months. Sudden death may occur when a bacterial clump breaks off and causes a fatal embolism. The most common cause of death results from congestive heart failure attributed to valve destruction or myocardial damage (Weinstein and Schlesinger, 1974; Kaye, 1983). The heart fails when the infected valve becomes incompetent, preventing the proper emptying of the heart chamber. The blood literally backs up because the valve is no longer able to close and permit the proper blood flow out of the heart to the rest of the body.

With early diagnosis and appropriate antibiotic treatment, 90% of patients survive subacute bacterial endocarditis (Durack, Kaplan, and Bisno, 1983). The clinician's role is to prevent the disease from occurring by screening susceptible patients with the comprehensive health history and providing the proper antibiotic protection prior to treatment.

In a recent study, 52 cases of endocarditis prophylaxis failure were reported to a national registry established by the American Heart Association (Durack, Kaplan, and Bisno, 1983). Forty-eight cases (92%) occurred after dental treatment. Only six patients (12%) had received the antibiotic treatment currently recommended by the American Heart Association. These data indicate that endocarditis prophylaxis failures may be more common than was previously believed, and most regimens used in patients with prophylaxis failure did not conform to current recommendations.

The American Heart Association's recommended prophylactic regimen (antibiotic premedication) for dental procedures is:

1. Standard regime—Oral Penicillin
   For adults and children over 60 lbs (27 kg): penicillin V 2.0 gm 1 hour before the procedure and then 1.0 gm 6 hours later.
   For children less than 60 lbs: 1.0 gm 1 hour before the procedure and then 500 mg 6 hours later.
2. Standard regime for patients allergic to penicillin—Oral Erythromycin
   For adults: erythromycin 1.0 gm 1 hour before the procedure and then 500 mg 6 hours later.
   For children: Erythromycin (20 mg/kg) 1 hour before the procedure and then 10 mg/kg 6 hours later (1 kg = 2.2 lbs).

Patients with a history of rheumatic fever without a residual organic heart murmur need not be premedicated. Patients classified as having "functional" heart murmurs or heart sounds not associated with structural defects do not need antibiotic protection. However, consulting the patient's physician for the exact nature of a cardiac condi-

tion is advisable. This can be accomplished by using a form of the medical release letter described later in this chapter.

Information gained through the comprehensive health history *aids in identifying the need for precautionary measures*. As mentioned in Chapter 3, disease transmission from patient to patient or patient to clinician can occur with some medical conditions. Hepatitis, venereal disease, and the common viral "cold" are examples. To prevent the transmission of such diseases the clinician is advised to wear a protective mask, gloves, and glasses; observe strict disinfection of the patient environment; and ensure proper sterilization of all instruments contacting the patient.

Undiagnosed conditions can also be detected as a result of the complete health history. A dental problem may be the one reason why a healthy person seeks any professional care over a period of years. A complete health history provides a unique opportunity to review the general health status of such a person. Perhaps, being unaware of its significance, the patient will discuss a symptom that could necessitate a medical consultation. Taking the blood pressure at each recall visit may reveal a jump in blood pressure levels or indicate a pattern worthy of medical advice. Additionally, taking the pulse and noting the ease and rate of respiration may help in assessing the patient's need to consult a physician. A discussion of vital signs, hypertension, and the role of the dental team in screening for these patients is contained in Chapter 10.

The health history *aids in diagnosis and treatment planning*. Questions related to dental status reveal the nature of the patient's chief complaint. For example, the patient may be aware of carious lesions in the posterior teeth but be most concerned about the appearance of a discolored front tooth. A patient may report sensitivity to hot or cold liquids in a particular area but be unable to locate the exact tooth that seems to be affected. Information such as this is helpful in guiding the dental team in performing diagnostic services (e.g., radiographs, vitality testing) and in directing care to satisfy patient concerns.

The overall physical and psychologic state of the patient can be assessed in general through the health history. The opportunity to talk candidly with the patient in discussing personal physical health allows the clinician to appreciate how the patient feels about himself or herself. Is the patient generally optimistic or pessimistic? Is the patient relaxed or anxious? The sensitive interviewer may be able to identify other significant tendencies. Is the patient cooperative or defensive? Compulsive or indifferent? In addition, the patient's ability and comfort in expressing himself or herself can be noted. Also, the patient's attitudes about dentistry are usually revealed during the interview. Evaluation of both the physical and psychologic factors will be helpful in providing individualized care.

Gathering the health history data is often the *first opportunity to establish professional interest*. Each patient desires to feel valued as an individual with special needs that the dental team will focus on. With an understanding of the patient's past and current health status and an appreciation of the patient's wants and needs, the dental care provider has guidelines on which to establish rapport and build a professional helping relationship. Within the framework of such a relationship, dental treatment issues become easier to address and trust in care increases.

Collecting detailed health information and updating the history at regular intervals provide a legal record as well as an important source of information about the patient when treatment is planned and delivered. The patient signs the health history to indicate that the information is accurate to the best of his or her knowledge. This record becomes an important reference when treating the patient over a period of time.

Occasionally, a patient may feel skeptical about the need for a comprehensive health history. Often this stems from feelings of privacy being invaded, defensiveness about medical problems, or a desire to simply get the dental visit over with as quickly as possible. Regardless of the reason for skepticism, it is important to dispel the patient's anxiety. The patient should be informed of the dental professional's responsibility to keep information confidential. The patient should be assured that the information is necessary to provide safe treatment, and examples may be given of the way health information can affect dental treatment. One can agree that gathering information is time consuming, but it can be explained that this time means consideration for the patient's benefit. On occasion, some practitioners may choose not to

provide elective treatment if the patient refuses to cooperate with the health history. Generally, most patients are agreeable and extremely helpful once the professional's sincere desire to provide the best possible care has been demonstrated.

COMMUNICATION: THE QUESTIONNAIRE/INTERVIEW

For gathering information, a questionnaire provides a thorough and timesaving tool for the professional. Fig. 5-1 is an example of one of the health questionnaires copyrighted by the American Dental Association. An interview provides a flexible and personal approach to obtaining and clarifying information. The combined questionnaire/interview technique is a practical and sensitive method for assessing the patient's health (Froelich and Bishop, 1977).

Although a lengthy interview or written health summary may not be necessary for every patient, the completed questionnaire should be closely examined prior to treatment. The patient may have missed an important question or misunderstood an item. Perhaps a medical condition was indicated that needs important follow-up information before dental care can begin. The following communication/interviewing principles will be helpful in conducting the review of the questionnaire with the patient.

The outcome of the comprehensive health history, using a questionnaire/interview technique, is determined to a great extent by the professional's ability to communicate. Conducting an interview demands a high level of communication skill. The interviewer must respond to both the attitudes and the behaviors of the patient. A good interviewer is nurturant, supportive, and helpful (Froelich and Bishop, 1977). It is not always easy for the patient to share highly private information about his or her personal or family history. The interviewer must listen and accept the patient's attitudes and perceptions without judging. As the interviewer responds to the patient by listening and clarifying statements, the patient begins to have a feeling that the problem is well understood. At this point, information may be shared with the patient to allay fears or anxiety. In this way, the good interviewer may be able to convey to the patient a conceptual model by which the patient can better understand his or her illness, problem, or disease (Froelich and Bishop, 1977). When acquiring the

Medical History

Date _____

Name _____ Address _____
    Last   First   Middle   Number, Street

City _____ State _____ Zip _____ Home _____ Business _____
                                 Code   Phone   Phone

Date of Birth _____ Sex ___ Height _____ Weight _____ Occupation _____

Social Security No. _____ Single _____ Married _____ Name of Spouse _____

Closest Relative _____ Phone _____

If you are completing this form for another person, what is your relationship to that

person? _____

Referred by _____

In the following questions, circle yes or no, whichever applies. Your answers are for our records only and will be considered confidential.

1. Are you in good health?. . . . .   Yes   No

2. Has there been any change in your general health within the past year? . . .   Yes   No

3. My last physical examination was on _____

4. Are you now under the care of a physician? . . . .   Yes   No
   If so, what is the condition being treated? _____

5. The name and address of my physician is _____
   _____
   _____

6. Have you had any serious illness or operation? . . . .   Yes   No
   If so, what was the illness or operation? _____

7. Have you been hospitalized or had a serious illness within the past five (5)
   years? . . . .   Yes   No
   If so, what was the problem? _____

8. Do you have or have you had any of the following diseases or problems?
   a. Damaged heart valves or aritifical heart valves, including heart murmur .   Yes   No
   b. Congenital heart lesions . . . .   Yes   No
   c. Cardiovascular disease (heart trouble, heart attack, coronary insuffi-
      ciency, coronary occlusion, high blood pressure, arteiosclerosis, stroke).   Yes   No
      1. Do you have pain in chest upon exertion?. . . . .   Yes   No
      2. Are you ever short of breath after mild exercise?. . . . .   Yes   No
      3. Do your ankles swell?. . . . .   Yes   No
      4. Do you get short of breath when you lie down, or do you require extra
         pillows when you sleep?. . . . .   Yes   No
      5. Do you have a cardiac pacemaker?. . . . .   Yes   No
   d. Allergy . . . .   Yes   No
   e. Sinus trouble . . . .   Yes   No
   f. Asthma or hay fever . . . .   Yes   No
   g. Hives or a skin rash . . . .   Yes   No
   h. Fainting spells or seizures. . . . .   Yes   No
   i. Diabetes . . . .   Yes   No
      1. Do you have to urinate (pass water) more than six times a day?. . .   Yes   No
      2. Are you thirsty much of the time?. . . . .   Yes   No
      3. Does your mouth frequently become dry?. . . . .   Yes   No

Continued.

Fig. 5-1. ADA health questionnaire.
(Copyright by the American Dental Association. Reprinted by permission.)

Medical History—cont'd

j. Hepatitis, jaundice or liver disease . . . .   Yes   No
k. Arthritis . . . .   Yes   No
l. Inflammatory rheumatism (painful swollen joints) . . . .   Yes   No
m. Stomach ulcers . . . .   Yes   No
n. Kidney trouble . . . .   Yes   No
o. Tuberculosis . . . .   Yes   No
p. Do you have a persistent cough or cough up blood? . . . .   Yes   No
q. Low blood pressure . . . .   Yes   No
r. Venereal disease . . . .   Yes   No
s. Epilepsy . . . .   Yes   No
t. Psychiatric problems . . . .   Yes   No
u. Cancer . . . .   Yes   No
v. AIDS or other immunosuppressive disorders . . . .   Yes   No
w. Other _____

9. Have you had abnormal bleeding associated with previous extractions, surgery, or trauma? . . . .   Yes   No
    a. Do you bruise easily? . . . .   Yes   No
    b. Have you ever required a blood transfusion? . . . .   Yes   No
       If so, explain the circumstances _____

10. Do you have any blood disorder such as anemia? . . . .   Yes   No

11. Have you had surgery, x-ray or drug treatment for a tumor, growth, or other condition of your head or neck? . . . .   Yes   No

12. Are you taking any drug or medicine? . . . .   Yes   No
    If so, what? _____

13. Are you taking any of the following:
    a. Antibiotics or sulfa drugs . . . .   Yes   No
    b. Anticoagulants (blood thinners) . . . .   Yes   No
    c. Medicine for high blood pressure . . . .   Yes   No
    d. Cortisone (steroids) . . . .   Yes   No
    e. Tranquilizers . . . .   Yes   No
    f. Antihistamines . . . .   Yes   No
    g. Aspirin . . . .   Yes   No
    h. Insulin, tolbutamide (Orinase) or similar drug . . . .   Yes   No
    i. Digitalis or drugs for heart trouble . . . .   Yes   No
    j. Nitroglycerin . . . .   Yes   No
    k. Oral contraceptive or other hormonal therapy . . . .   Yes   No
    l. Other _____

14. Are you allergic or have you reacted adversely to:
    a. Local anesthetics . . . .   Yes   No
    b. Penicillin or other antibiotics . . . .   Yes   No
    c. Sulfa drugs . . . .   Yes   No
    d. Barbiturates, sedatives, or sleeping pills . . . .   Yes   No
    e. Aspirin . . . .   Yes   No
    f. Iodine . . . .   Yes   No
    g. Codeine or other narcotics . . . .   Yes   No
    h. Other _____

Fig. 5-1 cont'd, ADA health questionnaire.

Medical History—cont'd

15. Have you had any serious trouble associated with any previous dental treatment? . . . .   Yes   No
If so, explain _____

16. Do you have any disease, condition, or problem not listed above that you think I should know about? . . . .   Yes   No
If so, explain _____

17. Are you employed in any situation which exposes you regularly to x-rays or other ionizing radiation?.   Yes   No

18. Are you wearing contact lenses? . . . .   Yes   No

19. Have you had anything to eat or drink in the last 4 hours?. . . . .   Yes   No

20. Are you wearing removable dental appliances? . . . .   Yes   No

Women

21. Are you pregnant? . . . .   Yes   No

22. Do you have any problems associated with your menstrual period? . . . .   Yes   No

23. Are you nursing? . . . .   Yes   No

Chief Dental Complaint

I certify that I have read and understand the above. I acknowledge that my questions, if any, about the inquiries set forth above have been answered to my satisfaction. I will not hold my dentist, or any other member of his/her staff, responsible for any errors or omissions that I may have made in the completion of this form.

_____
Signature of Patient

_____
Signature of Dentist

Fig. 5-1 cont'd, ADA health questionnaire.

comprehensive health history using a questionnaire/interview format, the health professional not only gathers information and builds rapport, but creates the environment and opportunity to educate and counsel the patient.

Interviewing skills

Awareness of and sensitivity to the kinds of messages communicated are important to counseling and interviewing. (See Chapter 7).

Communication involves words, facial expressions, gestures, body movements, tone of voice, rate of speech, and silence. The interviewer must become an active listener by being aware of the patient's total communication effort and being able to respond in a way that the patient will interpret as attentive and concerned (Froelich and Bishop, 1977).

Body communication signifies to the patient that the interviewer is listening. The interviewer should find a comfortable and relaxed position. The interviewer and patient should be at approximately the same eye level. Eye contact should be made with the patient when he or she is talking. Affirmative head nods also are used to indicate listening. Facial expressions should agree with the feelings being expressed by the patient.

The verbal communication and attitude of the interviewer can strongly influence the atmosphere of the interview. The following are techniques for verbal communication: Use a vocal tone that reassures the patient. Help the patient develop and pursue the topic using affirmative words to indicate understanding. Do not interrupt the patient if possible. Fit comments into the context of the topic. Use silence to aid the interview communication. For most inexperienced interviewers, silence is uncomfortable. Often, a question is hastily asked and may not be helpful. Interviewer-initiated silence can be used to communicate the desire for the patient to continue to provide information or to choose the topic. Silence allows the patient time to think about the response to the questions. Silence can be supportive and signify interest. Patient-initiated silence may mean that the patient needs time to think, is examining himself or herself, or wishes to avoid the topic. Each function of silence is important to the communication effort.

Interviewing suggestions (Froelich and Bishop, 1977)

1. Introduce yourself. Ask a direct, open question, such as "What situation brings you here today?"
2. Have a plan or order for obtaining information.
3. Guide the interview; do not dominate it.
4. Respond by showing support and empathy.
5. Restate or reflect a patient's response to clarify meaning.
6. Avoid questions that can be answered "Yes" or "No." Such questions permit the patient to avoid discussing a topic or allow the patient to give a response he or she thinks the interviewer is looking for. An appropriately phrased question is "When does this pain bother you?" as opposed to "Does it hurt when you eat something cold?"
7. Avoid antagonistic "why" questions that make the patient account for behavior, such as "Why didn't you seek care sooner?"
8. Direct the patient to information closely related with current thoughts. Do not jump from one topic to another.
9. Use verbal and nonverbal signals to encourage the patient to say more.
10. Complete the interview with a summary to clarify what has occurred and affirm mutual understanding.

COMPONENTS OF THE COMPREHENSIVE HEALTH HISTORY

Three areas of information are explored in the comprehensive health history: the patient profile, the patient's current health status, and the patient's historical health data.

The *patient profile* includes the patient's name, address, telephone number, date of birth, and physician's name and office telephone number. Each practitioner may develop his or her own version of the patient profile section of the chart. Items that may be included are the patient's occupation, business telephone number, marital status, number of children, and dental insurance or preferred billing plan; the name of the person who referred the patient; and weekdays/times preferred for appointments. The patient completes this information on the questionnaire. The interviewer should be familiar with this basic information before greeting the patient. Follow-up on this information is usually indicated only when a response needs clarification.

The patient's *current health status* and *historical health data* require more attention. The interviewer should take a few minutes to review the patient's questionnaire responses and note the questions to which an affirmative response has been indicated. These areas need specific follow-up during the patient interview. The following format with the accompanying descriptions is designed as a guide for directing the interview and organizing patient data.

Current health status

Chief complaint (CC). This usually is stated in the patient's own words and refers to the symptoms for which the patient is seeking treatment.

History of present illness (HPI). Signs and symptoms of the current problem should be described in this section, along with the location, onset, intensity, and duration of the problem. Additional probing questions may be in order to define and clarify the nature of the patient's needs, such as "When did this problem *first* occur?" "Describe the discomfort for me," "When does it bother you the most?"

Medications (Meds). It is important to note clearly the medications that the patient is currently taking. This includes over-the-counter remedies or preparations such as vitamins, aspirin, and weight control pills in addition to prescribed medications. State the reason for the medication and the dosage in which it is taken. The *Physicians' Desk Reference* (described later in the chapter) gives additional information. Note medication allergy or intolerance IN BOLD LETTERS. Inquiring into the patient's social habits, such as frequency of consumption of alcoholic beverages and coffee and tobacco use, is appropriate at this time.

Review of systems (ROS). This allows information from the questionnaire and interview to be organized into physical systems. At this point, the professional is interested in the current (within 6 months) status of each system. The past medical/dental history will be summarized later.

Following are the signs and symptoms related to each system. The patient should be asked if he or she is bothered by any of these.

General constitution (Gen). Includes recent significant weight gain or loss, weakness, fatigue, fever, chills, insomnia, irritability, and change in general vigor. If the patient has experienced any of these signs and symptoms, additional probing follow-up questions should be asked. The interviewer should summarize the patient's response. It is advisable to repeat the summary so that the patient can verify its content. Otherwise the interviewer may record "Patient denies" the specific symptoms.

Head, ears, eyes, nose, and throat (HEENT). Includes reports of headache, trauma, dizziness, disturbance of vision, loss of hearing acuity, ringing in ears, loss of balance, disturbances of smell, discharge, symptoms of obstruction, hoarseness, and difficulty in swallowing.

Respiratory (Resp). Includes difficulty in breathing, chest pain, coughing blood or sputum, wheezing, and effect of exercise.

Cardiovascular (CV). Includes chest pain, palpitation,

difficulty in breathing when lying flat, murmurs, and blood pressure.

Gastrointestinal (GI). Includes abdominal pain, nausea, vomiting, indigestion, food intolerance, hernia, and change in bowel habits.

Genitourinary (GU). Includes painful urination, blood in urine, frequency of urination, flank pain, and change in menstrual cycle.

Muscles, bones, and joints (MBJ). Includes pain, stiffness, swelling, limitation of movement, arthritis, and back problem.

Central nervous system (CNS). Includes fainting, seizure, stroke, paralysis, spasm, tremor, and loss of feeling.

Endocrine (Endo). Includes change in growth or development, thyroid function, change in appetite or tolerance to temperature, diabetes, and excessive urination, thirst, or hunger.

Hemopoietic (Hemo). Includes tendency to bruise or bleed excessively after injury, recent blood transfusion, and exposure to radiation.

Medical/dental history

Past medical history (PMH). Summarize the medical status previous to current history. Include general health and vigor, childhood diseases, past infectious diseases, chronic diseases, injuries, accidents, hospitalizations (include name of hospital and dates), history of immunizations, allergies and type of allergic reactions, and service-related disability.

Family history (FH). Summarize data regarding the state of immediate family members, past hereditary diseases, and the presence of infectious or chronic disease in the family.

Past dental history (PDH). Summarize the nature of dental care the patient has had in the past. Include type of clinic, treatment by specialist, experience with local and general anesthetics, degree of preventive education, and satisfaction with past treatment.

MEDICALLY COMPROMISED PATIENTS

The following section provides the dental hygienist with information regarding common medical conditions that should be identified by the health history. A basic definition of the problem is presented, along with common signs or symptoms the patient may report. In some cases examples of medications the patient may be taking are given by generic name. The significance of the disease

Comprehensive health history

Patient profile

NAME: Ms. Sample Case
ADDRESS: R.R. 10, Paradise, Pa.
TELEPHONE: 222-1234
OCCUPATION: Supermarket cashier and homemaker

PHYSICIAN: Dr. John D. Smith
PHYSICIAN TELEPHONE: 222-5678
REFERRAL: Neighbor, Ms. Mary Jones
DATE: May 1, 1988

Current status

CC: Patient is a 58-year-old woman who has come for treatment because of "bleeding gums for the past 3 months."

HPI: During the past 3 months patient noticed she expectorated blood each time she brushed her teeth. The bleeding would stop within 1 minute. Within the past 2 weeks her gingivae bled spontaneously 2 or 3 times.

MEDS: **Allergic to penicillin.** Reaction: immediate generalized body rash, and "My throat closed off."

1. Digoxin, 0.25 mg daily, for congestive heart failure
2. Hydrochlorothiazide (Hydrodiuril), 50 mg two times a day, for congestive heart failure
3. Chlordiazepoxide (Librium), 10 mg one to two times a week when she feels "nervous or upset"
4. Takes vitamin C and vitamin B_{12} supplement daily
5. Prefers acetaminophen (Tylenol) for headache, one to two times a week
6. Smokes cigarettes: one-half pack a day
7. Averages one to two alcoholic drinks a week

ROS:

Gen: Denies recent weight gain or loss, weakness, fever, insomnia, or change in general health

HEENT: Denies headache, dizziness, disturbance in vision, tinnitus, vertigo, nasal obstruction, difficulty in swallowing

Resp: Denies coughing blood or sputum; reports difficulty in breathing when walking one flight of stairs

CV: Reports difficulty in breathing when walking one flight of stairs and when lying flat; uses two pillows for sleeping at night; denies murmur

GI: Denies food intolerance, abdominal pain, change in bowel habits

GU: Denies pain or blood when passing urine, has nocturia due to diuretic (1 time); current menopause transition; experiences labile emotions; reports "hot flashes"

MBJ: Denies limitation of movement, back problems; reports "seasonal" stiffness and swelling of finger joints

CNS: Denies fainting, seizure, loss of feeling, stroke

Endo: Denies weakness, change in appetite, change in weight; reports occasional heat intolerance due to menopause

Hemo: Denies tendency to bruise or bleed, no recent blood transfusion or radiation exposure

Historical data

PMH: Patient denies history of rheumatic fever, diabetes, hepatitis, glaucoma, VD, TB, or bleeding disorders, Generally healthy childhood: measles, mumps, and chickenpox with no residual effects, all before age 10. Broken leg in car accident 1952. Hospitalized for normal childbirth, University of Pennsylvania, 1953, 1956, 1958. Myocardial infarction 3 years ago (see physician's letter); hospitalized for 3 weeks. Takes digoxin and Hydrodiuril for congestive heart failure. Sees physician every 3 months. Patient allergic to penicillin. Reports reaction of total body rash and swelling of mucosa after infection 10 years ago. Tolerates erythromycin well.

FH: Father: died age 74, myocardial infarction after history of hypertension 15 years. Mother: died age 79, cerebral vascular accident. Two brothers alive and well. Three children alive and well. Denies family history of diabetes, cancer, mental illness.

PDH: Had several restorations placed in childhood by private dentist, for past 30 years has been treated sporadically by several dental clinics, mostly for toothache or extraction. Tolerates local anesthesia well; brushes teeth one time a day; does not use floss or other home care aid; satisfied with dental care in past.

is presented followed by precautions recommended for dental treatment.

Heart disorders

Rheumatic heart disease. Rheumatic heart disease results from rheumatic fever and causes rigidity or deformity of the heart valves.

Patient reports: History of rheumatic fever or heart murmur. Patient may be taking antibiotics (e.g., penicillin) on a regular basis.
Significance: Patient is susceptible to subacute bacterial endocarditis.
Precautions:
1. Obtain consultation letter from physician concerning nature of heart involvement.
2. Antibiotic premedication necessary (Kaye, 1983; Prevention, 1985).
3. Be sure patient has taken antibiotic as prescribed before dental treatment.
4. Avoid unnecessary trauma to tissues during instrumentation.

Congenital heart defect. This term refers to structural defects of the heart (e.g., a hole in the common wall between heart chambers) that is present at birth.

Patient reports: History of heart murmur, "hole in heart," or other heart abnormality, corrective heart surgery, or valve replacement.
Significance: Patient is susceptible to subacute bacterial endocarditis.
Precautions:
1. Obtain letter from physician as to nature of defect and correction.
2. Antibiotic premedication may be necessary (Kaye, 1983; Prevention, 1985).

Surgical valve replacement. A diseased heart valve due to rheumatic heart disease or congenital heart defect is replaced with an artificial prosthesis.

Patient reports: History of heart surgery; may be taking anticoagulant.
Significance: Patient is susceptible to subacute bacterial endocarditis.
Precautions:
1. Obtain letter from physician as to heart status and surgical correction.
2. Antibiotic premedication necessary (Kaye, 1983; Prevention, 1985).
3. Patient may be taking anticoagulant (e.g., warfarin or coumarin). Consult physician. Test for bleeding time may be necessary before treatment,

or patient may be advised to stop medication for a few days before appointment.

Coronary artery disease. Coronary circulation is inadequate for metabolic demands on the heart; this disease is secondary to hardening of arteries (arteriosclerosis) which causes blockage or narrowing of vessels.

Patient reports: Episodes of substernal pain (angina pectoris), typically radiating to left arm and jaw. Pain is precipitated by activity and anxiety and is relieved by rest and certain medications. Patient may be taking vasodilators, nitroglycerin, or propranolol.
Significance: Patient may have angina attack in dental office.
Precautions:
1. Obtain letter from physician to clarify medical status.
2. Have patient's vasodilator medication accessible.
3. Use local anesthetic without vasoconstrictor, or keep vasoconstrictor use to minimum (less than 0.04 mg vasoconstrictor (Bennett, 1984).
4. Keep appointments to reasonable length, avoiding unnecessary stress and anxiety.

Coronary thrombosis (myocardial infarction). The blood supply through the coronary arteries is insufficient to meet the metabolic demands of the heart; this differs from angina pectoris in that damage is irreversible (i.e., a portion of the heart muscle dies).

Patient reports: History of angina pectoris, previous heart attack, taking vasodilators.
Significance: Patient may have angina attack or myocardial infarction.
Precautions:
1. Obtain letter from physician as to severity of disease.
2. Do not treat patient if heart attack occurred within 6 months.
3. Have vasodilator medication ready.
4. Avoid vasoconstrictors in local anesthetic or keep to minimum.
5. Keep appointments short.
6. Be prepared to resuscitate patient; should cardiac arrest occur, call emergency rescue team.

Congestive heart failure. Blood backs up behind a failing chamber, causing congestion of circulation and pooling of blood in organs. For example, if the left ventricle fails, blood backs up in the pulmonary circulation and lungs. Forward flow from the failing chamber is also diminished.

Patient reports: Shortness of breath, swollen ankles, sleeping on two or more pillows; may be taking diuretics and/or digitalis.

Significance: Patient may have difficulty in breathing when supine in dental chair. If inhalation anesthetics are used, oxygenation of blood may be poor because of fluid in lungs.

Precautions:
1. Obtain letter from physician concerning severity of disease.
2. Keep patient in semiupright position.
3. Keep appointments short.
4. Possible need for supplemental oxygen.

Cardiac arrhythmias. This is a disturbance of the heart's electrical conduction system. The heart beats at too rapid or too slow a pace or at an irregular pace (either continuously or with occasional odd beats).

Patient reports: Fast or irregular heartbeat, palpitations (awareness of rapid heart beats), recurrent fainting, surgical implant of pacemaker; may be taking digitalis or other antiarrhymic medication.

Significance: Patient may faint, a pacemaker device may be affected by electromagnetic interference (EMI). Dental office equipment such as ultrasonic scaling devices, pulp testers, electrodesensitizing equipment, electrosurgical instruments, and motorized dental chairs may adversely affect some devices.

Precautions:
1. Obtain letter from physician concerning severity of disease and/or surgical history. Inquire as to need for antibiotic premedication and type of pacemaker device implanted.
2. Avoid use of ultrasonic equipment or proximity to such equipment being used on other patients if pacemaker will be affected.

Hypertension

Hypertension is high arterial blood pressure (see Chapter 10).

Patient reports: History of elevated blood pressure, frequent dizziness, headaches, nosebleeds; may be taking antihypertensives or diuretics.

Significance: Patient may have a "stroke" (cerebrovascular accident). Disease can cause cardiac enlargement, impaired kidney function, and accelerate arteriosclerosis.

Precautions:
1. Take blood pressure at each appointment.
2. Obtain letter from physician if diastolic reading exceeds 95 mm Hg or systolic exceeds 160 mm Hg.
3. Do not provide dental treatment if diastolic blood pressure is greater than 115 mm Hg, or systolic blood pressure is greater than 160 mm Hg.
4. Determine if antihypertensive medication has been taken as prescribed.
5. Use local anesthetic without vasoconstrictor, or do not exceed 0.1 mg epinephrine (Bennett, 1984).
6. Avoid sitting patient up rapidly. This may cause fainting (orthostatic or postural hypotension), an effect of some antihypertensives.
7. Have patient remain sitting upright for several minutes before leaving the dental chair.

Diabetes mellitus (Kaye, 1983)

Diabetes mellitus is a disorder of glucose intolerance manifested by hyperglycemia (increased blood glucose). In general, there are two types of diabetes mellitus. Insulin-dependent (type 1) diabetes has its onset in young people. Hyperglycemia is due to a lack of insulin normally produced by the pancreas. Adult-onset (type 2) diabetes occurs in older patients and is often associated with obesity. Although the amount of insulin produced by the pancreas is adequate, this type of diabetes is characterized by insulin insensitivity of the tissues.

Patient reports: Personal or family history of disease; excessive thirst, hunger, urination; high birth weight children; may be taking injectable insulin or oral hypoglycemics.

Significance: Patient has low resistance to infection; is prone to periodontal disease and poor healing; may have episode of insulin shock, especially if meal was missed prior to appointment.

Precautions:
1. Determine if disease is under control (frequency of urine testing, medication taken as prescribed, recent incidents of diabetic coma, insulin shock, or diabetes-related hospitalizations). Obtain letter from physician to determine status of other diabetes-related conditions. Patient with severe diabetes may have compromised vascular system, renal impairment, or loss of vision.
2. Determine if patient has eaten. Schedule appointments around eating schedule.
3. Have sugar source available in case of impending shock, which patient can usually anticipate.

Epilepsy (Braham, 1977; Kaye, 1983)

Epilepsy is a disorder characterized by convulsions (seizures) or disturbances of consciousness (e.g., momentary inattentive staring), usually associated with a disturbance of electrical activity of the brain.

Patient reports: History of seizures. Examples: petit mal (trancelike state, fixed posture, blinking); grand mal (twitching, seizing, loss of consciousness, incontinence). Patient may report a peculiar sensation that heralds a seizure (aura), such as a specific odor or visual sensation; may be taking phenobarbital, phenytoin, or other anticonvulsant.

Significance: Patient may have a seizure. Phenytoin (Dilantin) may cause gingival hyperplasia or orofacial changes (Angelopoulous, 1975; Israel, 1974).

Precautions:
1. Determine if anticonvulsant medication has been taken.
2. Make appointments when patient is rested; keep them short.
3. If seizure occurs, do not try to restrict patient. Remove equipment from striking distance, and keep patient from injuring self. Keep airway open after the seizure when saliva, blood (from biting tongue), and/or dental materials may block airway, requiring suction or manual removal.

Allergies

Allergies are localized or systemic reactions caused by a variety of substances (allergens). The reaction may be mild, causing itching or a rash. A severe reaction may cause a rapid fall in blood pressure, airway obstruction from swelling of oral mucosa, and/or cardiac arrest (anaphylaxis).

Patient reports: Reaction to a known substance (e.g., penicillin).

Significance: Reaction may occur to substances used in dental treatment.

Precautions:
1. Determine exact cause and severity of previous reaction.
2. Avoid allergen or related substance.
3. Caution using anesthetics and antibiotics.
4. If patient is unsure of specific anesthetic agent that caused previous allergic reaction, request physician to perform skin patch test. (See Chapter 31 on local anesthesia.)
5. If anaphylaxis should occur, be prepared to support patient with cardiopulmonary resuscitation and to call emergency rescue team.

Kidney disease

In patients with kidney disease there is impairment of renal function with accumulation of waste products and fluid, resulting from congenital abnormalities, infection, diabetes, and other disease processes. The patient may be maintained on hemodialysis (an artificial kidney machine) or have a kidney transplant.

Patient reports: History of renal failure, hemodialysis, headache, swelling of extremities, fever, flank pain, nausea, mental dullness, excessive fatigue, easy bruising; or if kidney transplant, will be taking immunosuppressant medication.

Significance: Patient is prone to infection, poor healing, bleeds easily. Medications metabolized by kidney (e.g., local anesthetics of amide type) will remain in circulation longer.

Precautions:
1. Obtain letter from physician regarding extent of disease. If patient is immunosuppressed, obtain recommendations for precautions during dental treatment. These patients are susceptible to bacterial endocarditis at site of hemodialysis shunt or transplanted kidney graft, making prophylactic antibiotic coverage necessary.
2. If medication is to be administered, check with physician, *Physicians' Desk Reference,* or pharmacologist regarding renal metabolism.
3. Exercise care in instrumentation.

Infectious or contagious diseases

Hepatitis.* Hepatitis is an inflammation of the liver caused by several different viruses (see Chapter 3).

Patient reports: History of disease, fatigue, loss of appetite, nausea, fever, dark urine, tender liver, sore joints. Patient may appear jaundiced (yellow).

Significance: Patient may bleed excessively; may have impaired metabolism of drugs broken down in liver (e.g., local anesthetics of the ester type); excellent possibility for transfer of disease to dental professional or other patients.

Precautions:
1. Do not treat patient with active disease.
2. Wear gloves, face mask, and glasses; maintain strict sterilization and asepsis of all objects in contact with patient.
3. If medication is administered, consult physician, *Physicians' Desk Reference,* or pharmacologist regarding possible liver metabolism.
4. Determine status of office personnel for hepatitis B markers (hepatitis B antibody or hepatitis B surface antigen).

Tuberculosis. Tuberculosis most commonly

---

*Hepatitis may be used as a model for other types of liver dysfunction (e.g., cirrhosis).

affects the lungs; it is caused by the organism *My-cobacterium tuberculosis*.

Patient reports: History of disease, positive TB test, fever, weight loss, night sweats, cough, blood in sputum, tender lymph nodes; may be taking streptomycin, ethambutol, isoniazid, or other antituberculosis medication.

Significance: Patient may transmit disease to others. Documented TB patients are generally followed yearly for a sputum culture and chest x-ray examination. If medical clearance is given for patient being noncontagious, no special precautions are required for treatment.

Precautions:
1. Obtain letter from physician determining if disease is active. Additional TB tests may be necessary.
2. Wear gloves, face mask, and glasses; maintain strict sterilization and asepsis of all objects in contact with patient.

Venereal disease. Venereal disease is an acute or chronic infectious disease such as syphilis or gonorrhea, typically acquired through sexual intercourse or other close physical contact.

Patient reports: History of disease, painful urination, urethral or vaginal discharge, sore throat, skin eruptions, painless ulcer with firm rolled edges involving oropharyngeal mucosa or genitalia (chancre), mucous patch in oral cavity (gumma).

Significance: Patient may transmit disease to others.

Precautions:
1. Wear gloves, face mask, and glasses; maintain strict sterilization and asepsis of all objects in contact with patient.

Blood diseases

Anemia. Anemia is a deficiency of red blood cells (erythrocytes) in the circulating blood. Anemia may result from a vitamin or iron deficiency, bone marrow problems, excessive loss of blood, or red cell destruction.

Patient reports: Fatigue, weakness; appears pale; may be taking iron and vitamin supplements.

Significance: Lowered resistance to infection; possibly delayed healing.

Precautions:
1. Exercise care in instrumentation.
2. Advise patient to consult physician for further investigation of problem.

Leukemia. In the patient with leukemia, there is an excessive number of white blood cells (leu-

kocytes), which do not function normally; this disease is a type of blood cancer. Cells may overpopulate bone marrow and crowd out normal blood cells and other components such as red blood cells and platelets.

Patient reports: History of disease, fatigue and fever; bruises easily; may be taking medications directed at controlling proliferation of these abnormal leukocytes (chemotherapeutic agents).

Significance: Patient is extremely prone to infection; may have lesions of oral mucosa, xerostomia, more acidic saliva, and aggravated periodontal conditions as a result of chemotherapy. These conditions necessitate modifications in oral hygiene. Excessive bleeding due to bone marrow depression and decreased platelets may effect healing time. Consultation prior to periodontal treatment or extractions is indicated.

Precautions: Obtain letter from physician regarding disease status and recommended procedures for dental intervention.

Hemorrhagic disorders (hemophilia, other). (Grossman, 1975; Kaye, 1983). Hemophilia is a hereditary disorder characterized by excessive bleeding due to lack or deficiency of a coagulation factor. Types include classical hemophilia, (factor VIII, hemophilia A), Christmas disease (factor IX, hemophilia B), and Von Willebrand's disease. Other hemorrhagic disorders include (1) clotting factor deficiency (vitamin K deficiency, for example, can cause depression in certain clotting factors, as do certain drugs such as warfarin and heparin) and (2) platelet dysfunction (platelets are crucial to clotting; aspirin and certain drugs, including dipyridamole, interfere with platelet aggregation).

Patient reports: Family history of hemophilia, spontaneous or excessive bleeding, tendency to bruise easily.

Significance: Failure of blood to clot, danger of patient aspirating blood or even bleeding to death if bleeding is not arrested; medical measures necessary when large quantity of blood is lost. Patient may have received blood plasma factor replacement therapy and may carry hepatitis B antigen or have history of hepatitis (Evans, 1977).

Precautions:
1. Obtain letter from physician concerning severity of disease, possible need for medication prior to treatment (e.g., transfusion of deficient factor).
2. Limit treatment to a specific area per appointment. If factor replacement therapy has been nec-

essary prior to dental treatment, allow sufficient time for procedure to be completed in one visit/day to reduce risks and expense of multiple transfusions (Evans, 1977).

3. Do not prescribe aspirin or aspirin-related products for pain control. Substitute acetaminophen, codeine, propoxyphene hydrochloride, or other analgesic.
4. Wear gloves, face mask, and glasses; maintain strict sterilization because of hepatitis risk.

MEDICAL CLASSIFICATION

A medical classification system, as described in Table 5-1, is useful for identifying a patient's medical status. A standardized system of marking the medical classification in bold numbers on the chart provides a simple mechanism for conveying information quickly while preserving patient privacy.

UPDATING THE RECORD

A person's health is dynamic. Performing the comprehensive health history and classifying the medical status at the initial visit are only the first steps in providing safe treatment for the patient. Reviewing the chart at every visit is imperative. Should an emergency arise, precious time can be lost fumbling for information regarding medical problems or medications that would have been noted by a minute's review of the health history prior to beginning the day's treatment. Updating the chart at recall intervals is recommended. The dental professional should make a sincere inquiry about the patient's general health at every dental visit and note additional information.

Following are appropriate questions to ask the patient for updating the health history:

1. How has your health been lately?
2. What medications are you currently taking?
3. Have you been hospitalized for any reason since your last visit?
4. How has your (name specific medical condition) been since the last appointment?
5. How did you get along with the dentistry we did last time?

These questions are direct, but open, to allow the patient to respond with as much information as possible.

The dental professional should take the blood pressure for the day and compare it to previous entries. The health history form should have a

Table 5-1. Sample format for medical classification system

Classifi-cation	Description
1	*Minimal risk.* Patient in good health and all dental procedures may be carried out with no special precautions.
2	*Some precautions must be observed in treating this patient* (e.g., patients with drug allergies, rheumatic heart disease without decompensation, controlled diabetes, or controlled hypertension).
3	*Deferred classification.* Reserved for patients with questionable health status but who have given insufficient information regarding their ailment, abnormality, or treatment status. Consultation with local physician is usually required (e.g., patients taking unknown medications, patients with possible blood dyscrasias or with heart murmurs of unknown nature, and patients taking anticoagulants).
4	*Unable to withstand prolonged, difficult, or stressful dental procedures because of overall health status.* Ascertainment of degree of decompensation must be made on an individual basis.
5	*Should be hospitalized for treatment or referred for care by more qualified health care providers.* Experienced health care providers should exercise high-level precautions during treatment, preferably under hospital conditions (e.g., patients with uncontrolled hypertension, uncontrolled diabetes, severe congestive heart failure, or hemophilia).

specific update summary area, as important information can be easily missed when one is looking through a long series of treatment notes.

THE MEDICAL RELEASE LETTER

A medical release form is used for the patient to give consent for health professionals to exchange otherwise confidential information. This is necessary in acquiring pertinent medical details that the patient may be unable to provide regarding illness or medication. This is also useful in obtaining dental-related information when a patient transfers from one office or clinic to another.

A standard three-carbon copy format is practical (Fig. 5-2). A form such as this saves the staff from having to write individual letters. It allows the office to retain an original copy and the physician and/or dentist to mail back the reply copy and keep a copy for his or her own records.

```
Dentist_____    Patient_____

Address_____    Address_____

Phone_____    Phone_____




REQUEST  Date_____

Dear Dr._____,


The patient named above was recently seen in our office as a new patient.
Before dental therapy is initiated, I would appreciate information
regarding the patient's health status in the following areas.  Thank you.






                                        _____


I,_____ , hereby consent to the release of my medical/
dental records to the office of_____.
                                         (Patient signature)

REPLY  Date_____






                                        _____
                                           (Consultant signature)
```

Fig. 5-2. Sample medical release letter.

PHYSICIANS' DESK REFERENCE

The *Physicians' Desk Reference (PDR)* is published annually and is used as a reference by health professionals when seeking information about medications. The *PDR* is used to check such information as drug dosage, composition, contraindications, and the interactions of one drug with another. Today, with the huge number of medications available, a drug dictionary of this nature is essential for providing information about current and newly released medicaments.

It is important for dental professionals to use

the *PDR* to investigate medications being taken by their patients. In this way the dental professional will be familiar with the reason the patient is taking the medication and will be aware of possible contraindications or interactions between medication and dental treatment. For example, warfarin (Coumadin) is a blood anticoagulant, often prescribed for patients with phlebitis. Before a scaling procedure is performed, a consultation with the patient's physician may be necessary to change the patient's dosage to prevent prolonged bleeding during treatment.

Acetyl sulfisoxazole (Gantrisin) is an antibiotic used for the treatment of urinary tract infections. Procaine, once used as a primary dental local anesthetic, and sulfonamides (such as Gantrisin) are chemically related. Taken together, an antagonistic response occurs, rendering both medications ineffective.

Pharmacologic terms to be familiar with include *brand name, generic name,* and *drug classification.*

Brand name is the name given to a particular medication or product by its manufacturer. Many manufacturers make the same product but market it under their own brand name. *Generic name* is the chemical name of the product. The use of generic names is advised because these always remain the same, given more chemical information, and do not limit prescription to one commercial preparation.

Example: The product propoxyphene hydrochloride (generic name) is made by five manufacturers and marketed with these brand names: Darvon, Dolene Compound 65 capsules, Propoxyphene Hydrochloride capsules, Wygesic tablets.

Drug classification refers to the broad category to define drugs sharing similar actions.

Examples: Analgesics—products that alleviate pain
Diuretics—products that promote urination
Sedatives—products that induce a quiet, calm state

The *PDR* consists of cross-referenced indices of products arranged alphabetically by manufacturer, brand name, generic name, and drug classification. If a sample medication is available, a picture identification section is included. The largest portion of the book is the product information section. Each product is described as to its chemical composition, the form in which it is supplied, its action and suggested use, administration, recommended dosage, contraindications, precautions, and side effects. Other sections include information on diagnostic products and management of drug overdose. Between the yearly publication dates, quarterly supplements are issued to update product information or describe new products.

Procedure for using the *PDR*

Obtain as much information from the patient as possible. Perhaps the patient has brought the medication. Read the prescription; look at the product. Ask the following questions:
1. For what condition are you taking this medication?
2. How often do you take it?
3. How long ago was it prescribed for you?
4. Do you take the medication exactly as prescribed?
5. When did you last take the medication?
6. Besides the manner in which this medication helps you specifically, does it alter the way you feel in general?

Generally, patients are aware of the name and nature of the medication and the prescribed regimen for administration. Knowing the dosage is not as common; follow up by checking the prescription or the *PDR.*

Inquire whether the patient is taking the medication as directed by his or her physician. One may discover that the patient is altering the dosage in some way. This often happens when the patient "feels good" regardless of the state of the illness. Patient noncompliance in taking medications is a common problem. In a professional manner, reinforce the prescribed routine, and suggest that the patient check with the physician for approval of the alteration. Explain that not taking a medication as prescribed alters the control of the medical condition, which may create a risk to the individual and may affect reactions during dental treatment.

Often medications have minor effects that patients cope with readily. For example, antihistamines can make people sleepy; antibiotics can cause nausea; asthma medications can make people agitated or tremulous. The conditions may or may not affect dental therapy, but the clinician's understanding of these states may help put the patient at ease, making treatment more comfortable.

Following these questions, note the name of the medication, the reason for its prescription, and the patient's dosage in the appropriate history or update section. Check the *PDR* for drug action and any complication that might affect dental treatment.

SUMMARY

This chapter has discussed one part of the dental appointment: obtaining a comprehensive health history. It has been an introduction to some areas where medicine and dentistry are interrelated. Other courses such as anatomy/physiology and oral medicine/pathology will enrich the student's understanding of normal conditions and specific diseases in relation to dental care. In conclusion, the important points are recognizing the need for a thorough review of health conditions prior to dental treatment and detailing the contents of such a review to identify medical conditions that may necessitate changes in dental care. In addition, the history-taking experience provides an opportunity for the clinician and patient to interact in a way that can be the foundation of the professional relationship.

ACKNOWLEDGMENT

A special thanks to Donald C. Dafoe, M.D., for his critique and review of the information presented in this chapter.

ACTIVITIES

1. Provide sample health history information for small groups to discuss. Practice completing the patient write-up using this information.
2. Role play the medical interview. Discuss communication skills and hygienist/patient interactions observed.
3. Practice using the *Physicians' Desk Reference* by identifying medications, contraindications, side effects, and so on.
4. Observe and critique health histories (interviews or written documentation) completed by students during their final year of clinical education. Discuss the observations in small groups.
5. Complete a comprehensive health history for a student partner. Preserve the complete data for use in treatment planning (discussed in Chapter 18). Students should note that recording such data also ensures safe practice of intraoral procedures for a student partner.
6. Prepare a report summarizing the most recent research on hepatitis, AIDS, or heart disease.

REVIEW QUESTIONS

1. Respond to this situation: Mrs. Jones is a new patient. Partway through the health history interview she states, "This is just wasting time. I want my teeth checked."
2. Which of the following conditions should be followed up by a physician's consultation and why?
   a. Rheumatic heart disease
   b. History of myocardial infarction
   c. Blood pressure reading of 160/100
   d. Hemophilia
   e. All of the above
3. List the medical conditions that *require* antibiotic premedication prior to dental treatment to prevent bacterial endocarditis.
4. List several communication principles that help ensure a thorough medical history and a helping relationship with the patient.
5. How is the *Physicians' Desk Reference* useful to the dental hygienist?

REFERENCES

ADA Council on Dental Therapeutics: Accepted dental therapeutics, ed 40, Chicago, 1984, American Dental Association.

Angelopoulous AP: Diphenylhydantoin gingival hyperplasia: a clinicopathological review, J Can Dent Assoc 41:103, 1975.

Baltch AL et.al: Bacteremia following dental cleaning in patients with and without penicillin prophylaxis, Am Heart J 104:1335, 1982.

Bennett CR: Monheim's local anesthesia and pain control in dental practice, ed 7, St Louis, 1984, The CV Mosby Co.

Bodak-Gyovai LZ: Diagnostic center manual. Philadelphia, 1978, Department of Oral Medicine, University of Pennsylvania School of Dental Medicine.

Braham L, editor: The dental implications of epilepsy: report to the Commission for the Control of its Consequences, by the ad hoc committee of the Academy of Dentistry for the Handicapped. Pub (ASA) 78-5217. Washington, DC, 1977, Department of Health, Education and Welfare.

Butler RT, et. al: Drug-induced gingival hyperplasia: phenytoin, cyclosporine, and nifedipine, J Am Dent Assoc 114(1):56, 1987.

Durack DT, Kaplan EL, and Bisno AL: Apparent failure of endocarditis prophylaxis: analysis of 52 cases submitted to a national registry, JAMA 250:2318, 1983.

Evans BE: Dental care in hemophilia. New York, 1977, Cutter Laboratories and the National Hemophilia Foundation.

Froelich RE, and Bishop FM: Clinical interviewing skills: a programmed manual for data gathering, evaluation, and patient management, ed 3, St Louis, 1977, The CV Mosby Co.

Grossman R: Orthodontics and dentistry for the hemophilic patient. Am J Orthod 68:391, 1975.

Israel H: Abnormalities of bone and orofacial changes from anticonvulsant drugs, J Public Health Dent 34:104, 1974.

Kaye D, et al: Internal medicine for dentistry, St Louis, 1983, The CV Mosby Co.

Kerr D, and Ash Jr M: Oral pathology: an introduction to general and oral pathology for hygienists, ed 5, Philadelphia, 1986, Lea & Febiger.

Mohammad AR, et al: Assessment of dental patient's comprehension of health questionnaire, J Oral Med 38(2):74, 1983.

Physician's Desk Reference, ed 41, Oradell NJ, 1987, Medical Economics Co.

Prevention of bacterial endocarditis: A committee report of the American Heart Association, JADA 110:98,1985.

Small I: Introduction to the clinical history, ed 2, Flushing, NY, 1971, Medical Examination Publishing Co, Inc.

Sullivan BV, et al: The cardiac patient. Chemoprophylaxis considerations, Dent Hyg 60(10):462, 1986.

Tzukert AA, et al: Prevention of infective endocarditis: not by antibiotics alone, Oral Surg Oral Med Oral Pathol 62(4):385, 1986.

Weinstein L, and Schlesinger J: Pathoanatomic, pathophysiologic, and clinical correlations in endocarditis, I and II, N Engl J Med 291:832, 1122, 1974.

Woodall IR, editor: Curriculum guidelines, ed 3, Chicago, 1975, American Dental Hygienist's Association.

6 BASIC INSTRUMENTATION AND POSITIONING

OBJECTIVES: *The reader will be able to*

1. Describe the basic purposes of the following instruments in assessment phases of dental hygiene care:
   Mouth mirror
   Retractor
   Explorer
   Periodontal probe
2. Given an instrument, identify its handle, working end(s), shank, and terminal shank.
3. Given a variety of instruments, identify single-ended, double-ended, and paired instruments.
4. Give two reasons for the importance of being able to identify instruments by their shapes and recognize variations in shape and design.
5. Explain how proper positioning at the dental chair enhances proper instrumentation.
6. Describe the properly seated clinician, patient, and chairside assistant.
7. Adjust the positions of the clinician, patient, and chairside assistant for maximum access and visibility for any area in the dentition.
8. Given any tooth surface, adjust himself or herself to the proper position; adjust the patient's head position and the overhead light; use the mouth mirror to maximize access and vision; and establish a modified pen grasp, a fulcrum, and a wrist rock to generate vertical, overlapping strokes on a tooth.
9. Establish proper positioning, access, vision, grasp, fulcrum, wrist rock, and stroke for each area in the recommended sequence of positions.
10. Use proper positioning, grasp, wrist rock, instrument adaptation, and stroke for the following instruments:
    Periodontal probe
    Paired explorer (cowhorn, pigtail)
    Straight-shanked explorer (No. 17 or 20)
11. Use the shepherd's hook (No. 23) to explore for caries.

PURPOSE OF HAND INSTRUMENTS IN DENTAL HYGIENE CARE

The hand instruments used in dental hygiene care serve a variety of functions in the assessment, implementation, and evaluation phases of care. Before learning and performing any additional assessment procedures, it is important to develop basic skills in handling instruments and in learning to work at the chairside.

Mouth mirrors

One of the most important instruments in dental hygiene care is the mouth mirror. It is an instrument used to *enhance vision* in the recesses of the oral cavity. Mirrors are available in a variety of sizes and have a magnifying surface. The mouth mirror is used for retracting tissues such as the cheek and tongue, for reflecting light onto an area that otherwise would be in a shadow, for indirect vision of an area that cannot be seen directly (such as the distal aspect of the most posterior molar), and for transillumination (casting light through teeth to determine the presence of caries or calculus by detecting variations in translucency).

An essential prerequisite skill in learning to use

dental instruments is the effective use of the mouth mirror to ensure comfortable, adequate vision of all areas of the mouth. An exercise at the end of this chapter outlines a method for developing this skill prior to the introduction of "working instruments." The goal should be careful, assertive placement of the mirror to obtain a clear view of the operative site and adequate space to locate a firm fulcrum or finger rest for the working hand. This should be done without clanking the mirror against the teeth, without pinching the lip against the teeth, without pressing the mirror head against the gingiva, and without impinging soft tissue against bone.

Retractors

Another example of a dental instrument that enhances vision is the cheek retractor, most often

SINGLE END

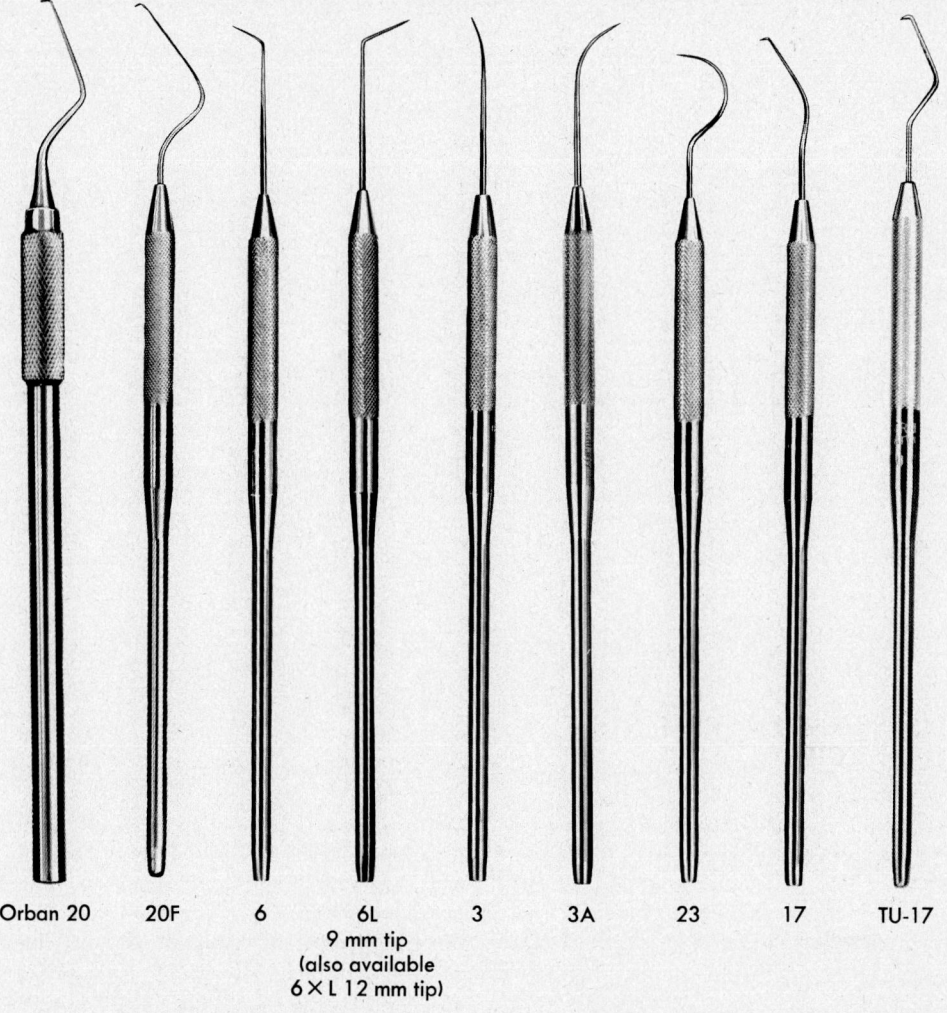

| Orban 20 | 20F | 6 | 6L
9 mm tip
(also available
6 × L 12 mm tip) | 3 | 3A | 23 | 17 | TU-17 |

Fig. 6-1. Explorers used for detection of caries and for examining teeth for calculus and other irregularities are available in a variety of shapes and sizes.
(Courtesy Hu-Friedy Co, Chicago.)

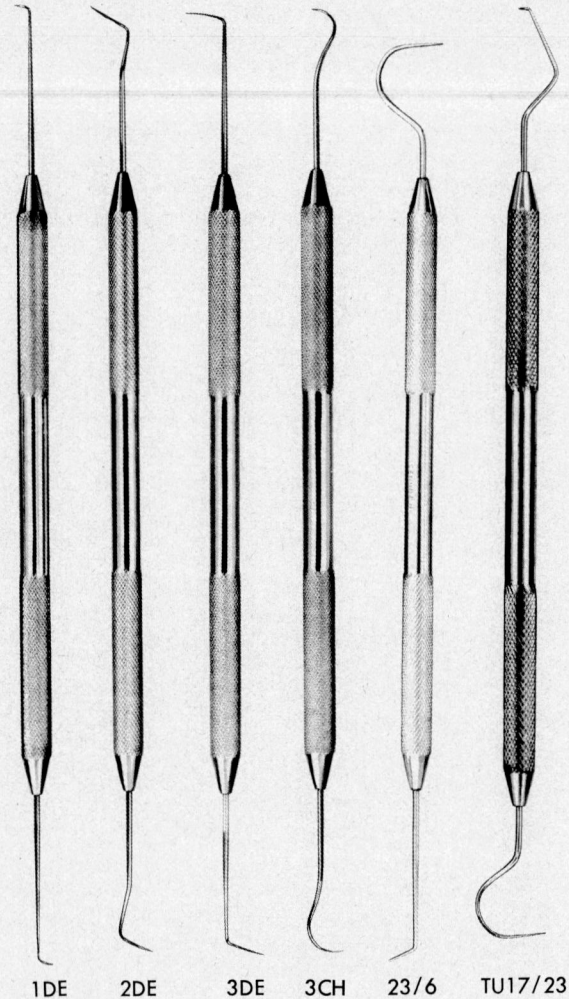

1DE   2DE   3DE   3CH   23/6   TU17/23

Fig. 6-2. Explorers are available in pairs, for instance, to gain access to a tooth from facial aspect with one end and from the lingual aspect with the other end. Double-ended instruments may have two entirely different styles of working designs, such as the 23/6.
(Courtesy Hu-Friedy Co, Chicago.)

used to extend the cheeks and lips away from the mouth to assist in intraoral photography. Other intraoral retractors can be used to keep the tongue from wandering toward the operative site, thus preventing accidental trauma.

Explorers and probes

Other instruments are used to *examine* teeth and tissues by exploring the teeth and by measuring the size and location of tissue entities. Explorers are instruments used primarily to examine the teeth for caries and for the presence of tooth irregularities such as calculus deposits, root roughness, anatomic defects, and margins of restorations. Explorers come in a variety of shapes and sizes—some best suited for exploring for caries and others for the detection of fine subgingival irregularities. (Figs. 6-1 and 6-2 show several common types of explorers.) Because the dental hygienist's role includes identifying tooth character-

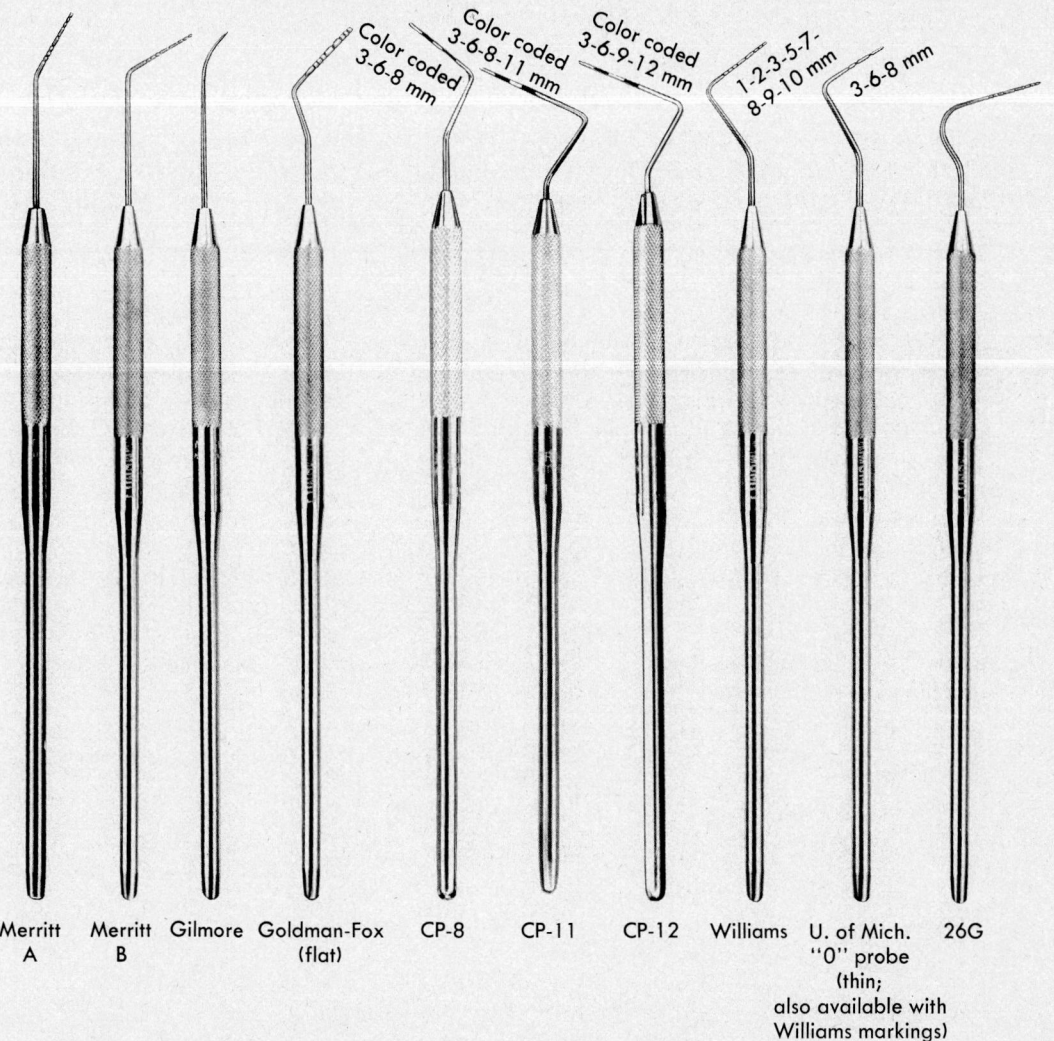

Fig. 6-3. Periodontal probes, used primarily for examining sulcus and measuring its depths, are calibrated in millimeters. Some are color coded to improve readability. Shank length, angle, and working tip shape vary. (Courtesy Hu-Friedy Co, Chicago.)

istics and monitoring a patient's oral health, it is important to master the use of explorers early in clinical practice.

The periodontal probe is used for examining oral tissues also. It is not used for caries detection, since it does not have a sharp point for retention in carious areas. Probes that are noted for their delicate design can be used for detection of root irregularities and hard deposits. However, the probe's primary use is for measuring the depth of the gingival sulcus or periodontal pocket (Pattison and Behrens, 1973; Ward and Simring, 1978). The periodontal probe's unique characteristic is its calibrations, marked in millimeters. How far the probe slides into the sulcus or a pocket indicates the level of the attachment of the gingiva to the tooth. The probe can trace the topography of the attachment around the tooth, providing the clinician with an idea of the extent of disease and the health status of the periodontium.

The calibrated probe also can be used to measure recession of the free gingiva, the amount of attached masticatory mucosa, or the size of a lesion. It is critical to know how the probe is calibrated, as some are marked in 3-mm increments and others are marked at 1, 2, 3, 5, and 7 mm and other variations (Fig. 6-3).

Exercises described in this chapter provide opportunities for using the mouth mirror for vision and the periodontal probe for exploring and measuring subgingival areas. A subsequent exercise advances the student to the use of a cowhorn explorer and a No. 17 explorer.

Once the mouth mirror, probe, and explorers can be used competently, the clinician is prepared to assess the intraoral dental findings for a patient.

Other instruments

Instruments used in the implementation of care are those used to *remove deposits* from teeth such as scalers and curettes and those used to *recontour or excise tissue*. Other working instruments, particularly those used in restorative dentistry, are used to *place materials on or in the teeth and the surrounding tissues* and to shape those materials. As each phase of implementation of dental hygiene care is addressed in later chapters, the design and use of each instrument are also discussed.

BASIC INSTRUMENT DESIGN

The basic terminology used to describe most dental instruments makes it easier for the student and faculty member or for the clinician and assistant to understand each other when discussing instrument selection and use. Refer to Fig. 6-4 as the parts of the instruments are described.

The *handle* is the part grasped by the clinician or assistant. Handles come in various shapes and sizes, including variations of hexagonal, round, and tapered. They can be smooth or have knurls or a grooved pattern to prevent the handle from slipping in the user's hand (Pattison and Behrens, 1973; Ward and Simring, 1978).

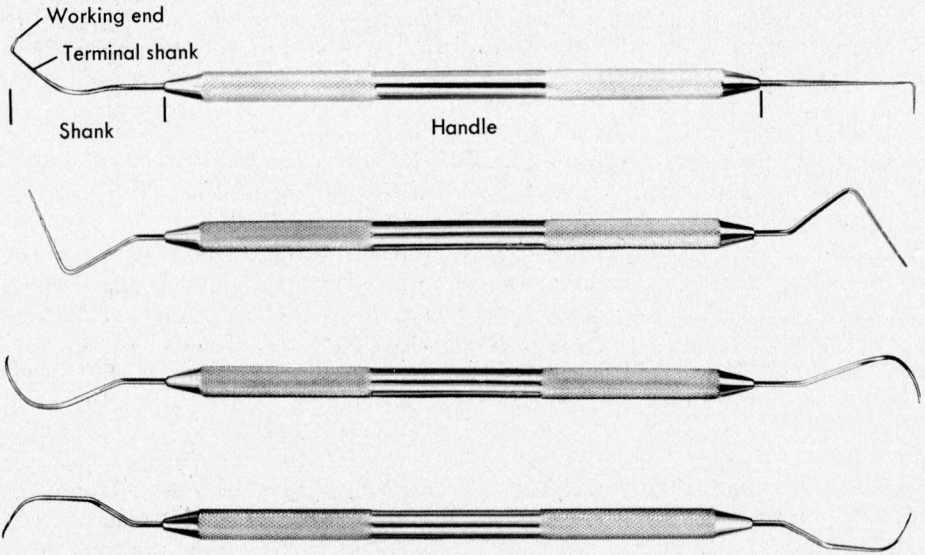

Fig. 6-4. Handle of instrument is connected to a thinner shank that is angled to permit access to various areas of the dentition. Working end is at tip of instrument. Part of shank closest to working end is called the *terminal shank*. All instruments shown are double ended. Bottom two instruments are paired. (Courtesy Hu-Friedy Co, Chicago.)

The *working end* of the instrument refers to the end of the instrument that contacts the tooth and performs the intended task. The working end can have a point, a blade, a blunt nib, pincers for grasping an object, or some other useful configuration (Pattison and Behrens, 1973; Ward and Simring, 1978).

Joining the working end and the handle is the *shank,* which determines the accessibility of the instrument to various places in the mouth and the flex and strength of the instrument. The angles and convolutions in the shank permit access to posterior areas and proximal surfaces while allowing the clinician's hand to enter from the front of the mouth. The thickness and tensile strength of the shank dictate the amount of stress that the shank can endure in intraoral procedures requiring considerable pressure. Shank shape and strength are therefore particularly important considerations when selecting instruments for removing particularly heavy, tenacious deposits from the teeth (Pattison and Behrens, 1973; Ward and Simring, 1978).

The *terminal shank* is the part of the shank that is closest to the working end. It is important to be able to locate the terminal shank on instruments with simple and complex shanks, since the terminal shank is one important cue in adapting the instrument to the tooth. This term is used frequently in this chapter in describing the procedure for selecting the correct end of the instrument and for ensuring that it is being used safely and correctly.

Instruments are available with two working ends, one at each end of the handle. These are referred to as *double-ended* instruments. Using double-ended instruments necessitates fewer instrument changes and minimizes the number of individual instruments on the tray, reducing clutter. However, when changing ends of an instrument, one must take care to prevent contacting the patient with the instrument. Instrument changes should occur away from the patient's face, usually over the patient's chest, as is the practice in four-handed dentistry. All the instruments in Fig. 6-4 are double ended.

Two of the double-ended instruments in Fig. 6-4 are also examples of *paired instruments*. The ends of a paired instrument are mirror images of each other. One end is intended for use on a proximal surface of a tooth from the facial aspect. Its pair is intended for entry from the lingual aspect. Thus the bends in the shank allow access to a given proximal surface from both aspects.

A more complete discussion of where instruments may be used and how pairs are identified is presented in later chapters. At this point in developing an awareness of instruments and their use, it may be helpful to remember that many instruments are used in pairs, permitting universal access to tooth surfaces.

As each instrument is introduced and used in assessing patient needs and implementing care, it may be helpful for the clinician to identify the parts of the instrument and to project what function it might serve and where it could be adapted. Such an approach to instruments will make it possible for the clinician to identify instruments on the basis of their shapes and sizes rather than by the numbers engraved in the handle. It also will help the clinician develop a working familiarity with instruments that will enable experimentation with a variety of designs as skill and experience grow.

Another important reason for knowing and analyzing instrument design is that the original shape must be preserved as instruments are sharpened. Strokes with a sharpening stone are more likely to sharpen without damaging the working end if the clinician has a clear concept of the proper shape.

HOLDING AND USING INSTRUMENTS: THE GRASP, FINGER REST, AND WRIST ROCK

Holding an instrument is different from the way most people hold writing implements. Fig. 6-5 shows a typical pen grasp with the thumb and first finger grasping the handle, supported by the middle finger under the handle. Fig. 6-6 shows the modified pen grasp, in which the first and second fingers are placed on the instrument, opposed by the thumb. This grasp is commonly used in holding dental instruments. Fig. 6-7 shows a common error made in grasping a dental instrument. The first two knuckles of the first finger should be flat on the instrument to improve stability and to ensure tactile sense. The third finger should serve as a *fulcrum,* or pivot point, often called a *finger rest.* With this grasp and fulcrum, it should be

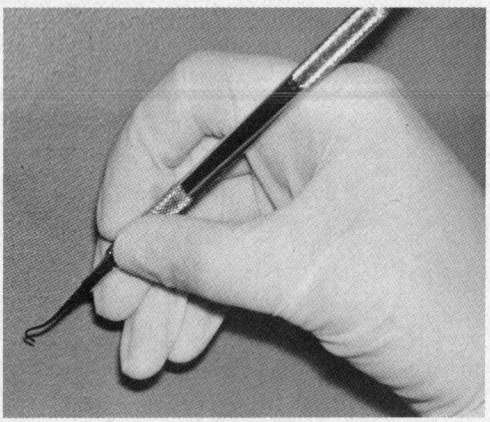

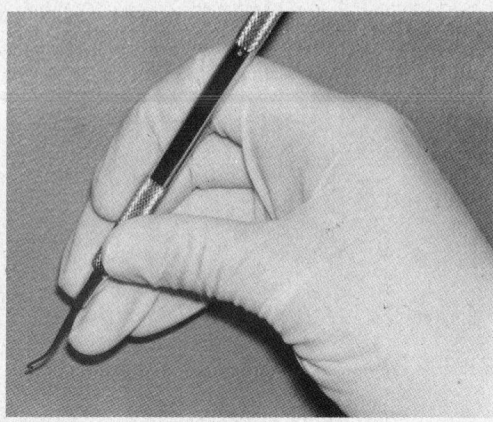

Fig. **6-5.** Typical pen grasp with thumb and first finger grasping handle. Middle finger supports instrument from underneath.

Fig. **6-6.** Modified pen grasp with both first and second fingers holding handle, opposed by thumb. Third finger is in position to rest on tooth structure to create stability and to create a fulcrum point for moving the instrument.

Fig. **6-7.** Incorrect modified pen grasp because knuckle of first finger is buckled. Handle should lie flat against first two sections of first finger as shown in Fig. 5-6.

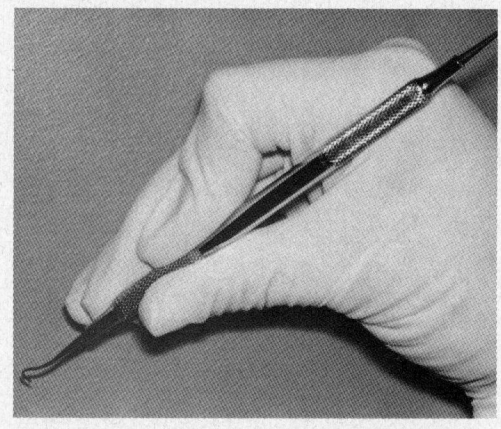

possible to see the palm of the hand when looking past the instrument from the thumb, as evident in Fig. 6-6. The wrist rock begins in this position and moves on the fulcrum point as a unified movement of arm, wrist, and hand in a side-to-side, rock-and-return oscillation (Fig. 6-8). With the wrist rock, the instrument should be moved up and down the tooth without changing the angle of the shank to the tooth with each stroke. A

heavily accentuated wrist rock that starts with the palm cupped downward can cause the shank to move in and out from the tooth, and this is undesirable.

Another motion that can be useful in areas where lateral rocking is difficult is the vertical, or forward-and-back, wrist rock (Fig. 6-9). The instrument is moved up and down the tooth in the same stroking pattern, but the hand movement is

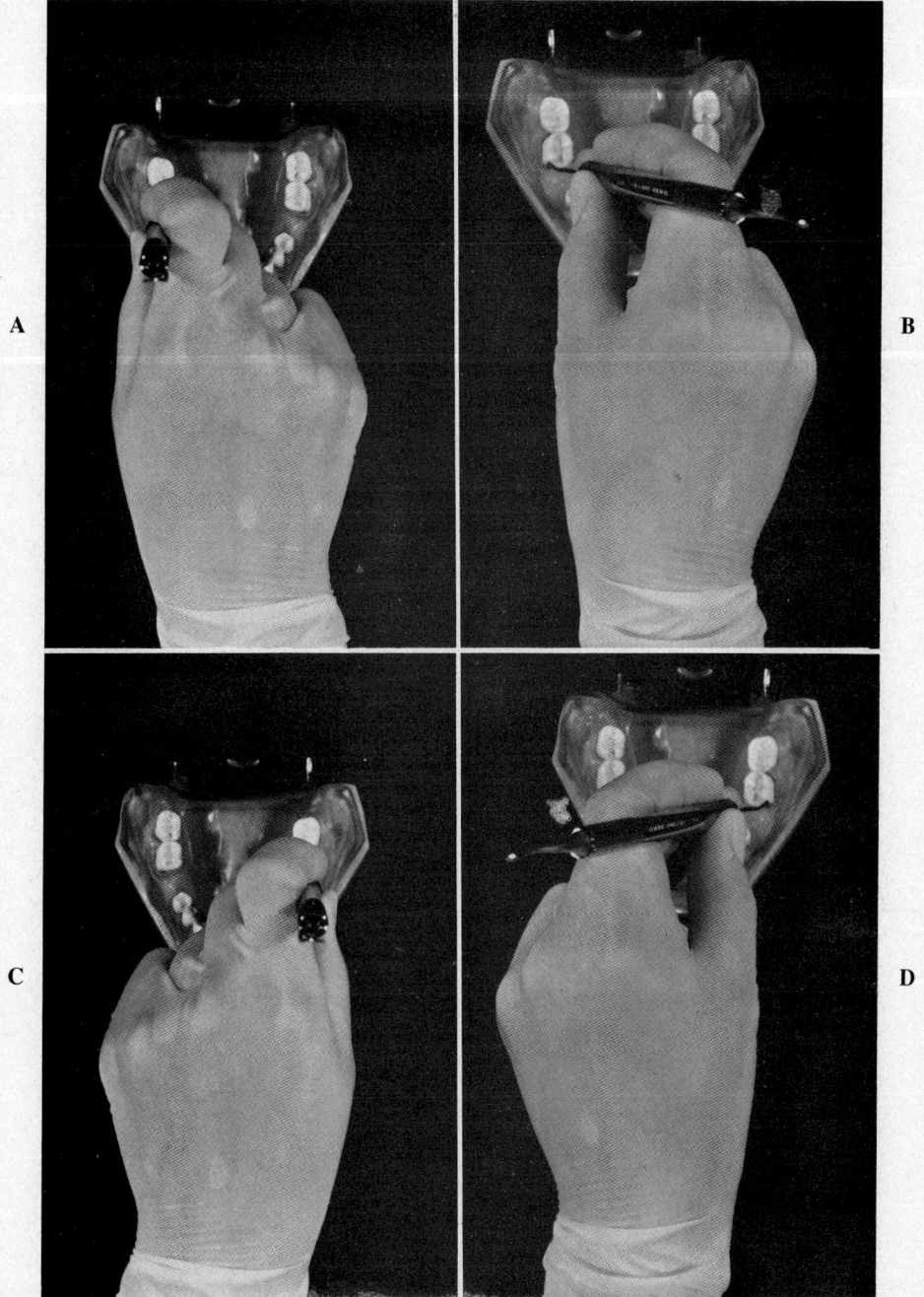

Fig. 6-8. **A,** Beginning position for lateral wrist rock, with pen grasp and solid fulcrum. **B,** Hand rocks laterally to the right, moving working end of instrument in coronal direction. Rocking back to position in **A** moves working end of instrument apically. Thus instrument strokes are accomplished by rocking the hand back and forth. **C,** Beginning position for left-handed clinician. **D,** Hand rocked laterally to the left.

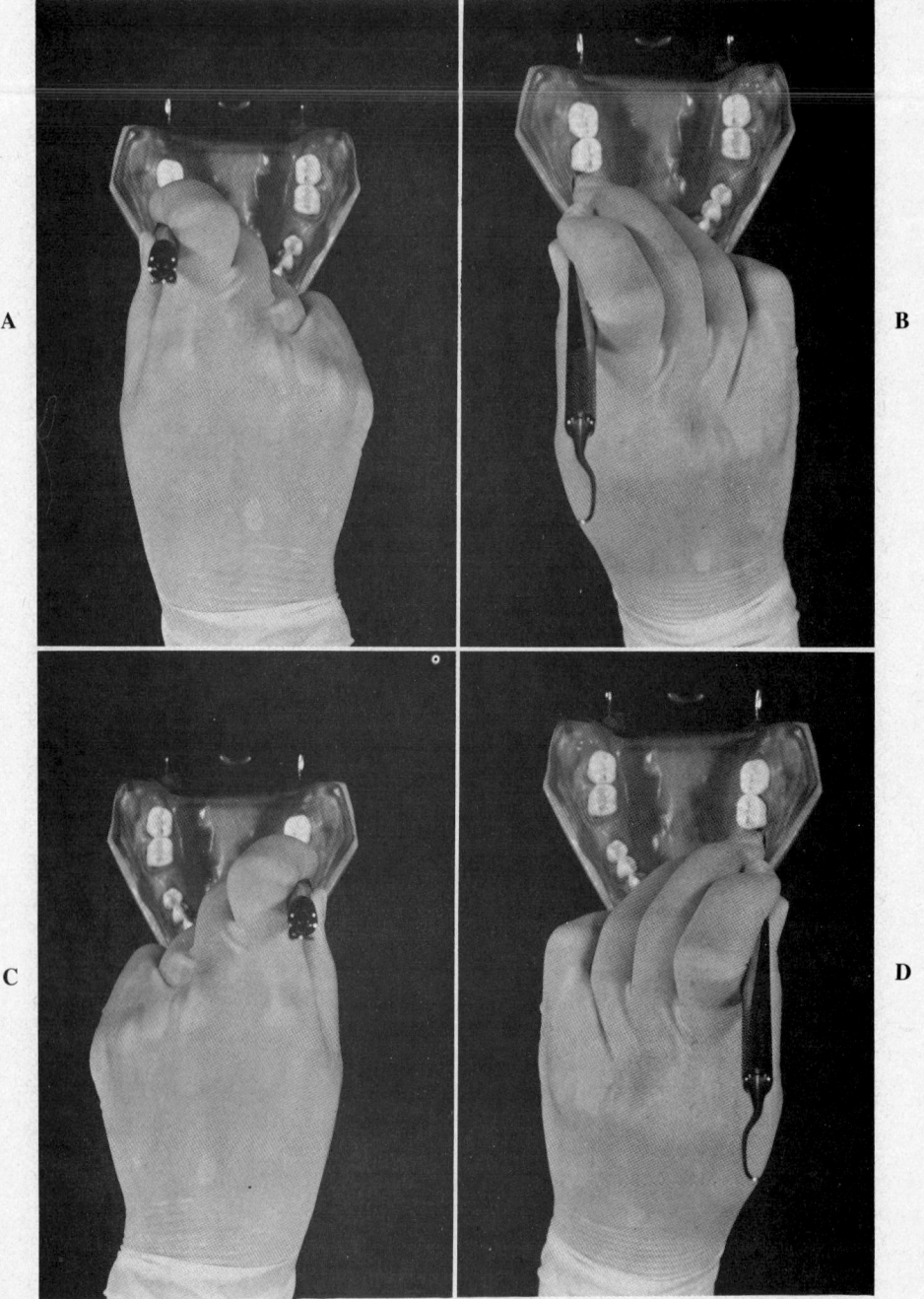

Fig. 6-9. **A,** Beginning position for vertical wrist rock. **B,** Hand moves in vertical plane by bending the wrist. Bending the wrist moves instrument tip coronally, and returning to position in **A** moves instrument tip apically. **C,** Beginning position for left-handed clinician. **D,** Hand moved by lowering the wrist while maintaining a fulcrum.

done by lowering the wrist while maintaining a fulcrum.

EFFICIENCY AND MOTION ECONOMY IN INSTRUMENTATION

When any instrument is used in performing intraoral procedures, effectiveness is improved and fatigue can be reduced if a few simple guidelines are followed. Proper positioning of the clinician, the patient, and the dental assistant during the very first efforts at instrumentation can help the dental hygienist develop safe practice habits that will enhance efficiency and aid in mastery of instrumentation skills.

Proper positioning at the chair makes it easier to see the operative site, to maintain a stable fulcrum or finger rest, and to adapt the instrument. Finally, good positioning reduces muscle strain and fatigue for the entire dental team, including the patient.

Therefore, as the basic principles of instrumentation are introduced and practiced, principles of motion economy, including proper positioning, will be implemented as well. The basic premises underlying this approach are that good instrumentation learned from detrimental or impossible clinician and patient positions does not transfer readily to a useful pattern of clinical practice, and instrumentation learned from ideal positions at the chair makes mastery of basic manipulation much easier, as it is enhanced by good vision, fulcrum placement, and access.

BASIC POSITIONS OF THE DENTAL TEAM

To begin instrumentation, the patient should be placed in a supine position. As described in Chapter 2, this is best accomplished by tilting the entire chair back to ensure seating the patient's hips in the angle of the chair. The back of the chair is then lowered to just above the lap of the seated clinician. The headrest should be adjusted, and a protective drape and napkin placed on the patient. The patient's feet should be at approximately the same height as the patient's head.

The clinician should be seated so that the thighs are parallel to the floor and the feet are flat on the floor. If the clinician's stool has an abdominal rest, the rest should be located just below the clinician's ribs to provide support as he or she inclines the upper body forward from the waist.

The chairside assistant should be seated so that his or her eye level is 4 to 6 inches above the clinician's eye level. Depending on the assistant's height, this may necessitate a foot support on the stool to enable the thighs to be parallel to the floor.

With the three members of the team in this basic seating arrangement, the clinician may move from a front to a rear position at the chair with the assistant making appropriate minor adjustments to ensure proper instrument transfers and visibility. The right-handed clinician's position is at approximately 8:30 to 10 o'clock at the chair for the front position and at 10:30 to 12 o'clock for the rear position. Left-handed clinicians occupy 3:30 to 2 o'clock and 2:30 to 12 o'clock positions for front and rear positions, respectively (Figs. 6-10 and 6-11).

In addition to the flexibility of moving from front to rear, there is additional flexibility and access as the patient turns his or her head toward or away from the clinician. Additionally, the patient can raise or lower the chin. The back of the chair can be raised or lowered 1 to 2 inches for access to specific areas.

The combination of clinician position, patient head movement, and the wisely used mouth mirror eliminates the need for contorted positions for adequate vision. It is possible to gain access to all areas of the mouth while maintaining a healthful posture.

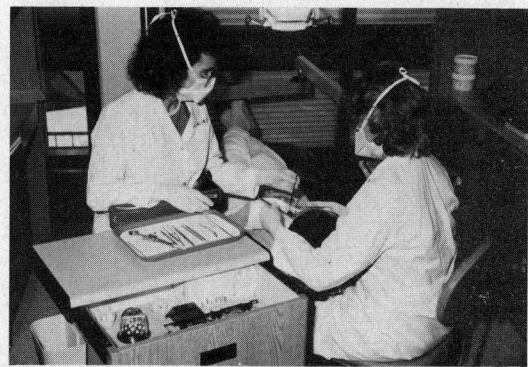

Fig. 6-10. Properly positioned patient, right-handed clinician, and assistant.

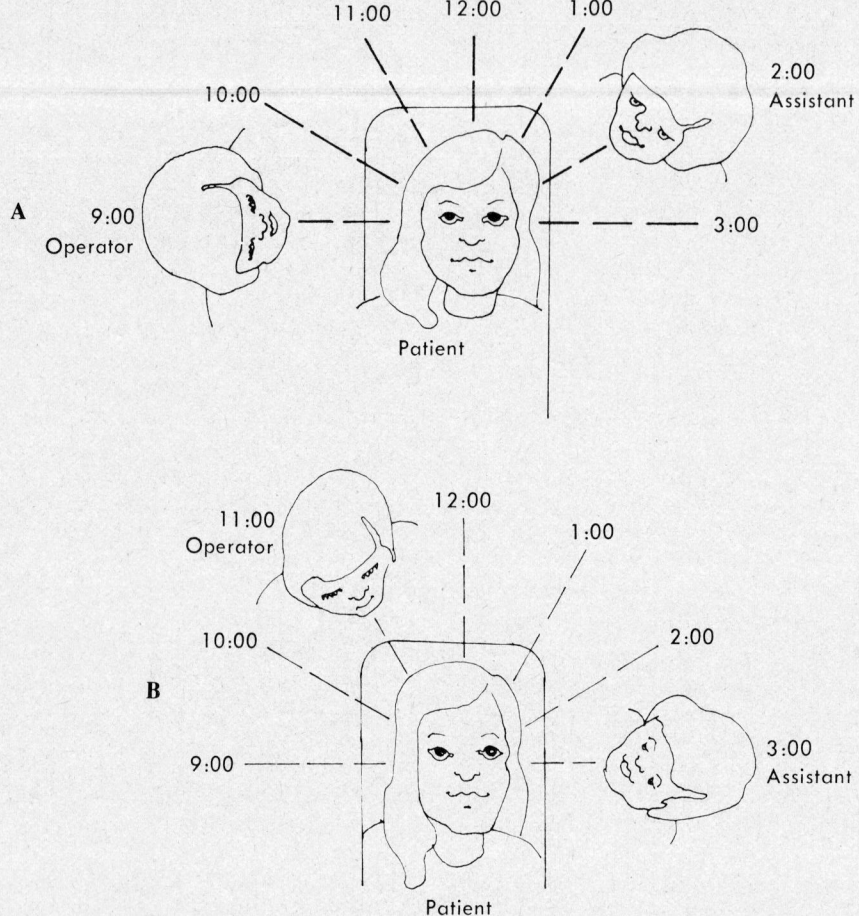

Fig. 6-11. **A,** Right-handed clinician seated at approximately 9 o'clock position with assistant at 2 o'clock position. **B,** Right-handed clinician seated at 11 o'clock position with assistant at 3 o'clock position. Left-handed clinician sits at 3 o'clock and 1 o'clock positions for front and rear positions, respectively.

POSITIONING EXERCISES

To develop skill in gaining access to all areas of the mouth, students should divide into groups of three to practice the basic positions, each serving once as patient, clinician, and assistant. The student who serves as chairside assistant should prepare the dental unit by disinfecting equipment and placing sterile instruments on the tray (including a mouth mirror and a cotton-tipped applicator), seat the patient in a supine position, and place the drape. The assistant should adjust his or her stool to the proper height in relation to the clinician and ensure an adequate view of each operative site by making minor adjustments in position.

The dental assistant should ensure proper adjustment of the overhead light by observing the target of the primary beam of light and adjusting the overall position and angle of the lamp so that the beam is on the operative site and is not blocked by a hand, the clinician's head, or some other obstacle. A general rule is to bring the lamp up over the patient's face and angle it downward (nearly perpendicular to the floor) for mandibular sites and to bring the lamp back over the patient's lap and angle it toward the mouth so that the primary beam is nearly parallel to the floor for maxillary sites (Fig. 6-12). From these two basic positions it is possible to angle the lamp from one

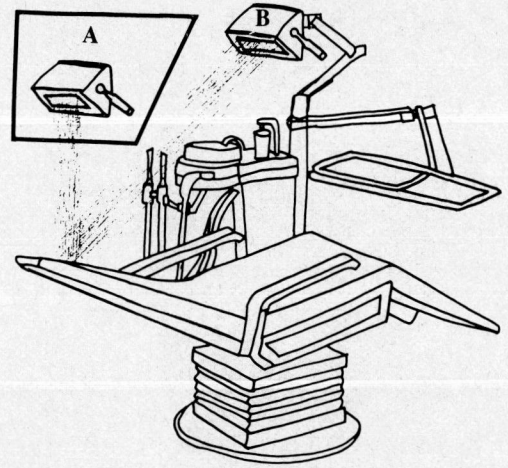

Fig. 6-12. A general rule in obtaining optimal intraoral illumination is to angle beam of overhead lamp nearly perpendicular to floor, **A**, for mandible and more parallel to floor, **B**, for maxilla. Range of angulation for maxilla is usually between 45 and 10 degrees to floor.

side or the other to eliminate shadows created by the hands.

The clinician should adjust his or her stool to the proper height and use the mouth mirror for retraction, indirect vision, and/or light reflection as appropriate for each area of the mouth. The mouth mirror should be held in the nonworking hand. The cotton-tipped applicator should be held in the working hand (right-handed people use the right hand; left-handed people use the left hand).

Moving sequentially from area to area of the dentition, the clinician should use the mouth mirror as indicated in Table 6-1 or 6-2. The clinician should establish a solid modified pen grasp with the working hand as shown in Figs. 6-13 and 6-14 for right- and left-handed clinicians, respectively, establish a fulcrum or finger rest on the teeth, and use the wrist rock so that the cotton tip rides up and down the tooth in a vertical pattern of overlapping strokes. Two or three teeth in each area should be traced to provide practice in maintaining retraction and in using a stable grasp, fulcrum, and wrist rock.

Figs. 6-15 to 6-26 show sample hand positions for right-handed clinicians; left-handed clinicians should follow Figs. 6-27 to 6-38. These hand positions should be referred to for this exercise. The student may progress to the probe and then to the cowhorn (as shown in these illustrations) after basic skill is achieved with the cotton-tipped applicator.

The student playing the role of patient should comply with requests to turn the head to the right or to the left or to tilt the head up or down to facilitate access. It is also appropriate for this student to provide feedback about the careful use of the mouth mirror (reporting pain or discomfort) and to comment on the sense of confidence inspired by the stability of the fulcrum and the clinician's caring approach to the "patient." From the beginning, the clinician should treat the patient as a person rather than as a mannequin or "object of care." The student playing the role of the patient may also hold the table of positions, areas and approaches for the clinician's reference as the sequence is learned. As the sequence is mastered and approaches become more comfortable, the student-patient may wish to observe the student-clinician in a hand mirror.

All three students should feel free to discuss comfortable ways of implementing each position. The instructor should circulate among the groups of students to check mirror use, pen grasp, fulcrum placement, and wrist rock as well as basic positions and the location of the overhead lamp.

In order to see how the mirror can be used to *reflect light through tissue (transillumination),* the clinician should place the mirror behind the teeth and angle it until the teeth brighten from the light being reflected through them. The clinician should look at the teeth rather than the image in the mirror. The shadow of restorations should be visible, as well as caries and interproximal or lingual calculus. The light passing through substances other than healthy tooth structure is not as easily transmitted. These substances or defects are thus usually visible as dark shadows.

As each clinician practices and completes the sequence of positions, the team should rotate to ensure each student an experience as clinician, assistant, and patient. All the basic principles of contamination control, including unit preparation, instrument sterilization, hand scrub, and aseptic chain should be practiced to reinforce previously learned skills.

After one or two practice sessions and study of the table of positions, students should be prepared to assume the proper position for any given area of the mouth and, also, to assume each position

Table 6-1. Positioning for right-handed clinicians

Area of operation	Patient's head position*	Clinician position	Finger rest	Vision	Use of mirror
Mandible					
Right buccal	Left	9 o'clock	Bicuspid/cuspid	Direct	Retract cheek
Left lingual	Left	9 o'clock	Bicuspid/cuspid	Direct	Retract tongue
Right lingual	Right	9 o'clock	Bicuspid/cuspid	Indirect	Retract cheek; indirect vision and illumination
Left buccal	Right	11 o'clock	Bicuspid/cuspid	Direct	Retract cheek
Anterior lingual	Straight†	11 o'clock	Cuspid	Direct	Reflect light; retract tongue
Anterior labial	Straight†	11 o'clock	Cuspid	Direct or indirect	Indirect vision; retract lip
Maxilla					
Right buccal	Left	9 o'clock	Occlusal surface of tooth posterior to area of operation	Direct	Retract cheek
Left lingual	Left	9 o'clock		Direct	Reflect light
Right lingual	Right	11 o'clock		Indirect	Indirect vision; reflect light
Left buccal	Right	11 o'clock		Direct	Retract cheek
Anterior lingual	Straight†	11 o'clock	Incisal edge	Indirect	Indirect vision; reflect light
Anterior labial	Straight†	11 o'clock	Incisal edge	Direct	None

*Patient is in the supine position.
†Patient is asked to turn his/her head slightly as clinician moves from cuspid to cuspid in the anterior areas.

Table 6-2. Positioning for left-handed clinicians

Area of operation	Patient's head position*	Clinician position	Finger rest	Vision	Use of mirror
Mandible					
Left buccal	Right	3 o'clock	Bicuspid/cuspid	Direct	Retract cheek
Right lingual	Right	3 o'clock	Bicuspid/cuspid	Direct	Retract tongue
Left lingual	Left	3 o'clock	Bicuspid/cuspid	Indirect	Retract cheek; indirect vision and illumination
Right buccal	Left	1 o'clock	Bicuspid/cuspid	Direct	Retract cheek
Anterior lingual	Straight†	1 o'clock	Cuspid	Direct	Reflect light; retract tongue
Anterior labial	Straight†	1 o'clock	Cuspid	Direct or indirect	Indirect vision; retract lip
Maxilla					
Left buccal	Right	3 o'clock	Occlusal surface of tooth posterior to area of operation	Direct	Retract cheek
Right lingual	Right	3 o'clock		Direct	Reflect light
Left lingual	Left	1 o'clock		Indirect	Indirect vision; reflect light
Right buccal	Left	1 o'clock		Direct	Retract cheek
Anterior lingual	Straight†	1 o'clock	Incisal edge	Indirect	Indirect vision; reflect light
Anterior labial	Straight†	1 o'clock	Incisal edge	Direct	None

*Patient is in the supine position.
†Patient is asked to turn his/her head slightly as clinician moves from cuspid to cuspid in the anterior areas.

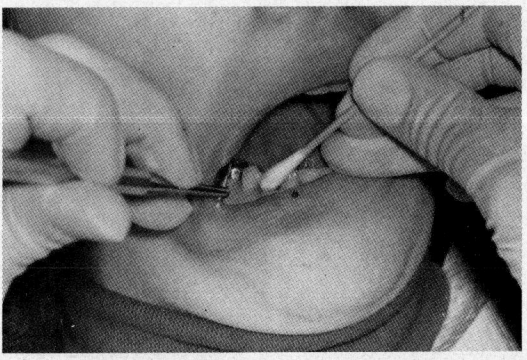

Fig. 6-13. Modified pen grasp for right-handed clinician, showing cheek retraction and stable third-finger fulcrum on teeth for access to mandibular right buccal area.

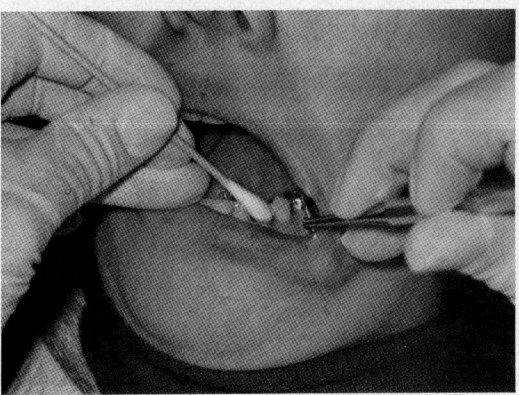

Fig. 6-14. Modified pen grasp for left-handed clinician, showing cheek retraction and stable third-finger fulcrum on teeth for access to mandibular left buccal area.

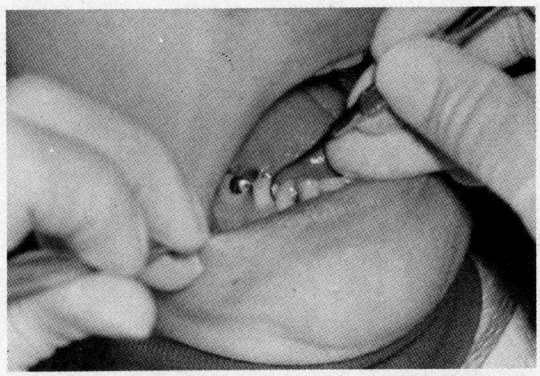

Fig. 6-15. Right-handed clinician: Hand position for instrumentation on mandibular right buccal aspect. Once cotton-tipped applicator has been used in each area, student may progress to periodontal probe to learn subgingival insertion and to explorer to learn adaptation. Mirror retracts cheek; fulcrum is anterior to operative site, resting on occlusal surfaces.

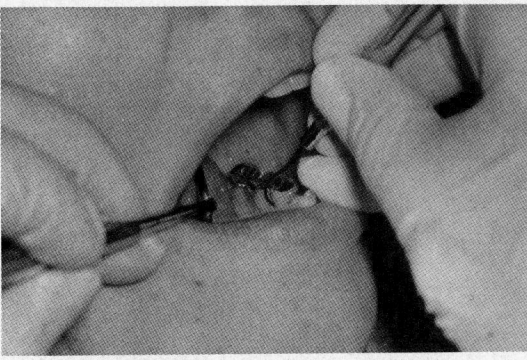

Fig. 6-16. Right-handed clinician: Hand position for instrumentation on mandibular left lingual aspect. Mirror retracts tongue. Fulcrum is on facial-occlusal aspect of teeth in that sextant.

in sequence. Skill with the mouth mirror should be considerable, and beginning skills for instruments used with the working hand should be apparent.

As the positioning exercise is implemented, the skills of the modified pen grasp, fulcrum, and wrist rock should improve.

Following the arbitrary sequence of positions found in Tables 6-1 and 6-2 allows integration of time and motion economy with mastery of most dental hygiene instruments as each instrument is learned. The sequence is designed to minimize position and instrument changes and to provide a systematic approach to completing each arch or quadrant. Experienced clinicians may have variations in approach to specific areas that complement or replace some of the suggested positions and sequence.

Typically difficult areas to master are (1) the lingual surfaces of the mandibular quadrant closest to the clinician (Fig. 6-17 or 6-29), (2) the buccal surfaces of the maxillary quadrant closest to the clinician (Fig. 6-21 or 6-33), and (3) the lingual surfaces of the quadrant (Fig. 6-23 or 6-35).

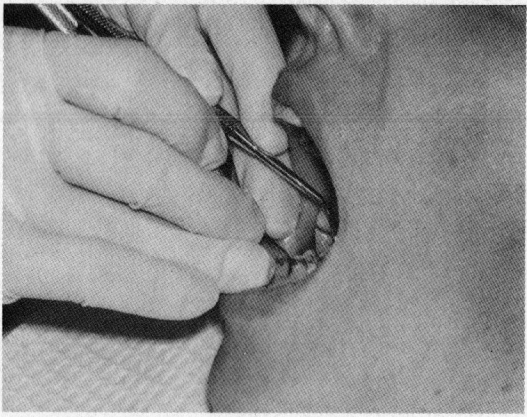

Fig. 6-17. *Right-handed clinician:* Hand position for instrumentation on mandibular right lingual aspect. Mirror retracts tongue but faces teeth, directing light onto area and providing indirect vision. Some clinicians prefer to approach this area from a rear position, with patient's head turned well toward clinician to enable direct vision.

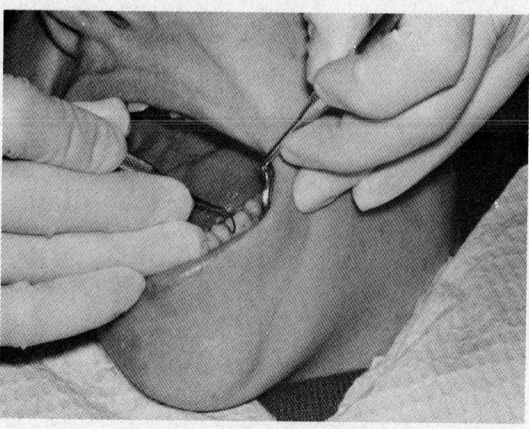

Fig. 6-18. *Right-handed clinician:* Hand position for instrumentation on mandibular left buccal aspect. With patient's head turned toward clinician, mirror retracts cheek, enabling direct vision. Clinician is seated in rear position.

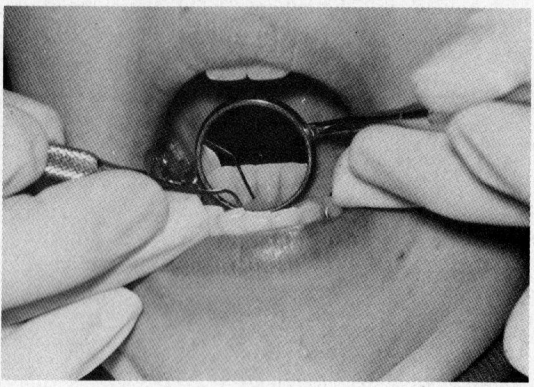

Fig. 6-19. *Right-handed clinician:* Hand position for instrumentation on mandibular anterior lingual aspect. Seated in rear position, clinician uses mirror to retract tongue and reflect light on area for direct vision.

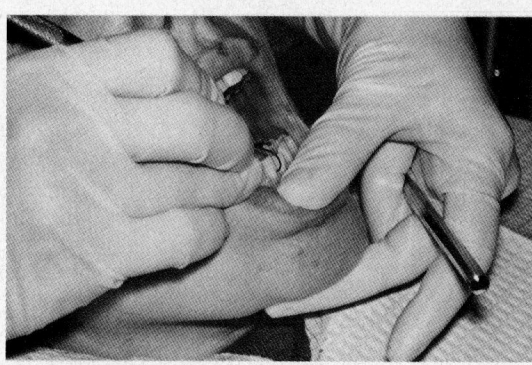

Fig. 6-20. *Right-handed clinician:* Hand position for instrumentation on mandibular anterior facial aspect. Clinician is seated in rear position. Lower lip is retracted by thumb, forefinger, or mouth mirror. Direct vision is used. When direct vision is difficult to achieve, mouth mirror can retract lip and provide indirect vision.

Problems with the positions shown in Figs. 6-17 and 6-29 usually arise from the dual role of the mouth mirror. It is both retracting the tongue and cheek and serving as a source of indirect vision. Many times it also acts to reflect light on an otherwise dark area. Therefore the beginning clinician needs to acquire a high degree of control with the mirror. The shank retracts the cheek, the back of the mirror head retracts the tongue, and the face of the mirror serves as the primary source of vision and illumination. The patient's head position is critical in enabling all this to happen. Many clinicians prefer to approach this area from a rear position, with the patient's head turned well toward them.

The maxillary right buccal (for right-handed clinicians) and the maxillary left buccal (for left-handed clinicians) are controversial as well as dif-

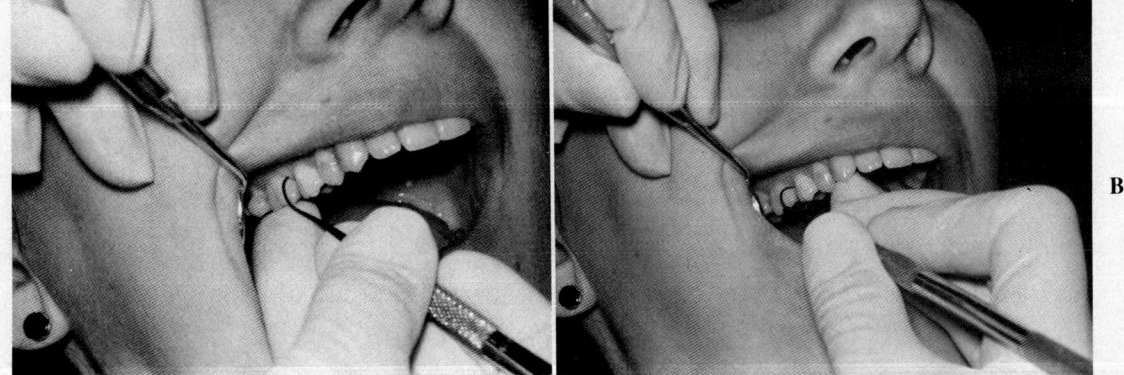

Fig. 6-21. *Right-handed clinician:* Two approaches to maxillary right buccal aspect. **A,** Palm up, fulcrum on or posterior to operative site, giving stability and greater leverage for deposit removal during scaling. Clinician is seated at approximately 9:30 position. **B,** Palm down, fulcrum anterior to area being explored. Clinician is seated in front position. While this technique is easier to learn and is adequate for exploring, it provides less control and leverage during scaling. A vertical wrist rock (see Fig. 6-9) is used for this approach.

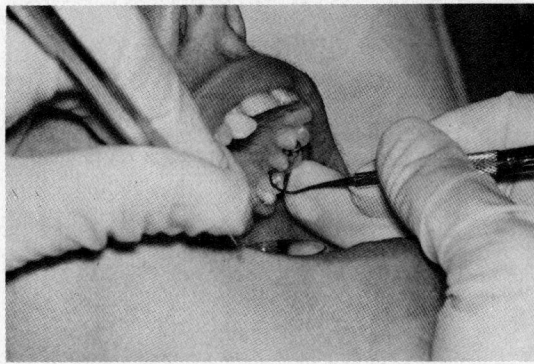

Fig. 6-22. *Right-handed clinician:* Hand position for instrumentation on maxillary left lingual aspect. Fulcrum is placed on occlusal surface of tooth or slightly on buccal aspect. All fingers are kept together as a single unit to ensure a solid wrist rock and stroke. Mirror reflects light onto area. Direct vision is used, with patient's head tilted away. Clinician is seated in front position.

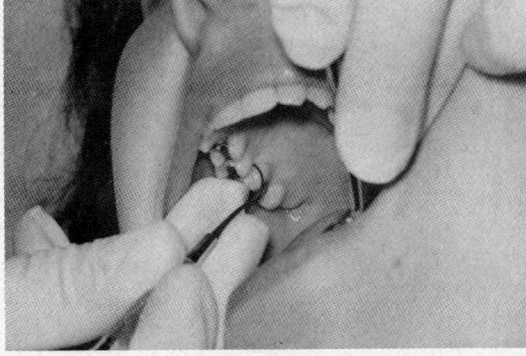

Fig. 6-23. *Right-handed clinician:* Hand position for instrumentation on maxillary right lingual aspect. Clinician is in rear position. Mirror reflects light and provides indirect vision. Fulcrum is on occlusal aspect of sextant. Maintaining good posture, clinician holds mirror so it is visible, then angles mirror until light is cast on area to be explored and image is visible in mirror.

ficult areas. Most people agree that the mirror retracts the cheek. The controversy centers around fulcrum placement and hand position. The easiest approach to learn is to place the fulcrum anterior to the area to be examined with the palm down. The wrist rock then becomes a back-and-forth vertical rock rather than a rock to the side (Figs. 6-21, *B,* and 6-33, *B).*

The more difficult position to learn is the placement of the fulcrum finger on the occlusal surface of the tooth posterior to the tooth being examined, with the palm up. Although the clinician is in a front position, it usually is at 9:30 o'clock, (or 2:30 o'clock for left-handed clinicians) with the body turned toward the patient. For beginners

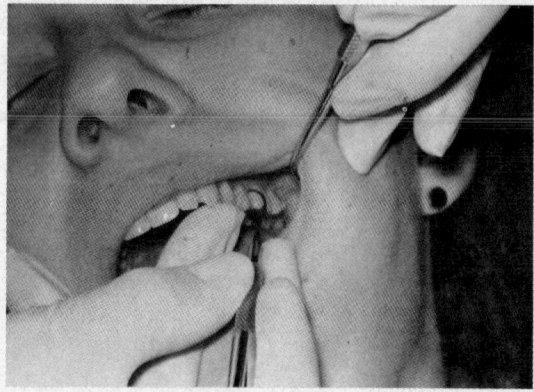

Fig. 6-24. *Right-handed clinician:* Hand position for instrumentation on maxillary left buccal aspect. Clinician is in rear position. Mirror retracts cheek, and fulcrum is on occlusal aspect of teeth, with patient's head turned toward clinician for direct vision.

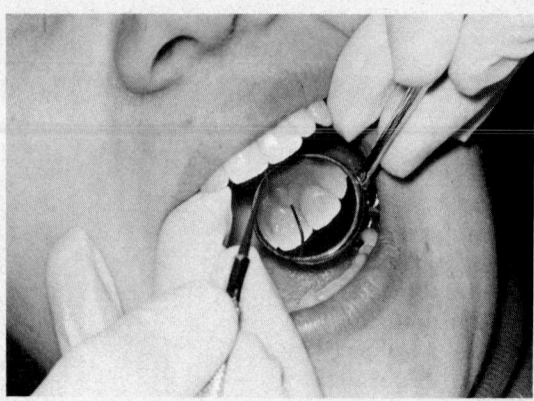

Fig. 6-25. *Right-handed clinician:* Hand position for instrumentation on maxillary anterior lingual aspect. Clinician remains in rear position and uses mirror to reflect light and provide indirect vision. Maintaining good posture, clinician holds mirror so it is visible, then angles mirror until area is illuminated and visible in mirror. Fulcrum is on incisal edge, with palm up for efficient wrist rock.

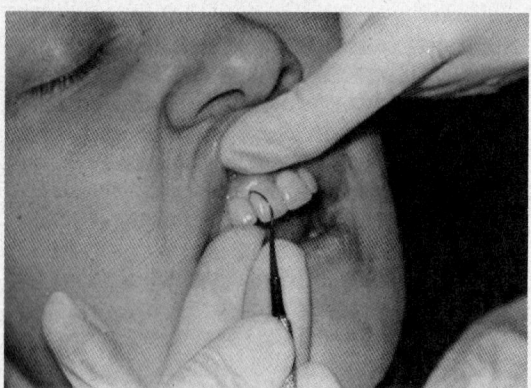

Fig. 6-26. *Right-handed clinician:* Hand position for instrumentation on maxillary anterior labial aspect. To ensure a stable fulcrum, rear position is preferred. Hand remains a solid unit, with all fingers resting on fulcrum, palm up. Direct vision is used, with forefinger retracting lip.

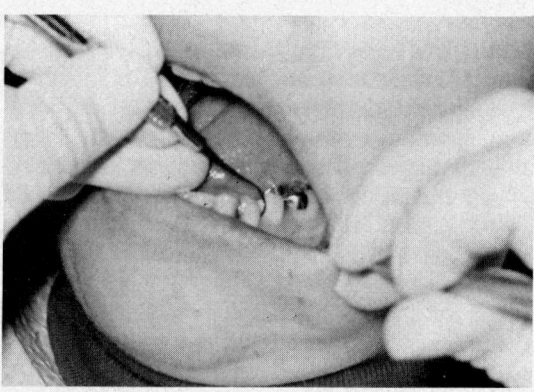

Fig. 6-27. *Left-handed clinician:* Hand position for instrumentation on mandibular left buccal aspect. Once cotton-tipped applicator has been used in each area, student may progress to periodontal probe to learn subgingival insertion and to explorer to learn adaptation. Mirror retracts cheek; fulcrum is anterior to operative site, resting on occlusal surfaces.

it is best to practice this position on the premolars, moving posteriorly tooth by tooth. As the clinician's hand moves back toward the last molar, the actual fulcrum is less on the fingertip on the tooth and more on the side of the finger on the muscular resistance of the obicularis oris (Figs. 6-21, *A,* and 6-33, *A).*

This palm-up position may be more difficult to master, but according to the laws of physics, it

increases control of the instruments, makes it possible to maintain proper terminal shank relation to the tooth, and allows for more efficient use of strength in engaging and removing hard deposits from the teeth and in root planing.

The difficulties encountered with the lingual side of that quadrant are simpler to identify and overcome. Usually, at first the student has difficulty working with a mirror image. This area re-

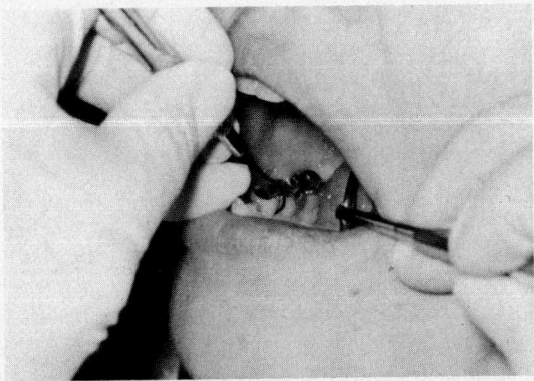

Fig. 6-28. *Left-handed clinician:* Hand position for instrumentation on mandibular right lingual aspect. Mirror retracts tongue. Fulcrum is on facial-occlusal aspect of teeth in that sextant.

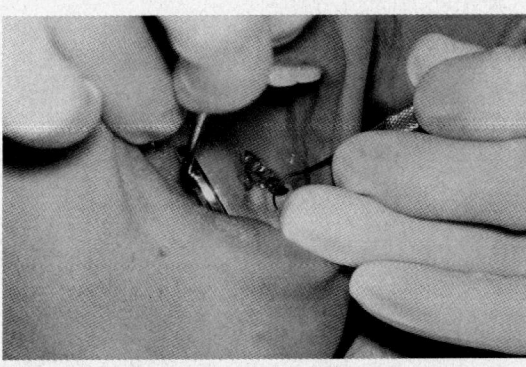

Fig. 6-29. *Left-handed clinician:* Hand position for instrumentation on mandibular left lingual aspect. Mirror retracts tongue but faces teeth, directing light onto area and providing indirect vision. Some clinicians prefer to approach this area from a rear position, with patient's head turned well toward clinician to enable direct vision.

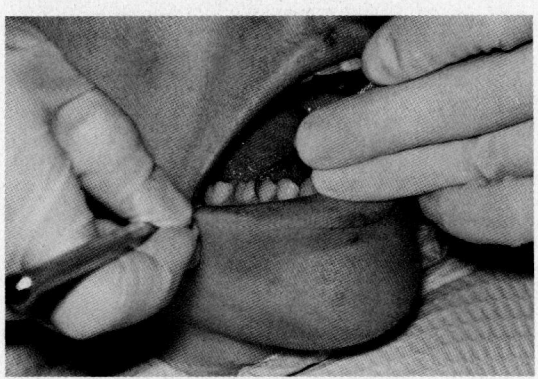

Fig. 6-30. *Left-handed clinician:* Hand position for instrumentation on mandibular right buccal aspect. With patient's head turned toward clinician, mirror retracts cheek, enabling direct vision. Clinician is seated in rear position.

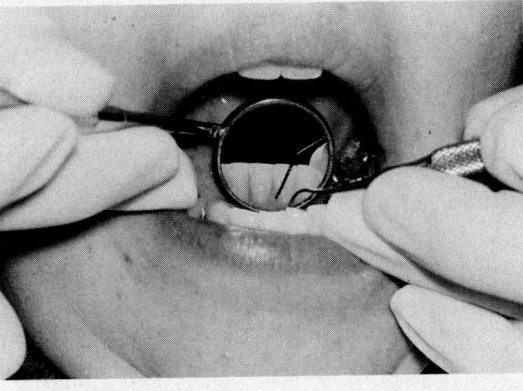

Fig. 6-31. *Left-handed clinician:* Hand position for instrumentation on mandibular anterior lingual aspect. Seated in rear position, clinician uses mirror to retract tongue and reflect light on area for direct vision.

lies heavily on indirect vision by means of the mirror. Ways to overcome this are to bring the mirror to the front of the mouth and to maintain good posture. With the mirror located in the anterior area, the reflective surface can be seen clearly by the seated clinician. The mirror head is then angled until the area to be examined is visible in the mirror. Skill in moving the working hand in the intended direction while looking at a mirror image will develop with practice. This is one reason why rubbing the cotton-tipped applicator up

and down the tooth structure is good practice. It is a safe instrument with which to learn indirect vision and instrument control.

Exercises with the periodontal probe

Once the student can move quickly and easily from area to area using the proper positioning, mirror function, grasp, fulcrum, and wrist rock, he or she is ready to learn to use the periodontal probe.

Since the periodontal probe can be used on all

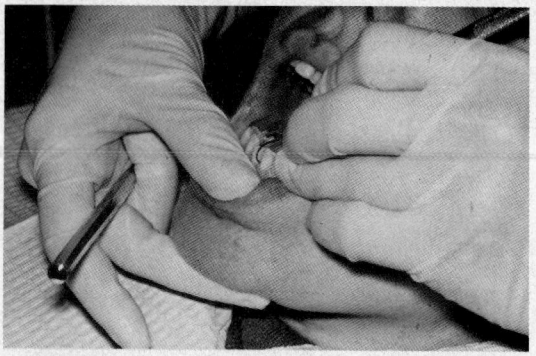

Fig. 6-32. *Left-handed clinician:* Hand position for instrumentation on mandibular anterior facial aspect. Clinician is seated in rear position. Lower lip is retracted by thumb, forefinger, or mouth mirror. Direct vision is used. When direct vision is difficult to achieve, mouth mirror can retract lip and provide indirect vision.

A 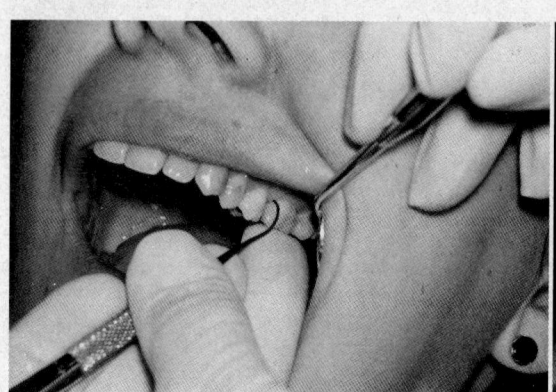 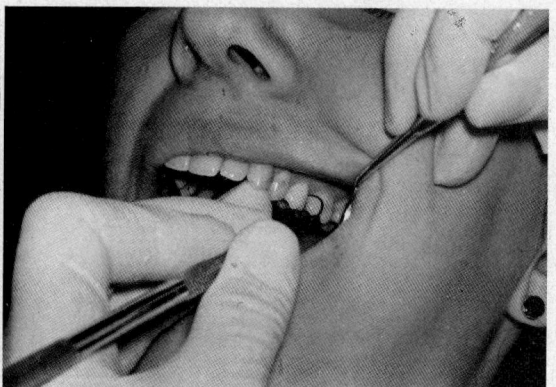 B

Fig. 6-33. *Left-handed clinician:* Two approaches to maxillary left buccal aspect. **A,** Palm up, fulcrum on or posterior to operative site, giving stability and greater leverage for deposit removal during scaling. Clinician is seated at approximately 2:30 position. **B,** Palm down, fulcrum anterior to area being explored. Clinician is seated in front position. While this technique is easier to learn and is adequate for exploring, it provides less control and leverage during scaling. A vertical wrist rock (see Fig. 6-9) is used for this approach.

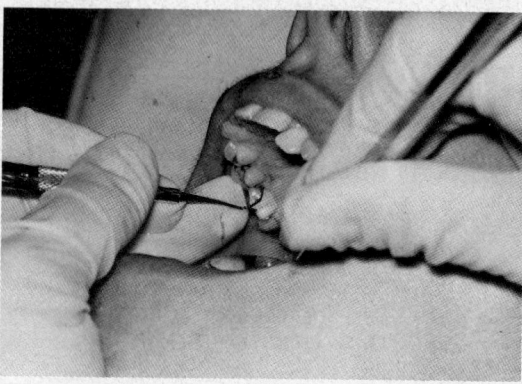

Fig. 6-34. *Left-handed clinician:* Hand position for instrumentation on maxillary right lingual aspect. Fulcrum is placed on occlusal surface of tooth or slightly on buccal aspect. All fingers are kept together as single unit to ensure a solid wrist rock and stroke. Mirror reflects light onto area. Direct vision is used, with patient's head tilted away. Clinician is seated in front position.

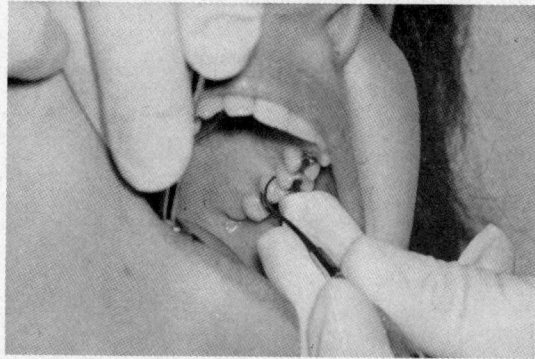

Fig. 6-35. *Left-handed clinician:* Hand position for instrumentation on maxillary left lingual aspect. Clinician is in rear position. Mirror reflects light and provides indirect vision. Fulcrum is on occlusal aspect of sextant. Maintaining good posture, clinician holds mirror so it is visible, then angles mirror until light is cast on area to be explored and image is visible in mirror.

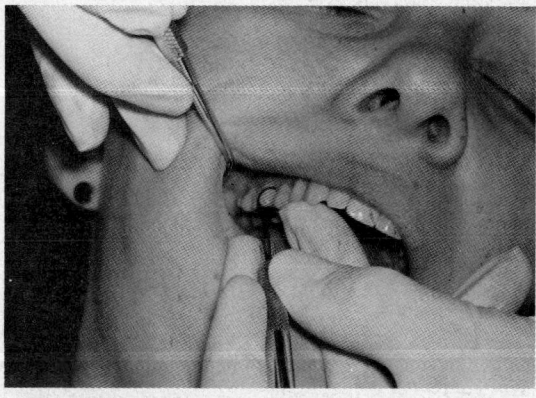

Fig. 6-36. *Left-handed clinician:* Hand position for instrumentation on maxillary right buccal aspect. Clinician is in rear position. Mirror retracts cheek, and fulcrum is on occlusal aspect of teeth, with patient's head turned toward clinician for direct vision.

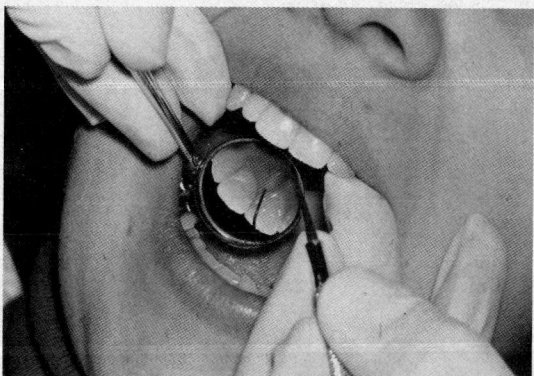

Fig. 6-37. *Left-handed clinician:* Hand position for instrumentation on maxillary anterior lingual aspect. Clinician remains in rear position and uses mirror to reflect light and provide indirect vision. Maintaining good posture, clinician holds mirror so it is visible, then angles mirror until area is illuminated and visible in mirror. Fulcrum is on incisal edge, with palm up for efficient wrist rock.

surfaces (universally) and has no cutting edge or sharpened point, it is a relatively safe beginner's instrument. In addition, it is a key instrument in assessing oral health. Sliding it into the gingival sulcus reveals the depth of the sulcus and the presence of root irregularities and hard deposits. Gently bobbing the instrument up and down in the sulcus (using an overlapping *stroke* pattern) as it travels around the tooth helps the clinician trace the topography of the attachment. Thus, even in the first phases of learning instrumentation, the clinician can learn about his or her partner's oral conditions.

Guidelines for using the probe include the following:

1. Using the same positioning, grasp, fulcrum, and wrist rock as was practiced in the previous exercise
2. Sliding the probe into the sulcus until it meets the elastic resistance of the epithelial attachment
3. Using approximately 1 mm of the tip of the calibrated portion of the instrument to feel the side of the tooth as it slides in and out of the sulcus and around the tooth
4. Keeping the calibrated portion of the instrument parallel to the long axis of the tooth, except for modifications necessary to accommodate the flare of the crown of the tooth

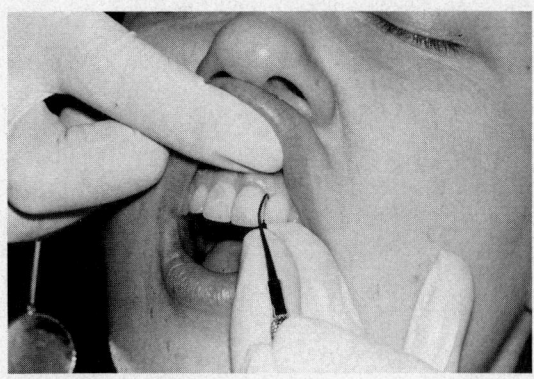

Fig. 6-38. *Left-handed clinician:* Hand position for instrumentation on maxillary anterior labial aspect. To ensure a stable fulcrum, rear position is preferred. Hand remains a solid unit, with all fingers resting on fulcrum, palm up. Direct vision is used, with forefinger retracting lip.

5. Using the wrist rock to move the instrument coronally for each stroke
6. Pivoting on the fulcrum finger and rolling the instrument slightly in the fingers to move the bobbing instrument around the tooth

The probe should slide in gently so as to avoid causing pain; yet it must travel the full depth of the sulcus or pocket to yield valuable, accurate information. One frequent error is failure to "instrumentate" far enough across the proximal surfaces (Ward and Simring, 1978). If the probe is not placed to the base of the sulcus at the middle portion of the proximal surface, the most frequent site of early periodontal disease will remain unexamined. Examining this area, particularly below contact areas, may necessitate a *slightly* angled approach with the probe.

One way to begin probing a tooth is to *insert* the probe into the sulcus at the distofacial line angle and *bob* or *walk* the instrument across the distal surface (at least slightly more than halfway); *retrace* the probing to the distofacial line angle and *across the facial* surface, past the facial line angle at least slightly more than halfway *across the mesial;* and *back out* to the mesial line angle. The probe should not emerge completely from the sulcus with each stroke. Rather, the probe should remain subgingival as it travels around the tooth (Fig. 6-39).

The student serving as the assistant should record millimeter readings for the distal, facial, and mesial surfaces and then for the distal, lingual, and mesial surfaces for each tooth as it is probed in sequence. Otherwise, the clinician should record findings for at least two teeth in each sextant. The faculty member should circulate to help students improve their grasp, fulcrum position, wrist rock, stroke (in and out of the sulcus), adaptation of the tip to the tooth, and pivot motion around the tooth.

By the end of the exercise, the student should have probed all areas of the mouth and measured two teeth for sulcus depth in each sextant of teeth. The student should have acquired entry-level competence in at least six of the following skills:

Proper positioning
Grasp of instrument
Fulcrum placement and use
Wrist rock
Adaptation of tip to tooth
Smooth sulcular bobbing and walking strokes around tooth
Maintenance of calibrated position in parallel relation to long axis of tooth
Guidance of instrument at least slightly more than halfway across proximal surfaces
Measurements of sulcus accurate within 1 mm

Further practice sessions should allow students to concentrate on those areas in which they are not yet skilled.

Exercises with the paired explorer

Many of the basics of instrumentation given in the previous two exercises will prove helpful in learning to use the paired explorer (such as the cowhorn or pigtail). The student will learn to (1) select the appropriate end of the explorer for adaptation in each area of the dentition, (2) adapt

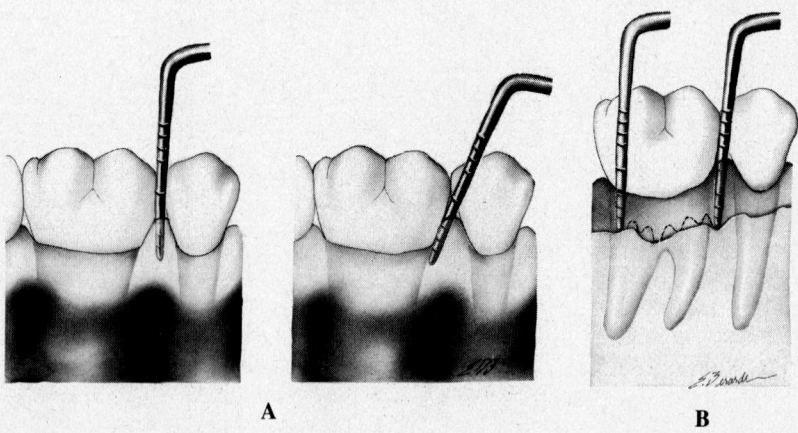

A   B

Fig. 6-39. A, Incorrect *(left)* and correct *(right)* adaptations of probe to tooth. Correct adaptation ensures that tip is adapted and is not free to engage soft tissue in sulcular wall. Walking, or bobbing, motion of probe in sulcus is shown in **B.** Note that probe follows topography of attachment.

the side of a sharp tip against the tooth to minimize discomfort, and (3) change (pivot) the direction of a tip moving out from the distal surface so that it can be guided in an anterior direction across a facial or lingual surface, around the mesial line angle, and across the mesial surface.

For this exercise the same positioning, use of the mouth mirror, pen grasp, fulcrum, and wrist rock are used. The stroke with the instrument is an overlapping pattern of vertical strokes around the tooth. The purpose for using the instrument subgingivally is to detect the presence of calculus, root irregularities, normal anatomic landmarks such as the cementoenamel junction (CEJ), and root furrows and contours. The thin shank and working end facilitate the transmission of vibrations to the clinician's fingers and thumb holding the shank and handle. It can be used supragingivally to examine the tooth for roughness and contours to confirm what is visible.

In selecting which end to use, it is helpful to (1) select either end of the paired explorer, (2) assume the proper position for the first sextant (mandibular facial area closest to the clinician), (3) establish a proper pen grasp and fulcrum, and (4) place the randomly selected end so that the tip is aimed across the mesial surface from the facial aspect in one of the teeth in the sextant. One of the two views in Fig. 6-40 should resemble this first effort.

The next step is to assess whether the instrument point is curling out toward the tissue as if ready to penetrate it if it were moved subgingivally. Depending on the selected end, the point will be directed either toward the soft tissue or toward the tooth. The latter, for obvious reasons, is preferable.

Another cue is whether the terminal shank (which is contiguous with the working tip) is horizontal or vertical. The point is curved toward the tooth when the terminal shank is vertical. Thus a handy guide for determining which end to use is to look at the direction of the point and the terminal shank's relation to the long axis of the tooth. The end that aligns the terminal shank with the long axis of the tooth will provide correct adaptation for distal, facial, and mesial surfaces on the first sextant of teeth. Fig. 6-40, *A,* meets these criteria.

Once the proper end is selected, the side of the tip (1 to 2 mm) should be placed on the distobuccal line angle. A wrist rock should be activated to move the instrument up and down. A pivot on the fulcrum finger and a slight rolling of the instrument in the fingers should guide the tip around the line angle and across the distal surface at least

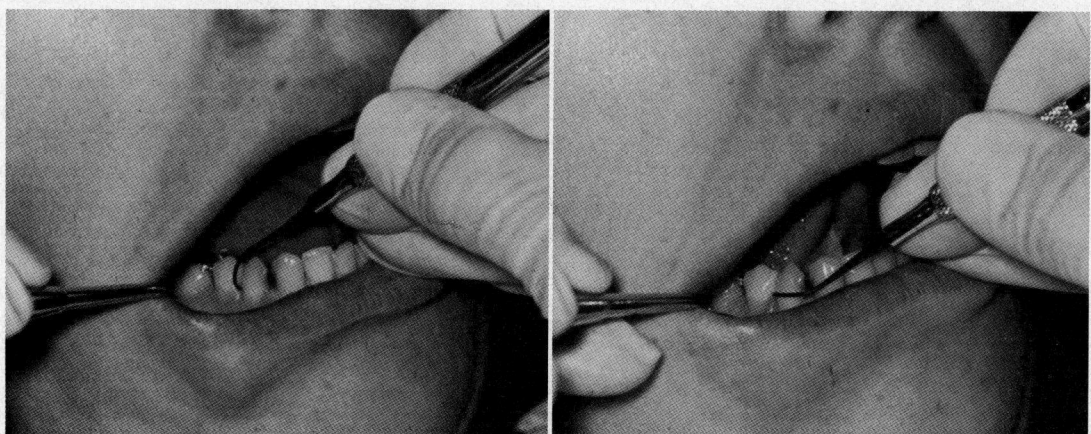

A   **B**

Fig. 6-40. **A,** Adaptation of one end of cowhorn explorer to mesial surface of tooth with point directed across mesial surface. Terminal shank is parallel to long axis of tooth; point is curved in toward tooth. **B,** Opposite end of explorer, which, although adapted in same area, has terminal shank in horizontal relationship with point curved toward gingiva. These cues help in selecting correct end of paired cowhorn explorer.

slightly more than halfway (Pattison and Behrens, 1973). The clinician should concentrate on what can be felt with 1 mm of the side of the tip. He or she should explore for calculus, the CEJ, rough margins of restorations, and the root shape.

Then the side of the tip should be bobbed back out to the distobuccal line angle. The tip should be pivoted so that it is aimed toward the anterior of the mouth, and the side of the tip should contact the facial aspect of the tooth. Again, a pivot of the hand on the fulcrum finger and a slight rolling of the instrument in the fingers should allow the side of the tip to move past the mesiobuccal line angle onto and across the mesial surface. The tip is then backed out to the mesiobuccal line angle and removed from the tooth (Figs. 6-41 to 6-46). It is critical to keep 1 to 2 mm of the tip in contact with the tooth. No more and no less should be used; otherwise (1) the tip may wander into the tissue, (2) it is less possible to determine exact locations of deposits, and/or (3) the point will merely scratch over the tooth, sending misleading vibrations to the clinician's hand (Pattison and Behrens, 1973).

It is also important to use overlapping strokes that cover the area. A few long sweeping strokes do not thoroughly evaluate a tooth surface for the presence of miniscule deposits and root roughness (Pattison and Behrens, 1973).

As with probing, exploring must drop to the attachment with each stroke to complete a thorough evaluation of subgingival areas (Pattison and Behrens, 1973). Gentle subgingival exploring does not allow the explorer to exit completely from the sulcus with each stroke. Reentry to the sulcus for each downward motion is unnecessary and may cause trauma to the margin of the gingiva.

A student exploring a partner's teeth should identify calculus, root irregularities, and margins of restorations while focusing on stroke and adaptation. The faculty member should circulate to help students improve form and approach. Each student should be able to identify all areas in the dentition where each end of the explorer can be adapted simply by testing the direction of the point and the relationship of the terminal shank to the tooth's long axis. If one end can be adapted on the facial aspect of teeth No. 28 to No. 32, where else in the dentition can the *same end* be used?

At the completion of the exercise the student should have improved performance in the following basic skills:

Positioning and maintenance of vision
Grasp
Fulcrum location and maintenance
Wrist rock
Exploratory stroke

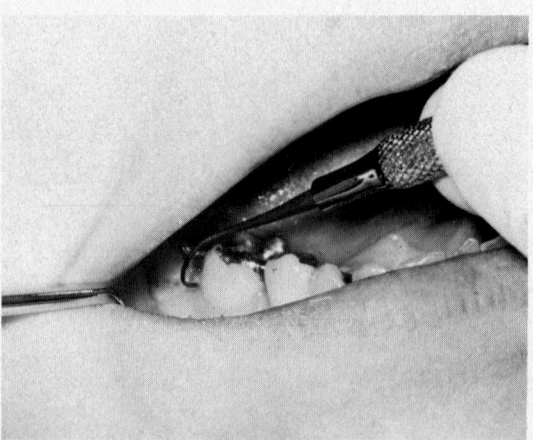

Fig. 6-41. Explorer is inserted on tooth's distobuccal line angle and is moved with vertical strokes around line angle into proximal area to fully explore distal surface.

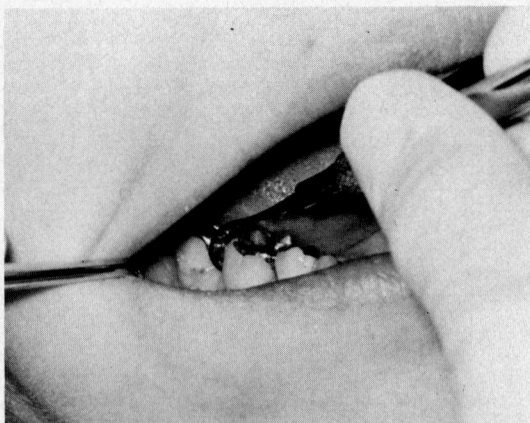

Fig. 6-42. Once explorer is more than halfway across distal surface and has explored from attachment to margin of gingiva, it should be backed out to distobuccal line angle with overlapping strokes.

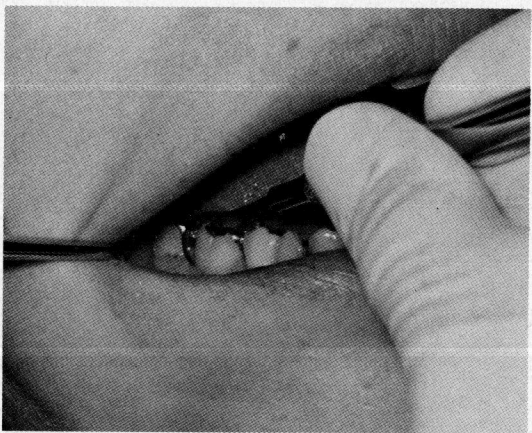

Fig. 6-43. At distolingual line angle the point is pivoted so that it is directed toward mesial aspect of tooth and stroked in overlapping pattern across facial surface.

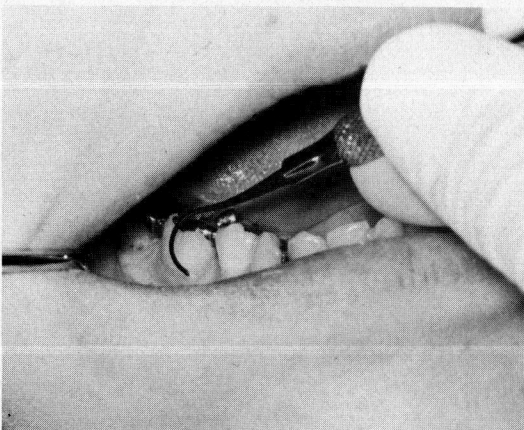

Fig. 6-44. When explorer reaches mesiobuccal line angle, tip is pivoted so that it stays in adaptation with tooth and does not wander into soft tissue. Stroking pattern continues around line angle and into mesial aspect to fully explore proximal surface.

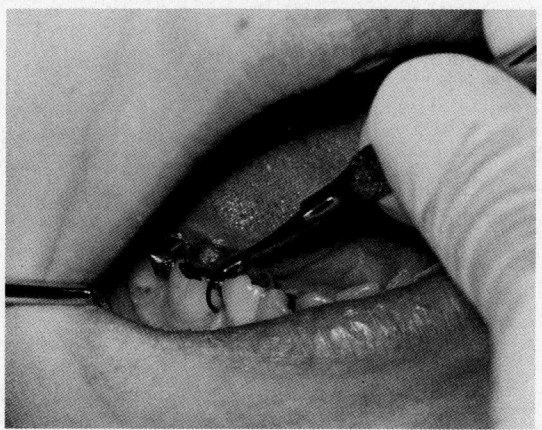

Fig. 6-45. Thorough exploration of mesial surface includes moving explorer in vertical and oblique pattern over all subgingival tooth surface, ensuring that area is fully explored to base of sulcus more than halfway across tooth.

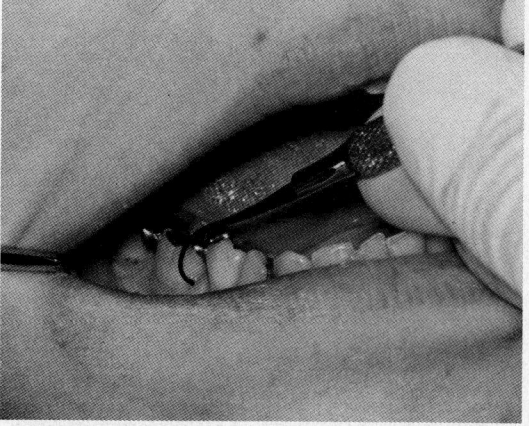

Fig. 6-46. After fully exploring mesial aspect of tooth, explorer is backed out to mesiobuccal line angle, where it is removed from sulcus. Tip of explorer should remain in subgingival position throughout its course around tooth to minimize trauma of reentering sulcus with each stroke.

The student should have learned how to select the correct end of a paired explorer for any sextant in the dentition and be able to adapt the tip safely and effectively. Safety and effectiveness should improve with practice.

Exercises with the "anterior" explorer

Once adaptation of the tip to the tooth has been added to the student's repertoire of entry-level skills, it is possible to move from the paired contra-angled explorer to the more simply designed "straight shanked" explorer such as the No. 17 or No. 20. The shanks for these explorers do have bends and angles, but they do not have the contra-angles that necessitate their use in pairs. The No. 20 explorer is shaped similarly to the No. 17; however, it is much finer and has a longer shank and thus more flex.

The No. 17 or No. 20 can be used almost universally; accessibility is limited to the relatively straight shank that makes it difficult to obtain a solid fulcrum and adaptation in posterior areas. For purposes of simplicity (and with the full acknowledgment that the instrument *can be* and *is* used in posterior areas), the instrument is referred to here as an *anterior* instrument. The maxim "the simpler the shank, the more anterior the intended use of the instrument," is applied here for explorers and later in those chapters in which scalers and curettes are discussed. Variations in areas of use can be added as the student gains experience and confidence.

One reason for calling the No. 17 or No. 20 explorer an *anterior* instrument is that it allows the student to learn some basic principles associated with adapting instruments into anterior teeth prior to learning about cutting edges.

When an anterior instrument is being used, the terminal shank is kept parallel to the long axis of the tooth. To do this, the fulcrum must be on the same tooth or on the immediately adjacent one (Fig. 6-47). Allowing the fulcrum to rest two or three teeth away causes the terminal shank to angle in the direction of the fulcrum rather than remaining parallel to the tooth's long axis.

Many straight-shanked instruments can be used with a circumferential or horizontal stroke (as opposed to a vertical stroke) on the facial and lingual surfaces of teeth, including posterior teeth. The tip is angled more apically, the shank is *not* parallel to the long axis of the tooth, and the tip moves in short overlapping oblique strokes from line angle to line angle (Fig. 6-48).

Another key factor is the need to accommodate the sharp line angles of the anterior teeth. If the tip is not carefully adapted to the tooth as the surface changes from facial to proximal, the sharp point will catch the gingiva, causing an iatrogenic hemorrhage point and its accompanying discomfort.

Therefore practice in adapting the instrument is the focus in learning anterior instruments. The exercise also allows the student to improve skills in the following:

Positioning and maintenance of vision
Grasp
Fulcrum location and maintenance
Wrist rock
Exploratory stroke
Detection of irregularities, landmarks, and calculus

At the completion of exploring the anterior teeth, the student should have achieved entry-level competence in all of the aforementioned skills and be able to explore anterior teeth and the direct facial and lingual surfaces of any tooth in-

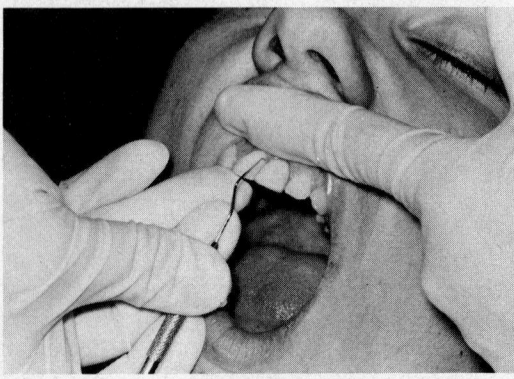

Fig. 6-47. When an anterior-design instrument is used, fulcrum must be on same tooth or nearby tooth to ensure that shank is parallel to long axis of tooth.

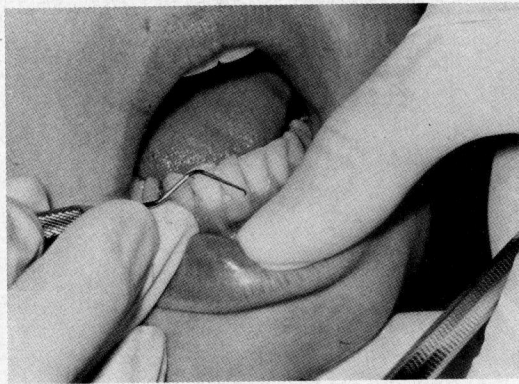

Fig. 6-48. Instruments may be used with a circumferential or horizontal stroke around tooth. Tip is placed so that it is inclined apically and with terminal shank at 45-degree angle to long axis of teeth. Care must be taken to adapt carefully at line angles when using this stroke on facial and lingual aspects.

the dentition without creating iatrogenic hemorrhage points or pain.

Another straight-shanked explorer is the shepherd's hook (No. 23). It can be used for calculus detection, but its use is frequently limited to caries detection because of the thickness of its tip and shank (Pattison and Behrens, 1973).

Fig. 6-49 shows the No. 23 explorer adapted for caries detection in the distal pit of tooth No. 28. The sharp point of the explorer is pressed into the pit to see if it sticks in soft tooth structure (caries). If resistance is felt as the explorer is removed from the tooth structure, the area is usually considered carious and worthy of further evaluation for restoration.

In addition to exploring pits for caries, the explorer can be used to check grooves, margins of restorations, and other caries-prone areas of the teeth, such as the gingival third of the facial and lingual surfaces and the proximal surfaces. While it is usually necessary to examine a patient radiographically in order to rule out proximal caries, large lesions can often be found with an explorer.

The student should explore a partner's teeth for caries and for defective margins of restorations by placing the point into the pits and grooves, applying pressure, and detecting *retention* of the point in a *soft area*. Similarly, gently tracing the margins allows the detection of caries and other defects around restorations.

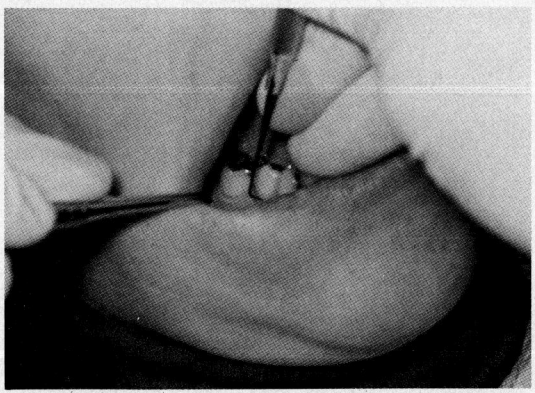

Fig. 6-50. Exploring for calculus with No. 6 explorer, a simply designed instrument with universal use.

ADJUNCT EXPLORERS

Refer again to Figs. 6-1 and 6-2 and note the variety of explorers available for calculus and caries detection. With greater experience a clinician can experiment with the variety that is available.

Fig. 6-50 shows the No. 6 explorer being adapted in the posterior teeth. It has a simple design with only one angle in the shank. The terminal shank is the portion that is in the same plane with the handle, and it is maintained in a nearly parallel relationship to the long axis of the tooth. The tip is angled slightly downward into the sulcus, but not so that it is pointed directly apically. This instrument can be used universally; its versatility makes it a popular choice.

SUMMARY

The probe and explorers are valuable tools for assessing dental health. They also provide a framework for learning basic positioning and instrumentation skills, which can be generalized to apply to the use of other instruments.

Once the student is familiar with the probe, a paired contra-angled explorer, and a straight-shanked explorer, other instruments used for exploring can be learned. Students should then use the instruments to prepare assessment data for partners or for the patients of more advanced students.

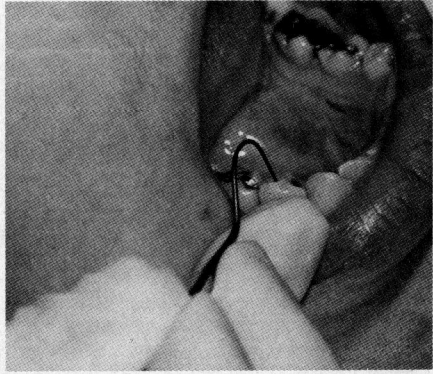

Fig. 6-49. Shepherd's hook (No. 23) explorer is usually reserved for caries detection because of its thick, resilient shank. Its sharp point is pressed into pits and grooves and suspicious margins of restorations to see if it sticks in soft tooth structure (caries).

ACTIVITIES

1. Compare a variety of instruments to determine the parts of the instruments, to distinguish between double-ended and paired instruments, and to examine shank shape and strength and the location of the terminal shank.
2. Ask a partner to grasp the handle of an instrument you are holding and try to move it while you are using each of the following grasps. Which grasp provides the most stability against movement? How would this grasp ensure best control of the instrument?
   a. A typical pen grasp used in holding a pencil
   b. The modified pen grasp, but with the knuckle buckled as shown in Fig. 6-6, *B*
   c. The modified pen grasp as shown in Fig. 6-6, *A*
3. *Exercises in positioning.* In groups of three, rotate from clinician to assistant to patient roles in completing the following procedures:
   a. As chairside assistant
      (1) Disinfect unit
      (2) Place sterile mirror and cotton-tipped applicator on covered tray
      (3) Clear pathway for patient entry to chair
      (4) Position patient:
         (a) Tilt chair back
         (b) Lower back of chair
         (c) Adjust headrest
         (d) Place drape
      (5) Adjust assistant's stool to proper height and location
      (6) Adjust overhead light to ensure illumination of each area
   b. As patient
      (1) Comment on seating comfort
      (2) Comment on comfortable use of mouth mirror and cotton-tipped applicator
      (3) Turn head as requested by clinician
      (4) Hold table of positions for clinician and assistant reference
   c. As clinician
      (1) Adjust stool properly (thighs parallel to floor; feet flat on floor; abdominal rest below rib cage)
      (2) Seat self at chairside at 9 o'clock position (for right-handed clinician) or at 3 o'clock position (for left-handed clinician)
      (3) Use Table 6-1 or 6-2 to guide position, mouth mirror use, and fulcrum placement for each of the following areas of the mouth:

Right-handed clinician	Left-handed clinician
Mandibular	Mandibular
Right buccal	Left buccal
Left lingual	Right lingual
Right lingual	Left lingual
Left buccal	Right buccal
Anterior lingual	Anterior lingual
Anterior labial	Anterior labial
Maxillary	Maxillary
Right buccal	Left buccal
Left lingual	Right lingual
Right lingual	Left lingual
Left buccal	Right buccal
Anterior lingual	Anterior lingual
Anterior labial	Anterior labial

      (4) Use mouth mirror as indicated for each area
      (5) Use cotton-tipped applicator as dental instrument to explore two teeth in each area, using
         (a) Modified pen grasp
         (b) Fulcrum
         (c) Wrist rock
         (d) Stroking pattern
      (6) Reflect light through anterior teeth with mirror and observe the presence of caries, restorations, or calculus
4. *Exercises with periodontal probe.* In dyads, serve as patient and as clinician in completing the following procedures:
   a. As patient
      (1) Comment on seating comfort
      (2) Comment on comfortable use of mouth mirror and probe
      (3) Monitor proper positioning of clinician
   b. As clinician
      (1) Use proper seating and positioning of self, patient's head, and mouth mirror for each area as described in Tables 6-1 and 6-2
      (2) With periodontal probe in working hand
         (a) Maintain modified pen grasp
         (b) Maintain firm fulcrum
         (c) Gently insert probe in sulcus
         (d) Explore each area with probe
            From distobuccal line angle to direct distal
            From distal to distobuccal line angle and across facial aspect
            Past mesiobuccal line angle to direct mesial and back to mesiobuccal line angle
         (e) Explore with 1 mm of tip adapted to tooth
         (f) Maintain calibrated working end parallel to long axis

(g) Bob or walk instrument from base of sulcus to free margin of gingiva while traveling around tooth

(h) Measure depth of sulcus in millimeters

(3) Record measurements of sulcus depth for at least two teeth in each sextant

5. *Exercise with paired explorer.* In dyads, serve as patient and as clinician in completing the following procedures:

a. As patient

(1) Comment on seating comfort

(2) Comment on comfortable use of mouth mirror and paired explorer

(3) Monitor proper positioning of operator

b. As clinician

(1) Use proper seating and positioning of self, patient's head, and mouth mirror for each area as described in Table 6-1 or 6-2

(2) With paired explorer in working hand

(a) Maintain modified pen grasp

(b) Maintain firm fulcrum

(c) Select proper end of explorer

(d) Adapt side of point (1 mm) to tooth at distobuccal line angle in first area

(e) Activate wrist rock to stroke instrument in overlapping vertical pattern around distal surface and back out to line angle

(f) Pivot point at line angle so that it is aimed anteriorly, stroking vertically across facial surface

(g) Continue stroking past mesiobuccal line angle and across mesial surface, using pivot on fulcrum finger and rolling instrument slightly with fingers

(h) Back instrument out of mesiobuccal line angle using vertical stroking pattern

(i) Remove instrument from sulcus

(3) Explore root anatomy, margins of restorations, and calculus deposits

(4) Watch for iatrogenic hemorrhage points, and correct adaptation to ensure that side of point is in contact with tooth

6. *Exercises with anterior explorer.* In dyads, serve as patient and as clinician in completing the following procedures:

a. As patient

(1) Comment on seating comfort

(2) Comment on comfortable use of mouth mirror and anterior explorer

(3) Monitor proper positioning of clinician

b. As clinician

(1) Use proper seating and positioning of self, patient's head, and mouth mirror for each area as described in Table 6-1 or 6-2

(2) With straight-shanked explorer in working hand

(a) Maintain modified pen grasp

(b) Establish fulcrum close to site of operation in anterior teeth

(c) Maintain terminal shank parallel to long axis of tooth

(d) Adapt 1 mm of tip at line angles and activate vertical overlapping strokes with wrist rock to move instrument across proximal surfaces

(e) Use horizontal or oblique stroke with terminal shank horizontal to long axis of tooth to explore direct facial and lingual surfaces of anterior and posterior teeth (tip toward base of sulcus)

(f) Explore tooth for normal anatomy, margins of restorations, calculus, and irregularities

(3) Using shepherd's hook explorer, explore for caries; direct point into pits, grooves, and around restorations with pressure to find areas of retention that feel soft

REVIEW QUESTIONS

1. What are four functions of a mouth mirror?

2. What are the functions (at least four) of a periodontal probe?

3. What are the functions (at least two) of explorers?

4. True or false:

a. The terminal shank is that part of the shank closest to the working end.

b. In exploring, the full length of the working end should contact the tooth.

c. Generally, the simpler the shank, the more anterior the use intended for the instrument.

d. In selecting one end of a paired instrument for a given area, one cue in selecting the right end is that the terminal shank is perpendicular to the long axis of the tooth.

5. Identify the proper clinician and patient's head position for each of the following areas. For each area, designate whether the positions are for a right-handed or a left-handed clinician.

a. Labial No. 8

b. Lingual No. 18

c. Buccal No. 3

d. Buccal No. 12

e. Lingual No. 5

f. Lingual No. 14

g. Buccal No. 31

REFERENCES

Carter LM, and Yaman P: Dental instruments, St Louis, 1981, The CV Mosby Co.

Nield JS, and O'Connor GH: Fundamentals of dental hygiene instrumentation, Philadelphia, 1983, WB Saunders Co.

Pattison AM, and Behrens J: Dental hygiene: the detection and removal of calculus, Reston, Va, 1973, Reston Publishing Co, Inc.

Pattison GL, and Pattison AM: Periodontal instrumentation, Reston, Va, 1979, Reston Publishing Co, Inc.

Ward HL, and Simring MR: Manual of clinical periodontics, ed 2, St Louis, 1978, The CV Mosby Co.

7 THE PATIENT'S PERCEPTIONS

OBJECTIVES: *The reader will be able to*

1. Describe briefly at least three possible motives for choosing a career as a health care provider that may influence the degree to which the patient is viewed as a partner in care.
2. Identify language patterns that may indicate to the patient the role he or she has in treatment.
3. Given case descriptions of two views of proposed treatment (the patient's and the hygienist's), identify discrepancies in wants, needs, and expectations.
4. Explain the probable impact of discrepancies in wants, needs, and expectations on the success of treatment.
5. Given case presentations, identify ways in which the dental hygienist can gather information regarding the patient's perspectives (wants, needs, and expectations).
6. Describe the helping relationship.
7. Differentiate between the helping relationship and a dependency relationship.
8. Differentiate between professional closeness and excessive familiarity.
9. Identify ways to blend responsiveness to patients' needs with professional responsibility to provide the "best" care.
10. Explain preliminary plans for assessment phases of care to a series of hypothetical patients who have a variety of wants, needs, and expectations regarding dental hygiene care.

As described in Chapter 1, there are many reasons for a person deciding to become a dental hygienist. The motivations related to self-esteem, a flexible working schedule, and a comfortable income and working environment form one basic group related mostly to "self" needs. A second group of motivations is based largely on the desire to perform technical kinds of procedures with one's hands and to work with fascinating equipment and instruments that can improve the function and appearance of teeth and their surrounding tissues. Although this second group is "other"-oriented, it focuses largely on the procedural aspects of practice. A third kind of basic motivation is that of helping persons experience positive health changes or of helping them maintain health. In most instances health care providers have traces of all three motivations that, in balance, can provide satisfaction with the profession as well as favorable outcomes for patients.

According to communication theory regarding the building of interpersonal relationships, the person with a major interest in helping people maintain and achieve health is most likely able to encourage and develop the patient's role as a cotherapist or as a partner in care. If the health care provider's major interests are self-oriented or procedure-oriented, the patient is more likely to be viewed as an object of care or as a means to an end.

THE PATIENT AS A PARTNER IN CARE

The health care provider who views the patient as a partner in care is more likely to be interested in finding out what the patient's wants, needs, and expectations are with regard to care rather than in creating an independent set of needs for the patient based solely on clinical data. The partner-in-care concept includes opportunities for the patient to self-assess personal needs, as well as oral conditions, under the guidance of the dental hygienist (Chapters 10 and 20). Partners in care arrive at mutually satisfying treatment plan configurations and appointment sequences that will best enable both members of the partnership to complete preventive and therapeutic phases of care (Clark and Morton, 1977).

Basic communications theory explains that people are more likely to feel a commitment to a project or a goal if they share in its development and if its development clearly meets their individual needs (Collins, 1977; Keltner, 1973). While sharing in the design of the plan, participants learn about needs they had not identified on their own and begin to feel some ownership of the entire proposal. Thus, in a partnership between the dental hygienist and the patient, the dental hygienist learns about the specific needs and limitations of the patient, and the patient learns about the needs and limitations of the hygienist (Cohen, 1975; Dworkin, Ference, and Giddon, 1978). Mutual respect for wants and needs can emerge, and a clear set of reasonable expectations can be defined, which both persons will be more likely to fulfill. Unshared expectations are difficult to meet. Unilateral treatment planning is often unrealistic, because it is focused on what may be low priorities in the patient's view (Dworkin, Ference, and Giddon, 1978). The classic example is the treatment plan that is based on carefully gathered clinical, radiographic, and laboratory findings prepared by the brightest, most incisive diagnostician, scheduled into logical, perfectly spaced appointments, and presented to the patient with beautiful slides and a well-ordered outline of objective findings and related plans, but for which the patient never appears. Regardless of how well prepared the health care provider's procedures are, if the patient does not believe his or her needs are addressed and being met, the likelihood of compliance in care is remote. The patient has the final say in whether care will be delivered. If it is not in the form of a "no" at the time of the case presentation, it may be a cancelled or "forgotten" appointment.

The patient is usually able to detect whether he or she is an object or a partner in care. The language that health care providers use is an indicator. Do health care providers perform a procedure *for* someone or *with* someone, or do they do it *to* someone? Which expression connotes partnership and which connotes object? Is the person scheduled for an appointment at 3:00 PM referred to as the "Class III prophylaxis" or as the "Class II

amalgam," or is that person referred to by name, with a diagnosis or planned treatment described as his or her condition? Compare the following two statements: "The upper denture case is in operatory 3." "Ms. Wolfe is in operatory 3, waiting for a try-in of the upper denture." While the second phrasing may be a few words longer, it does connote a different image of just what is residing in operatory 3. Patients often hear our descriptions of them; if they are viewed as partners in care, they are likely to be referred to as people and not as conditions (Collins, 1977).

PATIENT INVOLVEMENT IN PLANNING CARE

Involving the patient in the preparation of a treatment plan and in designing appointment sequences is a difficult concept for many health care providers to accept. The most frequent response to such an idea is that the patient does not really know what he or she needs; that is why the patient has come to the health care provider—to find out what is wrong and to have it fixed. Although it is certainly true that the health care provider has far greater knowledge of the objective, observable needs of the patient's conditions, the patient may have some important information or notions regarding health status or particular needs that can greatly influence the outcome of care. Such information may not emerge unless it is during a discussion of wants, needs, and expectations. Even if the patient has little to contribute to modify suggested care, inclusion in the decision-making process may improve the likelihood of the patient feeling a sense of commitment to the process and may help ensure that the disease state is avoided in the future (Clark and Morton, 1977; Collins, 1977; Keltner, 1973; Purtilo, 1984).

Evaluate the following two case presentations for the extent to which they include the patient in the decision-making process:

Presentation 1: Well, Mr. Brennan, I've taken a careful look at your examination findings and have decided that you need three appointments to completely clean your teeth and to complete four areas of soft tissue curettage. You have some problems with your gums, and the dentist and I concur that the best way to reverse that problem is to remove all the hard calculus from your teeth and to remove some of the necrotic lining of the gum tissue pockets around your teeth. Now, I know you are interested in having those front teeth turned so they are better looking, but I think your highest priority should lie with getting these gum problems under control. So, we have decided to delay discussing orthodontic treatment until these appointments are complete. If you'll see the receptionist, you can schedule those appointments some time in the next 2 weeks.

Presentation 2: As I remember our initial conversation, Mr. Brennan, your primary interest in dental care was to have those front teeth straightened. Is that still a primary concern for you? (Discuss with patient.) You may recall that during the guided self-assessment we did of your teeth and gums, we found a lot of red, swollen tissue and quite a bit of hard accumulations of calculus on your teeth. Well, the x-ray films confirm that you do have gum or gingival problems. Take a look at these films; I think if you compare the bone around the molars with the bone around your lower front teeth, you will see a difference in appearance and in height around the teeth. The bone around the molars appears to be in an active state of destruction. I consulted the dentist, and we agree that you may want to postpone the movement of the teeth until we modify the state of the supporting tissues for all your teeth. The bone and the gingiva should be made healthy before we put any additional stress on them. And even after their health has improved, we will have to decide whether tooth movement is advisable. The dentist has agreed that an orthodontist should completely review your case after the initial preparation is complete. We are suggesting that the efforts to move your teeth now might cause harm to the rest of your teeth if we don't attend to these other problems first. Is this set of priorities acceptable to you? Would you agree that we should proceed with the removal of these hard deposits? (Discuss with patient.) Once we have the irritants off your teeth, we'll show you a way to prevent their recurrence, since these gingival and bone problems will recur if plaque builds up on your teeth and if hard deposits form again. (Pause for response; check nonverbal response.) And, after the plaque is under control, we'll assess the gingiva to decide whether a soft tissue curettage is indicated to remove some of the lining of the gingival pockets around your teeth. Sometimes the gingiva are unable to heal completely unless necrotic tissue from those areas is removed and the root surfaces are hard and smooth. This will require three appointments, spaced over the next few weeks to allow time between each appointment for healing. Then, when all this is accomplished, we'll reevaluate orthodontic care. Does this sound reasonable to you? Do you have suggestions that could make it easier for us to accomplish our goal together? Are you as interested in having your supporting tissues heal and remain solid as you are in having those front teeth moved? (Discuss after each sample question.)

Which case presentation is more patient centered? Pick out the phrases that tell you the patient is viewed as a partner rather than a person expected to agree. In which case can you imagine the hygienist making eye contact frequently with the patient? What other differences in nonverbal behavior can you imagine would be evident between these two case descriptions? The differences intended between the two styles of case presentation are in the degree of opportunity the patient has to react to the suggested treatment plan and the extent to which the patient's need (tooth movement for esthetics) is kept in mind as a serious priority worthy of consideration. Patients may not necessarily value certain elements of dental health (or general health, for that matter) as much as health care providers do (Collins, 1977; Purtilo, 1984). Certainly, explanation regarding the rationale for an altered treatment plan and for including more in the plan than the patient expected is essential and valid. This explanation is given in patient-centered care with the underlying premise that the patient's wants and needs are equally important in designing the total plan and that the patient has the right to be involved in the discussion and in the decision making (Collins, 1977; Dworkin, Ference, and Giddon, 1978). The patient should always be asked if he or she is satisfied with the proposed treatment plan (Clark and Morton, 1977).

While this chapter focuses on the interpersonal responsibility and wisdom of keeping a patient fully informed and of seeking the patient's verbal consent, this responsibility is also a legal one. It is not enough to be right about what a patient needs. The attitude of engaging a patient as a partner in decision making is supported by the law as well as by the need for harmony and cooperation (Rosoff, 1981; ADA Council, 1987; Rozovsky, 1984; Broonten and Chapman, 1987).

An obvious outcome of sharing plans, discussing priorities, and asking opinions is that the patient may disagree with what the provider believes is right. There are times when the patient may not wish to compromise desires for care, despite the careful discussion of rationale to include other phases of care or to delay or eliminate the phases of care the patient believes are needed to improve appearance or health. A case in point may be the person who appears with perfectly healthy teeth and periodontium but who insists that he or she will have all the teeth extracted and dentures made. A patient who is convinced that this course of treatment is best certainly deserves discussion of some alternatives and a careful analysis of why and how the patient came to this conclusion. In some cases it may not be possible to convince the patient sufficiently that other approaches should be followed. The health care provider then has to decide whether to provide the procedures the patient wants or refuse care. Generally speaking, if a patient requests care that, in the opinion of the dentist or hygienist, is totally inappropriate or dangerous, the health care provider should refuse care. The alternative is to write out all the adverse possible outcomes of such care and have the patient sign the statement. Such a statement should relieve the health care providers from responsibility for the negative outcomes of such treatment and place full responsibility on the patient. Because of the critical nature of such a disclaimer, it is absolutely essential that an attorney draw up such a document.

The patient who demands unreasonable care is certainly a challenge to health care providers, since the only realistic decision may be to refuse care. The professional must then allow the patient to leave with untended real problems to seek another professional to solve the imagined problems. For the patient, however, the labels for those problems are just the opposite, and efforts to solve what the patient sees as imaginary problems and the health professional sees as real will probably result in further patient dissatisfaction.

Another challenge is the patient who says he or she is satisfied but who does not act that way. The patient may act resentful or miss appointments. If there is a discrepancy between what is said and what is done, the patient should be asked about it (Purtilo, 1984).

LISTENING

The first step in developing an attitude that will "let the patient in" as a partner is to practice good listening skills. Many new clinicians are concerned about what to say to a patient. A clinician's first priority is to *listen* to what the patient

says and to let the patient know the clinician understands. This is *not* accomplished by saying, "I understand." Even though these words of assurance are spoken, the patient is left wondering what it is the clinician thinks he or she understands.

Listening involves rephrasing (1) the *content* of the message the patient has sent and (2) the patient's *affect* or emotion behind it. Listening requires "immediate, genuine, concrete, and empathic reaction to verbal and nonverbal messages." Usually what people say—the actual words spoken—conveys an apparent message, but the way it is said and the subtle choice of words often provide an underlying message that should not be ignored (Okun, 1987). Reading those messages, reflecting them back accurately, and using those new insights is a highly refined, but essential, skill that helpers develop as they work with people (Gottschalk et al, 1986).

For instance, a new patient arriving for dental hygiene care says, "I sure hate coming to a dental office." Listening would involve reflecting back the content and affect by saying, "It sounds like you don't enjoy these visits very much and you'd rather be elsewhere right now." The patient responds to correct an inaccuracy, such as:

Well, no. I don't look forward to being here. But I know I should have this done. So here's the place to be.

Or the patient may confirm the hygienist's reflection and elaborate:

You bet. My mouth must be very sensitive, because I feel *everything*. Having my teeth cleaned really hurts.

Further listening would be:

So you've had your teeth cleaned many times before, and it always hurts.

The patient:

Yes, it does. Every time an instrument touches my teeth, I feel like a needle is touching the nerve.

The hygienist:

So what hurts is a metal instrument touching the tooth rather than your gums feeling sore.

The patient:

Yes. My gums don't bother me at all. It's the teeth. I

just have to hang on for fear of crying. I wish someone could do something so I wouldn't feel the pain.

The hygienist:

It sounds like having your teeth cleaned must be awful for you—like you're "white knuckling" it through the appointment. Anesthesia hasn't worked for you.

The patient:

Well, no one has given me anesthesia. I just put up with it and keep quiet.

After all that *listening* it may now be time for the hygienist to begin *talking*. It appears that the patient could benefit from anesthesia, and it could be suggested. But imagine that the hygienist had not used active listening. Typical responses to a patient's complaint about being in a dental office could be:

- Don't worry. I'll be gentle.
- Everyone hates to be in a dental chair—even I don't like it.
- Dentistry is an evil necessity, isn't it?
- Do you come to the dentist regularly?
- You should try relaxation exercises.
- Well, we're just cleaning your teeth today. It won't be bad.

Any one of those typical comments shuts off the communication. The patient either gives up and suffers again or has to start up with another entry to get the hygienist to listen. Even the question response shuts off communication because it redirects the patient to talk about what the hygienist suspects is behind the problem. The patient's message is lost, and thus a critical insight to the patient's needs and expectations is missed.

Poor communication with patients results in two important roadblocks. First, the patients will not understand what you are saying and cannot act appropriately on what you say even if they want to. Second, the patients become convinced that you don't care whether they understand or not—that you do not value their feelings and needs (Purtilo, 1984). Nonverbal behavior can close out communication as well. One example is the smile that conveys no warmth, acceptance, or respect. These negative "smiles" include those that say:

1. *I know something you don't know.* The hy-

gienist smiles this way when thinking, "You think you have good dentistry in your mouth, but it is really poor quality."
2. *Poor, poor you.* This smile accompanies the hygienist's intervention to change a person's flossing technique after smugly watching him try for 5 minutes.
3. *Don't tell me.* The hygienist asks how the patient is and smiles a "how wonderful" even before the patient speaks.
4. *I'm smarter than you.* This smile is a nonverbal reprimand, perhaps because a hygienist's recommendations were not followed, resulting in expensive treatment.
5. *I don't like you either.* This smile is given when the patient's beliefs are backed up by the dentist or some other authority, contrary to what the hygienist has said. The patient looks at the hygienist to note the "victory"; the hygienist smiles through his or her teeth.

These are destructive, nonverbal messages that hurt more than words, and are difficult to combat verbally (Purtilo, 1984).

Nonverbal messages reveal a great deal about what the communicator really means. "Negative smiles," a touch that carries anger or disinterest, failure to make eye contact, and other distancing behaviors can undo all the carefully selected phrasing. A person will see right through a beautifully prepared speech about warmth and caring and see the true feelings. Accepting people for who they are and learning to enjoy their foibles and to see the bright side of each encounter can help the hygienist learn how to feel warmth and caring and then communicate it naturally.

THE HELPING RELATIONSHIP

The first basic element of the helping relationship in which the patient is a partner in care is the patient *wanting* to be helped (Purtilo, 1984). Patients must have the freedom to refuse help (even if help is *good* for them). If help is requested as a result of discussions with the patient, the relationship can grow.

Second, the function of the helper is to meet the needs of the "helpee," not those of the helper. A true helper should not be working to change other people to fit an image of something better. The helper and helpee work together to seek the best solution and determine how to implement it.

Helping is a mutual learning process (Okun, 1987).

The third basic element is that the helping relationship should build toward patient self-reliance (Purtilo, 1984). A sound helping relationship enables the patient to accept responsibility for self-care, for preventing disease, and for seeking professional help to maintain health. The alternative is a dependency relationship in which the patient sees the health care provider as the one responsible for the patient's dental health.

The helper must be able to work with people in the affective domain (feelings and emotions), the cognitive domain (thinking), and the behavioral domain (actions) (Okun, 1987). This is important in dentistry, because people arrive for care with a basketful of emotions about what they expect will happen, previous experiences, and the appearance and health of their teeth. People arrive with misinformation, and they often have unhelpful health habits or omit ones that are necessary for their oral health.

In the practice of dental hygiene, it is common to encounter patients who believe that as long as they have their teeth checked and cleaned every 6 months, their responsibility toward good dental health is fulfilled; the rest is up to the dentist and hygienist. Having clean teeth 2 days out of the year (every 6 months) and having restorations placed year after year result in detrimental long-term effects. Periodontists who treat patients who have "graduated" to their care from years of such a routine refer to this kind of care as supervised neglect. The patient has become dependent on the professionals for something they cannot possibly provide. Daily self-care in removing plaque and debris and in monitoring diet are critical components in dental health that cannot be assigned to the dental hygienist or dentist.

Certainly, there is a degree of dependence on the health care provider in some early stages of care when considerable therapeutic time and skill are required to correct disease status. The goal throughout these early stages, however, should be to shift primary responsibility from the health care provider to the patient (Purtilo, 1984), beginning with (1) involving the patient in the diagnostic phases of care by means of a guided self-assessment of oral conditions, (2) including the patient in decision making regarding treatment, and (3)

facilitating the shift of responsibility for maintaining health by dental health education, nutritional guidance, and mechanisms for self-evaluation of oral status between appointments. Thus "constructive dependence" grows toward the interdependence of a partnership (Purtilo, 1984).

This relationship may be difficult to achieve for professionals whose major motives are self-oriented or technically oriented. Likewise, this may be a difficult relationship for the patient who would rather not be bothered with responsibility for health and who would rather say, "You're the doctor! Do what you need to." Usually the partnership relationship develops at different rates, depending on the perceptions and needs of the health care provider and the patient. In most cases it is the health care provider who leads the way in developing the partnership; in this era of consumer awareness, however, it may be the patient who leads the way by seeking information, input, and shared responsibility. Adopting these fundamental assumptions can help clinicians work more effectively with people:

1. People are responsible for and capable of making their own decisions.
2. People are controlled to some extent by their environment, but they do have control of their lives—often more than they realize. Even in the face of restricted options, they have the freedom to choose.
3. What people do is goal directed and purposive—even if the purposes seem unclear and vague.
4. People want to feel good about themselves; they want others to see them as worthwhile.
5. People are capable of learning new behavior if there are visible reinforcements for those changes that fit their own values and beliefs.
6. People's problems may arise from unfinished business (conflicts from the past) or by a perception that does not match with others' views of reality.
7. Problems can be due to environmental or societal conditions; those conditions can be managed or altered through personal choice and action (Okun, 1987).

Values are changing among patients in tandem with the emphasis on consumer rights that has grown over the last 15 years. Such values include a greater sense of independence (less reliance on a health care provider's words), self-determination, and egalitarianism. Patients look past the status-claiming medical or dental degree and seek second opinions, inquire about alternatives, and question the conclusions presented (Gallagher, 1976). Thus the patients a hygienist or dentist encounters may expect to be involved more than the health care provider expects they will be.

PROFESSIONAL CLOSENESS

Because relationships with dental patients in particular may last many years and involve families of patients as well as individuals, there is considerable opportunity for developing trust and refining ways to move in and out of a dependency relationship with each person, depending on the patient's social and economic needs and growth as well as on overall health status (Purtilo, 1984). This may well be among the most satisfying aspects of the practice of dental hygiene.

This high degree of trust with a patient is professional closeness. During a series of appointments, and especially over a period of years, the patient and dental hygienist may be able to share personal ideas and judgments and perhaps feelings and emotions. They may be able to share laughter, grief, solutions to the world's problems, a new recipe, or an easy method for adjusting the carburetor. In any case, they will have passed the stage of limiting conversation to cliches about the weather and facts about plaque levels and gingival conditions. The critical balance (professional closeness) is between aloofness and excessive familiarity (Purtilo, 1984). Both verbal and nonverbal expressions declare which side of the balance the hygienist has found. Aloofness is cold, factual, precise, and uncomplicated with human feeling. Excessive familiarity is inappropriately casual or chummy, filled with expressions or feelings that are seen as overreactions, but still uncomplicated with much true understanding of human feelings. It is the lack of awareness of the other person's boundaries and freedom to move toward an open relationship or to reserve such a response for somewhere other than the dental environment. Professional closeness, in contrast to both extremes, is largely in response to the patient's expressed needs and is, above all, a genuine expression of caring for a fellow human being

(Collins, 1977). It includes an interest in the patient as a person with values, needs, and beliefs that deserve respect (Collins, 1977; Goldberg, Plume, and Nacman, 1973; Murray and Weise, 1975; Purtilo, 1984), and it recognizes that efficiency and formality can express caring when they do not impose rigid limits on interaction. Issues regarding the use of white uniforms and the use of first names or last names with patients require individual judgment of outcomes based on the *expressed* preferences of the patients and a careful analysis of personal perference (Purtilo, 1984).

One useful guideline in developing a professional relationship with a patient is to ask what the patient prefers: "What would you prefer I call you?" or "Do you prefer to have me talk to you during the appointment, or do you like it better if I work quietly?" After a while, experience seems to help the health care provider know when to talk, when to remain silent, when to work efficiently with minimal verbal exchange, and when to set aside instruments and discuss an issue. In some ways, developing a professional relationship is much like establishing a friendship, but with the complicating factors of specifying wants and needs, which hopefully will be considered appropriate by the patient for inclusion in a plan of care.

The patient-professional relationship is a unique combination of closeness and distance. For all its genuine emotional content, closeness, and honesty of communication, the therapeutic relationship is peculiarly distanced, circumscribed, and asymmetrical. Most of the time, one person talks and the other listens. The client almost always talks about himself and the therapist almost never does. There is money exchanged. There are tight procedural, businesslike rules that limit the monetary exchange, the time spent, the scheduling of encounters, and sexual behavior or conventions of friendship. The therapist is not a moralist, but helps people make their own judgments. Still, the therapist is a model of behavior to the client (Bellah, et al, 1985).

INTRODUCING THE PATIENT TO INITIAL PHASES OF CARE

Often the dental hygienist's initial encounters with the patient center on the critical issue of what shall or shall not be included in care. This issue can be a major one if the patient thinks that one or two specific procedures will be completed to meet his or her needs. For instance, if the patient has been accustomed to having his or her teeth cleaned on request, the patient may not expect to have a complete medical history, a complete series of radiographs, and plaque and gingival indices recorded. The patient may be even more aghast at having a facial massage (actually an extraoral examination) and blood pressure taken.

For this reason, it is wise to describe for the patient exactly what is routinely included in the first visit, how long it will take, and how much it will cost. The "laundry list" of procedures should be prefaced by a few introductory comments regarding the need at the first appointment to gather some baseline information on the basis of which decisions regarding treatment can be made. As each procedure is begun, the patient should be told what the procedure is, why it is important to perform the procedure, how it is done, and how the patient can cooperate in the effort. A simple request to proceed should precede performance of the procedure.

Some patients may be put at ease if the health care provider describes aloud what he or she is doing as each phase is performed. The patient may wish to observe in a hand mirror. Significant findings can be shared with the patient as long as no definitive diagnostic conclusions are given until after the dentist has completely reviewed the data. For instance, the hygienist may say, "I can feel the muscles in the floor of your mouth, and I see the normal structures that carry saliva to your mouth and that attach your tongue to the floor of the mouth. There is some normal tonsillar tissue on the side of your tongue."

Once the assessment data have been gathered and a diagnosis has been confirmed by the dentist, the hygienist may discuss in greater detail the significance of the findings with the patient. Most patients would like to know more about themselves, including their oral health, as long as the technical language is kept to a minimum and the descriptions are clear and relevant.

At the conclusion of the first appointment, the dental hygienist should tell the patient what will occur at the next appointment and approximately how long it will take (Clark and Morton, 1977). If an additional charge will be made, an estimate of cost should be provided. Usually all subsequent needs are addressed in a treatment plan as discussed in Chapter 18.

What if the patient refuses a phase of care? As mentioned earlier, the patient does have the right to refuse. For preliminary procedures, it may be helpful to explain how the missing data will affect the accuracy of the diagnosis. If the patient still elects to refuse a specific phase of care, the health care provider can elect to terminate care, can have an attorney draw up a disclaimer similar to that suggested for patients who request care that is not in their best interests, or can postpone that phase of care until other aspects not reliant on the rejected procedure can be completed. Sometimes, after a few appointments and some low-pressure discussion, the patient will reconsider and decide to include the procedure, especially if the undesirable result of its exclusion becomes increasingly apparent.

If the patient has the opportunity to see the health care provider as a trustworthy person who accepts the patient as an individual with unique needs rather than as one who views the patient as an object for demonstrating technical prowess or as a means to a lucrative end, he or she may see the dentist and hygienist as partners in care rather than as necessary evils. The patient may ask to have the omitted procedure performed.

In some instances this relationship depends on an initial lowering of apparent control over the environment. Sharing a bit of the control may yield more freedom in the long run to suggest and implement care. Insisting on immediate, total control may send many patients away or may unintentionally foster a dependency relationship in which the patient hears the message, "Doctor knows best. Hygienist heals all."

ACTIVITIES
1. Tape record interactions between a health care provider and a patient, and listen to the recording to determine signs of:
   a. Listening
   b. Dependence/partnership
   c. Aloofness, closeness, familiarity
   d. Conflicts of wants, needs, and expectations
2. Role play vignettes to demonstrate:
   a. A helping relationship

b. A dependency relationship
3. Role play the explanation of preliminary assessment procedures to a patient who is:
   a. Interested only in restorative care
   b. Concerned about excess exposure to radiation from x-rays
   c. Convinced he or she will need dentures in another 10 years
   d. Accustomed to *no* preliminary procedures in a dental office other than two x-ray films and a caries charting
   e. Afraid he or she has oral cancer
4. Watch carefully for "negative smiles" during day-to-day interaction. Record what the circumstances were that resulted in the negative smile. Share those observations in a small group.

REVIEW QUESTIONS

1. The patient wants her front teeth polished so she will look nice for her son's wedding. The hygienist wants to do something about those inflamed gingivae and the heavy calculus on the molars. How might this discrepancy affect the outcome of care?
2. The patient wants his cavities filled. He does not want to hear the hygienist's eighteenth rendition of how to floss and the need to eat fewer sweets. The hygienist wants to end this string of recurrent caries that is evident from the patient's record. How might this discrepancy affect the outcome of care?
3. A hygienist's patient looks up and says contentedly, "I know that as long as you take care of me, I'll never lose my teeth." What might that statement imply?
4. Identify whether each of the following vignettes reflects professional aloofness, professional closeness, or excessive familiarity:
   a. Hygienist slaps new patient on the back and says, "Well Joe, how's tricks?"
   b. Hygienist decides she prefers to wear a clinic jacket over street clothes. To verify this decision, she asks several patients what they think of the new garb.
   c. A long-term patient complains that she has been under considerable tension lately and that she knows she has not taken proper care of her teeth. The hygienist elects not to discuss the unusually bad state of the gingivae other than to show the plaque index and a few selected papillae (by means of a mirror) to the patient. Later during the appointment, the hygienist gently asks whether the patient has been able to get some help for her tension.
   d. The dental hygienist checks a plaque index and sees that it is actually worse than that from the previous visit. The hygienist launches into her "plan B" speech on the merits of brushing and

flossing and states that care will fail if the patient does not comply with these directives.
5. What measures can a health care provider take if a patient refuses a phase of care that is essential for diagnostic or therapeutic purposes?
6. Give a listening response to each of these patient comments:
   a. "I don't think you are going to like the way my teeth look!"
   b. "I never have liked these dental chairs where I have to lie flat."
   c. "You really dig a lot deeper than other hygienists I've had."
   d. "I want the dentist and not some girl to clean my teeth."
7. How does each of these nonlistening replies to the statements in 6 cut off further communication and understanding?
   a. "Don't worry. I *always* like the way your teeth look!"
   b. "Well, these new ones are much better for posture than those old clunkers."
   c. "I could give you some anesthesia."
   d. "I'm not 'some girl.' I'm a licensed hygienist who is highly skilled at cleaning teeth and many other procedures."

REFERENCES

American Dental Association Council on Insurance: Informed consent: a risk management view, JADA **115:**630, 1987.

Bellah RN, et al: Habits of the heart: individualism and commitment in American life, Berkeley, 1985, University of California Press.

Broonten KE, and Chapman S: Malpractice: a guide to avoidance and treatment, Orlando, 1987, Grune & Stratton, Inc.

Clark JD, and Morton JC: Behavioral assessment: an appraisal of beliefs and behaviors relating to treatment, Dent Clin North Am **21:**515, 1977.

Cohen DW: Preventive periodontics, J Indian Dent Assoc (special issue), p 273, 1975.

Cohen LC, et al: Caring and controlling dimensions in patient relations: the dental student perspective, J Am Coll Dent **47:**180, 1980.

Collins M: Communication in health care: understanding and implementing effective human relationships, St Louis, 1977, The CV Mosby Co.

Dworkin SF, Ference TP, and Giddon DB: Behavioral science and dental practice, St Louis, 1978, The CV Mosby Co.

Faden RR, and Beauchamp TL: A history and theory of informed consent, New York, 1986, Oxford University Press.

Gallagher EB: The doctor-patient relationship in the changing health scene, Washington, DC, 1976, U.S. Department of Health, Education, and Welfare.

Goldberg HJ, Plume M, and Nacman M: The importance of attitude in the delivery of health services, J Public Health Dent **33:**35, 1973.

Gottschalk LA, Lolas F, and Viney LL: Content analysis of verbal behavior: significance in clinical medicine and psychiatry, New York, 1986, Springer-Verlag.

Keltner JW: Elements of interpersonal communication, Belmont, Calif, 1973, Wadsworth Publishing Co, Inc.

Murray BP, and Weise HJ: Satisfaction with care and the utilization of dental services at a neighborhood health center, J Public Health Dent **35:**170, 1975.

Okun B: Effective helping: interviewing and counseling techniques, ed 3, Monterey, Calif, 1986, Brooks/Cole Publishing Co.

Purtilo R: Health professional/patient interaction, ed 3, Philadelphia, 1984, WB Saunders Co.

Rosoff AJ: Informed consent, Rockville, Md, 1981, Aspen Systems Corp.

Rozovsky FA: Consent to treatment: a practical guide, Boston, 1984, Little, Brown & Co.

Weinstein P, et al: Oral self-care: a promising alternative behavior model, JADA **107:**67, 1983.

8 BASIC EMERGENCY PROCEDURES

OBJECTIVES: *The reader will be able to*

1. Explain briefly why a dental hygienist should:
   a. Be able to identify promptly early signs and symptoms of medical emergencies
   b. Follow an established emergency protocol system when managing a medical emergency
   c. Successfully complete a comprehensive course in medical emergency management, basic life support, and CPR at level C*
2. Identify drugs and equipment that would constitute a basic emergency kit for a dental clinic.
3. Identify and know the appropriate use of advanced emergency drug therapy.
4. Operate an oxygen tank and know the appropriate use for the various delivery systems demanded by various emergency situations.
5. Explain how a complete, reviewed medical history and knowledge of preoperative vital signs can help prevent and identify medical emergencies.
6. Explain the importance of stress management in preventing medical emergencies.
7. Indicate the appropriate management of specific medical emergencies in response to given signs and symptoms.
8. Develop an emergency protocol for a given clinical setting and explain how it will be implemented in a variety of emergency situations.
9. Identify the necessary considerations for emergency preparedness when working with the homebound and nursing home population.
10. Identify basic fire, accident, and personal injury prevention guidelines for a clinical setting.

Before beginning clinical practice, a dental hygiene student must be able to identify and respond to basic emergency signs that may occur during care of patients. It is also important for the student to recall significant patient assessment data that may indicate the likelihood and nature of an emergency situation. This chapter alerts the student to the rudiments of responsible attention to safety in practice. *A complete course in first aid and in basic life support, including cardiopulmonary resuscitation (CPR) and techniques for clearing the airway, is essential.*

*The American Heart Association recommends level C certification for health care providers. Level C certification includes one- and two-man CPR on the infant, child, and adult, as well as management of the obstructed airway for the infant, child, and adult.

THE HYGIENIST'S ROLE

A dental hygienist often is the first to recognize a potential medical emergency, as the dental hygienist may be the one to perform the medical history and record vital signs. Likewise, working with a patient in a private or semiprivate operatory frequently makes the hygienist the sole observer of the patient's condition and responses to various phases of care. It is the competent hygienist's responsibility to monitor the patient's responses throughout care, being constantly aware of changes in expression, skin tone, muscle tonus, respirations, and verbal expression. As intraoral procedures are performed, the clinician's peripheral vision should watch for signs of distress, relaxation, puzzlement, and other indications of the patient's state.

An additional responsibility is to be able to classify the kinds of responses and know when an emergency situation seems imminent. Prompt, appropriate reaction to a patient showing signs of distress may avert an emergency and even save a life. The hygienist's ability to provide complete descriptions of signs of distress to the dentist or attending medical team can hasten the provision of appropriate care.

A further responsibility that may be assumed following a comprehensive first aid and life-support course is that of administering care to reverse an emergency or to sustain life until help can be secured. This role is essential for hygienists who function in their own practice or under general supervision when a dentist or physician may or may not be present. All members of the dental team should be qualified to administer oxygen, record vital signs, perform basic life support procedures to open an airway, and perform CPR. As a primary provider of care, the dental hygienist certainly has this responsibility.

Once the signs of distress are noted, the clinician should be able to follow a logical, rehearsed pattern of behavior (emergency protocol) in response to the signs. The response may be simply to move instruments and other pieces of potentially harmful equipment away from the patient, to raise the back of the chair, to lower the back for a full supine position, to go for help calmly, to push the emergency signal button, or to let the patient rest quietly for a moment. The response may include preparing a syringe for an intramuscular (IM), intravenous (IV), or subcutaneous injection; performing CPR; or directing an emergency squad to the right location. For each possible situation, the clinician should be prepared to respond in a predetermined fashion, as there may be little time for contemplation or turning to references for suggested behavior.

BEING PREPARED TO ACT

Responding to a medical emergency involves many steps that can and should be divided among dental team members according to their skill levels and their abilities to react quickly and appropriately under stress. All team members should be aware of the possible problems and the proper responses to ensure that everyone participates knowledgeably and according to a well-rehearsed plan. While procedures should be divided and delegated to individual team members, the division should be flexible enough to ensure that all steps are taken even when a team member is missing or is the subject of the emergency care.

A rehearsal of one of the possible emergencies should be held monthly, according to a carefully delineated script. For instance, in the event of aspiration of a foreign object into the lung, the clinician would follow predetermined steps to assist the patient and alert another team member to notify the dentist and the emergency squad.

Emergency phone numbers must be readily accessible; ideally, they are attached to the phone itself. Procedures for alerting other team members of the occurrence of an emergency should be unmistakable, but a calm atmosphere should be preserved as much as possible.

Many tasks to be performed must be assigned and rehearsed. Eleven generic functions described by Kinne (1982) as part of any emergency are as follows:

1. Evaluate the vital signs
2. Diagnose the nature of the emergency
3. Decide on the appropriate treatment
4. Instruct others what to do
5. Phone for help
6. Prepare for treatment administration
7. Administer treatment
8. Monitor vital signs
9. Reassure the patient
10. Record events that occur
11. Ensure privacy and/or manage other patients

MEDICAL EMERGENCIES IN THE DENTAL ENVIRONMENT

Any medical emergency can occur in the dental office. Patients with a predisposition to a medical emergency (such as patients with high blood pressure, cardiac insufficiency, asthma, or angina) may be more likely to experience such an occurrence in a dental office, as anxiety levels may be high for a patient anticipating or experiencing dental care. The combination of a medical problem and the anxiety may trigger a physical response that can be classified as an emergency (Trieger, 1982). Accordingly, patient anxiety levels are of prime concern to the practitioner, even in the "healthy" patient. Preventive procedures must include the patient's ability to cope mentally with the dental procedure. In other words, consider the "total" patient *before* therapy begins. An effective means of assessing patient anxiety (see box) was developed by Corah (1969). Using this Dental Anxiety Scale as part of the total patient evaluation will allow the practitioner to recognize patient anxiety, modify dental therapy, and prevent an emergency.

Table 8-1 summarizes the signs, symptoms, and treatments for the medical emergencies presented in this section. The emergency situations are presented by disease or emergency (for example, syncope, cardiac arrest, angina pectoris). But when a medical emergency occurs, the clinician will be faced with the signs and symptoms of a patient experiencing a medical emergency, such as an unconscious or convulsing patient. It is strongly suggested that the reader complete activities 8 and 9 on p. 149 to prepare for responding to a medical emergency.

Emergency supplies and equipment

An integral part of any emergency protocol system is a strategically and conveniently located emergency kit. Even more important is the contents of the kit. What should the kit contain? At this time the experts cannot agree. The increasing numbers of medically compromised people seeking dental care, the frequently changing methods of managing emergencies, and the varied levels of skill and training in emergency management techniques make it difficult to develop prepackaged emergency kits that can meet all needs. Indeed, the ADA Council on Dental Therapeutics (1986) has refrained from endorsing any commercial kit, suggesting instead that emergency kits be "individualized to meet the special needs and capabilities of each practitioner."

Accordingly, where prepackaged kits are considered, practitioners should commit considerable time to developing knowledge of and familiarity and skill with the entire contents of their kits. Otherwise the practitioner may develop a false sense of confidence in his or her emergency management skills because of the presence of the kit. In certain cases, this could lay the groundwork for possible malpractice claims.

Ideally, the practitioner should prepare to select emergency kit items with an exhaustive research of current literature, a consultation with referral physicians, a review of pharmacologic texts, and an examination of community emergency medical systems. This procedure allows the informed practitioner to select only drugs and equipment that are effective, economical, and suited for the job. All clinicians should recognize their limitations in this area, however, and endeavor to enhance needed emergency skills.

In any medical emergency, time is of the essence. Seconds lost fumbling with unfamiliar drugs or equipment can compromise the outcome

---

Dental Anxiety Scale

1. If you had to go to the dentist tomorrow, how would you feel about it?
   a) I would look forward to it as a reasonably enjoyable experience.
   b) I would not care one way or the other.
   c) I would be very uneasy about it.
   d) I would be afraid that it would be unpleasant and painful.
   e) I would be very frightened of what the dentist might do.
2. When you are waiting in the dentist's office for your turn in the chair, how do you feel?
   a) Relaxed.
   b) A little uneasy.
   c) Tense.
   d) Anxious.
   e) So anxious that I sometimes break out in a sweat or almost feel physically sick.
3. When you are in the dentist's chair waiting for him or her to get the drill ready and begin working on your teeth, how do you feel? (Same choices as question 2.)
4. You are in the dentist's chair to have your teeth cleaned. While you are waiting and the dentist is getting out the instruments with which to scrape your teeth around the gums, how do you feel? (Same choices as question 2.)
5. In general, do you feel uncomfortable or nervous about receiving dental treatment?
   a) Yes
   b) No

From Corah, N.: J Dent Res 48:596, 1969.

Text continued on p. 141.

Table 8-1. Emergencies: signs, symptoms, and treatments

Emergency	Signs and symptoms	Treatment
Acute adrenal insufficiency (Adrenal crisis)	Confusion Weakness Nausea, vomiting Hypotension Severe pain in abdomen, lower back, legs Syncopal episodes Coma	*CONSCIOUS PATIENT* Terminate therapy Monitor vital signs Place in supine position Administer oxygen (5-10 liters per minute) *UNCONSCIOUS PATIENT* Recognize unconsciousness Place in supine position Provide basic life support* Emergency kit O_2 Summon medical assistance Transfer to hospital
Vasodepressor syncope	**Presyncope** EARLY Feeling of warmth Loss of color Heavy perspiration Complaints of feeling bad Nausea Blood pressure approximately baseline Rapid heart rate LATE Pupillary dilation Hyperpnea Coldness in hands and feet Hypotension Bradycardia Dizziness **Syncope** Loss of consciousness	EARLY Recognize signs and symptoms Terminate therapy Place in supine position, feet slightly elevated Reassure patient Waft ammonia vaporole under patient's nose Administer oxygen; patient may hold mask Attempt to determine cause of presyncopal signs LATE Terminate therapy Place patient in supine position, feet slightly elevated Establish patient airway using head tilt, chin lift method Check breathing Artificial ventilation (if necessary) Check circulation Monitor vital signs Support patient Waft ammonia vaporole under patient's nose Cold towels to forehead Blankets if cold and shivering Attempt to determine cause of syncope Arrange for transportation Modify future therapy
Insulin shock Insulin reaction (hypoglycemia)	RAPID ONSET Moist and pale skin Full and bounding pulse Respirations, normal to shallow Blood pressure baseline to normal Bizarre behavior; may appear intoxicated but with no odor of alcohol Loss of consciousness (sometimes) Tremors Convulsions (in late stages)	 Terminate therapy Recognize hypoglycemic symptoms *CONSCIOUS PATIENT* Assess ABCs** Administer oral carbohydrates *UNCONSCIOUS PATIENT* Provide Basic life support* Summon medical assistance Carbohydrate IV or IM

Continued.

Table 8-1. Emergencies: signs, symptoms, and treatments—cont'd

Emergency	Signs and symptoms	Treatment
Diabetic coma (hyper-glycemia)	GRADUAL ONSET	
	Dry, flushed skin	Terminate therapy
	Dry mouth	Recognize symptoms of hyperglycemia
	Intense thirst	Summon medical assistance
	Vomiting	Provide basic life support*
	Abdominal pains	Transport to hospital
	Rapid respiration (Kussmaul)	(This patient needs insulin; however, due to com-
	Acetone odor to breath	plications associated with injectable insulin, it
	Low BP	should *never* be a part of the emergency kit)
	Weak, rapid pulse	
	Loss of consciousness (sometimes)	
Respiratory problems		
Choking (aspiration)	**Upper airway obstruction**	
	Partial obstruction	Terminate therapy
	Good air exchange	Do not interfere
	Coughing	Allow patient to cough
	PARTIAL OBSTRUCTION	
	Poor air exchange	Treat as totally obstructed airway
	High-pitched, crowing sound	
	Cyanotic	
	Ineffective cough	
	Panic	
	TOTAL OBSTRUCTION	
	CONSCIOUS PATIENT	Perform Heimlich maneuver until obstruction is
	Ominous quiet	relieved***
	Patient clutches throat (universal	Reassure patient
	choking symbol)	Transport to hospital
	Cyanotic	Summon medical assistance
	Panic	Heimlich maneuver (6-8 times)
	UNCONSCIOUS PATIENT	Finger sweep to remove obstruction (adults only)
		Attempt to ventilate
		Continue sequence until obstruction is relieved
		Cricothyrotomy if obstruction cannot be relieved
		Monitor vital signs
		Artificial ventilation (if necessary)
		CPR (if necessary)
		Transport to hospital
	Lower airway obstruction	
	Not as immediately life-threatening	*Unless object is retrieved,* patient must be trans-
	Object usually goes to right main bronchi and	ported to hospital to locate and retrieve object
	into right lung	
	Patient may be unaware or may cough	
Hyperventilation	Acute anxiety	Terminate therapy
	Rapid breathing	Position patient comfortably (this patient usually
	Shortness of breath	does not want to recline)
	Tingling in extremities and perioral area	Have patient place a paper bag, full face mask,
	Dryness of mouth	or cupped hands over mouth and nose to breath
	Chest pain	CO_2-enriched air
	Palpitations	Drug management—Diazepam (only when the
	Muscle cramps and pain	above therapy is ineffective)
		Attempt to determine cause of anxiety

Table 8-1. Emergencies: signs, symptoms, and treatments—cont'd

Emergency	Signs and symptoms	Treatment
Acute asthmatic attack	Intense coughing Intense wheezing Perspiration Cyanosis of nail beds and mucous membranes Flushing Fatigue Mental confusion	Terminate therapy Position patient comfortably (sitting or standing) Administer bronchodilator (use patient's prescription whenever possible) or subcutaneous epinephrine Administer O_2 Summon medical assistance
Chest pain		
Acute congestive heart failure and acute pulmonary edema	Weakness and undue fatigue Dyspnea on exertion Cyanotic Skin cold and clammy Wheezing (moist rales) Frothy sputum Pulsus alternans	Terminate therapy Place patient in an upright position Administer O_2 Monitor and record vital signs Attempt to alleviate apprehension Summon medical assistance
Angina pectoris	Pain usually substernal, but may radiate Brought on by exertion or stress Patient may hold clenched fist over chest (Levine's sign) Elevated BP and heart rate Dyspnea Feeling of faintness	Terminate therapy Place patient in upright position Administer nitroglycerin (patient's prescription whenever possible) Administer O_2 If pain persists, administer nitroglycerin again Monitor vital signs Summon medical assistance Modify therapy at future appointments
Myocardial infarction	Severe, prolonged substernal pain (30 minutes or more); pain may radiate (nitroglycerin provides no relief) Dyspnea Weakness Nausea and vomiting Severe distress Heart rate bradycardia to tachycardia BP baseline to low (may drop precipitously in first few hours)	Terminate therapy Record vital signs Administer nitroglycerin Initiate basic life support* as needed Summon medical assistance Administer O_2 Reassure patient Administer an analgesic for pain Transport to hospital
Cardiac arrest	Ashen gray appearance Skin cold and clammy Absence of adequate pulse Absence of respiration Most common cause is cardiovascular disease May occur as a result of complications to other emergency situations (such as airway obstruction, overdose, anaphylaxis, asthma, seizure disorders)	Terminate therapy Provide basic life support* Summon medical assistance
Altered consciousness		
Hypoglycemia	See insulin shock	
Hyperglycemia	See diabetic coma	
Hypothyroidism	Dry skin Coarse hair Lethargy Weakness Slow speech Edema of eyelids Gain in weight	No special management Prior medical consultation Judicious use of drugs

Continued.

Table 8-1. Emergencies: signs, symptoms, and treatments—cont'd

Emergency	Signs and symptoms	Treatment
Hyperthyroidism (thyroid storm; life-threatening; extremely rare)	Hyperpyrexia Profuse sweating Nausea, vomiting Abdominal pain Tachycardia Disorientation Agitation Coma	Terminate therapy Supine position Provide basic life support* O$_2$ Summon medical assistance
Seizure disorders		
Epilepsy (tonic-clonic seizures)	PRODROMAL STAGE Increase in anxiety or depression Aura Loss of consciousness ICTAL STAGE Cyanosis Tonic and clonic movements Frothing Occasionally urinary and fecal incontinence POSTICTAL STAGE Deep sleep to comatose Disoriented Headache Muscle soreness	Terminate therapy Place in supine position Protect from injury Provide basic life support* Monitor vital signs Allow patient to recover If duration is longer than 5 minutes, summon medical assistance Continue to monitor vital signs
Cerebral vascular accident		
(Sudden onset)	Flushed Bounding pulse Paralysis Headache Dizziness Drowsiness Nausea, vomiting Loss of consciousness	Terminate therapy Provide basic life support* Manage signs and symptoms Monitor vital signs Summon medical assistance
Allergic reaction		
	One or more body systems must be affected Reaction may be mild or severe Itching Urticaria Wheezing Nausea, vomiting Abdominal cramps Urinary, fecal incontinence Cardiac dysrhythmias Obstructed airway	For mild reaction (slow onset—longer than 1 hour), administer antihistamine and arrange for medical consultation For severe reaction (anaphylaxis) administer epinephrine, provide basic life support,* summon medical assistance, and arrange medical consultation for future therapy
Toxic (Overdose)		
Reaction to local anesthetic or vasoconstrictor	MILD TO MODERATE OD Confusion Excitedness	Terminate therapy Reassure patient

Table 8-1. Emergencies: signs, symptoms, and treatments—cont'd

Emergency	Signs and symptoms	Treatment
	Slurred speech Headache Blurred vision Numbness in perioral area	Administer O_2 and instruct patient to hyperventilate Provide basic life support* Monitor vital signs Recovery Medical consultation for further therapy
	MODERATE TO HIGH OD Tonic-clonic seizures CNS depression Depressed BP, heart rate, and respiratory rate May lose consciousness	Supine position Manage seizure Provide basic life support* Monitor vital signs Summon medical assistance Transport to hospital Medical consultation for future therapy

*Basic life support (BLS) does two things: (1) prevents circulatory or respiratory arrest or insufficiency through prompt recognition and intervention, and (2) externally supports circulation and respiration of a victim of cardiac or respiratory arrest through CPR.
**ABCs refers to airway, breathing, and circulation.
***The Heimleich maneuver is performed differently in infants, children, and adults. A course in BLS provides information and practice for this procedure.
Data from American Heart Association (1985), Malamed (1987), Rose (1981), McCarthy (1982), and Braum (1979).

of most critical medical situations. Accordingly, actual medical emergencies are *not* the time for "trying out" or "practicing" emergency techniques for the first time.

Keep in mind when developing an emergency kit that consideration should also be given to the anticipated arrival time of backup advanced life support. A clinician must be able to manage a critical situation for at least as long as it takes for expert help to arrive. Thus, an emergency kit for a practice located in a large medical building or an emergency medical clinic is likely to differ in content from a kit for a rural practice that is dependent upon a volunteer ambulance department whose arrival time may be more than an hour.

Note that *most* emergency situations can be managed using basic life support (without use of drugs) until advanced life support can arrive. Therefore, keep the emergency kit simple and, whenever doubt exists, do *not* medicate. (An important exception for drug intervention is treatment for acute anaphylaxis, where epinephrine would be the drug of choice.) (Malamed, 1987)

A basic emergency kit should normally include aromatic ammonia capsules, portable oxygen (O_2) with delivery system (separate from the nitrous

oxygen unit), nitroglycerine, and epinephrine. Aromatic ammonia capsules are one of the most commonly used drugs in emergency management. They should be readily available in each operatory and in the emergency kit itself. An ammonia capsule taped to the back of the patient's chair can provide practitioners with quick and easy access to the medication in case of a syncopal episode (Malamed, 1987).

Oxygen is also used to manage many emergency situations, from minor to very serious. Portable equipment is essential here, as emergencies don't occur exclusively in the operatory. Patients may require oxygen in waiting rooms, hallways, restrooms, and other parts of the practice setting. Practitioners should acquire an "E" size portable cylinder, providing at least 30 minutes of oxygen, and an additional backup full cylinder, so that 1 full hour of total emergency oxygen is available for use in treatment and transport of the patient. Every staff member should know how to replace oxygen tanks under emergency conditions. In addition, a written record of oxygen use should be plainly presented on all tanks so that a verifiable and adequate supply is also ensured.

A reliable method of delivering oxygen is also important. If a patient is not breathing (that is, in respiratory arrest), the practitioner must have access to a mechanism capable of forcing air into the victim's lungs. One such device is the positive pressure mask (Robert Shaw). When attached to the oxygen tank, this mask will deliver 100% oxygen to the patient. Another device, the portable self-inflating resuscitation bag (Ambu bag), can be attached to the O_2 tank to deliver 100% O_2 or be used alone to deliver 20% atmospheric O_2. During a cardiac emergency, the patient will benefit more from 100% oxygen.

Masks for either of these devices should be clear, allowing the operator optimal visibility to monitor vomitus, blood, or other substances that may be expelled. Ensuring an airtight seal is also critical. Masks are sized adult, pedo, and infant to facilitate proper fit and seal. Accordingly, a complete kit should contain a full range of sized masks. Basic competence with any delivery system is, of course, realizable only through diligent and conscientious practice.

Nitroglycerin is a vasodilator and is used for the treatment of chest pain, such as angina pectoris and myocardial infarction. Nitroglycerin is available in spray or tablet; spray is recommended due to its longer shelf life. Whenever possible, a patient's own prescription should be used.

Epinephrine is used in the treatment of acute anaphylaxis. Because time is critical in this type of emergency, preloaded syringes are recommended. Hollister-Stier Laboratories offers a preloaded, metered syringe that allows only a preset or recommended dosage of epinephrine to be administered, thereby minimizing the risk of overdose; to administer an additional dose, the syringe plunger must be rotated. The importance of this built-in safety device cannot be overstated (Malamed, 1987).

Many other types of drugs and equipment could be included in any functional emergency kit. Primary drugs and equipment—those necessary for prompt, successful management of a crisis—should receive priority consideration. Secondary drugs and equipment, although important, would be less critical for crisis management and often require advanced training for use. A third group of drugs and equipment, designed for practitioners with ACLS (advanced cardiac life support)

training, would not be included in the normal makeup of an emergency kit unless an operator had received such training (Malamed, 1987).

A suggested list of primary drugs and equipment is as follows (see Table 8-2 for additional information):
1. Primary Injectable Drugs
   a. Epinephrine
   b. Antihistamine
   c. Anticonvulsant
   d. Narcotic antagonist
2. Primary Noninjectable Drugs
   a. Oxygen
   b. Vasodilator
3. Primary Emergency Equipment
   a. O_2 plus delivery system
   b. Suction and suction tips
   c. Tourniquets (for the practitioners skilled in venipuncture)
   d. Syringes for drug administration (Malamed, 1987)

Finally, a complete and plainly visible log of drugs should always be affixed to any emergency kit. This log should list and identify drugs by both generic and proprietary name and should include the expiration date of each, to minimize confusion in time of crisis and to prevent the use of outdated drugs.

Syncope, or simple fainting, can occur if the patient's brain fails to receive adequate oxygen and glucose as the result of vasodilation or loss of vasomotor tone. The signs of simple syncope are loss of color from the skin (pallor), perspiration, slight confusion, complaints of nausea or dizziness, and sometimes loss of consciousness from which the patient can be roused; in coma, the patient cannot be roused (Miller, 1982). Since most dental procedures are performed with the patient in the supine position, which facilitates adequate blood flow to the brain, syncope is probably a less likely occurrence now than in the era of the upright position (Miller, 1982). Sitting up rapidly after being in a supine or recumbent position can, however, bring on syncope.

If a patient does exhibit signs of syncope and complains of discomfort, instruments should be moved away, the chair should be adjusted to the full supine position, and another team member should be alerted. Oxygen should be readied for administration, a cool cloth may be applied to the

Table 8-2. Emergency drugs and equipment

Category	Drug of choice	
	Generic	*Proprietary*

I. Injectable drugs
PRIMARY DRUGS

Category	Generic	Proprietary
Allergy	Epinephrine	Adrenalin
Anthistamine	Chlorpheniramine	Chlor-Trimeton Maleate
Anticonvulsant*	Diazepam	Valium
Narcotic antagonist†	Naloxone	Narcan

SECONDARY DRUGS

Category	Generic	Proprietary
Analgesic	Morphine sulfate	
Vasopressor	Methoxamine HCl	Vasoxyl
Corticosteroid	Hydrocortisone succinate	Solu-Cortef
Antihypoglycemic	50% Dextrose	—
	Glucagon	Glucagon

ADVANCED CARDIAC LIFE SUPPORT INJECTABLES

Category	Generic	Proprietary
	Sodium bicarbonate	
	Atropine sulfate	
	Lidocaine	Xylocaine
	Calcium chloride	

*Anticonvulsant is a primary drug only when the practitioner is able to administer the drug intravenously.
†Narcotic antagonist is primary drug if any narcotic is employed in patient management. It need not be present if narcotics are never used.

II. Noninjectable drugs
PRIMARY DRUGS

Category	Generic	Proprietary
Oxygen	Oxygen	—
Vasodilator	Nitroglycerin	Nitrolingual spray

SECONDARY DRUGS

Category	Generic	Proprietary
Respiratory stimulant	Aromatic ammonia	—
Antihypoglycemic agent	Carbohydrate	Many available, plus juice, icing tubes
Bronchodilator	Metaproterenol	Alupent

III. Emergency equipment

Equipment	Description

PRIMARY EMERGENCY EQUIPMENT

Equipment	Description
Oxygen delivery system*	Positive pressure/demand valve or self-inflating bag-valve-mask *and* clear full face masks
Suction and suction tips	Large-diameter, round-ended suction tips or tonsil suction tips (high-volume suction)
Syringes for drug administration	Disposable syringes
Tourniquets	Rubber tourniquet or latex tubing or sphygmomanometer

SECONDARY EMERGENCY EQUIPMENT

Equipment	Description
Scalpel or cricothyrotomy device†	
Artificial airways†	Oropharyngeal airways
	Nasopharyngeal airways
Airway adjuncts†	Laryngoscope and endotracheal tubes

*Advanced training is required for safe and effective use of these devices. All dental personnel should be trained in their use.
†Advanced training is required for safe and effective use of these devices. *Do not* include in emergency kit if personnel are not trained to use properly.
Adapted from Malamed SF: Handbook of medical emergencies in the dental office, ed 3, St Louis, 1987, The CV Mosby Co.

patient's forehead, and an ammonia ampule should be ready for wafting under the patient's nose.

Many times, prompt action can avert loss of consciousness. If the patient does retain consciousness, he or she should be allowed to rest comfortably, essential procedures such as suturing an area should be completed, and the patient should be allowed to leave when fully recovered.

If the patient does lose consciousness, an ammonia ampule can be broken and wafted under the patient's nose (Dunn and Booth, 1975; Malamed, 1987; Miller, 1982). A quick whiff will usually restore consciousness. Oxygen can then be administered along with comforting words. When fully recovered, the patient should be allowed to leave. It may be necessary to escort the patient home.

If a woman in the late stages of pregnancy loses consciousness, the back of the chair should be lowered and the patient should be turned onto her side (Malamed, 1987). Placing a woman in the third trimester of pregnancy on her back, especially on a hard surface, can cut off circulation in the venous system; the weight of the uterus impinging on the vena cava can encourage loss of consciousness.

A patient recovering from syncope (or another emergency) may be frightened or even embarrassed. Care and comfort without undue solicitousness may be appreciated by the patient during the recovery stages.

Syncope is only one of the possible reasons for a patient lapsing into unconsciousness. In the beginning stages of syncope, the patient has a lowered blood pressure and increased pulse. Recovery is usually rapid if the actions previously described are taken. If the recovery is not immediate, the clinician should check for respirations. The mouth mirror can be placed close to the mouth or nose to check for fogging, or the clinician can listen for sounds of respiration by placing his or her ear close to the patient's mouth. The pulse can be checked by placing the fingers in the area of the carotid artery between the larynx and the anterior border of the sternocleidomastoid muscle. If either sign is absent, help should be summoned immediately. Someone should be directed to call a rescue team. Then the procedures of basic life support are begun. The clinician clears and maintains an airway, forcing oxygen into the lungs, and performs external cardiac massage if there is no pulse (Dunn and Booth, 1975; Malamed, 1987; McCarthy, 1982).

Acute adrenal insufficiency, wherein the adrenal gland does not produce sufficient amounts of cortisol, rendering the body incapable of coping with stress, is another possible cause of loss of consciousness. Patients likely to experience acute adrenal insufficiency fall into three groups: persons in the late stages of Addison's disease (adrenocortical insufficiency) who have not yet been diagnosed and are not yet taking medication; persons who are suddenly withdrawn from steroid hormones; and persons experiencing stress, particularly those with compromised functioning of the adrenal or pituitary glands (patients receiving corticosteroids) (Malamed, 1987). Many diseases (Addison's disease, asthma, herpes zoster, ulcerative colitis, rheumatoid arthritis, lichen planus, to name only a few) are treated with steroid hormones. Athletes and body builders often use self-prescribed steroids indiscriminately. A thorough dialogue review of the patient's medical history (Brady, 1980), including medications being taken or recently stopped, is imperative so that the clinician can be aware of factors that may predispose a patient to acute adrenal insufficiency. A patient experiencing acute adrenal insufficiency is in danger of death from shock and cardiac arrest. The hygienist should summon assistance, initiate CPR, and relate the symptoms to the dentist or physician, who may administer cortisone to counteract the crisis.

A person with *diabetes mellitus* may lose consciousness as a result of low blood sugar levels *(hypoglycemia)* secondary to a relative excess of insulin. This can happen if a meal is omitted, if the patient exercises heavily and uses available blood glucose, or if there is an overdose of insulin (insulin shock). For the conscious patient, orange juice or any carbohydrate can reverse the condition. For the unconscious patient, IV or IM glucose is indicated, accompanied by basic life support.

Hypoglycemia can occur in patients who do not have diabetes. Patients who skip meals before dental treatment and who are anxious about the dental visit may experience a drop in the blood glucose level. Alcoholics suffer from hypoglycemia because of a lack of stored glycogen in the liver and poor nutrition.

Hyperglycemia is a possible cause of loss of consciousness for the diabetic. In this case insulin levels are insufficient; the blood sugar rises above safe levels. Insulin is necessary to reverse this situation. If the patient has a history of insulin shock, this should be included in the medical history. The patient may carry a supply of insulin for injection, of which the clinician should be aware. Coma associated with hyperglycemia occurs most frequently in juvenile diabetics, usually when the case is first diagnosed. In most cases a comatose patient is hypoglycemic and needs glucose. The response to glucose should be immediate. The hyperglycemic patient will not improve with glucose.

Patients may experience respiratory difficulty in a number of ways. A patient may be *choking* on excess saliva, water, or a foreign object or may need to cough for some other reason. If the patient is able to cough, do not interfere. Coughing will aid in object removal and indicates good air exchange (American Heart Association, 1985).

If choking is due to a foreign object, such as a prophy cup in the oropharynx area, do not allow the patient to sit up. Instead, place the chair in a head-down position (Trendenlenberg), allowing gravity to return the object to the oral cavity where it can be retrieved by coughing or forceps. Do not allow the patient to sit up if the object has progressed into the trachea. Place the patient in the head-down position, lying on the right side. Encourage the patient to cough, if coughing does not occur spontaneously (Malamed, 1987). If the patient cannot cough and begins to express panic, assistance may be necessary to free the air passage. The recommended procedure is the Heimlich maneuver, in which the air in the lungs is forced out by upward compression on the diaphragm. This technique should be learned under supervision as part of a life-support course.

A second form of respiratory difficulty is *hyperventilation* (Dunn and Booth, 1975; Malamed, 1987), usually due to anxiety, in which insufficient carbon dioxide is present in the bloodstream because of prolonged rapid breathing. It is characterized by tingling fingers and toes, light-headedness, acute anxiety, and rapid breathing. Perioral tingling or numbness is characteristic also of hy-

perventilation. Usually, having the patient breathe in and out of a bag (a headrest cover, perhaps) will permit the patient to inhale sufficient amounts of carbon dioxide to reverse the problem. The patient should be calmed. A tranquilizer may be necessary in severe cases.

There are two kinds of *asthmatic attacks*. The mild form is more typical and is characterized by a feeling of thickness in the chest, coughing, wheezing, slow and labored breathing, heightened anxiety, a slightly elevated blood pressure, and an elevated heart rate. Treatment for a mild attack includes steps 1 to 3 and 8 below, which will usually be effective; steps 4 and onward can be taken in the case of a severe attack or if relief is incomplete (Malamed, 1987).

1. Terminate the dental therapy.
2. Position the patient comfortably (usually either sitting up or standing).
3. Administer an aerosol spray of epinephrine or similar drug. (Most patients who suffer from these attacks carry a bronchodilator for such emergencies.)
4. Administer oxygen.
5. Give IM or subcutaneous injection of aqueous epinephrine if necessary.
6. Summon medical assistance if steps 1 to 5 are ineffective.
7. Give IV medication if necessary.
8. After recuperation, reevaluate for continued therapy, recovery, and eventual dismissal.

Chest pain associated with cardiovascular problems can be caused by heart failure, angina pectoris, or myocardial infarction. Further discussion of these diseases is found in Chapter 5.

Heart failure will cause respiratory difficulty (Malamed, 1987). The signs of onset include chest pain and palpitation, a feeling of suffocation, coughing including bloody sputum, and sometimes cyanosis. The difficulty in breathing is due to the filling of the interstitial tissues of the lungs with serous fluid. As long as the patient is conscious, he or she should be positioned in an upright position, which allows the excess lung fluid to settle in the lower lung areas so that there can be some exchange of air in the tissues. Oxygen should be administered; avoid using a mask, if possible, to minimize the patient's sensation of suffocation. Emergency assistance and hospital transport must be summoned. Diuretics to reduce the fluid and digitalis to improve heart contractility may be administered as a part of medical treatment.

Angina pectoris is a temporary lack of oxygen in the heart muscle due to (1) narrowed coronary arteries; (2) exertion, excitement, or eating a heavy meal; or (3) an increased work load. The pain ranges from mild to severe and often radiates to the left shoulder or arm. It usually is not as intense as the pain caused by an infarction, wherein blood supply is cut off to a portion of muscle, causing tissue death. Vasodilators, such as nitroglycerin, are used to treat angina. The vasodilator allows the circulatory capacity of the heart muscle to dilate, improving flow and reducing the work load and thus the pain. Currently, nitroglycerin spray (developed in 1986) is most commonly used for the treatment of an anginal episode. At the onset of pain, one dose of nitroglycerin spray is administered sublingually. If the pain persists beyond 10 minutes and 3 doses of nitroglycerin, emergency medical help should be summoned (American Heart Association, 1985; Malamed, 1987; McCarthy, 1982).

Myocardial infarction, also called *coronary occlusion,* results when the coronary artery flow to some portion of the heart muscle is stopped. The affected muscle dies from lack of oxygen. About 75% of cases are caused by a thrombosis (blood clot). Symptoms are similar to those of angina pectoris, but the pain is more crushing and is not relieved by nitroglycerin. The patient is often in a cold sweat, weak, and restless. In contrast, the patient with angina stays still, knowing movement heightens the pain. An infarction often is accompanied by nausea, light-headedness, coughing, wheezing, and abdominal bloating (which may cause the patient to mistake the problem for indigestion) (McCarthy, 1982).

The first step in treating an infarction is to administer nitroglycerin and watch for pain relief. If the pain continues or increases, summon emergency assistance, administer oxygen, and monitor vital signs. Drugs for relief of pain can be administered. The emergency medical team should manage complications such as arrhythmia. In the event of cardiac arrest, CPR must be begun to prevent death (Blair, 1982; Malamed, 1987; McCarthy, 1982).

Cardiac arrest occurs when the heart has stopped beating or "circulation of blood is absent or inadequate to maintain life" (Malamed, 1987). Myocardial infarction is only one cause. Others are airway obstruction, drug overdose, anaphylaxis, seizure disorders, and acute adrenal insufficiency. The treatment is to restore circulation. In a dental office, the method of choice is CPR, where a heartbeat and respiration are created for the patient through external cardiac compression and ventilation.

All dental health care providers must complete a course in CPR. The American Heart Association recommends level C certification for health care providers and annual recertification (American Heart Association, 1985).

Altered consciousness can be observed in patients who are intoxicated, patients in early stages of hypoglycemia or hyperglycemia, patients with hypothyroidism or hyperthyroidism, or patients entering a convulsive state, such as epilepsy. The patients should be monitored to ensure they do not lose vital signs and should be escorted home (in the case of excess alcohol) or taken for physical evaluation by a physician. In severe cases, hospitalization may be indicated. In the case of epilepsy, it is important to ensure that a patent airway be maintained during tonic-clonic seizures. Obstruction often is caused by removable dental appliances or objects forced between the victim's teeth. Placement of any object in the oral cavity usually is NOT indicated during tonic-clonic seizures (Malamed, 1987).

An additional cause of altered consciousness is a *cerebral vascular accident* in which a blood vessel in the brain breaks or is occluded, preventing adequate blood supply to the brain. Accompanying signs are intense headache, weakness or paralysis of speech and extremities, dizziness, and nausea. The patient should be positioned in a semierect position. The symptoms should be managed until assistance can be summoned.

Reactions to a local anesthetic

Patients can have reactions to local anesthetics, ranging from syncope (psychogenic reaction) to a toxic reaction (overdose) to an allergic reaction (Malamed, 1987). It is extremely important that a member of the dental team who is capable of recognizing an emergency situation remains with a patient after he or she has received an injection, as a minor or severe immediate reaction can occur in 3 to 5 minutes. Most patients are anxious before and during an injection. Syncope is the most common reaction to a local anesthetic injection; its signs and symptoms and the methods for treating it have been described. Another stress-related reaction that can occur is hyperventilation, which also has been described.

A *toxic reaction* is due to an absolute or relative overdose of a local anesthetic agent or a vasoconstrictor. It is caused by the clinician injecting more solution than the patient's body can metabolize and excrete. This reaction can be prevented by aspirating before injecting, by injecting the solution slowly, by injecting only the recommended amount according to body weight, and by checking the patient's history for the presence of disease or previous reaction to local anesthetic. During a mild toxic reaction the patient will appear restless, talkative, and agitated. The clinician should stop administering the agent, instruct the patient to hyperventilate O_2 from the O_2 mask (Malamed, 1987), and allow the patient's system to remove some of the anesthetic; a mild toxic reaction can reverse itself. A severe toxic reaction is characterized by an excitatory stage (agitation or possibly convulsions), followed by a corresponding depression. A patient suffering from such an attack needs immediate medical attention. The clinician should begin life-support measures, alert the supervising dentist immediately, and have someone notify a rescue squad.

Another possible reaction is an *allergic reaction,* which can be a delayed mild reaction or an immediate severe reaction.

The immediate and severe reaction, called *anaphylaxis,* often begins with itching and urticaria but rapidly progresses to a life-threatening stage including muscle spasms, fluid accumulation, swelling in the throat causing inability to breathe, and cardiovascular collapse and death (Stroh and Johnson, 1982). Anaphylaxis requires immediate attention, including epinephrine IM or IV, an antihistaminic IM or IV, and a corticosteroid IM or IV. Further assistance from a medical team should be sought.

At the first signs of itching or urticaria, the clinician should stop dental treatment and retrieve the preloaded syringe of epinephrine (0.3 milliliters of 1:1000 aqueous) for subcutaneous injection

(Malamed, 1987). If the reaction progresses, this agent should be administered immediately. If the patient is already in shock, the quickest route for distribution of the drug is IV. Because peripheral veins may be collapsed at this stage, injection is best accomplished by injecting into the highly vascular underside of the tongue. Such injections have been shown to assist resuscitation (Stroh and Johnson, 1982; Shaber and Smith, 1982).

Following injection, the clinician should ensure that the airway is maintained, which may require an emergency cricothyrotomy. As the throat is occluded, and no air can circulate, an airway can be created by penetrating the neck with a large-bore needle into the trachea through the cricothyroid cartilage. As soon as the opening is created, the tubeway should be firmly stabilized and oxygen administered via that route.

A mild allergic reaction is characterized by a skin rash and itching; often this will be a delayed reaction. The patient may call the office several hours after the injection, complaining of a rash and itching. A mild allergic reaction is treated by administering an antihistaminic; the patient should be referred for further medical care.

It is extremely important to record accurately any untoward reaction of a patient during treatment. Many of the medical emergencies described could recur or may indicate a severe physical condition that needs prompt medical attention. The supervising dentist should refer a patient for a medical evaluation if a previously indicated medical condition seems apparent.

In addition to helping to ensure the patient's safety, accurate records are necessary in the case of later legal proceedings. Thorough, objective, accurate progress notes about a medical emergency are part of the dental personnel's best defense.

EMERGENCIES IN NONTRADITIONAL SETTINGS

As the role of the dental hygienist expands into nontraditional settings, so must the emergency management skill of the hygienist. The nursing home hygienist should inform the head nurse of her presence before therapy begins. It is important to be familiar with the emergency protocol of each facility and to review it thoroughly before entering the residence. This procedure should also be followed by the hygienists in industry, schools, elder care centers, and other nontraditional practice settings. The hygienist working with the homebound should invest in an emergency kit and create an emergency protocol for each home visited. It is important to know the location of phones and emergency numbers and to be familiar with the local emergency medical services before beginning dental therapy.

Accident, personal injury, and fire prevention

Although many emergencies in the dental office relate to the disposition of patient medical emergencies, other kinds of emergencies can be precipitated by negligence, carelessness, or unforeseeable circumstances.

To prevent accidents, it is important to ensure that all equipment is safe and functioning properly. A loose hinge, a missing bolt, or a short circuit can lead to unfortunate accidents that can harm the patient and the dental professional. It is the dental professional's responsibility to protect the patient from harm due to faulty equipment and to eliminate hazards that could cause harm, such as a tangle of cords in the patient's pathway or a wet, slippery floor.

Personal injury can result from criminal acts of intruders as well as from physical hazards in the office. It is always wise to have a co-worker available to summon assistance in the case of a medical emergency and to dissuade persons (including, perhaps, a patient) from assaulting the dental professional. Working alone in a quiet office in close proximity with a patient may stimulate a normal patient and may provoke erratic behavior in an emotionally disturbed patient.

Drugs and cash or checks should be locked away in an unnoticeable place to reduce the likelihoood of robbery during or after office hours.

The department of education and safety of local police forces provide many individualized programs, such as self-protection, personal safety for women in employment, single female safety, and crime prevention, to ensure the safety of the dental staff and office. The programs are free and of invaluable service.

Fire prevention is an additional factor in preventing emergencies. Flammable substances should be kept clear from the flame of a Bunsen burner and from the heat of a radiator. The laboratory, in particular, is a hazardous area, because the open flame of a Bunsen burner may ignite hair, electrical wiring, papers, or other materials. A fire extinguisher should be kept in the laboratory for prompt response to such occurrences. The natural gas supplied to operatories and the laboratory is a potential hazard if there is a leak or if a gas jet is left open. If such a leak goes undetected and fills the room, simply turning on a light switch and producing a spark or static electricity can cause a sudden explosion.

Fire departments routinely inspect public buildings; however, additional educational courses will be provided upon request to help ensure the safety of office personnel and patients. The courses are free.

Preparing for emergencies

Once the entire dental team has completed life-support and emergency management courses, the team should write out specific protocols for action in the event of medical emergencies. Specific assignments should be made to individuals to ensure that all designated procedures are completed. The protocols should be posted, reviewed monthly, and rehearsed.

Routes for fire escape, procedures for extinguishing fires that are contained, and procedures for summoning assistance should be drafted by the team, reviewed, and rehearsed. Smoke detectors should be installed. A main valve for natural gas should be installed and should be closed at the end of each working day. Again, procedures in the event of a police or fire emergency should be rehearsed. This preparation could save a person's life.

ACTIVITIES

1. Identify the location of the emergency kit in the clinic. Note the contents and purposes of each item included. Also note the expiration date of each drug. Discuss the security system for guarding against theft of drugs while ensuring ready access to drugs by the dental staff during an emergency.
2. Locate and operate the oxygen mask and supply for the conscious and unconscious patient.
3. Role play various emergency situations, such as the following:
   a. Cardiac arrest
   b. Syncope
   c. Hypoglycemia
   d. Respiratory difficulty
4. Design an emergency protocol for several different clinical settings. Consider office personnel, office

design, emergency equipment, and location. Your plan must consider contingencies in the event that a staff member is the victim or is out of the office.

5. Review a variety of medical histories of medically compromised patients. In groups of three or four, plan for potential medical emergencies and simulate the proper emergency responses for the entire class.
6. Refer to Absi EG: A cardiac arrest in the dental chair, British Dental Journal **163**:199, 1987, for a case history. As a group, discuss the protocol that was followed before, during, and after the incident.
7. Simulate a fire emergency evacuation from the clinical setting.
8. Refer to Malamed (1987): "Appendix/Quick-reference Section to Life-threatening Situations," pp. 392-397. Have your emergency team discuss each of the emergency situations contained in this appendix.
9. Refer to Blair (1982) and have your emergency team discuss each of the errors shown and described.
10. Locate your own carotid pulse by palpating with your fingers between your larynx and the anterior border of the sternocleidomastoid muscle. Check for respirations by using a stethoscope on a partner's larynx and by placing a dental mirror under the nose.
11. Refer to Fast TB: Emergency preparedness: a survey of dental practitioners, JADA **112(4)**:1986. Have a group discussion on the report.
12. Arrange for a local law enforcement body to provide a personal safety and crime prevention course for the class.

REVIEW QUESTIONS

1. Why is it essential for a dental hygienist to have completed a comprehensive course in first aid and in basic life support?
2. List the suggested primary drugs and equipment for an emergency kit and their use.
3. How can the dental team prepare for an emergency?
4. What do you do if:
   a. Your patient becomes ashen and agitated and complains of nausea and dizziness?
   b. Your patient complains of severe chest pain?
   c. Your patient suddenly loses consciousness?
5. Explain how oxygen delivery to the conscious victim will differ from oxygen delivery to the unconscious victim.

REFERENCES

ADA Council on Dental Materials, Instruments, and Equipment. Dentist's desk reference: materials, instruments and equipment. Chicago, 1981, American Dental Association.

ADA Council on Dental Therapeutics. Chicago, 1986, American Dental Association.

American Heart Association: Instructor's manual for basic life support, Dallas, 1985, American Heart Association.

Blair DM: Cardiac emergencies, Dent Clin North Am **26**:49, 1982.

Blair DM: Common errors in handling medical emergencies, Dent Clin North Am **26**:163, 1982.

Blitz P: Personal communication, 1979.

Bodak-Gyovai LZ: Oral medicine: patient evaluation and management, Baltimore, 1980, Williams & Wilkins.

Brady W, et al: Validity of health history data collected from dental patients and patient perception of health status, JADA **101**:642, 1980.

Braun R: Dentists' manual of emergency medical treatment, Reston, Va, 1979, Reston Publishing Co.

Capello J, et al: Medical emergencies: the dental team approach, Dent Surv **53**:24, Aug 1977.

Corah N, et al: Assessment of a dental anxiety scale, JADA **97**:816, 1978.

Dunn MJ, and Booth DF: Dental auxiliary practice: internal medicine and systemic emergencies, Baltimore, 1975, Williams & Wilkins.

Freeman NS, et al: Office emergencies: causes, symptoms, treatment, Oral Health **67**:60, Oct 1977.

Howell RB: Office emergency procedures: a self-study course, Chicago, 1979, American Dental Hygienists' Association.

Jaffe M: Teaching medical emergencies in a dental hygiene program, NY State Dent J **48**:456, 1982.

Kinne RD: Training for the effective management of medical emergencies, Dent Clin North Am **26**:147, 1982.

Lown B: Lidocaine to prevent ventricular fibrillation. New Eng J Med 33, 1985.

Maitland RI: Patient assessment in the dental office emergency, NY State Dent J **48**:442, 1978.

Malamed, SF: Handbook of medical emergencies in the dental office, ed 3, St Louis, 1987, The CV Mosby Co.

Martin M, et al: Skills in cardiopulmonary resuscitation: a survey of dental practitioners, JADA **112**:501, 1986.

McCarthy F: A new-patient administered medical history developed for dentistry, JADA 111, 1985.

McCarthy F: Vital signs—the six minute warnings. JADA **100**:682, 1980.

McCarthy, FM: Medical emergencies in dentistry, ed 8, Philadelphia, 1982, WB Saunders Co.

McCarthy F, and Malamed S: Physical evaluation system to determine medical risk and indicated dental therapy modifications, JADA **99**:181, 1979.

Miller AG Jr: Syncope, Dent Clin North Am **26**:119, 1982.

Morrow GT: Designing a drug kit, Dent Clin North Am **26**:21, 1982.

Perks ER: The diagnosis and management of sudden collapse in dental practice, I, Br Dent J **143**:196, Sept 1977.

Proy HG, et al: Minicomputer simulation of medical emergencies and advanced life support, J Dent Educ **46**:657, 1982.

Rose F, and Hendler B: Medical emergencies in dental practice, Chicago, 1981, Quintessence Publishing Co, Inc.

Rose L: Diagnosis and management of medical emergencies in the dental office, Cont Dent Educ (Self-instruction Series) **1**:3, 1977.

Rose LM, and Hendler BH: Medical emergencies in dental practice, Chicago, 1981, Quintessence Publishing Co, Inc.

Ryan DE, and Bronstein SL: Dentistry and the diabetic patient, Dent Clin North Am **26:**105, 1982.

Safar P: Cardiopulmonary cerebral resuscitation, Stavenger. Norway, 1981, Asmund S. Laerdal.

Sanger RG, et al: Training program in emergency medical service for the dental profession, JADA **98:**695, 1979.

Shaber EP, and Smith RA: Techniques of drug administration, Dent Clin North Am **26:**35, 1982.

Shannon ME: Strokes, Dent Clin North Am **26:**99, 1982.

Shijatshky M: Life threatening emergencies in the dental practice, Chicago, 1975, Quintessence Publishing Co, Inc. Translated by HM Koehler.

Solomon AL: Emergency treatment: local and general anesthesia, NY State Dent J **48:**447, 1982.

Stroh JE Jr, and Johnson RL: Allergy-related emergencies in dental practice, Dent Clin North Am **26:**87, 1982.

Trieger N: Special care of the medically compromised patient, NY State Dent J **48:**451, 1982.

Trieger N, et al: The art of history taking, J Oral Surg 36, Feb 1978.

Turner R: First aid in acute myocardial infarction, Br Med J **1:**356, 1976.

Woodworth JV, and Woodworth CE: Emergency! The dentist's role in prevention and treatment, I, Gen Dent, **26:**35, May-June 1978.

Woodworth JV, and Woodworth CE: Emergency! The dentist's role in prevention and treatment, II, Gen Dent **26:**46, July-Aug 1978.

Woodworth JV, and Woodworth CE: Emergency! The dentist's role in prevention and treatment, III, Gen Dent **26:**56, Sept-Oct 1978.

Zinman, EJ: Emergency care: some legal implications, Dent Surg **55:**46, Aug 1979.

9 INSTRUMENT SHARPENING

OBJECTIVES: *The reader will be able to*

1. State the advantages of using sharp periodontal instruments.
2. Discuss three ways to tell if cutting edges are sharp.
3. Describe the design features of universal curettes, Gracey curettes, and sickle scalers that must be maintained during the sharpening procedure.
4. Describe four different techniques for sharpening instruments.
5. State the rationale for sharpening the lateral surfaces of curettes and sickle scalers.
6. Discuss the care of an Arkansas sharpening stone.
7. Describe two techniques for sharpening curettes and sickle scalers using a hand-held sharpening stone.

RATIONALE FOR SHARPENING

A clinician's success at all instrumentation procedures is directly related to the quality of the instruments used. Effective scaling, root planing, and soft-tissue curettage depend on the use of sharp instruments for their success. There are a number of advantages to using sharp instruments. First, a sharp cutting edge is more effective in removing calculus and cementum from tooth surfaces. Dull instruments are more likely to smooth over or burnish calculus deposits than remove them cleanly from the tooth surface. A sharp cutting edge can shear off deposits and plane root surfaces with less effort and fewer strokes. A sharp cutting edge will also deliver more sensitive tactile feedback to the clinician during the scaling and root planing procedures so that more information is gained by exploring strokes.

Instruments should be sharp at the beginning of the appointment and should be resharpened frequently during scaling and root planing procedures. Tal et al. (1985) found that cutting edges of curettes had been slightly bevelled (dulled) after only 15 strokes on root surfaces of extracted teeth. Wider bevels were seen after 45 strokes. Depending on the condition of the root surfaces, this number of strokes may be needed to root plane only one or two teeth. This study underscores the need for continual resharpening during root planing procedures. The soft-tissue curettage

procedure requires an extremely sharp cutting edge, so that inflamed tissues can be sliced away from healthy gingiva, rather than being torn or ripped away. Using a dull instrument for soft-tissue curettage would be about as effective as trying to peel an apple with a plastic spoon—it could be done, but there would be little apple left when it was finished.

Hygienists who work with properly sharpened instruments are more effective and more efficient. When instruments are sharp, fewer strokes are needed to remove calculus deposits or diseased cementum from the tooth. A sharp cutting edge allows more effective exploration, which saves time by eliminating the need to constantly switch back and forth between an explorer and the scaling instrument. Both patient and clinician will benefit from the time saved during the appointment by using sharp instruments. An additional benefit to the professional is that instruments that are resharpened frequently require less recontouring than those which are allowed to get extremely dull. Only a small amount of metal must be removed from well-maintained instruments, so less time is required to sharpen them and they tend to last longer.

The use of a sharp instrument can also make scaling procedures a more pleasant experience for both the clinician and patient. Less effort is needed for a scaling stroke when sharp instru-

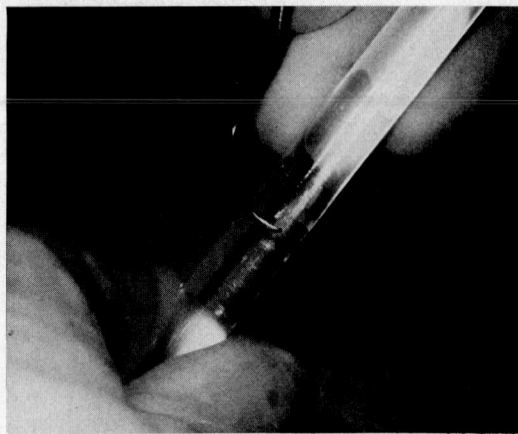

Fig. 9-1. Acrylic testing stick is used by applying light pressure against stick with the instrument at its working angle.

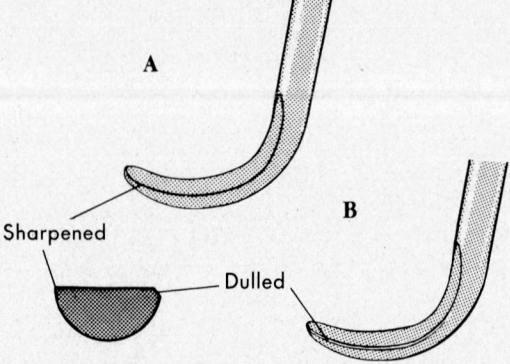

Fig. 9-2. A, A sharp cutting edge will not reflect light. **B,** A dull cutting edge will appear as a bright area at junction of face and lateral surface.

ments are used. The patient will appreciate a light and gentle approach to scaling and root planing. When dull instruments are used, working strokes must be repeated again and again in the same area until the deposits are finally removed. This repetition can be tiring for the hygienist and unpleasant for the patient. It is easy to understand that the short amount of time it takes to sharpen instruments effectively is certainly justified by the benefits that are gained.

IDENTIFICATION OF SHARP VERSUS DULL INSTRUMENTS

The first step in learning how to sharpen instruments is to develop the ability to determine whether or not an instrument is optimally sharp. There are a number of ways to evaluate instrument sharpness. Experienced clinicians can determine when their instruments are getting dull by the increase in the effort needed to remove calculus deposits and cementum. A beginning clinician, however, has not had the opportunity to develop a sense for what a sharp instrument can be expected to accomplish. Several other ways to detect a dull instrument are available that may be easier for the beginning clinician to use.

One of the best ways to test instrument sharpness is by applying the cutting edge to be tested against an acrylic or plastic rod. Special acrylic testing sticks have been designed for this purpose and are available from instrument manufacturers

(Fig. 9-1). Place the instrument's cutting edge against the surface of the testing stick at the same angle that would be used to implement a working stroke against the tooth surface. If the edge is sharp, it will "bite" into the plastic surface when light pressure is applied. If the instrument tends to drag, slide, or grate across the surface, it is not sharp. Evaluate the entire length of the cutting edge for dullness. If a commercial testing stick is not available, a plastic disposable cotton-tipped applicator or a disposable evacuation tip can serve the same purpose. Commercial testing sticks are made of materials that can be sterilized and can be included on each tray setup, so that instruments can be tested during treatment procedures.

Another way to detect a dull cutting edge is to examine it under a microscope or a magnifying lens. Hold the instrument so that the cutting edge faces a strong light source. A dull surface reflects light, so that a white area or a bright light line will be visible where the cutting edge should be (Fig. 9-2, B). If the cutting edge is truly sharp, there should not be a flat surface (bevel) at the junction of the facial and lateral surfaces. Only a thin, dark line will be visible where these two surfaces meet when the instrument is correctly sharpened (Fig. 9-2, A). This evaluation method is only useful when a specific time has been set aside to sharpen instruments and when a special work area with a good light source and a microscope or magnifying lens is available. This technique would take too much time during patient treatment. It should be noted that the reliability

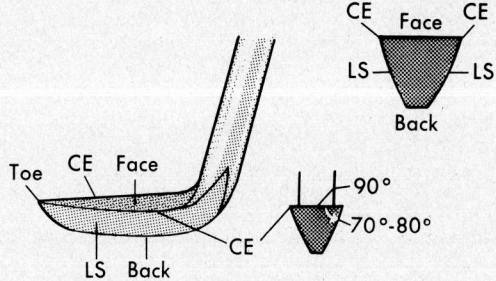

Fig. 9-3. Straight sickle. Face is basically flat; back surface is also flat.

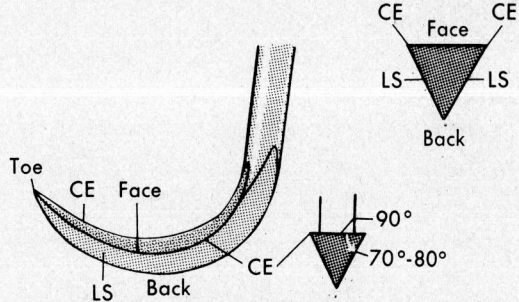

Fig. 9-4. Curved sickle. Note pointed back.

and validity of using the light reflection method to determine sharpness has been questioned. Sassie (1987) found that cutting edges that appeared to be dull using this method were judged to be clinically sharp when examined under much higher magnification using a scanning electron microscope (SEM). Therefore, instruments might appear to be dull when they are still clinically acceptable.

One method that should *never* be used to test instrument sharpness is to apply the edge to a fingernail. Not only is this damaging to the clinician's fingernail, but it is also a violation of aseptic technique. Instrument sharpening is often performed at the chairside during a patient appointment. If the clinician were to use this method to test the sharpness of scaling instruments, the instruments would be contaminated and no longer acceptable for patient treatment. All clinicians who perform intraoral procedures should wear disposable gloves to protect themselves and the patient from cross-contamination. It would be very time consuming and inconvenient to remove the gloves, wash the hands, test the instruments, sharpen them, wash the hands, and put the gloves back on each time instrument sharpening was necessary. It is much easier to use a sterile testing stick or one of the other methods discussed to evaluate instrument sharpness.

APPLICATION OF INSTRUMENT DESIGN TO SHARPENING TECHNIQUES

Each type of periodontal instrument has specific design characteristics that must be preserved during sharpening. The clinician must understand exactly how these design principles affect the use of each type of instrument so that sharpening techniques are employed that preserve original instrument contours. The two types of instruments used most frequently for scaling and root planing procedures are the sickle scaler and the curette. Design characteristics of both of these instrument types will be discussed.

Sickle scalers

Design features of sickle scalers are shown in Figs. 9-3 and 9-4. There are actually two different blade designs for sickle scalers: straight and curved blades. The straight blade design is shown in Fig. 9-3. The side view shows that two cutting edges of this sickle form a gentle arc that converges in a sharp tip. Both cutting edges are used, so both must be sharpened. The pointed tip of the sickle scaler provides access beneath tight contact areas. A significant design feature of the straight sickle blade is the squared-off back of the blade, which can be seen in the cross-sectional view of Fig. 9-3.

Fig. 9-4 shows the design characteristics of a curved sickle blade. The facial surface of the instrument forms a slight curve as it extends from the shank of the instrument to the pointed tip. The lateral surfaces of this sickle are flat and converge at the pointed back. Differences in the back design can be seen by comparing the cross-sectional views of these two sickle scalers.

In both of these instruments the lateral surfaces and the facial surface form an internal angle of approximately 70 to 80 degrees. When properly applied, the sharpening stone will form a complementary angle of 100 to 110 degrees with the base of the sickle blade.

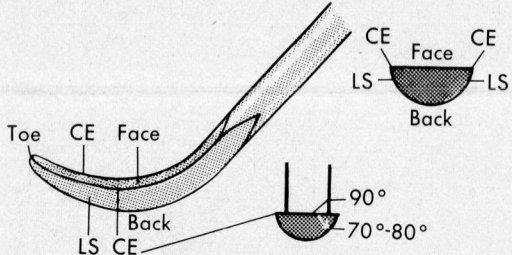

Fig. 9-5. Universal curette. Note that the two cutting edges are parallel. Rounded back and toe are important design features.

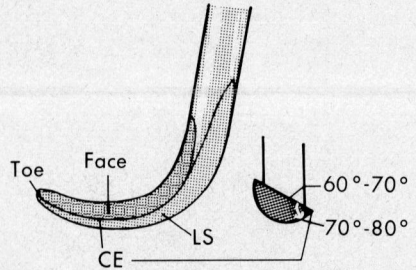

Fig. 9-6. Gracey curette. Note offset relationship of cutting edges so that one blade appears lower than the other.

Curettes

Design characteristics of the universal curette are shown in Fig. 9-5. The side view of the universal curette blade shows two parallel cutting edges, both of which are used during scaling and root planing. The two cutting edges converge in a rounded toe. It is important to maintain a rounded toe during the sharpening procedure, because this is one of the design features that allows this instrument to be used safely in subgingival areas. Failure to maintain this design could result in trauma to the soft tissues when the curette is inserted below the gingival margin.

Another important characteristic of the curette is that the lateral surfaces are curved, rather than flat, and form a rounded back surface. A cross-sectional view of the universal curette looks like a half circle. This is the second design feature that allows this instrument to navigate in tight pockets without damaging the adjacent soft tissues. The rounded back must be preserved during sharpening. The cross-sectional view of the universal curette shows that the facial surface of the blade forms a 90-degree angle with the shank of the instrument. The internal angle of the curette blade is the same as that of the sickle scaler—70 to 80 degrees.

The design features for the Gracey curette (Fig. 9-6) are the same as those of the universal curette with two notable exceptions. The blade is slightly offset at an angle of about 60 to 70 degrees from the shank of the instrument, so that the two cutting edges are not parallel to each other. Instead, one of the cutting edges appears to be lower than the other when the instrument is held so that the last bend in the shank (terminal shank) is perpendicular to the floor, as pictured in Fig. 9-6. Only

this "lower" cutting edge is used during periodontal procedures, so only one of the cutting edges should be sharpened on a Gracey curette blade. Other design characteristics of a curette blade described earlier for the universal curette (e.g., rounded back, rounded toe, internal angle of 70 to 80 degrees) are also present on a Gracey curette blade.

SHARPENING TECHNIQUES

Techniques for sharpening periodontal instruments vary according to the type of sharpening device used. The most commonly used technique uses hand-held sharpening stones. In other techniques smaller cylindrical or conical stones are mounted on slow-speed handpieces or flat or rounded stones are mounted on stationary sharpening (or honing) machines. Sharpening may also be accomplished using a rotating abrasive felt wheel (DeNucci and Mader 1983). Each method has certain advantages and disadvantages.

Instrument sharpening using a hand-held sharpening stone has the advantage that it can be performed anywhere in the dental office where there is adequate light and a good working surface. The use of a hand-held stone also allows the clinician to control the exact speed and pressure with which the instrument is being sharpened so that there is no unnecessary loss of instrument surface due to over-sharpening. This technique is recommended for routine sharpening of instruments.

There are two ways in which a hand-held stone can be used for sharpening. One method is to hold the instrument stationary while moving the stone against it; the second method is to stabilize the stone and drag the instrument blade across the

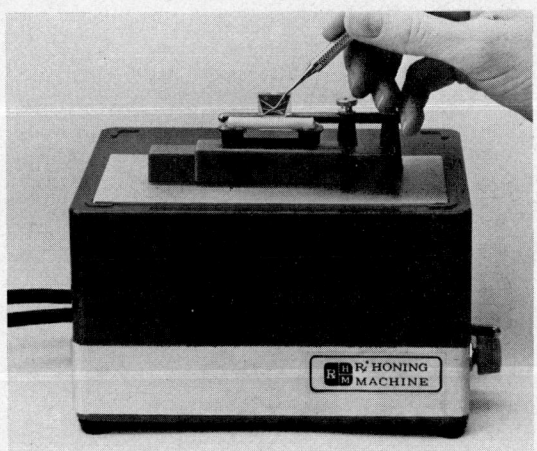

Fig. 9-7. Sharpening/honing machine.
(Courtesy Rx Honing Machine Co., Mishawaka, Ind.)

surface of the stone. Both techniques are discussed and shown in this chapter so that the clinician can decide which approach to use. Use of hand-held stones is a very practical approach to instrument sharpening because it can be accomplished easily at chair-side during patient treatment. It requires only commonly available, inexpensive equipment. In addition, hand sharpening techniques are easily mastered by beginning clinicians. Once the principles and skills of instrument sharpening have been mastered, the advanced clinician may choose to supplement the use of hand sharpening techniques with mechanical ones.

If hand-held sharpening is not preferred, a second instrument sharpening technique using small cylindrical or conical stones mounted on a slow-speed handpiece may be selected. The clinician must carefully control the speed of metal removal and the proper instrument/stone adaptation with this method. If implemented properly and with concern for preserving the original instrument design, this and other mechanical sharpening methods are timesaving approaches, useful for sharpening instruments that require a great deal of sharpening or recontouring. An added advantage of this method is that sterile sharpening stones can be available at the dental unit and readily mounted on a slow-speed handpiece for sharpening instruments during patient treatment. Sharpening equipment can be resterilized after use to pre-

vent cross-contamination. The clinician should always wear protective eye wear when using mechanical sharpening techniques due to the risk of flying metal, abrasive particles, and other debris.

Bench-type sharpening or honing machines are also available for sharpening periodontal instruments (see Fig. 9-7). The principles for preserving instrument design that apply to hand-sharpening techniques are also followed when using a sharpening machine. The main difference is that the sharpening stone is mechanically rotated or moved back and forth while the instrument blade is applied to it. The amount of metal that can be removed with this method depends on the amount of pressure applied and the length of time that the blade is in contact with the sharpening stone. These machines can be time-savers if the clinician is skilled in placement of the blade against the stone at the correct angle and if the instrument requires a great deal of contouring. Inexperienced clinicians or those unfamiliar with instrument design, however, can ruin instruments much more quickly with this technique than with a manual technique. In addition, the need for special equipment limits the clinician's access to sharpening during patient treatment; this method is more useful when a special time has been alotted specifically for instrument sharpening. The use of honing machines on facial surfaces of instruments may produce an undesirable side effect known as nonfunctional wire edges. These formations are thin, irregular, metal extensions of the cutting edges (Antonini et al. 1977). Whenever a facial approach to sharpening is employed, instrument blades should be carefully inspected for the presence of nonfunctional wire edges. Their presence could interfere with the smoothness of the surface produced by the cutting edges. A technique for removing wire edges is discussed later in the chapter.

A bench-mounted felt wheel machine has also been described as an effective method for sharpening periodontal instruments (DeNucci and Mader, 1985). In this technique a lateral surface of the instrument blade is held against a rotating felt wheel that has been impregnated with abrasive particles. The disadvantages of this method are the same as those discussed for other mechanical sharpening approaches. Appropriate measures should also be taken to control microbial cross-contamination when using this method.

Sharpening lateral versus facial surfaces

Sharp cutting edges can be created in one of two ways: by grinding the facial surface or by grinding the lateral surfaces. In one approach, the cutting edges are sharpened by applying a cylindrical or conical stone to the facial surface of the blade, thus sharpening both sides of the blade simultaneously. The second approach is to sharpen each cutting edge individually by applying a flat stone to each of the two lateral surfaces. Both methods can provide a fine cutting edge when properly implemented. The major advantage of sharpening the facial surface is that it is less time consuming because both cutting edges of the blade are sharpened simultaneously.

A number of authorities do not recommend grinding away the facial surface because reducing the depth of the blade decreases the strength of the instrument more quickly than grinding the lateral surfaces (Paquette and Levin, 1977; Carranza, 1984; Wilkins, 1983; Green, 1972). However, evidence against this position was discussed by Murray et al. (1984). They found that there was no difference in instrument strength when they compared facial sharpening to lateral sharpening. They also noted that both methods result in significant reductions in instrument strength when the size of the instrument blade had been reduced by 20% or more. Clinicians should exercise caution when using instruments that have been sharpened beyond this point because reduced strength could result in the tip of the blade breaking if it is applied with much force against heavy or tenacious calculus deposits, restorative materials, or tight contact areas. Removal of broken instrument tips, especially from subgingival areas, can be an arduous task and an unpleasant experience for both the patient and clinician. The clinician can prevent this situation from occurring by inspecting instrument blades and exercising good judgement in their use.

Selecting a sharpening stone

Sharpening stones come in a variety of materials and designs (Fig. 9-8). The most popular stone for sharpening periodontal instruments is a natural stone known as Arkansas oilstone. This stone is composed of abrasive crystals that are much finer than those of man-made stones. The quality of a cutting edge is determined by the fineness of the

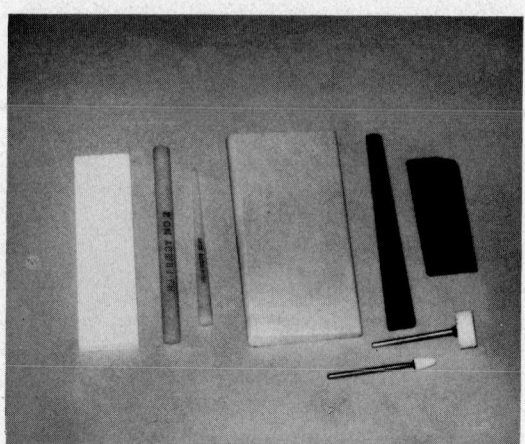

Fig. 9-8. Stones used to sharpen instruments.

stone with which it is sharpened. An Arkansas oilstone is capable of producing a high-quality cutting edge while not grinding away the metal surface of the instrument as fast as a coarser stone. Therefore, it is preferred over other sharpening stones for routine sharpening.

Several man-made stones are also available for use in dentistry, including the ruby stone, the India stone, the carborundum stone, and the diamond hone. These stones are impregnated with abrasive crystals such as aluminum oxide, silicon carbide, or diamond particles, all of which are coarser than those of the Arkansas stone. These man-made stones may be useful, however, if a great deal of recontouring is needed, because they grind a surface more quickly than the Arkansas stone.

Sharpening stones are available in rectangular, wedge, or cylindrical shapes. The choice of shape and size depends on clinician preference and on how the stone will be used. Small cylindrical or conical stones can be mounted for use in a slow-speed handpiece. Larger or tapered cylinders are used to sharpen the facial surfaces of instruments. Flat or rectangular stones are used to sharpen the lateral surfaces of instruments.

Preparation for sharpening

The most convenient way to sharpen instruments is to have a workbench or countertop reserved for that purpose so that there is easy access to all necessary supplies, including an effective light

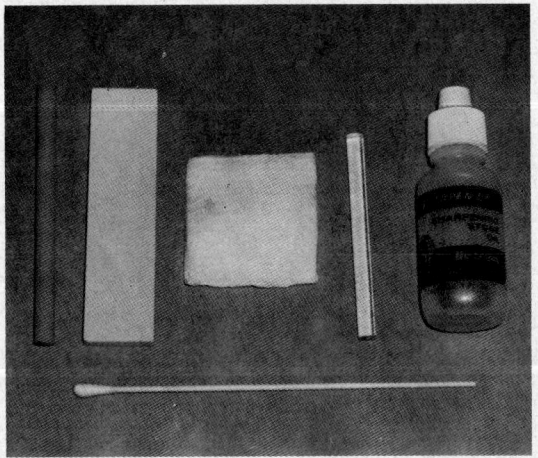

Fig. 9-9. Supplies used for instrument sharpening. *Left to right:* Cylindrical sharpening stone, rectangular Arkansas stone, alcohol gauze, testing stick, lubricating oil, and cotton-tipped applicator.

source, a magnifying lens, sharpening oil, applicators, and alcohol-soaked gauze. If space is not available for this purpose, the methods of sharpening discussed in this chapter can be used wherever an adequate light source and working surface are available.

The supplies needed for instrument sharpening are shown in Fig. 9-9. They include a cylindrical stone (optional), a rectangular or wedge-shaped Arkansas stone, gauze squares, a testing stick, light-grade oil, and a cotton-tipped applicator. Only sterile supplies should be used for instrument sharpening. These supplies must be resterilized after use on contaminated instruments. If all instruments are resharpened at one designated time—either before or after being sterilized—the same sterile stone and testing stick can be used for the entire batch and resterilized for later use. A sterile stone and testing stick should be included on each tray set-up if scaling and root planing are to be performed, because frequent resharpening during treatment may be necessary. A light coating of oil should be applied to the stone with the cotton-tipped applicator. The purpose of the oil is to prevent metal filings from the sharpening procedure from becoming embedded in the surface of the stone. The oil also has a lubricating effect, which reduces the heat produced during sharpening and enhances the ability of the clini-

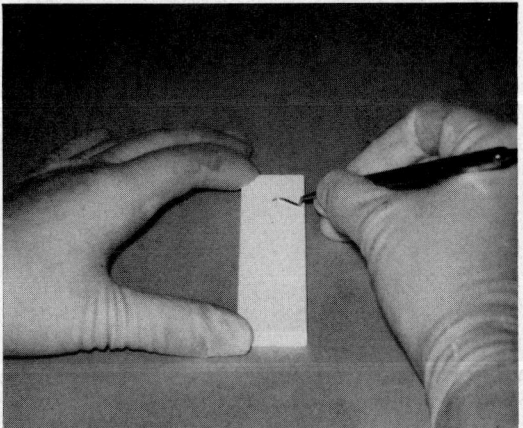

Fig. 9-10. Positioning of stone and instrument for sharpening with stationary stone.

cian to implement smooth, even strokes over the stone's surface. Other types of sharpening stones may require the use of water as a lubricant or no lubricant at all. Oil is the lubricant of choice for Arkansas stones and India stones. Water is used for ruby, composition, carborundum, and ceramic stones. Manufacturers' instructions should be followed regarding the choice of lubricant. The sterile gauze sponge is used to remove the oil and metal sludge from the sharpening stone and the instruments. To facilitate cleaning and asepsis, the sterile gauze squares may be moistened with an appropriate surface disinfectant solution.

Sharpening with a stationary stone and a moving instrument

The clinician should follow the following steps when using this approach to instrument sharpening. Place the Arkansas stone on a flat surface. Coat the surface of the stone with oil with a cotton-tipped applicator. Hold the instrument with a modified pen grasp, as shown in Fig. 9-10, with the third and fourth fingers providing support for the hand on the surface of the table. Grasp and stabilize the stone with the fingers of the other hand as shown. Gloves should be worn during sharpening procedures for maximal asepsis and operator protection. Place the instrument near the top of the stone so that the face forms a 90-degree angle with the stone's surface (Fig. 9-11), then rotate the instrument handle slightly away from

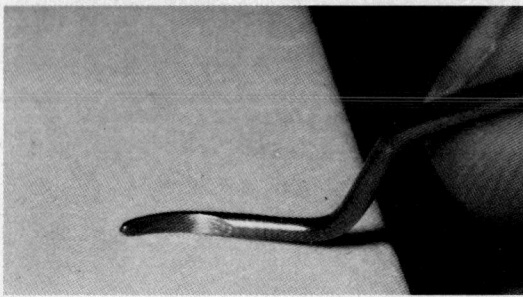

Fig. 9-11. Close-up view of facial surface of curette at 90-degree angle to stationary stone.

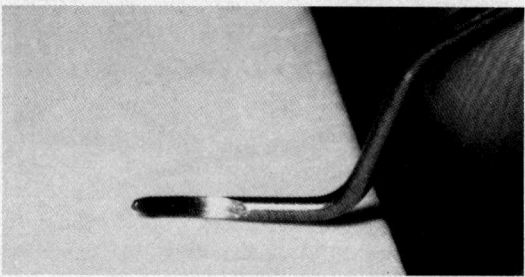

Fig. 9-12. Angle has been opened to 110 degrees prior to beginning sharpening stroke.

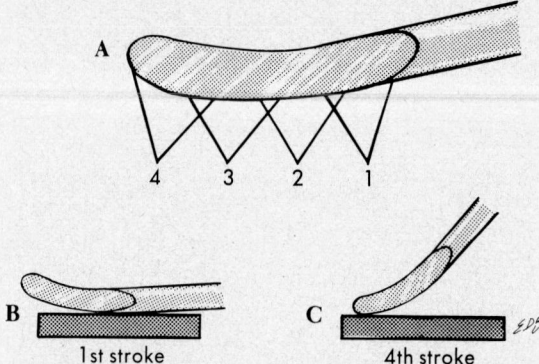

Fig. 9-13. A, Four different adaptations of stone are necessary to sharpen entire surface. **B,** First stroke should start at heel of blade. **C,** Last stroke should end at toe.

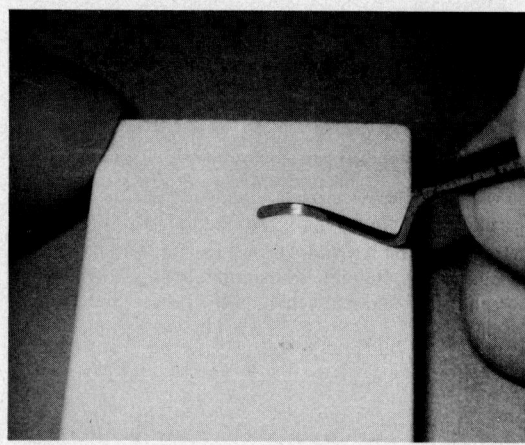

Fig. 9-14. Stationary stone and moving instrument; stroke begins at top of stone where heel of blade is in contact with stone at an angle of 100 to 110 degrees.

yourself until the angle between the face and the stone is 100 to 110 degrees (Fig. 9-12). This is the correct angle for sharpening all curettes and sickle scalers. This angle complements the internal angle of the instrument (70 to 80 degrees) so that the original design of the blade is maintained during sharpening. It is important to maintain this same angle for the entire length of the sharpening stroke. Until becoming experienced at identifying the correct angulation, it may be helpful to continue to place the instrument first so that the 90-degree angle is formed and then open it up slightly another 10 to 20 degrees. Figs. 9-11 and 9-12 show close-up views of the placement of the curette blade at both 90 and 110 degrees.

After the correct angle has been established, begin the stroke with the heel of the blade adapted to the stone. As you pull the instrument toward you, rotate the instrument blade toward the toe so that the entire blade is sharpened during each complete stroke. Fig. 9-13 shows that four different adaptations of the instrument to the stone

may be necessary to ensure that the entire cutting edge has been sharpened. Move the entire hand and arm as a single unit toward you while rotating the wrist. At the end of the stroke, rotate around the entire toe of the blade so that its curvature is maintained. Failure to grind the toe surface evenly may result in a toe that is flattened or pointed instead of curved. The steps involved in a single stroke are shown in Figs. 9-14 to 9-17. Several light strokes may be necessary to completely sharpen the entire cutting edge. After one cutting edge of the curette has been completely

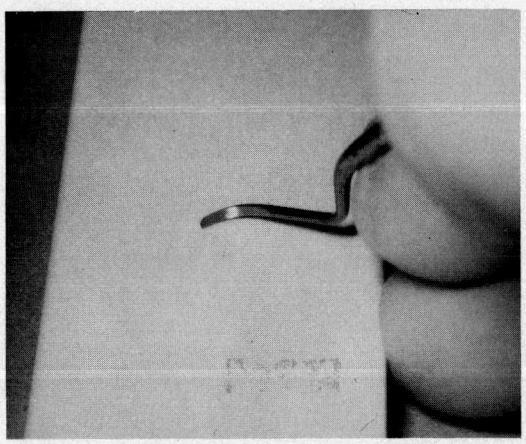

Fig. 9-15. As instrument is pulled forward across stone, blade is slowly rotated toward middle of cutting edge.

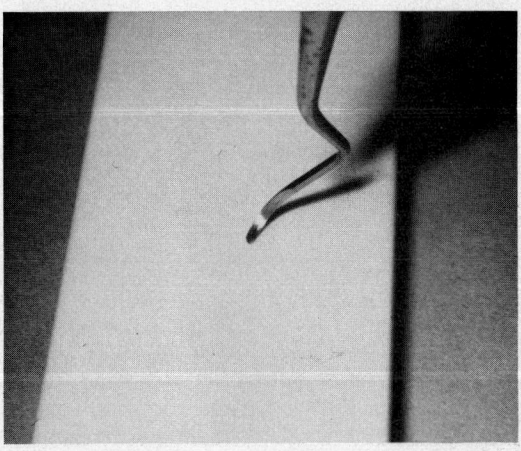

Fig. 9-16. As end of stroke approaches, back of cutting edge is lifted so that toe is in contact with stone.

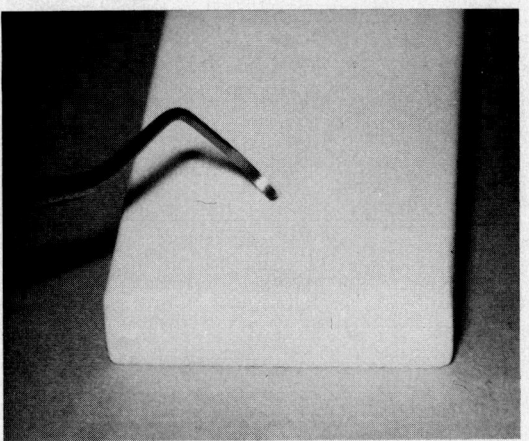

Fig. 9-17. Entire toe should be rounded off at end of stroke so that a sharp point is not created. Less pressure can be used at toe, since it is not a cutting surface.

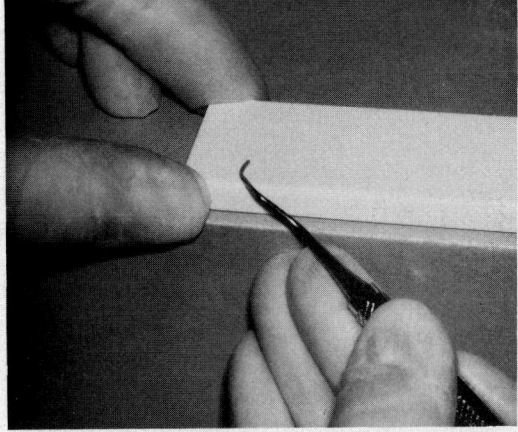

Fig. 9-18. Placement of stone at edge of table to facilitate sharpening of opposite edge of universal curette.

sharpened, sharpen the other cutting edge in the same way. You may need to reposition the stone at the edge of the table to facilitate the placement of the opposite cutting edge (Fig. 9-18). After sharpening, inspect the blade carefully to ensure that the original design has been preserved.

Gracey curettes are sharpened in the same way with only a few exceptions. Only one cutting edge of the Gracey curette should be sharpened. The clinician must first identify this lower cutting edge. Since the face of the Gracey is not perpendicular to the shank, care should be taken at first to align the facial surface at a 90-degree angle to the stone and then open the angle to the proper sharpening angle of 100 to 110 degrees.

Sickle scalers can be easily sharpened by this method. The same principles of instrument placement and angulation apply. The only major difference is that, because the lateral surfaces of this instrument are flatter and straighter than those of the curette, there is not as much rotation of the blade from heel to toe during each stroke. Stop

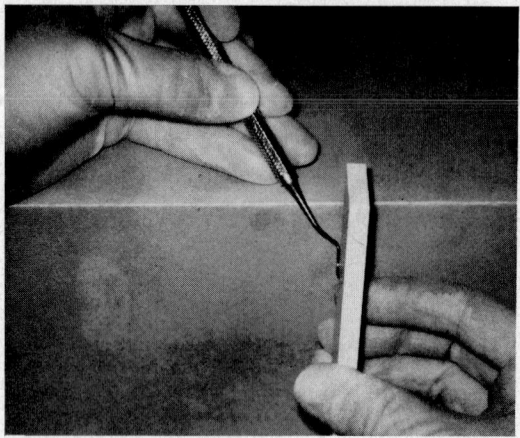

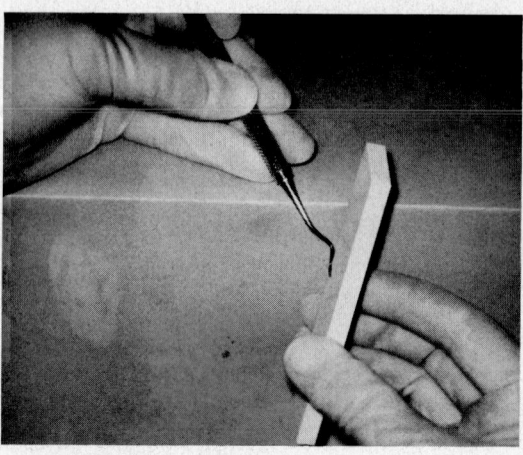

Fig. 9-19. Stationary instrument and moving stone technique. Note position of left hand, which is braced against tabletop. Facial surface of instrument is parallel to floor. Stone is placed at 90-degree angle.

Fig. 9-20. Stone is correctly oriented at an angle of 100 to 110 degrees to the facial surface. This exact angle must be maintained for all strokes.

the stroke at the tip of the instrument so that the sharp point is maintained. Repeat the sharpening strokes until the cutting edge is sharp, then reposition the instrument to sharpen the opposite cutting edge. After sharpening, remove the metal sludge from both the instrument blade and the stone with sterile gauze squares.

Sharpening with a stationary instrument and a moving stone

A second method of sharpening curettes and sickles with a hand-held stone is to hold the instrument in one hand and move the stone across the lateral surfaces with the other hand. The first step is to grasp the instrument to be sharpened firmly in the left hand (if the clinician is right-handed) and brace the hand against the top edge of a counter or table so that the instrument blade extends over the edge of the table with the toe pointing toward the clinician. Grasp the sharpening stone with the fingers of the other hand as shown in Fig. 9-19. Hold the instrument so that its facial surface is parallel to the floor. Fig. 9-19 shows the adaptation of the stone to the cutting edge of a curette at a 90-degree angle. Rotate the top of the stone slightly away from the instrument until the correct angle of 100 to 110 degrees is formed between the stone and the facial surface (Fig. 9-20). Apply short down strokes (½ to 1

inch) to the cutting edge of the blade, being careful to maintain the stone at exactly the same angle during each stroke. Apply pressure against the instrument only during downstrokes to avoid the formation of a wire edge.

Apply sharpening strokes first to the heel of the instrument and then rotate the stone slightly until the entire cutting edge has been sharpened. A separate stroke is needed to maintain the rounded toe of the curette. The stone should be adapted so that a 45-degree angle is formed between the bottom half of the stone and the facial surface of the curette (Fig. 9-21). Short downstrokes should be applied around the curvature of the toe.

The same technique can be used to sharpen sickle scalers and Gracey curettes. Again, sharpen only the lower cutting edge of a Gracey curette, taking care to position the instrument so that the facial surface is parallel to the floor before positioning the stone to begin the sharpening stroke.

If pressure is applied to both the upstroke and the downstroke using this technique, smoothing the facial surface with a cylindrical stone may be necessary if wire edges have been created (Antonini et al. 1977). Place the cylindrical or tapered sharpening stone squarely against the facial surface of the curette (Fig. 9-22). Stabilize the instrument and apply light, even pressure to the facial surface while the stone is rotated in a coun-

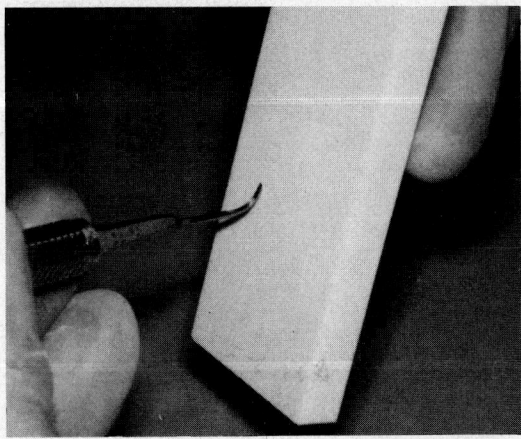

Fig. 9-21. To sharpen toe of curette using moving stone, place stone at 45-degree angle to back of blade.

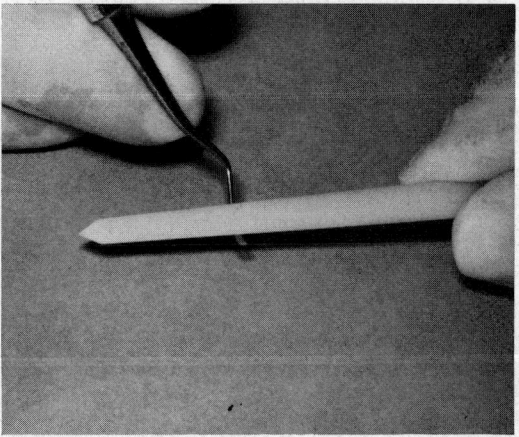

Fig. 9-22. Tapered cylindrical stone is applied to facial surface of curette to assist in removal of wire edges.

terclockwise direction (i.e., heel to toe). Facial grinding should be done only if wire edges are detected, because excessive grinding both here and on lateral surfaces could reduce the instrument size and strength unnecessarily.

Sharpening explorers

Explorers used for detection of decay (e.g., design #23 or "Shepherd's hook" explorer) should be kept sharp to maximize their effectiveness. Apply the stone to the tip of the explorer at an angle of about 15 to 20 degrees (Fig. 9-23). Use short strokes around the entire point until it becomes sharp. Extremely sharp points are not desirable for explorers that are used primarily for submarginal calculus detection, so these instruments do not need to be sharpened unless their tips require recontouring because of damage.

STERILIZATION EFFECTS

Following patient treatment, used instruments should be cleaned ultrasonically or scrubbed by hand before resharpening. Protective gloves should always be worn when sharpening nonsterile instruments to protect against accidental cuts or punctures. Instruments that have been used to treat patients who are known or suspected carriers of serious transmittable diseases should be sterilized before being handled for cleaning or sharpening procedures to protect the clinician from cross-contamination. Once they have been rendered

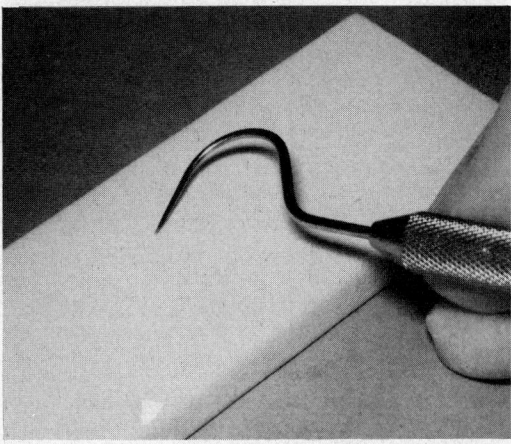

Fig. 9-23. Sharpen explorers by adapting tip to stone at an angle of 15 degrees.

harmless, they can then be cleaned, sharpened, and resterilized for use.

Except for these high-risk situations, instruments should be sharpened routinely before being sterilized. If instruments are sharpened after being sterilized and before patient treatment, the sterility of the instruments can be compromised. Contrary to some beliefs, commonly used sterilization procedures (e.g., steam sterilization at 250° F, chemical vapor at 270° F, dry heat up to 340° F) will not dull the cutting edge of stainless steel instruments (Parkes and Kolstad, 1981; Sassie,

1987). One study found that there was no significant loss of blade sharpness even after 240 sterilization cycles by either the autoclave or the chemical vapor sterilizer (Sassie, 1987). Carbon steel instruments, however, can be dulled slightly by steam or chemical vapor sterilization methods and should be sterilized in a dry heat oven to preserve blade sharpness (Parkes and Kolstad, 1981).

SUMMARY

Development of the clinical judgment to detect when instruments are dull and the technique required to properly sharpen and recontour instruments are skills that the hygienist must attain. The most well-executed scaling and root planing strokes will be ineffective and inefficient if dull instruments are used. Instrument sharpening skills are an indispensible step on the road to becoming a master clinician.

ACTIVITIES

1. Examine and compare the designs of the following types of instruments under a microscope:
   a. A new instrument
   b. A well-sharpened instrument
   c. A missharpened instrument
   d. A dull instrument
2. Compare the ease of scaling and root planing on extracted teeth when using an instrument that has been optimally sharpened versus using a dull instrument.
3. Inoculate a bacterial culture medium with shavings taken from a fingernail while testing instrument sharpness; incubate the test sample, and examine for bacterial growth.
4. Observe a demonstration of instrument sharpening using a handpiece-mounted stone or a honing machine and discuss the use of these techniques for routine instrument sharpening in terms of amount of metal removed, ability to control the application of the stone to the instrument, heat generated, contamination control, and access to equipment during patient treatment.

REVIEW QUESTIONS

1. Which of the following methods is not an acceptable way to determine instrument sharpness?
   a. Evaluation of the cutting edge during scaling procedures
   b. Evaluation of light reflection from the cutting edge when observed under magnification
   c. Evaluation of the cutting edge against a plastic testing stick
   d. Evaluation of the cutting edge against the clinician's fingernail
2. True or false:
   a. The Arkansas stone is a man-made, or artificial, sharpening stone.
   b. Sterilization by autoclaving will not dull the cutting edges of stainless steel instruments.
   c. Both cutting edges of a Gracey curette should be sharpened.
3. What is the internal angle formed by the facial and lateral surfaces of curettes and sickle scalers?
   a. 45 degrees
   b. 70 to 80 degrees
   c. 90 degrees
   d. 100 to 110 degrees
4. Identify two design characteristics of curettes that must be preserved during sharpening.
5. Routine sharpening of the _____ of a curette or sickle scaler will weaken the blade strength of the instrument and shorten its working life.
   a. Facial surface
   b. Lateral surfaces
   c. Back
   d. Toe
6. When a stationary instrument is being sharpened with a moving stone, pressure should be applied on the _____.
   a. Upstroke only
   b. Downstroke only
   c. Upstroke and downstroke

REFERENCES

Antonini CJ, et al: Scanning electron microscope study of scalers, J Periodontol **48**:45, 1977.

Carranza FA, ed: Glickman's clinical periodontology, ed 6, Philadelphia, 1984, WB Saunders Co.

DeNucci DJ and Mader, CL: Scanning electron microscopic evaluation of several resharpening techniques, J Periodontol **54**:618, 1983.

Green E and Seyer PC: Sharpening curettes and sickle scalers, ed 2, Berkeley, 1972, Praxis Publishing Co.

Murray GH, et al: The effects of two sharpening methods on the strength of a periodontal scaling instrument, J Periodontol **55**:410, 1984.

Paquette DE and Levin MP: The sharpening of scaling instruments: I. An examination of principles, J Periodontol **48**:163, 1977.

Parkes RB, and Kolstad RA: Effects of sterilization on periodontal instruments, J Periodontol **53**:434, 1982.

Sassie J: Cutting edges of curets: effects of repeated sterilization, Dent Hyg **61**:14, 1987.

Tal H, et al: Scanning electron microscope evaluation of wear of dental curettes during standardized root planing, J Periodontol **56**:532, 1985.

Wilkins EM: Clinical practice of the dental hygienist, ed 5, Philadelphia, 1983, Lea & Febiger.

10 GENERAL PHYSICAL EVALUATION AND THE EXTRAORAL AND INTRAORAL EXAMINATION

OBJECTIVES: *The reader will be able to*

1. State the purposes and advantages of performing a complete general and oral examination for each patient.
2. Identify the characteristics to observe in assessing a patient's general appearance and state why they may be significant to treatment.
3. Identify the four vital signs.
4. Demonstrate the technique for obtaining a patient's vital signs.
5. Discuss the role dentistry plays in identifying and monitoring hypertension.
6. Describe the extraoral and intraoral examination, including:
   a. The names of all structures to be visually inspected and palpated
   b. Normal landmarks associated with these structures
   c. The prescribed method of palpation for each structure
   d. Common abnormalities that may be detected
7. Given an illustration of an abnormal lesion, describe its location in the mouth, size, and clinical characteristics using medical descriptions of the type of lesion represented.
8. Define the four different methods of examination—inspection, palpation, auscultation, and percussion—and give an example of each method.

A complete head and neck examination is a vital component of comprehensive health services. The total procedure combines a subjective and objective appraisal of the patient's health and an examination of extraoral structures of the head and neck and all intraoral structures. In the appointment sequence, the clinical examination procedures described in this chapter should follow the gathering of all pertinent data in a comprehensive health history. Information recorded in the health history of the patient provides not only a summary of the patient's health background, but also valuable insight into potential health problems or clinical manifestations that might be detected during the head and neck examination.

The major objectives when performing a com-

plete head and neck examination for each patient are as follows:

1. To examine thoroughly structures of the head and neck in an effort to gather accurate and comprehensive assessment data for diagnosis and treatment planning
   a. To determine the goals and priorities of treatment
   b. To determine the need for additional consultations and referrals
   c. To assist in planning preventive programs designed around patient needs
2. To provide early detection of oral diseases and thus improve the prognosis for recovery
3. To detect systemic disturbances that have oral manifestations

4. To detect conditions which might contraindicate dental treatment
5. To provide baseline and continuing data of the patient's health status for evaluating the success of treatment and preventive education
6. To provide accurate descriptions of the patient's health status in the charts for potential use as legal records

The treatment plan designed for the patient must be based on a thorough identification and description of all observed and suspected health problems. At this point in treatment, the health history has already provided information regarding past health experiences and insight into current problems of which the patient is aware. The clinical examination will *supplement and update this history* with identification and/or descriptions of the current health status of the patient. The information gathered in the examination will also help the clinician determine what *preventive methods* and *education* are most appropriate for each patient's needs.

Potential need for further consultations with dental or medical specialists is also identified through information gathered in the head and neck examination. Cooperative efforts among health professionals are necessary to provide comprehensive care for the patient. The clinical examination will provide clues as to whether the services of specialists such as pathologists, periodontists, endodontists, oral surgeons, or the patient's physician are needed.

Total patient care involves a responsibility for more than just the patient's teeth and gums. It includes an awareness of other health problems that may be manifested during the head and neck examination. Often, systemic disorders can be identified through signs and symptoms that occur extraorally or intraorally. The complete examination may reveal signs of nutritional deficiencies or imbalances that may have dental implications.

Early detection of diseases that are progressive and irreversibly destructive in nature is a critical factor in determining the extent of the destruction that they might cause. This is especially true of oral cancer. A thorough head and neck examination performed at regular intervals could greatly reduce the incidence of deaths from oral cancer. It is estimated that in 1987 there were 29,800 new cases of oral cancer, 12,100 cases of cancer of

the larynx, and 25,800 cases of skin cancer (some of which may have been manifested on the head and neck area). The number of deaths each year due to oral cancer alone is estimated at 9,400 (American Cancer Society, 1987). Early detection and diagnosis of these malignancies is critical to reduce deaths caused by oral and other cancers.

It is the responsibility of every dental hygienist to apply the necessary skills and knowledge to ensure that all patients not only are examined thoroughly, but are educated to perform frequent and effective self-examination to increase the chances of early detection of cancer. The self-examination procedure is discussed in greater detail later in this chapter. As each patient will be seen at regular recall intervals, it is likely that the clinician will be able to detect health or tissue changes from one appointment to another and thus identify the need for prompt and early treatment of disease or malignancies. The clinician can also use this opportunity to revise or reinforce patient education and self-care methods based on new information gathered from each updated clinical examination. Frequent examinations enable the clinician to become familiar with a patient's normal oral manifestations and to identify deviations.

Throughout the clinical examination, the clinician should *identify contraindications* to dental treatment that would affect the health of the patient, the clinician, or both. Clinical signs of transmittable diseases (such as hepatitis B, AIDS, syphilis, or severe sore throat) or of other potentially dangerous conditions (such as uncontrolled hypertension) may be apparent at the time of the examination, even if they were not discussed in the health history. By referring these patients back to their physicians for care, both the patient's health and that of the dental team are protected.

The information gathered from the initial head and neck examination serves as valuable *baseline data* describing the patient's health status at the time of the initial appointment. These data form a standard by which the patient's progress through treatment and preventive procedures can be measured. They are the primary starting point from which the dental professional can measure effectiveness in treatment. If those problems identified in the clinical examination are not resolved through treatment and home care, the professional must reevaluate the current treatment plan to determine what factors may be causing the lack of success and whether or not those factors can be alleviated. Clinical examinations at recall appointments will provide additional data to be added to the patient's overall health profile and will ensure a constant reevaluation of present oral conditions.

It is important that the description of the patient's general health and oral conditions be noted as completely as possible in the patient's chart to facilitate the chart's use as a *legal record* if it should become necessary. Evaluation of information recorded in patient records is also becoming more and more prevalent in situations in which *third-party insurance carriers* are involved or in situations in which *peer review* is used to evaluate treatment.

In summary, the clinical head and neck examination is a necessary component of the total assessment of patient health care needs. It provides detailed information of disease, malignancy, or dysfunction that will help determine treatment planning and priorities. It identifies problems that necessitate further laboratory tests or consultation with other health practitioners. It provides data that will assist in patient education and self-care. When the clinical examination occurs frequently and regularly at recall appointments, continual monitoring of the patient's oral health care status and early detection of new disease processes are possible.

A thorough knowledge of head and neck anatomy and physiology, coupled with the mastery of comprehensive examination techniques as described in this chapter, will enable the clinician to identify deviations from normal and to report them accurately for diagnosis. As the health history data has already been gathered and recorded, that information can be correlated with clinical findings to provide a comprehensive review of all pertinent data.

CLINICAL HEAD AND NECK EXAMINATION

The clinical head and neck examination is divided into four basic components: (1) general appraisal, (2) vital signs, (3) extraoral examination, and (4) intraoral examination.

In the following descriptions of each compo-
nent, the tissues, structures, or functions to be examined are given, along with the suggested examination technique and sequence and possible significant findings that might be encountered during the examination. In most cases one of the following four methods of examination will be used to gather clinical information:

inspection A systematic visual assessment of body tissues, structures, or systems to identify normal and abnormal appearances and/or functioning.

palpation The use of the fingers or hands to examine the texture, form, and function of soft and hard tissue structures.

auscultation Listening for sounds produced within the body (such as clicking of the temporomandibular joint [TMJ], abnormal breathing sounds, or vocal fremitus).

percussion Striking tissues with the fingers or an instrument to hear the resulting sounds and patient response.

Objective information (signs) gained from one or more of these methods, combined with the patient's subjective responses (symptoms), provides a complete description of clinical findings.

General appraisal

Many aspects of the patient's health and general disposition may be detected from simple observation of overall appearance, movements, and responses. The examination methods used are inspection and auscultation. As the patient enters the office or operatory, *observe the general body weight, height, posture, and gait* for abnormal signs. For example, obesity or excessive height deviations not only may provide clues to possible nutritional or endocrine disorders but may indicate necessary alterations in patient positioning. The posture and gait may signal back problems or other handicaps that would also affect patient positioning in the chair. Does the patient limp or seem uncoordinated? Deficiencies of motor or sensory functions that include hand or arm movements would affect the type of home care the patient is capable of performing. Are there additional signs of paralysis, tremors, or other dysfunctions that will affect the patient's needs or treatment? What do the rate and character of the gait or gestures indicate about the patient's level of anxiety? While looking at the extremities, glance at the patient's legs and ankles for signs of swelling or other indications of poor circulation.

Observe the patient's face. Is the skin color normal, pale, or flushed? Does it appear dry or sweaty? What might the patient's facial expression indicate about his or her general attitude? Are there any signs of facial paralysis, tremors, asymmetry, or other abnormalities?

Monitor the patient's respiration rate. Is it shallow or deep? Is it fast or slow? Is it regular or punctuated with gasps, puffs, or wheezes? Are there signs that the patient experiences difficulty in breathing through either the nose or mouth? Does the chest cavity appear particularly shallow (caved in), or is the patient barrel-chested? Any deviation from normal breathing may be an indication of respiratory or cardiac problems or of an anxiety response to the dental appointment.

Once the patient is seated and engaged in a conversation, the clinician can take a closer look at the appearance of the skin, hair, eyes, and nose for signs of abnormalities. The clinician should also *evaluate the speech* for hoarseness, rate, pitch, and general quality. This information may assist in the recognition of problems of the larynx (voice box) and, again, the patient's anxiety level. A nervous patient may speak at a pitch and rate higher than normal.

Observe the patient's hands to acquire valuable information about general health and attitude. Does the patient bite or chew the nails? Are the palms dry or sweaty? Are the hands fidgeting and gesturing nervously? Look between the first and second fingers for signs of tobacco stain from cigarettes. A constant tremor or paralysis of the hands or fingers may indicate nerve damage. The hands may also manifest signs of systemic or local diseases. For instance, a patient with anemia may exhibit spoon-shaped nails. Clubbing of the fingers may be associated with cardiac or pulmonary disorders. Swollen, painful finger joints are observed in the arthritic patient. Any of these specific conditions of the hands would likely have an effect on the overall treatment plan and should be noted.

Because this general appraisal is the first clinical introduction to the patient, it is important to retain the impressions and information that are accumulated and use them to guide later discussion with the patient concerning the health history and reactions to dental treatment. As subjective observations become confirmed through the health questionnaire or discussion with the patient, the final objective findings should be recorded in the patient's chart.

After reviewing the health history with the patient and not finding any obvious contraindication to proceeding (such as a current contagious disease), the hygienist should explain the content and purpose of the clinical examination. Hopefully, the patient and hygienist will have developed a feeling of mutual trust and confidence and patients will feel free to ask questions about the procedures and will share responsibility by reporting any symptoms that occur as the examination progresses. When all examination procedures have been explained and agreed to by the patient, assuming there are no contraindications to treating the patient at this point, the hygienist is ready to proceed with the next portion of the examination—taking the vital signs.

Vital signs

Pulse rate, respiration rate, temperature, and arterial blood pressure constitute the patient's vital signs. Usually this part of the physical examination is performed as one of the initial procedures in the appointment. For some patients, however, apprehension about the dental appointment or rushing to be on time may increase the vital signs. An attempt should be made to relax the patient through conversation or a calm atmosphere to ensure accuracy of the findings. Repeating the pulse and blood pressure measurements near the end of the appointment may be helpful to ensure accuracy.

Pulse rate. An arterial pulse that reflects the count of heartbeats may be palpated at the following locations that are accessible to the clinician:

radial Located on the thumb side of the patient's wrist over the radial bone.
brachial Located in the antecubital fossa before the brachial artery branches into the radial and ulnar arteries in the lower arm.
carotid Located on the lateral aspect of the neck on either side of the trachea.
temporal Located slightly above and in front of the ear.
facial Located at the border of the mandible in the mandibular notch.

Because of its accessibility, the radial pulse in

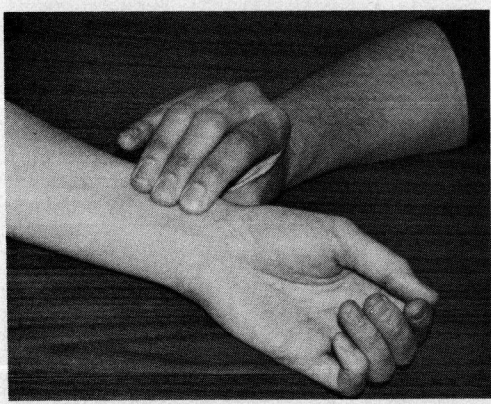

Fig. 10-1. Technique for pulse determination. Place fingers on radial artery. Gently compress artery against bone. Count pulse for 1 minute.

the wrist area is most commonly used for determining the pulse rate during the physical examination. The pulse rate may be affected by age, exercise, and emotional status. Generally, a rate of 60 to 80 beats per minute is considered normal for most adults. Patients accustomed to regular exercise may exhibit lower pulse rates because of the strength and efficiency of the heart muscle's pumping ability. The normal pulse rate for children is 90 to 120 beats per minute.

Technique (Klimaszewski and Grim, 1985; Malasnos et al, 1986). Seat the patient with the arm supported comfortably at the patient's side. Place the first three fingers on the patient's radial artery. (The clinican's thumb is not used to determine the pulse, because it contains a pulse and may create confusion when determining the patient's pulse rate.) Gently compress the artery against the underlying bone. Count the pulse for 1 minute while noting the rate, rhythm, and character of the beats (Fig. 10-1). If a pulse rate is abnormally fast, slow, irregular, or inconsistent in character, note this observation in the chart. Repeat the procedure a few minutes later to confirm the previous measurement. Be alert to unusual findings, and discuss the situation with the patient. A physician's consultation may be suggested.

Respiration rate. The hygienist should also note the quality and rate of respirations, especially for patients reporting a health history of respiratory symptoms such as asthma, congestive heart failure, or allergic reactions or for apprehensive patients prone to hyperventilation. Count the inspiration and expiration of air as one breath. Note the rate, rhythm (regular, irregular), type (strong, labored, weak), and depth (shallow, deep) of the patient's quiet breathing. Listen for wheezing sounds, and observe whether breathing occurs primarily through the nose or the mouth.

Record the findings on the chart. Notify the dentist of unusual or abnormal recordings.

Temperature. The average temperature of the body is 98.6° F (37° C) for most individuals. There is a certain amount of variation from one individual to another; the normal temperature may range from 97° F to 99.6 F (36.1° C to 37.6° C) (Malasanos et al, 1986). The temperature also fluctuates slightly depending on the time of day, the influence of hormones or drugs, and recent exercise, but for the most part it remains quite stable. When the temperature rises a full degree or more above normal, the patient is said to have a fever. This elevation usually is an indication of infection or tissue injury. Temperatures below normal may occur with shock or when the patient has been overly exposed to cold. The accepted normal temperature has been established by the oral method, but body temperature can be taken rectally or externally in the axillary or groin areas if the oral method is contraindicated (Kerr, Ash, and Millard, 1983). Standard normal temperature by the rectal method is 99.6° F and by the external methods is 97.6° F. The oral temperature method is contraindicated for infants, unconscious patients, those unable to breathe through the nose, or patients unable to hold the thermometer or understand the procedure.

Technique. Using an oral thermometer, shake the mercury indicator to below 96° F. Insert the thermometer under the patient's tongue. Ask the patient to hold the thermometer with the lips. Avoid taking the temperature immediately after the mouth has been rinsed with hot or cold liquids. Do not engage the patient in conversation when determining the temperature. Remove the thermometer after 3 minutes. Read the thermometer, and repeat the procedure if the accuracy of the reading is in doubt. Record the temperature in the chart. Unless the thermometer is disposable, wash it with detergent and water and disinfect it properly.

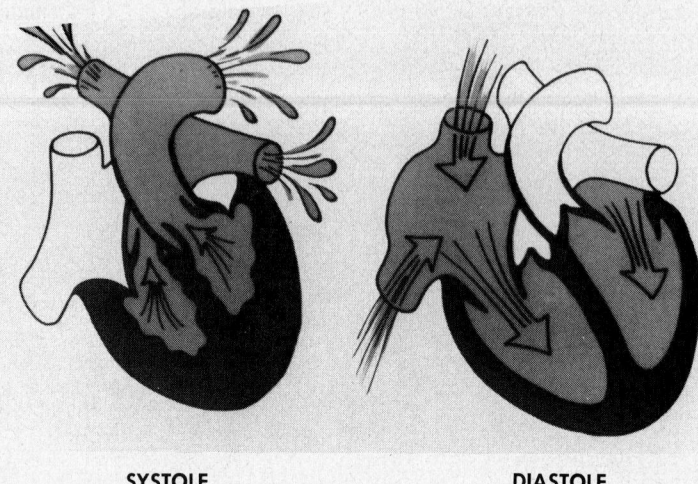

SYSTOLE   DIASTOLE

Fig. 10-2. Heart chamber during ventricular contraction (systole) and during ventricular relaxation (diastole). (From Anderson, J, and Geistfeld, NC: Hypertension . . . the silent killer, slide No. 14, self-instructional package. Minneapolis: University of Minnesota.)

As an efficiency measure, the pulse and respiration rate may be recorded while the thermometer is in the patient's mouth.

Arterial blood pressure. Blood pressure is the measurement of the force of the blood pushing against the walls of the blood vessels. The pressure is influenced by the physical condition of the heart, the volume of blood being pumped, and the resistance of the arteries to the flow of blood (peripheral resistance). The blood vessel most commonly used for blood pressure determination is the brachial artery in the arm. The normal adult blood pressure is 120/80 mm Hg. The top number refers to *systolic pressure*, the pressure in the blood vessel at the point of ventricular contraction of the heart. The systolic pressure is the maximal pressure that the arteries undergo when the heart is working. The bottom number refers to *diastolic pressure*, the pressure in the blood vessel during ventricular relaxation (Fig. 10-2). The diastolic pressure is measured when the heart is at rest and reflects the minimal pressure that is constantly sustained by the arteries. A diagnosis of hypertension is confirmed in adults when the average of two or more diastolic measurements on at least two subsequent visits is 90 mm Hg or higher or when the average systolic measurement on two or more visits is greater than 140 mm Hg (Joint Council, 1984).

Dental professionals can provide a valuable service for dental care consumers by detecting elevated blood pressure levels in individuals who are unaware of the problem. It is also important to detect uncontrolled hypertension before dental treatment because of the potential risk to the patient when the stress of dental treatment is added to an already stressed cardiovascular system. Detection of hypertension, patient education, and appropriate referrals and consultations with the patient's physician are all important aspects of the patient assessment procedures. The following information regarding hypertension will help the dental professional understand the nature of hypertension and its significance to dentistry.

Hypertension. Hypertension (high blood pressure) is a common disease found in approximately 20% of white and 30% of black Americans. Dental professionals can estimate that about 10% to 20% of their patients will suffer from hypertension and that about one-third of these will be unaware of the problem (Cutler, 1986). Hypertension is the second most common cardiovascular disease in this country. It is the principal risk factor in congestive heart failure, stroke, and kidney failure and a predisposing factor in the acceleration of arteriosclerosis. Undiagnosed or untreated hypertension can shorten a life by 10 to 30 years (Silverberg, 1976). The prevalence of this disease

Table 10-1. Classification of blood pressure readings and recommendations for individuals aged 18 years or over

Blood Pressure	Classification	Recommended Follow-up
Diastolic mm Hg		
<85	Normal blood pressure	Recheck at each appointment
85 to 89	High normal blood pressure	Inform patient that blood pressure reading was high and recommend medical evaluation
90 to 104	Mild hypertension	Refer patient for evaluation by physician within 2 months; request medical consultation; use routine dental management and stress reduction protocol
105 to 114	Moderate hypertension	Refer patient for evaluation within 2 weeks; request medical consult prior to dental therapy; use stress reduction protocol
≥115	Severe hypertension	Refer patient for medical evaluation immediately; postpone all elective dental procedures until blood pressure is controlled; request medical consultation
Systolic mm Hg		
(When DBP is <90 mm Hg)		
<140	Normal blood pressure	Recheck at each recall appointment; use routine dental management
140 to 159	Borderline isolated systolic hypertension	Refer patient for medical evaluation within 2 months; request medical consultation; use routine dental management and stress reduction protocol
≥160	Isolated systolic hypertension	Refer promptly for medical evaluation; request medical consultation before beginning dental therapy
≥200		Refer promptly for medical evaluation (within 2 weeks); postpone elective dental procedures until blood pressure is controlled; request medical consultation before beginning dental treatment

increases with age. Certain population groups are at a higher risk for developing hypertension; these include black Americans, obese individuals, and people with family histories of high blood pressure.

Blood pressure screening is an important part of the clinical examination of all dental patients. Many patients visit their dentists more frequently than their physicians, making the dental office a prime location for detecting patients who may require medical consultation and treatment. The American Dental Association has stated that blood pressure measurement for screening purposes is appropriate for all new patients, including children, and for recall patients once a year. The procedure should be part of the office routine for taking or updating the health history (ADA 1985.

Singer and others (1983) reported that during dental hygiene treatment, diastolic pressure fluctuated an average of 2.1 mm Hg for patients with normal blood pressure, 1.0 mm Hg for nonmedicated hypertensive patients, and 0.1 mm Hg for medicated hypertensive patients. These findings indicate that the stress of anticipated dental treatment does not significantly increase blood pressure and that blood pressure readings taken in the dental office are quite reliable.

Referral. Classification of blood pressure measurements and suggestions for appropriate referral and follow-up have been listed in Table 10-1.

Because an increase in diastolic pressure generally results from a narrowing of the arterioles throughout the body, this figure is considered more significant. A diastolic blood pressure of 90 to 104 mm Hg is considered mild hypertension; a diastolic pressure of 105 to 114 mm Hg is considered moderate hypertension; and a diastolic pressure greater than 115 mm Hg is considered severe hypertension (Joint Council, 1984). External factors that influence blood pressure include exercise, emotional status, and ingestion of stimulants (such as caffeine and nicotine) or depressants (such as alcohol). Systolic pressure tends to be more influenced by external factors than diastolic pressure. Systolic pressure may also be influenced by the age of the patient. The systolic pressure tends to rise 0.5 to 1.0 mm Hg per year until the seventh decade of life. Therefore, slightly elevated systolic readings may be within normal limits for an elderly adult, according to these guidelines (Cutler, 1986).

Patients whose diastolic blood pressure is between 85 and 89 should be informed that their blood pressure reading is higher than normal and that it should be checked annually. These individuals may have a higher risk for developing diagnosed hypertension. If the diastolic blood pressure is between 90 and 104 mm Hg or the systolic measurement is 140 to 199, the patient should be informed that the blood pressure should be checked by a physician within 2 months. If the diastolic blood pressure is between 105 and 114 mm Hg, the patient should be referred for a medical confirmation within 2 weeks. A telephone consultation with the patient's family physician is appropriate to determine whether dental treatment should be continued for the day and to establish communication for following the patient's medical status. If the diastolic blood pressure is greater than 115 mm Hg or the systolic blood pressure is greater than 200 mm Hg, the patient should be allowed to remain quiet for at least 5 minutes, and the reading should be confirmed. If the blood pressure is still elevated after two or more measurements, dental treatment should be delayed and immediate medical referral and confirmation obtained.

In most cases hypertension is an asymptomatic disease. Some patients with hypertension may complain of symptoms including severe headaches, dizziness, blurred vision, or signs of renal disease. Blood pressure readings should be correlated with findings such as these in the medical history.

When a medical referral is made, the patient should understand that: (1) his or her blood pressure exceeds normal limits; (2) hypertension is of-ten asymptomatic; (3) uncontrolled high blood pressure has serious consequences; (4) long-term follow-up and therapy are necessary; and (5) therapy will control but not cure high blood pressure (Joint Council, 1984).

In addition to the role of screening patients for untreated or uncontrolled hypertension, the dental professional must consider the implications of this disease for dental treatment. Recommendations for dental management of hypertensive patients and for medical consultation should be followed. Patients with uncontrolled high blood pressure may have a higher risk of suffering a medical emergency as a result of the stresses of dental treatment. The dental professional must assess whether these patients can safely tolerate the physical and psychological stresses of the planned dental procedures.

In addition to referring the patient for prompt diagnosis and treatment and obtaining a medical consultation, certain modifications of the dental appointment may also help to reduce the potential medical risks of dental treatment for hypertensive patients. Dental professionals should recognize signs of anxiety in these patients and work to eliminate their causes by taking time to explain all procedures to the patient and to provide reassurance and moral support during the dental treatment procedures. The dentist may prescribe premedication for anxious patients before the dental appointment. Nitrous oxide analgesia and adequate pain control measures will also help to reduce anxiety and discomfort during the dental visit. Appointments should be scheduled early in the day when patients are well-rested and should be kept as short as possible (Shapiro and Avery, 1984). Postoperative pain and anxiety control should also be implemented as needed.

Dental professionals should record the names and dosages of all medications that have been prescribed for treatment of hypertension. Dentists and hygienists should be aware of the side effects of these drugs and of potential contraindications or interactions with anesthetic solutions or other drugs used as part of dental treatment. The degree of patient compliance with the prescribed antihypertensive therapy should also be determined before dental treatment. Those diagnosed as hypertensive must understand the importance of complying with prescribed drug therapy in order to control this condition.

In a case tried by the New Jersey Supreme Court, a dentist administered a local anesthetic with epinephrine vasoconstrictor to a patient for a routine filling. The patient collapsed with a stroke and died a few days later. Negligence was alleged in this case due to the dentist's failure to make a physical evaluation or to complete a medical history before administering anesthesia. Because of these omissions the clinician was unaware of the patient's cardiovascular status. The court upheld the ruling of negligence. This is probably the most specific case on a dentist's failure to conduct a physical exam (Conway, 1980).

Treatment. In mild cases of hypertension, weight reduction and control of sodium intake may bring the blood pressure into normal range. When drug therapy is necessary, a "stepped-care" program is advisable. This approach entails initiating therapy with a small dose of antihypertensive medication, increasing the dosage of that drug, and adding one medication after another gradually as needed until the goal blood pressure is achieved, side effects become intolerable, or the maximum dose is reached (Joint National Committee, 1984). Depending on the patient, several medications may be necessary, making medical follow-up an important part of ongoing care. Generally, the need for treatment continues for life (Silverberg, 1976).

Diuretics are the first drug of choice for treating mild hypertension. These medications promote the renal excretion of water and sodium ions. Positive results occur in about 50% of mild hypertensive patients (Gaynor, 1983). Common diuretics include hydrochlorothiazide, furosemide, and spironolactone. The second step after diuretics is to prescribe adrenergic inhibiting agents, such as reserpine, methyldopa, clonidine, and propranolol hydrochloride. These agents deplete or inhibit norepinephrine. A vasodilator such as hydralazine may be added as the third step in medical therapy. For severe hypertension, the fourth step would include an additional adrenergic inhibiting agent such as guanethidine sulfate.

Implications for dental treatment. Antihypertensive medications often cause postural hy-

potension (positional low blood pressure), necessitating raising the patient slowly from the supine position to prevent dizziness or syncope. Antihypertensive medications may affect the fluid balance in the oral cavity, causing a dry mouth with resultant dental complications. Analgesic agents (cyclopropane, halothane) may produce a decrease in oxygen in the blood and may cause a rapid increase in blood pressure for these patients. Local and general anesthetics and vasopressor substances may potentiate the hypotensive effects of the antihypertensive medication, possibly causing cardiovascular collapse and shock. Epinephrine in the form of a gingival retraction cord or in a local anesthetic is contraindicated in patients taking guanethidine, reserpine, or methyldopa. It may potentiate the pressor effects of catecholamine, possibly causing a rapid increase in blood pressure. In a well-controlled hypertensive patient, 0.1 mg of epinephrine is allowed if necessary.

The dental team and physician need to work cooperatively in detecting, treating, and following the hypertensive patient. Noting the blood pressure at each dental visit is a preventive health service that cannot be overlooked. For the patient with a history of hypertension, the medical history should be updated at recall intervals by inquiring about the patient's current medications and recent visits to the physician in addition to recording the blood pressure for the day.

Technique. Obtain a stethoscope and a sphygmomanometer (blood pressure apparatus). This usually includes an inflatable bladder enclosed in an unyielding cuff, which will be wrapped around the patient's arm. The cuff must be the correct width for the diameter of the patient's arm. The width of the bladder should be slightly less than half the circumference of the arm and the length of the bladder should be at least 80% of the arm circumference. Approximately two-thirds of the upper arm should be covered by the cuff when it is in place. If the cuff is too narrow, the blood pressure reading will be erroneously high; if it is too wide, the reading may be too low. Several sizes of cuffs are available to fit small to obese patients. The circumference of the arm, not the age of the patient, is the determining factor in selecting the proper sphygmomanometer. Attached to the cuff is a rubber bulb to pump air into the

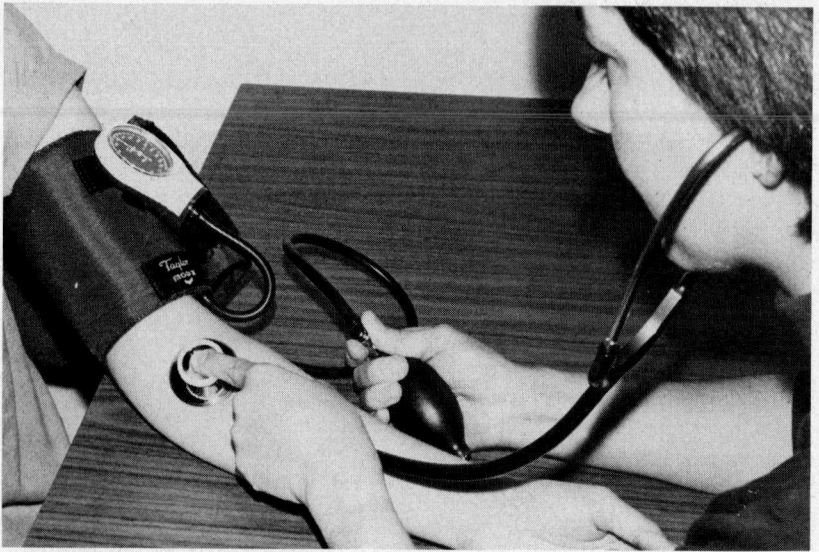

Fig. 10-3. Place cuff 1 inch above bend in arm with gauge in position for easy viewing.

bladder and a gauge (aneroid dial or mercury column) that reflects the pressure in the blood vessel as the air in the bladder is deflated by regulation of the air-release valve.

Also available is equipment that inflates and deflates the cuff automatically and displays a computerized digital readout of the blood pressure. Units that provide electronic digital readouts of blood pressure measurement are easy to use because a stethoscope is not needed. They are especially useful for individuals who are hearing impaired. Disadvantages of these units are (1) they are more expensive than standard manual equipment and (2) they are more likely to result in erroneous measurements, because they tend to provide readings which are sometimes inaccurate and because they are battery-dependent.

The following steps should be followed when taking a blood pressure measurement using a standard sphygmomanometer and stethoscope:

1. Allow the patient to relax in the chair for at least 5 minutes before taking the blood pressure in order to allow the blood pressure to stabilize. Seat the patient in a comfortable position in which the arm can be easily supported at heart level. Ask the patient to roll up a sleeve or to slip the arm out of the clothing to permit access to the brachial artery. Rest the arm in a slightly flexed position with the hand open and relaxed.

2. Wrap the cuff around the patient's arm with the arrows centered over the brachial artery. The lower border of the cuff should be 1 inch (or about the width of 2 fingers) above the bend in the arm. Place the manometer gauge (either a mercury gauge or an aneroid gauge) in a position where it can be viewed easily (Fig. 10-3). With a mercury manometer, the gauge should be viewed so that the meniscus is at eye level.

3. Find the radial pulse just above the thumb at the wrist joint. Close the valve of the pressure bulb (rotate clockwise until tightened) and inflate the cuff until the pulse is no longer felt. Note the pressure registering on the gauge. Open the air-release clamp until the cuff is completely deflated. Wait 30 to 60 seconds before reinflating.

4. Place the stethoscope comfortably in the ears with the earpieces directed forward. Place the diaphragm of the stethoscope over the brachial artery approximately 1 inch from the bend in the arm, toward the hand, and close to the inner aspect of the forearm (Fig. 10-4). The dia-

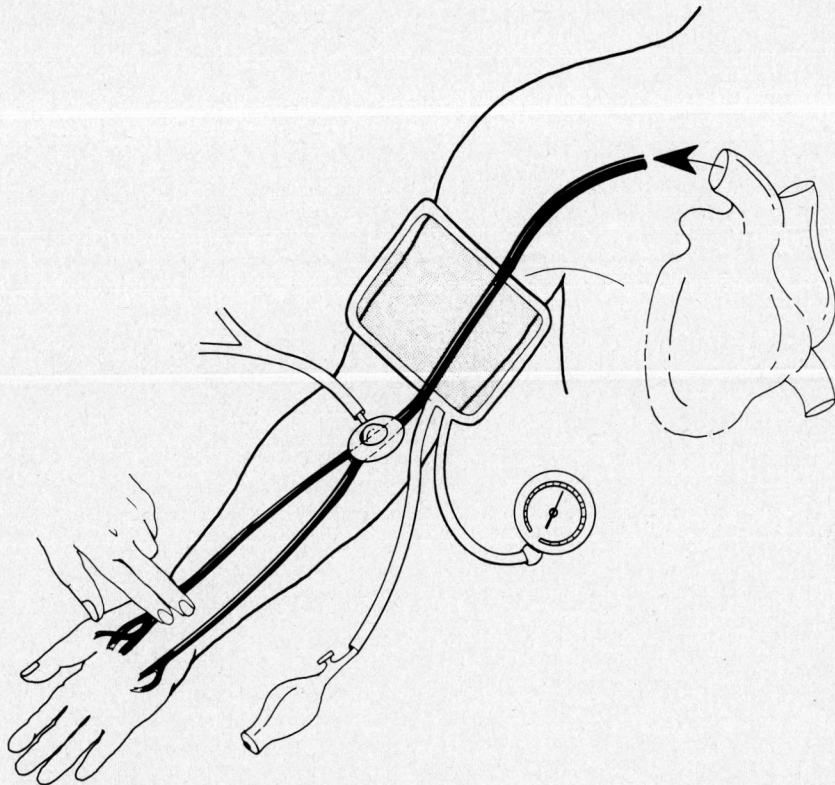

Fig. 10-4. Place diaphragm of stethoscope over branch of brachial artery. This is approximately 1 inch from bend in arm toward hand and close to inner aspect of forearm.

(From Boundy, SS, and Reynolds, NJ: Current concepts in dental hygiene, vol. 2, St Louis, 1979, The CV Mosby Co.)

phragm should be in total contact with the skin and should be positioned just below (but not touching) the cuff or tubing.

5. Inflate the cuff 20 to 30 mm Hg higher than the pressure at which the radial pulse disappeared, as noted in step 3.

6. Using the air-release valve, slowly deflate the cuff at a rate of about 2 to 3 mm Hg per heartbeat. Note the pressure at which the first pulse beat is heard. This is the systolic pressure. Continue to release the air in the cuff. The pulse sound will increase in intensity, then become muffled and disappear. Note the pressure at which the last sound occurred. This is the diastolic pressure. Continue listening during the entire range of deflation and at least 22 mm below the diastolic reading. On occasion there will be what is known as an "ausculta-

tory gap" in which the sounds disappear for 10 to 15 mm Hg and then return. Errors in measurement due to the "auscultatory gap" can be prevented if the clinician inflates the cuff beyond the point where the pulse is lost and listens to the entire range of sounds, continuing past the last sound.

If the sounds are too faint to take an accurate reading, they may be enhanced in the following ways. Ask the patient to open and close the fist 8 to 10 times *after* the blood pressure cuff is inflated above the systolic level; then take the readings as usual. Or elevate the patient's arm for several seconds before inflating the cuff; then inflate the cuff with the arm still elevated. Lower the arm and deflate the cuff in the normal manner while taking the measurement readings.

7. Record the blood pressure measurements as a fraction, as follows:

$$\frac{\text{systolic pressure}}{\text{diastolic pressure}} = \frac{120}{80}$$

This number is spoken as "120 over 80." Note the arm position of the patient (for example, 120/80 RAS, reg = right arm sitting, regular adult cuff).

8. Let the patient relax the arm once again before repeating the procedure for confirmation of the reading. Avoid repeating the procedure several times in a row without allowing the patient's circulation to return to normal. This may arouse anxiety in the patient and affect the reading, and the arm may become quite uncomfortable.

9. Compare the current reading with past blood pressure readings (if available). Consult the dentist and physician when the systolic pressure is greater than 160 mm Hg or the diastolic pressure is greater than 95 mm Hg. Note any unusual findings or changes in the pattern of blood pressure recordings as compared with past visits.

Table 10-2 shows the upper limits of blood pressure for children. When recording blood pressure readings for children, three numbers should be recorded (as in 110/80/70), compared with two numbers for an adult (as in 110/70). The first number (110) is the systolic reading that is recorded when the first two regular beats are heard. The second number (80) is recorded when the tapping sounds become muffled and lower in pitch. This point is the accepted diastolic reading for children. The third number (70) is the cessation or disappearance of all sound.

• • •

Table 10-2. Upper limits of normal blood pressure in children

Age (in years)	Arterial pressure (mm Hg) Systolic/diastolic
14-18	135/90
10-14	125/85
6-10	120/80
6	110/75

Once vital signs are recorded, the hygienist begins the extraoral examination.

Extraoral examination

For this part of the head and neck examination, the patient should be seated in an upright or semi-supine position. It is difficult to examine the deeper structures of the neck and submandibular area when the patient is in a full supine position because many of the soft tissue structures tend to fall back into the deeper structures of the head and neck and are less accessible for examination and palpation. The clinician will be working either in front of or behind the patient, depending on which structures are being examined. At all times, the patient should be positioned for maximum visibility. All necessary supplies that are needed for the examination procedure should be assembled and accessible to the clinician.

The following guidelines should be considered while the examination is being performed:

1. The clinician should be able to locate each structure in the head and neck region that will be examined.
2. All structures being examined should be accessible for observation or palpation.
3. The clinician should use a thorough technique to examine each structure.
4. The clinician should use a sequence of examination that is systematic and efficient in time and motion.

Patient considerations. The patient's needs for privacy and comfort should be given careful consideration during the head and neck examination. Patients appreciate a clinical attitude that demonstrates professional interest in their feelings and concerns. Before beginning the clinical examination, the clinician should explain the procedure and why it is an important part of dental health care. The clinician should speak in a quiet and friendly voice so that the conversation will not be overheard by other patients or personnel outside the operatory. Patients deserve to have all procedures explained to them and to be considered as partners in care rather than objects of care. During the head and neck examination, the clinician should display a confident attitude and a competent approach to the examination. Patients may not be used to being touched and examined in so close a manner and may feel some shyness or embarrassment until the clinician can put them at ease.

Many patients may avoid any type of physical examination because they fear the results of the procedure. The clinician can ease this apprehension by explaining the importance of regular professional examinations and self-examinations and by reinforcing this behavior in the patient. These same patient fears can be heightened if the clinician verbalizes clinical findings using technical jargon that the patient cannot understand. The clinician can accomplish a great deal of patient education on self-assessment of oral conditions if he or she uses language that is easily understood and carefully and thoroughly discusses the significance of diagnoses with the patient in lay terms. For instance, while examining the extraoral and intraoral structures, the clinician can describe what is being examined and why. This eliminates any guesswork and potential misunderstanding by the patient. An excerpt from such a conversation might sound like this:

Mrs. Willis, the next thing I will be examining is your tongue. Have you ever looked closely at your tongue? If you will watch me in the mirror you're holding, I'll show you how it can be examined and what to look for. First, I'd like you to place the tip of your tongue on this gauze square so that I can move it easily. Good! Now, as I look at the top of the tongue, I can see that it has a slight coating. This can be easily removed by brushing the tongue with a toothbrush. Otherwise, your tongue looks very pink and healthy. These bumps back here are normal papillae. Now I'm going to check the sides of the tongue for any areas that look like sores or for any white or red patches. The sides of the tongue and the floor of the mouth are two areas where oral cancer may sometimes occur, so you will want to take the opportunity to inspect these surfaces yourself at home. After seeing them here and at home, you'll have a good idea of what they normally look like and it will be easier for you to recognize any changes that might occur. These structures in the back of your tongue are also normal. They are the lingual tonsils. Now I'm going to feel your tongue for lumps or hard areas. Everything looks and feels fine, Mrs. Willis. Do you have any questions about what I've shown you?

In this way the patient will gain an understanding of the normal structures of the mouth while observing the clinician's examination and listening to the clinician's explanations. In addition, patients should be given the following instructions regarding their own oral self-assessments: (1) they should be looking for unusual lumps or bumps in the mouth; (2) they should check for unusual color changes that may appear as white, red, or bluish patches, or areas that appear to be speckled with both white and red areas; (3) they should establish a sequence for examining all parts of the mouth; (4) they should perform their own oral examination on a monthly basis; and (5) they should observe any unusual lesion for 2 weeks to see if it heals; if not, then it should be reported to a dentist or physician promptly (Glass et al, 1975).

Not only will patients benefit from the health information you have provided them about their own mouths, but they will also appreciate your interest in taking the time to answer their questions and discuss their concerns. This process will help make each patient a more educated and prevention-oriented health consumer. A more detailed explanation of self-assessment techniques for dental patients is described later in this chapter.

Visual inspection. The extraoral examination includes two components. The first is a visual inspection of each structure. It is followed by palpation and auscultation.

For the visual inspection the patient should be seated in an upright or semisupine position with the clinician seated facing the patient. Glasses should be removed, and clothing that restricts access to the neck (such as tight-fitting collars and ties) should be loosened. Starting from the top of the head and neck area and moving downward, *examine the hair* for texture, amount, and distribution. Note any apparent *scalp lesions,* such as scars, sores, or growths. Examine for the presence of lice or other transmittable conditions within the hair.

Next *examine the face* for symmetry, form, and profile. Observe the skin of the face for abnormal pigmentation, hair, texture, scars, or lesions. Facial asymmetry may be indicative of inflammatory conditions such as dental abscesses or mumps. Stroke victims or others who suffer from unilateral paralysis of facial muscles demonstrate an inability to produce normal facial expressions on the affected side. The muscles and soft tissues of the affected side may have a drooping or flaccid appearance.

Note the general color of the skin. An abnormal redness may indicate the presence of inflammation, fever, sunburn, or increased vascularity due to excitement or exertion. Abnormal paleness could indicate anemia, systemic illness, or shock. Patients with a history of heart or pulmonary disorders may exhibit a slightly bluish cast to the skin. Jaundice or yellow skin may be indicative of liver disease (hepatitis), red blood cell disorders, or drug toxicity.

Question the patient about the presence of any raised lesions, such as moles, to determine how long they have been present and whether they have undergone any changes in size, texture, color, or tendency to bleed. Malignant melanoma is a deadly type of skin cancer, which can appear as lesions similar to common skin moles. More than 25,000 new cases of malignant melanoma and almost 6,000 deaths from that cancer were predicted for 1987 (American Cancer Society, 1987).

The clinician should be aware of the risk factors and clinical characteristics of this cancer to aid in its detection during the head and neck examination. Factors that may increase the risk of this cancer include light-colored complexion or eyes; history of severe sunburn during childhood, teenage, and early adult years; extensive sun exposure due to occupation or recreational habits; presence of xeroderma pigmentosum or increased number of pigmented nevi in childhood; and a family history of malignant melanoma.

Malignant melanoma can result from an abnormal change in a preexisting pigmented nevus or it can develop as a totally new lesion, particularly in individuals 40 years or older. Because its appearance can be similar to that of other common, benign skin lesions, the clinician should be familiar with the characteristics that distinguish a benign lesion from a potentially malignant lesion. Most benign pigmented lesions (common moles) have round and symmetrical shapes, regular margins, and uniform color and are less than 6 mm in diameter. In contrast, early malignant melanomas have asymmetrical shapes with irregular borders, variegated color (multiple shades), and diameters greater than 6 mm.

The following changes in a raised skin lesion should be considered danger signs (Friedman et al, 1985):

Change in color to variegated shades of dark brown, black, red, white, or blue or a spread of color from lesion into surrounding skin

Change in size that is sudden or continuous

Change in shape resulting in irregular margins

Change in elevation

Change in surface, including scaliness, erosion, oozing, crusting, ulceration, or bleeding

Change in the surrounding skin, including redness or swelling

Change in sensation, including itching, tenderness, pain

Change in consistency, including softening or friability

If the clinical head and neck examination and the patient's report of relevant signs or symptoms indicate the possibility that skin lesions may be abnormal, a prompt referral should be made to the patient's physician for a definitive diagnosis. Early detection and treatment of malignant melanoma significantly increases the chances for survival.

Scars are indications of past trauma to the head or face. Discuss the cause of the trauma to determine its relevance to the patient's medical and dental history.

While examining the *eyes,* observe the following structures:

Scleras. Note color and signs of irritation.
Pupils. Note size and reactivity to stimuli such as light.
Eyelids. Note texture, form, color, and habits (blinking).
Conjunctiva. Note color, degree of moisture, and presence of foreign bodies; examine by retracting the lower lid in a downward direction with the tip of the index finger.

Examine the *nose* for form, symmetry, and obstructions. The airflow can be examined by placing the dental mirror underneath the patient's nostrils during normal respiration.

Examine the *lips* for symmetry, form, texture, color, and habits. Note signs of irritation, chapping, or breaks in the skin, especially at the corners of the mouth. Chapped lips should be protected with a coating of petroleum jelly or other lubricant to prevent the dried tissues from breaking open during the examination. Mouth ulcers or intact and healing vesicles on the lips should never be touched with unprotected hands. Herpes simplex virus can be transmitted from infected lesions to small breaks in the skin of the clinician, such as hangnails or torn cuticles. A recurrent viral infection, herpetic whitlow, can be established in the fingers of the clinician in this manner. Examine the function of the lips by asking the patient to open and close the mouth. Note lack of closure or mouth-breathing tendencies.

Examine the *ears* for form, texture, hair, symmetry, and color. Be sure to look behind the ears for possible lesions that would normally be shielded from view.

Check the *neck* area for symmetry of the structures in the neck. Examine the skin of the neck for pigmentation, texture, scars, obvious swellings, or lesions.

Description of significant findings. It is important that descriptions of all abnormal or unusual findings be recorded in the patient's chart in terminology that is clear, concise, and descriptive so that the dentist and/or oral pathologist has sufficient data on which to base a diagnosis. The color, morphology, surface texture, size in millimeters or centimeters, and symptoms of all lesions should be described. The patient should be questioned about the history of each lesion. Determine whether or not the patient has been aware of the lesion, how long it has been present, and what symptoms it has caused. The following descriptive categories and terminology may help the dental hygienist to describe the clinical findings accurately (McCann and Wesley, 1987):

1. *Morphology.* Note whether the lesion is localized or generalized, single or multiple, whether multiple lesions are separate or coalescing.
   a. Raised lesions
      Are lesions filled with clear fluid or pus (vesicles, pustules, bullae) or solid (papule, nodule, tumor, plaque)?
      Do lesions have a sessile or a pedunculated base?
   b. Depressed lesions (ulcers)
      Is there a regular or irregular border or outline?
      Is the margin raised or smooth?
      Is it superficial or deep?
   c. Flat lesions
      Are borders regular or irregular?
2. *Surface texture.* Describe the texture of the lesion as verrucous, papillomatous, fissured, corrugated, crusted, or smooth.
3. *Consistency.* Do raised or palpable lesions feel hard, firm, or soft?
4. *Size.* Measure the dimensions of visible lesions in millimeters or centimeters with a probe; estimate the size of palpable lesions that lie beneath the surface of the skin or mucous membrane.
5. *Color.* Does it display a single, uniform color or multiple colors or shades?
6. *Symptoms.* Is the lesion associated with pain, tenderness, itching, swelling, or other discomfort?

Lesions that are detected during the examination should be described using the following descriptive terms:

purpura Red-purple discoloration greater than 0.5 cm in diameter.

petechiae Red-purple discoloration less than 0.5 cm in diameter.

ecchymoses Red-purple discoloration of variable size.

macule Flat, nonpalpable circumscribed lesion of less than 1 cm in diameter (such as freckles, flat moles, rubeola, and rubella).

patch Flat, nonpalpable, irregularly shaped lesion greater than 1 cm in size.

papule Elevated, palpable, firm, circumscribed lesion less than 1 cm in diameter (such as warts or pigmented nevi).

plaque Elevated, flat-topped, firm, tough, superficial lesion greater than 1 cm in diameter.

nodule Elevated, firm, circumscribed, palpable, 1 to 2 cm in diameter (such as lipomas, traumatic fibromas, and lesions associated with rheumatoid arthritis, leprosy, and syphilis).

tumor Elevated, solid mass greater than 2 cm in diameter (such as tori, polyps, papillomas, and neoplasms).

vesicle Elevated, circumscribed, superficial, filled with clear fluid, less than 1 cm in diameter (blister).

bulla Vesicle greater than 1 cm in diameter.

pustule Similar to vesicle but filled with pus (as in acne).

cyst Elevated, circumscribed, palpable, encapsulated, filled with liquid or semisolid material.

fissure Linear crack or break (such as angular cheilosis).

erosion Depressed, moist, glistening, follows rupture of vesicle or bulla; larger than a fissure.

ulcer Defect in the skin or mucosa that extends beyond the surface epithelium and into the underlying tissues. Reddened border may be ragged or punched out; depressed bases may appear soft or indurated with a floor that is smooth, granular, glazed, pus-covered, or hemorrhagic; may be painless or extremely sensitive (as in acute necrotizing ulcerative gingivitis, traumatic injuries, certain types of oral cancer).

hyperplasia An increase in the number of cells resulting in an overgrowth of tissue.

keratosis Abnormal thickening of the outer layers of skin or mucosa that may appear as white, grayish-white, or brown lesions; may occur as localized or diffuse areas (as in linea alba, cheek biting, nicotine stomatitis, certain lesions of lichen planus, and leukoplakia).

Lesions may be further delineated through the use of the following descriptors:

confluent Blending or occurring together; originally separate but subsequently combined.

corrugated A rippled surface.

crusted A hard, scablike surface.

discrete Separate, not blending or occurring together.

induration Hardened area of tissue.

pedunculated Elevated papillary-type lesion attached to underlying tissue by a stem or narrow connector.

papillomatous Nipplelike growths.

sessile Attachment of a lesion by a broad base.

verrucose A wartlike surface.

Extraoral palpation. The clinician is now ready to continue the extraoral examination by palpating all extraoral structures. One of the following methods of palpation will be indicated for each structure, or several techniques may be combined.

digital palpation Use of a finger to examine tissues.

bidigital palpation Use of one or more fingers and the thumb to examine tissues by grasping the tissue between thumb and fingers.

manual palpation Use of all the fingers of one hand to examine tissues.

bimanual palpation Use of both hands by grasping tissues between them for examination.

bilateral palpation Examination of structures on both sides of the face or neck simultaneously to detect differences between the two sides.

circular compression Moving the fingertips in a circular pattern over a structure while simultaneously applying pressure to the tissue.

It is important for the clinician to palpate soft tissue structures against a harder structure such as underlying bone, other fingers, or hands. If the soft tissues are not supported by some means, there is greater possibility that abnormal masses might be displaced away from the examining fingers and not detected. Firm yet gentle pressure should be applied to the soft tissues to feel through all layers of skin and muscle. A hesitant examination technique that evaluates only the surface of the skin will not accomplish this goal.

Sequencing the palpation. The following sequence of the palpation procedure is designed so that all structures are examined in a logical and systematic order that avoids "hopping" from one area of the head to another. Following a set pattern of examination guarantees that the clinician always knows which structures have or have not been examined in case the procedure is interrupted and provides for efficient time and motion management. As you begin the examination, ask the patient to report any feelings of discomfort or tenderness in the areas being palpated.

The first structure to be palpated is the *mentalis muscle*. This muscle attaches to the lower lip and inserts into the symphysis of the mandible. Palpate it with digital compression, rolling the tissue over the mandible. Have the patient swallow and observe the function of this muscle in swallowing. Patients with abnormal swallowing habits often grimace and wrinkle the chin when using this muscle to assist in swallowing. (A glass of water may be useful to assist the patient in swallowing at various points during the examination.)

Examine the *anterior border of the mandible* next. From a position behind the patient, use bidigital and circular compression on the soft tissues, starting at the symphysis of the mandible and moving posteriorly along the borders of the mandible (Fig. 10-5). Through palpation, examine the soft tissues and underlying bone to locate normal bony landmarks, deviations in symmetry, tenderness, and crepitus (cracking sounds). Continue this method of palpation bilaterally until the angle of the mandible is reached.

The *occipital lymph nodes* are located at the base of the skull at the back of the head. Ask the patient to lean his or her head forward, and apply digital circular compression bilaterally with the fingertips. The palpation should begin at the back of the neck and extend horizontally to the sterno-cleidomastoid muscle (Fig. 10-6).

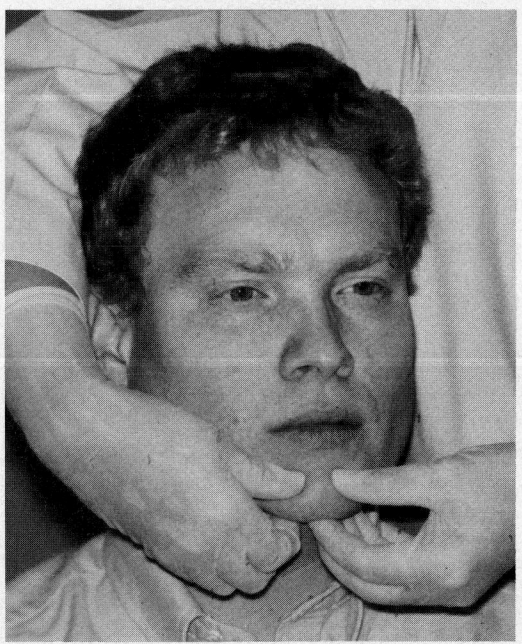

Fig. 10-5. Anterior border of mandible as it is palpated using bidigital compression and circular motion of soft tissues against bone.

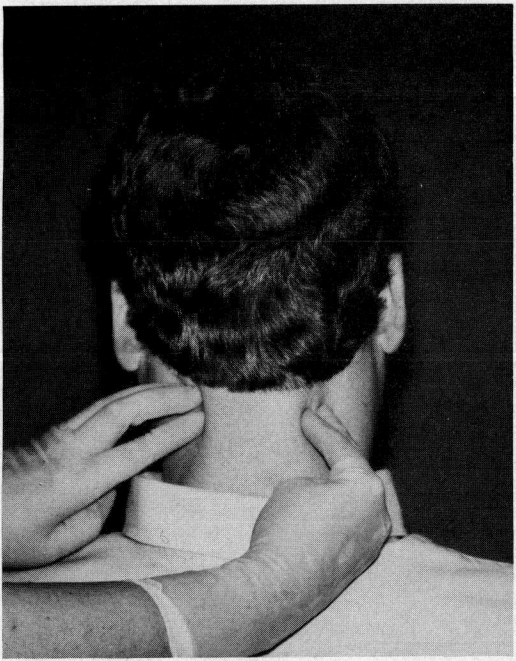

Fig. 10-6. Occipital nodes are being examined. Circular compression is applied at base of skull.

The *auricular and parotid lymph nodes* are located behind, beneath, and in front of the ears. Begin by applying the fingertips in digital compression and circular movement to the area of the posterior auricular nodes. The palpation should be done bilaterally to identify deviations from one side to another. Continue this palpation moving around the base of the ear and anterior to the ear, examining the parotid nodes and the anterior auricular nodes, located anterior to the tragus of the ear. Note enlargements, tenderness, degree of mobility, and firmness of nodes (Fig. 10-7).

Palpate the temporomandibular joint bilaterally by placing the index fingers of each hand just anterior to the outer meatus of the ear and asking the patient to open and close the mouth slowly several times. As the patient opens and closes, observe the face for deviations in the mandibular function. Feel for abnormal function of the joints and differences in function between the right and left sides (Figs. 10-8 and 10-9). Question the patient about any painful symptoms associated with these jaw movements. Auscultation of the joint

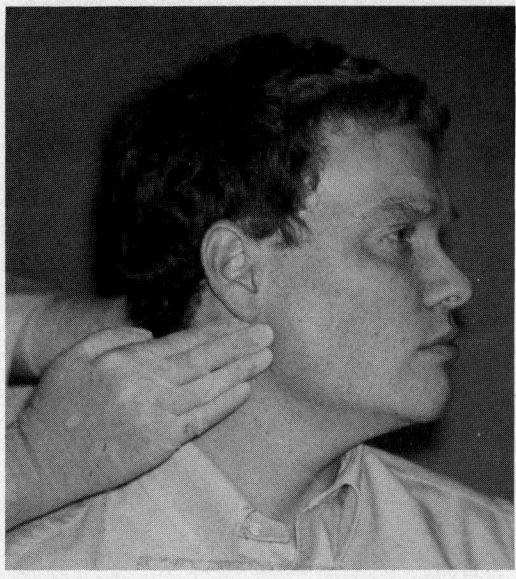

Fig. 10-7. Inferior auricular nodes are being examined by circular compression against tissues. Both anterior and posterior auricular nodes are examined in same manner.

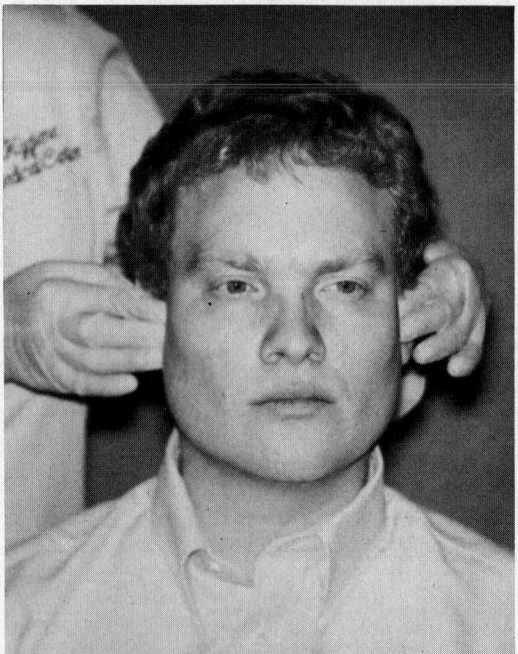

Fig. 10-8. Palpation of temporomandibular joint; fingertips are placed bilaterally just anterior to outer opening of ear.

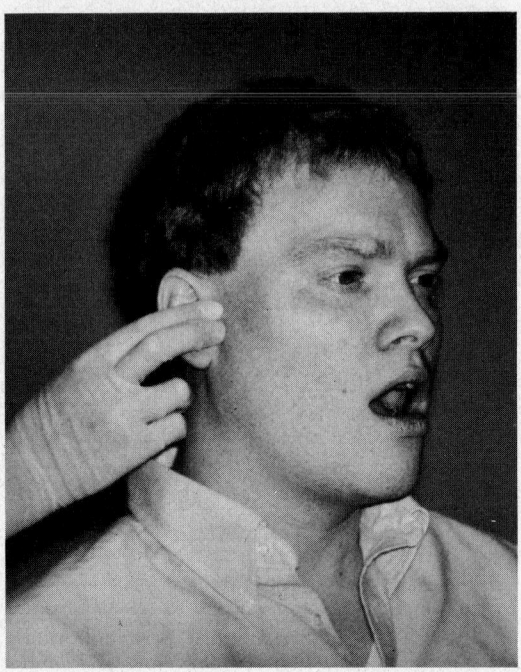

Fig. 10-9. Patient is asked to perform a variety of jaw movements as temporomandibular joint is palpated. Here patient is slowly opening his mouth as far as is comfortable while clinician feels for abnormal movement or clicking in joint.

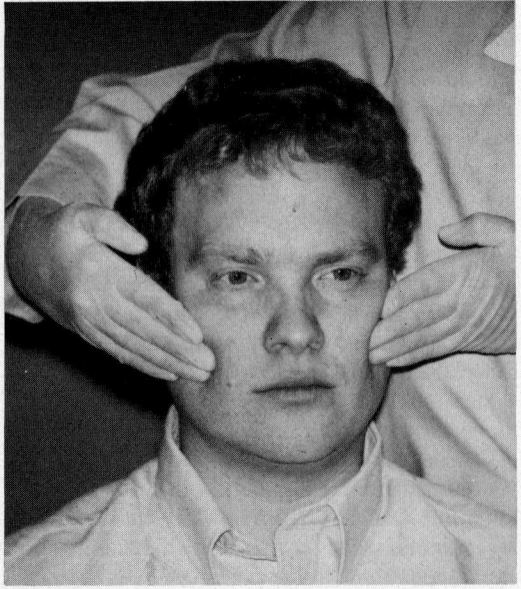

Fig. 10-10. Area of parotid gland is palpated with circular compressions over entire area of gland. This is a large gland and extends from in front of ear to cheek area and down to angle of mandible.

during movement is used to detect the presence of clicking, popping, or grating sounds. Also ask the patient to perform right and left lateral movements with the teeth apart and to make protrusive movements with the teeth together and then apart.

Palpate the area of the *parotid gland* (including the parotid nodes) bilaterally using digital compression and circular movement. Begin anterior to the tragus of the ear, and extend the palpation inferiorly to the angle of the mandible. Note any deviations in form, density, or size or tenderness in the area (Fig. 10-10).

Palpate the *masseter muscle* by placing the fingers of each hand over the angle of the mandible and extending the hand up onto the cheek. Then ask the patient to clench the teeth together several times, and examine the muscle bilaterally for size, function, and deviations between the two sides.

Examine the *temporalis muscle* in much the same way as the masseter muscle. Place the hands bilaterally across the muscle on the patient's tem-

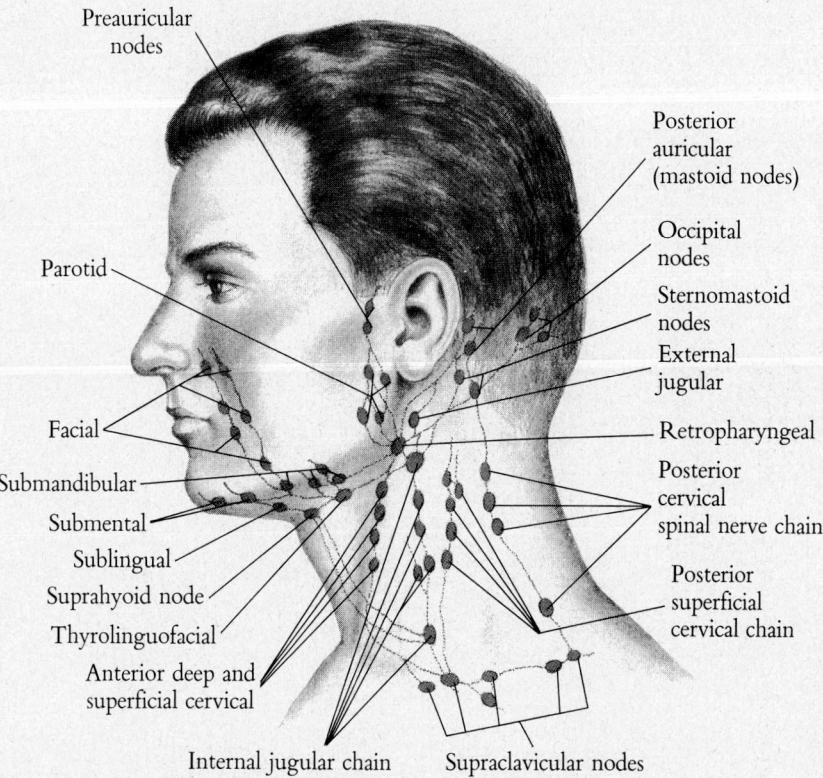

Preauricular
nodes

Posterior
auricular
(mastoid nodes)

Occipital
nodes

Sternomastoid
nodes

External
jugular

Parotid

Facial

Retropharyngeal

Posterior
cervical
spinal nerve chain

Submandibular

Submental

Sublingual

Posterior
superficial
cervical chain

Suprahyoid node

Thyrolinguofacial

Anterior deep and
superficial cervical

Internal jugular chain   Supraclavicular nodes

Fig. 10-11. Lymphatic drainage system of head and neck. If the group of nodes is often referred to by another name, the second name appears in parentheses.
(From Seidel, HM, et al: Mosby's guide to physical examination, St Louis, 1987, The CV Mosby Co.)

ples, and ask the patient to clench the teeth together several times. Check for muscle function and tenderness.

Examine the *submental region* (including lymph nodes) using digital compression and circular motion behind and beneath the symphysis of the mandible. Examine for swelling, enlargements, tenderness, firmness, and mobility of lymph nodes. For locations of lymph nodes of the head and neck see Figs. 10-11 and 10-12.

Palpate the *submandibular region* (including glands and nodes) using bidigital compression and circular movements. Ask the patient to lower the head so that the skin and muscles beneath the chin are not taut. This adjustment will make it easier to gain access to the deeper soft tissues of the submandibular area. Starting at the anterior border of the mandible, push the tissue from the

left submandibular area over to the right and grasp it with the fingertips of the right hand. The examining fingers should be cupped slightly to grasp the tissues effectively. Then use the fingertips to roll the soft tissue over the right border of the mandible, feeling for swelling or enlargements, tenderness, mobility, and firmness of lymph nodes. Reverse this procedure for the left submandibular area. Finally, use the fingertips to compress the soft tissues of the submandibular region bilaterally. Start this palpation at the midline of the submandibular area, and proceed outward to the borders of the mandible and posteriorly to the angle (Fig. 10-13).

To examine the structures of the neck, start with the *sternocleidomastoid muscle.* Ask the patient to turn the head to the left and lower the chin. This will cause the muscle on the right side

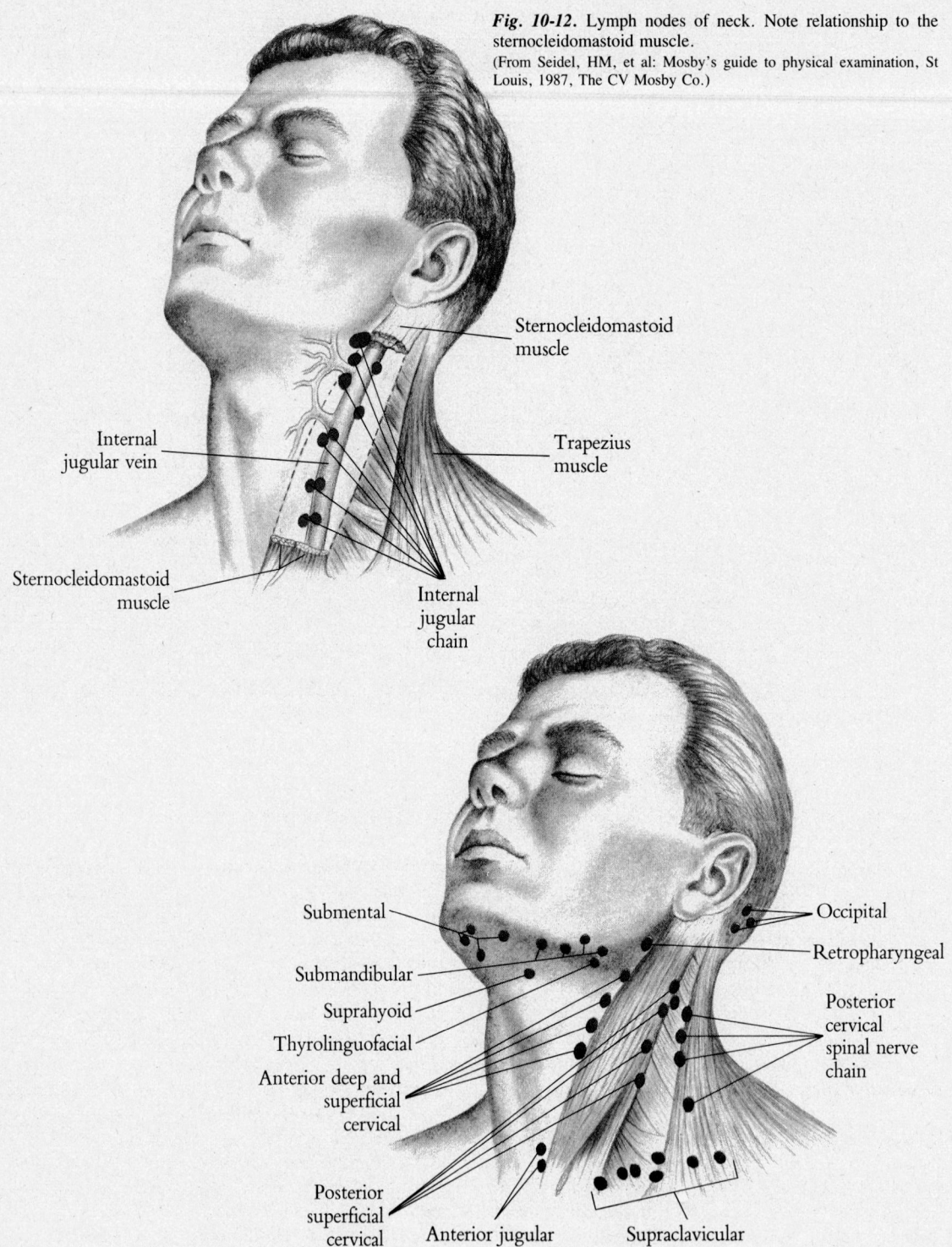

Fig. 10-12. Lymph nodes of neck. Note relationship to the sternocleidomastoid muscle.
(From Seidel, HM, et al: Mosby's guide to physical examination, St Louis, 1987, The CV Mosby Co.)

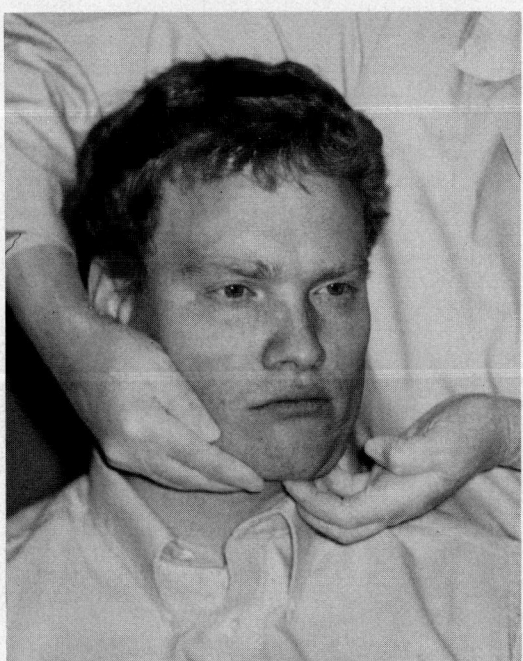

Fig. 10-13. Palpation of submandibular area. Note that clinician has pushed tissue from patient's left side over to opposite side where it is being grasped and rolled over angle of mandible. Opposite side will be examined in same way.

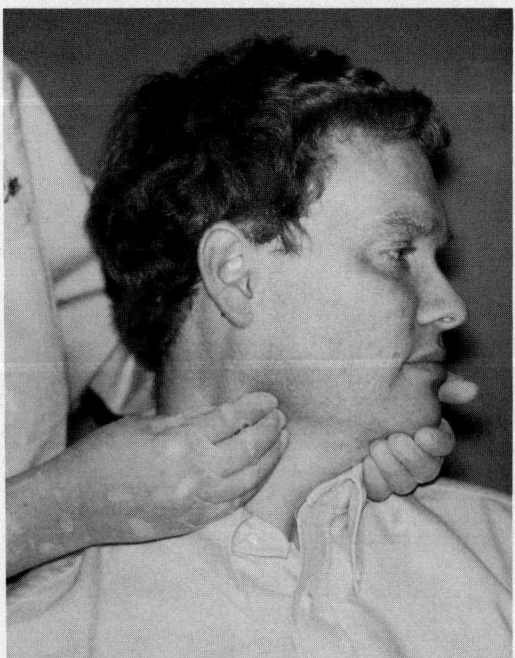

Fig. 10-14. Note patient positioning for palpation of sternocleidomastoid muscle. His head is turned to side and slightly down while chin rests in clinician's free hand. This causes muscle to protrude so that it is easily seen. Palpation is bidigital compression starting from below ear and continuing whole length of muscle to clavicle.

of the neck to be more prominent and will increase its accessibility for the examination. The left hand of the clinician should support the patient's head at the chin, and the right hand should grasp the muscle between the thumb and fingers.

Begin bidigital palpation, starting from behind the ear and continuing all the way down the muscle until you reach the clavicle. Remember that for thorough examination of the structures of the neck, the patient should have loosened tight collars or ties so that the neck area is exposed. Repeat the examination on the left side of the neck. Examine the muscle for rigidity, tenderness, induration, presence of masses, and difference in function from one side to the other (Fig. 10-14).

The *superficial cervical lymph nodes* are located anterior and posterior to the sternocleidomastoid muscle. Apply digital compression and circular movement to this area, extending from the angle of the mandible in a downward direction along the anterior and posterior aspects of

this muscle (Fig. 10-15). The patient's head should be in an upright and forward position. Palpate the area bilaterally to examine for deviations from normal. Look for enlarged lymph nodes, and note their tenderness, degree of mobility, and firmness.

The *deep cervical lymph nodes* are located along and behind the sternocleidomastoid muscle. The technique of palpation is the same as for the anterior cervical lymph nodes but with an increased effort being made to locate the thumb and fingers behind the muscle to locate nodes in the deeper, less accessible tissues.

The *thyroid gland* normally is not visible. It is located vertically between the cricothyroid ligament and the fourth tracheal ring and horizontally between the sternocleidomastoid muscle and the trachea. It can be palpated from behind or in front of the patient. With one hand place the fingers on

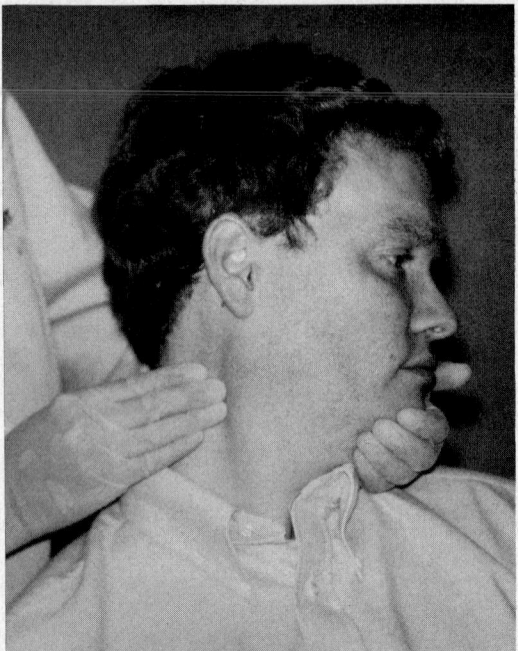 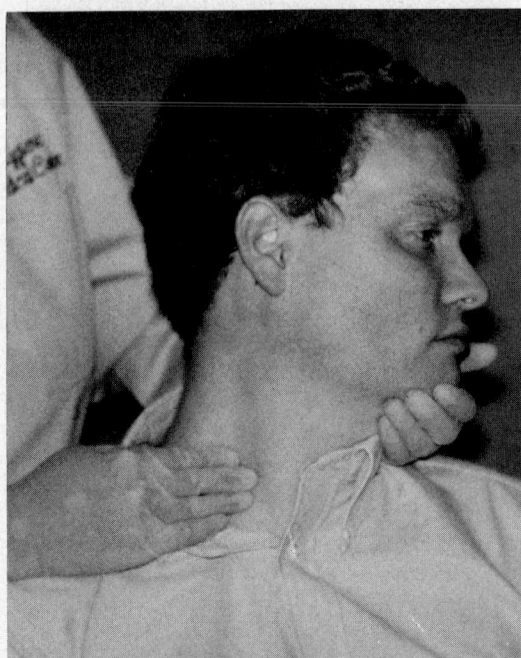

Fig. 10-15. Circular, digital compression is used to examine cervical chain of lymph nodes anteriorly and posteriorly to sternocleidomastoid muscle.

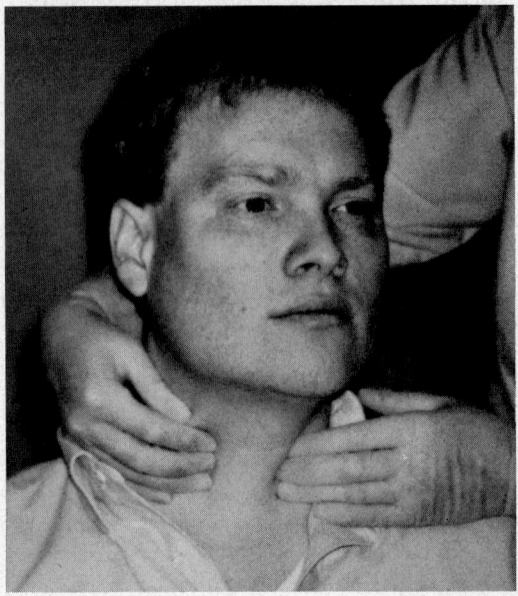

Fig. 10-16. Thyroid is being palpated from rear of patient. One hand gently displaces tissue to one side while fingers of other hand carefully feel for enlargements or abnormal masses.

one side of the trachea and gently displace the thyroid tissue over to the other side of the neck. With the opposite hand apply gentle circular digital compression to the tissues. Palpate the thyroid gland for enlargements, tenderness, and mobility. Ask the patient to swallow, and examine the gland for signs of masses or lack of movement during swallowing (Fig. 10-16).

Examine the *larynx* by placing the fingertips of one hand bilaterally over the larynx and applying alternate pressure in a medial direction against the structure. A normal larynx should be freely movable and should ascend and descend during the process of swallowing. A slight fremitus (palpable vibration or movement) may be noted when the normal larynx is displaced during palpation (Fig. 10-17).

This completes the description of the extraoral examination. All significant findings should be described and recorded in the patient's chart to aid in diagnosis and treatment planning. Significant inclusions in the chart may be summarized from the palpation as follows:

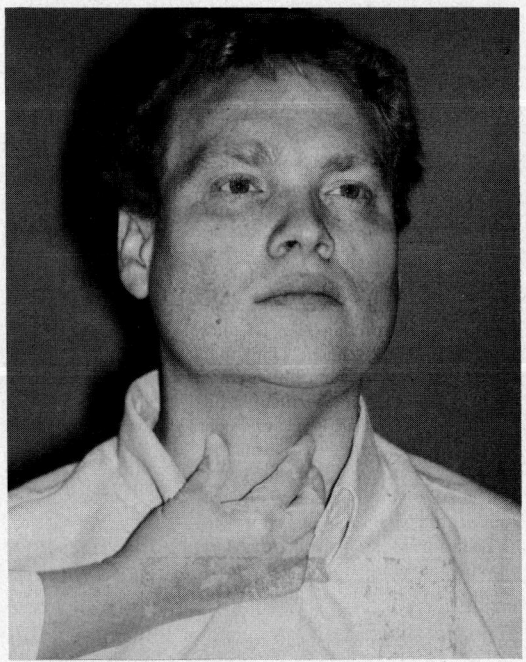

Fig. 10-17. Gentle medial pressure is used in area of larynx to check for mobility of larynx and trachea. Inability to move this structure slightly might indicate problems.

bony structures Record abnormal anatomy, growths, fractures, crepitus, and pain.

muscles Record hyperfunction or hypofunction, deviations between the two sides, swellings, masses, indurations, and tenderness.

glands Record abnormal swellings, tenderness, and hard masses.

lymph nodes Record palpable nodes and describe their size (estimate diameter), firmness (hard or soft), mobility (fixed or freely movable), tenderness (sensitive or painless), and how long they have been present. Determine if presence of lymph nodes can be traced to current manifestations of disease or recent history of disease.

skin Describe all lesions using the terminology discussed earlier.

Significance of lymph node examination

Normal lymph nodes are not visible or palpable during the head and neck examination. When the presence of swollen lymph nodes can be detected by either of these methods, the clinician should continue the evaluation of the patient to determine what the cause of the abnormality might be.

Lymph nodes of the head and neck area can become swollen and tender from infections that originate in the areas that they are draining. The clinician must have a clear understanding of human anatomy and the lymph node system in order to trace a detectable lymph node back to its associated cause. Enlargement of lymph nodes as a result of acute or chronic infections is known as *lymphadenitis*. Lymph nodes may become temporarily enlarged because of localized infections such as a dental abscess, regional infections such as tonsillitis, or systemic infections such as tuberculosis or syphilis. In most cases of acute inflammation, resolution of the infection allows the lymph nodes to return to their normal state. In some cases chronic infections will cause enlargement of affected lymph nodes because of the presence of scar tissue, so that they remain palpable as nontender firm or fibrotic single masses even after the source of the infection has been removed. Because many of these same characteristics might be found in nodes associated with malignant or metastatic diseases (cancer), the patient's medical history should be explored, and the patient should be interviewed to determine possible explanations for the presence of these nodes. In general, nodes that arise from acute inflammatory conditions are tender, soft, enlarged, and freely movable.

Lymph node involvement due to malignant diseases may display different characteristics. Detection and examination of these nodes reveals that they are often hard, nontender, and fixed to underlying tissues, and they may involve multiple nodes that are matted together. The patient may indicate no recent history of local or systemic infection in these cases to explain the presence of the detectable nodes. Bilaterally enlarged nodes may indicate the presence of systemic infection or an advanced malignancy. The presence of unilateral node enlargement may indicate either localized infection or possibly early metastatic disease. The alert clinician will combine information from the patient's medical and dental history, the oral examination, the lymph node examination, and an up-to-date knowledge of the demographics of patients who are at high risk for malignant diseases in order to evaluate the potential significance of detectable lymph nodes. When lymph node involvement suggests malignant changes, the clinician should examine the areas served by those nodes for signs of abnormal tissues. Although many detectable nodes may be easily explained by the presence of local, regional, or systemic infections, the dental professional should refer all questionable findings to the patient's physician or a specialist for a definitive diagnosis (Kerr, Ash, and Millard, 1983; Kutcher et al, 1981).

Intraoral examination

The supplies and instruments that are needed for the intraoral examination include a mirror, explorer, probe, gauze squares, and a tongue depressor. For this treatment procedure and all other intraoral procedures, the clinician should wear disposable gloves, a face mask, and safety glasses to prevent disease transmission.

The following factors will help ensure optimal examination technique: (1) lighting, (2) positioning, (3) tissue retraction, and (4) sequence. A complete and thorough examination cannot be performed without optimal consideration of all of these factors.

Direct lighting is provided by directing the central beam of the overhead light onto the area being examined. Care should be taken not to direct the light into the patient's eyes. Readjustment of the light beam is necessary as different areas of the mouth are examined. This responsibility should be assumed by the chairside assistant if one is present. Supplementary *indirect lighting* is also provided by the mouth mirror. This is especially useful for the posterior parts of the mouth, where it is difficult to use the direct beam of the overhead light.

Patient and clinician positioning should be such that both parties are comfortable and all areas are accessible to the clinician for complete examination. When necessary, the patient must be given instructions as to where to turn the head or place the tongue so that all areas are visible. The clinician should follow the principles of good positioning, discussed in previous chapters. Whenever possible, the clinician should seek a direct view of the structure to be examined. If a direct view cannot be obtained without violating the principles of effective positioning, such as in the maxillary tuberosity area, the dental mirror should be used to examine that area thoroughly.

The third factor for good examination technique is thorough, but gentle, *retraction* of soft tissues so that the entire area can be observed. There is no guarantee that lesions will not occur behind folds of tissue or at the hidden corners of the mouth. Failure to examine all tissues completely regardless of their accessibility can only be considered negligent.

The establishment of an efficient *sequence* is also an important factor. Optimal time and motion management, use of a logical order, and asepsis should all be considered in determining the sequence of examination. Because the examination of some intraoral structures, such as the labial and buccal mucosa and the floor of the mouth, requires external retraction or palpation technique, these structures should be done consecutively as a group. In this way the need for repeated handwashing can be minimized. Thus, the sequence presented in this chapter will be as logical and efficient as possible while still preserving maximal asepsis.

The clinician must be fully acquainted with the hard and soft tissue anatomy of the head and neck and especially of the oral cavity. To perform an examination that is comprehensive, it is necessary to be able to discriminate normal appearances from abnormal ones. For records to be universally understandable, the clinician must be well acquainted with the specific names and terminology associated with the structures to be examined and record all findings accurately.

To begin the intraoral examination procedure, the back of the dental chair should be lowered to a semisupine position. The clinician should be seated at the 9 o'clock (3 o'clock for left-handed clinician) position, where a direct view of the oral cavity and structures can be obtained. The patient should be asked to *remove all dental appliances* that are not permanent, and they are placed in appropriate containers until they can be examined. Radiographs should have been reviewed before the appointment, if they were available. Information from the radiographs will be correlated with the head and neck examination to aid in the detection of clinical findings. All necessary forms and supplies should be assembled and placed within easy reach of the clinician and assistant. Because this is the first intraoral procedure that the clini-

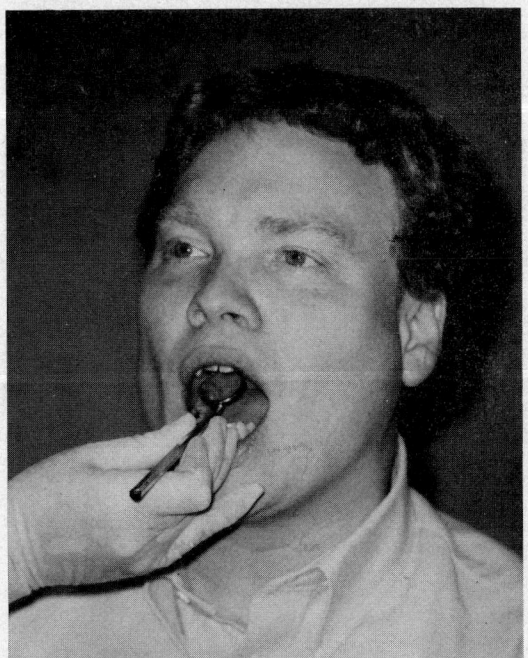

Fig. 10-18. A quick but thorough inspection of all areas of the mouth should be made before clinician begins more comprehensive examination of intraoral structures. In this view, a mirror is being used to examine palate and back of mouth.

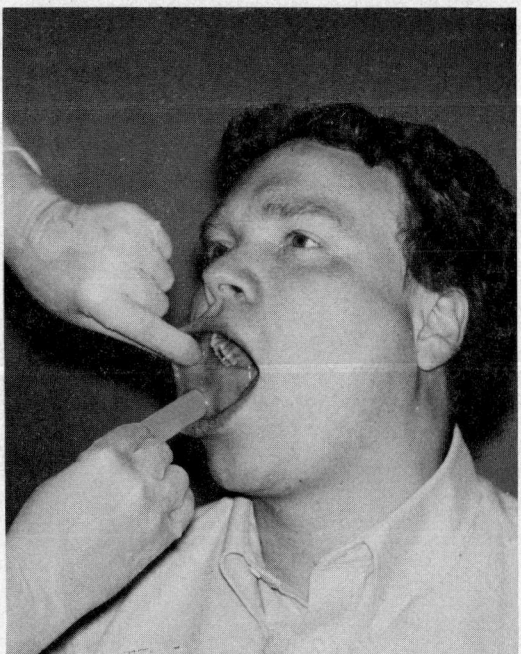

Fig. 10-19. A tongue blade may also be used to assist in tissue retraction during intraoral inspection.

cian is likely to perform, the hands should have been thoroughly scrubbed and gloved before the examination.

Before beginning a detailed examination of each structure, it is wise to *perform a cursory screening* of the intraoral tissues with a mouth mirror or tongue blade. This screening is to determine whether or not there are contagious lesions present that should not be contacted because of the risk of disease transmission (as with herpes simplex or syphilis) or patient discomfort (as with mouth ulcers or other traumatic lesions). The clinician should briefly inspect the following structures: lips, labial mucosa, buccal mucosa, hard palate, soft palate, tongue, floor of mouth, and alveolar ridges (Figs. 10-18 and 10-19). The clinician should also check the throat for signs of severe sore throat or other manifestations that would suggest that the patient should be seen or treated by a physician before any intraoral procedures are performed. A serious consequence of performing

an examination of oral tissues in the presence of a severe sore throat could be the introduction of multitudes of streptococci into the bloodstream. If the patient has a history of heart disease, a subacute bacterial endocarditis could result. The dental professional should postpone additional treatment until any acute infections have subsided or until infective lesions have healed. This will provide protection not only for the patient but also for dental personnel and other patients who could encounter the disease pathogens indirectly from contaminated surfaces or supplies.

When the initial screening is complete and no contraindications to continued treatment have been detected, the clinician should start the inspection and palpation of all intraoral structures using the following sequence:

1. *Lips.* Inspect the clinical appearance of the lips before retracting them. The skin should be intact and have a semimoist, firm texture. They should be free of all lesions, discolorations, growths, or swellings. Common abnormalities that might be detected include chapped lips,

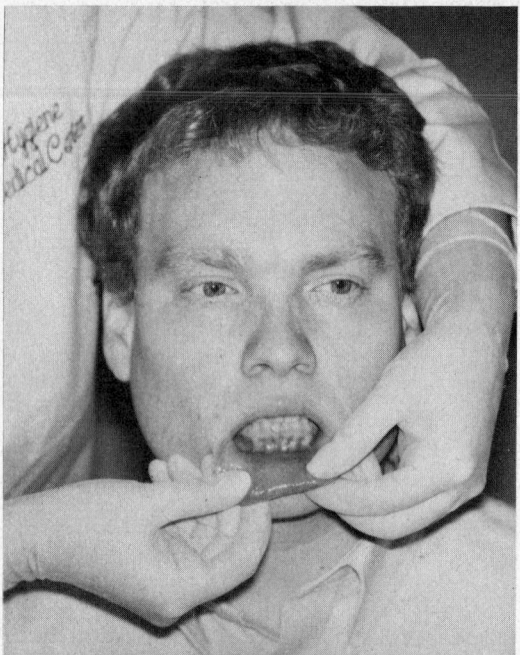

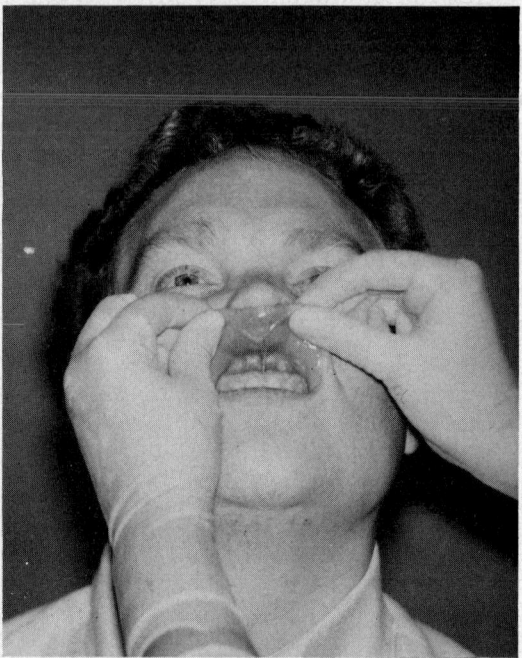

Fig. 10-20. Mandibular labial mucosa is retracted and examined. General appearance of gingiva and frenum attachments are also assessed.

Fig. 10-21. Maxillary labial mucosa is retracted; clinician should try to use same fingers intraorally at all times if possible, or wash hands before proceeding.

cracks at the corners of the mouth, traumatic lesions such as from lip biting and blisters, ulcers, and cold sores. Protect dry and cracked areas from further trauma by applying petroleum jelly to lubricate the area during retraction. Avoid touching ulcers or blisters.

2. *Labial mucosa.* Retract the mandibular labial mucosa down and away from the teeth. Grasp the tissues so that the thumb is placed intraorally and the fingers are kept extraorally. Try always to use this same arrangement so that the fingers used extraorally do not go back inside the mouth at any time unless the hands have been washed again; this will help reduce contamination during the examination. On the labial mucosa, check for a moist red surface that does not demonstrate any abnormal lesions, masses, or color deviation. You might notice small white or yellowish bumps located just below the mucosal lining. These are probably the labial sebaceous glands and are normal for this tissue. Examine the labial frenum for any tissue tags or lesions. Check also to make sure that this muscle attachment is

not pulling on the gingival tissues and causing recession. Continue this inspection and retraction around the corners of the mouth and up onto the maxillary labial mucosa. Palpate this tissue using bilateral, bidigital compression, feeling the tissues between the thumb and fingers. Note any swelling, hard masses, or tenderness (Figs. 10-20 to 10-22).

3. *Buccal mucosa.* Retract the buccal mucosa out and slightly away from the teeth so that its surface can be inspected from the labial mucosa back to the retromolar area. Alternately extend and examine the vestibular areas. As with the labial mucosa, the tissue should be moist and red. The soft tissue structure visible opposite the maxillary molar area is the parotid papilla. It houses the opening of Stensen's duct of the parotid salivary gland. Check the salivary flow by drying the duct opening with a gauze square and applying light, intermittent external pressure to the parotid gland. Watch for evidence of salivary flow from the duct opening. Examine the tissues for swelling, lesions, breaks in the mucosa, or abnormal

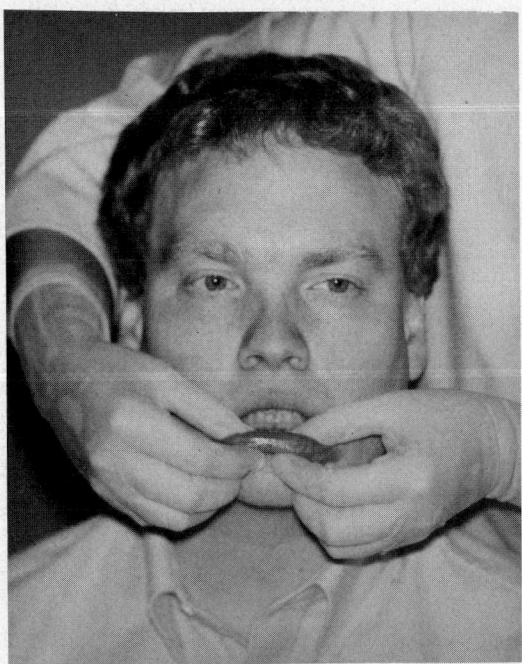

Fig. 10-22. Labial mucosa is palpated with bilateral bidigital compression, moving from midline to corners of mouth.

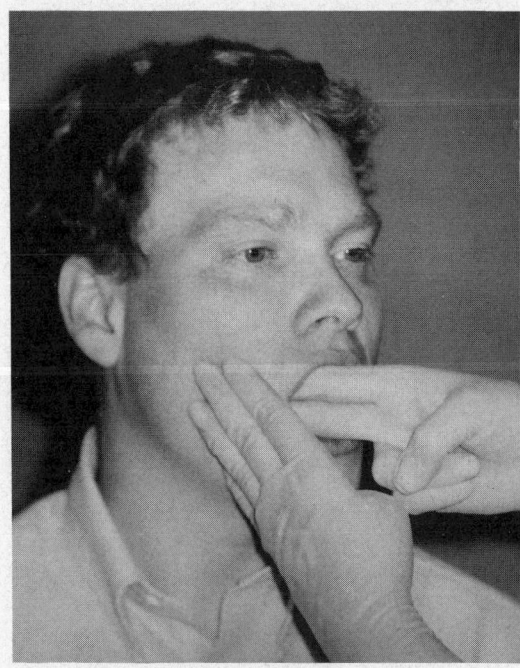

Fig. 10-23. Buccal mucosa is palpated bimanually with fingers of one hand inside mouth and fingers of other hand supporting tissues extraorally.

color changes, including white or red patches. There will be variable amounts of brown melanin pigmentation in this tissue, depending on the race of the patient. Palpate this area bimanually by placing the fingers of one hand intraorally while the other hand supports the tissues extraorally. Palpate the tissue between the two hands from the front of the mouth all the way back to the retromolar area. Note all abnormal swellings, masses, or tenderness (Fig. 10-23). Common findings may include Fordyce's granules, xerostomia, scarring, cheek biting, and linea alba.

4. *Floor of the mouth.* Before washing hands and proceeding with the rest of the intraoral examination, examine the floor of the mouth. Ask the patient to lift the tongue to the roof of the mouth. This area should appear moist and extremely vascular. Examine the following structures of the floor of the mouth:

lingual vein This vein courses up either side of the ventral surface of the tongue. Varicosities may be seen in the older patient.

plica fimbriata These are small hairlike projections of tissue that lie along the lingual vein.

lingual frenum This is the muscle attachment between the tongue and the floor of the mouth. An extremely short lingual frenum will restrict the movement of the tongue (ankyloglossia or "tongue-tied"). This is often detected when the tongue cannot touch the palate. It may also be manifested in abnormal speech patterns.

sublingual caruncle This is located at the base of the frenum and appears as a small rounded projection. It houses the opening of Wharton's duct for the submandibular salivary gland. Test the action of this duct by drying the floor of the mouth with a gauze square and then applying intermittent compression to the submandibular tissue between the ducts. Observe the floor of the mouth for the rate and amount of saliva flow entering the area.

sublingual folds These appear as two elevations or ridges that run along the floor of the mouth on either side of the tongue. These tissues house the ducts of Rivinus that service the minor sublingual salivary gland in the floor of the mouth.

plica lingualis These are small hairlike projections of tissue that lie along the crest of the sublingual folds.

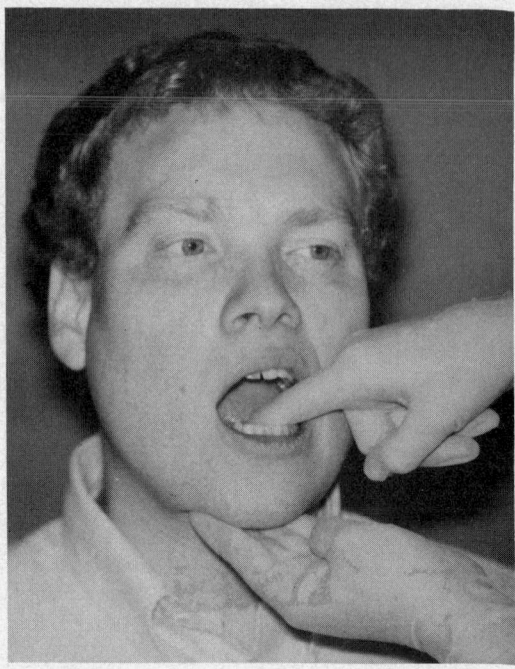

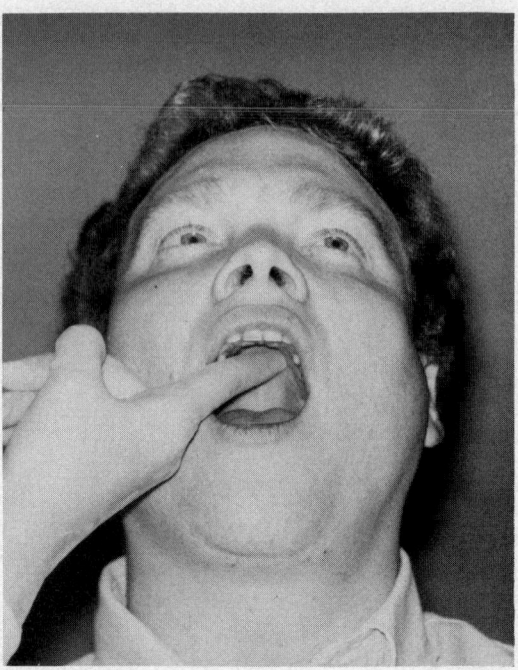

Fig. 10-24. Floor of mouth is palpated bimanually by placing one hand intraorally and supporting tissues against extraoral hand. Entire floor of mouth should be examined in this way.

Fig. 10-25. Hard palate is palpated using firm digital pressure against hard tissues.

While inspecting these structures, inspect the floor of the mouth for lesions or abnormal color changes. Palpate the area by placing the right hand intraorally and the left hand extraorally and feeling the tissues between the two hands (bimanual palpation) (Fig. 10-24). Note any swellings, masses, white or red patches, the comparative size of glands, and any tenderness described by the patient.

As the remainder of the examination will involve only intraoral structures, at this point the clinician should stop and wash both hands before proceeding.

The next area to be examined is the *hard palate*. With the light source directed up onto the palate, inspect the surface for lesions, swellings, and color deviations. A normal palatal surface will appear light pink and will have the following anatomic structures:

incisive papilla A protuberance of soft, firm tissue located between the two central incisors. It covers the incisive foramen, which is the opening for the blood and nerve supply to this area of the palate. This papilla is normally slightly redder than the surrounding palatal tissue because of increased blood supply.

medial palatal raphe A white line extending from the incisive papilla to the soft palate.

palatal rugae Irregular ridges of tissue radiating from either side of the raphe.

palatine foveae Two small depressions, one on either side of the midline, at the junction of the hard and soft palate.

Inspection of these structures may reveal abnormalities such as nicotine stomatitis, inflamed incisive papilla, ulcerations, palatal tori, or redness and irritation due to dentures.

Palpate the palate using digital compression of one or two fingers against the palatal surface (Fig. 10-25). Take care not to extend this technique onto the soft palate, as this could initiate gagging in some patients. Firm on-and-off pressure against the tissue is more comfortable than light circular pressure, which tends to "tickle" the palate. Pal-

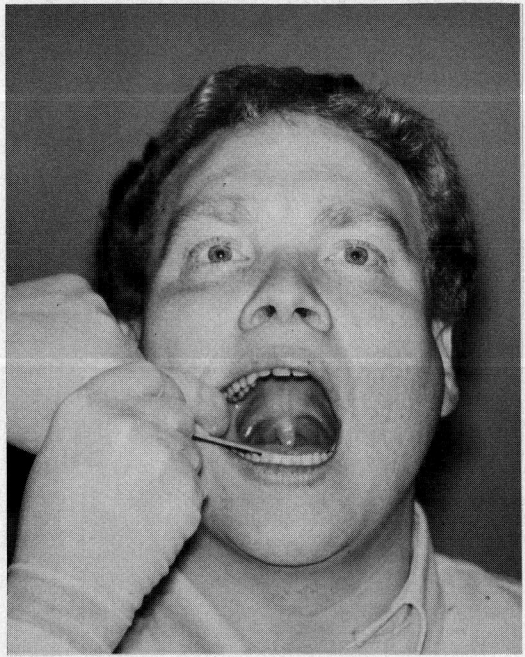

Fig 10-26. Since the tongue normally shields the oral pharynx from view, this area is examined by placing a mirror or tongue blade on anterior third of tongue and asking patient to say "ah."

pate for swellings or hard masses (for example, palatal tori), tenderness, and continuity of the underlying bone.

Next inspect the back of the mouth and examine the *soft* palate for color and lesions (Fig. 10-26). Observe the *palatine uvula* for deviations in form or color. To examine the oral pharynx, place a tongue depressor on the middle third of the dorsum of the tongue and ask the patient to say "ah." As the patient does this, the posterior third of the tongue should lower, providing a full view of the entire area. Observe also the movement of the uvula as the patient is saying "ah." Note any deviation of movement to either the right or the left. With the pharynx clearly visible, locate the following structures and examine them for color and signs of abnormal lesions or form: posterior wall of the pharynx, posterior pillars, palatine tonsils, and anterior pillars. Note any redness, signs of exudation, lesions, or tenderness.

The examination of the tongue is specific for

each of four surfaces: the dorsal (top), ventral (bottom), and the two lateral borders. Examine the dorsal surface first for color, lesions, symmetry, and form. The normal structures of this surface of the tongue include:

filiform papillae Plentiful hairlike papillae covering the dorsal surface of the tongue. These generally have a whitish color, although they often are stained extrinsically from food, tobacco, or medication.
fungiform papillae Flat, broad papillae that appear as red, mushroom-shaped elevations and are scattered among the filiform papillae. They house taste buds for sweet, sour, or salty stimuli.
circumvallate papillae A series of large papillae located in a V-formation on the posterior dorsal surface. They contain taste buds that respond to bitter stimuli only.

Retract the tongue by wrapping a gauze square around the anterior third to obtain a firm grasp and pulling it anteriorly as far as it will extend comfortably. Palpate the dorsal surface using digital compression over the entire surface (Figs. 10-27 and 10-28). Feel for abnormal masses, indurations, or swellings. Common abnormalities that may be detected on the dorsal surface of the tongue include a coated tongue, black hairy tongue, geographic tongue, and fissured tongue.

While still retracting the tongue out from the mouth, inspect the lateral borders by turning the tongue slightly over on its side so that a full view of the border can be seen (Fig. 10-29). Examine this area carefully for abnormal redness, red or white patches, swellings, ulcerations, or masses, because it is a common site for oral cancer. The normal structures found on the lateral borders of the tongue are the foliate papillae, which appear as a series of vertical ridges on the posterior borders. These papillae house taste buds for sour and acidic stimuli. Inspect the other side of the tongue in the same way. Palpate the lateral borders using bidigital compression of the tissue between the thumb and fingers, beginning at the posterior borders and moving to the anterior borders after removing the gauze (Fig. 10-30). Inspect and palpate the entire ventral surface of the tongue using digital compression (Fig. 10-31).

Use the mirror to aid in the inspection of the maxillary tuberosity and retromolar area. Note any deviations in form, color, or size; presence of abnormal growths of tissue; or lesions. Palpate

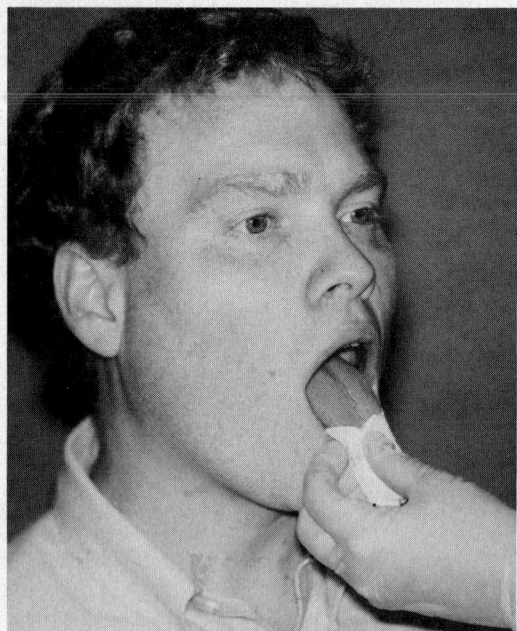

Fig. 10-27. Tongue is grasped by holding it with a folded gauze square and retracted so that entire dorsal surface can be examined.

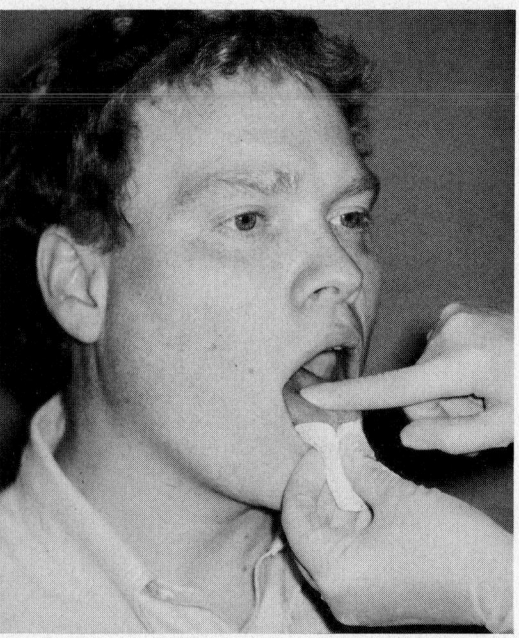

Fig. 10-28. Palpation of dorsal surface of tongue is done with digital compression over entire surface.

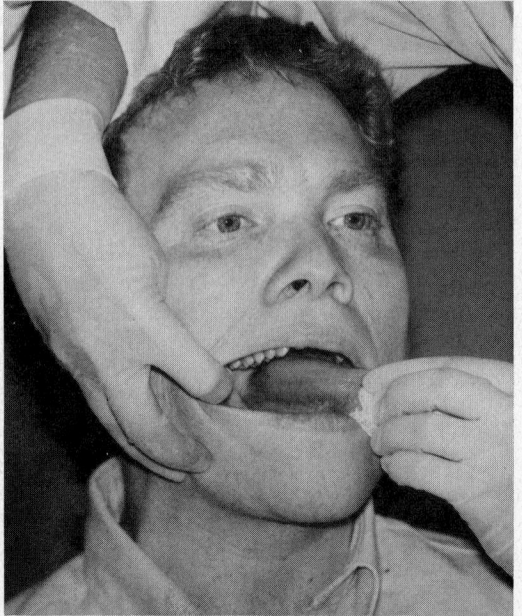

Fig. 10-29. Inspection of lateral borders of tongue involves retracting tongue out using a gauze square and turning it slightly over on its side so that entire lateral border can be closely examined. This is a common site for oral cancer.

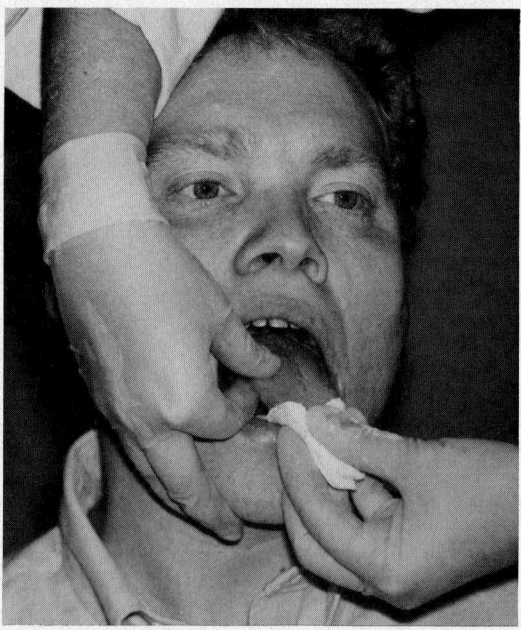

Fig. 10-30. Lateral borders of tongue are palpated with bidigital compression. While one hand stabilizes tongue, the other palpates. This procedure is repeated for other side.

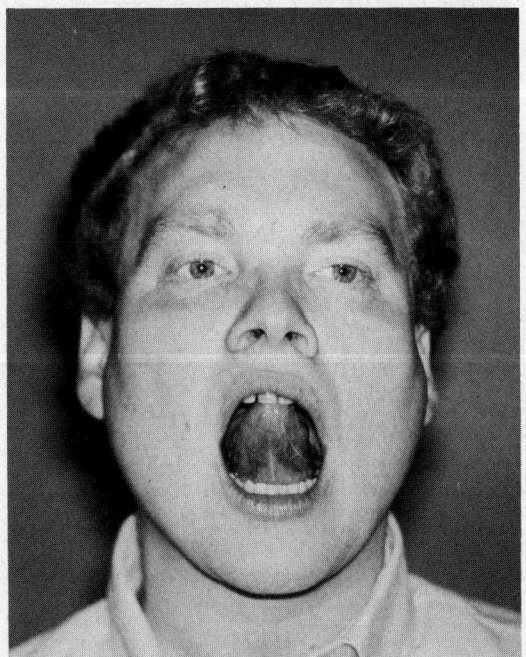

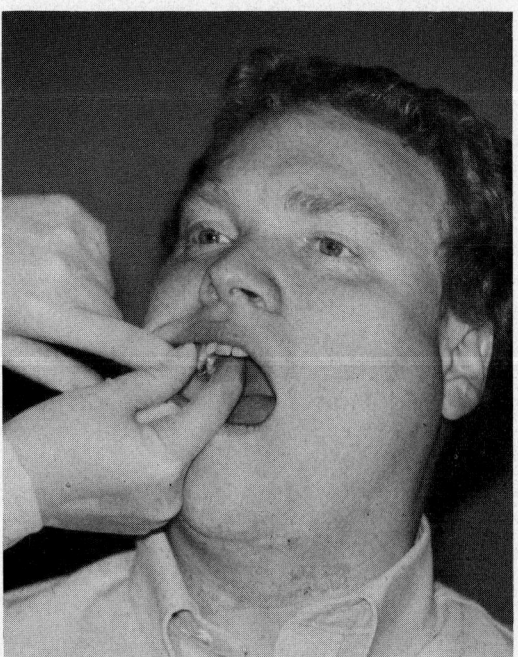

Fig. 10-31. Ventral surface is inspected by asking patient to lift tip of tongue to roof of mouth. With use of a mirror or tongue blade, the floor of the mouth can be examined simultaneously. Palpate the surface.

Fig. 10-32. Alveolar ridges are shown being palpated with bidigital compression. Any signs of abnormal masses or lack of continuity in the bone should be noted. Patient should also be requested to report any symptoms experienced during palpation.

the retromolar areas and maxillary tuberosities using digital compression. Common findings may include scarring from third molar extractions, overgrowth of tissue, inflammation, or tenderness due to erupting third molars.

Examine the *alveolar ridges* thoroughly for signs of redness, color deviations, swellings, or lesions. Retraction of the buccal mucosa and tongue is necessary for good visibility of these structures. Palpate the ridges using bidigital compression with thumb and index finger opposing each other. Examine the ridges for hard masses (tori), swellings, or crepitus, and note any tenderness experienced by the patient (Fig. 10-32).

• • •

The general and oral examination of the patient is now complete. After all significant findings are recorded, the clinician can continue the examination and assessment of the patient with more specific assessments of the dental and periodontal structures in the mouth, which, together with the

information obtained from this portion of the examination, will be used to construct a total picture of the patient's needs so that treatment planning and implementation can be accomplished.

IDENTIFICATION OF PATIENTS WITH SPECIAL NEEDS

During the examination of patients for dental treatment planning, the dental professional may encounter signs and symptoms of conditions that demand the attention of medical and other professionals. As health professionals, the dentist, hygienist, and dental assistant should be alert to the presence of conditions that require referrals. Specific situations discussed in this chapter include nutritional disorders, anorexia nervosa, and child neglect or abuse.

Nutritional disorders

A number of conditions that may be observed during the physical evaluation of the patient may indicate nutritional disorders. For example, the hair may lack luster and be thin and sparse; the fingernails may appear spoon shaped, dry, and brittle; the skin may lack color and appear dry and flakey; bruised areas may be visible under the skin because of subdermal bleeding; there may be an abnormal lack of body fat; the face may appear red and swollen; areas under the eyes may appear dark and shadowed; the eyes may appear dull or bloodshot; and the corners of the eyes and lips may be dry, red, and fissured.

Intraoral signs that may indicate nutritional deficiencies include gums that bleed easily and a tongue that appears deep red and raw, abnormally smooth, and glossy. The tongue may also exhibit sores or hypertrophy of papillae on the dorsal surface. The teeth may show evidence of decay or abnormal eruption patterns.

Other signs that the nutritionally deficient patient may exhibit include an increased heart rate, hypertension, enlargement of the abdominal cavity due to liver or spleen enlargement, mental irritability, loss of normal reflexes in the knees and ankles, and muscle weakness. This list of signs and symptoms is by no means specific only to nutritional disorders, as other medical conditions could produce similar effects. The clinician should combine these findings with information gathered during the patient interview, however, to assess the need for including a nutritional survey in the preventive treatment plan. Additional data from that survey may provide sufficient information that will allow the dental professional to ascertain the role of nutrition in contributing to these conditions.

Anorexia nervosa/bulimia nervosa. Individuals suffering from anorexia or bulimia nervosa may be seen in the dental practice. Dental care providers may be the first ones to suspect these conditions because of the presence of certain oral complications. In general, these individuals do not recognize their condition as a health hazard, and they need support and understanding to encourage them to seek professional help. Patients most likely to display signs of anorexia and bulimia nervosa are teenage or young adult women who have poor self-images and preocupation with weight control.

Anorexia nervosa causes avoidance of eating, leading to a significant loss of weight and signs of malnutrition. Anorexics may exhibit any of the following physical symptoms: electrolyte imbalance, insomnia, constipation, skin disorders, brittle or thin hair and nails, hypotension and/or a low pulse rate (Rollins and Piassa, 1978). Untreated cases have been known to result in death, usually due to cardiac failure or suicide.

Patients with bulimia alternate between eating "binges" and "purges" (induced vomiting). Reports indicate that known bulimics may binge and purge an average of 12 times a week. These episodes are often precipitated by emotional stress. In addition to inducing vomiting, these individuals may use laxatives, diuretics, and cathartics to effect weight loss. The resulting physical complications may include acute stomach dilation, electrolyte imbalance, alkalosis, hypochloremia, edema, kidney disorders, and cardiac arrhythmias. Oral symptoms and signs include dental caries, gingivitis, parotid gland enlargement, erosion of enamel, and dental hypersensitivity brought on by the presence of gastric acids in the mouth (Roberts and Li, 1987).

Patients suffering from these problems will usually deny that the problems exist and deny vomiting. They do not respond positively to criticism, so an empathetic yet direct approach to the problem is needed. The treatment of this condition is not within the dental professional's area of training, so referral is necessary. The dental professional can be instrumental, however, in providing information and encouragement to convince the affected individual of the need to seek professional help. The dentist or hygienist can also help by telling the patient how to minimize the oral complications of frequent vomiting until the condition is brought under control. Patients should be advised to use a sodium bicarbonate or magnesium hydroxide rinse after vomiting to neutralize the effects of excess acids. In addition, the use of daily fluoride rinses or fluoride gels may be indicated to prevent the occurrence of decay and to minimize enamel erosion and related hypersensitivity. Patients should also be advised not to brush immediately after vomiting, because doing so might increase the eroding effect of the acids. Usual approaches to plaque control should be encouraged, although these individuals do not seem to be more susceptible than the general population to periodontal destruction (Roberts and Li, 1987).

Child neglect or abuse

The general appraisal and head and neck examination of children may lead to suspicions regarding the presence of child neglect or abuse. Dental professionals are especially likely to detect the signs and symptoms of maltreatment during their examinations because an estimated 50% of these injuries occur to the head, face, and intraoral areas (Becker et al, 1978; Kittle et al, 1981).

There is a difference in the meaning of the terms *child neglect* and *child abuse*. *Child neglect* refers to physical or emotional negligence relative to a child and usually represents a case of omission (failure to provide shelter, food, and medical and dental care). Child neglect in terms of dental care might include such findings as untreated rampant caries, untreated dental pain or infection, or a lack of continuity of dental care in the presence of known pathology (Davis et al, 1979).

Child abuse includes any physical, sexual, or emotional act that is directed against a child. During the general appraisal of the patient, the dental professional might notice that the child appears fearful, withdrawn, or watchful and provides no eye contact or spontaneous smiles. There may be signs of malnutrition, uncleanliness, limping, or a slumped or withdrawn posture. During the extraoral examination, signs of bruises, slap marks, bite marks, black eyes, cigarette burns, or abrasions and lacerations in unusual places should be noted. The ears should be examined for signs of trauma that might have been caused by twisting, pulling, or pinching. Marks on the neck that might have been caused by strangling may be detected (Davis et al, 1979).

Intraorally, signs of child abuse may include teeth that have been fractured or displaced; scars on the lips, mucosa, or tongue; binding marks at the corners of the mouth where the child has been gagged; darkened or nonvital teeth; or laceration to the maxillary frenum. Jaw fractures also might result from abuse.

More than 1 million cases of child abuse or neglect are reported each year in the United States; at least 2,000 deaths are caused annually by child abuse or neglect (Kittle et al, 1981; Winters, 1985). Those numbers translate into six deaths a day or one every 4 hours (Stimson, 1984). It is believed that the true incidence of child maltreatment is actually much higher than these figures indicate, as only about half of all child abuse cases are reported to authorities (Sopher, 1977).

Surveys of abused children have shown that there are no reliable predictors for its occurrence. The age distribution varies from birth to 17 years. Children from all socioeconomic groups are affected (Davis et al, 1979; Kittle et al, 1981). Schwartz and others (1977) have noted little difference in the incidence of the problem based on racial, religious, economic, or educational grounds. Obviously, this problem is a serious one that deserves the attention and action of the dental community to assist in its detection and solution.

Dental professionals as well as others in the community are mandated by law to report suspected cases of child abuse or neglect to the appropriate local authorities. It is not the responsibility of dental professionals to prove that maltreatment has occurred, only to report that it is suspected. Other health and welfare authorities must then investigate.

The dentist or dental hygienist should follow several steps prior to reporting suspected child maltreatment. First, the presence of unexplained or unusual injuries must be recognized and documented in the dental record. Color photos of suspicious injuries may also be taken to document their appearance. The child and/or parents should be asked how injuries occurred, and the explanations should be correlated with the appearance of the wounds. Parents should be approached not in an accusatory or critical manner but in a manner demonstrating genuine concern for the child (Stanley, 1981). The dentist or hygienist should explain to the parents the legal responsibility of health professionals to ask about unusual injuries. If explanations seem unsatisfactory to account for the nature of the injuries, the dental professionals may seek assistance through consultation with the family's physician or with special agencies set up to deal with these problems.

Information regarding procedures for reporting suspected child abuse usually can be obtained from state or local welfare or health departments. Laws in most states require dental professionals to report suspected cases of child abuse or neglect to the appropriate state agency for investigation. Failure to do so can result in a fine, imprisonment, or both. In addition, all states and the District of Columbia protect dental professionals and others from civil and criminal lawsuits when the reports of child abuse or neglect are made in good faith (Schwartz et al, 1977).

SELF-EXAMINATION FOR ORAL CANCER
Oral cancer self-examination: teaching approach

The first time the patient performs the examination, the clinician can guide the patient through the steps of the examination and confirm the patient's findings. Ideally, the patient should sit in front of a large mirror, and the clinician should stand behind the patient or sit at the patient's side; from either of these positions, both the patient and the clinician can see into the patient's mouth. At the beginning of the examination, it may be helpful to remind the patient that he or she is examining the face, neck, and mouth to become familiar with the normal forms and structures so that any changes can be noticed during subsequent examinations. Also, the clinician will be helping the patient identify the normal structures within the mouth. The patient should follow the outline or pamphlet that he or she will be using at home and should perform as much of the examination on his or her own as possible. This is a difficult balance to strike, because the clinician is playing the dual role of teaching the procedure and fostering some independence in the patient. Ultimately, at the end of the session, the patient will have learned the examination and be confident enough to perform the examination at home at regular intervals. In addition, the clinician has the challenging task of motivating the patient to want to perform the examination at regular intervals. The approaches for motivating a patient to perform the oral cancer self-examination are the same as the approaches for motivating a patient to perform home care procedures. In this situation, however, the potential benefits to the patient are even greater—his or her life.

The oral cancer self-examination is composed of several steps in which the face, neck, and mouth are examined (Atterbury, 1979; Burzynski, Moore, and DeJean, 1970; Carl et al., 1982; Engelman and Schackner, 1966; Glass, Alba, and Wheatley, 1975; Olszewski, 1976). A pamphlet such as *Early Detection of Oral Cancer May Save Your Life,* published by the American Cancer Society (Eastern Great Lakes, 1976), can be given to the patient. Many dental and dental auxiliary schools also have pamphlets outlining the steps of the oral cancer self-examination that can be used by the patient.

While the patient is learning to perform the examination, the clinician should point out the normal structures in each area and review with the patient the kinds of changes that should be noted.

At the completion of the examination, it should be emphasized to the patient that the earlier any changes are brought to the attention of the dentist the better. Any change or lesion that is present for 2 weeks should be checked by the dentist; waiting even until the next 6-month checkup may be too risky. It may be helpful to reassure the patient that the dentist would prefer to be asked to check a thousand changes in the patient's mouth that turn out to be normal rather than not being asked to check the one change that may lead to cancer.

The following outline for the lay person describes one way a dental hygienist can teach oral cancer self-examination (Eastern Great Lakes, 1976; Glass, Alba and Wheatley, 1975).

Oral cancer self-examination: outline for the lay person

This outline is to be used as a guide when you perform the oral cancer self-examination. The outline lists each of the areas to be examined and the kinds of changes that may be significant and should be brought to the dentist's attention. In general, you are looking for any of the following changes:

1. Any sores on the face, neck, or mouth that do not heal within 2 weeks
2. Any white, red, or dark patches in the mouth
3. Any swelling, lump, bump, or growth
4. Repeated bleeding for no apparent reason
5. Pain or loss of feeling in any area of the face, neck, or mouth

A mirror and good lighting are needed for the examination. Following are the steps of the oral cancer self-examination.

1. *Facial symmetry.* Look at yourself in the mirror. Both sides of your face and neck should be the same size, shape, and form. No person's face is absolutely symmetrical, but the two sides are basically the same. Any swell-

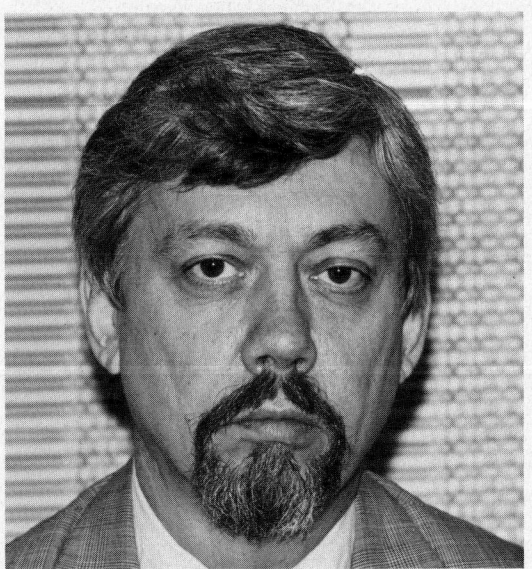

Fig. 10-33. Examining facial symmetry visually.

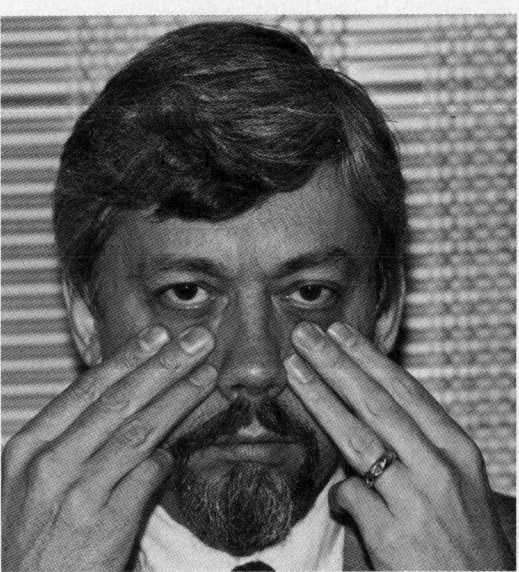

Fig. 10-34. Palpating face with both hands.

ings, lumps, bumps, or growths that appear on one side of your face should be noted; if they appear on both sides of your face, they are probably normal (Fig. 10-33).

2. *Face*. Look at the skin on your face and neck. You are looking for any changes in skin color, moles that have changed, lumps, or sores. If you wear glasses, take them off and examine the areas covered by them—the bridge of the nose. Finally palpate your face by gently pressing fingers from each hand against all areas of your face. By palpating both sides of your face at the same time, you will notice any differences between one side of your face and the other (Fig. 10-34).

3. *Side of neck*. With fingers of both hands, palpate both sides of your neck at the same time. As with your face, you are feeling for any lumps, bumps, or swellings that appear on one side of your neck but not on the other (Fig. 10-35).

4. *Center of neck*. Gently place your fingers against your "Adam's apple" and swallow; it should move when you swallow. Then grasp your Adam's apple and gently move it from side to side (Fig. 10-36). Once again check for any lumps or bumps, and note any hoarseness that does not clear up within 2 weeks.

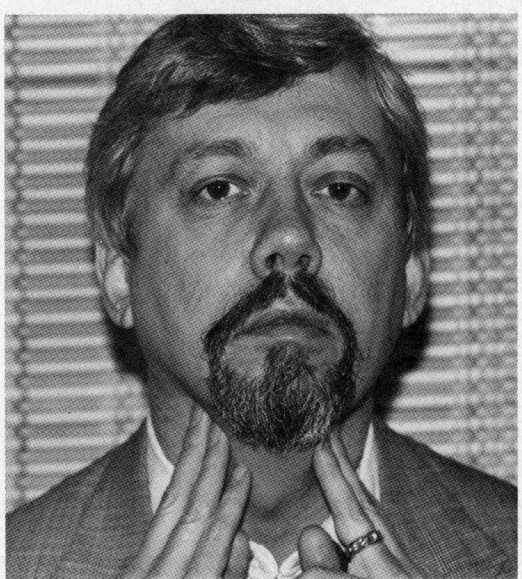

Fig. 10-35. Palpating neck with both hands.

Any dentures or partial dentures should be removed at this point.

5. *Lips*. Pull your lower lip down and look for any sores or color changes. Gently squeeze your lip with your fingers to feel for any

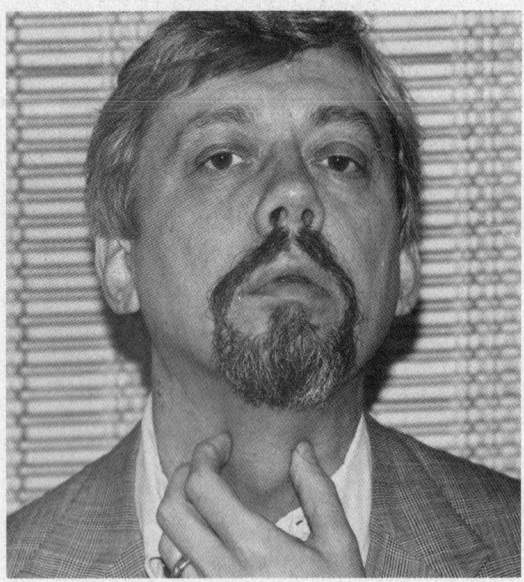

Fig. 10-36. Palpating center of neck ("Adam's apple").

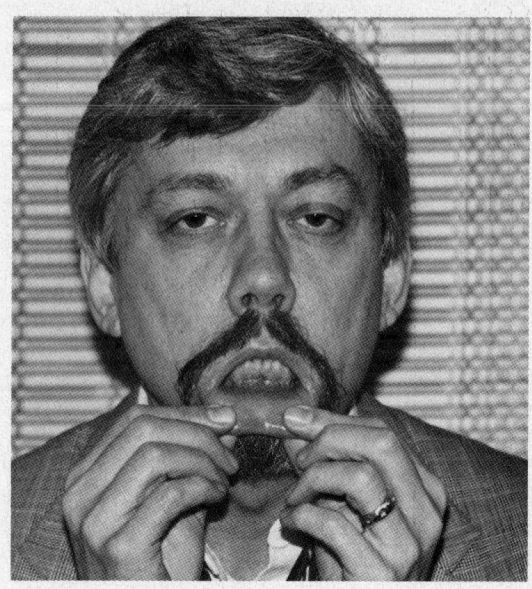

Fig. 10-37. Examining inner surface of lips.

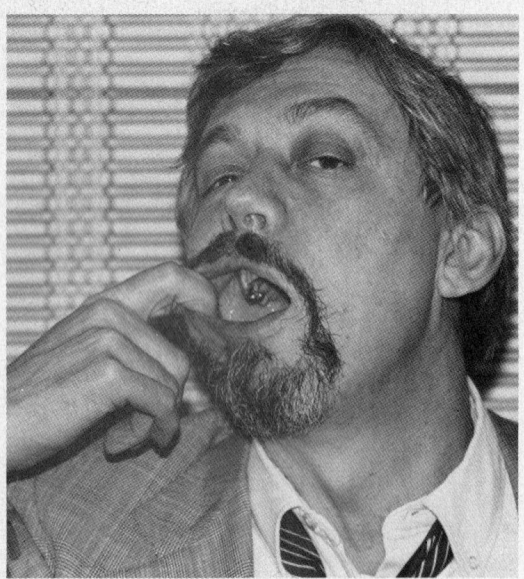

Fig. 10-38. Examining inner surface of cheek.

swellings, lumps, bumps, or tenderness. Repeat this procedure for your upper lip (Fig. 10-37).

6. *Cheek.* Pull back your cheek with your fingers so you can see the tissue inside your cheek. Look for any color changes—red, white, or dark areas. Place your thumb on the outside of your cheek and your index finger inside your cheek, and gently squeeze your cheek. Note any swellings, lumps, or bumps. Repeat this procedure for your other cheek (Fig. 10-38).

7. *Roof of mouth.* Tilt your head back and look at the roof of your mouth. Note any color changes—white, red, or dark areas—or any lumps. With your index finger gently press against the roof of your mouth to feel any lumps, bumps, or swellings (Fig. 10-39).

8. *Gums.* Look at your gums for any color changes—red, white or dark areas—lumps, bumps, or growths. Are there any sores that have not healed for longer than 14 days? Any areas that bleed without cause (Fig. 10-40)?

9. *Tongue and floor of mouth.* Place the tip of your tongue to the roof of your mouth. Look at the underside of your tongue and the floor of your mouth for any color changes, lumps, bumps, or growths. Palpate the floor of your mouth by gently pressing your finger against the floor area to feel any lumps, bumps, or growths. Extend your tongue and look at the

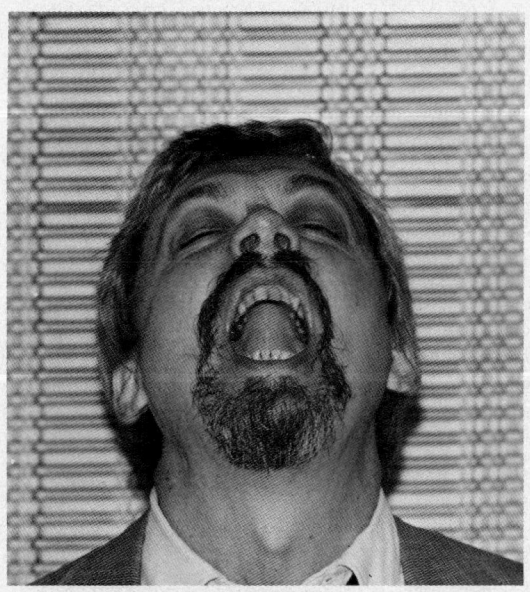

Fig. 10-39. Examining roof of mouth.

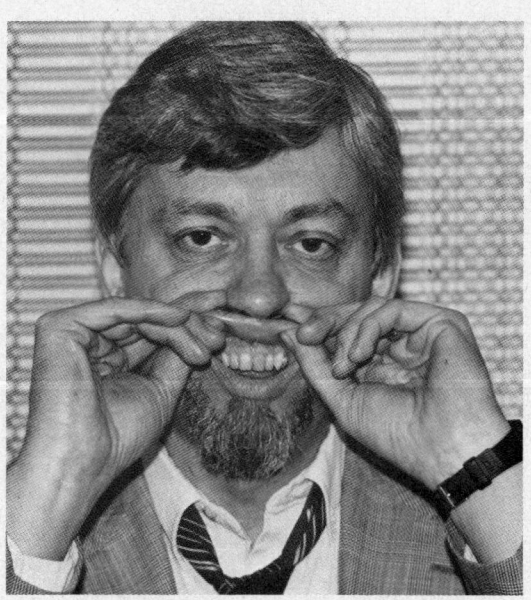

Fig. 10-40. Lifting lip to examine gums.

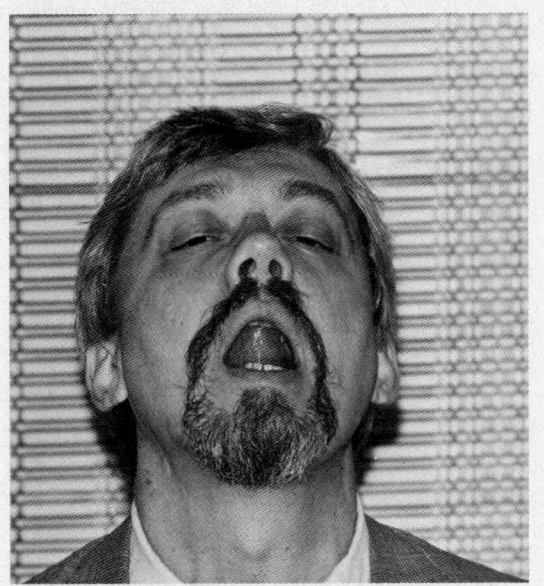

Fig. 10-41. Raising tongue to examine its undersurface and floor of mouth.

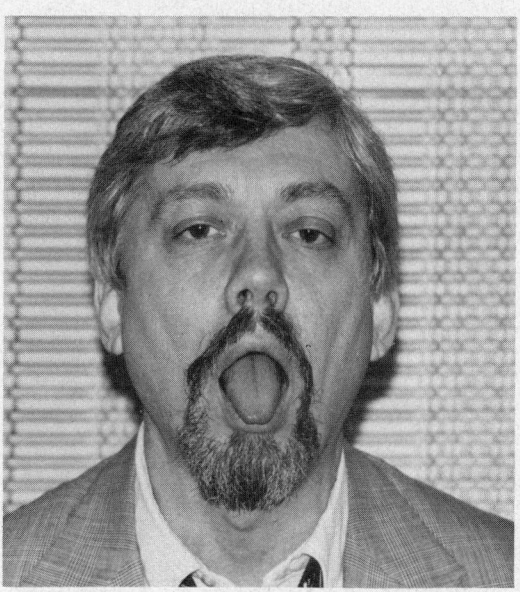

Fig. 10-42. Examining upper surface of tongue.

top side of your tongue. Using a gauze square, grasp the tip of your tongue and gently pull your tongue to one side. Look at the side of your tongue and palpate your tongue. Note any color changes, lumps, bumps, or sores that have not healed. Repeat this procedure on the other side of your tongue (Figs. 10-41 to 10-44).

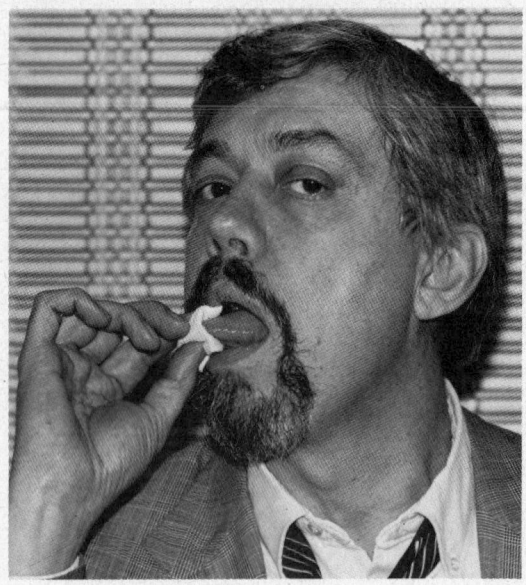

Fig. 10-43. Grasping tip of tongue with gauze and examining side of tongue.

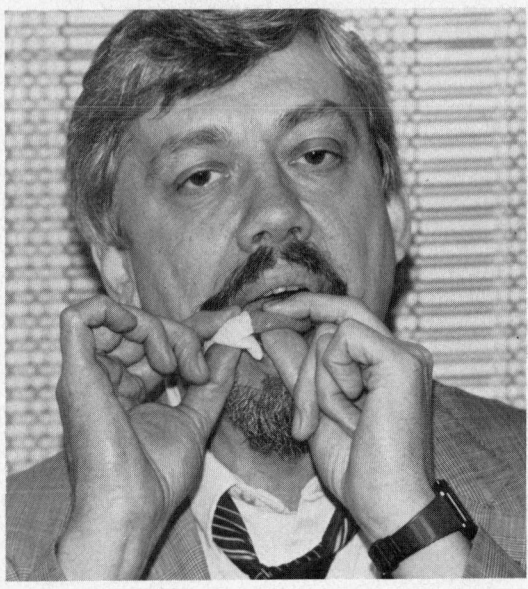

Fig. 10-44. Palpating tongue.

Summary

At the completion of the examination, the clinician can ask if there are any questions about the procedure. This is also a good time to ask patients if they have any concerns or hesitations about performing the examination. The clinician should be sensitive to patients' responses; some patients may express their concerns about actually finding oral cancer. Perhaps the patients' fears can be acknowledged and discussed as is appropriate. The patients should be encouraged to perform the examination routinely and to call the office as needed.

Conclusion

Teaching the guided self-assessment and oral cancer self-examination are important preventive adjuncts in dental hygiene treatment. The procedures and findings of the examination will need to be reviewed with patients at subsequent visits to ensure proper completion of the examinations. These examinations benefit both the patients and the dental health professional. The patients become knowledgeable about their oral conditions and able to detect oral cancer in its early stages.

The professional is able to work with patients who are truly partners in care.

ACTIVITIES

1. Obtain a presentation designed to teach the concepts of blood pressure screening and hypertension, such as *Hypertension . . . The Silent Killer:* "Screening" (14:41) B-1460 and "Practice in Blood Pressure Reading" (13:40) B-1315.*
2. Practice the procedures for determining each of the four vital signs on a lab partner or clinic patient.
3. Practice the procedures for intraoral and extraoral examination on a lab partner or clinic patient. To sharpen tactile perceptions during the palpation of hard and soft tissues, work in pairs and practice palpating individual structures on a lab partner with your eyes closed. Concentrate on the different anatomic structures and textures that you feel and describe these to your partner.
4. Arrange for a guest speaker from the oncologic department of a nearby hospital to speak on the inci-

*Written by Jane Anderson, G.D.H., B.S., and Nancy Champlin Geistfeld, G.D.H., B.S. Produced by Health Sciences Learning Resources, Dental Audio-Visual, Biomedical Graphic Communications, University of Minnesota, Minneapolis.

dence of oral cancer in your area; check with the local American Cancer Society to get the latest pamphlets, statistics, and public information on oral cancer.

5. Have a group discussion about students' feelings regarding touching another person's body as in the head and neck examination. Some students react at first with embarrassment at having to perform this procedure on strangers. Discuss ways in which these feelings might be dealt with. Role-play explaining the purpose and use of the oral examination to a patient. Include in the role-play a situation in which a suspicious lesion that might be cancerous is detected. What would be said to the patient in that situation? When discussing the role-play, ask the "patient" what feelings or reactions he or she had to a thorough examination.

6. Contact the state or local child welfare department to find out the exact procedures required for reporting child neglect or abuse in your state.

7. Show slides of a variety of intraoral and extraoral lesions and have students write a clinical description of each lesion.

REVIEW QUESTIONS

1. Give five reasons for performing a complete general and oral examination.
2. List the four vital signs.
3. State the normal range for each of the following:
   a. Adult pulse
   b. Adult respiration rate
   c. Adult temperature
   d. Adult blood pressure
   e. Borderline temperature for fever
   f. Borderline blood pressure for hypertension
4. Describe the procedure for obtaining the following from a patient:
   a. Pulse rate
   b. Blood pressure
5. State the four methods of examination described in the text and give an example of how each method is used.
6. Describe the palpation technique recommended for the following structures:
   a. Submandibular lymph nodes
   b. Floor of the mouth
   c. Buccal mucosa
7. Why is the initial inspection of the mouth necessary before the clinician's hands enter the mouth?
8. What chain of lymph nodes is located near each of the following structures?
   a. Ear
   b. Sternocleidomastoid muscle
   c. Base of the skull
   d. Floor of the mouth

REFERENCES

Abbey LM, et al: A resurvey of hypertensive patients detected in a dental office screening program, J Public Health Dent 36:244, 1976.

Abbey LM, et al: Hypertension screening among dental patients, JADA 93:996, 1976.

American Cancer Society: Cancer Statistics 1987. CA 37:13, 1987.

American Dental Association Council on Dental Health and Health Planning and Bureau of Health Education and Audiovisual Services: Breaking the silence on hypertension: a dental perspective, JADA 110:781, 1985.

Atterbury RA: Self-examination of paraoral tissues for detection of early oral cancer, Dent Surv 55:18, 1979.

Baden E: Prevention of cancer of the oral cavity and pharynx, CA 37:49, 1987.

Barkmeier WW, et al: Anorexia nervosa: recognition and management, J Oral Med 37:134, 1982.

Becker DB, et al: Child abuse and dentistry: orofacial trauma and its recognition by dentists, JADA 97:24, 1978.

Burzynski NJ, Moore C, and DeJean E: Basic steps in mouth-throat examination for cancer detection, J Am Dent Assoc 81:932, 1970.

Carl W et al: Early detection of oral cancer: another aspect of preventive dentistry, Quintessence Int 13:1179, 1982.

Conway BJ: High blood pressure screening and referral by dentists; legal implications of blood pressure measurement in the dental practice, R I Dent J 13:16, Dec 1980.

Cutler LS: Evaluation and management of the dental patient with cardiovascular disease II: hypertension, J Conn Dent Assoc 60(4):230, 1986.

Davis GR et al: The dentist's role in child abuse and neglect, J Dent Child 46:185, 1979.

Eastern Great Lakes Head and Neck Cancer Control Network and Department of Oral Medicine: Early detection of oral cancer may save your life. New York, 1976, American Cancer Society.

Engelman MA and Schackner JS: Oral cancer examination procedure. Poughkeepsie, N.Y., 1966, St. Francis Hospital.

Friedman RJ, et al: Early detection of malignant melanoma: the role of physician examination and self-examination of the skin, CA 35:130, 1985.

Gaynor AM: Commonly used drugs in dentistry and the hypertensive patient, W Va Dent J 57(1):18, 1983.

Glass RT, et al: Teaching self-examination of the head and neck: another aspect of preventive dentistry, JADA 90:1265, 1975.

Glass RT, Abla M, and Wheatley J: Teaching self-examination of the head and neck: another aspect of preventive dentistry, J Am Dent Assoc 90:1265, 1975.

Joint National Committee on Detection, Evaluation and Treatment of High Blood Pressure: 1984 Report. Washington, DC, June 1984, US Department of Health and Human Services, Public Health Service, National Institutes of Health, pub. No. 84-1088.

Kerr DA, Ash MM, and Millard HD: Oral diagnosis, ed 6, St Louis, 1983, The CV Mosby Co.

Kittle PE, et al: Two child abuse/child neglect examinations for the dentist, J Dent Child 48:175, 1981.

Klimaszewski DL, and Grim CM: Blood pressure measurement: standardization and certification program manual, Indianapolis, 1985, Indiana University Hospitals.

Kutcher MJ, et al: Oral medicine in general dental practice I: Physical evaluation of the dental patient, Compend Contin uc Dent 2:79, 1981.

Malamed SF: Blood pressure evaluation and the prevention of medical emergencies in dental practice, J Prev Dent 6:183, 1980.

Malasanos L, et al: Health assessment, ed 3, St Louis, 1986, The CV Mosby Co.

McCann AL, and Wesley RK: A method for describing soft tissue lesions of the oral cavity, Dent Hyg 62:219, 1987.

Olsqewski V: The role of the dental hygienist in oral cancer detection, Dent Hyg 50:169, 1976.

Rawson RD: Child abuse identification, CDA J 14:21, 1986.

Rollins N and Piazza E: Diagnosis of anorexia nervosa: a critical reappraisal, J Am Acad Child Psychiatry, 17:126, 1978.

Roberts MW, and Li H: Oral findings in anorexia nervosa and bulimia nervosa: a study of 47 cases, JADA 115:407, 1987.

Schwartz S, et al: Oral manifestations and legal aspects of child abuse, JADA 95:586, 1977.

Shapiro S, and Avery K: An office protocol for treating patients with hypertensive disease, Ark Dent J 55(4):15, 1984.

Silverberg DS: The dentist's role in hypertension detection, J Can Dent Assoc 42:549, 1976.

Singer J, et al: Blood pressure fluctuations during dental hygiene treatment, Dent Hyg 57:24, Aug 1983.

Sopher I: The dentist and the battered child syndrome, Dent Clin North Am 21:113, 1977.

Stanley RT: Child abuse—what's a dentist to do? Ohio Dent J: 16, 1981.

Stimson PG: Battered child syndrome, Tex Dent J 101(9):10, 1984.

Winters R: Child absue digest. Tampa, Fla., 1985, Winters Communications.

11 COMPREHENSIVE CARIES, RESTORATIVE, TOOTH CHARACTERISTIC, AND RADIOGRAPHIC CHARTING

OBJECTIVES: *The reader will be able to*

1. Identify the basic purposes of preparing dental chartings.
2. Describe the advantages and disadvantages of anatomic, geometric, and numerically coded charting forms.
3. Given examples of tooth numbering systems, including universal, international, and Palmer's notation, identify which tooth is being referred to and specify from which system the notation is derived.
4. Given a variety of carious lesions or restorations, identify the proper classification number using G. V. Black's classification system.
5. Complete comprehensive chartings for a variety of patients, including identifying and recording the following from clinical and radiographic findings:
   a. Sound teeth
   b. Missing or unerupted teeth
   c. Removable prostheses
   d. Restorations (including all classifications of single-tooth restorations, crowns, bridgework, sealants, and endodontic treatment)
   e. Caries
   f. Decalcification and hypocalcification
   g. Developmental anomalies
   h. Attrition, abrasion, erosion
   i. Malposed teeth
   j. Periapical pathology
   k. Calculus
   l. Changes in supporting bone
6. Read aloud recorded notations concisely and accurately, using proper dental terminology for verification by a second clinician.

A comprehensive dental charting provides an accurate description of the patient's dental status. It is a valuable tool in the assessment phase of care, because it provides, in most instances, a graphic representation of the active or repaired disease process and the unique clinical problems related to the patient's teeth. As a combined record of clinical and radiographic findings, it is a comprehensive diagnostic tool. Dental chartings are valuable legal records, as they show the dental conditions of the patient at the beginning of care and a pictorial review of how those conditions changed over a period of months and years.

Depending on the format and manner in which a patient's treatment is documented, the dental charting can depict the maintenance of health or the progression of disease.

It also provides a useful check against financial records. Entries in financial records indicating the placement of specific restorations should be re-

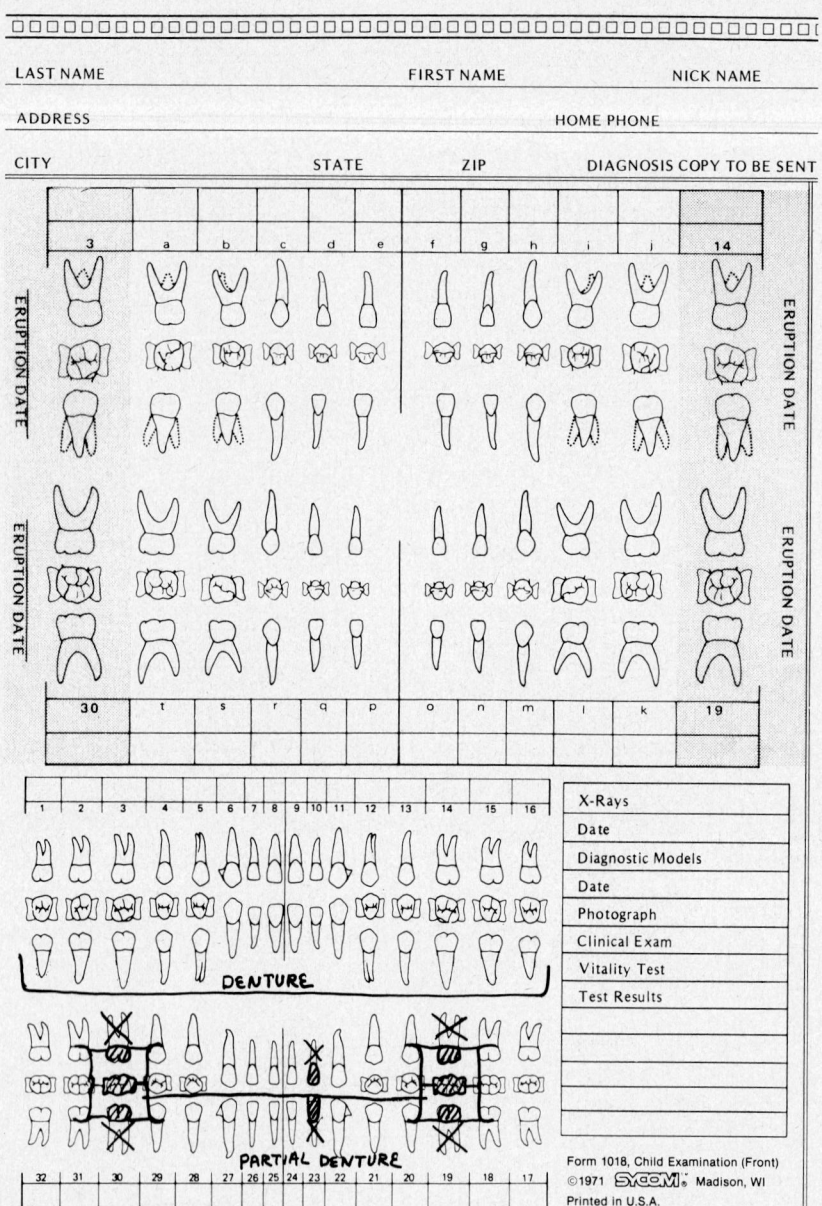

Fig. 11-1. Anatomic charting form that accommodates chartings of adult, primary, and mixed dentitions. A complete maxillary denture and mandibular partial denture are charted to illustrate one method of symbol use. (Courtesy Sycom, Madison, Wis.)

flected in the updated charting of the patient's teeth.

Because the comprehensive charting is most often used in establishing a basis of entering needs for purposes of treatment planning, the most comprehensive charting procedures occur at the initial patient visit. The initial data should be updated as treatment progresses and at subsequent recall visits when the patient returns for periodic diagnosis of new needs.

CHARTING FORMS

Fig. 11-1 is an example of an anatomic charting form. The anatomy of the crown and root(s) of each tooth is shown with facial, occlusal, and lingual views. Anatomic charting provides the most realistic graphic description, as the anatomic features of each tooth can be used to denote specifically the presence of lesions and restorations. This particular form allows for charting both permanent and primary teeth.

Fig. 11-2 provides an example of a geometric charting, with stylized "anatomy." The tooth surfaces are divided by lines to indicate marginal ridges and line angles so that the extent of disease or a restoration can be shown without attempting to replicate the exact design. As precise anatomy is not required, it is usually a neater, more easily read charting.

To follow the patient's progress, a comprehensive charting must be completely redone at each visit, or changes at each 6-month visit will become lost in the original charting. The original generally becomes increasingly cluttered and unreadable if there are many clinical changes. One way to preserve the original charting, to show progress at each assessment visit, and to avoid the time-consuming and tedious process of recharting the entire dentition is to photocopy the original charting. Findings at the second visit can be marked in colored pencil or pen on the photocopy to highlight recent changes. At the beginning of a third course of treatment in which a charting is indicated, the charting from the second course is photocopied with the new photocopy updated in color. This procedure results in a highly specific time line of conditions and care. It also results in many additional pages in the patient record. Eventually, microfilm or microfiche will be necessary to permit long-term storage.

The numeric coding system requires less paper for showing progress through time. Because number codes rather than drawings are used to indicate conditions of the teeth, the pictorial quality of anatomic and geometric chartings is lost. Fig. 11-3 shows a numeric code charting. As conditions change, markings are made in the next line above (for the maxillary teeth) or below (for the mandibular teeth). The lines are dated so that changes are identified along a time line.

TYPES OF CHARTINGS

The vast majority of chartings focus on the presence of caries, restorations, and missing teeth. Depending on treatment protocols in a given practice setting, the routine charting may be limited to these three conditions or may be expanded to include malposed teeth, attrition, erosion, abrasion, developmental anomalies, and other findings.

In addition to chartings of the clinical and radiographic conditions of the teeth, protocols may call for charting calculus deposits, periodontal conditions, plaque and hemorrhage points, and occlusal assessment. This section focuses on charting clinical and radiographic findings of the teeth. Charting the other conditions is explained in subsequent chapters.

TOOTH NUMBERING SYSTEMS

Regardless of the selection of anatomic, geometric, or numerically coded chartings; it is essential to adopt a consistent method of denoting each of the teeth. The *universal* system numbers each of the permanent teeth from *1* to *32* and the primary teeth from *a* to *t,* beginning with the last molar on the maxillary right quadrant and progressing sequentially around the arch to the last molar (Project ACORDE, 1974). The next tooth counted (or lettered) is the last molar on the mandibular left quadrant, progressing sequentially around the mandible to the last molar on the mandibular right. The "last molar" for permanent dentition (1 to 32) is the third molar; for children (a to t) it is the second primary molar. This system is widely accepted in the United States and is frequently used in denoting teeth. (See Figs. 11-1 and 11-2 for the numbering of each tooth.)

An older system, *Palmer's notation,* numbers or letters each of the teeth in the quadrant from *1* to *8* for permanent dentition and from *a* to *e* for primary teeth. Therefore a permanent central is always No. 1. A permanent cuspid in any quadrant is labeled No. 3. The quadrant position of the tooth under consideration is identified by using the appropriate quadrant of a graph created by two intersecting perpendicular axes. Using the quadrant denotation, the second permanent premolar in the maxillary left quadrant would be

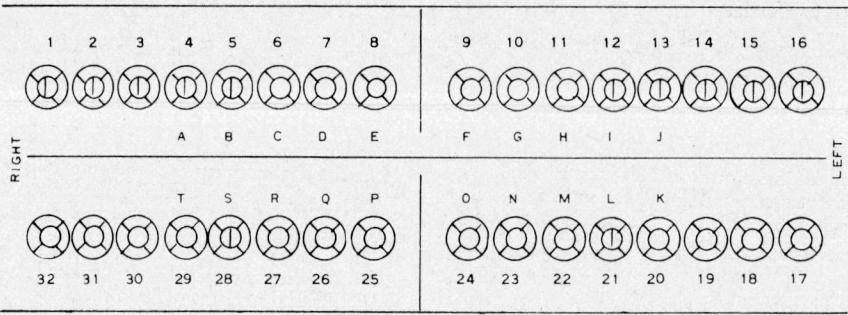

Fig. 11-2. Geometric charting form with stylized teeth. This form accommodates charting adult, primary, and mixed dentition.

written ⌊5 . The second primary molar on the mandibular right would be written e̅⌋.

The *international system* is similar to Palmer's notation, since each tooth in the quadrant is numbered *1* to *8* from central to third molar. However, the quadrant location is designated by a prefix number *1, 2, 3,* or *4* for the maxillary right, maxillary left, mandibular left, and mandibular right, respectively. The quadrant prefix is followed by the tooth number (Project ACORDE, 1974). Thus the second permanent premolar in the maxillary left quadrant shown as an example in the previous paragraph would be written 25. For distinguishing primary and permanent teeth, primary quadrants are numbered *5, 6, 7,* or *8,* respectively, with numbers (not letters) used for primary teeth. Therefore the second primary molar on the mandibular right, shown as an example in the previous paragraph, would be written 85.

Table 11-1 summarizes the differences among the three numbering systems. In practice it is important to determine what system has been adopted to enable all co-workers to identify the tooth under discussion. Because the universal system is still the most widely understood and used, the detailed procedures for preparing a charting are described with *1* to *32* and *a* to *t* tooth designations. To ensure an accurate, complete charting, a sequence moving from the maxillary right third molar to the mandibular right molar (1 to 32) will be followed.

PROCEDURE FOR CHARTING

To prevent confusion and error, the first condition that should be charted is *missing teeth*. The teeth may have been extracted or may not yet have erupted. It is also possible that the tooth buds for the teeth were missing congenitally. In most instances it is not possible, with clinical data alone, to determine why the tooth is not present. A radiographic series can add data; a patient's dental history also provides information to help determine the cause of missing teeth.

Missing teeth should be crossed out with a single vertical line or an X. Some practitioners prefer for box or color in missing teeth.

Fig. 11-4 shows three ways in which No. 32 can be marked as missing. A partially erupted tooth can be marked so that it is obvious which portion of the tooth is exposed clinically. (See tooth No. 16 in Fig. 11-5.) Marking *all missing teeth first* is especially important when charting mixed dentition.

Once all missing teeth are marked, removable prostheses, such as partial dentures, complete dentures, and removable bridges should be marked with brackets. Fig. 11-1 (on the adult dentition) shows a maxillary denture and a mandibular partial denture replacing Nos. 23, 30, and 19. The clasps are shown on Nos. 31, 29, 18, and 20.

After marking all missing teeth and removable prostheses, the clinician should return to the first chartable tooth in the maxillary right quadrant. The tooth number should be identified, and the tooth should de examined for existing restorations.

Marking restorations

The basic shape of the restoration should be drawn on the appropriate tooth on the charting form. There are a number of ways to further des-

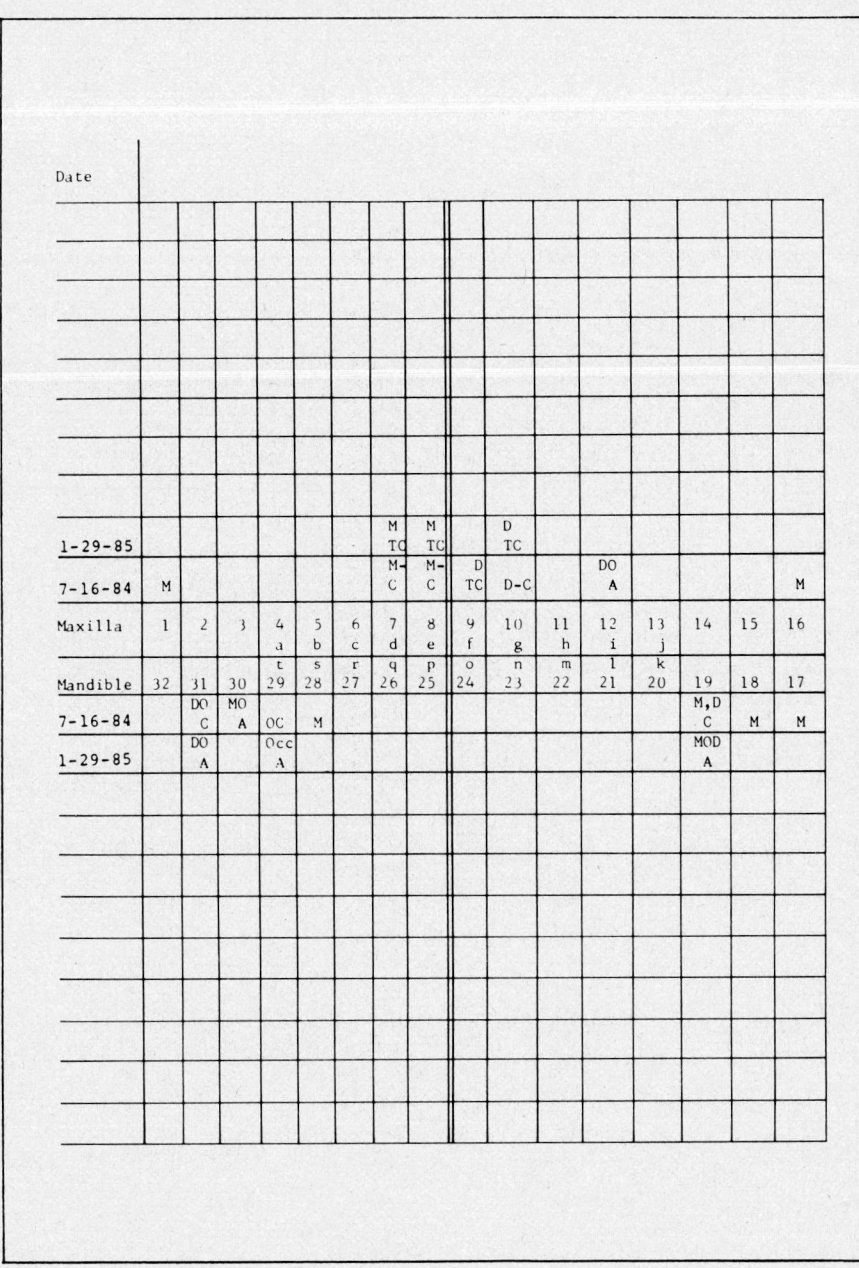

Date																
1-29-85							M TC	M TC		D TC						
7-16-84	M						M- C	M- C	D TC	D-C		DO A				M
Maxilla	1	2	3	4 a	5 b	6 c	7 d	8 e	9 f	10 g	11 h	12 i	13 j	14	15	16
Mandible	32	31	30	t 29	s 28	r 27	q 26	p 25	o 24	n 23	m 22	l 21	k 20	19	18	17
7-16-84		DO C	MO A	OC	M									M,D C	M	M
1-29-85		DO A		Occ A										MOD A		

Fig. 11-3. As each examination is performed, entries of charting symbols are made in the boxes above the maxilla entry and below the mandible entry. As defects are treated, corrections are entered in the next row of boxes above or below the corresponding teeth needing treatment. As no anatomic drawings of caries and restorations are used, charting symbols must be explicit regarding location of specific condition.

Table 11-1. Summary of tooth numbering systems

System	Permanent dentition	Primary dentition
Universal	Each tooth is designated by a number *(1 to 32)*	Each tooth is designated by a letter *(a to t)*
International	Each tooth is designated by a quadrant number prefix *(1 to 4)* and a tooth number suffix *(1 to 8)*	Each tooth is designated by a quadrant number *(5 to 8)* and a tooth number *(1 to 5)*
	$\dfrac{1 \mid 2}{3 \mid 4}$	$\dfrac{5 \mid 6}{8 \mid 7}$
Palmer's notation	Each tooth is numbered *(1 to 8)* and positioned within intersecting axes to designate the quadrant	Each tooth is lettered *(a to e)* and positioned within intersecting axes to designate the quadrant

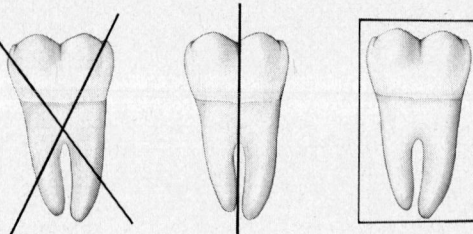

Fig. 11-4. Three symbols to indicate a missing tooth.

ignate that the area defined is an existing restoration—including filling in the area with a designated color or simply leaving the restoration outlined and using a letter code to indicate the material used in the restoration, such as amalgam, resin, gold foil, cast gold, or silicate.

For a precise charting, these letter designations for the type of restorative material may be used even if shading or otherwise filling in the outline is the preferred method. Thus an amalgam restoration may be designated by an anatomic outline of its shape, which is shaded in a color and marked *A* for amalgam. (See tooth No. 2 in Fig. 11-5 for an example.)

To draw and identify single-tooth restorations, a knowledge of G.V. Black's system of classifi-

cation of carious lesions is helpful. Fig. 11-6 provides a summary of the system.

Class I lesions are located in pits and fissures of the occlusal two thirds of posterior teeth or on the lingual surface of anterior teeth.

Class II lesions are located on the proximal surfaces of premolars and molars.

Class III lesions are located on the proximal surfaces of central and lateral incisors and cuspids.

Class IV lesions are located on the proximal surfaces of anterior teeth and involve the incisal edge.

Class V lesions are located at the gingival third of the facial or lingual surfaces of anterior or posterior teeth.

Class VI lesions are located on cusp tips.

The same classification system applies to restorations that replace the tooth structure lost to dental caries.

In identifying restorations for chartings, the classification of restoration (I, II, III, IV, V, VI) is noted, especially where idealized drawings are used. When orally describing the restorations to

---

Fig. 11-5. Composite charting of most commonly used charting symbols with provisions for clinical and radiographic findings.
(Courtesy Sycom, Madison, Wis.)
Key to symbols (numbers refer to teeth):

1—Facially inclined; drifted mesially
2—Occlusal amalgam; drifted mesially
3—Mesioocclusal, gold inlay; caries on distobuccal margin; mesially inclined and drifted mesially
4—Missing
5—Three-quarter gold crown; distally inclined
6—Class III, mesial gold foil
7—Class III, distal tooth-colored restoration
8—Porcelain jacket crown; periapical disease
9—Temporary crown; root canal

10—Peg lateral
11—Lingually inclined; watch for distal caries
12—Distal pit caries
13—Decalcification in gingival third on facial aspect; supernumerary tooth between 13 and 14
14—Decalcification in gingival third on facial aspect
15—Full gold crown
16—Partially erupted
17—Abutment tooth for fixed bridge; full gold crown

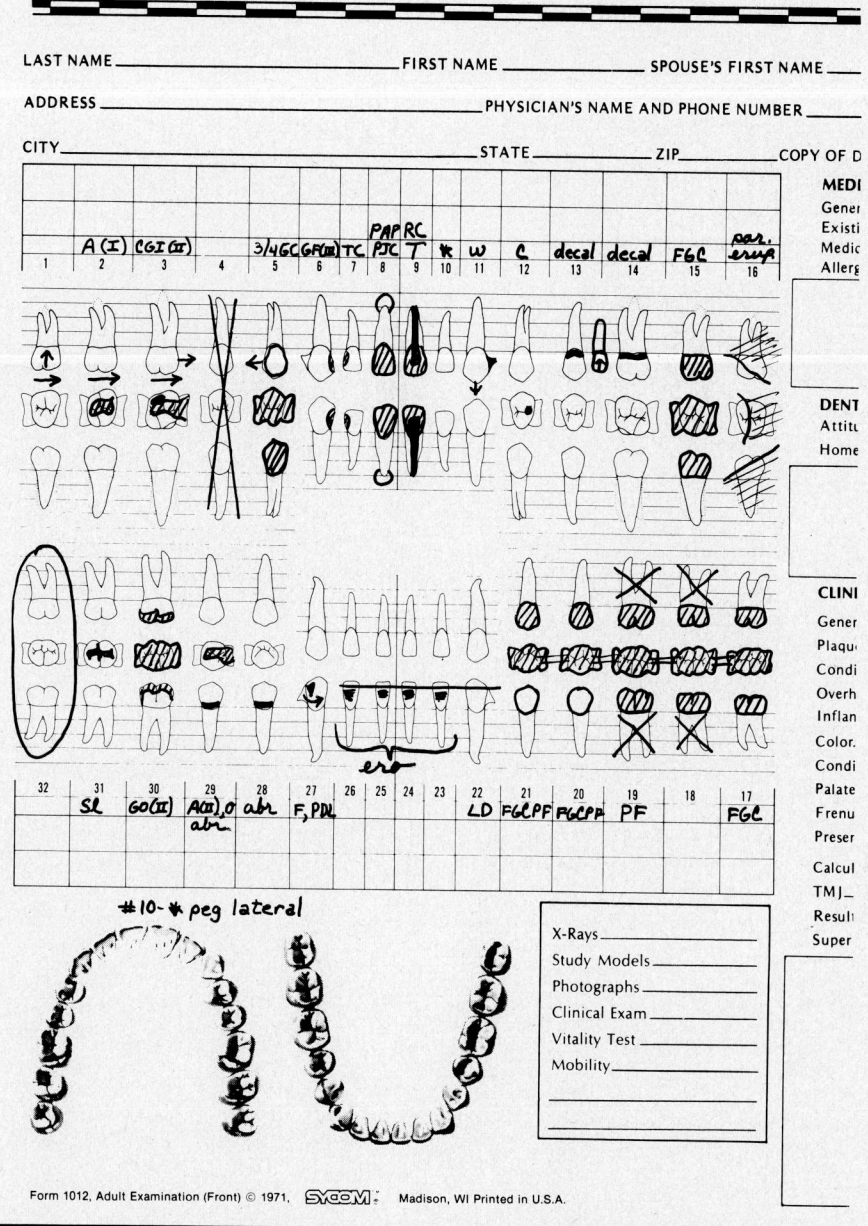

Form 1012, Adult Examination (Front) © 1971, SYCOM. Madison, WI Printed in U.S.A.

18—Pontic
19—Pontic with porcelain facing
20—Full gold crown with porcelain facing
21—Full gold crown with porcelain facing
22—Attrition; loss of continuity of lamina dura
23—Attrition; erosion
24—Attrition; erosion
25—Attrition; erosion
26—Attrition; erosion

27—Facet on distal third of facial surface; distal surface rotated toward facial; widened periodontal ligament (PDL)
28—Abrasion
29—Abrasion; mesioocclusal amalgam; overhang on mesial surface
30—Mesioocclusodistal gold onlay
31—Sealant
32—Unerupted

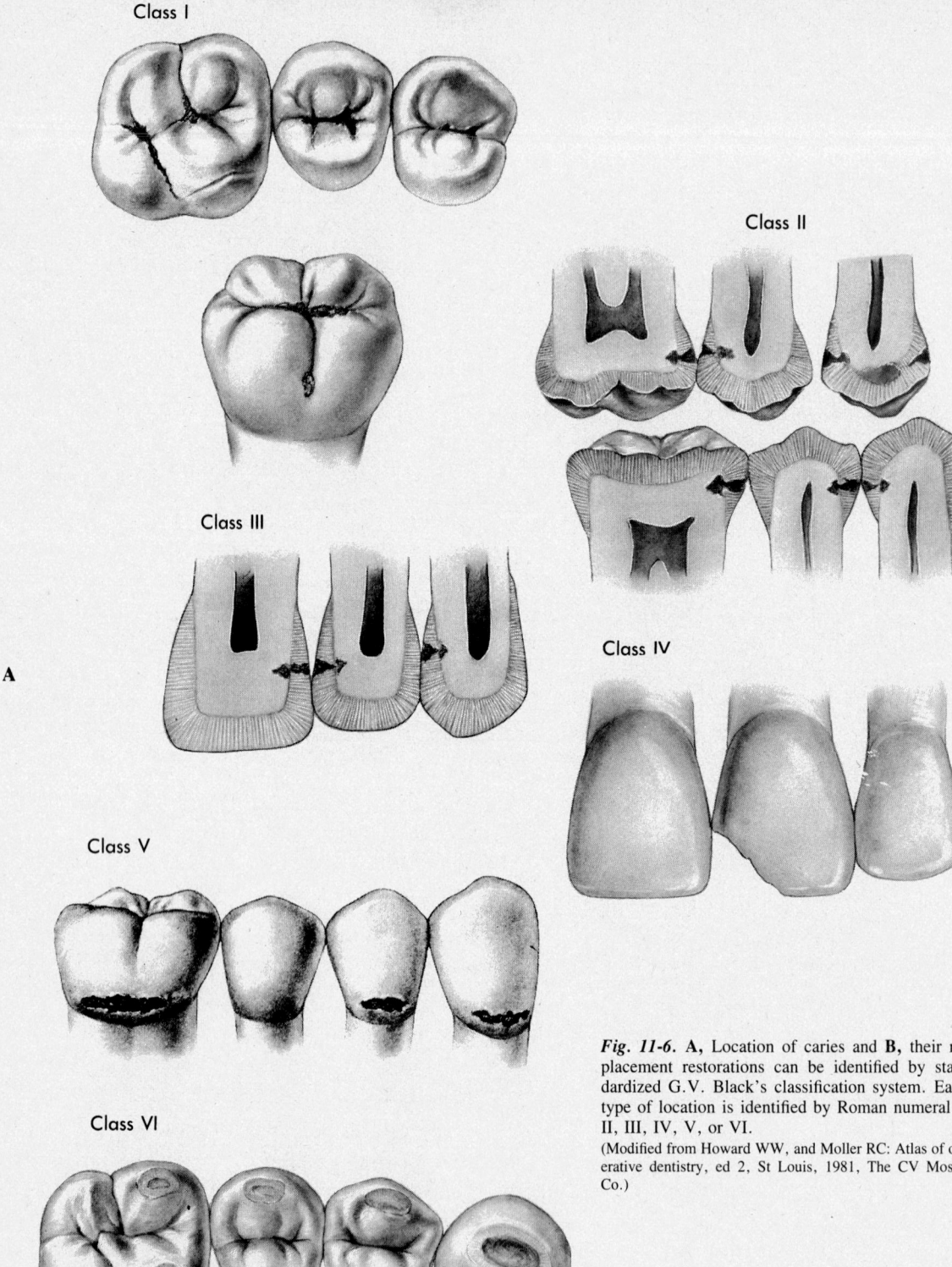

Class I

Class II

Class III

Class IV

Class V

Class VI

Fig. 11-6. **A,** Location of caries and **B,** their replacement restorations can be identified by standardized G.V. Black's classification system. Each type of location is identified by Roman numeral I, II, III, IV, V, or VI.

(Modified from Howard WW, and Moller RC: Atlas of operative dentistry, ed 2, St Louis, 1981, The CV Mosby Co.)

A

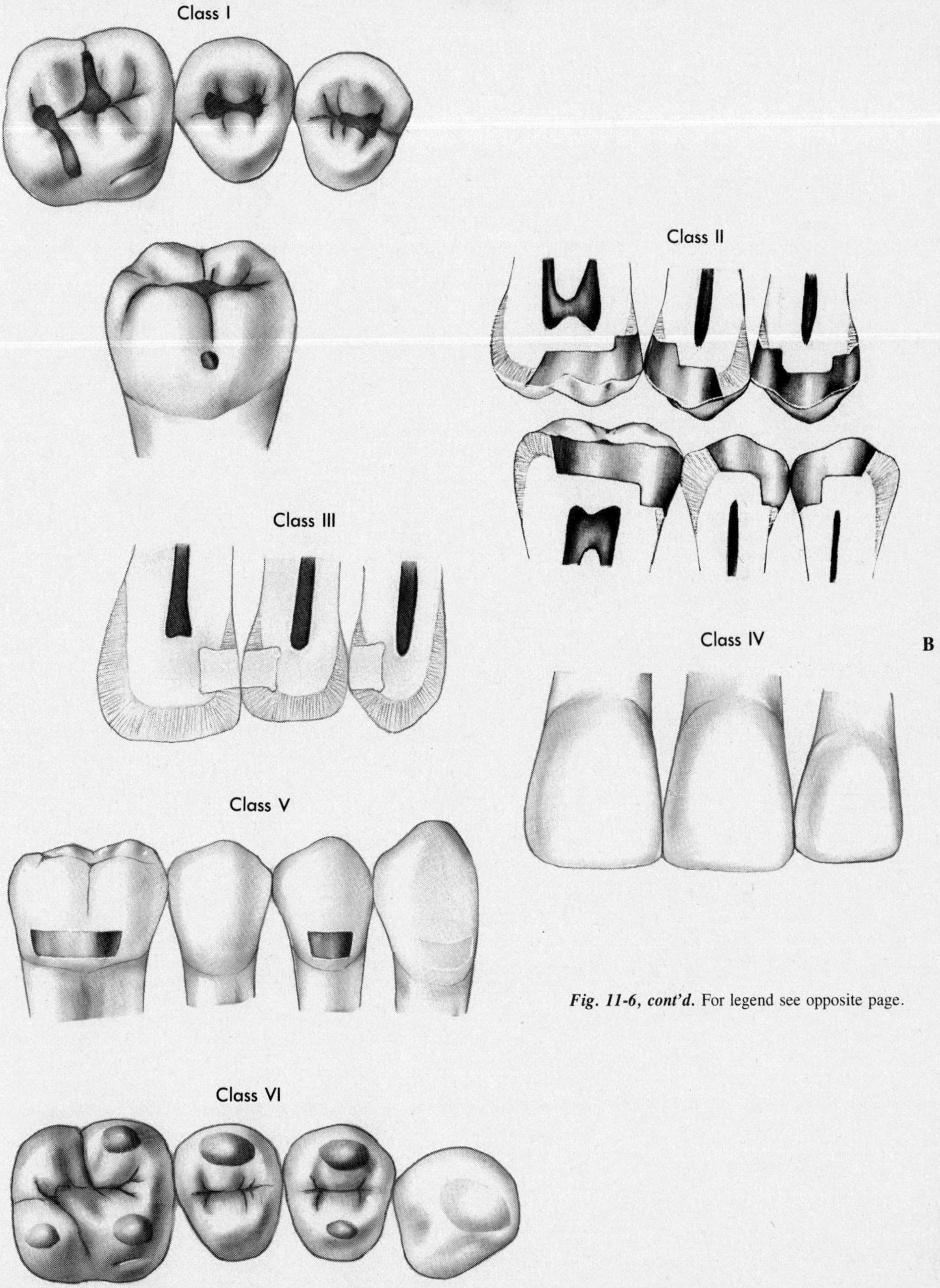

Class I

Class II

Class III

Class IV

B

Class V

Class VI

Fig. 11-6, cont'd. For legend see opposite page.

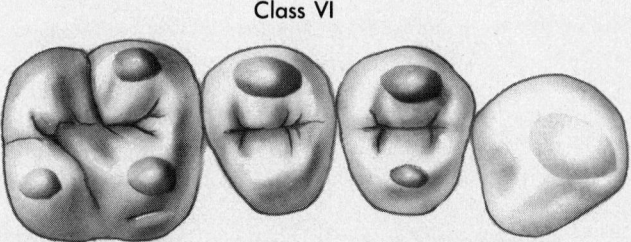

an assistant who is recording the data on the charting, describing the classification of restorations helps the recorder picture the likely shape. As restoration shape and size are dependent largely on the physics of retention and resistance to masticatory stress and strain as well as to the maintenance of esthetics, restorations follow predictable patterns, most of which are shown in the comprehensive charting (Fig. 11-5) and in Fig. 11-6. Therefore the procedure for marking a restoration is to outline its shape according to G.V. Black's classification system, to shade in the outline carefully, and to label it according to the type of restorative material.

Amalgam restorations. Plate 3, *F* through *G*, illustrates a variety of amalgam restorations. They are identifiable by their dark grey (unpolished) or bright silver (polished) appearance. Amalgam is commonly used for Class I, II, and V restorations.

Gold restorations. Gold is easily distinguished from amalgam by the obvious color difference. Gold has no grey cast; it resembles gold jewelry in color and shine. It is designated with a *G*. (Compare the restorations in Plate 3, *E* and *F*.)

The most frequently seen gold restoration is cast gold. A wax pattern of the exact shape and size of the needed restoration is prepared and then replaced by molten gold alloy in a laboratory process of casting similar to the manner in which jewelry is made. The result is a solid piece of gold that fits exactly into the prepared tooth. It is polished in the laboratory and cemented into the tooth as a permanent restoration when the fit is exact.

Such a cast gold restoration feels hard to the touch of the explorer. As with the amalgam restoration, the outline is drawn to match the shape and size of the restoration, and it is shaded and labeled, in this case with a *G*.

A single-tooth cast gold restoration can be either an *inlay (GI)* or an *onlay (GO),* so more detail is necessary to differentiate gold restorations. Tooth No. 3 in Fig. 11-5 has a gold inlay. It lies within the marginal ridges of the occlusal table, except where it crosses the mesial marginal ridge to include the mesial surface. It is a Class II gold inlay. Tooth No. 30 shows a Class II *mesioocclusodistal (MOD)* gold onlay, which includes all

cusp tips and thus covers all the marginal ridges of the tooth. However, the onlay rarely extends below the occlusal third of the facial or lingual surfaces of the tooth. (See Plate 3, *J,* for two gold onlays, a DO inlay, and an MO amalgam.)

The three-quarter crown, in contrast, includes the full occlusal table and extends to the gingiva on the mesial, distal, and lingual aspects of the tooth. The facial marginal ridge is included, along with a small portion of the facial surface, to ensure strength and retention while allowing the natural tooth structure on the facial aspect to preserve esthetics.

The three-quarter gold crown is designated with an outline, shading, and the label *3/4 GC,* as is shown for tooth No. 5 in Fig. 11-5.

The three-quarter gold crown should be differentiated from the full gold crown with a porcelain or acrylic facing. The full gold crown covers and replaces all visible enamel tooth structure and considerable underlying dentin. It is used to restore badly broken-down teeth. Although it is stronger than the three-quarter gold crown, it may result in less than desirable esthetics if the facial aspect is visible when the patient speaks or smiles. Thus when the crown is cast, an area is created on the facial aspect where white porcelain or acrylic may be added to simulate white tooth structure. A full gold crown is outlined, shaded, and labeled *FGC.* (See tooth No. 15 in Fig. 11-5.) A gold crown with a facing is labeled *GCPF* for porcelain and *GCAF* for acrylic.

Another type of single-tooth gold restoration is *gold foil.* This restorative material is quite different from cast gold. It lacks the strengthening alloys that make cast gold hard and able to endure stress and strain. Gold foil is soft and is condensed or packed into the tooth preparation until the void area is completely filled and the anatomy can be carved. The material (1) feels softer to the touch of an explorer than does cast gold, (2) is a lighter or more yellow gold color because of the purity of the material, and (3) is used in Class I, II, III, IV, V, or VI restorations where occlusal wear is minimal. When identified on a tooth, the outline should be drawn, shaded, and labeled *GF.* (See tooth No. 6 in Fig. 11-5.)

Gold is also used for multiple-tooth restorations such as *fixed bridges* (fixed partial dentures) that replace one or more missing teeth or *splints* that join several teeth together with a series of soldered or cast-together gold crowns intended to strengthen the ability of individual teeth to absorb occlusal forces. The teeth absorb the forces collectively by virtue of their joined crowns.

A bridge enables two or more healthy adjacent teeth to support a *pontic* (dummy tooth) so that an open space in the arch can be preserved with a functional tooth replacement. Usually the supporting teeth have full crowns or three-quarter crowns. The crowns to which the pontics are attached are *retainers*. They are seated or anchored on *abutment* teeth. The pontics are made of cast gold also; they can be distinguished from the abutment teeth because they have no roots. They are either cast in one piece with the abutments or soldered to the abutment teeth. In either case, the contacts are sealed together.

The easiest way to locate and chart a bridge is first to identify the location of the missing teeth. The roots of the missing teeth should be charted as absent (by a vertical line, an *x,* or boxing the roots). The crowns replaced by pontics can be outlined and shaded. The abutment teeth are then identified by examining the location of permanently joined contacts. The crown restorations on the abutment teeth are outlined, shaded, and labeled (¾ GC, FGC, GCPF, etc.). Then horizontal lines should be drawn between the attached abutments and pontics to show the size and location of the entire bridge. Fig. 11-5 shows a five-unit bridge (three abutments and two pontics) extending from Nos. 17 to 21. No. 17 has a full gold crown; Nos. 18 and 19 are pontics, with No. 19 having a porcelain facing; and Nos. 20 and 21 are full gold crowns with porcelain facings.

If the pontics are in close contact with the gingiva and cannot easily be differentiated clinically from rooted teeth, reference to a radiographic survey will quickly identify pontics and abutments. Also, threading dental floss underneath one of the closed contacts should enable the clinician to pass the floss under the pontics and to identify the presence or absence of the root structure. Palpating the alveolar process should also help distinguish between edentulous areas where pontics replace the teeth and areas where abutments are present. The shape of the roots of the natural teeth can be felt in the alveolar bone.

Tooth-colored   restorations. Tooth-colored restoration (designated *TC*) is the generic term for silicate, composite, and resin single-tooth restorations that restore the tooth functionally and esthetically. They are used primarily in anterior teeth but may be also found in posterior teeth, depending on the location and size of the area to be restored. If it is possible and desirable to distinguish the material used, the labels *S* for silicate, *R* for resin, and *CR* for composite resin can be used in conjunction with the shaded-in outline of the restoration. Otherwise, the label *TC* is sufficient. (See tooth No. 7 in Fig. 11-5.)

In addition to tooth-colored restorations that restore a portion of a tooth, porcelain and acrylic jacket crowns (designated *PFC* and *AJC*) provide full coverage of teeth, usually where maintenance of esthetics is critical. (See tooth No. 8 in Fig. 11-5; for a radiographic example, see tooth No. 9 in Fig. 11-7; and for a clinical example, see tooth No. 9 in Plate 3, *A, B,* and *D.*)

Temporary restorations. Temporary restorations are usually easily identified as a chalky yellow, white, or pink substance placed in a prepared tooth or by an aluminum preformed or nonanatomic "can" fitted over a posterior tooth prepared for a full crown. Sometimes relatively crude-looking acrylic crowns are used as temporary restorations also, particularly for anterior teeth undergoing crown preparation. The label *T* is used to designate a temporary restoration. It is usually outlined and shaded as a permanent restoration would be (See tooth No. 9 in Fig. 11-5.)

Sealants. Sealants are thin, transparent plastic coatings that are chemically and physically bonded to posterior teeth that have pits and fissures that would be highly susceptible to decay (caries). Therefore sealants are usually found on occlusal surfaces of posterior teeth. They are detected as a shiny narrow clear filling when felt with the tip of an explorer. Sealants can be clear or lightly colored pink or yellow or some other shade that enhances detection. When detected, they should be outlined, shaded, and labeled *Sl.*

Sealants are being used with increasing frequency, both for purposes of preventing caries and for restoration of areas that have beginning caries. The clinician can simply remove the carious portion of the tooth, without having to remove any additional tooth structure, to make a boxlike preparation as is commonly done for the

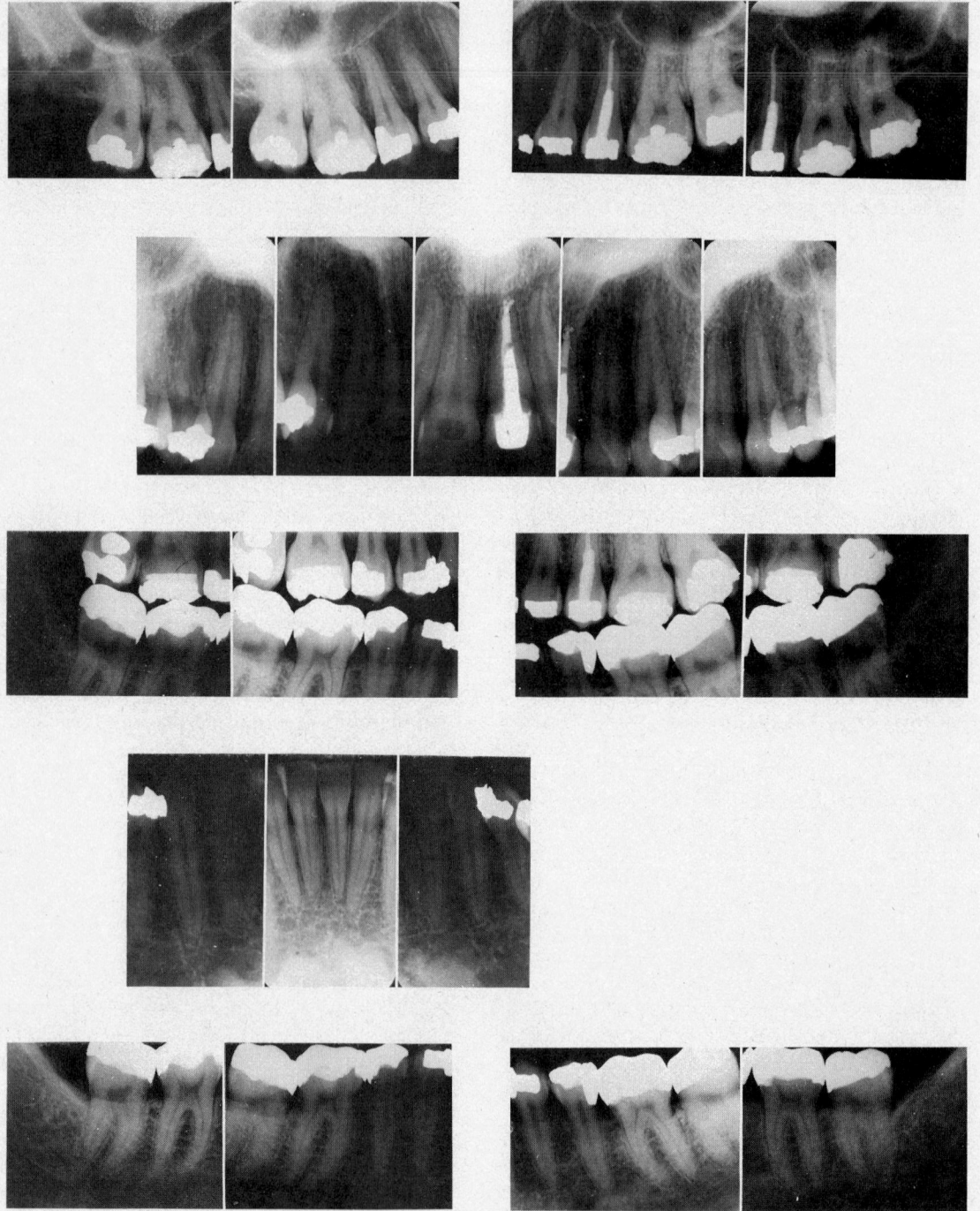

Fig. 11-7. Complete set of radiographs, including 4 bitewing films (teeth occluded, apices not visible) and 16 periapical views.

previously introduced restorations. Research has shown that, if the teeth and type of sealant are carefully selected, these preventive resin restorations (PRR) give excellent results (Simonson, 1980, 1982).

Using the abbreviations described and being anatomically specific about the size and location of restorations and sealants leads to an accurate, detailed charting of the clinical conditions of the teeth.

Charting for other conditions

As each tooth is charted for the presence of restorations, the margins of each restoration should be explored to evaluate for the presence of *recurrent caries* or an open area that may eventually become carious. *Overhanging margins* should be identified (with an *O*), as the overhangs should be removed or the restoration replaced. The prefix of *C* for caries and *D* for defective should be added to the letter label for the restoration. Therefore a carious amalgam would be labeled *C-A*. (See tooth No. 3 in Fig. 11-5 for a carious gold inlay.) A defective composite resin would be labeled *DCR*. When colored pencils are used to differentiate carious areas from existing restorations, the carious margin can be marked simply with the color designated for caries, and the prefix letter is then unnecessary.

Likewise, all the exposed surfaces of the teeth should be felt for soft, *carious areas,* particularly in pits and grooves, at contact points, and on exposed root surfaces. If the sharp explorer tip sticks in a pit (it seems to be retained by the pit or groove) and the area feels soft, then it should be marked for caries with either the designated color or by outlining the area of caries, shading it in, and marking it *C*. Incipient or beginning caries or suspicious pits and grooves can be marked "watch," *W*. (See Nos. 11 and 12 in Fig. 11-5.)

Obvious areas of tooth breakdown, such as large craters, do not require exploration, and exploring them may cause the patient considerable pain.

Closely related to caries are areas of *decalcification*. In these areas there is evidence of demineralization of the tooth structure with an enamel surface that is whiter than the surrounding tooth and that may be chalky and soft. If such an area is likely to become carious or needs to be noted for some other reason, such as esthetics, it can be noted on the chart by shading in the area and labeling it *decal. Hypocalcification,* which rarely is clinically significant and thus is rarely charted, can be labeled *hycal.* (See Plate 1, *D,* for a clinical example.)

A *supernumerary tooth* can be drawn in its general location (See Fig. 11-5 in the maxillary left quadrant.) Other developmental *anomalies* are usually marked with an asterisk near the tooth involved, with a full notation included on the charting page to explain the observed characteristics. (See tooth No. 10 in Fig. 11-5.)

Attrition, the loss of tooth structure due to normal mastication, is often seen on the incisal edges of anterior teeth (Fig. 11-5). This can be noted with a horizontal line drawn across the facial aspect of the drawings of the teeth to illustrate the amount of lost tooth structure. (See the mandibular anterior teeth in Plate 4 for a clinical example.) Closely related to attrition, but far more clinically significant, is the presence of *wear facets*. These highly polished wear areas often show the pattern of wear associated with malocclusion. Wear facets are boxed in to show the plane of wear on each tooth. They are marked with an *F*.

Abrasion is caused by mechanical wear other than that associated with mastication. Vigorous horizontal strokes with a toothbrush cause abrasion, as does improper flossing, opening hairpins with the teeth, and other habits that wear the tooth structure. The area is outlined and shaded and marked *abr*. Colored pencils are useful to distinguish this characteristic from a Class V restoration or other defect. (See Plate 2, *H,* especially the maxillary right quadrant, for a clinical example.)

Erosion, in contrast to attrition and abrasion, is caused by chemical wear of the teeth. Sucking lemons, for instance, can cause generalized erosion of the anterior facial surfaces. Since this feature is more generalized over a broad surface and involves several teeth, the teeth involved can be bracketed and marked *ero*. (See Fig. 11-5 for a graphic description of these characteristics on Nos. 22 to 29.)

Malposed teeth should be charted on a comprehensive dental charting including rotated, extruded, and inclined teeth. Rotated teeth are marked by drawing an arrow on the proximal surface that is rotated toward the facial. The arrow is then arced across the facial view of the tooth to suggest the direction of rotation of the tooth. Fig. 11-5 shows No. 27 as having the distal suface rotated toward the facial. The arrow starts on the distal and arcs across the facial surface. It would be just as valid to show an arrow starting on the mesial surface and arcing across the lingual view. For purposes of consistency, facial views are used for rotations. Because of the different perceptions persons have when viewing a two-dimensional drawing and attempting to visualize a three-dimensional characteristic, it is best for all persons who may record or interpret a dental charting to agree on one way to chart malpositions.

This is true not only for axial rotations, but also for lingual and labial versions (inclinations), which may cause equal confusion if a variety of methods are used to chart the condition. One easily understood rule is to mark a vertical arrow pointed from the incisal edge away from the facial aspect of the tooth to show *lingual version* (see tooth No. 11 in Fig. 11-5) and to show the vertical arrow starting at the incisal edge and traveling vertically up or down the facial aspect of the drawing of the tooth to depict *labial version*. Mesial or distal inclination is shown with a straight, horizontal arrow pointing toward the midline of the arch from the mesial surface to show mesial inclination and pointing posteriorly from the distal surface to show distal inclination.

Drifting of the teeth either mesially or distally with or without rotation or inclination is shown with a horizontal arrow pointed in the direction of the drift, above the occlusal table or incisal edge. Fig. 11-5 shows the distinction in recording version and drifting. Tooth No. 5 is distally inclined; tooth No. 3 is mesially inclined and drifted; and Nos. 1 and 2 are positioned mesial to their usual locations but are not inclined. This is probably due to the loss of tooth No. 4.

Locating all these malpositions is accomplished best by sitting in a rear position (11 o'clock, for instance) and observing the curve of the maxillary arch in the dental mirror. Careful observation should help contrast rotations and versions from the natural curvature of the maxillary arch. The curve of the arch on the mandible should reveal deviations from normal arch curve. (See the anterior rotations evident in Plate 3, *C,* and the more

obvious malpositions in Plate 2, *G.*). Having the patient close his or her teeth and retracting the cheeks should reveal patterns of drift and version.

Radiographic chartings

Radiographs are a necessary and helpful adjunct to the clinical examination. The radiographs provide information about the teeth and supporting structures that cannot be collected during a clinical examination. Most practitioners require a complete series of radiographs consisting of 16 to 18 periapical views or a panoramic radiograph and bite-wing radiographs at the beginning of treatment (Wuehrmann and Manson-Hing, 1981). (See Fig. 11-7 for a complete set of radiographs.) The radiographs are updated according to individual patients' needs.

Under guidelines developed in response to a growing concern regarding overexposure of patients to radiation, the clinical examination typically precedes the prescription for the number and type of radiographs to be exposed. Some patients may require a complete set, while others may require only one or two exposures in order to support clinical evidence of pathology (American Dental Association, 1981).

The radiographs should be viewed on a back-lit view box or other device; they should not be held up to the room light for examination. The films should be mounted on dark, nontranslucent mounts, and extra light around the mount should be masked so that glare does not interfere with accurate observations. The room light should be dim. Magnification helps in detecting subtle changes (Rumberg, 1987).

If a panoramic film is available (shown on the viewbox in Fig. 11-8), read it first, as it lacks detail but provides an overview of the maxilla and mandible. Then review bitewing or caries detection films and finally the periapicals (Rumberg, 1987).

The *radiographic findings* are charted on the comprehensive charting form using the same symbols and codes explained earlier in this section. Several additional symbols and codes, which are unique to a radiographic charting, are described here. The radiographs are viewed and charted in a sequence that is slightly different from the sequence used during a clinical examination. The radiographs are viewed for kinds of changes

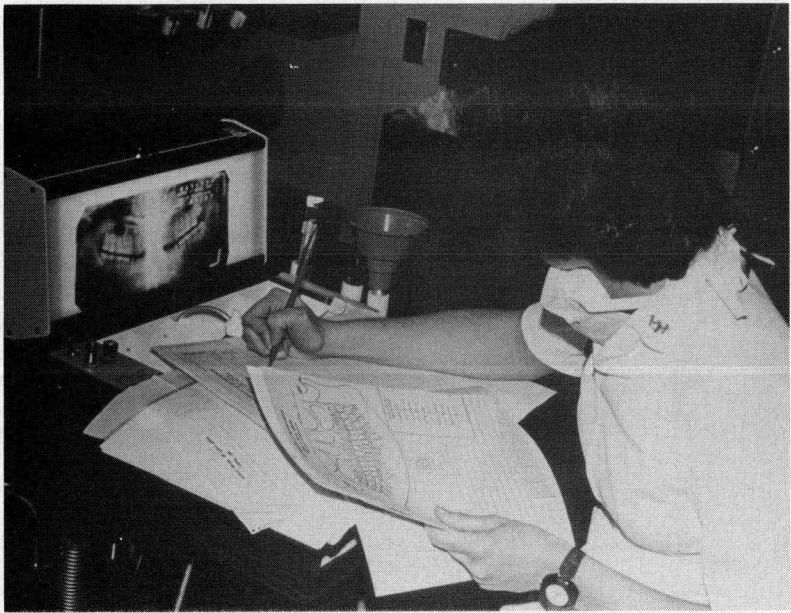

Fig. 11-8. Radiographic chartings should be prepared as a separate procedure before completing an intraoral charting.

rather than tooth by tooth (Wuehrmann and Manson-Hing, 1981). For example, first the radiographs are viewed for missing teeth; the clinician scans the radiographs moving from tooth No. 1 to tooth No. 32 and charts missing teeth. Then the radiographs are viewed for the next change, such as caries. (Plate 3 and Fig. 11-7 are of the same patient.)

The first radiographic finding to be charted is missing or unerupted teeth. Missing teeth are charted using the previously mentioned line, *X*, or box. Unerupted teeth are circled. Most practitioners differentiate between missing and unerupted teeth; this differentiation is especially important for pedodontic chartings. Notice that all four third molars are missing in Fig. 11-7, but all other permanent teeth are present.

Existing restorations, including crowns, bridges, and root canal fillings, are charted next. The same symbols used previously are used for the restorations, although it is difficult to distinguish the type of metallic restorations radiographically. The interproximal extensions of the restorations and pontics can be readily identified from the radiographs; it is important to use the radio-

graphs to detect these findings. Root canal fillings are recorded by darkening the root canal and pulp chamber on the charting and by placing the letters *RC* in the appropriate box. (See tooth No. 9 in Fig. 11-5.)

Note that in Fig. 11-7 there are numerous restorations and two teeth showing endodontic treatment: Nos. 9 and 13. Note the lower right quadrant restorations, as shown in the bitewing films (where the teeth are occluded and the apices are not visible). The knife-edge restoration margins on Nos. 29 and 30 and the mesial aspect of No. 31 indicate that these are cast gold restorations. The restorations appear to provide cuspal coverage, suggesting that these are gold onlays. Compare the shape and the exact margins of the gold onlays with the shape of the restorations on Nos. 5, 6, 11, 12, and 28. The restoration margins on these teeth are less precise, and they appear to be set into the occlusal grooves and pits of the posterior teeth and into the direct distal surfaces of the cuspid teeth.

Some tooth-colored restorations appear radiolucent and can be confused with carious lesions; newer materials have additives to make them ra-

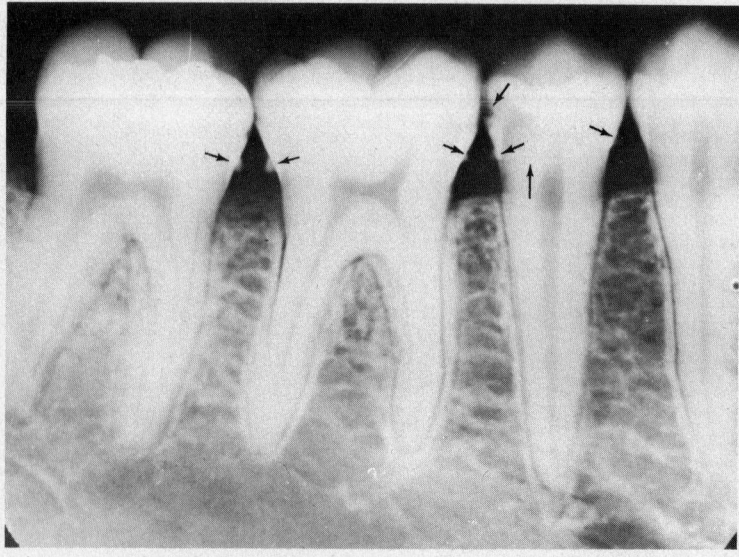

Fig. 11-9. Arrows show calculus extending from proximal surfaces into interdental spaces and ringing the crown of the second premolar. Caries has penetrated proximal surfaces at or below contact points on second premolar and the two molars. Loss of bone height is observable between the two molars, and a widened periodontal ligament space is most apparent along distal root of first molar and distal root of first premolar. (From Wuehrmann AH, and Manson-Hing LR: Dental radiology, ed 5, St Louis, 1981, The CV Mosby Co.)

diopaque. Usually a restoration will have well-defined margins, so there will be a well-defined distinction between the radiopaque and radiolucent areas; a carious lesion will not have well-defined margins. Temporary restorations may also be radiolucent and may or may not have well-defined margins.

Tooth No. 8 in Fig. 11-7 shows two tooth-colored restorations, one located either facially or lingually and one on the mesial surface. Tooth No. 23 also shows a tooth-colored restoration, located on the distal surface (see Plate 3, *B* and *C*).

When the radiographs are viewed, for existing restorations, overhangs can also be recorded. An overhang will appear as an extension of the metallic restorations beyond the tooth. Overhangs are most commonly observed in the gingival third of the tooth (see Chapter 21). It is difficult to detect tooth-colored restoration overhangs radiographically, as the restorations usually appear radiolucent.

Carious lesions can be charted next. Caries appears radiolucent and can be seen as a new lesion or a lesion recurring around a restoration. When detecting caries radiographically, it is important to view each tooth carefully and to check the interproximal areas and around all of the margins of restorations. Lesions can be extremely small or extremely large; some carious lesions will affect the pulp, with this advanced pathology detectable radiographically. (See Fig. 11-9 for interproximal caries and Fig. 11-10 for caries that has advanced to the pulp.)

After the teeth have been surveyed for carious lesions, the radiographs are surveyed for supernumerary teeth, other developmental disturbances, and retained root tips. These findings are recorded as explained previously.

A key to finding pathology is to carefully observe the border characteristics of suspected carious lesions, bone resorption, abscesses, or cysts or tumors. This becomes particularly important in identifying the signs of periodontal involvement.

Next the radiographs are surveyed for *periodontal findings*. The height of the bone level, width of the periodonal ligament space, and continuity of the lamina dura of each tooth are viewed. The *height of the bone* can be drawn on the comprehensive chart or possibly on the periodontal charting (see Chapter 14). The numbers

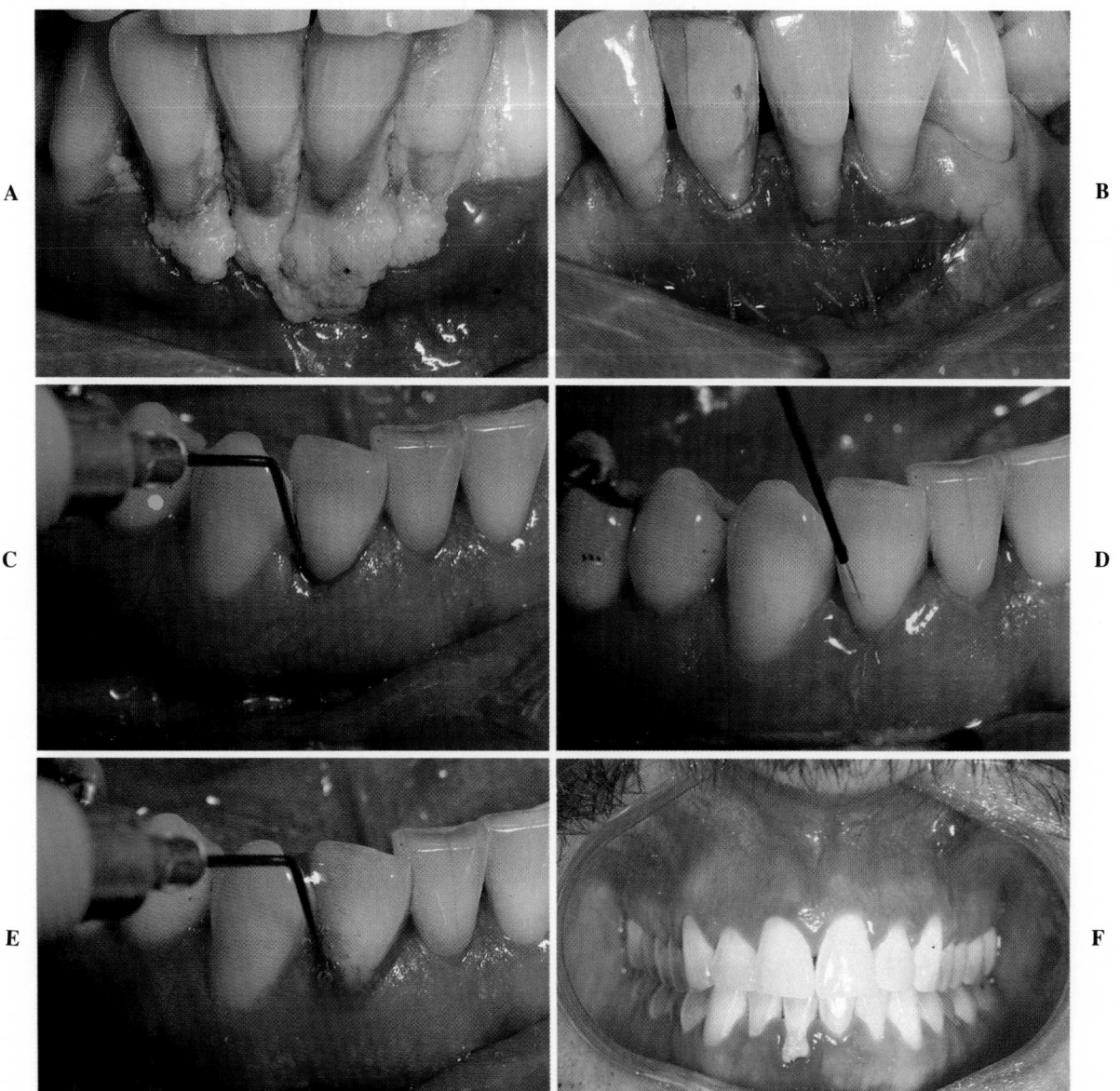

Plate 1. **A,** Continuous bridge of calculus covers anterior teeth facially (and lingually) and is covered with materia alba. **B,** Teeth in **A** were scaled and tissue resected; note residual ledge on mesiofacial of No. 24 despite careful instrumentation. **C,** Subgingival cannula placed in the periodontal pocket to deliver antimicrobial following scaling. **D,** Gentle stream of liquid emerging from end-port cannula. **E,** Liquid emerges from the pocket as the tip is activated subgingivally. **F,** Obvious pathology on No. 25 but remainder of tissue shows minimal inflammation.

Plate 1, cont'd. **G,** Probing prompts sulcular and papillary bleeding, indicating ulcerated lining of pockets. **H,** Probing reveals generalized soft tissue bleeding. **I,** Disclosed plaque is visible on most teeth. Using Turesky modification of Quigley-Hein plaque index, the teeth would be scored as follows, starting with the mandibular premolar and moving anteriorly: No. 20, "0"; No. 21, "1"; No. 22, "2"; No. 23, "5"; No. 24, "2"; No. 9, "2"; No. 10, "2"; No. 11, "4"; No. 12, "5"; No. 13, "5"; No. 14, "1." **J,** Fluoroscein dye seen under blue light reveals plaque as a green adherent mass on teeth. This disclosant is preferable for people who do not want to have lips and gingivae stained red. **K,** Four types of plaque. **L,** Relationship of the four types of plaque to the periodontal pocket.

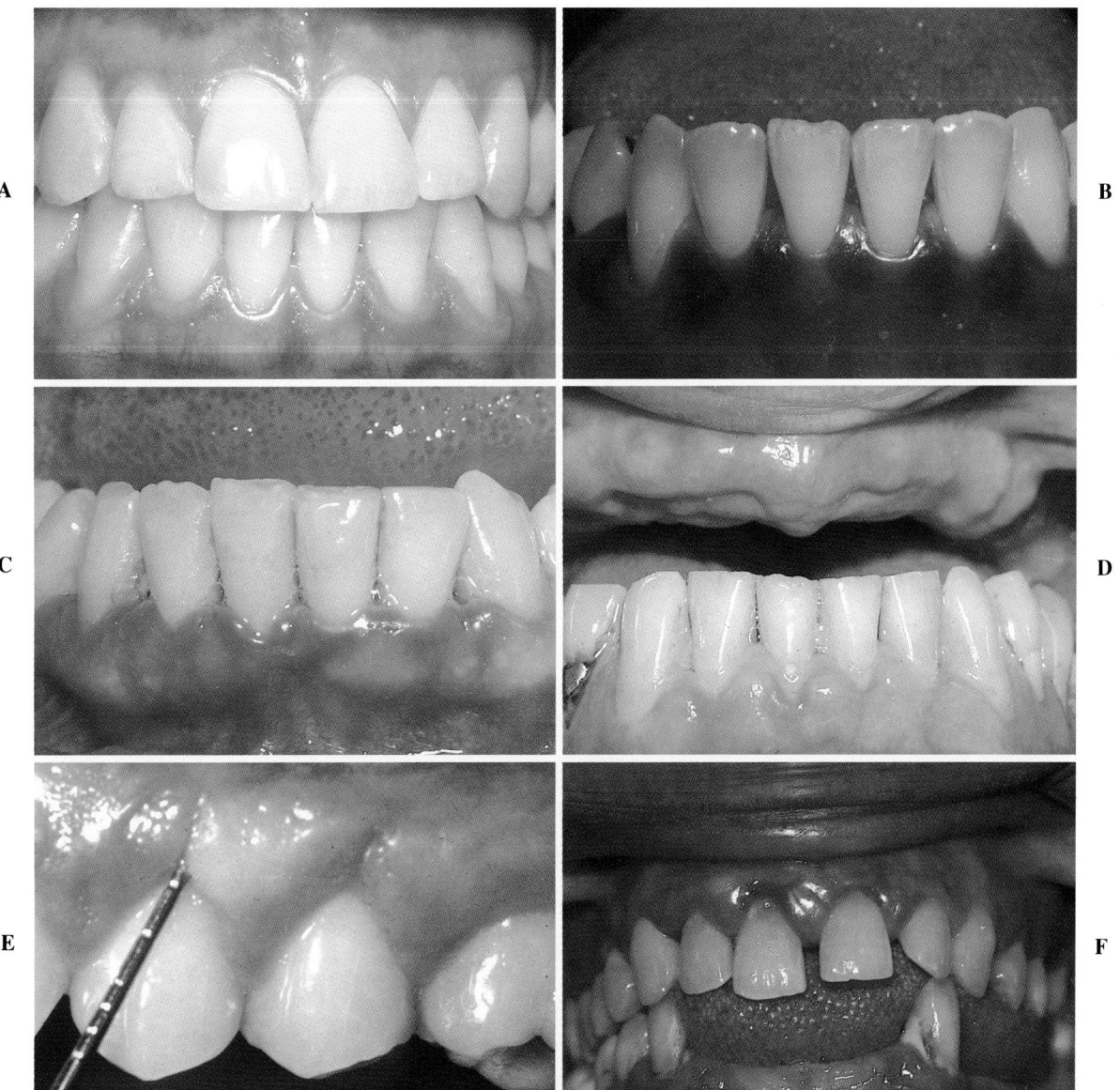

Plate 2. **A,** Clinically healthy gingiva. **B,** Normal melanin pigmentation is visible on free and attached gingiva of this patient. **C,** Signs of marginal inflammation are visible, including redness, rolled margins, and loss of contour. Papillae appear blunted and swollen. Note differences in appearance between attached gingiva and alveolar mucosa. **D,** Fibrotic (hyperplastic) tissue, as seen in mandibular arch of this patient, may appear normal or near normal in color and has a very firm, hard consistency. **E,** Gingival clefting is evident on facial surfaces of premolars. **F,** Marginal gingivitis and periodontitis. Clinical signs of inflammation are visible, especially around Nos. 6 to 10. Note open contacts between teeth and extrusion of maxillary right central incisor, indicating loss of periodontal support. Melanin pigmentation can also be seen in this patient's gingiva.

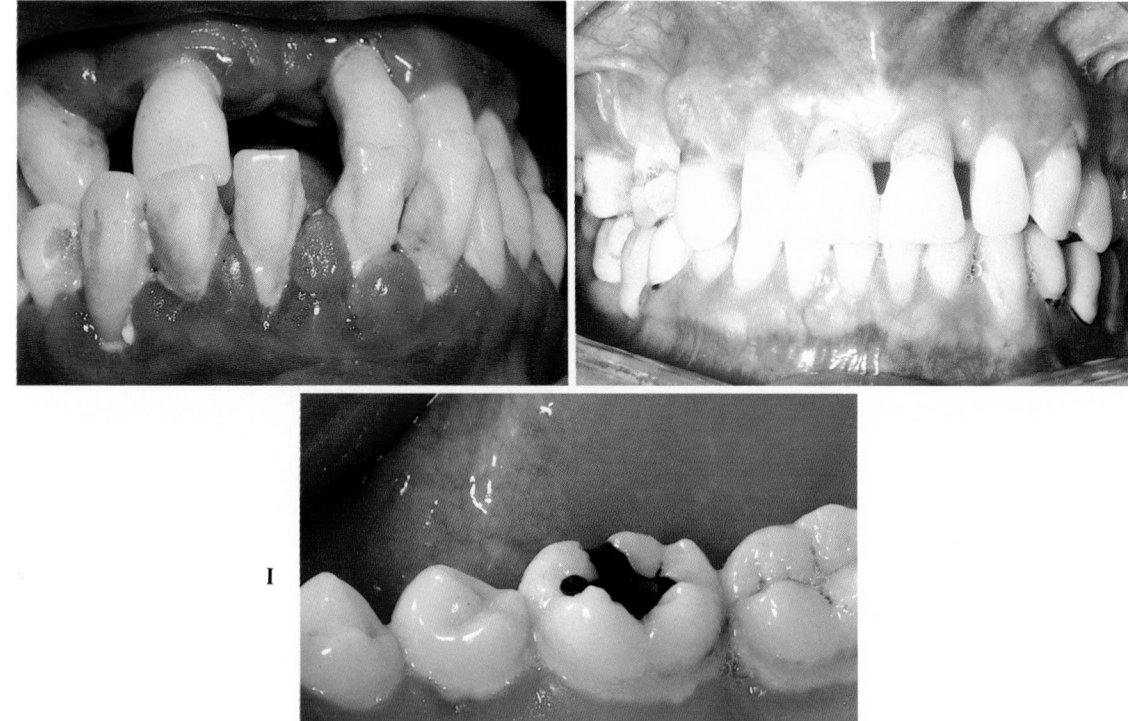

Plate 2, cont'd. **G,** Severe periodontal disease. Presence of heavy hard and soft deposits can be seen. Gingiva exhibits signs of both acute (redness, edema) and chronic inflammation (hyperplasia). Note presence of extruded and shifted teeth and recession due to periodontal destruction. Anterior teeth are clinically mobile. **H,** Generalized recession of maxillary gingivae due to periodontal disease. **I,** Clinical signs of acute necrotizing ulcerative gingivitis can be seen. Tissues are red, swollen, and extremely painful. Necrotic ulceration, which began in interdental papillae, now includes marginal gingiva in this patient. Yellowish "pseudomembrane" is actually a collected mass of bacteria, dead inflammatory cells, and necrotic tissue.
(Courtesy Catherine Schifter, R.D.H., Ph.D.)

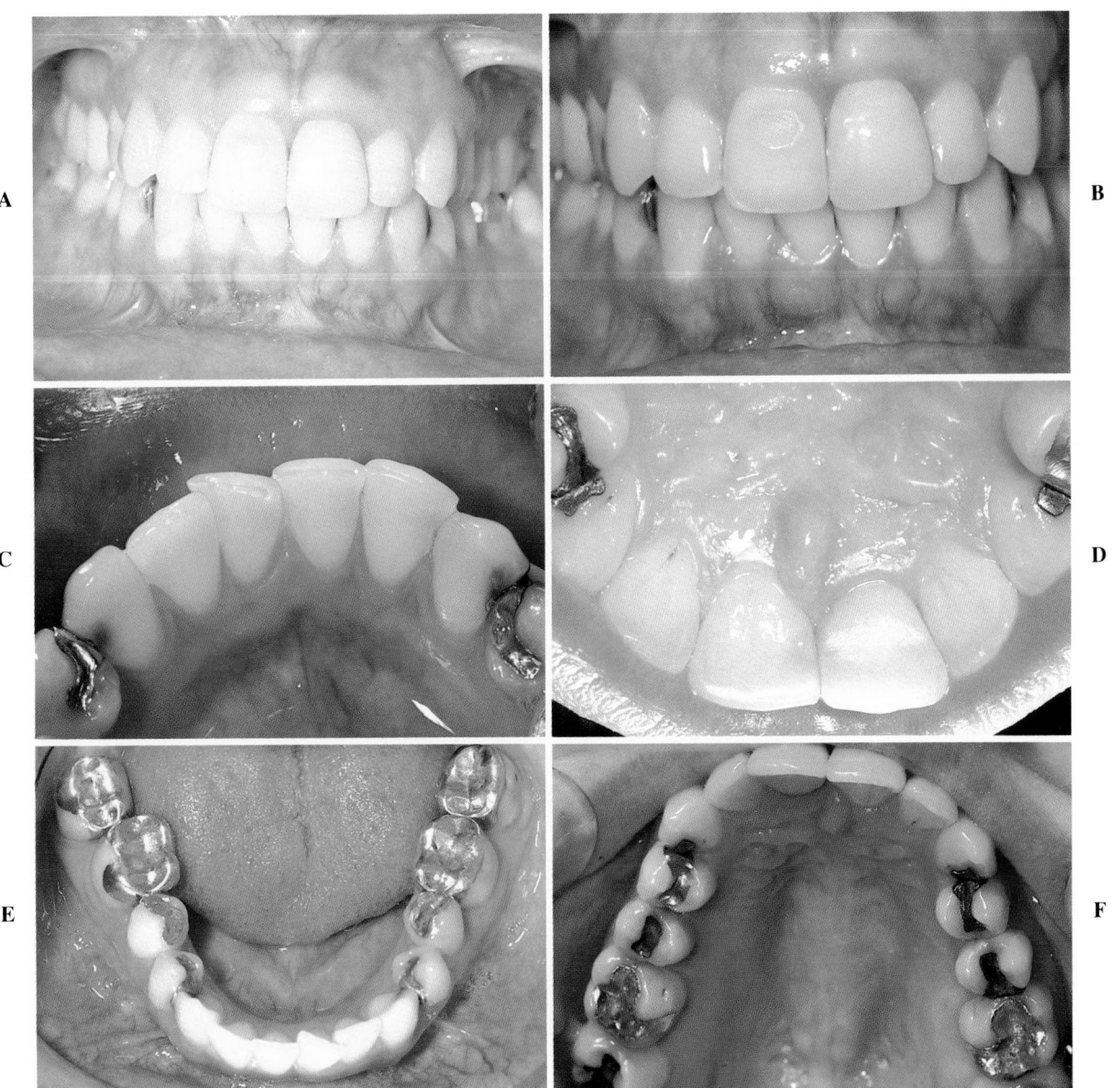

Plate 3. Complete intraoral series. **A,** Full direct view. **B,** Anterior direct view. **C,** Mandibular anterior lingual view. **D,** Anterior palatal view. **E,** Mandibular occlusal view. **F,** Maxillary occlusal view.

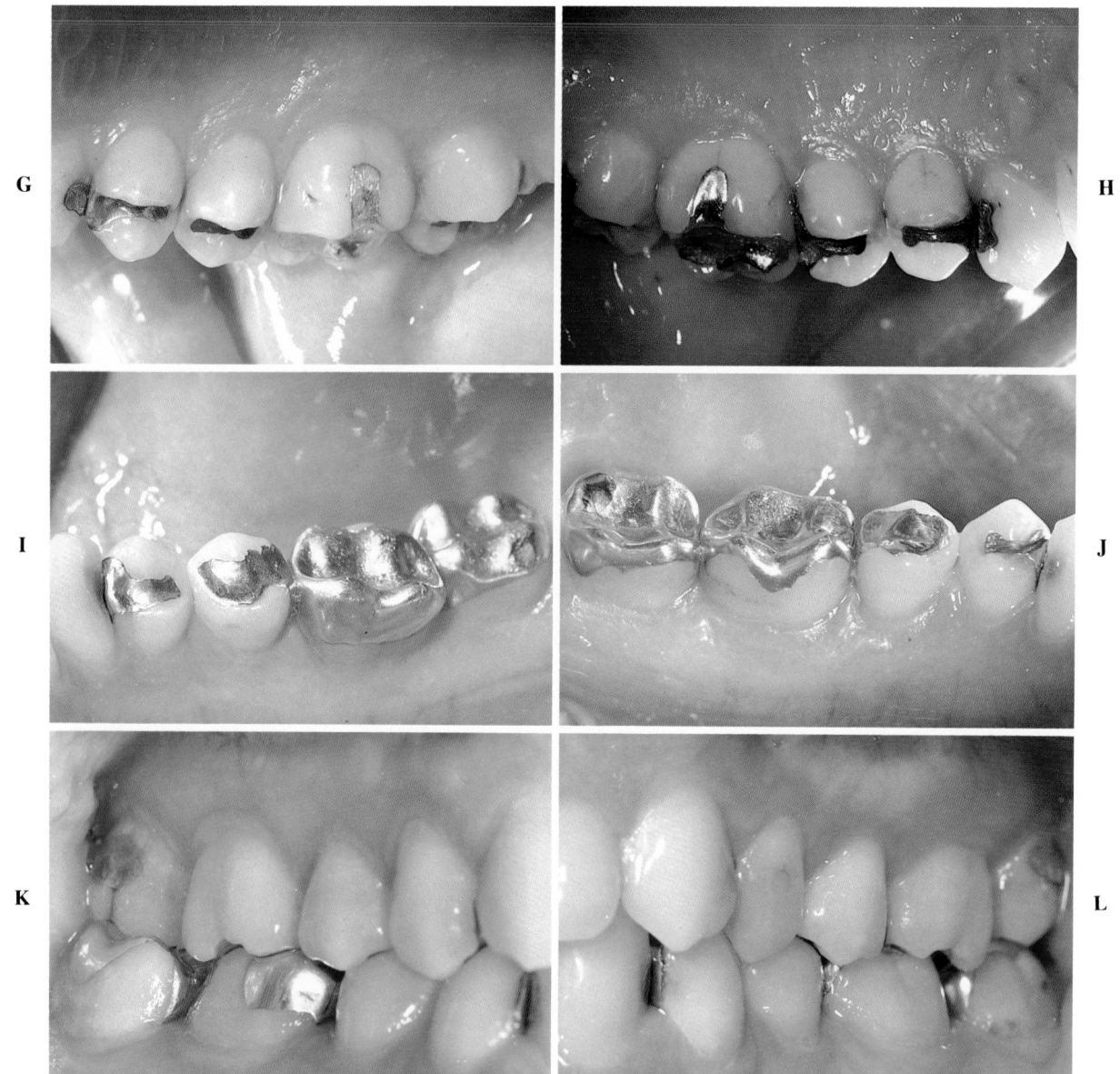

Plate 3, cont'd. **G,** Right posterior palatal view. **H,** Left posterior palatal view. **I,** Right posterior lingual view. **J,** Left posterior lingual view. **K,** Right buccal view. **L,** Left buccal view.

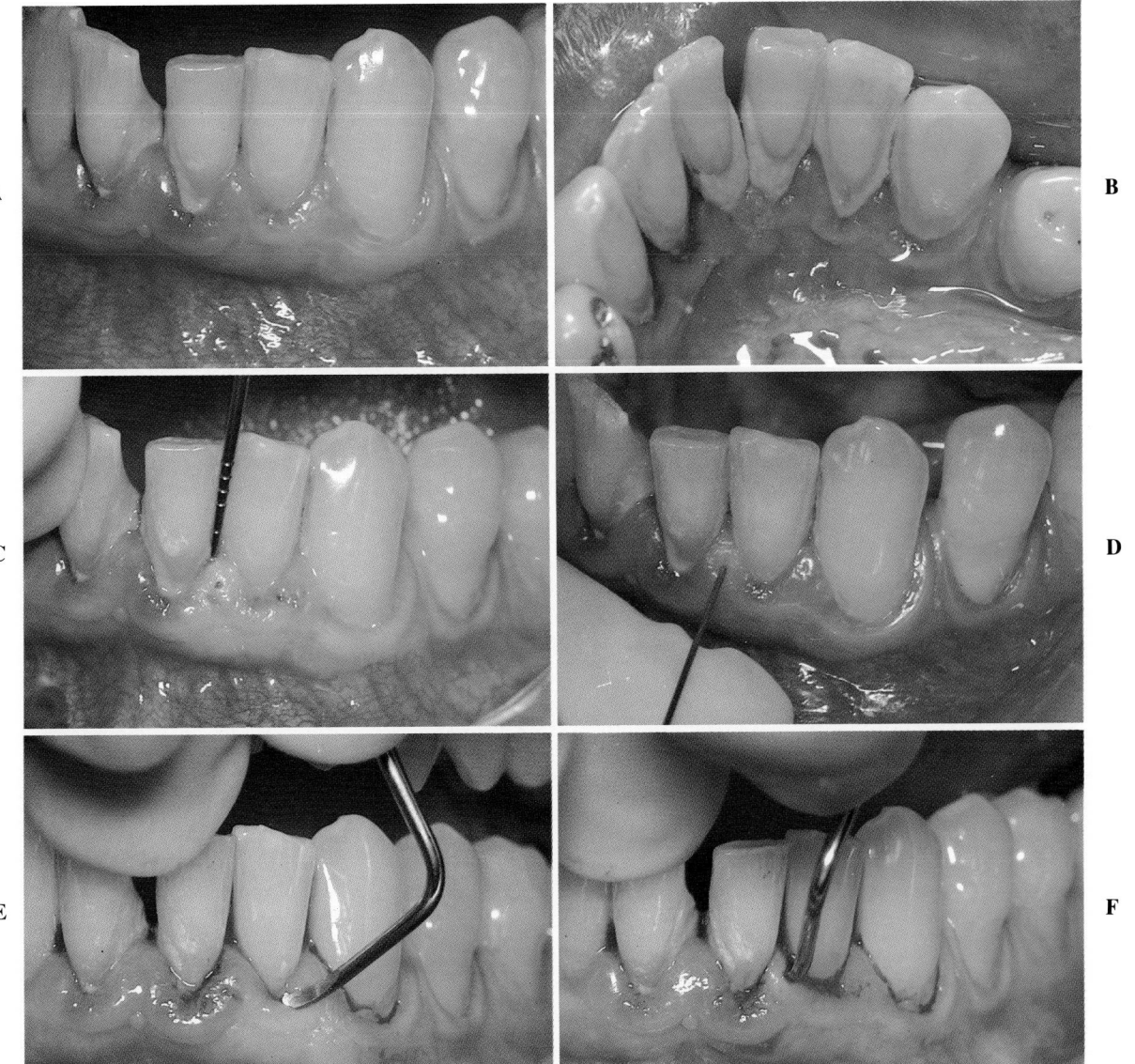

Plate 4. Series depicting steps involved in treatment of selected teeth by scaling and soft tissue curettage. **A,** Pretreatment condition of patient prior to scaling and soft tissue curettage. Clinical examination reveals signs of marginal gingivitis. Gingival tissues are red and edematous. Plaque and calculus are clearly visible. **B,** Lingual view of mandibular incisors shows heavy calculus deposits. Removal of these deposits must precede soft tissue curettage procedure. For this patient scaling and curettage were performed during same appointment. **C,** Clinical pocket depth of 3 mm is measured on distal surface of tooth No. 24 prior to treatment. **D,** Interpapillary injection is given to each interdental papilla. Blanching of tissues can be seen. Local anesthetic will not only make curettage procedure more comfortable for patient but will also provide control of bleeding (hemostasis). **E,** Close-up view of Gracey curette as it is inserted shows that lower cutting edge will be adapted against soft tissues during curettage. **F,** Gracey curette is shown correctly positioned to perform vertical curettage strokes against distal aspect of interdental papilla on tooth No. 23.

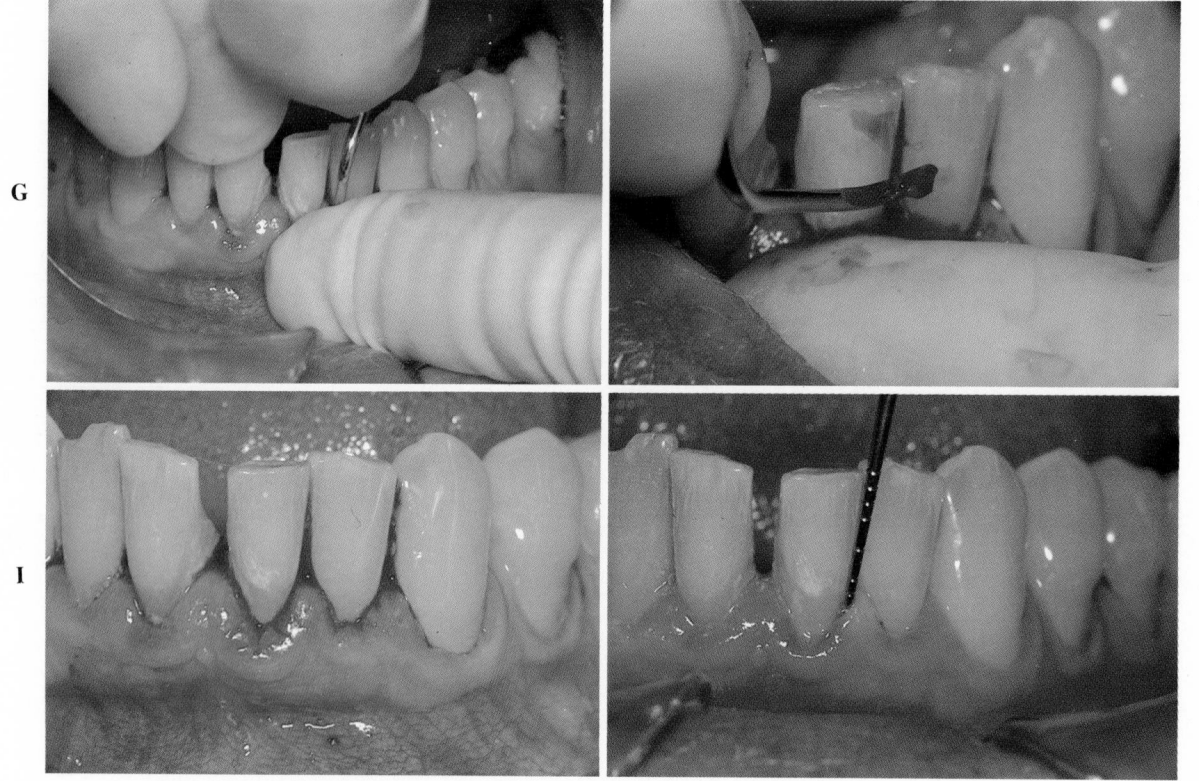

Plate 4, cont'd. **G,** External finger support against gingiva should be applied opposite cutting edge of curette for all strokes. This position stabilizes soft tissues and prevents them from being deflected away from cutting edge so that strokes will be more effective. Gloves are worn to protect both clinician and patient from disease transmission. **H,** Sample of inflamed epithelial lining and connective tissue that was removed during curettage procedure. **I,** Appearance of soft tissues immediately after scaling and curettage can be seen on teeth No. 22 to No. 24. **J,** After only 1 week of healing, reduction of gingival inflammation can be seen. Gentle probing reveals clinical pocket depth reduction of more than 1 mm on distal aspect of tooth No. 24.

(Courtesy Catherine Shifter, R.D.H., Ph.D., and Robert Benedon, D.M.D.)

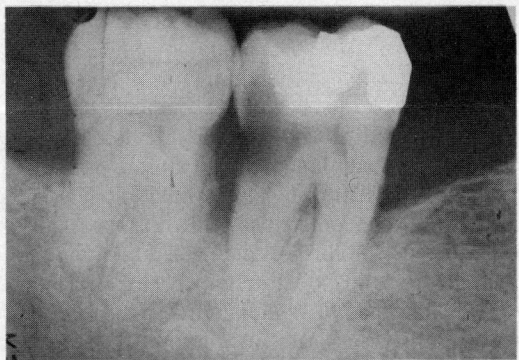

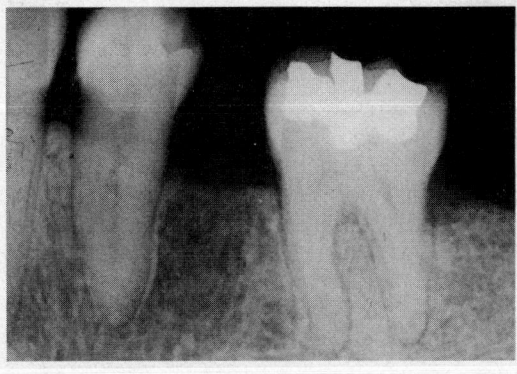

Fig. 11-10. Obvious advanced caries on distal of No. 31; root structure appears carious on mesial of No. 32. Calculus visible on mesial of No. 31 root. Periodontal furcation involvement on No. 31.

Fig. 11-11. Calculus on mesial and distal of molar and mesial of premolar.

of the teeth with *widened periodonal ligament* spaces and *loss of lamina dura* continuity should be recorded. The letters *PDL* or *LD* can be placed in the boxes corresponding to the teeth.

In Fig. 11-9 the bone between the two molars does not have a defined radiopaque line showing the crest of the bone. That line is the lamina dura, and it is lost or less evident in this area of dentition. Compare the crest shown here with those depicted in Fig. 11-7, where loss of lamina dura is not evident.

Teeth No. 19 and No. 30 in Fig. 11-7 show evidence of a widened periodontal ligament space on the mesial aspect as seen in the periapical films. Note that this finding is less evident in the bitewing films, which is one reason why clinicians prefer having both bitewing and periapical films in order to minimize diagnostic errors due to the differences in the angle of the x-ray beam when the film was exposed.

Calculus can be noted next. Figs. 11-9, 11-10, 11-11, and 11-12 show calculus, loss of bone level, and a widened periodontal ligament space. Calculus will be observed as radiopaque projections from the cervical areas of the teeth. Not all calculus will be visible in radiographs, even to the trained eye; there is an error rate of approximately 63% in detecting deposits (White et al, 1984). However, deposits that are observable should be charted so that they will be sought and removed clinically.

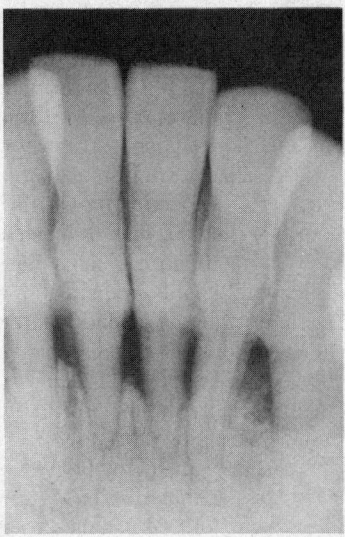

Fig. 11-12. Heavy ledge of calculus bridging the lower anteriors; minimal supporting bone. See Plate 1, view *A* for a photo of this deposit.

Some clinicians chart calculus according to location by drawing triangles corresponding to the location of the calculus. An equally effective method of noting the calculus is to write a statement such as "Radiographic calculus is visible in the maxillary and mandibular posterior areas" in the summary of findings.

Periapical disease and other changes in the bone are viewed last. Periapical disease usually

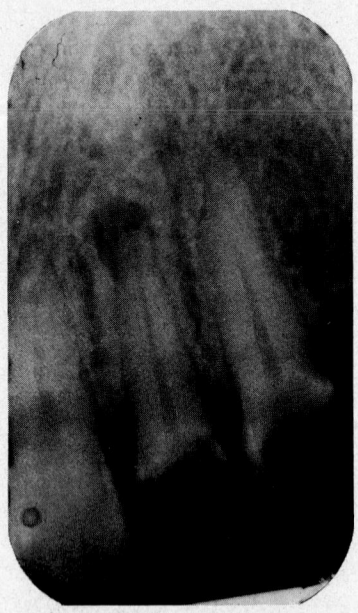

Fig. 11-13. Periapical film of Nos. 10 and 11 showing gross caries and periapical pathology.

appears as a radiolucent area around the apex and can be noted with the letters *PAP* or by drawing a circle around the apex of the affected tooth. While the radiographs are being reviewed for periapical disease, any other abnormalities, radiopaque or radiolucent, should be noted with an asterisk and then described.

Fig. 11-7 shows radiolucencies near the root tips of Nos. 21, 22, 28, and 29. These are not signs of periapical pathology. They are the shadows caused by a normal anatomic landmark of the mandible: the mental foramen through which the mental nerve and blood vessels pass. Fig. 11-13 shows periapical pathology at the tip of No. 10. The pathology is undoubtedly the result of the extensive caries the crown has suffered. Clinically, only a stub of a tooth would be visible. Such pathology can be seen surrounding root tips of clinically healthy teeth and is often the result of trauma.

The radiographic charting is an involved procedure, but it provides invaluable information to augment other assessment data and help make quality treatment a reality.

• • •

All teeth to which none of these clinical or radiographic characteristics apply are described as *sound*.

Fig. 11-5 describes all the usual charting symbols, with the key to each symbol given in the legend. They are probably never all used for any one patient. However, over the course of charting the dental conditions of a wide variety of patients, each of these charting symbols will probably prove useful.

Describing the charting orally

In some instances the person observing the oral conditions will also be marking the symbols on the charting form, which, of course, does not involve an oral description of the characteristic noted. Far more frequently, an assistant will record what is described aloud. In addition, often the observer or the recorder will need to describe to another person each of the recorded findings for verification.

In order to expedite the charting and/or verification approach, an explicit and systematic approach should be used in describing aloud each charted characteristic.

Moving sequentially from 1 to 32 or a to t is the best organizational guideline, with all charted characteristics for each tooth described completely as each tooth is identified. The *tooth number* should be called first. If a restoration is present, the classification, the type of restorative material, and its anatomic location should follow. For example, "Tooth No. 2 has a Class I occlusal amalgam." In identifying anatomic locations, the basic structure (MOD, DO, MO) should be followed by a description of lingual or buccal extensions and the inclusion of complete cusps. For example, "Tooth No. 2 has a Class II MO amalgam with a buccal extension."

Any defective or carious margins should be described following the description of the restoration in question. For example, "Tooth No. 3 has a Class II MO gold inlay with recurrent caries on the distobuccal margin."

When describing a bridge, it is best to first call the number of units (abutments plus pontics) and then call each involved unit as an abutment or pontic and state the type of restoration present on the unit. For example, "There is a five-unit bridge from tooth No. 17 to tooth No. 21. No. 17 is an abutment with a full gold crown. Nos. 18 and 19 are pontics with gold crowns and a porcelain facing on No. 19. Nos. 20 and 21 are abutments with full gold crowns with porcelain facings."

Caries, decalcification, hypocalcification, attrition, facets, erosion, and abrasion are located anatomically. For example, "Tooth No. 12 has caries in the distal pit. Nos. 13 and 14 have decalcification on the gingival third of the facial surface. No. 27 has a vertical facet on the distal third of the labial surface."

Anomalies are called as the tooth is encountered. For example, "No. 10 is a peg lateral."

Malposed teeth are described by naming the tooth and indicating the direction in which it is inclined. For example, "No. 1 is buccally inclined (or verted)." Rotations are described by stating the proximal surface that is directed facially and describing the rotation. For example, "No. 27—the distal surface is rotated labially."

Proceeding around the mouth in this fashion allows for rapid, precise cross-evaluation of findings.

PEDODONTIC CHARTINGS

For most purposes, the preparation of pedodontic chartings is similar to the preparation of adult chartings. Differences include the fact that primary dentition chartings usually use the lower case letters of the alphabet *(a* to *t).* Also, mixed dentition chartings may pose a challenge, as permanent teeth must be differentiated from primary teeth and described with the *1* to *32* system. For instance, a 6-year-old child may have four permanent first molars (Nos. 3, 14, 19, and 30) and four permanent centrals (Nos. 8, 9, 24, and 25), with all the rest being primary teeth (a, b, c, d, g, h, i, and j on the maxilla and k, l, m, n, q, r, s, and t on the mandible). It should be apparent that assessing present and missing teeth *must* precede the attempt to mark restorations, caries, and other characteristics. A guidline never to be forgotten is that *the first permanent molar appears posterior to the second primary molar; it does not replace a primary molar, and it closely resembles the second primary molar.*

Tooth characteristics that may be encountered in pedodontic findings include space maintainers and preformed stainless steel crowns. A space maintainer should be identified by drawing the retaining band on the abutment tooth and drawing a bar to show the space being saved. Stainless steel crowns are marked like full gold crowns, except they are labeled *SSC.*

Practice in reading aloud mixed dentition chartings is particularly helpful, as it is easy to confuse the sequence of teeth to be described and to err in identifying teeth.

In all cases, precision in identifying and recording comprehensive chartings is extremely important, since the chartings serve as legal records and as one basis for treatment planning.

ACTIVITIES

1. Practice reading aloud from a completed anatomic or geometric form a variety of comprehensive chartings to a partner who will record the described findings on a blank form. Compare the chartings for accuracy.
2. Record comprehensive chartings for an advanced student who is assessing his or her patient's oral conditions. Read the findings back to a clinical instructor for verification.
3. In groups of three, take turns (1) observing and describing aloud each tooth's significant characteristics, (2) recording the findings on a charting form, and (3) sitting as a patient observing in a mirror.
4. Translate anatomic or geometric charting symbols to a numerically coded charting form.
5. View a complete series of periapical and bitewing radiographs to practice identifying, recording, and reading aloud the findings.
6. Chart a set of radiographs that has a variety of restorations. Compare the radiographic charting with what you see during an oral examination of the patient. Compare how the restorations look radiographically with their clinical appearance.
7. Compare the radiographic appearance of the teeth and restorations in Fig. 11-7 with the photographs in Plate 3. Some photographs are mirror images. Tooth numbering will be backward in those.
8. Read the article by Johnson and Silvers titled "Attrition, abrasion, and erosion: diagnosis and therapy." Find clinical evidence of each of these phenomena among the group members or clinical patients.
9. Complete the training module: Dental Auxiliary Education Project: Normal radiographic landmarks. New York, 1982, Teachers College Press. Locate normal landmarks on several sets of periapical, bitewing, and panographic radiographs.

REVIEW QUESTIONS

1. Identify at least four basic uses of a comprehensive dental charting.

2. Give one advantage of each of the following charting formats:
   a. Anatomic
   b. Geometric
   c. Numerically coded
3. Following are three columns for the three types of systems used for numbering the teeth and a column for the description of the designated tooth. How would the remaining blanks be filled in so that the designations for a given tooth are identified according to each system and a description of the tooth is included?

	Universal	Palmer's notation	International	Description
a.	—	6|	—	—
b.	29	—	—	—
c.	—	—	28	—
d.	—	|6	—	—
e.	—	—	—	Maxillary left second premolar

4. What is the likely Black classification for a restoration on the following:
   a. DO #12
   b. M #6
   c. B #28
   d. O #18
   e. cusptip of #5
   f. MI of #24
5. Identify each of the following commonly used symbols in charting:
   a. A
   b. T
   c. TC
   d. FGC
   e. GF
   f. C
   g. SSC
   h. DGO
   i. RC
   j. PAP

6. Describe how each of the following findings should be marked:
   a. Tooth anomaly
   b. Pontic
   c. Drifting
   d. Rotation
   e. Attrition
   f. Unerupted teeth
   g. Calculus
   h. Overhang
7. List at least nine conditions, not readily identified clinically, that can be charted from radiographic surveys.

REFERENCES

American Dental Association Council on Dental Materials, Instruments, and Equipment: Recommendations on radiographic practices, JADA 103:103, 1981.

Brand RW, and Isselhard DE: Anatomy of orofacial structures, ed 3, St Louis, 1986, The CV Mosby Co.

Ekstrand K, Qvist V, and Thylstrup A: Light microscope study of the effect of probing in occlusal surfaces, Caries Res 21:368, 1987.

Johnson GK, and Silvers JE: Attrition, abrasion and erosion: diagnosis and therapy, Clin Prev Dent 9(5):12, 1987.

Project ACORDE: Restoration of cavity preparations with amalgam and tooth-colored materials: instructor's manual. Washington DC, 1974, U.S. Department of Health, Education, and Welfare.

Rumberg H: Differential interpretation of radiographic images. Presented at the Arizona State Dental Hygienists' Association meeting, Tucson, Ariz, 1987.

Simonson RJ: Preventive resin restorations: three-year results, JADA 100:535, 1980.

Simonson RJ: Preventive resin restoration: innovative uses of sealants in restorative dentistry, Clin Prev Dent 4(4):27, 1982.

White SC, Gratt BM, and Hollender L: Comparison of xeroradiographs and film for detection of calculus, Dentomaxillofac Radiol 13:39, 1984.

Wuehrmann AH, and Manson-Hing LR: Dental radiology, ed 5, St Louis, 1981, The CV Mosby Co.

12 CALCULUS DETECTION

OBJECTIVES: *The reader will be able to*

1. Explain the importance of accurate calculus detection.
2. Complete calculus chartings for patients exhibiting various amounts of dental calculus in various locations.
3. Describe the types and locations of calculus usually identified intraorally and radiographically.
4. Describe the role of calculus in the progression of periodontal disease.
5. Identify current theories of calculus formation.

Because removing calculus deposits and planing root surfaces are functions dental hygienists perform regularly in most practice settings, developing basic skills in locating and removing deposits is crucial. Chapter 5 introduces the beginning manual skills. This chapter describes the "target" we are seeking when we explore for calculus deposits.

Finding and removing *all* deposits, both above and below the margin of the gingivae, is the ideal toward which clinicians strive. The more closely a clinician approaches accurate detection and complete removal, the more likely it is that the patient will be able to regain and maintain periodontal health. Failure to find calculus, especially when it is several millimeters subgingival or hiding in a root furrow or furcation, can result in the persistent, insidious advance of disease.

TYPES OF DEPOSITS

Calculus deposits are varied in shape, size, and color. The deposits may be chalky and relatively soft, or they may be extremely hard and firmly attached to the root structure (Schroeder, 1969). Calculus is frequently found in children. From 56% to 85% of children examined in one study had supragingival deposits; 30% to 67% had subgingival deposits. The occurrence was greater for children 12 to 14 years old than for those 9 to 11 years old. Calculus is more extensive in adults, particularly in those over 30 years old. In children as well as adults, calculus was most commonly found on the lingual aspect of mandibular anterior teeth and on the facial aspect of maxillary molars (Turesky, 1970).

The most common visible deposits are chalky yellow or white, rough *crustaceous* deposits that are located on the lingual aspect of the mandibular anteriors and on the facial aspect of maxillary molars (Alexander, 1971; Baumhammers et al, 1973). These two sites are adjacent to major salivary ducts. As many of the elements known to exist in calculus are found in saliva, the flow of saliva over the teeth is believed to influence the deposition of the hard material on the teeth (Alexander, 1971; Listgarten and Ellegaard, 1973; Mandel, 1972; Mislowsky and Mazzella, 1974). Drying the teeth with air and feeling the teeth with the side of the explorer or probe will make it possible to find these deposits. Patients who have not had their teeth cleaned for extended periods of time may have a bridge of calculus covering the lingual surfaces of the mandibular teeth, filling the interdental spaces and literally splinting the teeth from cuspid to cuspid. Similar large deposits are sometimes seen on the facial aspect of the maxillary molars as well (Alexander, 1971). (See Plate 2, *G*, and Plate 4 for clinical examples.) One case in the literature reports a calculus deposit so large that a referring dentist mistook it for a bone tumor; it actually aided the patient's mastication (Subash, 1985).

These visible deposits are referred to as *supragingival*, or *supramarginal*, calculus because they are located coronally to the gingiva. In many instances, a deposit that is visible extends subgingivally into the sulcus or pocket and therefore is both supramarginal and submarginal by location.

The visible deposits are usually softer than the subgingival deposits. They are usually amorphous or follow a pattern on the teeth that is molded by the pressure of the tongue or cheek. Efforts to remove the deposits often cause them to crumble. Complete removal of these types of deposits depends on persistence, good visibility, and frequent use of a stream of air to dry the teeth so that remaining particles are apparent. These fine residual deposits will often be visible only with a disclosant solution. If polishing does not remove the disclosant solution and the surface feels rough, the surface of the tooth should be scaled, as the remaining deposit is calculus and not plaque or stain.

Subgingival or submarginal deposits take on a variety of characteristics. They usually are dark brown, green, or black in appearance. They are usually harder then supragingival deposits, and they have a more identifiable form. Their microscopic structure is quite different from that of supragingival calculus (Mislowsky and Mazzella, 1974; Schroeder, 1969).

The calculus deposits can be long *fernlike* or *fingerlike projections* that are relatively flat against the root surface. Or they can be hard spurlike *spicules* that extend outward from the tooth. A deposit can be a ledge or ring of calculus that encircles all or a part of a tooth. Deposits can also be found as hard *nodules* on the tooth surface (Turesky, 1970) (Fig. 12-1). In most instances the calculus is firmly embedded in the tooth surface (cementum) (Singh, Manhold, and Volpe, 1972) and is removed in chunks rather than in crumblings.

Because the deposits are subgingival, they are rarely visible. It is sometimes possible to direct a stream of air into the sulcus and see the calculus deposits located subgingivally if the tissue is loose around the tooth. If the tissue is relatively tight to the tooth and is not overly fibrous, the shadow of the dark calculus can sometimes be seen through the tissue. This is a particularly useful observation when a patient is being seen for a final evaluation of deposit removal, and the tissue is healing well. The signs of localized continued

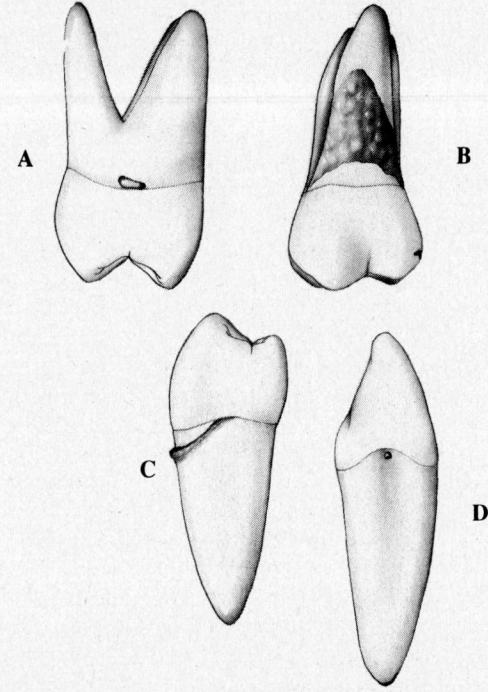

Fig. 12-1. Subgingival calculus can take many forms, including, **A,** small spicule or portion of a ledge of calculus in depression on root, especially at cementoenamel junction; **B,** fingerlike or fernlike projection of calculus down the root; **C,** ledge or ring of calculus surrounding all or part of tooth; and, **D,** small nodules of calculus.

inflammation and the dark "shadow" on the tissue stand out as signals that calculus remains in that particular area.

Veneer, or burnished calculus, is a deposit located subgingivally that has been shaved away rather than fractured away from the tooth in a chunk. With dull instruments or insufficient pressure against the tooth, it is possible simply to shave away the rough parts, leaving a very thin sheet of calculus that is still firmly attached to the tooth and now much more difficult to remove, as there is little possibility of engaging the blade of an instrument against it for removal.

CLINICAL SIGNIFICANCE OF CALCULUS

The presence of calculus is a significant aspect of the data to be gathered in assessing a patient's needs. It has long been associated with diseases of the periodontium, although there is still controversy regarding its role in the initiation and/or the advancement of the disease process (Baer, 1970; Hazen, 1970; Schroeder, 1969; Tuersky, 1970).

It is undisputed, however, that one phase of reducing and eliminating gingivitis and periodontitis includes complete removal of calcareous deposits. These rough deposits harbor volumes of active microorganisms in a covering of dental plaque; these microorganisms irritate the adjacent soft tissues with their byproducts (Baumhammers et al, 1973; Turesky, 1970). Some researchers believe that the bulk of the deposit limits the free flow of gingival/sulcular fluids and reduces the natural blood circulation to the gingiva, thereby contributing to the advancement of the disease (Schroeder, 1969; Turesky, 1970). However, in an experiment using rats in which 2% chlorhexidine gluconate, together with brushing and interdental cleaning, was used over a period of time, junctional epithelial cells formed an attachment to the calculus deposits, perhaps because of decreased plaque formation and decreased toxicity of calculus (Listgarten and Ellegaard, 1973).

Patients with calculus typically will have those deposits removed before other periodontal or preventive procedures are begun. The removal of subgingival deposits creates a smooth environment and disturbs the bacterial plaque colonized subgingivally. Typically, scaling procedures (to remove chunks of calculus) are augmented by definitive root planing to remove necrotic cementum and curettage to reduce granulation tissue so that connective tissue reattachment is possible. Leaving calculus makes healing more difficult, and it provides a place for additional plaque to adhere and proliferate.

STAGES OF CALCULUS FORMATION

Calculus is composed of an organic matrix of bacterial plaque in which calcium (Ca^{2+}) and phosphate (PO_4^-) ions crystallize to form a hard mass (Armitage, 1974; Goldman and Cohen, 1980; Lustmann, Lewis-Epstein, and Shteyer, 1976; Schroeder, 1969). The formation is not simply a precipitation of ions, but rather an orderly deposition of layers of crystals into the matrix (Armitage, 1974; Goldman and Cohen, 1980; Lustmann, Lewis-Epstein, and Shteyer, 1976; Mislowsky and Mazzella, 1974; Schroeder, 1969). Mineralization occurs with the initiation of

crystal growth at nucleation sites in the organic matrix (Lustman, Lewis-Epstein, and Shteyer, 1976; Mislowsky and Mazzella, 1974; Schroeder, 1969). The bacteria themselves may calcify intracellularly. Scanning electron photomicrographs show the patterns of microorganisms, which are both hollow and solid with the hydroxyapatite and other calcium-phosphate minerals (Lustmann, Lewis-Epstein, and Shteyer, 1976; Schroeder, 1969; Ruzicka, 1984; Sakae et al, 1985).

Filamentous organisms are layered over supragingival calculus, whereas subgingival calculus is covered by a mixture of cocci, rods, and filaments. These forms can be seen by examining calculus with a scanning electron microscope. When the filamentous organisms are destroyed with sodium hypochlorite, the calculus shows the patterns of where those microorganisms were attached, which further supports the conclusion that bacteria serve as a matrix for calcification (Friskopp and Hammarström, 1980).

The plaque layer contains small "islands of calcified material"; in some observations, a thin band of calcified plaque material is separated from the calculus by a layer of soft, noncalcified plaque. When viewed with polarized light, supragingival calculus shows "large crystals arranged in rosettes." The border of the calculus shows microorganisms surrounded by needle-shaped crystals (Friskopp, 1983).

Subgingival calculus is not stratified but homogenous. It is covered with a thin layer of microorganisms not as densely packed as supragingival plaque. It does not contain the crystals characteristic of supragingival plaque associated with calculus (Friskopp, 1983). Supragingival calculus mineral content is approximately 37% by volume; subgingival calculus mineral content is approximately 58% (Friskopp and Isacsson, 1984).

Hydroxyapatite constitutes approximately 55% of the inorganic components, with octacalcium phosphate (31%), whitlockite (25%), and brushite (5%) being the remaining salts (Armitage, 1974). Supragingival calculus is comprised mainly of platelet-shaped crystals of octacalcium phosphate and needle-shaped crystals of hydroxyapatite. Subgingival calculus is mainly comprised of bulk crystals of whitlockite (Sundberg et al, 1985). A wide variety of trace elements have been identified in calculus (Retief et al, 1972, 1973; McDougall, 1985), including copper (Knuuttila, 1983).

Supragingival and subgingival calculus have about the same amounts of calcium, but subgingival calculus has greater zinc and strontium concentrations, and supragingival calculus has higher concentrations of manganese (Knuuttila et al, 1979).

The first stage of calculus formation requires, according to many researchers, the presence of acquired pellicle on the teeth (Canis et al, 1979; Schroeder, 1969). Schroeder (1969) has defined the pellicle as the *exogenous dental cuticle* and describes it as an unstructured, homogenous layer that adheres directly to and penetrates into the crystalline tooth structure, and also to all other firm surfaces in the oral cavity, as well as to old dental calculus. It is rapidly formed and renewed constantly. It is presumably formed by microbially altered salivary glycoproteins and is thin (Schroeder, 1969). Bacterial plaque attaches to this exogenous dental cuticle. Given the appropriate conditions, calcification begins. When the plaque pH rises above the pH in the saliva, calcification occurs. The rise may be due to the production of urea, ammonia, and amines produced through protein breakdown in the plaque (Driessens et al, 1985). Bacteria become encased in the forming calculus. Gram-negative cocci have been seen containing "spherules of amorphous calcium phosphate within the cytoplasm" as they are converted to the hard calculus substance (Sidaway, 1980).

Brushite is formed during the initial stages of calcification. It is slowly transformed into the less porous form of calculus: whitlockite. Thus calculus close to the tooth is harder and less porous, whereas calculus at the outer layers of the deposit that is exposed to saliva is porous (Kani et al, 1983). Calculus close to the cementum often is hardly distinguishable from the tooth structure when viewed microscopically because of its solid structure and its mechanical interlocking with the microscopic topography of the cementum (Canis et al, 1979).

Hard deposits may be detected as early as 2 days after thorough cleansing, although it may require as long as 12 days or more for undisturbed deposits of plaque to calcify and mature (Schroeder, 1969). There is great variability among individuals regarding how rapidly deposits form (Mandel, 1972). The saliva of calculus formers seems to have a higher phosphate precipitation rate (Mukherjee, 1986). Higher levels of calcium ions and urea in the saliva of the submaxillary salivary gland correlate with rapid deposit formation (Mandel, 1972; Schroeder, 1969). Studies indicate that smokers are more likely to have calculus deposits than nonsmokers (Kowalski, 1971; Feldman et al, 1987).

As the calculus matures, the deeper layers of microorganisms calcify. Additional layers of plaque accumulate, and the process continues as the deposit grows. Subgingival calculus contains fewer microorganisms than supragingival deposits. The current theory, as originally suggested by Black about 1900, is that subgingival calculus draws its calcium phosphate crystals from the exudate of the inflamed tissue that covers it rather than from saliva (Schroeder, 1969). As mentioned earlier, subgingival calculcus is extremely hard and is often a dark green or brown in color in contrast to the yellow color of most supragingival calculus.

Microorganisms are directly related to calculus formation. Greater numbers of microorganisms are associated with the presence of calculus (Singh, Manhold, and Volpe, 1972). The role of microorganisms appears to be largely one of providing a matrix of mineralization (Mislowsky and Mazzella, 1974). Devital microorganisms calcify more readily, since acid byproducts of microorganisms are antagonistic to crystal nucleation (Schroeder, 1969).

One study suggests that calculus formation is enhanced by the enzymes contained in the layers of dental plaque that cover the forming deposit (Friskopp and Hammarström, 1982). Protease activity (perhaps derived from epithelial cells in salivary sediment rather than from plaque microorganisms) seems to be higher in subjects who tend to form supragingival calculus (Morita and Watanabe, 1986).

People who are heavy calculus formers show about 60% more lipid weight in their saliva as compared with light calculus formers. Light calculus formers have much higher levels of free cholesterol and triglycerides in their saliva, whereas the saliva of heavy calculus formers contains more free fatty acids and cholesterol esters.

Thus researchers suspect that salivary lipids play a role in calculus formation (Slomiany et al, 1981). The calculus matrix actually contains fatty acids, probably contributed from saliva and microorganisms (Slomiany et al, 1983).

Two distinct types of mineralization centers are seen in calculus: type A, which is initiated by and formed with microorganisms, and adjacent type B centers, which appear unrelated to microorganisms (Lustmann, Lewis-Epstein, and Shteyer, 1976; Schroeder, 1969).

Calculus can form without the presence of any microorganisms, but its nature is quite different. Such sterile calculus is much like mother-of-pearl and does not have the extremely rough surface characteristics of naturally occurring calculus (Theilade et al, 1964).

Calculus deposits penetrate the irregularities of the tooth surface, creating a mechanical lock between the deposit and the tooth (Canis et al, 1979; Selvig, 1970). This is particularly true in areas where a preceding carious process, resorption lacunae, planing grooves, and other defects have created pathways for attachment. One investigator found "minute, atypical crystals within the surface layer of enamel and carious dentin immediately underneath calculus . . .[that] were similar in size to the crystals seen in the adjacent concrement, and characteristically different in size and orientation from the normal crystals of these hard tissues" (Selvig, 1970). When the calculus was chipped off, long needlelike crystals remained. This explains the difficulty frequently encountered in removing mature deposits and points out the importance of planing root structures after calculus removal if the reattachment of future deposits is to be minimized.

Research into the causes and clinical significance of calculus continues. As the many questions about it are finally answered, the clinician's role continues to be, in part, to locate and remove the deposits in combination with helping the patient achieve a high degree of personal control over factors affecting calculus reaccumulation.

Several dentifrices and oral rinses are available for consumer use to minimize calculus formation. Pyrophosphate (Schiff, 1987) and zinc chloride (Lobene et al, 1987) are demonstrated to have an anticalculus effect if used daily as a part of normal oral hygiene. These ingredients do not reduce plaque formation; rather, they inhibit the calcification of the plaque. They can be recommended to patients who have a propensity for heavy calculus build-up.

PREPARING A CALCULUS CHARTING

A comprehensive charting of oral conditions may include the identification and recording of oral deposits such as calculus and stain. This procedure is particularly useful for beginning students who have had limited experience in detecting calculus and in observing and "feeling" different formations and locations of hard deposits. It also helps the student begin to differentiate calculus deposits from normal anatomic characteristics, such as contact points, the cementoenamel junction, and cementum. It provides an opportunity for students to compare the "feel" of a margin of a restoration with the "feel" of calculus. Finally, a comparison of the results of the charting with the instructor's findings will show how well the student is mastering the art of detection.

As with all other initial assessment procedures, a calculus charting can provide valuable baseline data about the patient's oral conditions, which can then be compared with subsequent evaluations.

In dental hygiene practice, a calculus charting can be a useful tool in developing a dental hygiene treatment plan. A graphic description of the extent of deposits located in the mouth can help the clinician determine the amount of time needed to complete the removal of deposits and can assist in determining which instruments are most appropriate to accomplish the task. A complete calculus charting is probably performed only when a second clinician (hygienist, periodontist, dentist) is likely to perform the deposit removal. In most instances the hygienist who plans and completes the dental hygiene care, including complete scaling, will perform a cursory review of surfaces known to harbor deposits and make an overall assessment based on those findings. This can easily be accomplished during the phase of assessment when pocket depths are assessed. A periodontal probe can readily detect the presence or absence of calculus deposits—particularly those located close to the attachment of the soft tissue to the tooth and those located in furcation areas. Thus, as the probe is used to assess sulcus and/or pocket

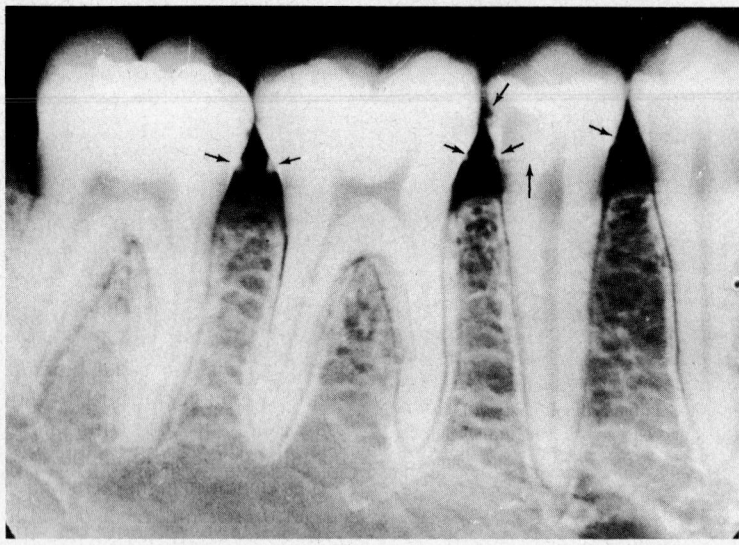

Fig. 12-2. Calculus is observable as spicules extending outward into proximal spaces and as ring around crown of second premolar. Compare radiopacity of calculus with radiolucency of caries on distal aspect of premolar.
(From Wuehrmann AH and Manson-Hing LR: Dental radiology, ed 5, St Louis, 1981, The CV Mosby Co.)

depth, it can be serving the dual function of assessing the presence or absence of hard deposits.

Most instances of heavy subgingival calculus can be seen radiographically, especially deposits that extend from the proximal surfaces into the interdental spaces. They are seen as radiopaque spicules (spurs) or chunks of calculus, usually at or apical to the cementoenamel junction. Radiographs can be useful adjuncts in preparing a calculus charting and in determining the extent of deposits in the pocket (Fig. 12-2).

Because radiographs can provide such useful information for assessing the presence or absence of calculus, it is wise to review the radiographic survey first, charting the presence of deposits on the standard charting form. Calculus is usually indicated by drawing its shape and size on an anatomic charting form. It can be marked in a color to distinguish it from caries, restorations, and other findings if the calculus charting is to be combined with the comprehensive charting on one form.

In assessing the radiographic survey for calculus, one tooth at a time should be reviewed, focusing on the proximal and cervical areas of the teeth. Observing the most apical aspect of the margins of restorations that extend on the proximal surfaces can often reveal small deposits, otherwise often missed in clinical chartings.

Once the radiographic charting of calculus is complete, the clinician should then begin the clinical charting by exploring each tooth surface, using the basic principles of instrumentation described in Chapter 5, being certain to extend the instrument well across the proximal surfaces from both the facial and lingual aspects, and ensuring that the instrument drops to the base of the sulcus or pocket. Failure to cover all surfaces that are exposed to the oral environment will probably result in an inaccurate charting. It is particularly important to ensure that when the instrument meets resistance in the sulcus, it is because it has reached the elastic resistance of the attachment and not the hard resistance of a piece of ledge calculus. There is a distinct difference in the feeling of the resistance. If the stopping point feels hard, the instrument should be moved out and around the deposit so that it can continue to the bottom of

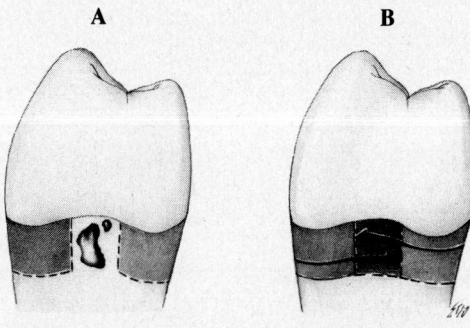

Fig. 12-3. When proximal area is being explored, explorer must cover tooth surface past midpoint of proximal surface. **A,** If exploratory strokes are stopped short of midpoint, calculus that is frequently found in furrows of root and directly below contact area will not be detected. **B,** Exploring past midpoint of tooth from both facial and lingual aspects will ensure that this critical portion of the tooth is thoroughly examined.

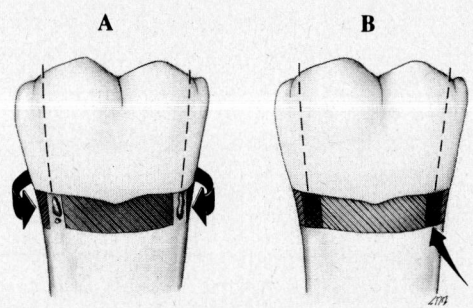

Fig. 12-4. A, Calculus remains undetected on line angles of teeth, **B,** unless exploratory strokes used to cover facial aspect overlap with strokes covering proximal aspects. Undetected calculus at "corners" of teeth is a common error beginning clinicians.

the sulcus or pocket. This is a frequent mistake in calculus detection.

Other frequent mistakes in detecting deposits follow:

1. Failure to move the instrument sufficiently across the proximal surface to ensure that the center of the proximal surface is explored from both aspects of the tooth (facial and lingual). Calculus tends to attach in the furrows and other indentations on the teeth, particularly on the mesial and distal aspects. Exploring short of the midpoint of the proximal surface will probably result in undetected deposits (Fig. 12-3).

2. Failure to explore adequately the corners or line angles of the teeth. A clinician frequently will explore the proximal surfaces thoroughly and then, when turning the instrument to explore the direct facial and lingual surfaces, miss the corner of the root (Fig. 12-4). Spicules of calculus are then left uncharted.

When patients have a low prevalence of plaque and gingivitis, the role of irregular or malposed teeth in the formation of calculus becomes more obvious. There is a positive correlation between malposed teeth and calculus formation (Buckley, 1980, 1981); thus careful exploring for calculus in these areas is important and often challenging because of the limited access caused by the malpositions. Even for patients who practice good oral

hygiene, deposits are likely to form in these areas.

As each tooth is explored, it should be examined for the presence of supragingival calculus as well, using air and light and by tracing the tip of the explorer over the visible tooth structure. As deposits are located on each tooth, they should be recorded on the chart form. Being anatomically specific in calling these findings to an assistant will ensure the accuracy of the finished charting. The finished charting should be helpful in planning care and in showing the patient the extent of the deposits present in his or her mouth.

SCORING CALCULUS

It may be necessary in clinical practice to attempt to quantitate the amount of calculus present on teeth. The most widely used indices in epidemiologic studies are the Periodontal Disease Index (PDI) (Ramfjord, 1959) and the Oral Hygiene Index (OHI) (Greene and Vermillion, 1960) or OHI-simplified index (OHIS) (Greene and Vermillion, 1964) in which only six teeth are scored. Calculus is an important component in these indices. In the PDI, presence of calculus is described as *slight, moderate,* or *abundant* for grades *1, 2,* and *3,* respectively. In the OHI indices, both supragingival and subgingival calculus are evaluated, as shown in Table 12-1. Both the PDI and OHI require the use of an explorer to detect the

Table 12.1. Calculus scoring criteria in the OHI or OHIS systems

	Calculus	
Score	Supragingival	Subgingival
0	None	None
1	Less than one third of crown	None
2	Less than two thirds of crown	Single or isolated deposits
3	More than two thirds of crown	Continuous band

amount and/or location of calculus deposits. These indices are recommended for routine use because of their widespread acceptance and reproducibility (Volpe, 1974).

These methods have been developed to quantitate calculus on specific tooth surfaces. When these methods were compared with determining the effect of unsupervised toothbrushing on calculus formation after 1 to 2 weeks, all scoring methods showed significant effects; the greatest reduction was scored using the Volpe-Manhold probe method (Turesky, 1970).

This method measures the extent of a supragingival deposit in three planes (vertical, and diagonally across the deposit from the mesioincisal and distoincisal edges) on the lingual surfaces of the six mandibular anterior teeth with a periodontal probe graduated in millimeters. This technique is most useful in doing clinical surveys but is of limited value in planning care for individual patients, since it assesses only selected teeth, does not address subgingival deposits, and requires that the examiner be highly trained (Volpe, 1974).

ACTIVITIES

1. Examine extracted teeth for the presence of calculus, identifying each type of deposit for its shape, location, consistency, and color.
2. Explore the calculus on extracted teeth, tracing its shape and differentiating it from the cementoenamel junction and margins of restorations. Compare the feel of calculus with the feel of cementum and enamel.
3. Prepare a calculus charting for a more advanced student's patient. Compare findings with those of the advanced student's charting. Observe as heavy deposits are removed by the advanced student.
4. Review Moskow's case description (1978) of a patient with unusual calculus formation. Note the radiographic indications of calculus and bone loss and the shape of the gingivae after calculus was removed.
5. Review the 1985 article by Moskow, Tannenbaum, and Bloom showing the periodontium with serial thin section contact radiography. Note the calculus shown in Fig. 14 and 15.

REVIEW QUESTIONS

1. In what ways is a calculus charting a useful assessment tool in clinical practice?
2. Describe the shape and location of the following types of calculus:
   a. Ledge
   b. Veneer
   c. Crustaceous
   d. Fingerlike projections
3. What is the role of calculus in the progression of periodontal disease?
4. True or false
   a. Calculus forms a mechanical lock with the cementum by molding itself to the irregularities of the tooth.
   b. Plaque is mineralized to form the hard deposit, calculus.
   c. The outer surface of a calculus deposit is less porous than the portion next to the tooth.
   d. There is one kind of mineralization center seen in forming calculus, which is initiated by and formed with microorganisms.
   e. Hard deposits can form within 2 days of a thorough cleaning.

REFERENCES

Alexander AG: A study of the distribution of supra and subgingival calculus, bacterial plaque and gingival inflammation in the mouths of 400 individuals, J Periodontol 42:21, 1971.

Allen D, and Kerr D: Tissue response in the guinea pig to sterile and nonsterile calculus, J Periodontol 36:121, 1965.

Armitage GC: Selected lectures in periodontology, San Francisco, 1974, University of California.

Baer PN: What is the role of subgingival calculus in the etiology of and progression of periodontal disease? J Periodontol 43:284, 1970.

Baumhammers A, et al: Scanning electron microscopy of supragingival calculus, J Periodontol 44:92, 1973.

Buckley LA: The relationships between irregular teeth, plaque, calculus and gingival disease, Br Dent J 148(3):67, 1980.

Buckley LA: The relationships between malocclusion, gingival inflammation, plaque, and calculus, J Periodontol 52:35, 1981.

Canis MF, et al: Calculus attachment, J Periodontol 50:406, 1979.

Driessens FCM, et al: On the physiochemistry of plaque calcification and the phase composition of dental calculus, J Periodont Res 20:329, 1985.

Feldman RS, Alman JE, and Chauncey HH: Periodontal disease indexes and tobacco smoking in healthy aging men, Gerodontics 1:43, 1987.

Fischman SL, and Picozzi A: Review of the literature: the methodology of clinical calculus evaluation, J Periodontol 40:607, 1969.

Friskopp J: Ultrastructure of nondecalcified supragingival and subgingival calculus, J Periodontol 54:542, 1983.

Friskopp J, and Hammarström L: A comparative, scanning electron microscopic study of supragingival and subgingival calculus, J Periodontol 51:553, 1980.

Friskopp J, and Hammarström L: An enzyme histochemical study of dental plaque and calculus, Acta Odontol Scand 40:459, 1982.

Friskopp J, and Isacsson G: A quantitiave microradiographic study of mineral content of supragingival and subgingival dental calculus, Scand J Dent Res 92:25, 1984.

Greene JC, and Vermillion JR: The oral hygiene index: a method for classifying oral hygiene status, JADA 61:171, 1960.

Greene JC, and Vermillion JR: The simplified oral hygiene index, JADA 68:7, 1964.

Hazen SP: What is the role of subgingival calculus in the etiology and progression of periodontal disease? J Periodontol 43:285, 1970.

Kani T, et al: Microbeam x-ray diffraction analysis of dental calculus, J Dent Res 62:92, 1983.

Knuutila M, et al: Concentrations of Ca, Mg, Mn, Sr, and Zn in supra- and subgingival calculus, Scand J Dent Res 87:67, 1979.

Knuuttila M, et al: Copper in human subgingival calculus, Scand J Dent Res 91:130, 1983.

Kowalski CJ: Relationship between smoking and calculus deposition, J Dent Res 50:101, 1971.

Listgarten MA, and Ellegaard B: Electron microscopic evidence of a cellular attachment between junctional epithelium and dental calculus, J Periodont Res 8:143, 1973.

Lobene RR, et al: Reduced formation of supragingival calculus with use of fluoride-zinc chloride dentifrice, JADA 114:350, 1987.

Lustmann J, Lewis-Epstein J, and Shteyer A: Scanning electron microscopy of dental calculus, Calcif Tissue Res 21:47, 1976.

Mandel ID: Biochemical aspects of calculus formation, J Periodont Res 10(Suppl):7, 1972; also 9:211, 1974.

McDougall WA: Analytical transmission electron microscopy of the distribution of elements in human supragingival dental calculus, Arch Oral Biol 30:603, 1985.

Mislowsky WJ, and Mazzella WJ: Supragingival and subgingival plaque and calculus formation in humans, J Periodontol 45:823, 1974.

Morita M, and Watanabe T: Relation between the presence of supragingival calculus and protease activity in dental plaque, J Dent Res 65:703, 1986.

Moskow BS: What is the role of subgingival calculus in the etiology and progression of periodontal disease? J Periodontol 43:283, 1970.

Moskow BS: A case report of unusual dental calculus formation, J Periodontol 49:326, 1978.

Moskow BS, Tannenbaum P, and Bloom A: Visualization of the human periodontium using serial thin section contact radiography, J Periodontol 56:223, 1985.

Mukherjee S: The state of calcium phosphate in saliva of caries susceptible and calculus susceptible children and adults, J Pedo 11:76, 1986.

Ramfjord SP: Indices for prevalence and incidence of periodontal disease, J Periodontol 30:51, 1959.

Retief DH, et al: Quantitative analysis of Mg, Na, Cl, Al, and Ca in human dental calculus by neutron activation analysis and high resolution gamma spectrometry, J Dent Res 51:807, 1972.

Retief DH, et al: The quantitative analysis of Sb, Ag, Zn, Co, and Fe in human dental calculus by neutron activation analysis and high resolution gamma spectrometry, J Periodont Res 8:263, 1973.

Ruzicka F: Substructure of sub- and supragingival dental calculus in human periodontitis: an electronic microscopic study, J Perio Res 19:317, 1984.

Sakae T, Yamamoto H, and Hirai G: Scanning electron microscopy of dental calculi, J Nihon Univ Sch Dent 27:181, 1985.

Schiff TG: The effect of a dentifrice containing soluble pyrophosphate and sodium fluoride on calculus deposits, Clin Prev Dent 9(2):13, 1987.

Schroeder HE: Formation and inhibition of dental calculus. Berne, Switzerland, 1969, Hans Huber Publishers.

Selvig KA: Attachment of plaque and calculus to tooth surfaces, J Periodont Res 5:8, 1970.

Sidaway DA: A microbial study of dental calculus, IV: an electron microscopic study of in vitro calcified microorganisms, J Periodont Res 15:240, 1980.

Singh S, Manhold JH, and Volpe AR: Definitive determination of clinical relationship between dental plaque and calculus, J Periodontol 43:39, 1972.

Slomiany A, et al: Lipid composition of human parotid saliva from light and heavy dental calculus-formers, Arch Oral Biol 26:151, 1981.

Slomiany A, et al: Lipids of supragingival calculus, J Dent Res 62:862, 1983.

Spencer AJ, et al: Periodontal disease in five and six year old children, J Periodontol 54:19, 1983.

Subash G: An unusual deposition of calculus—a case report, J Indian Dent Assoc 57:180, 1985.

Sundberg M, and Friskopp J: Crystallography of supragingival and subgingival human dental calculus, Scand J Dent Res 93:30, 1985.

Suomi JD, et al: Oral calculus in children, J Periodontol 42:341, 1971.

Theilade J, Fitzgerald RJ, and Scott DB: Electron microscopic observation of calculus in germfree and conventional rats, Arch Oral Biol 9:97, 1964.

Turesky SS: What is the role of subgingival calculus in the etiology and progression of periodontal disease? J Periodontol 43:285, 1970.

Villa P: Degree of calculus inhibition by habitual toothbrushing, Helv Odontol Acta 12:31, 1968.

Volpe AR: Indices for the measurement of hard deposits in clinical studies of oral hygiene and periodontal disease, J Periodont Res 9(Suppl 14):31, 1974.

13 PLAQUE AND GINGIVAL INDICES

OBJECTIVES: *The reader will be able to*

1. Differentiate among nonmineralized deposits of pellicle, materia alba, debris, and plaque.
2. Describe the nature and formation of plaque and its importance in the etiology of caries, gingivitis, and calculus.
3. Describe the purposes and usefulness of each of the plaque and gingival indices available.
4. Show and describe to patients the differences among the various soft dental deposits and methods for their detection.
5. Select and use one or more of the indices more appropriate for particular dental practice needs as compared with needs for clinical or epidemiologic studies.

It is essential for the dental hygienist to be able to recognize and evaluate soft and hard deposits that accumulate on the surfaces of the teeth. Chapter 12 described calculus as a hard deposit that forms as a result of the mineralization of bacterial plaque. When you are able to recognize the nature, formation, and location of other deposits, you will be able to provide information to your patients that will guide them toward the prevention and management of dental disease.

SOFT DEPOSITS

Soft, or nonmineralized, dental deposits can occur on all supragingival and subgingival surfaces of the teeth and sometimes on the gingival tissues. They can cause discoloration of the teeth, halitosis, and inflammation of the gingival and periodontal tissues.

Acquired pellicle, plaque, materia alba, and food debris are specific terms used to identify these deposits.

While there have been many in-depth reviews of the nonmineralized dental deposits (Dawes, 1968; Gibbons and Van Houte, 1973; Goldman and Cohen, 1980; Jenkins, 1965; Katz, McDonald, and Stookey, 1979), the general definitions have not significantly changed since the World Health Organization (WHO) report in 1961 on periodontal disease. The intervening years have seen increased knowledge of histologic, chemical, microbiologic, and pathogenic information about the

effects of these deposits (Armstrong, 1967; Lie, 1978; Osterberg, Sudo, and Folke, 1976; Socransky, 1977). Definitions of deposits according to the guidelines of the WHO report are summarized in Table 13-1.

Of all the soft dental deposits that have been mentioned, plaque is considered the most important and has been referred to as the primary etiologic factor in the initiation of both caries and periodontal disease (Fig. 13-1). It is one factor that, if eliminated, will eliminate the cause of the majority of the diseases currently treated in dental practice. With conscientious home care by the patient, most plaque can be removed or at least minimized.

PLAQUE
Description, microorganisms, metabolic activity, reactions, and retention

Plaque is a structured, yellow-gray nearly transparent mass of colonizing bacteria that adheres firmly to the teeth. Microorganisms from the oral environment attach firmly to the salivary glycoproteins and extracellular polysaccharides to form a matrix. This intermicrobial matrix or plaque consists of inorganic and organic components. Initially, plaque is comprised of gram-positive cocci. As the plaque matures, an increased number of gram-negative filamentous bacteria and rods appear (Löe et al, 1965). When oral hygiene practices are insufficient or discontinued, the ex-

Table 13-1. Nonmineralized dental deposits

Tooth Deposit	Characteristic
Acquired Pellicle	A translucent film composed of salivary glycoproteins. The pellicle cannot be removed by rinsing or brushing. It can be removed by professional prophylaxis; however, these acellular deposits will reform within minutes to hours. A disclosing agent will stain the pellicle; it appears much lighter than disclosed plaque or calculus. The acquired pellicle is the initial attachment site for bacteria that will eventually form the organized matrix defined as plaque.
Plaque	A dense coherent mass of bacteria in an organized intermicrobial matrix which adheres to surfaces of the teeth or restorations and remains attached despite muscle action, water rinsing, or irrigation. The primary sources of microbial plaque are oral microorganisms and salivary components.
Materia Alba	A loosely adherent complex of bacteria and cellular debris that covers plaque deposits. It is white or gray in color with no uniform structure. Materia alba can be removed by vigorous water rinsing or irrigation.
Food Debris	Loosely attached particulate matter that can be dislodged by muscular movements, water rinsing, and proper home care. Food debris can become impacted in plaque, between the teeth, or subgingivally and can be broken down by enzymes from plaque or saliva.

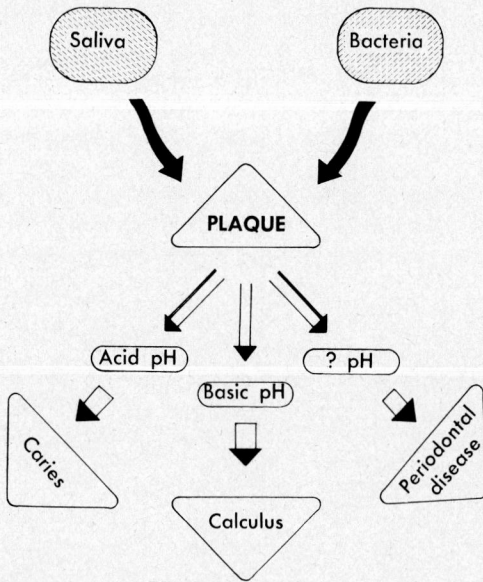

Fig. 13-1. Relationship of plaque to development of oral diseases.

isting microorganisms multiply and different types of bacteria begin to form within the existing supragingival and subgingival plaque.

Microorganisms forming supragingival plaque differ from those organisms that exist in subgingival areas. Gram-positive bacteria are more predominant in supragingival plaque, whereas more than 75% of the microorganisms existing in subgingival plaque are gram-negative. On a relatively clean tooth surface, more than 90% of the bacteria are gram-positive. As the plaque matures, the gram-positive microorganisms proliferate, and it is unusual for more than 25% of the plaque sample to contain gram-negative flora. This is not true for the subgingival plaque. More than 75%

of the microorganisms in the subgingival plaque are gram-negative. This percentage generally increases in rapidly progressing lesions (Löe et al, 1965; Loesche et al, 1985; Socransky, 1986).

Plaque that forms coronally at and above the gingival margin is referred to as *supragingival plaque*. *Subgingival plaque* forms apically beneath the gingival margin within the sulcus. Supragingival plaque that is one to two days old is comprised mainly of *Streptococcus mutans*. *Streptococcus sanguis,* and *Actinomyces* (gram-positive cocci). *Streptococcus mutans* are considered to be acidogenic microorganisms and are responsible for enamel caries. They synthesize carbohydrates into extracellular polysaccharides (dextrans, glucans, and fructans) and intracellular polysaccharides. The dextrans facilitate the plaque's adherence to the tooth's surface.

Plaque that is 3 to 4 days old consists primarily of cocci. There is a significant increase in filamentous bacteria that adhere to the surface of the colonized cocci at the gingival margin. These microorganisms will eventually become the predominate species. As the supragingival plaque matures, 6 to 10 days later more complex forms of mixed bacterial flora that are gram-negative and anaerobic begin to appear. Fusobacteria, rods, and spirilla increase in numbers during this time; eventually vibrios and spirochetes will prevail as the plaque becomes older. Ten to twenty-one-day-old plaque is composed of densely packed spirochetes and vibrios. Inflammation of the gingivae becomes apparent. (Listgarten et al, 1975, Rateitschak et al, 1985).

The subgingival region provides a different environment for microorganisms. When the plaque extends beneath the gingival margin it exists in two forms, adherent and nonadherent plaque. Although both gram-positive and gram-negative microorganisms exist in this area and the microbial composition is similar to supragingival plaque, these organisms can be identified by their location on the tooth surface. Adherent plaque develops within the sulcus on the root surface. It is composed primarily of *Filaments* and *Actinomyces* with decreased numbers of gram-positive cocci. This layer becomes mineralized to form subgingival calculus (see Chapter 12). Nonadherent plaque consists of gram-negative anaerobic microorganisms that are partially motile. These species include black pigmented *Bacteroides, Fusobacterium, Treponema, Acidaminococcus, Wolinella, Selenomonas,* and *Actinobacillus.* These organisms move around freely near the soft tissues and play an important role in inflammatory lesions (Fine et al, 1978; Rateitschak et al, 1985). These organisms are cultured and incubated in an anaerobic atmosphere (anaerobic chamber). When the petri dishes are removed from within the chamber, a foul-smelling odor is apparent due to the decomposition of proteins. This odor is the same as that found in people with periodontal disease.

Microorganisms have been found to invade tissues and bone not as colonies but as separate organisms. Individual microorganisms are often seen in histologic sections of tissue and bone. Therefore, the disease is referred to as an infection rather than simple inflammation. Toxins produced by subgingival microorganisms penetrate the cementum, impeding healing and reattachment. The host's response to the presence of microorganisms is a critical factor in the progression of the disease from gingivitis to periodontitis. In the rate of healing, a person with impaired abilities to combat the virulent pathogens will be more susceptible (Christersson et al, 1986, 1987; Pertuiset et al, 1987).

Although periodontitis was once believed to be a slow, chronic, progressive disease, it is now believed to occur in "bursts" of activity (Socransky, 1984) and to be site-specific, affecting one or two areas and not necessarily the entire mouth in each cycle of activity.

The metabolic byproducts of plaque and the invasive nature of some organisms produce continuous changes in the gingiva, resulting in both edematous (size) and erythematous (color) changes. These changes are usually accompanied by bleeding and pocket formation (separation of the attachment apparatus between the gingiva and tooth) and can proceed to other signs of periodontal disease (Loe, Theilade, and Jensen, 1965).

When carbohydrate materials, primarily simple sugars such as sucrose and glucose, are metabolized by plaque, an acid situation is produced that can lead to demineralization of enamel, commonly referred to as *caries.* When plaque metabolism develops or results in basic pH, calcification of the plaque occurs.

Plaque becomes mineralized by salts from the saliva forming calculus (see Chapter 12), which enhances plaque attachment (Driessens et al, 1985).

1. Anatomic, physiological, and iatrogenic factors that favor plaque retention include the following:
2. Supragingival and subgingival calculus is not pathogenic by itself. However, its surface irregularities and roughness provide an ideal foundation for plaque retention.
3. Tooth malalignment, such as crowded, rotated, or partially erupted teeth, contributes to the accumulation of plaque.
4. Mouth breathing produces drying of the gingiva and teeth. This causes the plaque to be adhesive.
5. Tooth contours, such as the cementum overlapping the enamel, altered tooth structure, abrasion, and erosion, make removing plaque more difficult.
6. Restorative dentistry affects plaque retention if fillings, crowns, and clasps are not contoured properly.
7. Gingival recession and enlarged, inflamed gingiva favor plaque accumulation.

INDICES

The growth and development of microbial plaque, gingivitis, and periodontitis may be measured in several ways (Barnes et al, 1986). These measures are typically applied in research and are reported in the literature. They can also be applied in clinical practice to assess the presence of plaque, gingivitis, and periodontitis and they can be applied in community-wide assessments of disease prevalence (epidemiological studies). It is important to be familiar with these indices in reviewing scientific literature and in selecting appropriate measures for clinical practice.

Plaque scoring methods

Plaque scoring is used to quantitate supragingival plaque occurrence on teeth. Following are descriptions of two indices used in scoring plaque.

Silness and Löe plaque index (PLI). The *plaque thickness* at the gingival margin is measured, on the assumption that plaque in contact with the gingival margin is the most clinically relevant accumulation. To examine the plaque, the teeth are carefully dried with air. The examiner first looks to see if plaque is visible; if so, it is scored as either a 2 or 3 (see box). If plaque is not visible, the examiner runs a periodontal probe along the tooth at the margin of the gingiva and examines the probe tip for plaque. If none is seen, the score is zero. If there is plaque on the probe, the score is 1. This index is useful for epidemiological studies and clinical trials. Figure 13-2 is a suggested scoring form.

Turesky modification of the Quigley-Hein. The *plaque area* covering the crown of the tooth is measured without attention to plaque thickness. To examine the plaque, the teeth are disclosed (usually with erythrosine) and dried with air. The examiner looks at the area covered and scores from 0 to 5 (see box on p. 237 and Fig. 13-3,A). See Plate 1, I, for a clinical view of how the index is scored.

Two other area scoring indices that have placed emphasis not only on the gingival margin but also on the interproximal areas are the Modified Navy Plaque Index (Elliott et al, 1972) (Fig. 13-3,B) and the Martens and Meskin (1972) adaptation of the Podshadley and Haley index (Fig. 13-3,C). In these modified indices, the tooth is divided into nine or five segments respectively, and each segment is assigned a letter and a score of 0 to 1.

The O'Leary Plaque Control Record (O'Leary, Drake, and Naylor, 1972) was designed as a simple method for the dental professional to use in scoring areas of plaque accumulation for individ-

---

Silness and Löe

0 = No plaque
1 = A film of plaque adhering to the free gingival margin and adjacent areas of the tooth; the plaque may be seen *in situ* by using a probe on the tooth surface or by disclosing it
2 = Moderate accumulation of soft deposits within the gingival pocket or on the tooth and gingival margin that can be seen with the naked eye
3 = Abundance of soft matter within the gingival pocket and/or on the tooth and gingival margin

From Silness J and Löe H: Periodontal disease in pregnancy, II. Correlation between oral hygiene and periodontal condition, Acta Odont Scan 22:121, 1964.

---

ual patients. An oval symbol, representing each permanent tooth, has been divided into four segments to represent the mesial, distal, facial, and lingual surfaces. The use of this form to record baseline and recall plaque scores allows both the patient and the professional to visualize exactly where plaque remains. This visualization is valuable during plaque control instruction, as specific problem areas can be pointed out and discussed with the patient, along with possible solutions. In addition, both the professional and the patient can see visual evidence of progress at recall appointments when improved plaque records are compared with the initial record. This objective measure of patient progress can provide a sense of accomplishment and motivation for the patient.

The record is scored by disclosing the patient's teeth and then examining each tooth surface, using an explorer or the tip of a probe, for the presence of soft stained accumulations on the cervical third of the tooth at the dentogingival junction. If a soft deposit is visible, the corresponding surface is marked on the plaque control record by shading it or placing a dash in the area. Only plaque accumulation that occurs at the dentogingival junction is recorded on the form. Those surfaces that have soft accumulations that are not at the distogingival junction are not recorded. No attempt is made to differentiate between varying amounts of plaque on the tooth surfaces. Teeth that are not present in

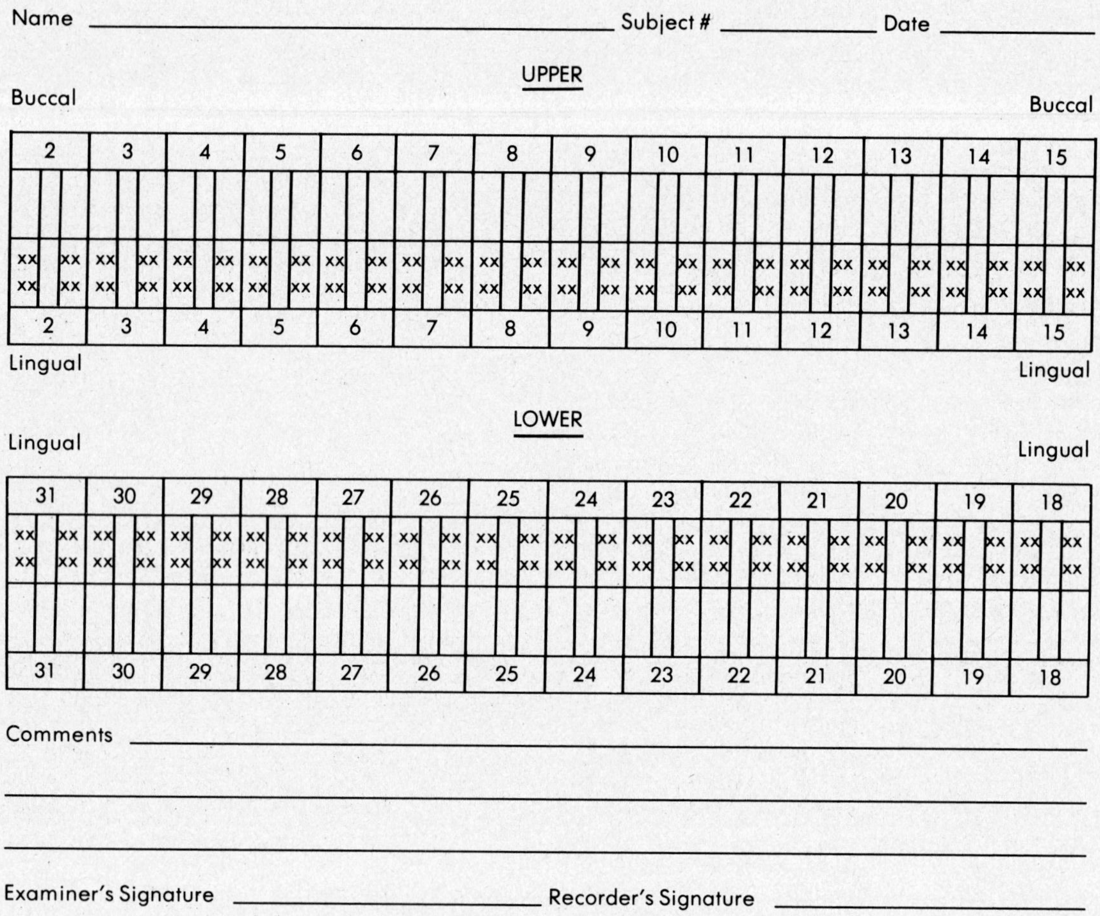

Name _____ Subject # _____ Date _____

UPPER

Buccal   Buccal

2	3	4	5	6	7	8	9	10	11	12	13	14	15
xx xx	xx xx	xx xx	xx xx	xx xx	xx xx	xx xx	xx xx	xx xx	xx xx	xx xx	xx xx	xx xx	xx xx
2	3	4	5	6	7	8	9	10	11	12	13	14	15

Lingual   Lingual

LOWER

Lingual   Lingual

31	30	29	28	27	26	25	24	23	22	21	20	19	18
xx xx	xx xx	xx xx	xx xx	xx xx	xx xx	xx xx	xx xx	xx xx	xx xx	xx xx	xx xx	xx xx	xx xx
31	30	29	28	27	26	25	24	23	22	21	20	19	18

Comments _____

_____

_____

Examiner's Signature _____ Recorder's Signature _____

Fig. 13-2. Suggested plaque index scoring form.

the mouth should be crossed out on the recording form (Fig. 13-4).

After all teeth have been examined, an index can be calculated by dividing the number of plaque-containing surfaces by the total number of available surfaces (total number of teeth $\times$ 4 surfaces). This procedure is repeated at each appointment; the percentages of plaque-covered surfaces are compared to evaluate the patient's progress.

Plaque area measurements require that plaque be visualized by the use of disclosing agents (Yankell and Emling, 1978). There are several commercially available plaque disclosing preparations that have been accepted by the American Dental Association. Following is a brief description of several available materials.

The most widely used disclosing agent has been erythrosine, or FD & C (Food, Drug, and Cosmetic) red No. 30 (Arnim, 1963). The primary problem with this material is that, because of its red color, it can be difficult to distinguish between stained deposits and stained gingiva. This agent stains the gingiva and other oral soft tissues, including the lips; it also has a potential for staining silicate fillings, clothing, and sink materials.

Another visible colorant used is FD & C green No. 30 (Mandel, 1974). This agent readily distinguishes plaque from the gingiva; however, it has

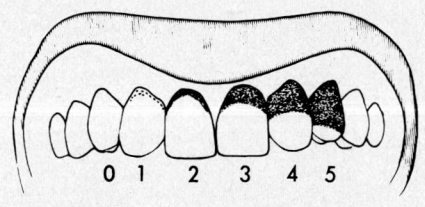

Quigley-Hein

The Turesky modification of this index was described in the article cited below. Plaque will be disclosed.

0 = No plaque

1 = Separate flecks or a discontinuous band of plaque at the gingival margin

2 = Thin (up to 1 mm) continuous band of plaque at the gingival margin

3 = Band of plaque wider than 1 mm but covering less than 1/3 of the gingival third of the tooth surface

4 = Plaque covering more than 1/3 but less than 2/3 of the tooth surface

5 = Plaque covering 2/3 or more of the tooth surface

From Turesky S, Gilmore, ND, and Glickman, I: Reduced plaque formation by the chloromethyl analogue of victamine C, J Periodontol 41:41, 1970.

CROWN AREA COVERED BY PLAQUE

A

0 — None

1 — Separate flecks

2 — Continuous band to 1 mm

3 — >1 mm and <⅓

4 — >⅓ and <⅔

5 — >⅔

Fig. 13-3. **A,** The plaque area scoring method, developed by Turesky, Gilmore, and Glickman.

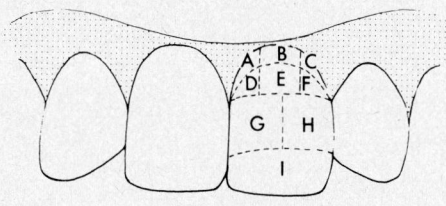

B

CROWN AREA COVERED BY PLAQUE

A,B,C — Continuous band to 1 mm

D,E,F — >1 mm and <⅓

G,H — >⅓ and <⅔

I — >⅔

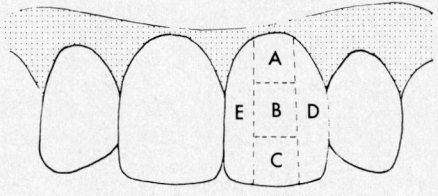

C

CROWN AREA COVERED BY PLAQUE

Middle area:

A — Gingival ⅓

B — Middle ⅓

C — Incisal ⅓

D — Distal area

E — Mesial area

Fig. 13-3. **B,** Modified Navy plaque index. **C,** Martens and Meskin adaptation of Podshadley and Haley index.

the same staining drawbacks as erythrosine. There are no commercially available products containing this colorant, and 2% to 5% solutions must be prepared by the researcher.

A commercially available combination of FD & C red No. 30 and FD & C blue No. 1 differentiates between old and newly formed plaque (Bloc, Lobene, and Derdivanis, 1972; Gallagher, Fussell, and Cutress, 1977). This differentiation is

due to differences in plaque penetration or permeability of these two different colorants. Again, this combination of food colors has the disadvantages of discoloring soft tissues and undesirable staining.

A different type of plaque disclosing system is Plak-Lite.* This system uses sodium fluorescein,

*Plak-Lite, Brilliant International, Bala-Cyrwyd PA

Name _____

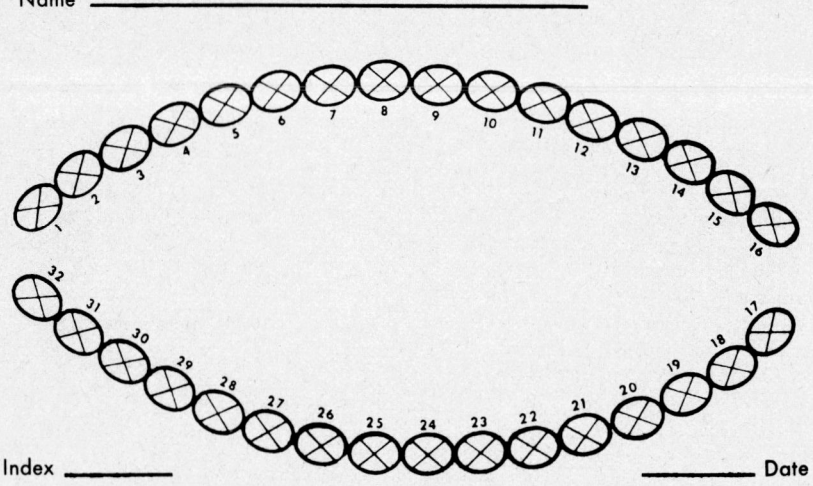

Index _____   _____ Date

Fig. 13-4. O'Leary plaque control record.
(From O'Leary TJ, Drake RB, and Naylor, JE: J Periodontol **43**:38, 1972.

which is not visible under normal light. Plaque stained with sodium fluorescein becomes visible only under a properly blue filtered light source (Lang, Ostergaard, and Löe, 1972). In laboratory studies, uptake of sodium fluorescein by plaque bacteria has been shown to be more specific than uptake of erythrosine (Landay et al, 1974).

Measurement of gingival inflammation

Gingivitis. Following are descriptions of several methods for measuring gingival inflammation.

Löe and Silness gingival index. Each gingival unit (the buccal, lingual, mesial, and distal aspects) of the individual tooth is scored. The gingiva is scored in four grades judged according to inflammation, color change and bleeding (see box). Fig. 13-5 provides a sample scoring form.

Lobene modification of the Lö and Silness. The Lobene modification produces a more sensitive scale in the first three grades of the index. The gingiva is scored in five grades (see box p. 239).

Gingival health has also been assessed by monitoring *gingival crevicular fluid (GCF) flow*. Flow of GCF begins before clinical signs of gingivitis can be ascertained (Borden, Golub, and Klein-

---

Gingival Indices: Löe and Silness

0 = Absence of inflammation, normal gingiva
1 = Mild inflammation: slight change in color and little change in texture
2 = Moderate inflammation: moderate glazing, redness, edema and hypertrophy; bleeding on probing
3 = Severe inflammation: marked redness and hypertrophy; tendency to spontaneous bleeding; ulceration

From Löe H: The gingival index, the plaque index, and the retention index systems, J. Periodontol 38:610, 1967.

---

berg, 1977; Löe and Holm-Pedersen, 1965; Pashley, 1976). Although GCF may not be related to preexisting gingival conditions, such as single measurements in the dental office, GCF flow can be used to monitor progress or control of gingival inflammation (Cimasoni, 1974; Golub and Kleinberg, 1976). A commercial digital unit to monitor GCF (Periotron*) is available. Following is a de-

*Periotron, Harco Electronics Winnipeg, Canada.

Name _____ Subject # _____ Date _____

UPPER

Buccal   Buccal

2	3	4	5	6	7	8	9	10	11	12	13	14	15
xx xx	xx xx	xx xx	xx xx	xx xx	xx xx	xx xx	xx xx	xx xx	xx xx	xx xx	xx xx	xx xx	xx xx
2	3	4	5	6	7	8	9	10	11	12	13	14	15

Lingual   Lingual

LOWER

Lingual   Lingual

31	30	29	28	27	26	25	24	23	22	21	20	19	18
xx xx	xx xx	xx xx	xx xx	xx xx	xx xx	xx xx	xx xx	xx xx	xx xx	xx xx	xx xx	xx xx	xx xx
31	30	29	28	27	26	25	24	23	22	21	20	19	18

Comments _____

_____

_____

Examiner's Signature _____ Recorder's Signature _____

Fig 13-5. Sample gingival index scoring form.

Gingival Indices: Lobene Modification of Löe and Silness

(Mesial-buccal, buccal, mesial-lingual, and lingual surfaces)

0 = Absence of inflammation

1 = Mild inflammation; slight change in color, little change in texture of any portion of, but not the entire, marginal or papillary gingival unit

2 = Mild inflammation: criteria as above but involving the entire marginal or papillary gingival unit

3 = Moderate inflammation: glazing, redness, edema, and/or hypertrophy of the marginal or papillary gingival unit

4 = Severe inflammation: marked redness, edema and/or hypertrophy of the marginal or papillary gingival unit; spontaneous bleeding, congestion, or ulceration

From Lobene RR et al: A modified gingival index for use in clinical trials, Clin Prev Dent **8**:3, 1986.

Sulcular Bleeding Index: Mühlemann and Son

0 = Healthy appearance of P and M, not bleeding on sulcus probing
1 = Apparently healthy P and M, showing no change in color and no swelling, but bleeding from sulcus on probing
2 = Bleeding on probing *and* change of color due to inflammation; No swelling or macroscopic edema
3 = Bleeding on probing *and* change in color and slight edematous swelling
4 = (1) Bleeding on probing *and* change in color *and* obvious swelling (2) Bleeding on probing and obvious swelling
5 = Bleeding on probing and spontaneous bleeding *and* change in color; marked swelling with or without ulceration.
Note: P = Papillary gingivae, M = Marginal gingivae. Score 4 has been subdivided into score 4 and 5 and redefined since the first communication (Mühlemann and Mazor, 1958).

From Mühlemann HR and Son S: Gingival sulcus bleeding — a leading symptom in initial gingivitis, Helv Odontol Acta 15:107, 1971

Papillary Bleeding Indices: Mühlemann

The periodontal probe used is rounded and dull (blunted) in order not to provoke traumatic bleeding.
0 = No bleeding after probing
1 = One singular point of bleeding after probing
2 = Several points of bleeding after probing
3 = The interdental triangle fills with blood after probing
4 = Blood flows immediately along the gingival groove after probing

From J Prev Dent **4**:6, 1977. Mühlemann HR: Psychological and chemical mediators of gingival health.

scription of the procedure for taking sample of GCF:

1. Isolate with cotton rolls and dry with gauze the region of the mouth under examination.
2. Place a dry paper strip in the facial crevice of the tooth to be monitored for 5 seconds to empty the crevicular pool of fluid; remove with tweezers and discard this strip.
3. Wait 30 seconds, and insert a dry paper strip in the crevice; wait for 5 seconds.
4. Remove the paper strip and immediately place in the Periotron for recording the crevicular fluid in this strip.

This procedure could be of value to the clinician monitoring treatment procedures or provide an incentive to the patient to improve home care of critical gingival areas.

Because of the difficulties involved in using

*Modified from Borden AM, Golub LM, and Kleinberg I. IDAR Abstract No. 482, 1974.

gingival indices, investigators should be trained in following standardized procedures before conducting clinical studies. Unfortunately, training of the dental professional today does not always include gingival indices. These indices are valuable to demonstrate to the patient those areas that require more attention during home care procedures. Even if only an all-or-none type of index is recorded, it is strongly recommended that the practitioner maintain a record of location of gingival problems as this parameter may often forecast major periodontal disease problems.

Sulcular bleeding index. This index considers color, contour, inflammation, and bleeding with probing. The index is scored in six grades (see box at left).

Papillary bleeding index (PBI). Papillary bleeding is an excellent indicator of gingival inflammation. This index is well suited for monitoring individual patients in clinical practice as well as for clinical research. Papillary inflammation is scored in five grades (see box above). A blunt probe is used to sweep the sulcus from the base to the tip of the papilla on the mesial and distal aspects.

The maxillary right and mandibular left quadrants are probed lingually, and the maxillary left and mandibular right quadrants are probed from the facial aspects. After probing each quadrant, which takes about 10 to 15 seconds, evaluate the bleeding scores of the probed sulci beginning from the first papilla probed. If no bleeding oc-

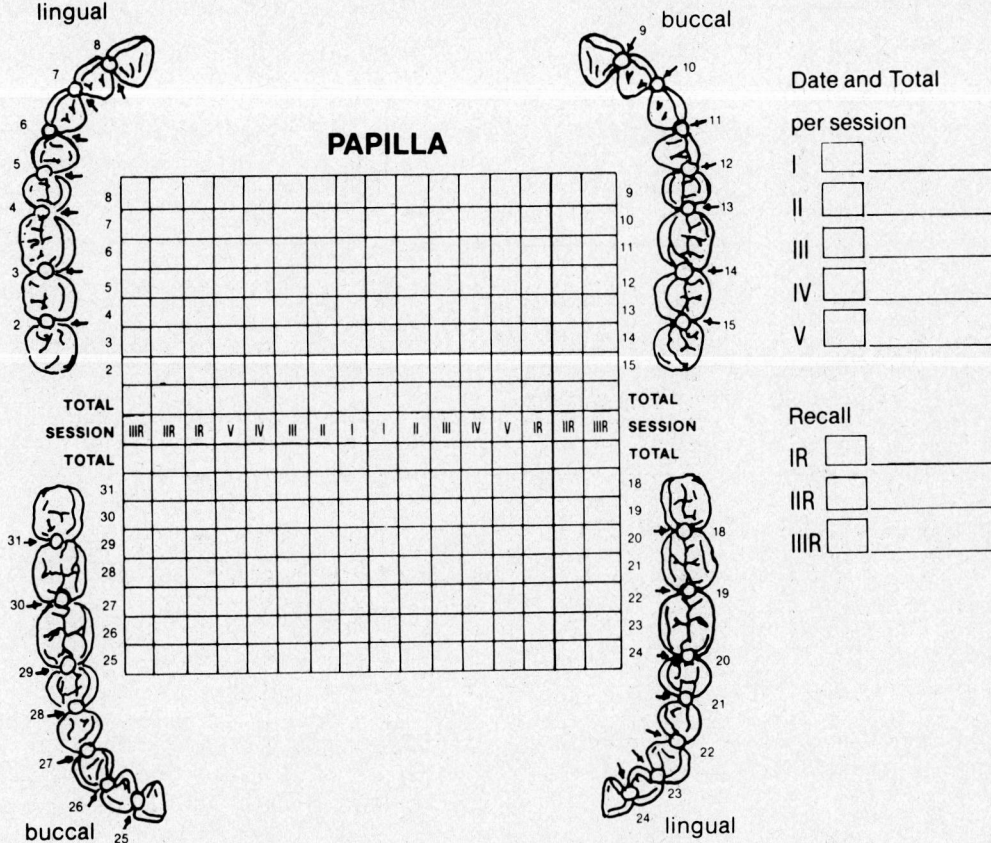

Fig. 13-6. Papillary Bleeding Index form.
(Courtesy University of Pennsylvania, Philadelphia.)

curs within 10 to 15 seconds, repeat the probing on individual papillae. Assessment of bleeding intensity is based on the criteria shown in the box.

Bleeding scores as they are evaluated at each visit are filled in on the PBI form (Fig. 13-7). When all teeth are present, 28 papillae can be scored. All papillae in the mouth are scored except between Nos. 8 and 9 and 24 and 25 and the distal aspects of third molars if present. If a tooth is missing, its corresponding papilla is crossed out on the form. After the individual scores are recorded, the scores for the four quadrants are added together and a total value is recorded for that session and entered to the right of the form.

The use of this index from a hygienist's point of view has recently been reported (Craig and Du-

hamel, 1981). In addition to its usefulness in the dental office, the PBI scoring method has been demonstrated to be effective in both school-based and public health programs (Saxter, Turconi, and Elsasser, 1977).

SUMMARY

The use of soft deposit and gingival indices in the dental office is important for several reasons. Initially, they are used as the basis for the patient's permanent record. From information obtained, the professional will be better able to establish a diagnosis and design the treatment plan. Indices also should be used to educate and motivate the patient.

Use scoring criteria in which the characteristic

Name _____ Subject # _____ Date _____

UPPER

Buccal   Buccal

2	3	4	5	6	7	8	9	10	11	12	13	14	15

2	3	4	5	6	7	8	9	10	11	12	13	14	15

Lingual   Lingual

LOWER

Lingual   Lingual

31	30	29	28	27	26	25	24	23	22	21	20	19	18

31	30	29	28	27	26	25	24	23	22	21	20	19	18

Comments _____

Examiner's Signature _____ Recorder's Signature _____

Fig. 13-7. Sample papillary bleeding index scoring form.

being examined can be clearly stated by the professional and understood by the patient. Indices properly used can measure the success of treatment and preventive home care programs and the long-term benefits of disease control.

ACTIVITIES

1. Examine plaque microscopically, identifying the kinds of microorganisms present.
2. Conduct a 3- to 5-day no-oral-hygiene study in the class, observing changes in the mouth. After using a plaque disclosant, document changes with intraoral photographs or by exposing several frames of 8 mm movie film each day to record and condense the progression of disease. Reverse the process by instituting brushing and flossing; record with photographs or daily exposure of movie film.
3. Use each of the described plaque and gingival indices on a student partner. Determine which methods are most easily incorporated in clinical practice for purposes of documentation and patient instruction.
4. Use a variety of disclosing solutions and evaluate each for its effectiveness, acceptability to the patient, and ease of use.

REVIEW QUESTIONS

1. Match the following terms with the appropriate descriptions. More than one answer may be correct.
   _____ Acquired pellicle
   _____ Materia alba
   _____ Food debris
   _____ Plaque
   a. Cannot be dislodged from the teeth with muscle action and vigorous water rinsing or irrigation

b. A dense coherent mass of microorganisms in an intermicrobial matrix

c. Primary source is oral microorganisms and salivary components

d. Can become impacted interdentally or mechanically in the plaque

e. A loosely adherent complex of bacteria and cellular debris that covers plaque

f. Will stain with a disclosant but appears lighter than disclosed plaque or calculus

g. Can be dislodged with muscular movements and water rinsing or irrigation

h. Reforms in a few hours after professional prophylaxis; cannot be brushed away

i. Major etiologic factor in dental caries and gingivitis

2. When plaque metabolizes or develops a basic pH, _____ of the microbial content occurs.

3. When plaque metabolizes carbohydrates, a(n) _____ pH occurs that leads to _____.

4. In no-oral-hygiene procedures, describe the plaque formation that occurs in the following organized and orderly fashion:
a. Days 1 to 2
b. Days 3 to 4
c. Days 6 to 10
d. Days 10 to 21

5. Identify 7 types of microorganisms found in loosely adherent, subgingival plaque.

6. Identify 4 types of agents used for disclosing plaque.

7. In gingival indices, the primary determinant in scoring is usually _____ and/or _____ in several aspects of each tooth or considering each tooth as a unit.

8. Why should plaque and gingival indices be incorporated routinely into clinical practice?

REFERENCES

Armstrong WG: The composition of organic films formed on teeth, Caries Res 1:89, 1967

Armin SS: The use of disclosing agents for measuring tooth cleanliness, J Periodontol 34:227, 1963

Barnes GP et al: Indices used to evaluate signs, symptoms, and etiologic factors associated with diseases of the periodontium, J Periodontol 56:643, 1986.

Block PL, Lobene RR, and Derdivanis JP: A two-tone dye test for dental plaque, J Periodontol 43:423, 1972.

Borden AM, Golub LM, and Kleinberg I: An intracrevicular technique for monitoring gingival crevicular fluid, IADR Abstract No. 482, 1974.

Borden AM, Golub LM, and Kleinberg I: The effect of age and sex on the relationship between crevicular fluid flow and gingivitis index in humans, J Periodont Res 12:160, 1977.

Christersson L et al: Tissue localization of actinobacillus acti-

nomycetemcomitans in human periodontitis, II. Correlation between immunofluorescence and culture techniques, J Periodontol 58(8):540, 1986.

Christersson L et al: Tissue localization of actinobacillus actinomycetemcomitans in human periodontitis, I. Light, immunofluorescence and electron microscopic studies, J Periodontol 58(8):529, 1987.

Cimasoni G: The crevicular fluid, ed 3. Basel, Switzerland, 1974, S Karger AG.

Craig D and Duhamel L: The papillary bleeding index: a new aspect in motivation. Eighth International Symposium on Dental Hygiene, Brighton, England, 1981.

Dawes, E: The nature of dental plaque, films, and calcareous deposits, Ann NY Acad Sci 153:102, 1968.

Driessens, FCM et al: On the physiochemistry of plaque calcification and the phase composition of dental calculus, J Perio Res 20:329, 1985.

Elliott, JR et al: Evaluation of an oral physiotherapy center in the reduction of bacterial plaque and periodontal disease, J Periodontol 43:332, 1972.

Fine, DH et al: Studies in plaque pathogenicity, I. Plaque collection and limulus lysate screening of adherent and loosely adherent plaque, J Periodont Res 13:17, 1978.

Fine DH et al: Studies in plaque pathogenicity, II. A technique for the specific detection of endotoxin in plaque samples using the limulus lysate assay, J Periodont Res 13:127, 1978.

Gallagher, IHC, Fussell, SJ, and Cutress, TW: Mechanism of action of a two-tone plaque disclosing agent, J Periodontol 48:395, 1977.

Gibbons, RJ and Van Houte J: On the formation of dental plaques, J Periodontol 44:347, 1973.

Goldman, HM and Cohen DW: Periodontal therapy, ed 6. St. Louis, 1980, The CV Mosby Co.

Golub, LM, and Kleinberg, I: Gingival crevicular fluid: a new diagnostic aid in managing the periodontal patient, Oral Sci Rev 8:49, 1976.

Jenkins, GN: The chemistry of plaque, Ann NY Acad Sci 131:786, 1965.

Katz, S, McDonald JL, and Stookey, GK: Preventive dentistry in action, ed 3. Upper Montclair, NJ, 1979, DCP Publishing.

Landay, MA, et al: A fluorescent microscopic study of human bacterial plaque smears stained with the plaklite fluorochrome, Calif Dent Assoc J 2:60, 1974.

Lang NP, Ostergaard E, and Löe: A fluorescent plaque disclosing agent, J Periodont Res 7:59, 1972.

Lie T: Ultrastructural study of early dental plaque formation, J Periodont Res 13:391, 1978.

Listgarten, MA, Mayo, HE, and Tremblay R: Development of dental plaque on epoxy resin crowns in man, J Periodontol 46:10, 1975.

Lobene, RR et al: A modified gingival index for use in clinical trials, Clin Prev Dent 8:3, 1986.

Löe H: The gingival index, the plaque index, and the retention index systems, J Periodontol 38:610, 1967.

Löe H and Holm-Pedersen P: Absence and presence of fluid from normal and inflamed gingivae, Periodontics 3:171, 1965.

Löe H, Theilade E, and Jensen SB: Experimental gingivitis in man, J Periodontol 36:177, 1965.

Loesche WJ et al: Bacterial profiles of subgingival plaques in periodontitis, J of Periodontol 56:8, 1985.

Mandel, ID: Indices for measurement of soft accumulations in clinical studies of oral hygiene and periodontal disease, J Periodont Res 9:7, 1974.

Martens LV and Meskin LH: An innovative technique for assessing oral hygiene, J Dent Child 39:12, 1972.

Mühlemann, HR: Psychological and chemical mediators of gingival health, J Prevent Dent 4:6, 1977.

Mühlemann HR and Mazor ZS: Gingivitis in Zurich schoolchildren, Helv Odontol Acta 2:3, 1958.

Mühlemann HR and Son S: Gingival sulcus bleeding —a leading symptom in initial gingivitis, Helv Odontol Acta 15:107, 1971.

O'Leary, TJ, Drake RB, and Naylor JE: The plaque control record, J Periodontol 43:38, 1972.

Osterberg SK-A, Sudo, SZ, and Folke LEA: Microbial succession in supragingival plaque of man, J Periodont Res 11:243, 1976.

Pashley, DH: A mechanistic analysis of gingival fluid production, J Periodont Res 11:121, 1976.

Pertuiset JH et al: Recurrent periodontal disease and bacterial presence in the gingiva, J Periodontol 58(8):553, 1987.

Rateitschak KH et al: Color atlas of periodontology. New York, 1985, Georg Thieme.

Saxer UP, Turconi B, and Elsasser CH: Patient motivation with the papillary bleeding index, J Prevent Dent 4:20, 1977.

Silness J and Löe H: Periodontal disease in pregnancy, II. Correlation between oral hygiene and periodontal condition, Acta Odontol Scand 22:121, 1964.

Socransky SS et al: New concepts of destructive periodontal disease, J Clin Periodont 11:21, 1969.

Socransky SS et al: Bacteriological studies of developing supragingival dental plaque, J Periodont Res 12:90, 1977.

Socransky SS et al: New concepts of destructive periodontal disease, J Clin Periodont 11:21, 1984.

Socransky SS and Haffajee AD: Frequency distribution of periodontal attachment loss—computer simulation, J Clin Periodontol 13(6):617, 1986.

Turesky S, Gilmore ND, and Glickman I: Reduced plaque formation by the chloromethyl analogue of vitamine C, J Periodontol 41:41, 1970.

Yankell SL and Emling RC: Understanding dental products: what you should know and what your patient should know, Cont Dent Ed, Univer of Penn School of Dental Medicine 1(7):1, 1978.

14 PERIODONTAL EXAMINATION AND CHARTING

OBJECTIVES: *The reader will be able to*

1. Discuss seven uses of the periodontal examination and charting.
2. Identify the significance of the following factors to the periodontal examination: missing teeth; unerupted, impacted, or supernumerary teeth; malpositioned teeth; open contacts; poorly contoured restorations and crowns; prosthetic devices; and carious lesions.
3. Discuss the procedure for examining and charting each of the following:
    a. Pocket depths
    b. Gingival height/recession
    c. Masticatory mucosa
    d. Attached gingiva
    e. Mobility
    f. Furcations
4. Describe four complications of periodontal probing and explain how to handle them.
5. Discuss the characteristics of effective probing in terms of adaptation and angulation of the tip, amount of pressure needed, and number and location of probe readings on each tooth.
6. Discuss the limitations of the various types of data collected to document periodontal disease.
7. Describe appropriate records and documentation of periodontal diagnosis, treatment, and referral.

PERIODONTAL DISEASE

The major purpose of the periodontal examination is to correlate the clinical signs and patient symptoms that point to either the presence of or the potential for periodontal disease. Periodontal disease may be inflammatory in nature, such as in gingivitis and periodontitis, or it may be noninflammatory, as in occlusal trauma. A basic understanding of these conditions is necessary to distinguish among their clinical signs and to understand the significance of collecting data for periodontal examination.

Gingivitis

Gingivitis is an inflammation of the gingiva and is the most common form of gingival disease. Its primary cause is the presence and composition of bacterial plaque in and around the gingival sulcus. Secondary causes include factors that contribute to the accumulation of supragingival plaque, in-terfere with its removal, or enhance the susceptibility of gingival tissues to infection (such as tooth position and anatomy, malocclusion, calculus, mouth breathing, dental restorations, and prostheses, systemic disease, pregnancy, stress, and trauma).

Gingivitis can be either *acute* or *chronic*. An acute inflammation is one which occurs suddenly, is associated with pain, and is of short duration. Acute necrotizing ulcerative gingivitis and acute herpetic gingivostomatitis are examples of acute inflammatory reactions in the gingiva. Chronic gingivitis, in contrast, begins slowly, is of a long duration, and is usually painless unless the tissues become secondarily infected. Gingivitis may also be *recurrent,* meaning that it returns following treatment or disappears spontaneously and then reappears.

Gingivitis may vary in severity in different sites in the mouth and may show varying patterns of distribution within the mouth, depending on the presence and composition of bacterial plaque. *Localized gingivitis* is confined to a specific area of the mouth, while *generalized gingivitis* involves the entire mouth. *Papillary gingivitis* involves the interdental papillae and may extend onto adjacent marginal gingiva. Most gingivitis develops first in the interdental papilla and then spreads to adjacent tissues. *Marginal gingivitis* involves the gingival margins of the teeth in addition to the papillae and may also include a portion of the attached gingiva. *Diffuse gingivitis* involves inflammation of all involved gingival tissues including papillae, marginal gingiva, and attached gingiva.

Epidemiology of gingivitis. Marginal gingivitis begins in early childhood, increases in prevalence and severity through the teenage years, and then levels off and becomes less severe in young adults. Although there is very little data regarding the prevalence of gingivitis in adults, estimates are that it affects from 50% to 100% of adults who still have natural teeth. The elderly do not appear to have higher prevalence rates than the rest of the adult population. Overall, the prevalence of gingivitis appears to be declining.

Males usually have higher amounts of gingival inflammation than females, although a significant number of women experience more severe gingivitis (pregnancy gingivitis) during pregnancy. Blacks tends to have a higher prevalence of gingivitis than whites, although these higher rates are likely to be more related to other factors such as oral hygiene, socioeconomic status, and access to dental care (Stamm, 1986).

Clinical signs of gingivitis. Clinical detection of gingivitis depends on recognition of inflammatory signs within the gingival tissues. In the early stages of inflammation, these signs may be subtle and difficult to discern; they become more obvious as the inflammation becomes established. The gingival tissues should be examined for signs of bleeding, exudate, or abnormal color, size, contour, consistency, surface texture, position, or pain. Table 14-1 lists characteristic signs of normal and abnormal (inflamed) gingival tissues. Each of these clinical characteristics will be discussed in detail later in the chapter in relation to their significance to the periodontal examination.

Acute forms of gingivitis. Although chronic gingivitis is the more common type of gingival inflammation, the dental hygienist should also recognize signs and symptoms of acute gingival inflammation. The presence of pain and rapid destruction of affected tissues makes it imperative that these conditions receive prompt diagnosis and treatment. The hygienist is responsible for recognizing acute infections during the periodontal examination, gathering assessment information, recording significant findings in the patient's record, and reporting those findings to the dentist for diagnosis and treatment. In many cases the hygienist is also qualified to implement part or all of the prescribed treatment.

Acute Necrotizing Ulcerative Gingivitis (ANUG). This acute gingival inflammation is also known as trench mouth, Vincent's gingivitis, Vincent's gingivostomatitis, and necrotizing gingivitis. It is most prevalent in young adults between the ages of 18 and 30 and is associated with factors other than those that cause chronic gingivitis. Three specific factors seem to be most frequently implicated in the occurrence of this condition: (1) poor oral hygiene in the presence of an existing chronic gingivitis; (2) smoking (Goldhaber and Giddon, 1964); and (3) emotional stress (Giddon et al, 1964).

The most obvious clinical signs of ANUG is ulceration of the marginal gingiva and interdental papilla. This destruction begins with the appearance of a necrotic ulcer on the papilla that rapidly progresses until the entire papilla is destroyed, leaving a central depression or crater where the intact papilla once stood. The necrosis spreads to the adjacent marginal gingiva and other papillae. The affected gingiva is often covered with a greyish or yellowish "pseudomembrane," composed of necrotic tissue, bacteria, and destroyed blood cells, which forms over the red, raw, exposed connective tissues. This lesion is extremely painful to the patient, so that the situation is exacerbated by a continued lack of plaque control. Spontaneous bleeding and a characteristic foul odor are also common findings. In advanced cases swelling of the regional lymph nodes (regional lymphadenitis) may also be present.

The initial treatment of ANUG involves relief of the acute symptoms by removing local etiologic factors. Gross scaling, preferably accomplished with an ultrasonic scaler, will help relieve the acute symptoms. This initial debridement can

Table 14-1. Gingival assessment: clinical characteristics

Clinical characteristic	Ideal/Normal	Abnormal
Color	Uniformly coral pink Variations may occur depending on patient's complexion and race	Acute—bright red Chronic—red, bluish red, dark pink Color changes may be restricted to papilla or extend to marginal and attached gingiva
Contour	Margins are knifelike Contour of free margin forms regular parabolic curve as it goes around teeth Papillae are pointed and fill embrasure space	Margins become rolled, bulbous, enlarged; irregular contour may be noted; clefting, festooning Papillae may be flattened, bulbous, blunted, or cratered
Size	Free margin is near cementoenamel junction (CEJ) Margin adheres closely to tooth	Enlarged because of excess fluid in tissues (edematous) or buildup of collagen fibers (fibrotic) Margin may be retracted away from tooth with air or instrument
Consistency	Firm	Edematous, soft, spongy; pressure on tissues with an instrument will leave a dent Fibrotic, firm, hard tissue
Surface texture	Smooth free gingiva Stippled attached gingiva	Acute—loss of stippling; smooth, shiny Chronic—stippling present; may increase in occurrence
Position of gingival margin	1 to 2 mm above CEJ in fully erupted teeth	May be enlarged so that margin is more coronal than CEJ May show apical recession so that root surface is exposed
Position of junctional epithelium	At CEJ in fully erupted teeth	Apical migration onto root surface
Mucogingival junction	Clear distinction between appearance of attached gingiva (pink, stippled, immobile, firm) and alveolar mucosa (red, shiny, smooth, mobile)	Lack of attached gingiva determined by 1. Loss of junctional line 2. Mobility of all existing tissues 3. Probing extends beyond mucogingival junction
Bleeding	No bleeding detectable with palpation or probing	Spontaneous bleeding Bleeding resulting from probing
Exudate	No exudate with palpation or probing	Increase in amount of clear crevicular fluid Presence of white fluid (pus) with palpation

Data from Examination and Diagnosis, 1975; Goldman and Cohen, 1980; Wilkins, 1983.

be followed at a later appointment by fine scaling and curettage when the pain and discomfort have been reduced. Patients should be instructed to perform gentle but thorough plaque control in all areas. As it is painful to touch the inflamed tissues, brushing and frequent rinsing should be instituted first, followed by flossing after some healing has occurred. The patient should rinse the mouth frequently with equal parts of hydrogen peroxide and warm water as a supplement to plaque control.

Following removal of all local etiologic factors, the other cause-related factors (such as poor oral hygiene habits, smoking, and stress) must be addressed to avoid recurrence. After initial therapy has been completed, periodontal surgery may be indicated to restore a normal contour to the gingiva; this will support the patient's plaque removal efforts (Goldman and Cohen, 1980; Lindhe, 1983; Johnson and Engel, 1986).

Acute herpetic gingivostomatitis. Acute herpetic gingivostomatitis is an infection of the oral tissues caused by the herpes simplex virus. Clinically, this infection appears as diffuse redness of the mucosa with associated edema, gingival bleeding, and pain. Vesicles form initially and later rupture to form small painful ulcers, which make chewing, eating, or drinking extremely uncomfortable for the patient until the ulcers have healed. The disease runs a course of about 7 to 10 days, with the most acute stages lasting for 2 to 3 days. This disease is seen most commonly in children under the age of 6, but it can also occur in older children and adults.

Desquamative gingivitis. Desquamative gingivitis is the term used to describe the gingival manifestations of a variety of systemic disturbances, most notably lichen planus or mucous membrane pemphigoid. Mild forms occur most often in young females and appear as diffuse painless redness (erythema) of the gingival tissues. Moderate forms occur most often in persons between the ages of 30 and 40 and are accompanied by burning sensations and sensitivity to temperature changes. Individuals may be unable to tolerate spicy or rough-textured foods and may experience pain during toothbrushing. Clinically, the tissues may appear smooth and shiny, with patches of bright red and gray areas. The surface epithelium may peel away from the underlying tissues exposing a raw, bleeding, and extremely painful surface. These signs and symptoms are worse as more severe forms of the infection develop.

Treatment of this condition is mainly palliative and involves careful plaque control with a soft brush and oxidizing mouthwashes (such as one part hydrogen peroxide to two parts warm water) (Carranza and Perry 1986). Careful examination of the patient's medical history and oral condition is necessary to identify the exact nature of the infection or infections which are contributing to the symptoms. Once the contributing factors have been identified, the dentist can determine the need for systemic therapy or other treatment.

Pericoronitis. A localized gingivitis that occurs around a partially erupted tooth, such as an erupting third molar, is called pericoronitis. The gingival tissue which lays over the partially erupted crown is a prime area for accumulation of plaque and food impaction. The nature of the inflammation may be acute, subacute or chronic. Acute inflammation of these areas is characterized by swelling, redness, exudate, and pain that may radiate to areas in the ear, throat, or floor of the mouth. Tenderness of lymph nodes, facial swelling, inability to close the mouth, fever, and malaise may also be associated with the acute form of the infection.

Treatment involves local removal of the bacterial and other irritants, use of antibacterial or antiseptic rinses. Systemic symptoms may require antibiotic treatment.

Acute gingival abscess. A gingival abscess is a localized, painful, and rapidly progressing lesion that develops suddenly and appears as a red, swollen, smooth, shiny, and painful area. Within 24 to 48 hours, the inflammatory process has resulted in a localized accumulation of pus, causing the lesion to "point" so that exudate can be expressed from its orifice. An abscess can develop in response to a puncture or irritation by a sharp object, such as a toothbrush bristle, or when foreign substances, such as popcorn hulls, become embedded in the tissue. These lesions usually rupture spontaneously, expelling the foreign materials, and heal.

Inflammation due to systemic factors. The following systemic factors may cause inflammation of the gingival tissue.

Pregnancy gingivitis. Changes in the hormonal balances and tissue metabolism in pregnancy can result in exaggerated responses of gingival tissue to local irritants and plaque. The clinical response to irritants under these conditions may result in generalized signs of gingivitis, including gingival enlargement, redness, and bleeding upon probing or spontaneously. Gingivitis related to pregnancy may also be manifested as localized enlargements of gingiva, known as "pregnancy tumors." These tumors appear as raised spherical lesions that extend from the gingival margin or the interdental papillae and are attached by a sessile or pedunculated base to the underlying tissues. Treatment includes removal of local irritants through professional and personal plaque control methods.

Puberty gingivitis. Enlargement of gingival tissues may also occur as an exaggerated response to local irritation in both males and females during puberty. The interdental papillae are the areas most often affected. Treatment involves individual plaque control and professional removal of calculus and other local irritants. Once the hormonal changes associated with puberty have moderated, the exaggerated response of the gingival tissues to plaque and calculus also subsides.

Other systemic factors that may affect the gingival response to inflammation include use of oral contraceptives, diabetes mellitus, diseases that affect the immune response, nutritional deficiencies, allergy, and metal poisoning.

Gingival hyperplasia. Use of the anticonvulsant drug Dilantin can lead to chronic enlargement (hyperplasia) of the gingiva. The initial lesion begins as a firm, pale pink, resilient enlargement of the gingival margin and interdental tissues that shows no bleeding tendency unless aggravated by secondary inflammation. Enlargement occurs gradually and can continue until a large portion of the crowns of the teeth are covered by tissue overgrowth, which can interfere with the occlusion. The presence of local irritants is not necessary for this enlargement to occur, but such irritants can result in a secondary inflammation that further complicates the exiting hyperplasia. When this condition becomes a functional or esthetic problem the tissue can be surgically removed, but the condition will recur unless use of the drug is discontinued.

PROGRESSION OF CHRONIC GINGIVITIS AND PERIODONTITIS
Gingivitis

The progression of gingival and periodontal inflammation has been described in terms of four progressive phases. The first phase is called the *initial lesion* and is the normal response of these tissues to the early plaque colonization. It occurs within 4 days of plaque accumulation. It includes increased vascular response and increased permeability of tissues to allow the passage of fluid and cells from the blood into the affected area. As almost everyone normally has some plaque accumulation in the mouth, there is some disagreement as to whether or not this category can be said to include healthy tissues as well as the initial stages of inflammation. Clinically, there is no clear-cut line of demarcation between the two situations. The *early lesion* is the second phase. It begins about 1 week after the formation of plaque. It includes the clinical signs of gingivitis in addition to the presence of lymphocytes and macrophages. The *established lesion* follows and is characterized by the further destruction of connective tissue fibers, the formation of a gingival pocket, and a predominance of plasma cells in the tissues. Some cases of established gingivitis remain stable and do not progress for months or even years, while other cases may convert to pro-

gressive destructive lesions. The last phase of inflammation, the *advanced lesion,* is characterized by the destruction of supporting tissues as well as gingival tissues and is also known as *periodontitis.* Although these levels of disease are described as stages, it is important to remember that activities within these stages can be stabilized for long periods or arrested, and that reversals can occur either spontaneously or as a result of treatment.

Chronic gingivitis and periodontitis are associated with the presence of microbial plaque. The plaque microorganisms contain or release substances that cause inflammatory reponses in the gingival and periodontal tissues (Lindhe, 1983). Even a healthy gingival sulcus may have a small number of bacteria and a slight inflammatory reponse (connective tissue infiltrate) at all times (Page and Schroeder, 1976), but the body's defense mechanisms and the ability of the microorganisms to cause infection are in balance; in other words, an equilibrium exists that allows both entities to coexist without a battle. When this equilibrium is maintained, there is no need for the body to initiate a full-scale inflammatory reaction in order to control the microorganisms; therefore, there are no inflammatory signs within the tissues.

The body has four major biological mechanisms for controlling infection. First, an intact epithelium of mucous membrane and skin prohibits access of the bacteria into the deeper tissues. The second mechanism is an army of inflammatory cells, including polymorphonucleocytes and macrophages, that localize and destroy the pathogens that may have gained entry into tissues before they can spread into adjoining tissues. The third mechanism of control is the body's immune response, whereby chemicals are produced to neutralize bacterial byproducts and toxins and to assist in the removal of bacteria from the infected area. The final mechanism is the varying ability of tissues to undergo repair and/or regeneration to restore their natural barriers and functions that may have been damaged as a result of infection and the inflammatory process (Listgarten, 1986; Page, 1986).

The equilibrium between existing microorganisms and body tissues can be maintained over an indefinite length of time as long as both the host tissue and the bacteria remain balanced in strength. A situation that overchallenges these mechanisms or a weak link in the system, however, will upset the equilibrium established between pathogens and the body, resulting in infection, inflammation, and associated tissue destruction.

Before the onset of disease, the tooth surface adjacent to the gingival sulcus is generally colonized by a thin layer of microorganisms that are predominantly gram-positive; they are found normally in the oral flora and are compatible with health. The normal residents of the healthy sulcus include *Streptococcus* and *Actinomyces* as well as other microbial species. An intact epithelial lining and frequent epithelial cell turnover within the sulcus prevent bacteria from entering the soft tissues adjacent to the tooth. Any bacterial toxins are easily neutralized and removed by the individual's normal defense mechanisms.

If plaque is allowed to accumulate beyond acceptable levels, however, or if it matures to a more pathogenic composition, these changes present an additional challenge to the body's defense. The result is an increased inflammatory reaction between the body's defense cells and the bacterial invaders. Polymorphonucleocytes begin to pour into the junctional epithelium, and lymphocytes enter the underlying connective tissues. Plasma cells may dominate the inflammatory infiltrate, and the ensuing battle between host and microorganisms may result in the destruction of gingival connective tissue fibers.

Clinical signs of the inflammation, such as redness, swelling, exudate, and bleeding, become more apparent as the reaction continues. The body may be able to adapt to the changed conditions so that a new equilibrium is established without resolution of the existing tissue responses to inflammation; thus, the condition becomes chronic in nature. As the equilibrium between the body and the microbes continues to shift, cycles of increased or diminished inflammation occur. In some cases the tissues may be able to repair spontaneously, in others they undergo continued damage and destruction.

Periodontal disease

When the destruction reaches the level of the connective tissues that form the attachment to the root of the tooth, gingivitis becomes periodontitis. It is important to note that not all sites affected by gingivitis will progress to periodontitis and that periodontitis can occur without a previous gingivitis. Periodontal disease is an inflammation and destruction of the supporting tissues of the tooth, including loss of connective tissue attachment to the root surface; loss of periodontal ligament fibers; and loss of alveolar bone. Over time, continued periodontal destruction is associated with the development of deep pockets, gingival recession, exposure of furcations, mobility, secondary occlusal trauma, and the ultimate consequence of tooth loss. Periodontal disease is a chronic condition that is progressive and destructive. The severity of the condition increases with age.

Although most cases of periodontitis fall into the category of *adult periodontitis,* a number of other categories of periodontitis which affect younger individuals have been categorized under the following names: *juvenile periodontitis, prepubertal periodontitis,* and *rapidly progressing periodontitis* (Page and Schroeder 1976). This chapter will focus on the detection and documentation of the most common type of periodontal disease, adult periodontitis.

As periodontal disease progresses, the composition of the microbial plaque begins to change. Bacteria associated with a healthy sulcus are predominantly nonmotile, gram-positive cocci and rods. More complex compositions of bacteria are associated with gingivitis and periodontitis and include an increasing proportion of motile, gram-negative, and anaerobic species. Although evidence does not implicate specific microorganisms as the major pathogens in adult periodontitis, certain microorganisms seem to be more strongly associated with this disease than others; among these are *Bacteroides intermedius, Bacteroides gingivalis, Wolinella recta, Actinobacillus actinomycetemcomitans,* and spirochetes (Loesche et al, 1985; Slots, 1986).

Periodontal disease is currently considered to be a group of infections rather than a single infection with a single etiology. Each periodontal infection is associated with different and specific groups of microorganisms (Newman, 1985). No single bacterial species has been identified as the primary cause of active periodontal disease. It appears instead that different bacteria that are already present in the mouth combine to produce the pathogenic potential necessary to initiate the progression from gingivitis to destructive periodontitis (Theilade, 1986). The exact nature of these microbial combinations is likely to differ depending on the person and the specific site. Pathogenicity is also related to the host response, so that bacteria which are pathogenic to one person may not be destructive in another person. The complexity of the interrelationships of all these factors explains why attempts to determine the exact bacterial etiology of periodontal disease and the conditions that must exist in order to predict disease activity have not yet been successful (Socransky et al, 1987).

Active periodontal destruction occurs with differing levels of severity and at different rates in selected sites in the same person. Periodontal disease is site-specific, meaning that the onset of the disease can occur in some areas of the mouth without affecting others (Haffajee et al, 1983; Socransky et al, 1984). The disease is cyclical in nature and does not progress in a linear fashion over time. Instead, it occurs as short bursts of intense activity and destruction that are followed by periods of remission, which can last months or years (Lindhe, 1983). Each burst of activity, however, results in additional destruction of the periodontal tissues, so that the apparent result over a long period of time appears to be a steady progression of disease.

The progression from health to gingivitis to periodontitis is characterized by long periods of remission and spontaneous reversals of disease interspersed with short bursts of destructive activity (Lindhe 1983; Page 1986). Some individuals are more susceptible to periodontal disease, as are specific sites within the mouth of the same individual. Even after treatment, some individuals remain more susceptible than others to recurrence of the disease as only a small percentage of treated patients account for most of the disease recurrence.

The prognoses for gingivitis and periodontitis are quite different. The damaged epithelium and connective tissues that form the gingival unit can regenerate if the cause of the inflammation, called the *etiologic agent,* is removed from the soft tissue environment. Therefore, simple gingivitis can often be treated quite successfully and the tissues

brought back to normal form and function. This is not the case with periodontitis, because supporting bone does not have the same ability to repair and restore the bone that has been destroyed by the inflammatory process. Another result of this disease is the apical migration of the junctional epithelium, which results in the formation of deep periodontal pockets that are difficult, if not impossible, for the patient to maintain free of plaque. If the disease process has spread to involve the supporting structures, there is permanent loss of tissues and an increased potential for the condition to persist or recur. It is painfully clear that the only effective method of curbing this disease and restoring the tissues to complete health is to recognize early signs of gingival inflammation and to eliminate the etiologic factors that cause it to occur. It is especially important to teach the patient to control etiologic factors, mainly dental plaque, before the condition develops into periodontitis.

The third form of periodontal disease is not inflammatory but degenerative in nature. This condition, known as *occlusal trauma,* is one in which the supporting structures of affected teeth are damaged because they cannot withstand the occlusal forces that act on them. The result is a breakdown of the periodontal ligament fibers, loss of supporting bone, widening of the periodontal ligament space, and tooth mobility. When this destruction is caused by excessive occlusal forces acting on an otherwise normal periodontium, the condition is referred to as *primary occlusal trauma.* The sources of the pressure may include bruxism, night grinding, malocclusion, or poorly constructed dental restorations. These factors can produce more stress than the supporting structures can withstand, and the result is that they are slowly destroyed. *Secondary occlusal trauma* is the result of normal occlusal forces on an attachment apparatus that has already been damaged and weakened by periodontitis. Some of the clinical signs of occlusal trauma include a widened periodontal ligament space, root fractures, loss of lamina dura, mobility, and signs of attrition or facets on the crowns of teeth (Grant et al, 1988).

It is not our purpose to provide detailed descriptions of these three forms of periodontal disease; a periodontal text will best serve that need. However, a basic understanding of their similarities and differences will help the beginning student understand the purpose for gathering as much data describing the periodontal condition of each patient as possible to ensure that accurate diagnosis and effective treatment planning will follow.

PURPOSE OF THE PERIODONTAL EXAMINATION

This chapter describes the complete periodontal examination and gives suggestions as to how it may be recorded on the periodontal charting form. The information gathered and recorded during the periodontal examination will assist the clinician in correlating all factors that might aid in assessing and describing the level of periodontal health or disease present in each patient. Without the information from a complete periodontal examination, diagnosis and treatment planning could be a hit-and-miss proposition, based on conjecture and not on reliable observed data.

In addition to the periodontal charting, many other diagnostic aids contribute vital information to the clinician. These aids include medical and dental histories, a head and neck examination, dental chartings, radiographs, study models, bite registration, photographs, and plaque and gingival indices. All of these assessment tools together provide a total picture of the patient's periodontal condition and permit comprehensive treatment planning. Exact descriptions of these other components are contained elsewhere in this text. The information they provide is supplemental to the periodontal examination, and specific situations in which they may be used are mentioned as the periodontal examination is described.

USES OF PERIODONTAL CHARTING

The data that are collected and recorded in a periodontal charting serve a number of purposes for both the patient and clinician. As part of an initial examination, periodontal charting provides a record of *baseline data* that describes the patient's periodontal condition before initial therapy is instituted. These data will later serve as a means for evaluating the success of treatment and preventive practices. Over a period of time, changes in the patient's periodontal status can be noted to trace the control of disease and restoration of health. The periodontal charting provides *information*

that is necessary to establish a diagnosis of the patient's condition. It consolidates a comprehensive collection of clinical data that, along with other components of the periodontal examination, allows for a careful analysis of all observable conditions so that an accurate diagnosis can be made. Because the periodontal charting represents the clinical conditions in written form, this analysis can occur without the patient's presence. The accumulation of all available clinical signs and symptoms will help the dental professional identify early signs of inflammatory disease while it still may be reversible.

After a diagnosis is made and confirmed, the periodontal charting continues to serve as a *resource for treatment planning*. Its information assists in establishing treatment priorities and in answering the following questions:

1. What areas show the most acute signs of disease and appear to have the highest potential for causing pain and/or destruction?
2. Which conditions demand additional examination or testing?
3. What types of treatment might be most effective?
4. What etiologic factors are present?
5. What combination of patient and professional efforts will be necessary to restore the tissues to health?

Data that have been recorded as part of a complete periodontal charting can be used to formulate treatment plans for restorative, periodontal, and preventive therapy. During the presentation of the treatment plan, the periodontal charting and other diagnostic aids provide visual evidence of the clinical findings to the patient, so that the diagnosis and its treatment can be understood.

The periodontal chart also serves as a valuable aid for the clinician during *implementation of the treatment plan*. During probing, scaling, root planing, and curettage, the chart can be used as a road map for instrumentation. Information such as the depth of pockets, root morphology, exposure of furcation areas, and mobility will affect the clinician's choice of instruments and the approach to scaling and root planing. When it is known from the chart that deep and complex pocket morphologies are present, the clinician can be more alert to tactile clues during exploring and probing and can plan effective approaches to areas in which access may prove challenging. Information recorded during the periodontal charting will help identify the need for special treatment procedures, such as temporary ligation of mobile teeth to facilitate scaling and root planing. It may also identify a need to recontour restorations so that their plaque-retentive characteristics are eliminated or at least reduced. The description of the pocket morphology and degree of destruction incurred by the soft and hard tissues will assist the clinician in determining indications for subsequent root planing and soft tissue curettage.

After treatment is completed, the periodontal chart serves as a valuable *reference for evaluating treatment success*. A posttreatment charting, when compared with pretreatment records, will indicate in which areas the soft tissues have been restored to some degree of normal form and function. It will also serve as a point from which referrals for more advanced treatment, such as periodontal surgery, may be made. The periodontal chart should be updated during recall appointments to document the patient's periodontal status over a period of time. If the gingiva remains healthy and shallow probing depths are maintained, it is an indication that home care, professional treatment, and recall intervals have been effective in health maintenance. If, on the other hand, subsequent chartings show that periodontal destruction is continuing, this evidence is a flagrant signal that one or all of these criteria need additional assessment and modification.

This permanent record of periodontal status is valuable not only for the clinician but also for the patient who is receiving verification of the success of treatment at the same time. Periodontal charting can be useful as *legal evidence* to support a diagnosis and to justify subsequent treatment. In addition, a periodontal chart can provide information about the rationale for proposed or actual treatment in cases involving a third-party payer such as an insurance carrier. A less familiar use of dental records, including periodontal charts, is their application in *forensic dentistry*. A periodontal chart may be used to identify deceased individuals. Their dental and periodontal conditions are as specific to them as their fingerprints; thus, dental records can be invaluable for making or confirming positive identification.

PREAPPOINTMENT CHARTING

Before the actual clinical examination of a patient, many factors relevant to the periodontal diagnosis may be assessed and charted from study models and radiographs. The advantage of studying these records is twofold. First, they provide information that can be reviewed when the patient is not present. The clinician can take the time needed to examine both the study models and radiographs carefully and in detail for possible etiologic factors that might affect the periodontal diagnosis and final treatment plan. Second, information from the study models and radiographs alerts the dental professional to search for particular clinical signs and symptoms which might be otherwise overlooked. This preparation can save time during the appointment and can reduce the time required to reach a diagnosis. The following paragraphs identify factors of the periodontal charting and examination which can be assessed in advance with the aid of radiographs and study models. The significance of each factor to the periodontal examination is described. Many of these factors have already been identified as components of a comprehensive charting (see Chapter 11).

Missing teeth should be noted, whether they are congenitally missing, extracted, or unerupted. This factor can be assessed from both the radiographs and the study models. Radiographs can help the professional determine whether the teeth are actually missing or simply unerupted. Radiographs will also provide the clinician with a view of root morphology and will assist in tooth identification. Study models assist in the identification of missing teeth by providing the clinician with the coronal anatomy of all erupted teeth. Missing teeth are significant in a periodontal examination because they may indicate a past history of periodontal disease. Areas left vacant by missing teeth also affect the distribution of teeth. The imbalanced forces can result in periodontal breakdown and occlusal trauma (Goldman and Cohen, 1980).

Malpositioned teeth should be noted during the periodontal examination. Malpositioned teeth are not only susceptible to occlusal trauma but may also point to previous destructive disease because the shifting may have been caused by breakdown of periodontal support (see Plate 2, *F* and *G*).

Other signs of abnormal occlusal stresses or wear can be detected in radiographs and study models. The radiographs will reveal signs of occlusal trauma such as periodontal ligament spaces that are abnormally wide because of increased pressures on the teeth. There may be signs of root fracture or loss of lamina dura. Attrition patterns on occlusal or incisal surfaces (wear facets) may be detectable on the radiographs but can be seen more clearly on the study models as flattened areas on the cusp tips or occlusal surfaces resulting from constant wear of opposing teeth. Wear facets are charted by shading on either the facial or occlusal views of the teeth that portion of the tooth that has undergone the wear.

Teeth that are *impacted* or *supernumerary* can be detected in radiographs. An unerupted tooth is one that is incomplete in its formation or not yet visible in the mouth. An impacted tooth is one that may be completely formed but is obstructed from normal eruption by an adjacent tooth or because of its position in the dental arch. A superumerary tooth is an "extra" tooth. These teeth are usually formed after the permanent dentition, and they remain apical to the erupted teeth in the alveolus. A common area for supernumerary teeth is apical to the maxillary central incisors. The significance of these conditions is that unerupted teeth can develop infections that affect the surrounding tissues. The constant pressure of an unerupted or impacted tooth against other hard tissues, such as an adjacent tooth or bone, can cause resorption or permanent destruction of these tissues. *Partially erupted teeth* should also be noted on the charting form. If, for some reason, full eruption is not completed (as in impaction), it becomes difficult for the patient to keep these teeth clean and to keep the surrounding soft tissues healthy. These areas become prime sites for food impaction and gingival inflammation (e.g., pericoronitis).

An *open contact,* called a *diastema,* can be detected on radiographs and study models. A good-quality radiograph will show the space between the adjacent teeth, and this can be confirmed by the study models. Clinically, the presence of a diastema can be determined visually if the diastema is wide (see Plate 2, *F* and *G*). Open or deficient contacts can also be detected by passing a piece of dental floss between the teeth. When the contact areas do not offer sufficient resistance to the floss, a deficient contact should be charted. Open or deficient contacts may be significant because of the potential for food impaction in these areas. They may also indicate tooth movement from periodontal destruction if the patient reports that they have not always been present. The presence of *plunger cusps* should also be noted during the periodontal examination. This situation involves cusps of teeth in one arch that fit directly into the area between two teeth in the opposing arch. The significance of this phenomenon is that the plunger cusps can push food directly into the space between the opposing teeth, causing trauma to the soft tissues in the area (Pennel and Keagle, 1977). A plunger cusp should be detectable in the study models if the occlusal relationships have been properly reproduced in the wax bite (see Chapter 15).

Abnormal crown and root morphologies may be detected radiographically or on the study models and should be charted by drawing the existing anatomic shape over the symbol of the affected tooth so that the drawing represents reality as closely as possible. Examples of these deviations are teeth that are exceptionally large or small in relationship to other teeth in the dentition, teeth with dilacerated roots, abnormal distances from the CEJ to furcations, and teeth with roots that are spread abnormally or with more or fewer roots than normal. The discovery of any of these deviations is significant for the determination of a tooth's susceptibility to disease, its roots' "anchoring" ability, and how its roots should be treated during root planing or surgical procedures.

Two anomalies that may affect a tooth's susceptibility to disease are the *distopalatal groove* and *cervical-enamel projections*. The former is a groove that extends apically along the root on some maxillary incisors. Most distopalatal grooves are found on maxillary lateral incisors (Withers et al, 1981). Their presence as plaque-retentive areas increases the chances of periodontal destruction. Enamel projections occur in mandibular furcation areas, causing a lack of normal attachment and a predisposition for the buildup of plaque in those locations (Pennel and Keagle, 1977). Areas affected by *abrasion* or *erosion* are also significant in the periodontal examination because of their potential as etiologic factors in the harboring of plaque. This loss of tooth structure affects the normal self-cleansing abilities of the dentition.

Other conditions that are plaque-retentive and serve as etiologic factors include *poorly contoured crowns and restorations, prosthetic devices,* and *carious lesions.* Until these problems are either removed, replaced, or restored, the patient will find it difficult to practice optimal plaque control, and periodontal disease will persist.

The quality of the proximal tooth surface plays an important role in the periodontal condition of adjacent soft tissues. Proximal surfaces that have caries or poorly contoured restorations are more likely to experience plaque accumulation and increased probing depths than similar proximal surfaces that are intact (Claman et al, 1986).

Periapical conditions should be carefully examined on the radiographs and charted in the location where they appear. Any radiopacities or radiolucencies in the periapical regions or supporting bone should be noted, and a tentative diagnosis should be made. In order to reach a final diagnosis, however, the dentist may require additional tests and questioning of the patient during the clinical examination.

Bone levels and the appearance of *bony defects* should be carefully examined on the radiographs. The topography of the bone should be scrutinized for the presence of vertical or horizontal defects. The extent of these defects should be estimated to guide periodontal probing during the clinical appointment. At that time, the clinical readings and the appearance of bone levels on the radiographs should be correlated to ensure that deep bony defects have not been overlooked. The crestal bone patterns should be examined for loss of definition or loss of lamina dura to determine the level of bone destruction. The presence of bony craters can also be observed on the radiographs (Newman and Moran, 1980).

Dental hygienists and dentists should be aware of the limitations of using radiographs as a primary source of evaluating bone levels and attachment loss. It has been shown that radiographs, especially bitewings, cannot be depended upon to identify early periodontal disease and bone loss

(Mann et al, 1985). Even if radiographic technique is excellent and a long-cone paralleling method is used to maximize the accuracy of tooth and bone relationships, early signs of bone loss may not be detected from radiographic images.

Many of the aforementioned conditions may have already been charted as part of the comprehensive charting. If so, they need not be included on the periodontal chart; the time and effort of duplication are unnecessary as long as the other chart is available for consultation when the periodontal treatment plan is being considered. The dental professional may also consider combining the periodontal and restorative charts into one form rather than having two separate ones. The purpose of identifying these elements as part of a periodontal examination is that they are pertinent not only in ascertaining a restorative treatment plan but also in determining the etiologies of periodontal conditions and in selecting the best sequence of priorities to meet patient needs during comprehensive treatment planning.

After a close examination of the radiographs and study models and after all pertinent findings have been reviewed from the restorative chart and/or charted on the periodontal charting form, the dental professional who will be conducting the clinical periodontal examination should make notes to indicate any special evaluations or tests that might be helpful in verifying diagnoses suggested by this initial assessment of data. When the patient is seated, the clinical examination should assess all characteristics of the soft and hard tissues that could not be evaluated from the radiographs, study models, or restorative charting and confirm clinically any details that are in question.

CLINICAL EXAMINATION

Before the periodontal examination is begun, the patient's medical history should be reviewed and confirmed with the patient so that any potential complications in treatment can be detected. Information gathered from the medical history of the patient can assist the clinician in identifying medical reasons for certain gingival and periodontal conditions. Systemic diseases such as diabetes, blood dyscrasias, and hormonal imbalances can affect the ability of the body to resist and repair

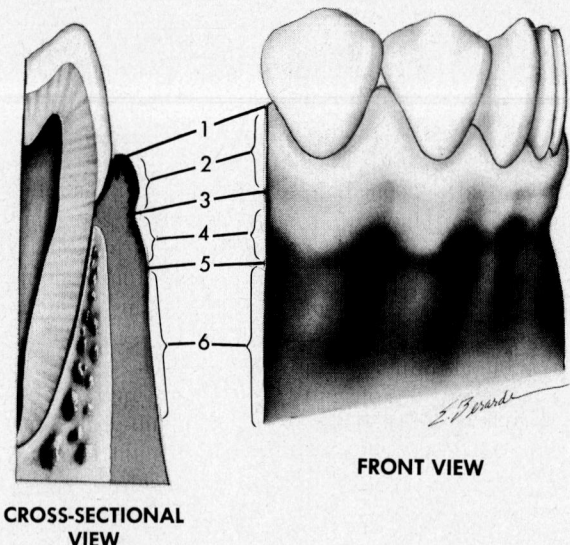

FRONT VIEW

CROSS-SECTIONAL
VIEW

Fig. 14-1. Normal landmarks and boundaries of gingiva and alveolar mucosa. *1,* Free gingival margin; *2,* free gingiva; *3,* free gingival groove; *4,* attached gingiva, *5,* mucogingival junction; *6,* alveolar mucosa. Clinician should be able to relate these landmarks to their appearance in patient's mouth.

damage that occurs as the result of inflammatory conditions. These patients may be more susceptible to periodontal destruction. Medications may also affect the periodontal tissues. Patients who take sodium dilantin for control of seizures often exhibit hyperplasia or fibrotic overgrowth of gingival tissues. Patients who use oral contraceptives may exhibit gingival changes similar to those seen during pregnancy. Corticosteroids are antiinflammatory drugs, and their use can mask the usual signs of inflammation in the gingival soft tissues even though the inflammatory process is active. Poor nutrition and emotional stress can also exacerbate the inflammatory response in the gingival and periodontal tissues.

Patients who require antibiotic premedication to prevent infection due to bacteremia should be premedicated for all periodontal procedures. Periodontal probing can cause a bacteremia in a susceptible patient, as can any other periodontal or dental procedure.

Information taken from the dental history will indicate past dental or periodontal treatment that might affect the present periodontal examination, such as surgical treatment or explanations regarding tooth loss. The dental history will also reveal information about the patient's attitudes regarding

periodontal and preventive therapy; this information will aid in treatment planning.

The purpose of the periodontal examination and charting should be discussed with the patient, and the procedure should be explained to answer any questions the patient might have. The patient must understand that this is an exacting procedure that must be done carefully. The patient may experience some discomfort, depending on the severity of inflammation. The need for pain control (either topical, local or nitrous oxide) should be considered. After the purpose of the clinical periodontal examination has been explained to the patient and consent for treatment has been obtained, the procedure can begin.

Gingival assessment

The first areas to be studied during the clinical examination are the free and attached gingiva. Fig. 14-1 and Plate 2, *A,* show the normal structures of the gingiva and alveolar mucosa. The clinical appearance of the gingiva in all parts of the mouth should be closely examined for signs of inflammation. Table 14-1 contrasts the appearance of normal gingiva and inflamed gingiva. A careful examination is necessary to determine subtle changes in the gingiva because the patient's prognosis for treatment is much improved if gingivitis is recognized and treated in its earliest stages. Deviations from normal gingival characteristics should be noted and described as part of the periodontal examination. This description should include not only the appearance of the gingiva, but also the location and extent of the condition so that later comparisons and evaluation of the success or failure of professional treatment or home care procedures can be made.

The clinician should assess the condition of the gingiva by examining it for each of the following characteristics: color, contour, consistency, and texture. Normal characteristics and changes that may be visible as a result of inflammation should be well known to the clinician, so that exact descriptions of the character of the gingiva can be recorded. The extent of gingival change due to inflammation can vary. Signs of inflammation may extend into all attached and free gingiva, or they may be restricted to the marginal gingiva or interdental papillae. Specific changes may also be localized around one or several teeth, or generalized to an entire arch. The clinician must evaluate the degree of inflammation and extent of tissue involvement to determine if the inflammation can be considered as slight, moderate, or severe in quality.

The *color* of normal gingiva is usually a uniform, coral-pink shade. The light pink color should extend all the way from the mucogingival attachment to the gingival margin (see Plate 2, *A*). Shape variations will occur among different individuals, much the same as facial complexions differ. The amounts of normal melanin pigmentation present in the gingiva will also vary. This pigmentation may be visible as brown patches of color distributed in varying degrees throughout the tissue. This type of pigmentation is prevalent in black individuals. An example of melanin pigmentation is shown in Plate 2, *B* and *F*.

The earliest color change associated with gingival inflammation often begins as a subtle change in the interdental papilla from light pink to a darker pink or red. This color change will extend to the marginal gingiva and into the rest of the free and attached gingiva as the inflammation becomes more severe. Acutely inflamed gingiva will have a red color (see Plate 2, *G*), whereas chronically inflamed gingiva may take on a bluish or

cyanotic cast. This blue color change may be discernible around the margins of poorly contoured crowns (see Plate 3, *D*, No. 8). In many cases the color of fibrotic, chronically inflamed gingiva may be close to normal in appearance. Both chronic and acute signs of gingival inflammation may exist simultaneously within the same patient.

The *contour* of normal gingival tissues also can be seen in Plate 2, *A*. The interdental papillae fill the embrasure spaces and come to a sharp point at the contact area. The free gingival margins are knifelike and hug the coronal surface of the tooth. The margins also create a regular series of parabolic curves as the eye moves from tooth to tooth. The level of the free gingival margin should be at or slightly coronal to the CEJ of the tooth.

A number of changes occur in the contour of the gingiva as a result of inflammation. The interdental papillae become swollen and edematous. In later stages of the disease, they may become flattened, blunted, or cratered. This "punched-out" appearance caused by loss of papilla is characteristic in patients who have had ANUG. The marginal gingiva may also appear bulbous and swollen with rolled margins. As the edema increases, other gingival changes may occur such as clefting (see Plate 2, *E*) or festooning. The inflamed marginal gingiva also loses its elastic ability to adhere closely to the contour of the tooth. The inflamed tissues may stand away from the tooth, or they can be easily displaced with air or instrument retraction (see Plate 2, *G*). When gingival tissues undergo a change in the inflammatory response from acute to chronic inflammation, the constant destruction of the tissues results in the appearance of scar tissue or fibrotic tissue that is extremely firm and often enlarged and irregular in contour (see Plate 2, *D*).

Normal gingival tissues have a *consistency* that is firm and resilient. With the onset of inflammation, the consistency becomes edematous, soft, and spongy. This situation can be detected by applying slight pressure on the dried tissues with the tip of side of a probe or other blunt instrument. A "dent" will remain visible in the edematous tissues. The consistency of chronically inflamed, fibrotic tissues is very firm, hard, and unyielding because of the buildup of excessive amounts of repair or scar tissue.

The *surface texture* of normal free gingiva is

smooth. The attached gingiva may exhibit a smooth or stippled appearance. Stippling will appear as tiny indentations in the surface of the attached gingiva, similar to the appearance of an orange peel (see Plate 2, *A* and *B*). Although many individuals display this normal characteristic, its absence is not necessarily an indication of disease (Goldman and Cohen, 1980). Stippling may be easily detected if the tissues are dried with a stream of air. Acute inflammation usually results in the loss of stippling because of the increase in tissue edema. The surface texture becomes very smooth and glossy (see Plate 2, *C* and *F*). During chronic inflammation, stippling will often be present and may actually increase in prevalence.

Evaluation of the external appearance of the gingiva is useful as an assessment tool for describing the presence of gingival inflammation. It can be less reliable as a means of assessing inflammation within the sulcus or pocket area. Waerhaug (1978a, 1978b) demonstrated that inflammatory changes that affect the marginal gingiva may occur independently of inflammatory changes in the sulcular areas. Patients who performed effective supramarginal plaque control displayed normal-appearing gingiva in spite of the presence of submarginal plaque and sulcular inflammation. Waerhaug warned clinicians not to be misled by the overt appearance of the gingival tissues, especially when the patient has been effective in plaque control removal.

Although assessment of the clinical signs of gingival inflammation may be helpful in determining the presence of gingivitis, these measures are of little help in identifying periodontitis, and their presence cannot predict the onset of periodontitis (Morrison et al, 1982; Ryan, 1985). It has been shown that the clinical signs of inflammation are actually poor indicators of ongoing periodontal disease activity. While active periodontal destruction is taking place in the supporting tissues, the gingival tissues may exhibit no clinical signs of inflammation (Haffajee et al, 1983). An additional problem with the use of clinical signs to determine the extent of disease is that it requires subjective interpretation of the appearance of the tissues rather than objective measures, leading to disagreements over and variations in the interpretation of these signs. More objective methods of clinical assessment, such as the presence of bleeding or exudate from the pocket or sulcus, should complement the gingival assessment to provide a more accurate clinical evaluation.

The soft tissue that covers the supporting bone should be examined for signs of swellings, such as those that might be caused by periapical or periodontal abscesses, granulomas, or cysts. Initial signs of bone destruction caused by these lesions might have been detected during the radiographic examination, and the clinical examination can confirm the tentative diagnosis. The clinician should never rely solely on the use of radiographs to diagnose these lesions as they are not always detectable radiographically. Signs of openings or breaks in the gingiva or mucosa (such as draining fistulas) should be carefully examined and noted.

Gingival bleeding. The presence of sulcular bleeding can be detected during periodontal probing. One of the first signs of gingival inflammation is bleeding during gentle probing of the sulcus area (Meitner et al, 1979; Muhlemann and Son, 1971), and this is an immediate indicator of the need for improved home care and possibly for professional treatment. Bleeding is the result of an ulcerated epithelial lining in the sulcus or pocket and may occur to varying degrees. An acutely inflamed sulcus will bleed spontaneously from finger pressure against the tissue or from probing. Bleeding from incipient gingival inflammation may not be apparent at the surface of the free margin of the gingiva for as long as 30 seconds after complete probing of the entire sulcus depth (Carter and Barnes, 1974). Fibrotic tissues, because of a long-standing inflammation, may bleed little or not at all. All areas of gingival bleeding should be charted according to where they occur in the mouth as a method of assessing the extent and location of the inflammation. In Fig. 14-2, a check mark indicates the presence of bleeding when each area is probed. The amount of gingival bleeding may also be translated into a bleeding index by assigning a numeric value to its occurrence (see Chapter 13).

The presence of bleeding upon probing is considered to be the most sensitive indicator available in clinical practice for the determination of gingival inflammation (Polson and Goodson, 1985). One major advantage of this method of assessment is that it is an earlier sign of gingivitis than

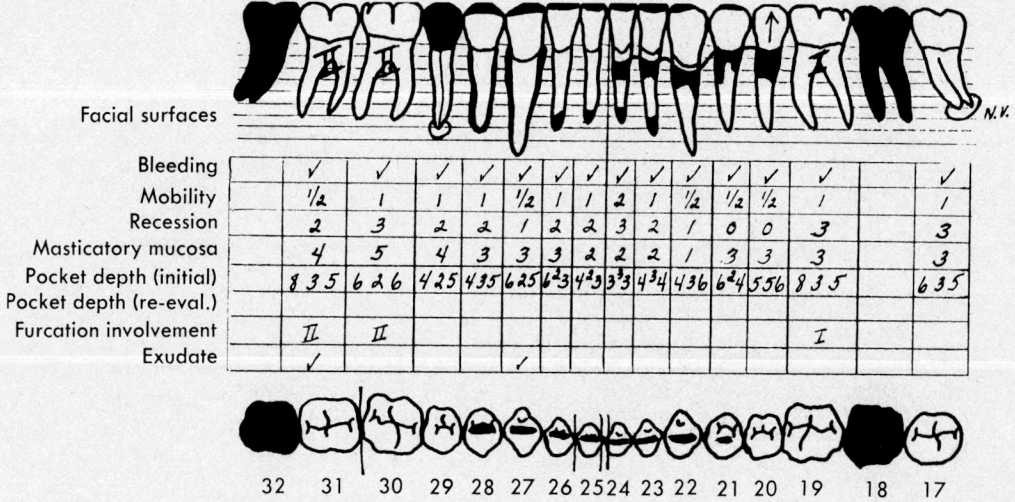

Fig. 14-2. Periodontal charting—sample section.

visual signs of inflammation. This method also permits assessment of inflammation at the base of the lesion, which is a critical area for diagnosis. Presence or absence of bleeding upon probing also provides a more objective means of assessing inflammation in contrast to interpretation of clinical signs of inflammation. The presence of clinical bleeding has been correlated with histological evidence of the presence or absence of inflammation, meaning that presence of bleeding can be considered an accurate indication of the presence of inflammation within the pocket (Greenstein, 1984, Abrams et al, 1984; Ryan, 1985; Polson and Caton, 1986).

Several researchers have used a wooden interdental cleaner (Stim-U-Dent®) to detect interproximal bleeding. The cleaner is inserted horizontally between the teeth from the facial in such a way that it depresses the gingival papilla 1 to 2 millimeters. It is then inserted and removed four times and the area observed for 15 seconds to determine bleeding tendencies. This method has been shown to correlate with histologic evidence of inflammation and has been recommended as a useful method for monitoring the success of periodontal treatment and as an aid to patients for monitoring of plaque control measures (Polson and Caton 1986; Abrams et al, 1984; Amato et al, 1986).

Gingival fluid. Gingival crevicular fluid flow and composition have also been studied as possible indicators of inflammation and disease activity. Measurements of the amount of gingival fluid within the pocket are considered to be an indirect way to measure gingival inflammation objectively. The fluid may be gathered and measured using calibrated microcapillary tubes or filter paper strips or by an electronic meter (Harco Periotron®). Currently, none of these methods is practical for widespread use in clinical practice. Although it is generally felt that the rate of flow of gingival fluid may indicate the severity of the gingival inflammation, researchers are still uncertain how exactly to interpret the measured gingival fluid flow rates (Polson and Goodson, 1985).

The composition of the gingival fluid has also been studied for its potential as an indicator of early inflammatory changes that could indicate the onset of disease. Gingival fluid contains elements of host response and bacterial factors that could be analyzed to determine onset and severity of inflammation. Levels of local antibody present in gingival fluid may help identify areas of active periodontal disease. At the present time, however, additional research and long-term studies are necessary to show which antibodies are reliable predictors of disease activity (Ryan, 1985).

The presence of inflammatory exudate or pus is an obvious sign of acute inflammation and infection. This exudate is composed of white blood cells and other inflammatory debris. Exudate may be noticed during probing, or it may be expelled from the pocket by applying gentle finger pressure to the adjacent gingiva. The presence of exudate should be noted for each tooth involved as part of the periodontal assessment.

Periodontal probing

Periodontal charting is the culmination of a variety of characteristics of the dentition and attachment apparatus. These characteristics are either measured or observed and then recorded with symbols on paper. Those aspects of the periodontium that are commonly measured are sulcus or clinical pocket depth, masticatory mucosa, gingival recession, and mobility. The first three are measured with a periodontal probe. As explained in Chapter 6, the probe is an instrument whose working end is calibrated in millimeters to facilitate clinical measurements. There is a wide variety of probe designs, and the choice of design is based mainly on individual preferences. The diameter of the working end is important for detection during insertion into tight pockets. It should be long enough and narrow enough so that it can be easily inserted without causing undue distension of the soft tissue side of the sulcus. The tip, however, should be blunt so as not to puncture or damage the soft tissues of the sulcus base.

Calibrations of probes vary; some are calibrated at each millimeter up to 10, and others are calibrated in millimeter increments, with the markings at 4 and 6 left off for ease of reading. A probe that is even less complex has calibrations only at 3, 6 and 8 mm. Some clinicians prefer color-coded probes to assist reading. Examples of several different probe designs are shown in Fig. 6-3. No matter what type of probe is chosen, the accuracy of probing pocket depths depends on the skill and clinical judgment of the dental professional.

Other instruments that are necessary for periodontal charting include a mouth mirror, a writing implement, and a form on which the charting will be recorded. In addition, it is helpful for an assistant to record the findings as they are detected clinically. This enables the clinician to work more efficiently and makes it easier to prevent cross-contamination, because it is no longer necessary to keep moving from the mouth to the chart and back again. If an assistant is not available, the hy-

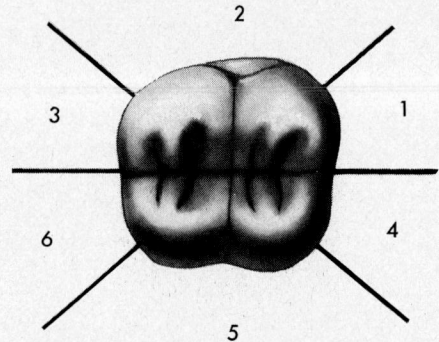

Fig. 14-3. Occlusal view of this molar shows areas where periodontal pocket depth readings are usually taken. Highest reading within each area is the one that should be recorded on charting form.

gienist should minimize cross-contamination by disinfecting the writing implement before and after each patient.

Periodontal probing may be painful for some patients, especially in the presence of advanced periodontal disease and acute inflammatory responses. In these situations a local anesthesia setup may be required to make the patient more comfortable. A saliva ejector and tri-syringe (air-water syringe) should be used during the procedure to keep the field clear of saliva and blood. Two other instruments that are helpful in special situations are a shepherd's hook explorer for detecting exposed furcation areas that are not accessible to the straight design of the periodontal probe and a curette for gross removal of heavy calculus pieces that might interfere with probing.

It is important to establish an effective and efficient order of instrumentation as in any dental procedure involving more than one tooth. This order is helpful to the hygienist working with an assistant because recording the location where the hygienist is working is then unnecessary due to the pattern's predictability. It is also helpful for the clinician who is personally recording results because it is easier to recall which segments of the mouth have been done and which have not. The order of instrumentation prevents unnecessary motion and time spent moving back and forth from one position to another. A recommended order of instrumentation is described in Chapter 6.

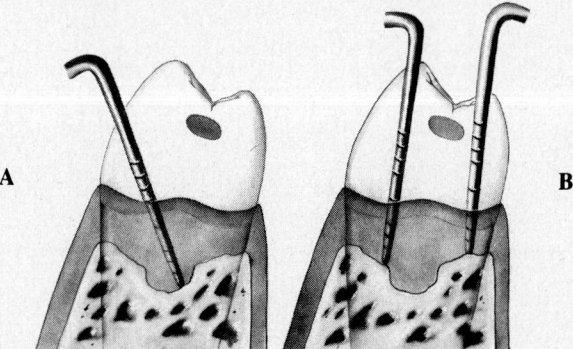

Fig. 14-4. **A,** Correct interproximal adaptation of probe. Both facial and lingual readings should detect this crater if probe is angled in this manner. **B,** Deep interproximal bony defects are missed if probe is not angled below contact area interproximally. No matter how hard this clinician tries, neither facial nor lingual reading will be accurate representation of disease present in this area.

The actual adaptation and activation of the periodontal probe within the sulcus is described in Chapter 6. It is important to remember, however, that only six probe readings will be taken for the periodontal charting, and they are in the areas shown on the molar tooth in Fig. 14-3. Although only six readings are recorded, the pockets are not probed at only six points around the tooth. The technique for probing involves carefully "walking" the probe around the entire circumference of the tooth and recording the greatest depth reading for each of the areas defined. If, for instance, the pocket reading is deeper near the distobuccal line angle on the buccal surface of the tooth than it is on the exact center of the buccal surface, the correct reading for this area would be the deeper of the two readings. The technique of "walking" the probe tip around the tooth allows the examiner to explore carefully the morphology of the entire pocket so that all defects are noted (Hassell et al, 1973; Tibbetts, 1969) (see Fig. 6-39).

For the most part, the probe's working end is kept as closely parallel to the long axis of the tooth as possible, with the tip in close contact with the tooth surface at all times. The tip must always be kept snug against the tooth to prevent damage to soft tissues. As the mesial and distal surfaces are approached, the probe should be moved proximally until it touches the contact and then should be angled slightly into the proximal area so that the tip is measuring directly beneath

the contact. This position is shown in Fig. 14-4, *A.* A common error is keeping the working end of the probe too straight with the long axis of the tooth when the interproximal area is reached and therefore failing to measure the entire proximal surface adequately. This error is shown in Fig. 14-4, *B.* (To review correct adaptation of the probe to the tooth, see Fig. 6-39.) Success with this adaptation depends on the tactile sense of the clinician in keeping the tip against the tooth. The *col* area, which is apical to the contact, is a frequent site for periodontal breakdown and destruction (Goldman and Cohen, 1980), and it is important to probe it carefully from both facial and lingual aspects. When the procedure is done correctly, there will be a slight overlap between the area probed for the mesiofacial and the area probed for the mesiolingual. In Fig. 14-4, *A,* the probe has gone slightly beyond the midline of the tooth to obtain its reading. If a choice must be made, it is better for the probe to be slightly overangled than underangled. With the former there is a slight risk of getting a deeper pocket reading than is accurate, but with the latter there is the possibility of missing a deep vertical defect altogether. With some clinical judgment and practice, the clinician will be able to visualize the distance and angle that will ensure that this vital area has been thoroughly explored and accurately measured.

When the probe is being maneuvered around the tooth and a reading is taken, it is easiest to read the correct pocket or sulcus depth from the top of the probe down to the free gingival margin. The deepest reading for each of the six probed areas of the tooth should be recorded on the periodontal charting form. Fig. 14-2 shows pocket depths recorded for the buccal surfaces of the mandibular teeth; there is one box for all three buccal readings. It should be noted that the three readings for tooth No. 31 are: distobuccal = 8 mm; buccal = 3 mm; and mesiobuccal = 5 mm. The readings are taken for each tooth in the mouth. When a pocket depth falls between two millimeter marks, it should be rounded off to the higher of the two numbers and recorded only as whole millimeters. In most situations it is not necessary to spend the time and effort required to estimate within less than a millimeter. A more graphic method of charting periodontal depths is shown for teeth No. 20 to No. 24 in Fig. 14-2. Here the recorded depths have been shaded onto the picture of the tooth so that pocket morphology can be clearly visualized.

Significance of pocket depth measurements. The periodontal probe is a valuable clinical tool for exploring and measuring the extent of the healthy gingival sulcus and its pathologic counterpart, the periodontal pocket. For years it has been assumed that this measurement of a clinical sulcus or pocket was an accurate representation of the actual histologic attachment of soft tissues to the tooth surface at the dentogingival junction. Based on this assumption, clinicians measured the depths of inflamed pockets prior to their treatment and compared these measurements with those obtained following treatment. The resultant decrease in pocket depth was interpreted and described as a gain in attachment level. More recent reports, however, have demonstrated that the probe does not measure the exact extent of the dentogingival junction in either health or disease (Listgarten, 1980). A number of factors contribute to this discrepancy, including the degree of inflammation present in the tissues, the amount of pressure used during probing, and the diameter of the probe (Ryan, 1985; Polson and Goodson, 1985).

As the inflammatory lesion of chronic periodontitis advances from early to established to advanced stages, there is a progressive disruption in the soft tissues of the dentogingival attachment. The junctional epithelium becomes more permeable to inflammatory cells and eventually loses its attachment to the tooth surface. The underlying and adjacent connective tissue fibers undergo destruction of the dense collagen network of supportive tissues that were present in health. These inflamed tissues cannot resist the normal forces of probing, so that the probe tip will usually penetrate past the junctional epithelium and not come to rest until the increased resiliency of healthy connective tissue fibers is detected. The probe tip penetrates through the partially destroyed fibers and comes to rest approximately 0.25 to 0.4 mm apical to the termination of the junctional epithelium according to a number of investigators (Listgarten et al, 1976; Powell and Garnick, 1978; Saglie et al, 1975; Sivertson and Burgett, 1976; Spray et al, 1978). Because the clinician cannot feel the presence of the inflamed tissues that are being penetrated, the resulting measurement of the pocket depth might be overestimated by as much as several millimeters (Listgarten, 1980).

Armitage and others (1977) studied the penetration of the probe tip in the gingival tissues of beagle dogs. They found that in healthy gingiva the probe tip stopped before reaching the apical termination of the junctional epithelium. When areas of gingival inflammation were probed, the probe came near, but not to, the apical termination of the junctional epithelium, and when areas displaying periodontitis were probed, the probe tip consistently went past the most apical junctional epithelial cells and into the underlying connective tissue. This study demonstrated that there is a relationship between the amount of inflammation present in the tissues and the level of probe penetration. Other investigators have studied the extent of probe tip penetration in healthy tissues and have reported that the probe usually comes to rest within the junctional epithelium (Hancock et al, 1978) or coronal to the junctional epithelium (Hancock and Wirthlin, 1981). The results of these studies demonstrate that clinical probing measurements seldom are reliable in predicting the actual histologic or anatomic sulcus or pocket depth, although they are closer to that prediction when a healthy, shallow sulcus is being measured than when an inflamed sulcus or pocket is being measured.

When pockets are treated with scaling, root planing, curettage, and daily plaque removal, the inflammatory conditions subside and the soft tissues of the dentogingival junction undergo repair. The clinical result, when measured by the periodontal probe, may be reported as a decrease in probing depth caused by an apparent gain in the level of the attachment and tissue shrinkage. Investigators have taken a closer look at the reported "gain" of attachment and have found that a decrease in pocket depth does not necessarily represent a gain of new attachment. Instead, the healed periodontal tissues can regain their dense collagen network and provide resistance to the penetration of the probe tip so that it can no longer extend as far apically into the soft tissues (Fowler et al, 1982; Magnusson and Listgarten, 1980). In these cases there has been no actual change in the level of connective tissue attachment, as determined histologically. The only change is that the healthy dentogingival fibers are able to resist penetration by the probe, which they were unable to do when they were inflamed. The actual levels of attachment, however, have not been altered as a result of treatment. In addition, a common healing response to initial therapy (scaling, root planing, curettage) is the formation of a long junctional epithelium that forms a new biologic attachment to the tooth. The length of the new junctional epithelium has been estimated in one study to range from 1.0 to 4.5 mm (Listgarten and Rosenberg, 1979). The long junctional epithelium will resist penetration by the probe in a healthy sulcus or pocket. Clinical pocket measurements following initial therapy are more likely to estimate the actual anatomic or histologic pocket depths than were the initial pocket measurements in the presence of inflammation.

In summary, then, clinical probing measurements seldom represent the actual anatomic sulcus or pocket depths. When baseline periodontal examinations are performed on new patients who demonstrate signs of inflammation, the pocket measurements may overestimate the actual pocket depths by 1 to 2 mm (Listgarten, 1980). Following treatment, resolution of the inflammation may result in a decrease in the pocket measurement, but the clinician has no way of knowing whether the decrease is due to new connective tissue attachments, decreased penetrability of repaired connective tissue fibers, or the presence of a new long junctional epithelium on the basis of pocket measurements alone. Listgarten (1980), in his re-

view of this topic, suggests that clinicians would be more accurate in referring to pocket measurements as "clinical pocket depths" rather than simply as "pocket depths."

The amount of pressure that is applied to the tip of the probe may also affect the accuracy of the clinical pocket depth measurements. Only a light pressure is necessary to determine these measurements. Additional error is introduced into the procedure when differing amounts of pressure are used in different areas of the mouth, usually because of access problems, or at different examination times. For research purposes, a special pressure-sensitive probe has been developed so that the pressure delivered can be standardized (Gabathuler and Hassell, 1971; van der Velden and de Vries, 1978). As this equipment is not available or practical for general clinical practice at this time, the problem of obtaining reliable probing measurements remains unsolved.

The size of the tip of the probe will also affect the pocket measurements. Probes that are extremely thin can gain easier access into narrow or tight pocket areas but can also penetrate the soft tissues more readily. Less pressure is required to direct a thin tip into soft tissue, and the clinician should evaluate and control the amount of probing force applied to thin probes. In contrast, a very thick probe can become wedged between healthy dense tissues and the tooth before it has reached the base of the sulcus. The use of these thick probes can also be painful for the patient if they are forced into tight, healthy sulci.

Complications of probing. Some of the complications that may interfere with periodontal probing include bleeding, sensitivity, saliva, and calculus. A patient with any degree of inflammation in the soft tissues is likely to exhibit bleeding with probing. If the principles of adaptation are being followed and probing is accomplished with only gentle pressure, the clinician can be assured that signs of bleeding represent an inflammatory response rather than poor probing technique. Bleeding areas should be noted carefully because they are one of the first signs of inflammation and appear before other clinical changes in the gingiva can be detected. If a bleeding index is to be taken, it is wise to incorporate it with the periodontal probing and to record signs of gingival bleeding as they occur. It is also important to use this opportunity to explain the cause and significance of bleeding to the patient so that it is not associated with the probing technique but rather with the inflammatory state of the soft tissues. This method of assessment is one that the patient should be encouraged to use at home to detect areas where home care may not be optimal. Many patients have experienced bleeding from toothbrushing or flossing and may regard this sign as a normal occurrence rather than as a sign of inflammatory disease. This discussion is an excellent opportunity to educate patients by showing them which areas need special attention during their home care practices.

Sensitivity from the probing procedure may result from two sources. If the clinician uses an excessive amount of pressure against the soft tissues at the base of the sulcus or pocket, the patient is likely to experience unnecessary sensitivity. Studies have shown that even gentle probing by an experienced clinician can send the tip of the probe through the junctional epithelium and down to the connective tissue attachment below it. This phenomenon is even more likely to occur when the sulcular and junctional epithelium is inflamed and lacks its usual resiliency and tissue firmness.

Another source of sensitivity may be entirely unrelated to poor technique but may simply be the normal response of acutely inflamed tissues to any type of contact by the probe. Inflamed tissues are ulcerated and bleeding, and they have an exaggerated response to any kind of instrumentation, whether it be probing or scaling. In situations like these, the clinician should be prepared to give an anesthetic for patient comfort to complete this procedure. An alternative is to postpone probing and give home care instructions that may lead to healing of the acutely inflamed tissues. A reduction of inflammation will serve to decrease the pain response to probing at a later appointment.

Visibility of the sulcus area is important during probing to ensure that the probe can be seen and read accurately. Excessive saliva in the area can make reading the probe difficult; patients may require the use of a saliva ejector during the procedure if they are salivating excessively. The use of the tri-syringe can also help clear the area of blood and saliva and dry the teeth and tissues that are being examined.

Another factor that can inhibit periodontal probing of pockets is calculus. If the deposits are

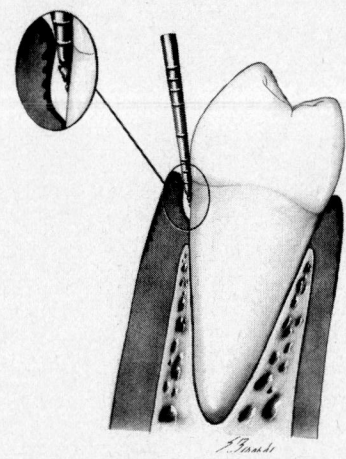

Fig. 14-5. Often calculus ledges prohibit tip of probe from reaching base of pocket. An inexperienced clinician may mistake hard unyielding pressure offered by calculus as the pocket base. If piece is small enough, it may be possible to navigate probe out and around it and continue on down to more resilient texture of pocket base. If calculus piece is too large, it must be removed before accurate probing can be done.

small and scattered throughout the mouth, it is usually possible simply to move the probe away from the deposit and then to continue apically into the pocket. One of the traps into which an inexperienced clinician might fall is that of mistaking a calculus deposit for the base of the sulcus or pocket (Fig. 14-5). A good tactile sense will help the clinician determine the difference between the hard resistance of the calculus and the more elastic resiliency of the pocket or sulcus base. If the calculus deposits that are encountered are large and prohibit convenient access to the probe, these gross deposits should be removed by means of ultrasonic or hand scaling to facilitate the probing procedure. There is no need to put the patient through the discomfort of a time-consuming probing procedure if the accuracy of the reading might be questionable. Instead, periodontal probing should be postponed until after these gross deposits have been removed.

Gingival enlargement or recession. Another measurement that must be made and recorded on the periodontal charting form is the height of the gingival margin on each tooth. The gingival height is the distance of the free gingival margin from the cementoenamel junction (CEJ). If the height of the gingival margin is above the CEJ, it

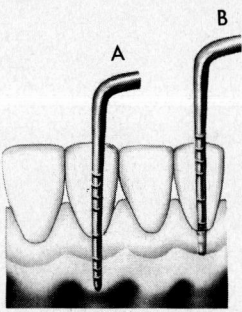

Fig. 14-6. The two measurements necessary to estimate amount of attached gingiva present. Probe *A* is measuring from mucogingival junction to free gingival margin on facial aspect of tooth. Probe *B* is measuring pocket depth. A comparison of the two readings, both taken on facial aspect of same tooth, will indicate amount of attached gingiva that is present.

is measured by placing the tip of the probe at the CEJ and measuring in millimeters to the free margin of the gingiva. If the free gingival margin has receded apically from the CEJ, the amount of recession is measured by placing the probe tip on the level of the free gingival margin and measuring to the level of the CEJ. Areas of gingival enlargement are recorded by noting a plus sign (+) in front of the number; areas of apical recession are recorded by placing a minus sign (−) before the number; areas where the free gingival margin lies at the level of the CEJ are noted as zero (0) recession. Usually only one reading is taken on the buccal surface of each tooth, and another one is taken on the lingual surface. The highest readings obtained for each of these two areas are then recorded in the appropriate box on the charting form (Fig. 14-2).

Another method of depicting gingival height is to draw a line representing the height of the gingival margin on the pictures of the teeth. This provides visual information for those reading the chart which is much easier to interpret than numeric millimeter readings alone. This method of charting gingival height is shown for teeth No. 20 to No. 24 in Fig. 14-2.

It is important that the clinician realize that pocket depth readings alone have little or no significance unless they can be compared with the level of the free gingival margin. For instance, a pocket reading of 3 mm on the buccal surface of a mandibular first molar may not sound significant

by itself, but when the same area has 4 mm of apical recession, the situation is one of exposed root surfaces, possible furcation involvement, and bone destruction. If the periodontal charting is to be used for diagnosis and treatment planning, the total picture must be represented. Simply recording pocket depths alone reveals insufficient information about the true status of the periodontal structure.

Amount of masticatory mucosa. Measurement of the amount of masticatory mucosa on each tooth is necessary for a complete periodontal charting. Masticatory mucosa is measured by placing the tip of the probe at the mucogingival junction and measuring the width of the masticatory mucosa, including all attached and free gingiva up to the free gingival margin. This measurement is being shown by probe *A* in Fig. 14-6. Usually it can be made by simply identifying the difference in the appearance of the darker, shinier alveolar mucosa and the light pink, stippled attached gingiva (see Plate 2, *C* and *H*). If this line is not clearly demarcated because of lack of attached gingiva or color changes due to inflammation, it may be helpful to retract the lip or cheek and move it coronally to determine where the junction lies. Tissue that is freely movable is alveolar mucosa, and tissue that is fixed is attached gingiva (Kopczyk and Saxe, 1974; Vincent et al, 1976). This test is also valuable in determining whether or not frena or muscle attachments are pulling attached gingiva and causing recession. After the junction has been identified, one measurement can be taken for the buccal surface of each tooth and another for the lingual surface. The measurement representing the smallest amount of masticatory mucosa for any one tooth surface should be recorded on the charting form (Fig. 14-2). This measurement is not necessary on the palatal surfaces of maxillary teeth because the attached gingiva is continuous with the masticatory mucosa of the hard palate.

From the information recorded for pocket depths and masticatory mucosa, the amount of attached gingiva can be calculated. If the buccal pocket depth for a given tooth is subtracted from the masticatory mucosa measurement, the result is the amount of attached gingiva. These two measurements are depicted in Fig. 14-6 as they are being taken on two different teeth. This information is important for determining the periodontal prognosis of a given tooth. To be maintained in a healthy state, a tooth must have an adequate amount of attached gingiva. Experts disagree on exactly how much is "adequate," but studies have shown that as little as 1 mm may be sufficient to maintain gingival health. Less than that may be a significant factor in the etiology of periodontal destruction. The delicate, moveable, elastic alveolar mucosa cannot withstand the rigors of mastication and the trauma of brushing as well as the tougher masticatory mucosa. If forced to do so, the result will be loss of gingival height and destruction of periodontal tissues (Bowers, 1963; Lang and Loe, 1972; Hall, 1977, 1981).

The amount of attached gingiva on each tooth is also an important factor when considering root planing, curettage, and periodontal surgery. Often the treatment of choice will vary, depending on the amount of attached gingiva present. Root planing and curettage are frequently contraindicated for areas where there is inadequate or no attached gingiva. Surgical techniques are necessary for successful treatment of these areas.

Mobility

After completing the periodontal probing and soft tissue measurements, the clinician should continue to document the degree of bone destruction and loss of periodontal support by checking the mobility of all teeth. This can be accomplished with two single-ended instruments by placing the flat end of the handle of each instrument against opposite sides of the tooth and attempting to move them alternately in a buccolingual and then mesiodistal direction. Any mobility that is more than the normal amount should be noted on the charting in the following manner (Periodontal Syllabus, 1975):

1 = Slight mobility
2 = Mobility of up to 1 mm in any direction
3 = Mobility of greater than 1 mm in any direction; tooth may be depressed in the socket

The amount of mobility should be noted in the box for each tooth on the charting form (Fig. 14-2). This box should be left empty if no pathologic mobility has been detected.

Furcation involvement

It is important to detect the presence and severity of root furcations that have become exposed as a result of periodontal disease. The presence of furcation exposure is a significant factor both for the patient and hygienist or dentist. The patient should be aware of the presence and location of furcations that are exposed to the oral cavity and should be shown supplementary methods for plaque removal that can gain access to these concavities (as by wooden toothpick or interproximal brush). The hygienist must implement precise instrumentation of these areas to remove as much as possible of the plaque and endotoxins that are not accessible to the patient's plaque control measures. The prognosis of periodontal treatment is closely related to the presence of exposed furcations because these teeth represent a large proportion of the teeth lost to periodontal disease in spite of therapeutic attempts.

Detection of furcations that lie within the submarginal area of the pocket and are not clinically visible relies on the clinician's understanding of root morphology and the evaluation of tactile sensations with the use of a probe or explorer. Areas where loss of bone has caused detectable furcations should be charted. As suggested earlier, it may be helpful to use a curved instrument such as a curette or a shepherd's hook explorer to enter these areas because of the difficulty of access with a straight periodontal probe. A specially designed curved probe, called the *Naber's probe*, is also available for this purpose (Fig. 14-7). Once the furcation is explored, the extent of destruction should be classified as follows:

Class 1. The explorer or probe can detect the concavity of the furcation but cannot enter it. This amount of involvement cannot be detected radiographically.
Class II. The explorer or probe can enter the furcation area but not extend through to the opposite side. A slight radiolucency in the furcation area may be detected with this amount of involvement.
Class III. The explorer or probe can pass all the way through the furcation to the opposite site. An obvious radiolucency should be visible, showing the total destruction of bone in the furcation area.

The classification Roman numeral I, II, or III should be placed over the picture of the affected tooth in the area of the furcation. This notation

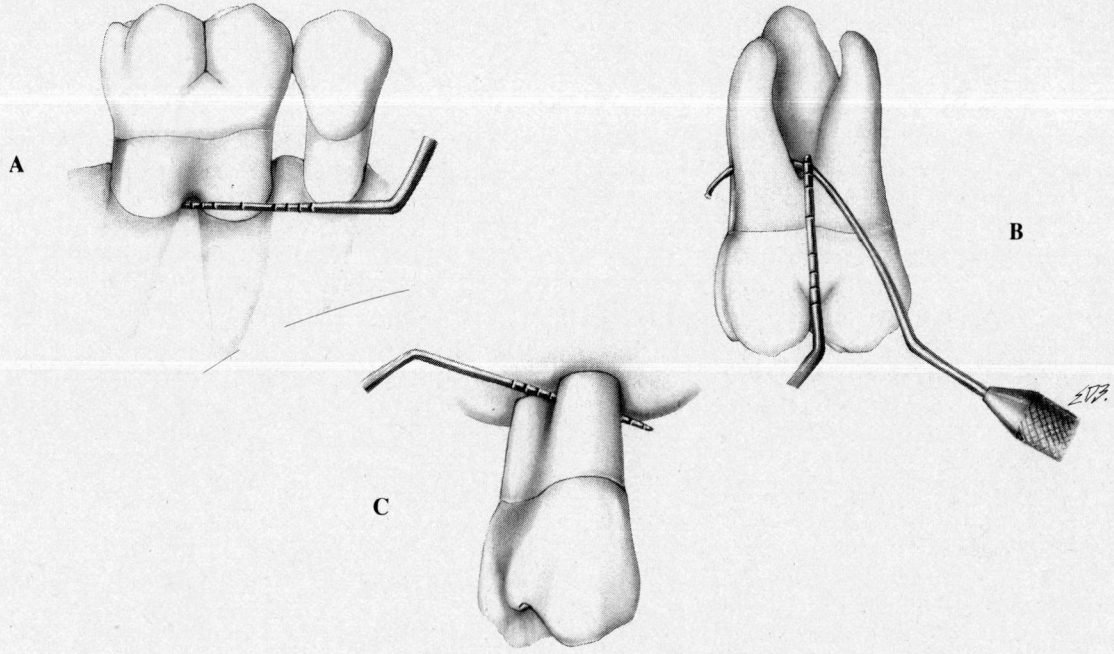

Fig. 14-7. Three teeth with furcation involvements. **A,** Tooth shows Class I involvement where probe can barely detect entrance to furcation. **B,** Tooth shows advantage of having a curved instrument, such as Naber's probe for detection of furcations. **C,** Tooth has Class III involvement going all the way through to other side. (From Matarazzo, F., and Casullo, D. 1978. Continuing Dental Education, University of Pennsylvania School of Dental Medicine **1:**No. 7.)

can be seen on teeth No. 31, No. 30, and No. 19 in Fig. 14-2.

The limitations of current assessment methods

Most of the currently available assessment tools indicate with varying degrees of accuracy the presence of gingival inflammation or provide evidence of past periodontal destruction. None of the measures available at the present time can reliably predict the onset of periodontitis or the presence of actively destructive periodontal disease. Consider the limitations of each of the following measures which are commonly used in the documentation of gingival and periodontal disease.

Periodontal probing. Measurement of probing depth or loss of attachment is the most commonly used and most sensitive measure of periodontal destruction. Probing depths cannot be used, however, to predict which sites are most susceptible to future destruction, nor can they be

used to identify sites that are currently undergoing active periodontal destruction. They can only document the extent of previous destruction and assist in monitoring the success of therapeutic attempts to restore periodontal tissues to levels compatible with the maintenance of health.

Gingival assessments. Clinical signs of gingival inflammation—including color, contour, consistency, bleeding, and crevicular fluid—are accurate in varying degrees for identifying the presence or absence of gingival inflammation, but have generally not been shown to be accurate as predictors of progression of gingivitis to periodontal disease or of the presence of active periodontal disease. The only gingival assessment factor that currently shows promise in this area is gingival fluid flow and composition. At present, the tools and techniques required to perform this assessment are too complicated or impractical for widespread use in clinical practice; it remains confined primarily to the research arena.

Plaque assessments. Quantitative measures of plaque do not provide information regarding periodontal disease activity at specific periodontal sites. They are useful only as educational aids and motivating tools for teaching patients how to be more effective with their supragingival plaque control. It has been clearly established that the qualitative aspects of plaque (composition of plaque bacteria) rather than the quantitative measures (amount of tooth surface covered with disclosed plaque) are significant in determining the potential for disease activity.

Microbial monitoring. One area of research that has drawn the interest of a number of researchers is the study of which bacterial species and compositions act as etiological agents in the progression of periodontal disease. Interest is also focused on methods for measuring the bacterial compositions of specific periodontal sites to identify active periodontal destruction and predict further disease activity.

Listgarten and Hellden (1978) investigated the use of dark-field microscopy to examine the bacterial composition of submarginal plaque in both healthy and diseased periodontal pockets. They found that the distribution of bacteria in the healthy sites was primarily coccoid (90%) and straight rods, with a small percentage of the bacteria being spirochetes (1.8%). In addition, most of the bacteria at these healthy sites were nonmotile rather than motile. When periodontally diseased sites were examined, the distribution of bacteria was very different. In these sites spirochetes made up 37.7% of the total bacterial flora of the pocket, and coccoid and rod types made up only 40% of the bacterial flora. There were also equal numbers of motile and nonmotile bacteria. These investigators proposed that the simple technique of collecting bacterial samples from the pocket areas, examining them under the dark-field microscope, and counting the relative distribution of different types of bacterial cells would allow clinicians to determine exactly which sites were undergoing periodontal disease activity at any given point in time.

Listgarten and others (1978) found that the numbers of spirochetes were reduced in pockets following treatment by tetracycline and/or scaling, as were other clinical parameters of disease, demonstrating the identification of the proportion of spirochetes and motile rods by dark-field microscopy could be used as a means of evaluating treatment effectiveness. Singletary and others (1982) confirmed that microscopic evaluation of the subgingival flora was accurate and convenient as a means of evaluating periodontal disease activity and to monitor the progress of treatment.

Listgarten and Levin (1981) continued to expand the usefulness of this method of periodontal evaluation by testing the reliability of dark-field bacterial analysis in predicting which patients were more likely to experience periodontal breakdown. They concluded that this method provided the clinician with a practical test to determine the susceptibility of patients to periodontal destruction as a result of chronic periodontitis.

Listgarten and Schifter (1982) demonstrated that differential dark-field microscopy could be used as a method for determining the length of the recall interval for an adult population. Patients were assigned "customized" recall intervals based on the relative proportion of spirochetes and motile rods in pooled samples of their subgingival pocket flora. Many patients in the experimental group did not receive a regular prophylaxis for as long as 15 to 18 months, yet the periodontal health of these patients was found to be no different than that of those who were seen at regular 6-month intervals.

These results indicate that dark-field microscopy may be valuable as a method for assessing periodontal disease activity, for evaluating the success of initial therapy, and for predicting which patients and which intraoral sites are most likely to suffer periodontal destruction. Access to this information would be valuable to the clinician in all aspects of periodontal treatment. In addition, it may offer a more scientific and effective way to determine how frequently patients should receive professional maintenance care, rather than basing this decision on the subjective judgment of the clinician, as has been done in the past.

Microbial monitoring cannot yet be considered an accurate predictor of periodontal disease activity. Although it does yield information about the presence of certain types of bacteria associated with diseased and healthy periodontal sites, the pathologic potential of these microorganisms and the thresholds or numbers of these bacteria that are needed to cause disease are still undetermined

(Greenstein and Polson, 1985). We do not know what bacterial populations are associated with a conversion from gingivitis to periodontitis, and there is evidence that spirochete counts alone may not be accurate predictors of attachment loss (Listergarten et al, 1984; Lindhe et al, 1983). Until investigators can identify the microorganisms directly associated with the etiology of gingivitis and periodontitis and the bacterial levels or combinations most likely to result in disease in a given person or a given site, the results of microbial monitoring should be interpreted with caution (Greenstein and Polson, 1985).

Ideally, methods of periodontal assessment would identify the individuals and teeth that are at risk for developing periodontal disease so that appropriate treatment could be implemented. Unfortunately, current clinical diagnostic methods permit only the assessment of past destruction from periodontal disease rather than the prediction of future periodontal breakdown or even the determination of current levels of activity. There are no accurate and practical ways of determining when and where periodontal disease activity will occur in a patient's mouth. Until such methods are developed, the dental hygienist must have a current knowledge of periodontal disease and must master the skills of recognition of healthy and diseased tissues, documentation of all evidence of periodontal disease, and use of that information in designing a preventive and therapeutic treatment plan to control existing disease and prevent future destruction.

LEGAL CONSIDERATIONS REGARDING PERIODONTAL ASSESSMENTS

Bailey (1987) reported that the failure to diagnose and properly treat periodontal disease may be one of the leading causes of dental malpractice. The most common claim arising out of periodontal treatment procedures is that of negligence, indicating a failure on the part of the dentist or hygienist to meet a standard of care which is ordinarily used under similar circumstances by other members of the profession who are in good standing. Bailey also noted that dental hygienists are commonly named as codefendents with the dentist based on their combined failure to diagnose and treat periodontal disease.

A number of suggestions for protecting dentists and hygienists against lawsuits as a result of periodontal treatment have been given. Dentists and dental hygienists must accept their legal responsibility to detect, diagnose, and treat (or refer to specialists) periodontal disease in their patients. They must perform these duties in ways that are consistent with the current standards of care set forth by the dental profession. When claims of negligence, breach of warranty, or fraud are made against the dentist or hygienist, it is the patient who must prove the standard by which periodontal care should be rendered, that the professional did not meet that standard, and that injuries were suffered by the patient as a result of the dental professionals' actions.

Routine documentation in the patient's record of all aspects of periodontal diagnosis and treatment is necessary to protect dental professionals against unfounded legal claims. Dental records are often the deciding evidence when such claims are made. The following information should be entered in the dental record in ink, dated, signed, and retained in the dental office for a minimum of 10 years (Bailey, 1987):

1. A detailed clinical description of the patient's periodontal condition at the initial visit and each subsequent visit, including all documentation discussed in this chapter as well as a plaque index, radiographs, and clinical impressions
2. A description of recommended treatment, alternatives, and the risks and benefits associated with each alternative as discussed with the patient and entered into the record at that time
3. A description of all home care instructions given to the patient, as well as the level of compliance that the patient demonstrated
4. Recommendations for referral and the dates on which these recommendations were discussed with the patient, as well as the patient's response to the recommendations
5. A signed treatment consent form
6. A record of all treatment procedures performed and their outcomes

Proper documentation is not only useful in planning, implementing, and evaluating periodontal treatment for the patient but is also important as a means of protecting the professional against claims of malpractice.

SUMMARY

A method of periodontal examination and charting has been presented to aid the clinician in performing and recording this assessment data. Although only one method of charting has been illustrated and described in detail, other symbols, figures and criteria may be used to achieve the same goals. It is important for the student to realize that the emphasis in periodontal examination and charting is more on the criteria of comprehensiveness, accuracy, and clarity than on the exact way the information is represented on paper. These data, as well as all the other patient assessments discussed in this chapter, must be as complete and easy to interpret as possible, so that those responsible for diagnosis and implementation of treatment can optimally perform their responsibilities to meet the patient's needs.

ACTIVITIES

1. View slides of actual clinical cases and describe and record the most accurate and specific gingival assessments possible of what is seen. Discuss descriptions in small groups and resolve discrepancies by reviewing the slides and discussing the most appropriate descriptions.
2. Watch slides depicting various factors that should be included on the periodontal charting form, such as the clinical appearance of tissues, radiographic findings, and study model records. (Study models could also be available for inspection.) Chart what is seen individually while the faculty member charts findings on an overhead transparency. When the faculty member projects the transparency and slides together, check the accuracy and consistency of your chartings.
3. Research the literature and private offices for charting forms and compare samples for similarities and differences. Review the Computerized Periogram* charting method for accurate graphic data depiction.
4. In small groups, discuss the many different ways in which periodontal findings can be recorded. For example, in how many different ways can the periodontal pocket depths be depicted? Use the same approach for gingival height, mobility, masticatory mucosa, and furcations. After the discussion, analyze these alternative methods in terms of *clarity* (could anyone understand what was being depicted?), *simplicity* (how complicated is it to reproduce?), and *efficiency* (can it be charted quickly?).

*Rhelco, Inc., Easton, Conn.

REVIEW QUESTIONS

1. Identify seven uses of the periodontal examination and charting.
2. How is the amount of attached gingiva on a given tooth surface measured?
3. Is it better to overangulate or underangulate the probe in interproximal areas?
4. On a charting, are pocket depths alone sufficient to describe the presence or absence of disease?
5. True or false:
   a. The calibrated end of the probe is adapted exactly parallel to the long axis of the tooth in all areas of the mouth
   b. Periodontal charting will always be completed before any scaling is performed
   c. Periodontal pocket readings are taken at the same points on every tooth

REFERENCES

Abrams K, et al: Histologic comparisons of interproximal gingival tissues related to the presence or absence of bleeding, J Periodontol 55:629, 1984.

Aeppli DM, et al: Measuring and interpreting increases in probing depth and attachment loss, J Periodontol 56:262, 1984.

Amato R, et al: Interproximal gingival inflammation related to the conversion of a bleeding to a nonbleeding state, J Periodontol 57:63, 1986.

Armitage GC, et al: Microscopic evaluation of clinical measurements of connective tissue attachment levels, J Clin Periodontol 4:173, 1977.

Armitage GC, et al: Relationship between the percentage of subgingival spirochetes and the severity of periodontal disease, J Periondontol 53:550, 1982.

Bailey BL: Malpractice and periodontal disease, JADA 115:845, 1987.

Bowers GM: A study of the width of attached gingiva. J Periodontol 34:201, 1963.

Carranza FA, and Perry DA: Clinical periodontology for the dental hygienist. Philadelphia, 1986, WB Saunders.

Carter HC, and Barnes GP: The gingival bleeding index, J Periodontol 45:801, 1974.

Caton JG, and Polson AM: The interdental bleeding index: a simplified procedure for monitoring gingival health, Compend Cont Educ Dent 6:88, 1985.

Claman LJ, et al: Proximal tooth surface quality and periodontal probing depth, JADA 113:890, 1986.

Examination and diagnosis of periodontal disease. Bethesda, Md, 1975, US Department of Health, Education and Welfare.

Fine DH, and Mandel ID: Indicators of periodontal disease activity: an evaluation, J Clin Periodontol 13:533, 1986.

Fowler C, et al: Histologic probe position in treated and untreated human periodontal tissues, J Clin Periodontol 9:373, 1982.

Gabathuler H, and Hassell T: A pressure-sensitive periodontal probe, Helv Odontol Acta 15:114, 1971.

Giddon DB, et al: Acute necrotizing ulcerative gingivitis in college students, JADA 68:381, 1964.

Goldhaber P, and Giddon DB: Present concepts concerning the etiology and treatment of acute necrotizing ulcerative gingivitis, Int Dent J 14:468, 1964.

Goldman HM, and Cohen DW: Periodontal therapy, ed 6, St Louis, 1980, The CV Mosby Co.

Goodson JM: Clinical measurements of periodontitis, J Clin Periodontol 13:446, 1986.

Grant, DA, et al, eds: Periodontics in the tradition of Gottlieb and Orban. St. Louis, 1988, C.V. Mosby.

Green JC: Discussion: natural history of periodontal disease in man, J Clin Periodontol 13:441, 1986.

Greenstein G: The role of bleeding upon probing in the diagnosis of periodontal disease—a literature review, J Periodontol 55:684, 1984.

Greenstein G, and Polson A: Microscopic monitoring of pathogens associated with periodontal diseases: a review, J Periodontol 56:740, 1985.

Haffajee AD, et al: Comparison of different data analyses for detecting changes in attachment level, J Clin Periodontol 10:298, 1983.

Hall WB: Present status of soft tissue grafting, J Periodontol 48:587, 1977.

Hall WB: The current status of mucogingival problems and their therapy, J Periodontol 52:569, 1981.

Hancock EB: Determination of periodontal disease activity, J Periodontol 52:492, 1981.

Hancock EB, and Wirthlin MR: Histologic assessment of probing in the presence of gingivitis, J Dent Res 58(Special Issue A):239, 1979.

Hancock EB and Wirthlin MR: The location of the periodontal probe tip in health and disease, J. Periodontol 52:124, 1981.

Hancock EB, et al: Histologic assessment of periodontal probes in normal gingiva, J Dent Res 57(Special Issue A):309, 1978.

Hangorsky U: Early detection of periodontal disease by the general practitioner, Compend Cont Dent Educ 1:409, 1980.

Hassell TM, et al: Periodontal probing: interinvestigator discrepancies and correlation between probing force and recorded depth, Helv Odontol Acta 17:38, 1973.

Johnson BD, and Engel D: Acute necrotizing ulcerative gingivitis: a review of diagnosis, etiology and treatment, J Periodontol 57:141, 1986.

Kopczyk RA, and Saxe SR: Clinical signs of gingival inadequacy: the tension test, J Dent Child 41:22, 1974.

Lang N, and Hill RW: Radiographs in periodontics, J Clin Periodontol 4:16, 1977.

Lang NP, and Loe H: The relationship between the width of keratinized gingiva and gingival health, J Periodontol 43:623, 1972.

Lang NP, et al: Bleeding on probing: a predictor for the progression of periodontal disease?, J Clin Periodontol 13:590, 1986.

Lindhe J: Textbook of clinical periodontology, Copenhagen, 1983, Munksgaard.

Lindhe J, et al: Critical probing depths in periodontal therapy, Compend Cont Dent Educ 3:421, 1982.

Listgarten MA: A perspective on periodontal diagnosis, J Clin Periodontol 13:175, 1986.

Listgarten MA: Pathogenesis of periodontitis, J Clin Periodontol 13:418, 1986.

Listgarten MA: Periodontal probing: what does it mean: J Clin Periodontol 7:165, 1980.

Listgarten MA, and Hellden L: Relative distribution of bacteria at clinically healthy and periodontally diseased sites in humans, J Clin Periodontrol 5:115, 1978.

Listgarten MA, and Levin S: Positive correlation between the proportions of subgingival spirochetes and motile bacteria and susceptibility of human subjects to periodontal deterioration, J Clin Periodontol 8:122, 1981.

Listgarten MA, and Rosenberg M: Histological study of repair following new attachment procedures in human periodontal lesions, J Periodontol 50:333, 1979.

Listgarten MA, and Schifter C: Differential dark field microscopy of subgingival bacteria as an aid in selecting recall intervals: results after 18 months, J Clin Periodontol 9:305, 1982.

Listgarten MA, et al: Comparative differential dark-field microscopy of subgingival bacteria from tooth surfaces with recent evidence of recurring periodontitis and from non-affected surfaces, J. Perio 55:398, 1984.

Listgarten MA, et al: Periodontal probing and the relationship of the probe tip to periodontal tissues, J Periodontol 47:511, 1976.

Listgarten MA, et al: Effect of tetracycline and/or scaling on human periodontal disease, J Clin Periodontol 5:246, 1978.

Loesche WJ, et al: Bacterial profiles on subgingival plaques in periodontitis, J Periodontol 56:447, 1985.

Magnusson I, and Listgarten MA: Histologic evaluation of probing depth following periodontal treatment, J Clin Periodontol 7:26, 1980.

Mann J, et al: Investigation of the relationship between clinically detected loss of attachment and radiographic changes in early periodontal disease, J Clin Periodontol 12:247, 1985.

Meitner SW, et al: Identification of inflamed gingival surfaces, J Clin Periodontol 6:93, 1979.

Morrison EC, et al: The significance of gingivitis during the maintenance phase of periodontal treatment, J Periodontol 53:31, 1982.

Muhlemann HR, and Son S: Gingival sulcus bleeding—a leading symptom in initial gingivitis, Helv Odontol Acta 15:107, 1971.

Newman MG: Current concepts of the pathogenesis of periodontal disease—microbiology emphasis, J Periodontol 56:734, 1985.

Newell DH: Current status of the management of teeth with furcation invasions, J Periodontol 52:559, 1981.

Newman PS, and Moran JM: Aspects of bone in periodontal disease, Dent Update 7:453, 1980.

Page RC: Gingivitis, J Clin Periodontol 13:345, 1986.

Page RC, and Schroeder HE: Pathogenesis of inflammatory periodontal disease: a summary of current work, Lab Invest 33:235, 1976.

Page RC, and Schroeder HE: Periodontitis in man and other animals: a comparative review. Basel, 1982, S Karger.

Parr RW: Examination and diagnosis of periodontal disease, DHEW Pub. No. (HRA) 74-36. Washington, DC, 1975, US Government Printing Office.

Pennel BM, and Keagle JG: Predisposing factors in the etiology of chronic inflammatory periodontal disease, J Periodontol 48:517, 1977.

Periodontal syllabus. Bethesda, Md, 1975, Naval Graduate Dental School, US Navy Dental Corps.

Polson AM, and Caton JG: Current status of bleeding in the diagnosis of periodontal diseases, J Periodontol 57:1, 1986.

Polson AM, and Goodson JM: Periodontal diagnosis: current status and future needs, J Periodontol 56:25, 1985.

Powell B, and Garnick JJ: The use of extracted teeth to evaluate clinical measurements of periodontal disease, J Periodontol 49:621, 1978.

Ralls SA, and Cohen ME: Problems in identifying "bursts" of periodontal attachment loss, J Periodontol 57:746, 1986.

Ramfjord SP, and Ash M: Significance of occlusion in the etiology and treatment of early, moderate and advanced periodontitis, J Periodontol 52:511, 1981.

Repine KD: Periodontal procedures for the general practitioner, I. Periodontal diagnosis, patient education, and referral procedures, Compend Cont Dent Educ 4:125, 1983.

Rodriguez-Ferrer HJ, et al: Effect on gingival health of removing overhanging margins of interproximal subgingival amalgam restorations, J Clin Periodontol 7:457, 1980.

Ryan RJ: The accuracy of clinical parameters in detecting periodontal disease activity, JADA 111:753, 1985.

Saglie R, et al: The zone of completely and partially destructed periodontal fibres in pathological pockets, J Clin Periodontol 2:198, 1975.

Schifter CC, and Levin SI: Dark field microscopy: adjunct in assessment, RDH 4:52, 1984.

Setchell DJ, and Shaw MJ: The graduated periodontal probe, Dent Update 7:431, 1980.

Singletary MM, et al: Dark-field microscopic monitoring of subgingival bacteria during periodontal therapy, J Periodontol 53:671, 1982.

Sivertson JF, and Burgett FG: Probing of pockets related to the attachment level, J Periodontol 47:281, 1976.

Slots J: Bacterial specificity in adult periodontitis—a summary of recent work, J Clin Periodontol 13:912, 1986.

Socransky SS, et al: Changing concepts of destructive periodontal disease, J Clin Periodontol 11:21, 1984.

Socransky SS, et al: Difficulties encountered in the search for the etiologic agents of destructive periodontal diseases, J Clin Periodontol 14:588, 1987.

Spindel LM, et al: Plaque reduction unaccompanied by gingivitis reduction, J Periodontol 57:551, 1986.

Spray JR, et al: Microscopic demonstration of the position of periodontal probes, J Periodontol 49:148, 1978.

Stamm JW: Epidemiology of gingivitis, J Clin Periodontol 13:360, 1986.

Theilade J: An evaluation of the reliability of radiographs in the measurement of bone loss in periodontal disease, J Periodontol 31:143, 1960.

Theilade E: The non-specific theory in microbial etiology of inflammatory periodontol diseases, J Clin Periodontol 13:905, 1986.

Tibbetts LS: Use of diagnostic probes for detection of periodontal disease, JADA 78:549, 1969.

van der Velden U, and de Vries JH: Introduction of a new periodontal probe: the pressure probe, J Clin Periodontol 5:188, 1978.

Vanooteghem R, et al: Bleeding on probing and probing depth as indicators of the response to plaque control and root debridement, J Clin Periodontol 14:226, 1987.

Vincent JW, et al: Assessment of attached gingiva using the tension test and clinical measurements, J Periodontol 47:412, 1976.

Waerhaug J: Subgingival plaque and loss of attachment in periodontosis as evaluated on extracted teeth, J Periodontol 48:125, 1977.

Waerhaug J: Healing of the dento-epithelial junction following subgingival plaque control, I. As observed in human biopsy material, J Periodontol 49:1(a), 1978.

Waerhaug J: Healing of the dento-epithelial junction following subgingival plaque control, II. As observed on extracted teeth, J Periodontol 49:119(b), 1978.

Wilkins E: Clinical practice of the dental hygienist, ed 5, Philadelphia, 1983, Lea & Febiger.

Withers JA, et al: The relationship of palato-gingival grooves to localized periodontal disease, J Periodontol 52:41, 1981.

15

THE ROLE OF OCCLUSION IN DENTAL HEALTH AND DISEASE

OBJECTIVES: *The reader will be able to*

1. Describe Angle's classification system.
2. Define overbite and overjet and demonstrate how to measure each.
3. Explain why it is important to examine the occlusion of a child with primary or mixed dentition.
4. Define the following terms:
   a. Occlusal trauma
   b. Occlusal traumatism
   c. Primary occlusal trauma
   d. Secondary occlusal trauma
   e. Centric stops
   f. Centric relation
   g. Centric occlusion
   h. Lateral and protrusive excursions
   i. Working and nonworking interferences
5. Recognize the differences between periodontitis and occlusal traumatism.
6. List, recognize, and record etiologic factors of occlusal trauma.
7. List, recognize, and record the subjective, clinical, and radiographic signs and symptoms of occlusal trauma.
8. Complete an occlusal screening for a partner.

The study of occlusion requires the student to examine the anatomy of the teeth, supporting structures, temporomandibular joint (TMJ), muscles of mastication, and the blood and nerve supply to those areas. Many common complaints such as headaches, sore muscles, toothaches, and sensitivity to temperature changes can be traced to occlusal or TMJ problems.

Occlusion is important throughout the patient's life. Even a newborn has an occlusal relationship. When the infant closes his or her mouth, occlusion is obtained by placing the tongue between the maxillary and mandibular gum pads (Borell, 1980). From infancy onward, the patient's occlusion is important to necessary functions such as suckling, swallowing, chewing, speaking, and even smiling.

It is no wonder that occlusal relationships are important in each dental specialty: pedodontics,

orthodontics, periodontics, prosthodontics, restoratives, oral surgery, and endodontics. Pedodontists examine children's occlusion and growth patterns. If a primary tooth is lost prematurely, the pedodontist will recommend placement of a space maintainer to preserve the needed room for the succeeding permanent tooth. Through such use of space maintainers (see Fig. 27-4), normal occlusal relationships are encouraged. Pedodontists and orthodontists evaluate the growing child's occlusion. Pedodontists examine children's occlusions during their development to detect early signs of malocclusions. If a malocclusion is detected early, treatment may be possible with a minimal amount of therapy. More severe malocclusions must be treated by orthodontists who have additional education in this area. Periodontists are interested in occlusion because some patients' occlusions can exacerbate the damage to supporting structures of the teeth, which complicates periodontal treatment. Dentists performing prosthetic and restorative dentistry are concerned because each restoration placed will affect the patient's occlusion either positively or negatively. Prosthodontists are especially concerned as they may replace one or more missing teeth, requiring them to restore occlusal relationships, especially when making full maxillary and mandibular dentures. These relationships must create occlusion compatible with the patient's TMJ and neuromusculature to ensure the patient's comfort and function. Oral surgeons must be aware of these relationships when performing facial reconstruction procedures. Even endodontists must be careful to avoid traumatic occlusion on an endodontically involved tooth.

The hygienist's awareness and knowledge of occlusion must increase to keep pace with the increasing responsibilities of dental hygienists in all of the specialties. The hygienist treating periodontal patients should be aware of the effects occlusion can have on periodontal treatment. The hygienist who performs restorative care affects the occlusion with the restorations placed.

This chapter provides the student with basic information about occlusion as well as some methods for detecting problematic occlusal conditions. The hygienist's role is to detect potential or current occlusal problems and to alert the dentist to the findings.

APPROACHES TO OCCLUSION

The study of occlusion can be confusing because it is complex and there are various approaches to its study. Presently, there are three commonly accepted approaches to the study of occlusion and treatment of occlusal problems: the prosthetic concept, the orthodontic concept, and the concept of dynamic individual occlusion (Mosteller, 1980; Ramfjord and Ash, 1971). Each of these approaches, or concepts of occlusion, has a particular set of understandings to guide occlusal treatment.

The *prosthetic concept* of balanced occlusion was developed to guide the construction of full dentures. The word *balanced* is very crucial to this approach. The underlying principle is that the occlusion should be balanced: there should be simultaneous, bilateral contact of the teeth during

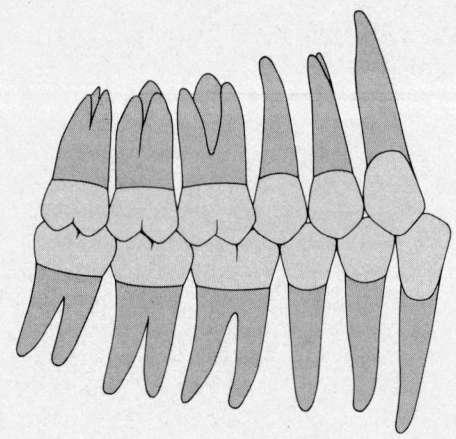

Fig. 15-1. Class I occlusal relationship. Mesiobuccal cusp of maxillary molar aligns with buccal groove of mandibular molar; maxillary cuspid rests between mandibular cuspid and first premolar.
(From Thurow RC: Atlas of orthodontic principles, ed 2, St Louis, 1977, The CV Mosby Co.)

mandibular lateral and protrusive movements. This balance is necessary to prevent full dentures from tilting or becoming dislodged. The prosthetic approach is applicable to persons with full dentures, rather than to persons with natural dentitions (Mosteller, 1980; Ramfjord and Ash, 1971; Weisgold, 1975).

The *orthodontic concept* of occlusion is most concerned with tooth-to-tooth, particularly the cusp-to-fossa, relationships between the teeth. Angle's classification and the positions of supporting cusps, discussed later in this chapter, are elements of the orthodontic concept. When orthodontia is performed, teeth are moved to approximate pre-established concepts of ideal occlusal relationships, such as a Class I molar relationship (Mosteller, 1980; Perry, 1976; Ramfjord and Ash, 1971). The issue has been raised of orthodontists' excessive concern with cusp-to-fossa relationships, without enough regard for the neuromuscular and vascular components of occlusion and the TMJ (Perry, 1976).

The concept of *dynamic individual occlusion*, as reflected by its name, considers each person's particular occlusion and recognizes that the systems affecting occlusion are in a continual state of flux. Dynamic individual occlusion considers all factors, such as the neuromusculature and vascu-

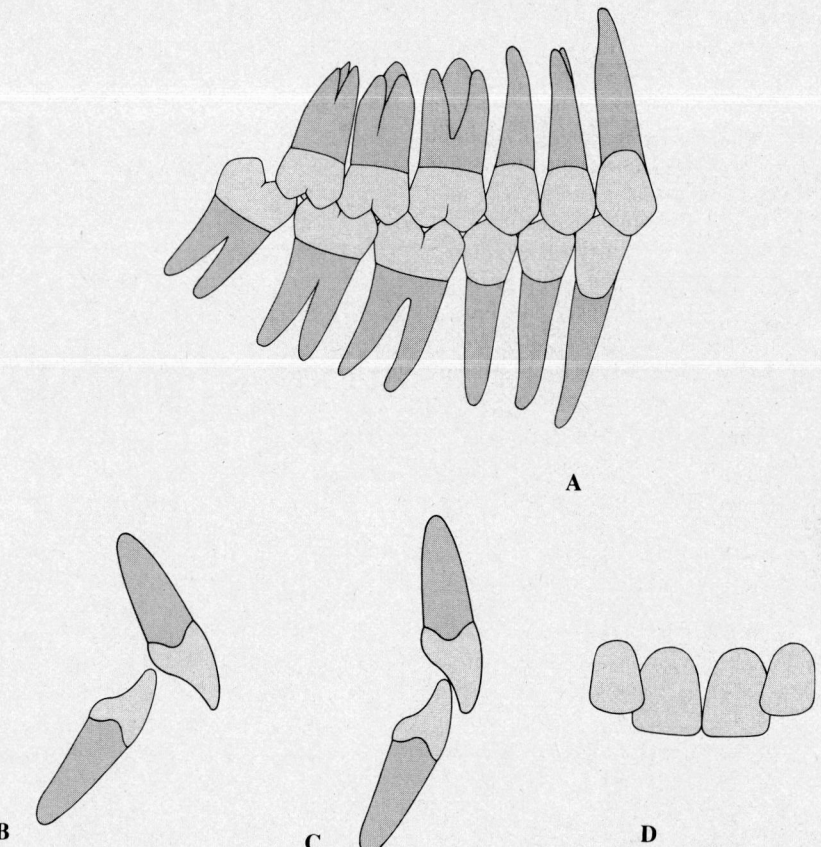

A

B   **C**   **D**

Fig. 15-2. **A,** Class II occlusal relationship. Mesiobuccal cusp and maxillary cuspid are mesial to mandibular landmarks. **B,** Class II, division 1. Anterior teeth are flared. **C** and **D,** Class II, division 2. Anterior central teeth are verted lingually.
(From Thurow RC: Atlas of orthodontic principles, ed 2, St Louis, 1977, The CV Mosby Co.)

lar systems associated with the TMJ and occlusion; stress and other psychologic conditions; tooth-to-tooth relationships; and other oral conditions such as restorative, periodontal, and endodontic health (Mosteller, 1980; Ramfjord and Ash, 1971).

The dynamic individual concept of occlusion is presented in this chapter. The discussion of the relationship between occlusal and periodontal health, the occlusal screening exam, and the occlusal analysis are all drawn from this concept. Occlusal screening and analysis are beginning steps to evaluating the person's occlusion. Elements of the orthodontic approach, such as Angle's classification, overjet, overbite, and posi-

tions of supporting cusps, are widely accepted and used measures of occlusion.

ANGLE'S CLASSIFICATION: IDEAL OCCLUSION

In 1899 Dr. E.H. Angle proposed a classification system of malocclusion designed to help identify occlusions that needed treatment (Jago, 1974). Angle's classification evaluates the mesiodistal relationship between the first molars (Thurow, 1977). Currently, practitioners evaluate the cuspid relationship as well. There are three classifications in this system—I, II, and III. Class II is subdivided into division 1 and division 2. (See Figs. 15-1 to 15-3 for a description of the classi-

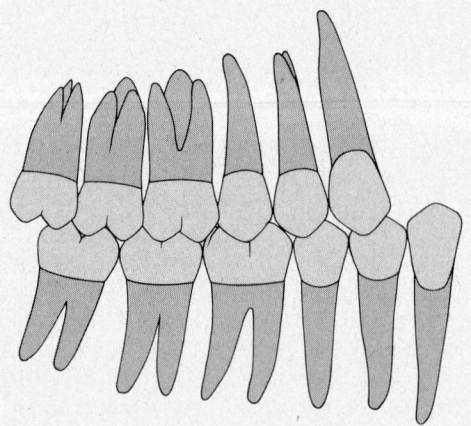

Fig. 15-3. Class III occlusal relationship. Mesiobuccal cusp and maxillary cuspid are distal to mandibular landmarks. (From Thurow RC: Atlas of orthodontic principles, ed 2, St Louis, 1977, The CV Mosby Co.)

fications.) According to this classification, only Class I is the ideal occlusion. Any other type is considered a malocclusion or a "bad" occlusion that could require treatment to become normal. The terms *occlusion* and *malocclusion* are used synonymously for Class II, division 1; Class II, division 2; and Class III. So a Class III occlusion may be the same as a Class III malocclusion. The terms can also be used synonymously, although they usually are not, for Class I. It is possible for a patient to exhibit ideal first molar and cuspid relationship and to have crowded anterior teeth. Many practitioners would call that type of condition a *Class I malocclusion,* although calling it *Class I occlusion with anterior crowding* would also be acceptable.

It is obvious that Angle's classification has limited meaning. It uses information about only a few teeth to classify the entire occlusal relationship. The Angle's classification is subject to the clinician's judgment. For example, if the first molars are more than a half-cusp from the ideal Class I, the occlusion is considered a Class II or Class III, although practitioners vary in the interpretation of half a cusp. Attempts have been made to develop new classification systems to overcome shortcomings of Angle's system, but none has received the universal acceptance of Angle's classification (Thurow, 1977). Therefore, Angle's classification will continue to be used until a more precise and descriptive system is developed.

Angle's classification can also be used to evaluate the molar relationship in the primary and mixed dentition. The primary second molars are used to determine the relationship in the primary dentition and in the mixed dentition until the permanent first molars are sufficiently erupted.

During the clinical examination, Angle's classification should be noted and the patient's overjet and overbite should be measured with a periodontal probe.

Overjet is the distance between the labial or lingual surface of the maxillary incisors and the facial surface of the lower incisors (Thurow, 1977). It is measured while the patient's teeth are fully occluded. The probe is placed perpendicular to the long axis of the teeth with the point against the facial surface of the lower incisor and the side resting against the incisal edge of the maxillary incisor. The measurement may be made from the facial surface of the lower incisor to the labial or lingual surface of the maxillary incisor, depending on the particular clinic's or office's preference. If the measurement is to the labial surface of the maxillary incisor, the labiolingual width of the incisal edge is included; it would seem that measuring to the lingual surface would provide a more meaningful measure. It is important to know which method is being used (Fig. 15-4, *A*).

Overbite is the amount that the maxillary anterior teeth overlap the mandibular anterior teeth in a vertical plane (Thurow, 1977). If a patient has an edge-to-edge relationship between the maxillary and mandibular teeth, the amount of overbite is 0 mm. Usually the overbite is 2 to 3 mm. In a severe overbite the incisal edge of the mandibular teeth may occlude with the soft tissue of the hard palate. The overbite is measured in two steps. First, the probe is placed as if the overjet were being measured. Then the probe is held in that position as the patient slowly opens the mouth. When the patient's mouth is open, the probe is placed upright. The distance from the tip of the

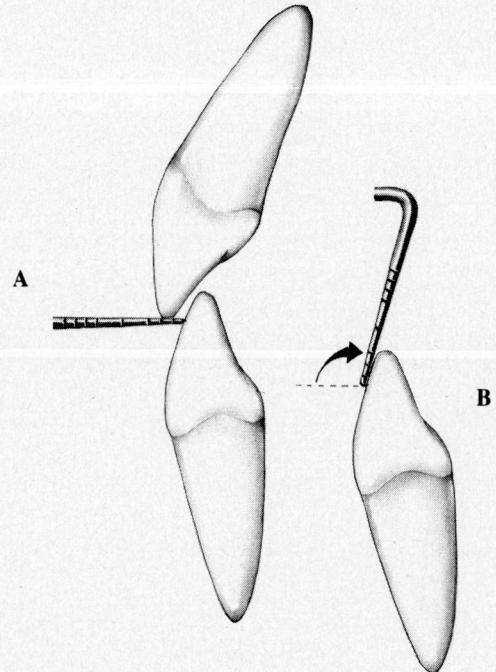

Fig. 15-4. **A,** Overjet is measured. **B,** Overbite is measured.

probe to the incisal edge of the lower anterior tooth is the amount of overbite (Fig. 15-4, *B*). Malaligned teeth may cause the overjet and overbite to vary, so more than one measurement may be taken and recorded.

As an alternative method for measuring an overbite, place a pencil, instead of a probe, against the tooth. A pencil mark is made, the pencil is removed, and the patient is asked to open his or her mouth. The clinician then can measure the amount of overbite by placing the probe upright against the mandibular tooth with the point at the level of the pencilmark.

Overjets and overbites are measured the same way for the primary and mixed dentitions. Severe overbite is more common in the primary dentition than in the permanent dentition.

DEVELOPMENT OF OCCLUSION

As mentioned earlier, even the infant has an occlusal relationship. From the start of life until its end, occlusion is important to well-being. This section briefly describes the development of occlusion from birth through the primary, mixed, and permanent dentitions. The characteristic occlusal relationships during each of these periods are discussed. Several influences on the development of occlusion must be kept in mind. The influences are biologic, anatomic, physiologic, pathologic, and environmental (Levine and Pulver, 1979).

Biologically, jaw size, tooth size, and the pattern of growth are believed to be inherited. Thus the development of a person's occlusion will be affected by genetic endowment. Development is not solely determined by genetics. Environmental and other factors play an important role (Levine and Pulver, 1979).

Anatomic influences include the craniofacial, vascular, muscular, neural, and endocrine structures and systems of the person. In particular, the systems composing the head, neck, face, and TMJ are of concern.

Physiologic influences include differential growth patterns. Chronologic and physiologic ages do not always coincide. Differential growth is a concern in evaluating the development, because the maxilla and mandible grow at different rates. At birth it is normal for a child to have a retrognathic mandible because its growth is slower in utero. The coincidence of chronologic and physiologic age is to be considered in evaluating eruption of the teeth. Tooth eruption varies for each person. Physiologic age is not always on schedule with chronologic age. So, even though permanent first molars are "6-year" molars, very few children's molars erupt on schedule. It is necessary to consider the child's overall physiological development when assessing occlusal development (Levine and Pulver, 1979).

Pathologic influences include physical and developmental disabilities or abnormalities that may interrupt, accelerate, or delay growth and development. These can range from very minor problems such as a congenitally missing tooth to more complex problems such as a cleft lip and palate. Both would affect the person's occlusion, but to much different extents (Levine and Pulver, 1979).

The final influence is *environmental,* including factors such as habits, carious lesions, traumatic injuries, iatrogenic dental treatment, and systemic disease. Habits such as finger or thumb sucking, improper swallowing, mouth breathing, bruxism, or tongue thrusting can affect the alignment of the teeth and growth of the jaws. Carious lesions can cause tooth breakdown, which in turn encourages tooth migration and loss of adequate space for succeeding teeth. Teeth can drift and tilt contributing to abnormally directed force on the teeth. Traumatic injuries can cause tooth fracture or loss with sequelae similar to those from carious lesions. Iatrogenic problems, such as improperly placed restorations or neglect of appropriate treatment, can damage or interfere with occlusion. Finally, systemic diseases can retard the growth and development of the jaws, teeth, or the entire skeletal system (Levine and Pulver, 1979).

In summary, these influences should be considered in assessing a child's or adult's occlusion. Once again, a thorough medical history in order to fully understand a patient's condition is important.

Primary dentition and occlusion

By the time the child is 2½ years old, a full set of primary teeth should be erupted. The teeth usually begin to erupt from the age of 4 to 6 months, and a deep overbite and overjet are common (Borell, 1980) due to the slower growth rate of the mandible. The growth of the mandible should be sufficient by the time the primary second molars erupt to reduce the overbite and overjet to approximately normal ranges. If not, the Class II molar relationship is likely to persist into the permanent dentition (Borell, 1980). The characteristics of the primary dentition include spaces between the teeth, upright teeth, and either a straight or mesial-step terminal plane between the opposing second molars (Borell, 1980; McDonald and Avery, 1983). Fig. 15-5 illustrates the difference between a straight and a mesial-step terminal plane. The planes are important because the permanent first molars are guided into position by the distal surfaces of the second primary molars. The configuration of the plane, in conjunction with the presence or absence of the primate space, the space between the primary cuspids and the first molars, influences the likelihood of the development of a Class I molar relationship in the permanent denti-

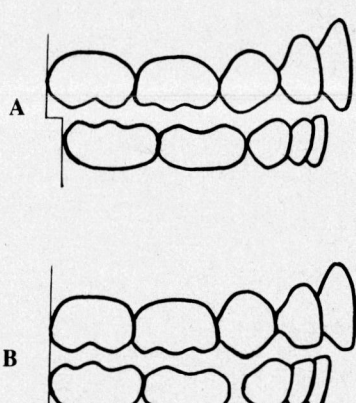

Fig. 15-5. Terminal plane is relationship between distal surfaces of maxillary and mandibular primary second molars. **A,** Mesial-step terminal plane: mandibular molar is mesial to maxillary molar. **B,** Straight terminal plane: molars are even. (From McDonald RE and Avery DA: Dentistry for the child and adolescent, St Louis, 1983, The CV Mosby Co.)

tion (Borell, 1980; McDonald and Avery, 1983). The development of a Class I relationship is possible with any combination of terminal plane and absence or presence of the primate space, but it is most likely if there is a mesial-step plane and a primate space (McDonald and Avery, 1983).

Mixed dentition and occlusion

The mixed dentition is characterized by the presence of both primary and secondary teeth. Permanent teeth are either *successional* (replacements for primary teeth) or *accessional* (new additions to the posterior portions of the dental arches) (Borell, 1980). The age span of the mixed dentition is usually 6 to 12 years. This period of time during the mixed dentition is of great importance to the development of normal occlusion. It is important for children to have their dentitions and occlusions evaluated and steps taken to enhance normal development. Eruption patterns should be assessed by the dentist and timely extraction of primary teeth performed. The *leeway space* (the sum of the mesiodistal widths of primary teeth from the cuspid to the second molar) should be evaluated. Leeway space is usually wider than the widths of the successional teeth, and the maxil-

Table 15-1. Centric stops during centric occlusion

Supporting cusps	contact with	Fossae or marginal ridges
Maxillary lingual cusps		**Mandibular ridges or fossae**
Lingual cusps of premolars		Marginal ridges of second premolar and first molar
Mesiolingual cusps of molars		Central fossae of mandibular molars
Distolingual cusps of molars		Marginal ridges of mandibular molars
Mandibular incisal edges and buccal cusps		**Maxillary ridges or fossae**
Incisal edges		Lingual fossae of incisors
Cusp of canine		Mesial marginal ridge of first premolar
Buccal cusps of premolars		Marginal ridges of premolars
Mesiobuccal cusps of molars		Distal marginal ridge of second premolar and marginal ridges of molars
Distobuccal cusps of molars		Central fossae of maxillary molars

Compiled from Ramfjord SP, and Ash MM: Occlusion. Philadelphia, 1983, WB Saunders Co.

lary leeway space is greater than the mandibular space. This enhances the development of a normal molar relationship in the permanent dentition (Borell, 1980).

The path of closure, lateral, and protrusive movements of the mandible should also be evaluated. These characteristic movements of the mandible are likely to continue with the permanent dentition. If problems or interferences are present in the mixed dentition, it is important that they be detected and treated (Borell, 1980). Evaluation of the path of closure and movements of the mandible were described in the section on occlusal analysis.

Permanent dentition and occlusion

By the time a person has reached the age of 12, the permanent dentition, excluding the third molars is usually present. Normally there are no interproximal spaces. There are axial tilts to the teeth to foster a trituration chewing stroke (Borell, 1980). There is a Class I molar relationship. It can be reemphasized that "normal" does not mean "ideal." The previous description of normal is close to ideal, but normal covers a wide range. Occlusal screening and analyses determine if the patient's occlusion can be considered normal (that is, not causing damage to the supporting structures). Many dentists refer to an occlusion not causing harm as a physiological occlusion.

Centric occlusion, or maximum intercuspation, is the position of the mandible that is guided by the teeth (Ramfjord and Ash, 1983). Centric occlusion is the position assumed when a person is asked to close his or her mouth "as usual." It is the position in which the teeth best fit together and usually is the position of the mandible during the last stages of chewing and swallowing. The supporting cusps are the buccal cusps of the mandible posterior teeth and the lingual cusps of the maxillary posterior teeth. They occlude with either the opposing marginal ridges or fossae. These occluding surfaces—cusp tips, marginal ridges, and fossae—are referred to as centric stops (Ramfjord and Ash, 1983). Table 15-1 lists the centric stops. In order to visualize the relationships among the centric stops, the reader is encouraged to look at a set of study models of a normal occlusion while studying the table.

Centric relation is the most retruded position of the mandible (that is, of the condyles) (Mostellear, 1980; Ramfjord and Ash, 1971). It is guided by ligaments and the structure of the condyles, articular disks, and glenoid fossae. Because centric relation is guided by anatomic structures other than the teeth, it is said to be a reproducible relationship between the jaws. Centric relation is used to determine the occlusion when full dentures or fixed partial dentures are constructed. For most persons with natural dentitions, centric relation and centric occlusion are not the same; rather, centric occlusion is about 1 to 2 mm anterior to centric relation (Mostellear, 1980; Ramfjord and Ash, 1971). A discrepancy between centric relation and centric occlusion is noteworthy for the patient's chart, but it does not denote occlusal problems in and of itself (Mostellear, 1980; Ramfjord and Ash, 1971).

Protrusive excursion is the forward movement of the mandible from centric relation or centric occlusion until the anterior teeth are in an edge-to-edge relationship. During a protrusive excursion (that is, once the anterior teeth are edge to edge) there should be no contact between the posterior teeth (Mosteller, 1980).

Lateral excursion is the movement of the mandible from centric occlusion or centric relation to the right or left until the cuspids on that side are in a cusp-to-cusp relationship. Some persons will not be able to achieve contact between the cuspids only; rather, they will have cusp-to-cusp contact with the premolars or molars as well. In lateral excursion, the teeth on the opposite side, the *nonworking side,* should be out of occlusion. For example, if the patient moves the jaw to the right, he or she has performed a right lateral excursion. The right side is the *working side,* and the left side is the *nonworking* side. If any of the teeth, other than the right cuspids, are occluding, they may be *interferences: working interferences* if on the right side and *nonworking interferences* if on the left side. Nonworking interferences are much more likely to cause destruction to the supporting structures than are working interferences. In fact, if more than one tooth other than the cuspid occludes evenly on the working side, the effect may be beneficial (Mosteller, 1980; Ramfjord and Ash, 1983).

Thus far in the chapter, the development of normal occlusion has been described and its characteristics discussed. Many patients have occlusal problems that cause them great pain, discomfort and tooth loss. The remainder of the chapter addresses occlusal trauma and assessment of occlusion.

TRAUMA FROM OCCLUSION

Ideally, the teeth are well aligned within each arch; contacts are present between adjacent teeth; marginal ridges of adjacent teeth are even; there are no rotated or malposed teeth (Krauss et al, 1969); and the teeth occlude in a Class I relationship (Thurow, 1977). This ideal arrangement of teeth permits the occlusal forces to be directed along the long axis of the teeth and permits forces to be shared by adjacent teeth (Carranza, 1979; Goldman and Cohen, 1980; Krauss et al, 1969; Ramfjord and Ash, 1971; Thurow, 1977). The supporting structures of the teeth—the periodontal ligament, cementum, and bone—accept and absorb the forces directed along the long axis of the tooth. The supporting structures can be damaged from forces that are in an oblique or horizontal direction to the long axis. In addition to permitting the forces to be directed along the long axis, this ideal arrangement also reflects a balance between the forces applied to the teeth by the tongue with the forces applied by the lips and cheeks (Carranza, 1979; Goldman and Cohen, 1980; Krauss et al, 1969; Ramfjord and Ash, 1971; Thurow, 1977). When forces are not directed through a normal arrangement, the supporting structures may be damaged; this damage is called *occlusal traumatism* (Glossary of Terms, 1977). *Occlusal trauma* is defined as "that force or forces . . . capable of producing pathologic changes in the periodontium" (Glossary of Terms, 1977).

There are two types of occlusal trauma: primary and secondary. *Primary occlusal trauma* is defined as excessive occlusal force applied to a tooth with normal supporting structures (Glossary of Terms, 1977); and *secondary occlusal trauma* is defined as "normal occlusal forces causing trauma to the attachment apparatus of a tooth or teeth because of inadequate support structure" (Glossary of Terms, 1977).

Occlusal trauma is a noninflammatory, destructive disease that affects the supporting structures; it is independent from periodontitis. Occlusal trauma does not cause periodontal pockets (Carranza, 1979; Goldman and Cohen, 1980; Zander and Polson, 1977). However, a tooth that is periodontally involved may be adversely affected by occlusal trauma. Occlusal traumatism is reversible if the etiologic factor(s) is removed or if the tooth moves away from the forces (Ramfjord and Ash, 1981). Therefore it is important to recognize and record the possible etiologic factors of occlusal trauma.

There are many possible *etiologic factors* of occlusal trauma. Any disturbance that interferes with the occlusal forces being directed normally or frequent, continuous, excessive forces exerted on one or a few teeth can cause destruction of the supporting structures (Carranza, 1979; Goldman and Cohen, 1980). The etiologic factors can be divided into several categories: tooth position, tooth-to-tooth habits, foreign object-to-teeth habits, oral musculature habits, and iatrogenic factors (Carranza, 1979; Goldman and Cohen, 1980; Krauss et al, 1969). Following is a summary of the etiologic factors that may affect occlusion:

1. Tooth position
   a. Rotated teeth
   b. Malposed teeth
   c. Extruded or submerged teeth
   d. Drifted teeth
   e. Missing teeth
   f. Other malocclusion
2. Tooth-to-tooth habit
   a. Clenching
   b. Grinding
3. Foreign object-to-teeth habit
   a. Biting pipe, pen, pencil, or other objects
   b. Biting or chewing fingernails
   c. Sucking thumb or fingers
4. Oral musculature habits
   a. Tongue thrust
   b. Tongue resting position
   c. Lip or cheek biting or sucking
   d. Mouth breathing
5. Iatrogenic factors
   a. Improperly contoured restorations
   b. Improperly fitted removal appliances

Etiologic factors causing occlusal traumatism or with the potential to cause occlusal traumatism should be noted in the patient's record during the oral examination.

In addition to etiologic factors, specific subjective, clinical, and radiographic signs and symptoms of occlusal traumatism should be detected and recorded by the clinician.

OCCLUSAL SCREENING

The subjective signs and symptoms reported by the patient are important in detecting occlusal traumatism. The patient will notice aching muscles, teeth that move, pain when biting, or pain with temperature changes. It is important to question the patient about grinding or clenching the teeth, holding a pipe in one area, chewing objects in one area, biting the lip, sucking a finger or thumb, and other possible habits. Sometimes a patient may be unaware of the habit or unaware of its significance until questioned.

Clinical and radiographic signs should also be recorded. Important clinical signs are mobility; wear patterns; changes in tooth position; poorly contoured restorations; plunger cusps; excessive overbite or overjet; overdevelopment of the muscles of mastication; clicking, pain, or improper movement of the TMJ; and tooth sensitivity (Carranza, 1979; Goldman and Cohen, 1980; Ramfjord and Ash, 1971). Remember that the presence of one or more of these signs does not mean that occlusal traumatism is present. All are indicators of potentially destructive forces, but the intensity, duration, and frequency of these forces and the resistance of the host to these forces are important factors in the development of occlusal traumatism. A force that causes destruction of the supporting structures of one person may not affect the supporting structures of another person. The key to occlusal traumatism is whether the force is causing, or is likely to cause, damage to the supporting structures. The destruction is best seen radiographically or histologically (Carranza, 1979; Goldman and Cohen, 1980; Zander and Polson, 1977).

Ramfjord and Ash (1981) have emphasized the role of plaque as an etiologic factor in periodontal disease associated with occlusal trauma. Destruction of the supporting structure due to plaque must be differentiated from occlusal traumatism.

The destruction of supporting structures from occlusal trauma includes widening of the periodontal ligament space, necrosis of the periodontal ligament, cemental tears, loss of the lamina dura, bone resorption, and root resorption (Carranza, 1979; Goldman and Cohen, 1980; Zander and Polson, 1977). Widening of the periodontal ligament spaces, loss of the lamina dura, and bone or root resorption can be detected radiographically and should be recorded.

These signs and symptoms are important and, if detected, should be brought to the attention of the supervising dentist. A suggested format for an occlusal screening is shown in the box. Note the suggested questions for gathering the subjective data from the patient. Once an occlusal screening

---

SAMPLE

Occlusal screening form

Patient's subjective findings

1. Are you pleased with the way your teeth look?
2. Have you noticed if any of your teeth have moved?
3. Do you have any problems speaking or eating because of your teeth?
4. Are any of your teeth bothering you? Are any of your teeth sore?
5. Do you clench or grind your teeth?
6. Do you bite or chew your lips, cheeks, or fingers?
7. Do you bite or chew any objects such as pencils or pipes?
8. Do you feel a "click" or "bump" when you open or close your jaw?

Clinical findings: record the tooth number of any tooth that exhibits

1. Mobility
2. Wear patterns
3. Malposition
4. Faulty restoration

and note the presence of

5. Pain or clicking in TMJ
6. Excessive overjet or overbite
7. Malocclusion

Radiographic findings: record the tooth number of any tooth that exhibits

1. Widened periodontal ligament space
2. Loss of continuity of lamina dura
3. Bone or root resorption

---

has been performed, the dentist may decide that an occlusal evaluation that examines the tooth-to-tooth relationships, the TMJ relationship, and the movements of the mandible must be performed.

OCCLUSAL ANALYSIS

Several formats for performing an occlusal analysis are available (Nasedkin, 1978; Ramfjord and Ash, 1971; Rieder, 1975; Shore, 1980). An occlusal analysis involves palpation and auditory examination of the TMJ and palpation of the mus-

cles of mastication in addition to examination of the tooth-to-tooth relationships. The occlusal analysis is presented here in a step-by-step format. It is recommended that a form such as the one shown opposite be used to record findings. The patient's subjective and radiographic findings discussed in the section on occlusal screening are also included in the occlusal analysis but do not need further discussion.

Extraoral findings

The clinician should examine the TMJ by placing his or her fingers over the joint and having the patient open and close his or her mouth. The clinician should record any clicking or excessive lateral movement of the TMJ. The TMJ can also be palpated by placing the little fingers into the patient's ears and having the patient open and close his or her mouth. This will allow the clinician to feel the posterior portion of the TMJ as the patient opens and closes the mouth (Nasedkin, 1978).

The lateral pterygoid muscle is palpated in two steps. If a patient is experiencing TMJ dysfunction, the lateral pterygoid muscle will be extremely sensitive. First, the patient opens the mouth, and the soft tissue posterior to the maxillary tuberosity is palpated. Then palpation buccal to the maxillary tuberosity is performed. The patient may have to close part way. If the muscle is in spasm, the patient will experience pain during the palpation. Pain or tenderness should be recorded. Other muscles of mastication–the temporalis, masseter, and buccinator—can also be palpated. Tenderness, swelling, or spasm should be recorded. At the minimum, the lateral pterygoid muscle should be palpated.

The clinician should note if the swallowing pattern is normal. It should also be noted if the mentalis muscle is used during swallowing. If so, the patient may have an abnormal swallowing pattern that is affecting the occlusion.

Intraoral findings

The patient's Angle's classification, overbite, and overjet should be determined and recorded. The patient's *maximum opening* must be recorded while the patient's mouth is open as wide as possible. The opening from incisal edge to incisal

SAMPLE
Occlusal Analysis Form

Extraoral findings

1. TMJ
   a. Pain
   b. Clicking
   c. Lateral movement
2. Lateral pterygoid muscle
3. Other muscles
   a. Masseter
   b. Buccinator
   c. Temporalis
   d. Mentalis
4. Swallowing pattern

Intraoral findings

1. Angle's classification
2. Overbite
3. Overjet
4. Maximum opening
5. Pathway of closure
6. Amount of movement from centric relation to centric occlusion
7. Direction of movement from centric relation to centric occlusion

Initial contact(s) in centric relation

1	2	3	4	5	6	7	8		9	10	11	12	13	14	15	16
32	31	30	29	28	27	26	25	24	23	22	21	20	19	18	17

Right lateral excursion

1	2	3	4	5	6	7	8		9	10	11	12	13	14	15	16
32	31	30	29	28	27	26	25	24	23	22	21	20	19	18	17

Left lateral excursion

1	2	3	4	5	6	7	8		9	10	11	12	13	14	15	16
32	31	30	29	28	27	26	25	24	23	22	21	20	19	18	17

Protrusive excursion

1	2	3	4	5	6	7	8		9	10	11	12	13	14	15	16
32	31	30	29	28	27	26	25	24	23	22	21	20	19	18	17

edge is measured (Fig. 15-6). The usual maximum opening is about 40 mm (Nasedkin, 1978). As the patient closes, the path of the mandible should be observed to note any deflection to the right or the left. An unusually small maximum opening or a large deflection may indicate a problem in the TMJ.

Centric relation must be determined next. If a patient is having occlusal problems, the muscles and ligaments guiding the mandible into centric relation may be in spasm. Centric relation may be difficult to establish. It can be determined if the patient relaxes the lower jaw allowing the clinician to guide it into centric relation. First stabilize the patient's head by holding the maxillary arch and grasping the chin to guide the mandible (Fig.

15-7, *A*). Then the clinician should try to move the mandible gently up and down until it feels relaxed. Once the mandible is relaxed, the clinician can guide the mandible upward and backward into centric relation (Fig. 15-7, *B*). Then the clinician can watch the mandible and direct the patient to bite together into centric occlusion. While the patient is biting from centric relation into centric occlusion, the clinician should note the approximate distance from centric relation to centric occlusion and the direction the mandible deflects. This information should be recorded.

Again, the patient is guided into centric relation and asked to indicate which teeth contact first during centric relation. Once the patient has indicated the area, it is dried with a stream of air

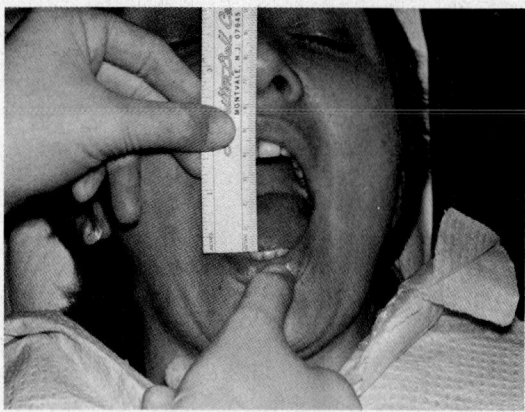

Fig. 15-6. Patient's maximum opening of mandible is measured.

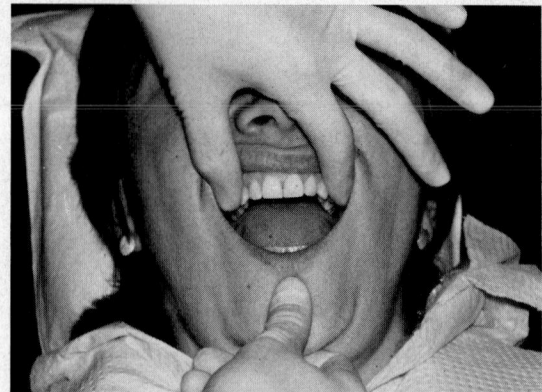

A

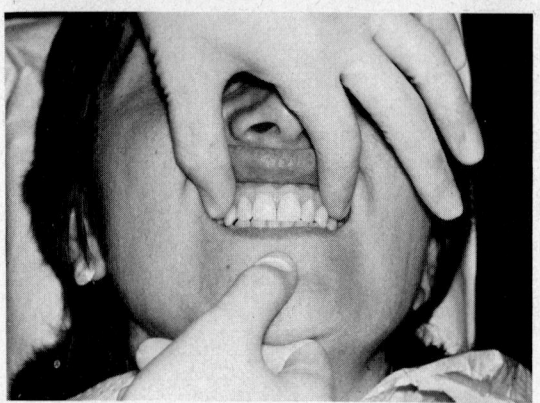

B

Fig. 15-7. Establishing centric relation. **A,** Patient's head is stabilized. **B,** Mandible is guided into centric relation.

(Fig. 15-8, *A*) and articulating paper is placed in the area. The patient is guided into centric relation with the paper in place; the patient then opens the mouth, and the initial contacts are recorded on the form. The initial contact or contacts are the teeth marked by the articulating paper (Fig. 15-8, *B, C*).

The lateral excursions are examined next. The patient starts from centric occlusion. The clinician guides him or her into a left lateral excursion (Fig. 15-9), observing the excursion to see which teeth may be contacting on the working as well as on the nonworking side. Interferences should be marked with articulating paper and recorded (Figs. 15-10 and 15-11). The same procedure is repeated for the right lateral and protrusive excursions (Fig. 15-12).

Once the teeth have been examined, the occlusal analysis is complete and can be analyzed. All of the findings must be considered as a whole. An interference may or may not be significant. If the interference is accompanied by other findings, such as bone loss, widened periodontal ligament space, tenderness of the lateral pterygoid muscle, or soreness of the tooth, the interference is probably significant.

SUMMARY

Occlusion is a complex human system that must be examined and considered as a whole. This chapter has presented information about the de-velopment of normal occlusion as well as occlusal trauma and occlusal analysis.

ACTIVITIES
1. Perform an occlusal screening for a partner.
2. Perform an occlusal screening as part of the baseline data collection for a patient.
3. Complete an independent project on any of the following topics:
   a. Centric relation versus centric occlusion
   b. Relationship of TMJ anatomy and occlusion
   c. Interrelationships among the TMJ, muscles of mastication, nerve supply, and teeth
4. Perform an occlusal analysis for a partner.

REVIEW QUESTIONS
1. Define the following terms:
   a. Overbite
   b. Occlusal trauma
   c. Occlusal traumatism

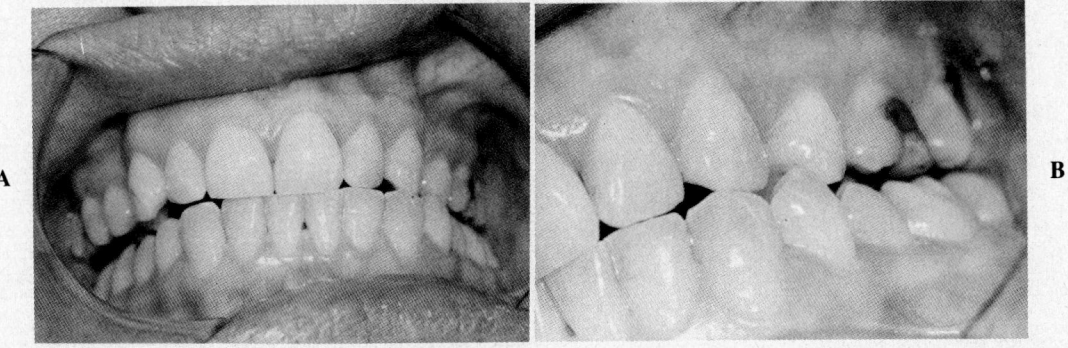

Fig. 15-8. Identifying initial contacts in centric relation. **A,** Drying teeth. **B,** Placement of articulating paper. **C,** Initial contact identified by markings.

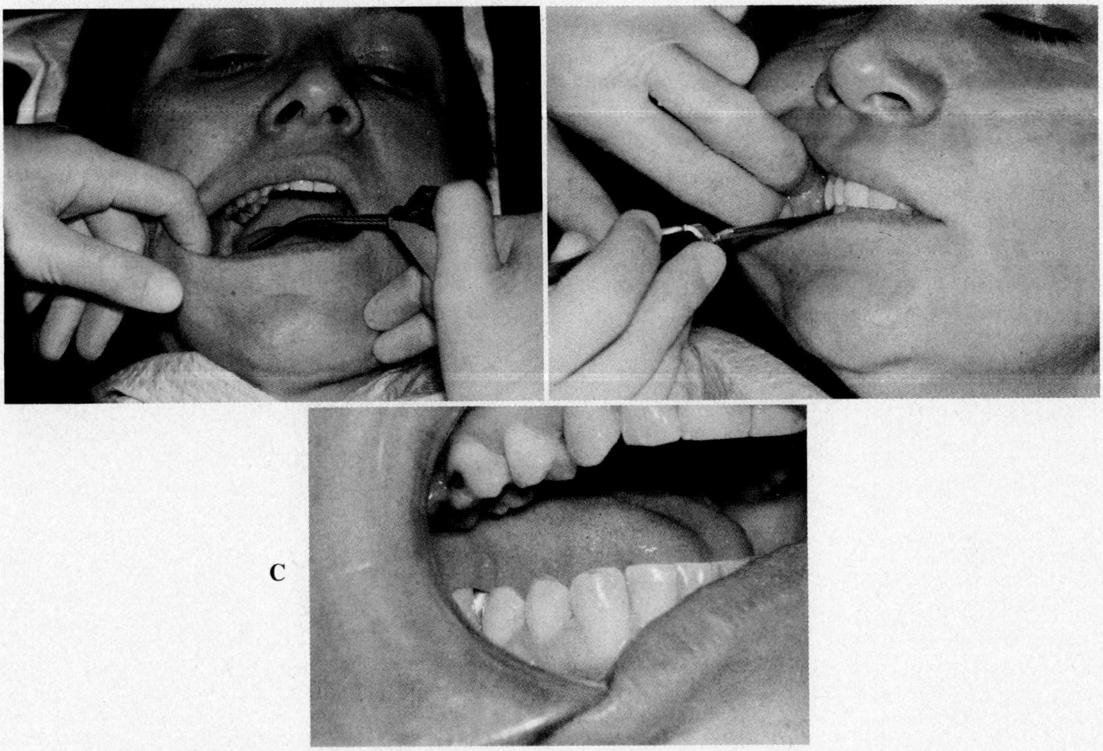

Fig. 15-9. Left lateral excursion. Mandible is shifted to left **A,** until cuspids are edge to edge, **B.**

2. List five etiologic factors of occlusal traumatism.
3. List the subjective, clinical, and radiographic signs and symptoms of occlusal traumatism.
4. True or false (correct each false statement):
   a. A patient may suffer from occlusal traumatism even though there is no damage to the supporting structure.
   b. Occlusal traumatism is serious because it causes the formation of periodontal pockets.
   c. If the force causing occlusal traumatism can be

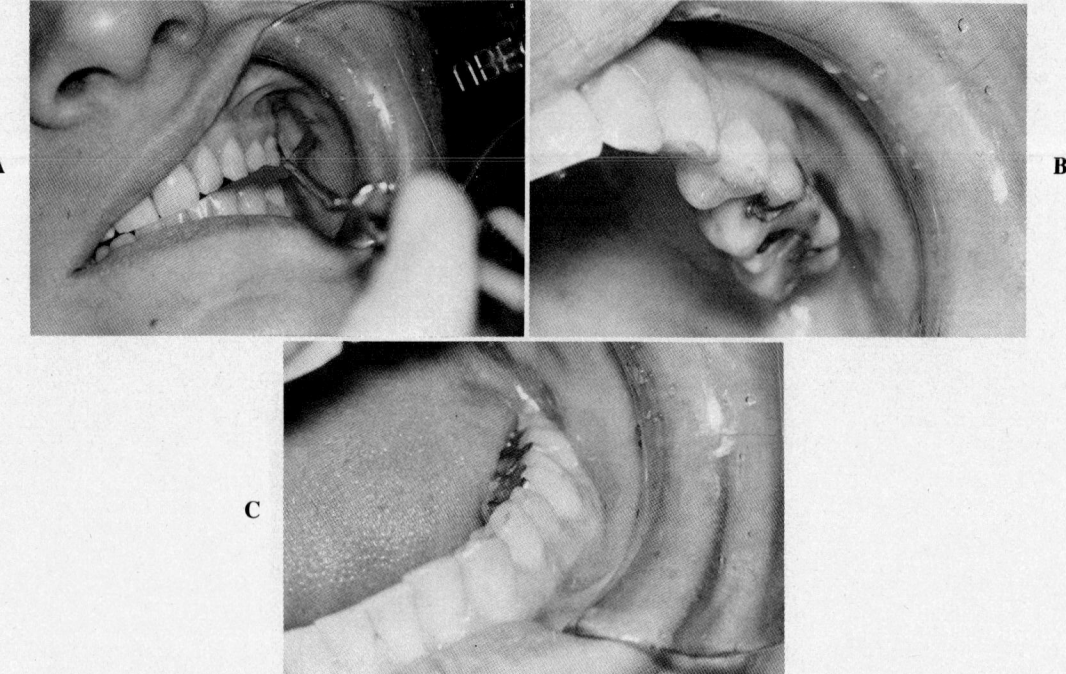

Fig. 15-10. Identifying working interferences of left lateral excursion. **A,** Articulating paper placed on dry teeth; left lateral excursion. Markings indicate interferences on maxilla **B,** and mandible, **C.**

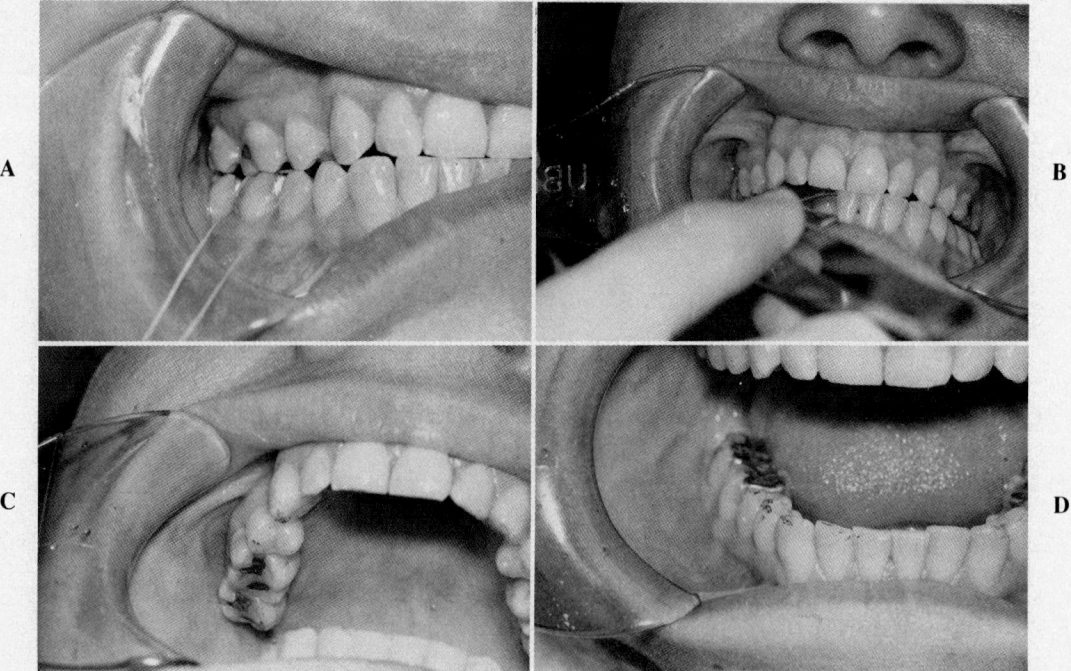

Fig. 15-11. Identifying nonworking interferences for left lateral excursion. **A,** Loop of floss is pulled from posterior to indicate interference. **B,** Articulating paper is placed. **C** and **D,** Interferences are shown by markings.

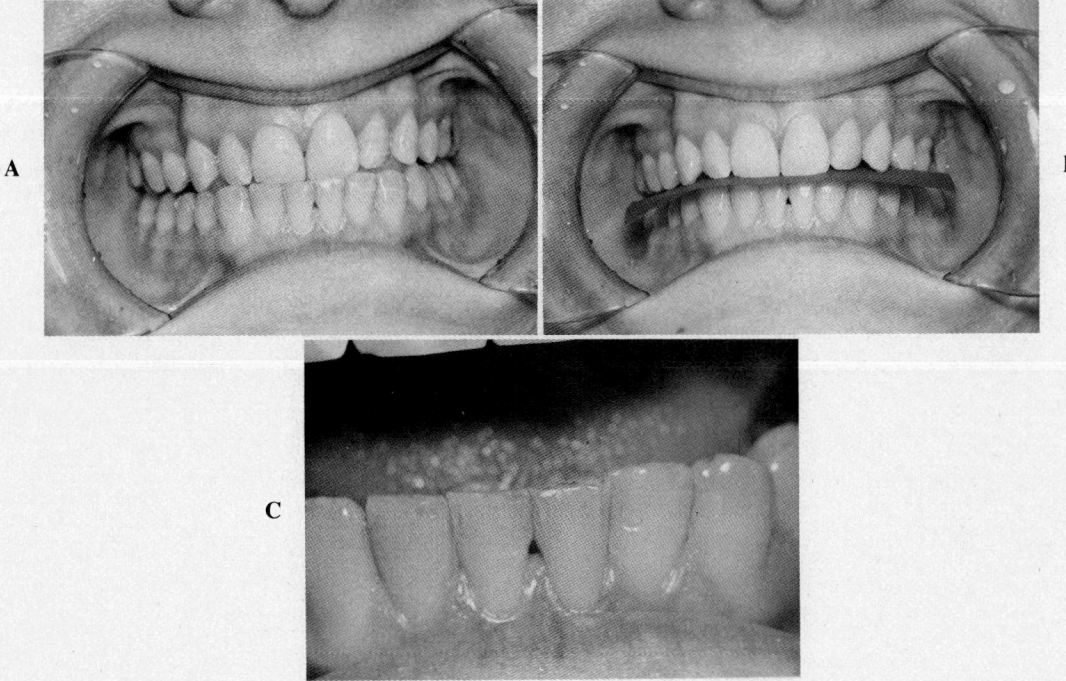

Fig. 15-12. **A,** Protrusive excursion. Articulating paper, **B,** shows markings of interferences, **C.**

removed from the tooth, the supporting structures will in many instances repair themselves.

REFERENCES

Ash MM, and Ramfjord SP: An introduction to functional occlusion, Philadelphia, 1982, WB Saunders Co.

Borell G: The development of normal occlusion, Alpha Omegan 73:15, 1980.

Carranza FA: Glickman's clinical periodontology, Philadelphia, 1979, WB Saunders Co.

Ericsson I, and Lindhe J: Effect of longstanding jiggling on experimental marginal periodontitis in the beagle dog, J Clin Periodontol 9:497, 1982.

Glaros AG, and Rao SM: Effects of bruxism: a review of the literature, J Prosthet Dent 38:149, 1977.

Glossary of terms. J Periodontol 48(Suppl):19, 1977.

Goldman HC, and Cohen DW: Periodontal therapy, ed 6, St Louis, 1980, The CV Mosby Co.

Hoople S: Occlusal evaluation module, Seattle, 1976, University of Washington.

Jago JD: The epidemiology of dental occlusion: a critical appraisal, J Pub Health Dent 34:80, 1974.

Krauss BS, et al: Dental anatomy and occlusion, Baltimore, 1969, Williams & Wilkins.

Levine N, and Pulver F: Guiding the developing occlusion in children, Alpha Omegan 72:49, 1979.

McDonald RE, and Avery DR: Dentistry for the child and adolescent, St Louis, 1983, The CV Mosby Co.

Mosteller JH: Occlusion of the natural dentition, J Ala Dent Assoc 64:36, 1980.

Nasedkin JN: Occlusal dysfunction: screening procedures and initial treatment planning, Gen Dent 26:52, 1978.

Perry HT: Temporomandibular joint and occlusion, Angle Orthod 46:284, 1976.

Ramfjord SP, and Ash MM: Occlusion, Philadelphia, 1983, WB Saunders Co.

Ramfjord SP, and Ash MM: Significance of occlusion in the etiology and treatment of early, moderate, and advanced periodontitis, J Periodontol 52:511, 1981.

Rieder CE: A simplified occlusal and temporomandibular examination procedure, CDA J 3:56, 1975.

Robinson, et al: Nocturnal teeth-grinding: a reassessment for dentistry, JADA 78:1308, 1969.

Schifter CC: Occlusal analysis module, Philadelphia, 1979, University of Pennsylvania.

Shore NA: Temporomandibular joint dysfunction: a review of successful diagnostic and therapeutic techniques, Alpha Omegan 73:67, 1980.

Stallard RE: Periodontal disease and its relationship to pulpal pathology, Periodontol Acad Rev 2:80, 1968.

Thurow RC: Atlas of orthodontic principles, ed 2, St Louis, 1977, The CV Mosby Co.

Waerhaug, J: The angular bone defect and its relationship to trauma from occlusion and downgrowth of subgingival plaque, J Clin Periodontol 6:61, 1979.

Weinberg LA: The role of stress, occlusion and condyle position in TMJ dysfunction—pain, J Prosthet Dent 49:532, 1982.

Weisgold AS: Occlusion: review of various concepts, Probe 16:373, 1975.

Wirth CG: Occlusion. In Boundy SS, and Reynolds NJ, editors, Current concepts in dental hygiene, vol 1, St Louis, 1977, The CV Mosby Co.

Woerth JH: Detecting occlusal dysfunction, Dent Hyg 53:456, 1979.

Zander HA, and Polson AM: Present status of occlusion and occlusal therapy in periodontics, J Periodontol 48:540, 1977.

16 PREPARATION OF STUDY MODELS

OBJECTIVES: *The reader will be able to*

1. List and describe the four uses of study models.
2. Identify the armamentarium used for making alginate impressions and gypsum models.
3. Discuss the health hazards associated with alginate, alginate impressions, and gypsum casts.
4. Briefly describe the significance of each of the following factors for alginate and for gypsum:
   a. Water-to-powder ratio
   b. Water temperature
   c. Method of manipulation
5. Justify the use of beading wax.
6. Describe how to prepare a patient who is to have an alginate impression.
7. List and evaluate the possible approaches to assist a patient with a gagging problem.
8. Describe how to determine if a tray is the proper size.
9. List and describe the steps for making maxillary and mandibular impressions.
10. Define the term border *molding*.
11. Discuss the proper way to remove an alginate impression from a patient's mouth.
12. State the rationale for making an interocclusal record and describe the technique.
13. Identify three methods for producing a properly formed base.
14. List the steps for pouring an alginate impression with plaster or stone.
15. Describe the effects of separating the impression too soon or too late from the cast.
16. List and describe the steps for trimming maxillary and mandibular casts.
17. Perform the following procedures for a partner:
    a. Assemble the armamentarium
    b. Prepare the patient
    c. Prepare the alginate impressions
    d. Prepare the interocclusal record
    e. Pour the models
    f. Trim the models

STUDY MODELS

Study models, or diagnostic casts, are exact plaster or stone replicas of the patient's mouth. The models are constructed from impressions of the patient's mouth that are filled with plaster material. When the hardened plaster is separated from the impression, the resulting model is referred to as a study model or a diagnostic cast (Fig. 16-1). After these models are trimmed and finished, they can be used as permanent records, diagnostic aids, and educational aids, as well as for the fab-

rication of temporary appliances (Craig, O'Brien, and Powers, 1983; Goldman and Cohen, 1980; Rudd, 1968).

Permanent records

Study models may be included in the initial records collected to document the conditions existing in a patient's mouth at the beginning of treatment. These three-dimensional records of the patient's mouth are a helpful addition to the two-dimensional charts and radiographs normally in-

289

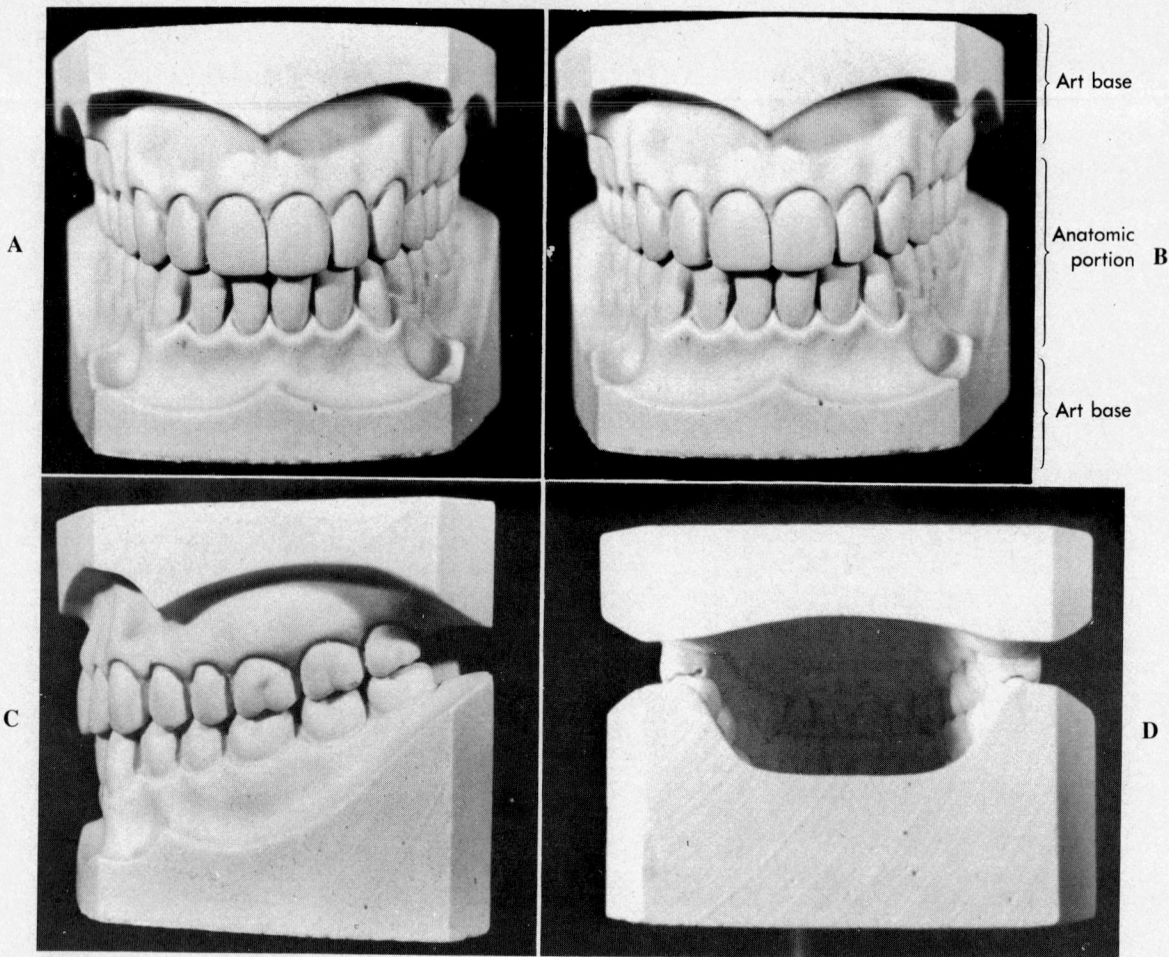

Art base

Anatomic portion **B**

Art base

Fig. 16-1. Trimmed study models. **A,** Anterior view. **B,** Anterior view with anatomic portion and bases indicated. **C,** Side view. **D,** Posterior view.

cluded in an initial set of records. Study models can be used to document the progress of involved and/or long-term treatment. Models are made periodically during treatment and again at the conclusion of treatment. Several of the dental specialties (orthodontics, prosthodontics, periodontics, and oral surgery) as well as general dentistry routinely include models in patient records.

Diagnostic aids

Study models permit the clinician to examine conditions in the patient's mouth from all views, including those impossible during a clinical examination (as from the lingual or the direct distal aspects) (Fig. 16-1). The relationships between ad-

jacent teeth and opposing teeth can be examined, measured, and analyzed as needed without discomfort to the patient. The clinician can draw or perform proposed treatments on the study models. Occlusal relationships can also be examined on the models. To demonstrate the precise movements of the mandible, the models can be mounted on an articulator (Rudd, 1968) (Fig. 16-2); in this way, the patient's mandibular movements can be replicated. The dentist can consider those movements when designing appliances and restorations for the patient.

Study models are also useful during charting procedures, particularly periodontal chartings (Goldman and Cohen, 1980; Hirshfeld, 1933).

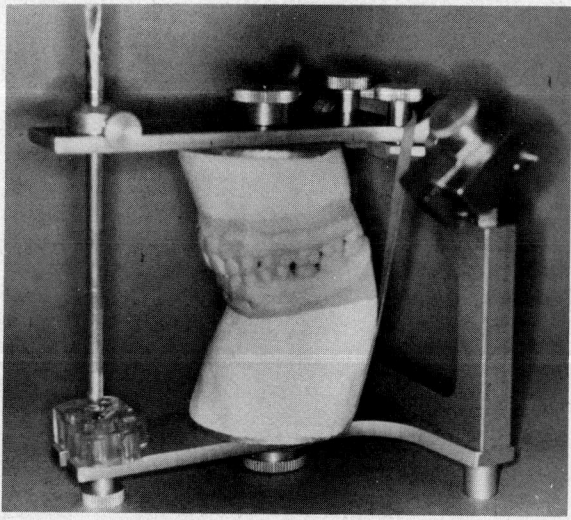

Fig. 16-2. Models mounted on an articulator.
(From Gilmore, HW et al: Operative dentistry, ed 4, St Louis, 1982, The CV Mosby Co.)

Wear facets, open contacts, rotated teeth, recession, and other such findings can be viewed on the models and recorded on the chart. The use of study models for recording these findings can save valuable chairside time.

Educational aids

During case presentations and patient education sessions, study models can be used as an educational tool to illustrate the patient's existing conditions and various possible treatments. The patient can become a partner during these sessions because she or he is able to view the mouth in the same way the clinician does. Study models are an excellent tool for describing and demonstrating individualized home care procedures to patients (Hirshfeld, 1933). Patients can practice the techniques on the models before performing them.

Fabrication of temporary appliances

Study models can be used in the making of temporary appliances such as mouth guards and some orthodontic appliances (Craig, O'Brien, and Powers, 1983; Rudd, 1968). When used for this purpose, they may be called *working models*. They are constructed of a harder gypsum product than are regular study models (Fig. 16-3).

An increasing number of states' dental practice acts permit dental hygienists and dental assistants to make alginate impressions and construct study models (see Table 1-1). This chapter describes the procedures for making alginate impressions and constructing study models. Brief descriptions of each of the materials used are presented. The reader should consult a dental materials textbook for in-depth discussions.

OVERVIEW OF THE PROCEDURES

The making of study models includes assembling the armamentarium, preparing the patient, making the alginate impressions, making the interocclusal record, pouring the models, and trimming and finishing the models. It is an involved process that can be mastered in stages.

Assembling the armamentarium

The armamentarium needed is as follows:

Making the impression	*Pouring the model*
Rubber bowl and spatula	Rubber bowl and spatula
Alginate with powder and water measures	Plaster or stone
	Vibrator
Impression trays	Buffalo knife
Beading wax	Model base formers or
Baseplate wax	boxing wax, glass
Buffalo knife	slab, or other materi-
Mouthwash	al(s) to form the base
	Model trimmer

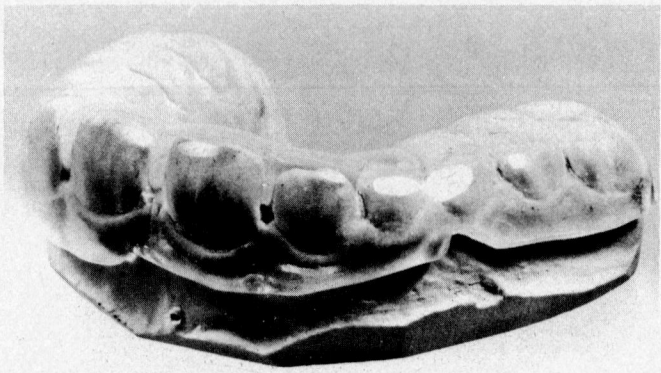

Fig. 16-3. Working model with clear plastic mouth protector in place.
(From Craig RG, O'Brien WJ, and Powers JM: Dental materials: properties and manipulation, ed 3, St Louis, 1983, The CV Mosby Co.)

Alginate is a flexible irreversible hydrocolloid impression material. It is composed of sodium alginate salt (derived from marine kelp); calcium sulfate; potassium sulfate, zinc fluoride, silicates, or borates; sodium phosphate, diatomaceous earth or silicate powder; and flavoring and coloring agents (ADA Council, 1983; Craig, 1980). The material is supplied as a powder in either premeasured pouches or a bulk-pack can to be measured as used, with a scoop and vial to measure the water and powder in the proper proportions. When the powder is mixed with water, it forms a gel that will flow around the oral structures and harden. When the alginate is removed from the mouth, it stretches slightly to pull over the structures and then springs back to the form it had in the mouth. Alginate is relatively pleasant tasting, easily mixed, inexpensive, and relatively accurate, making it the material of choice for study model impressions (Craig, O'Brien, and Powers, 1983).

Important factors to keep in mind when manipulating alginate are water-to-powder ratio, water temperature, and mixing method (Craig, O'Brien, and Powers, 1983; Roswick and Simon, 1974a). Follow the manufacturer's directions for each of these factors.

Too much water results in a runny, slow-setting, weakened mix; too little produces a stiff, fast-setting, hard-to-manipulate mix. The water temperature also affects the setting time of the alginate mix. The method used to mix the alginate should minimize the amount of air incorporated into the mix. This can be accomplished by adding the powder to the water and by using a mixing motion that wipes the spatula against the side of the bowl while the bowl is rotated (Fig. 16-4). A well-mixed alginate should be homogenous, smooth, and creamy (Fig. 16-5).

Alginate is available in fast-set or normal-set formulas. Fast-set alginate gels in 1 to 2 minutes from the beginning of the mix; normal-set alginate gels in 2 to 4½ minutes (ADA Council, 1981). Fast-set alginate is ideal for use with patients who have a tendency toward gagging and with children. It is recommended that both types of alginate remain in the mouth for 2 minutes, whenever possible, to allow sufficient flowing of the material around the structures and then time to gel (ADA Council, 1983).

Alginate impressions lose water when exposed to air, causing the impression to dry out, shrink, and eventually become very brittle. If the impression is not going to be poured immediately, it should be wrapped in a wet paper towel until it is poured (ADA Council, 1981; Craig, O'Brien, and Powers, 1983).

Impression trays. Various types of metal, plastic, and Styrofoam trays are available to use with alginate (Fig. 16-6). The type of tray used depends on convenience and the clinician's preference. The metal trays can be sterilized and re-

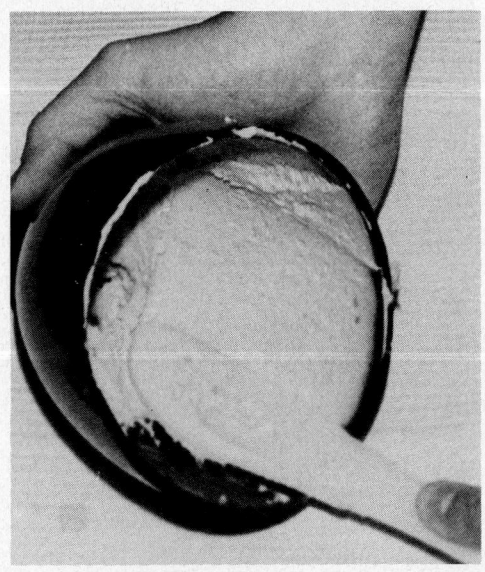

Fig. 16-4. Spatula is wiped against side of bowl to minimize air bubbles during mixing.

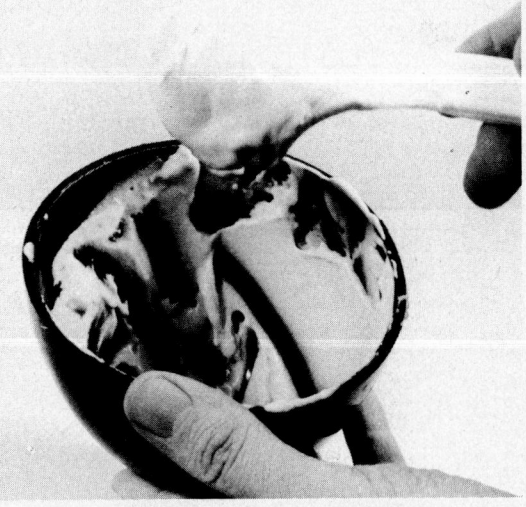

Fig. 16-5. Proper consistency of mixed alginate.
(From Craig, RG, O'Brien WJ, and Powers JM: Dental materials: properties and manipulation, ed 3, St Louis, 1983, The CV Mosby Co.)

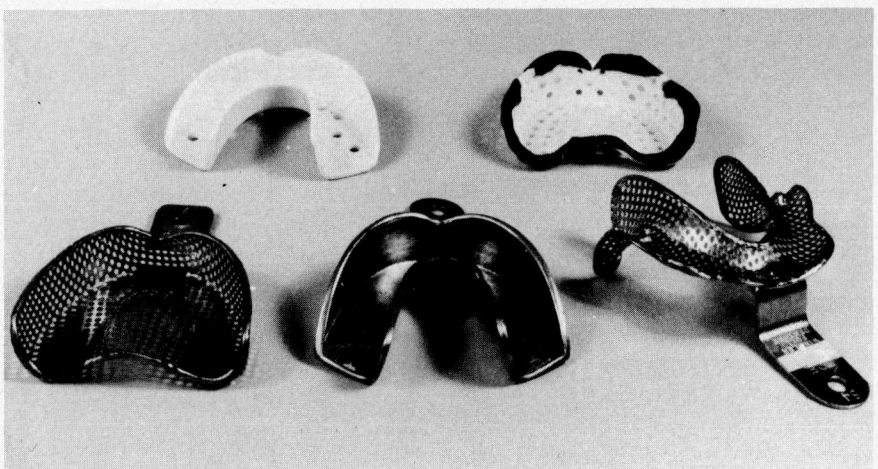

Fig. 16-6. Examples of impression trays: disposable and Styrofoam trays are also available. Note beading wax applied to upper right plastic tray.
(From Craig RG, O'Brien WJ, and Powers JM: Dental materials: properties and manipulation, ed 3, St Louis, 1983, The CV Mosby Co.)

used; the plastic trays cannot be sterilized with heat. With increasing knowledge of disease transmission and asepsis, it seems highly inappropriate to use a tray that cannot be sterilized (Greenlee, 1983). The Styrofoam trays are designed to be used once and then discarded. The trays can be imperforate or perforated, as long as there is some means of mechanically locking the alginate into the tray to prevent dislodgement when the impression is removed from the mouth. Some

Styrofoam trays may require an adhesive. All types are available in several sizes to accommodate any size mouth.

Beading wax. Beading wax, a soft wax available in strips, is placed around the edges of metal and plastic trays (Fig. 16-6). The wax extends the trays to include the vestibule and posterior areas in the impression. The wax also makes the trays more comfortable for the patient (Craig, O'Brien, and Powers, 1983).

Plaster and/or stone. Plaster and stone are two materials used to construct study models. They are derived from the mineral gypsum, the dihydrate form of calcium sulfate (Craig, O'Brien, and Powers, 1983). Plaster is less dense and easier to trim and finish. Some practitioners prefer stone because it is stronger and less likely to fracture or abrade. As with alginate, it is important to remember the following three factors when working with plaster and/or stone: water-to-powder ratio, water temperature, and mixing technique (Craig, O'Brien, and Powers, 1983; Roswick and Simon, 1974). Follow the manufacturer's recommendations for the water-to-powder ratio. The recommended ratio for plaster ranges from 40 to 50 ml of water for each 100 g of plaster; the range for stone is from 30 to 40 ml of water for each 100 g of stone (ADA Council, 1981). If scales and vials to measure the proper amount of each component are not provided, the clinician must learn to recognize the proper consistency through experience. Too much water increases the setting time and produces a weak final product. Too little water decreases the setting time and produces a stronger final product; however, the mix is extremely difficult to manipulate, and will not flow into the impression readily. Water temperature below 70°F (21°C) increases the setting time; water between 70°F (21°C) and 98.6°F (37°C) decreases the setting time; but a reaction will not occur in water above 98.6°F. As can be seen, water temperature and water-to-powder ratio are very important when trying to mix plaster and/or stone (Craig, O'Brien and Powers, 1983; Roswick and Simon, 1974b).

The gypsum product is mixed by placing the water in the rubber bowl and adding the powder. Craig, O'Brien, and Powers (1983) recommend that the powder be allowed to sit in the water, undisturbed, for about 30 seconds before mixing to decrease the amount of air incorporated into the gypsum. The mixing technique is similar to that recommended for the alginate: rotary and wiping strokes are used. Once the gypsum is mixed, the bowl can be placed on the activated vibrator so that the air bubbles will rise to the surface and burst. Eliminating air from the gypsum at this stage will lessen the possibility of air bubbles, which cause voids in the final study models. After mixing, the material should be homogeneous, smooth, and about the consistency of sour cream (see Fig. 16-17).

Vibrator. The vibrator is used to flow the gypsum into the impression, spreading it evenly throughout the impression. It is especially useful to eliminate air bubbles. The use of the vibrator is discussed further in connection with pouring the model.

Model trimmer. The model trimmer is used to trim the hardened gypsum into the proper form. Only the base and borders of the model are trimmed; none of the anatomic structures recorded on the model are trimmed.

Considering health hazards

Seemingly harmless materials such as alginate, the impressions, and gypsum models present health risks that must be considered and guarded against. The health hazards fall into three categories; cross-contamination from gypsum models, release of fluoride from alginate, and airborne particles from alginate.

Cross-contamination can occur between patients and dental personnel by means of gypsum models. Microorganisms have been recovered from stone casts, showing that the casts may be a medium for transmitting disease from patients to dental personnel, especially personnel working with the casts in a laboratory (Leung and Schonfeld, 1983).

Many diseases can be transmitted in the dental office. Viral hepatitis presents the most likely danger. In recent years, acquired immune deficiency syndrome (AIDS) has created great concern among both patients and health care workers. Although it is undeniably a deadly disease, AIDS is not transmitted by casual contact and does not pose a significant threat if routine precautions are taken. These precautions to prevent the spread of microorganisms are relatively easy to observe and do provide a high level of protection for office and laboratory personnel as well as patients.

All metal impression trays should be sterilized along with other instruments. Plastic and styrofoam trays should be used once and discarded. The impression itself can be disinfected after removal from the mouth. First, rinse it with water to remove saliva, blood, and/or debris. Then soak it for 10 minutes in either an iodophor solution or a solution of hypochlorite (household bleach) at a ratio of 1/4 cup of hypochlorite to 1 gallon of water. (Dum and Novak, 1987). Although neither of these solutions provides true sterilization, both decrease the activity of microorganisms significantly. The accuracy of the impression is not adversely affected by either spraying the impression or by soaking it in the solution used (Herrera and Merchant, 1986, Matyas et al, 1986). Other researchers (Rowe et al, 1978) have suggested soaking the impression for 1 minute in chlorhexidine. This reduces the level of bacterial contamination but does not eliminate the hepatitis virus.

The models formed from the impression, as well as any prosthesis or other appliance, should be soaked in either the iodophor or hypochlorite solution to further discourage the growth and spread of microorganisms that are transferred from the impression to the model. Any prosthesis or other appliance formed on the model can also be soaked in one of the solutions.

Other disinfecting and sterilizing agents are available, but they distort the impression, rendering it valueless. Additional information about the sterilization of impressions and casts should be sought.

Office personnel must wear rubber gloves and a mask when making the impressions and when pouring and trimming the casts. Such steps will decrease the chances of cross-contamination during these procedures (Leung and Schonfeld, 1983).

Fluoride is a component of alginate. It is released from the alginate and absorbed by patients (Hattab, 1981; Hattab et al, 1978). This fact caused concern because high blood levels of fluoride can be toxic. Hattab has indicated, however, that fluoride absorbed from alginate has caused a significant increase in the blood plasma level of fluoride in only one instance.

If alginate is swallowed, the fluoride level increases significantly. This is particularly important if the patient is a child; therefore, caution patients not to swallow alginate material. Hattab (1981) measured the amount of fluoride absorbed by personnel exposed to alginate during mixing and found it to be negligible.

The final health hazard to be considered is exposure to *airborne particles* from alginate. Most manufacturers recommend that the alginate be shaken before it is measured, but this shaking introduces particles of the alginate into the air when the can or pouch is opened. Dental personnel are exposed to powders, lead, and silicone particles (Brune et al, 1978). It has been found that masks do not filter out the particles; no adequate protection is available. The concentration of the airborne particles is greatly reduced after 10 minutes. The precise effect of breathing these particles is unknown, but working in a well-ventilated area is recommended (de Freitas, 1980).

Preparing the patient

One of the most important keys to obtaining acceptable impressions and, ultimately, acceptable study models is proper patient management. Explaining the procedure and offering reassurance usually puts the patient at ease and increases his or her confidence in the clinician. A brief explanation of what will be done and how the patient can help is appropriate. This is important for both adult and pedodontic patients. Children want to know what is to be done and how they should help. It is helpful to liken the materials to be used to objects with which the child is familiar—for example the tray is like a big spoon (Hill and Gellin, 1970). (Point out that, unlike with a spoon, the material in the tray *should not* be swallowed.) As with any procedure, the patient will have confidence in a clinician whose work is thorough, efficient, and done with confidence.

The patient may be seated in either an upright or a supine position for the alginate impression procedure. When working without an assistant, many practitioners seat the patient in an upright position to prevent patient gagging (Chasteen, 1988). With four-handed dentistry procedures used to make the impression, the patient can be placed in a supine position. Gagging may be less of a problem when the patient is in a supine position, because the tongue is then in a relaxed position. It rests against the soft palate, closing off the oropharynx (Hill and Gellin, 1970). If gagging is a problem for some patients, several approaches can be used to minimize it.

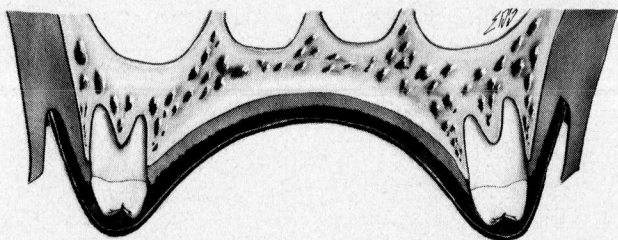

Fig. 16-7. Alginate flows between tray and oral structures. Note that there is about ¼ inch (6 mm) of material between tray and structures. Some of the alginate extends into mucobuccal fold area.

One approach is to encourage the patient to breathe through the nose rather than through the mouth when the tray is in place. The patient can practice breathing through the nose before the tray is placed; this may help the patient feel less panicky if gagging occurs. A patient who is a known gagger can hold an ice cube in the mouth or rinse with an anesthetic mouthwash before the tray is placed. These will have a slight numbing effect on the patient's mouth. Some clinicians use topical anesthetic ointment or spray to avert gagging. The use of a topical anesthetic spray is not recommended, however (see Chapter 31), because a patient with a numb soft palate may experience a gagging sensation. In addition, gagging is a reflex to prevent aspiration of a foreign object; eliminating the reflex can be dangerous. In a few instances a patient may have such a severe gagging problem that the dentist may decide to prescribe an agent such as nitrous oxide sedation for the procedure (Chasteen, 1988). Another approach is to have the patient concentrate on something other than the gagging sensation, such as looking at a spot on the wall or holding one leg up. These strategies will help. It is very important for the clinician to remain calm and to reassure the patient. The alginate should not be removed until it has set; removing it too soon would worsen the situation since the material would be very gooey. Fortunately, severe gagging problems are rare.

Making the impression

The tray selected should be large enough to permit ¼ inch (6 mm) of alginate to flow between the tray and the oral structures (Fig. 16-7); however, it should not be so large that it impinges on the soft tissues or causes the patient pain (Fig. 16-8). Once the proper tray has been selected, add beading wax to the borders of the tray. The

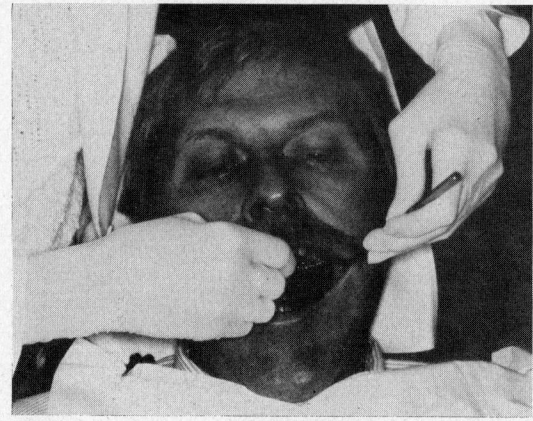

Fig. 16-8. After initial fitting of tray, beading wax has been applied to lower tray and tray is fitted once more.

wax should be added in a strip not more than 5 to 6 mm wide (the wax is supplied in a strip of this width). More wax would prevent the tray from being inserted or seated far enough over the teeth. The alginate material can then be mixed for the lower impression.

While it is being mixed (or before), the patient can rinse with the diluted mouthwash. The tray should be filled up to the level of the beading wax and smoothed with damp fingers (Fig. 16-9) to produce better gypsum models (Morris et al, 1983). Overfilling the tray will cause an excessive amount of material to flow out of the tray and into the patient's mouth; underfilling the tray may cause voids in the impression. When the mandibular tray is properly filled, invert the tray, retract one of the cheeks with the side of the tray, and rotate the tray into the mouth while retracting the other cheek with a mirror (Fig. 16-10). Once the tray is centered in the mouth and the posterior

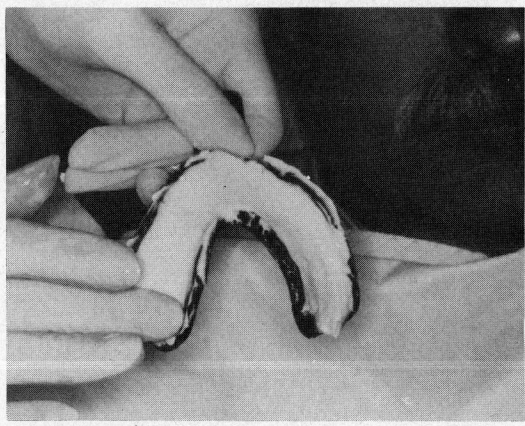

Fig. 16-9. Tray is filled to level of beading wax with alginate and smoothed with a damp finger.

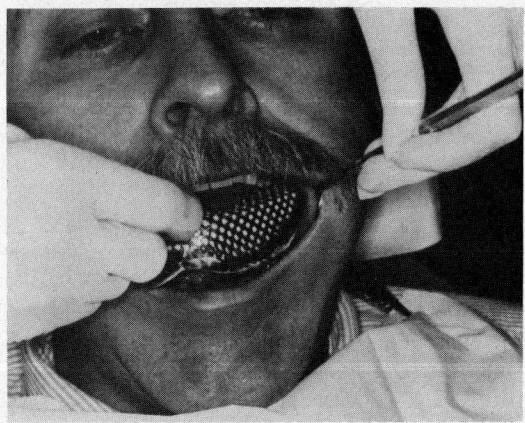

Fig. 16-10. Tray is inverted; one side is used to retract patient's right cheek while clinician retracts left cheek with a finger and rotates tray into mouth. Note that clinician is between 10 o'clock and 12 o'clock positions.

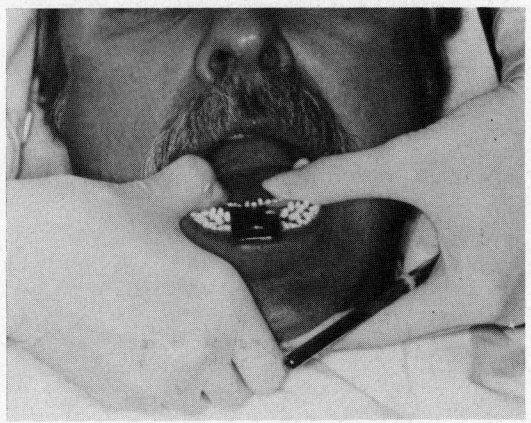

Fig. 16-11. Tray is centered, posterior border is seated, and tray is completely seated and stabilized until alginate sets.

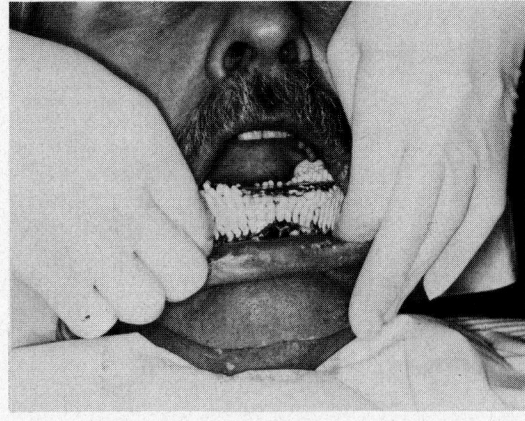

Fig. 16-12. Seal is broken with index fingers, and tray is removed with thumbs protecting upper teeth from contact with tray.

borders are seated over the arch, ask the patient to raise the tongue. The tray can then be completely seated (Fig. 16-11). Take care not to push the tray against the teeth. This could displace all the impression material, resulting in an inaccurate impression. The tray is held in position with a light pressure, while the lip is pulled up to ensure the inclusion of the frenum and the muscle attachments. This procedure of pulling the patient's lip is called *border molding* or *muscle trimming* and is performed to record the patient's muscle attach-

ment and mucobuccal fold in the impression (Roswick and Simon, 1974). When the alginate is set, the tray, with the impression, is removed with a quick, steady, upward motion. This can be accomplished by placing the thumbs on the occlusal portion of the tray to insulate the opposing teeth from the tray, placing the index fingers in the vestibule to break the seal around the tray, and lifting the tray upward (Fig. 16-12). An alternative method of removing the tray is to use the handle to pull the tray upward and the fingers

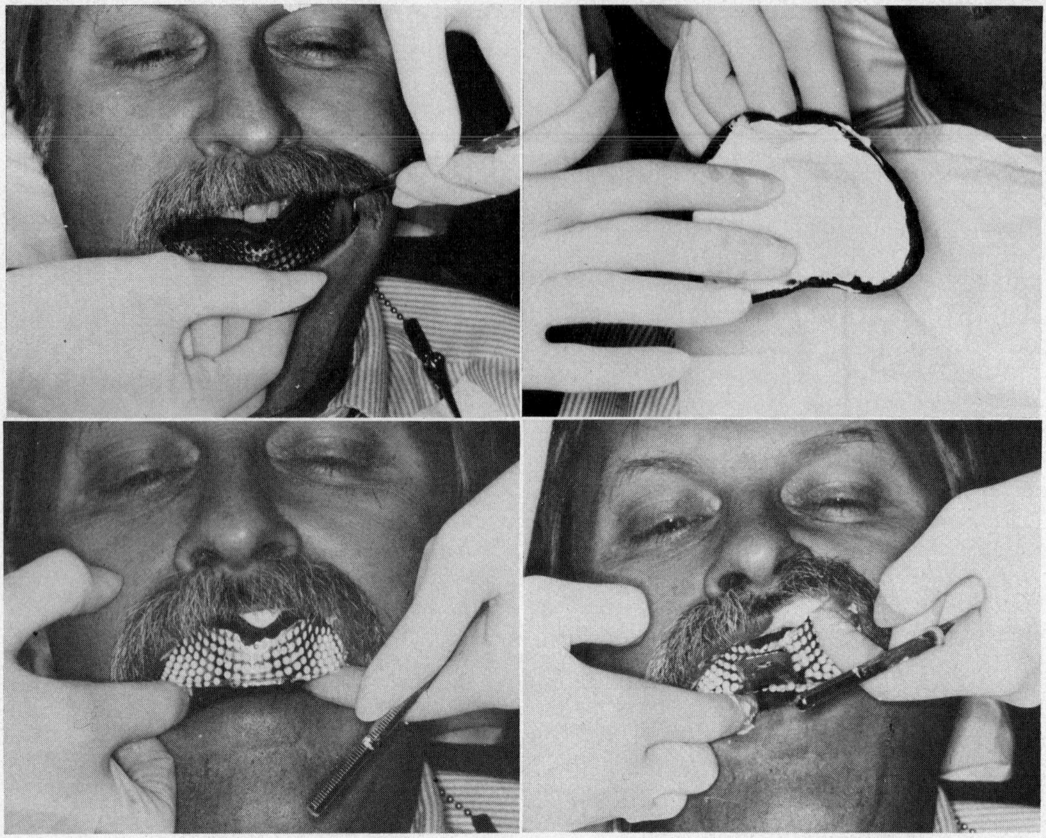

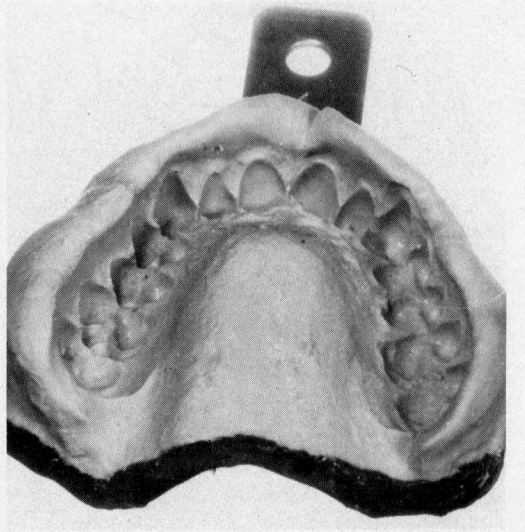

Fig. 16-13. Making maxillary impression. **A,** Tray is fitted. **B,** Alginate is wiped into tray and smoothed with damp fingers. **C,** The tray is rotated into mouth and the posterior border is seated; then remainder of tray is seated. **D,** Clinician muscle molds by pulling lip downward.

Fig. 16-14. Acceptable alginate impression.
(From Craig RG, O'Brien WJ, and Powers JM: Dental materials: properties and manipulation, ed 3, St Louis, 1983, The CV Mosby Co.)

from the other hand to insulate the opposing teeth. It is important to use a quick motion to reduce distortion of the material. Rocking the alginate impression during removal will cause permanent distortion of the material (Craig, O'Brien, and Powers, 1983; Roswick and Simon, 1974a).

Similar techniques (Fig. 16-13) are employed to make and to remove the maxillary impressions. The possibility of a gagging problem is greater for the maxillary impression procedure, so it is important to employ methods to reduce gagging. Avoid excess alginate in the posterior region to lessen chances of gagging.

An acceptable impression is shown in Fig. 16-14. The alginate impressions should be poured as soon as possible to prevent distortion. If they are not poured immediately, they can be wrapped in damp paper towels for brief storage.

Making the interocclusal record

An interocclusal bite record is needed for correct relation of the mandibular model to the maxillary model during the trimming. Many techniques and materials are available for making the bite record; one simple, common technique uses a soft, moldable wax such as pink baseplate wax. The wax is folded double and trimmed to the shape of the patient's dental arch using a Buffalo knife. It is then softened in warm water and held against the maxillary arch while the patient is guided into the desired occlusal relationship (Fig. 16-15). In this way, the patient's centric occlusion is recorded by

the indentations into the wax. It may help to tell the patient to bite on the back teeth (check to be sure the patient is biting "as usual"). While the patient's mouth is closed, use a cold water spray to harden the wax to avoid distortion when the wax is removed (Graber, 1972).

At the completion of the impression and the interocclusal record procedures, reassure the patient and thank him or her for being cooperative. Wipe the patient's face with a damp towel to remove any excess alginate.

As previously suggested, soak the impression for 5 minutes or longer in a disinfecting solution.

Pouring the study models

The maxillary and mandibular models are each composed of a base and an anatomic portion. The anatomic portion, formed by the impression, consists of the teeth and the soft tissues recorded in the impression. The base can be formed by several methods: base formers, boxing wax, and single-pour or double-pour techniques. Base formers, boxing wax, and the single-pour technique are described in this section. The base formed should be large enough to give the trimmed models a ½-inch (12.5-mm) base and borders that extend about ¼ inch (6 mm) beyond the recorded vestibule.

Before pouring, the impression can be gently rinsed with plain or soapy water to remove debris and saliva. A gentle stream of air can be used to dry the impression to reduce the excess moisture.

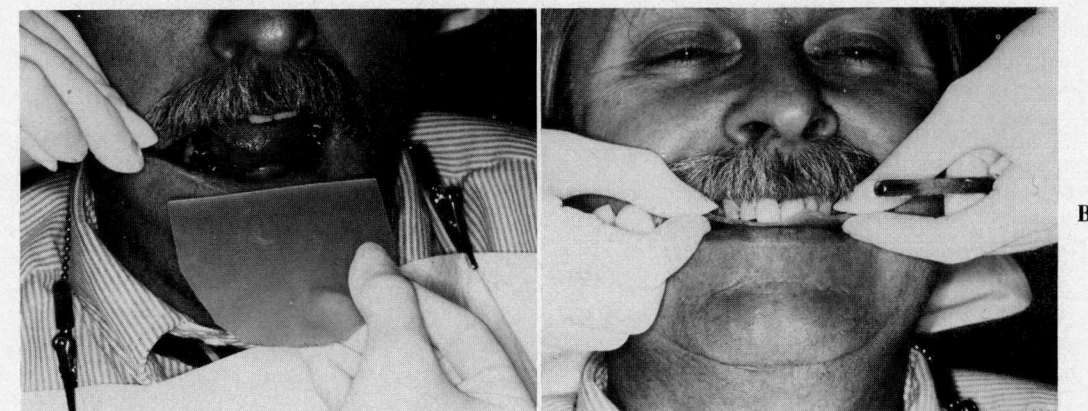

A   B

Fig. 16-15. Making interocclusal record. **A,** Trimmed baseplate wax. **B,** Softened wax is held against upper arch as patient bites.

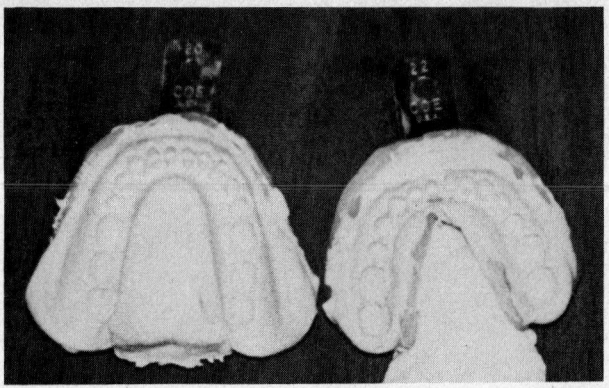

Fig. 16-16. Mandibular impression on left has had tongue area filled in with alginate; impression on right is ready for alginate to be smoothed into tongue area. This procedure eliminates void area in mandibular impression and prepares it for accepting stone or plaster during the pouring process.

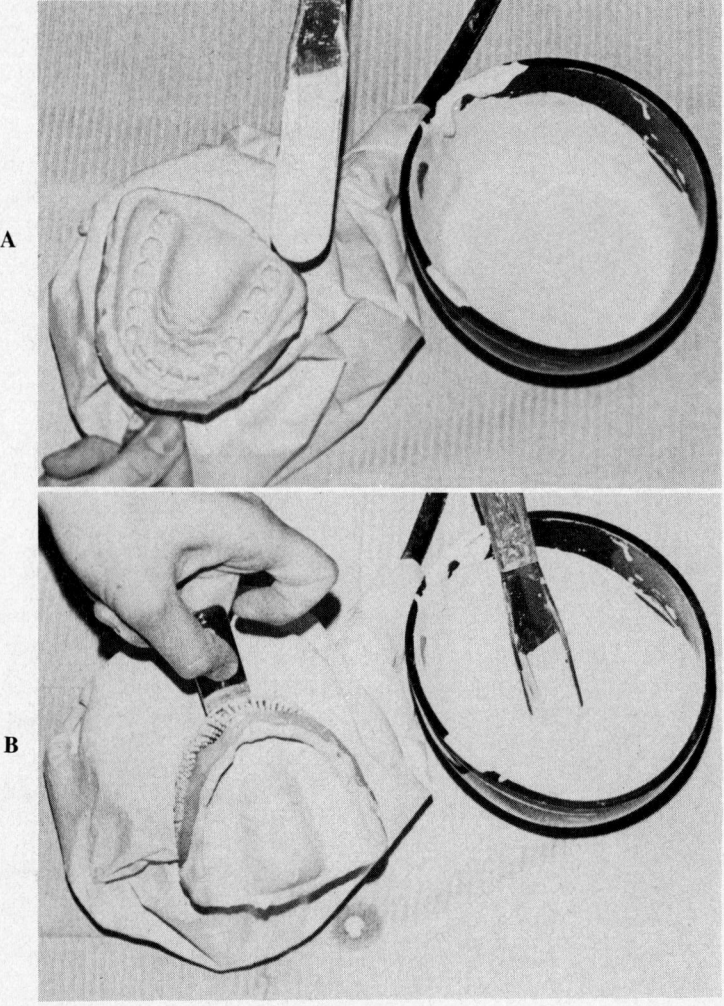

A

B

Fig. 16-17. A small increment is flowed into maxillary impression. **B,** Gypsum has been flowed around tray to fill all teeth. Note sour cream consistency of gypsum.

Excess water or saliva pooled in the impression can cause air bubbles and/or voids in the final study model.

That part of the mandibular tray that is open for the tongue must be filled in with alginate before the model is poured (Fig. 16-16). The tray is placed on a flat surface, and a damp paper towel is folded and placed in the opening at a level about one-half the height of the tray. One measure of alginate is mixed and is placed in the opening over the paper towel. The clinician must be careful not to allow the alginate to flow into any of the teeth. Once the alginate has hardened, the impression is ready to be poured.

After the plaster or stone is mixed, a small increment is flowed from one end of the impression to the other by rolling the tray on the vibrator (Roswick and Simon, 1974b) (Fig. 16-17). Increments of the gypsum are added and manipulated, as described previously, until all of the teeth are filled. Press the tray against the vibrator to eliminate air bubbles in the gypsum (Fig. 16-18). Throughout mixing and pouring, try to prevent and/or eliminate air from the mix. Once all of the

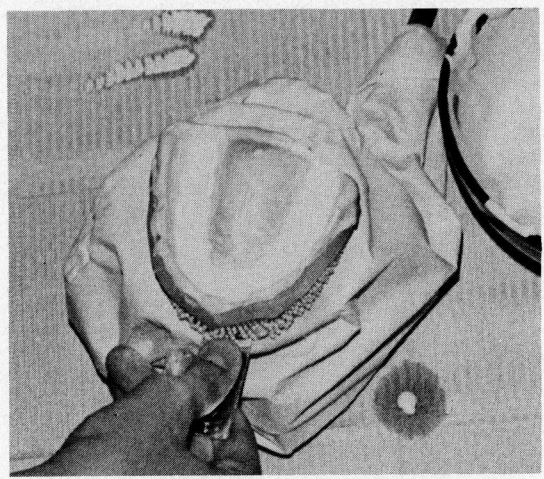

Fig. 16-18. Gypsum is added, and downward pressure is applied to tray on vibrator.

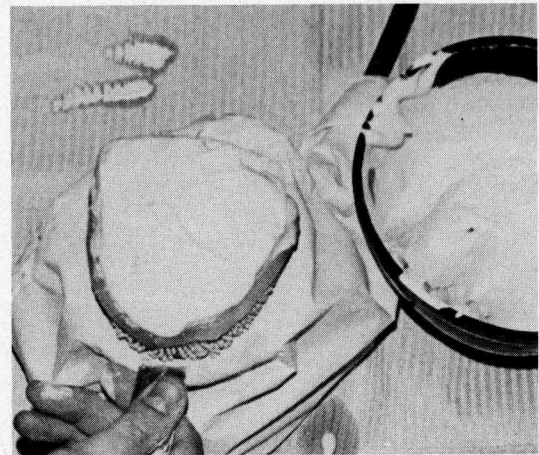

Fig. 16-19. Larger increments are added to fill tray.

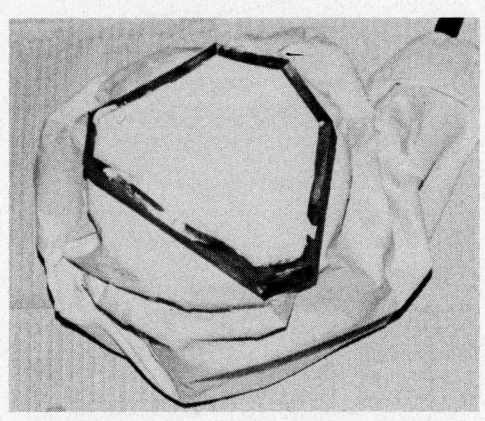

Fig. 16-20. Base former is filled with gypsum and vibrated to remove bubbles.

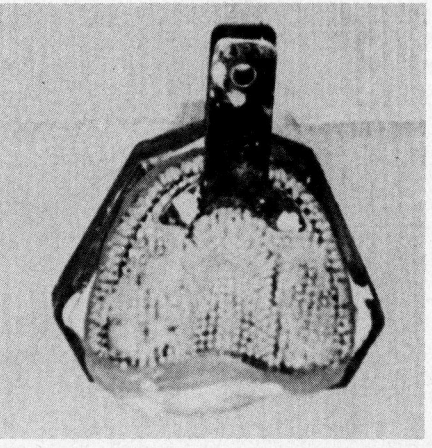

Fig. 16-21. Impression is inverted and joined with gypsum in base former.

teeth are filled, larger increments can be added, and the base can be formed by one of the methods described below (Fig. 16-19).

The use of a *base former* is a simple way to obtain a base of acceptable shape and size. The base former is filled with the gypsum and placed on the vibrator for a few seconds to remove any air bubbles (Fig. 16-20). It is then moved to a flat surface away from the vibrator. The impression filled with gypsum is inverted, centered, and gently pressed into the gypsum in the base former (Fig. 16-21). The tray should be placed into the gypsum so that the occlusal plane of the impression is approximately parallel to the table. The tray and base former should be inspected to be sure that the gypsum in the tray has joined the gypsum in the former. The gypsum should not extend up and around the sides or top of the impression tray. If it does extend onto the tray, the tray will be "locked into" the gypsum and will be difficult to separate from the hardened model.

The single-pour technique is commonly used to form the base. After the tray is filled, the remaining gypsum is formed into a ¾-inch-thick mass that approximates the tray dimensions and placed on the glass slab. Once the gypsum is placed, invert the tray to unite the gypsum in the tray with that on the slab. Adjust the tray so that the occlusal plane of the teeth is approximately parallel to the glass slab (Figs. 16-22 to 16-24).

A third way to form the base is with *boxing wax*. This method is popular in prosthodontics, for working casts used to construct dentures or bridges. Before the tray is filled with gypsum, a row of beading wax is attached to the outside of the tray. Sometimes the posterior portion of the alginate must be trimmed with a Buffalo knife, with care not to remove any anatomical features. Once the beading wax is applied, boxing wax is molded around the tray, extending above the tray to hold the gypsum and form the base (Figs. 16-25 to 16-27). The gypsum is then flowed into the tray with the boxing wax attached.

A fourth way of forming the base is with the double-pour method. The double-pour method is more involved than the other methods described; for a thorough description, consult Roswick and Simon (1974b).

Once the base is formed, the model should be left undisturbed for approximately 45 minutes while the gypsum hardens and sets. When the

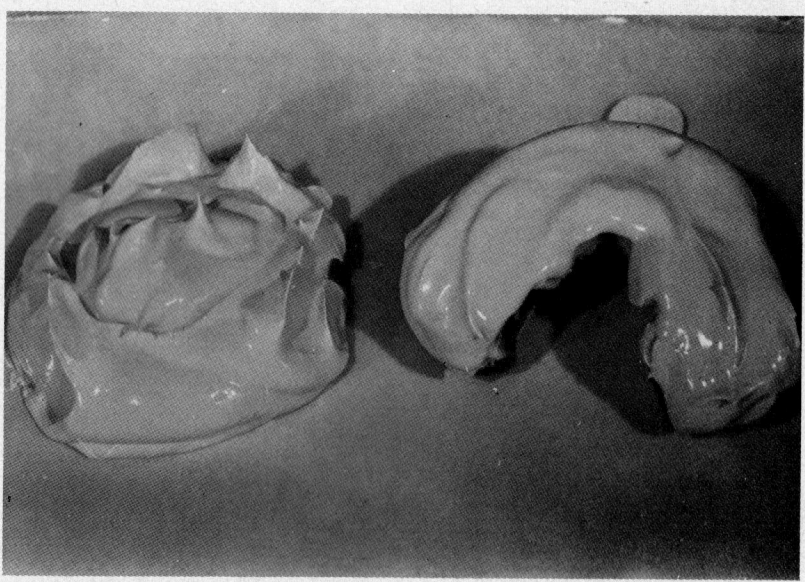

Fig. 16-22. Single-pour method. A mound of gypsum approximating shape of tray has been formed. Filled tray on right is ready to be inverted and joined to base.

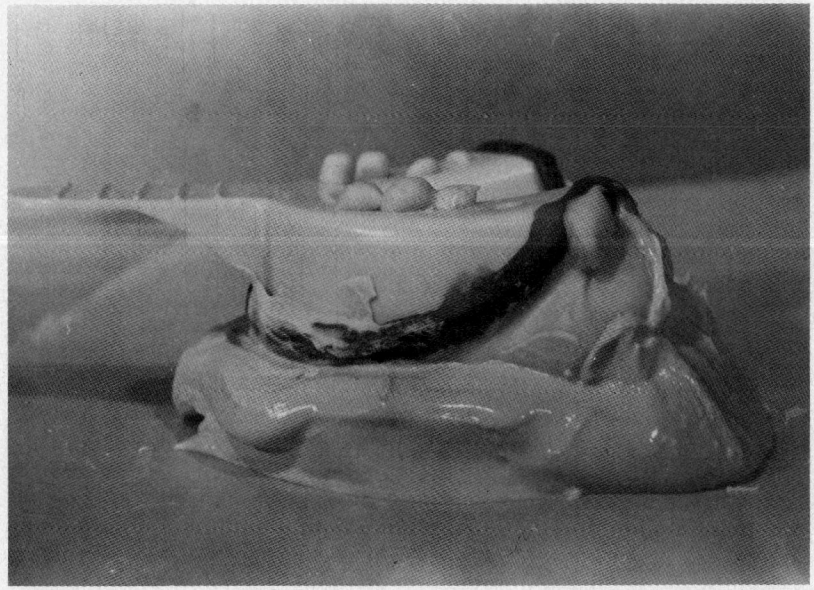

Fig. 16-23. Filled tray is joined to base so that tray and occlusal plane are parallel to table.

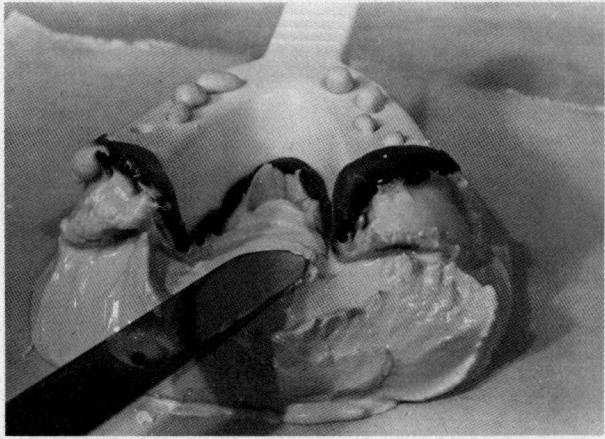

Fig. 16-24. As tongue area was not filled in with alginate, gypsum from that area is cleared with spatula.

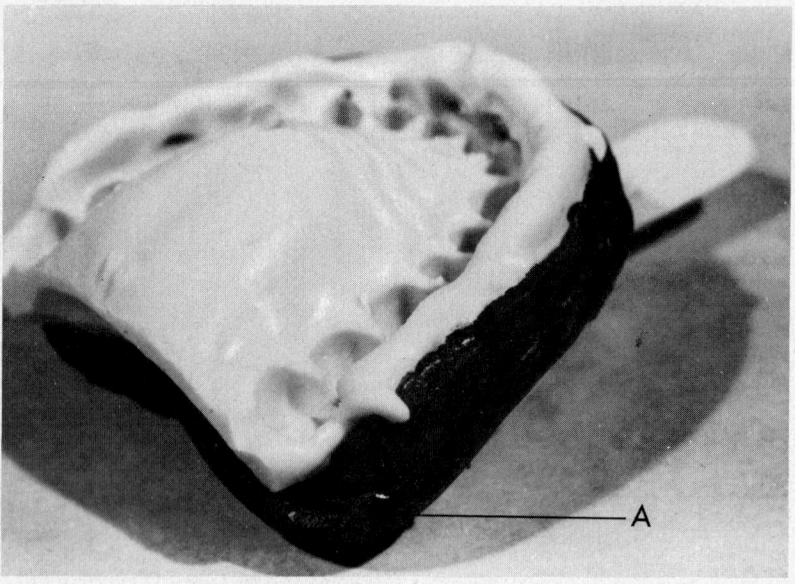

Fig. 16-25. Boxing wax method: an extra row of beading wax *(A)* has been applied to tray.

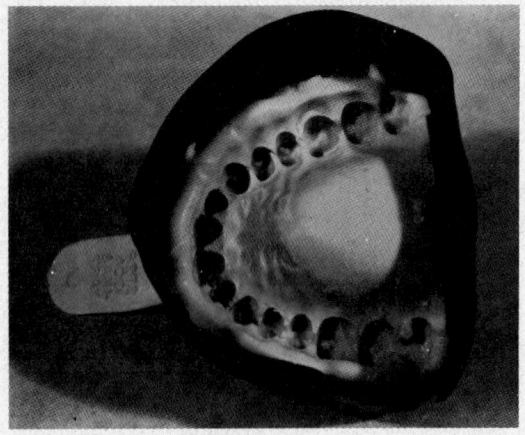

Fig. 16-26. Boxing wax is molded around tray and joined to beading wax.

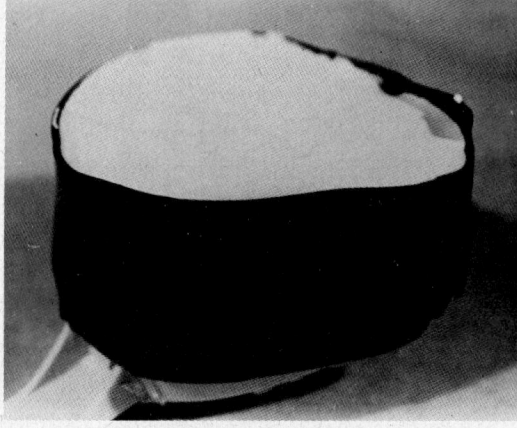

Fig. 16-27. Tray with boxing wax is filled with gypsum.

gypsum is no longer warm (the setting process is exothermic) to the touch, the model can be separated from the impression. If the model is removed from the impression too soon, it may break; if it is left in the impression too long, its surface will be rough (Craig, O'Brien, and Powers, 1983; Phillips, 1982) and the dehydrated im-

pression will harden, making it more difficult to separate the model without fracturing the model or abrading the surface.

Trimming and finishing the study models

If no base former is used, the base and borders of the models are trimmed to form the base shapes

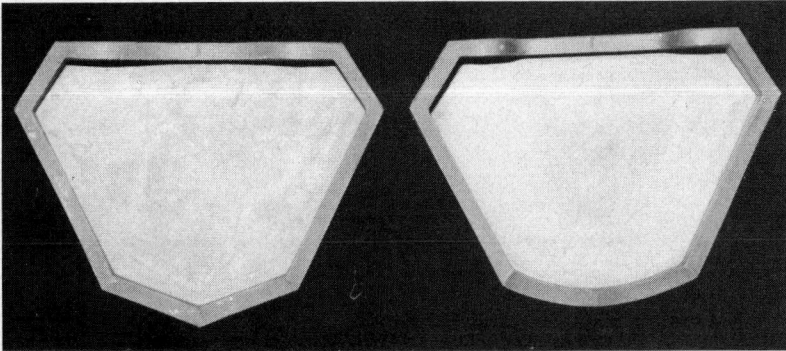

Fig. 16-28. These base formers show outline shapes of properly trimmed models. Pointed former on left is shape of maxillary model. Rounded former on right is shape of mandibular model.

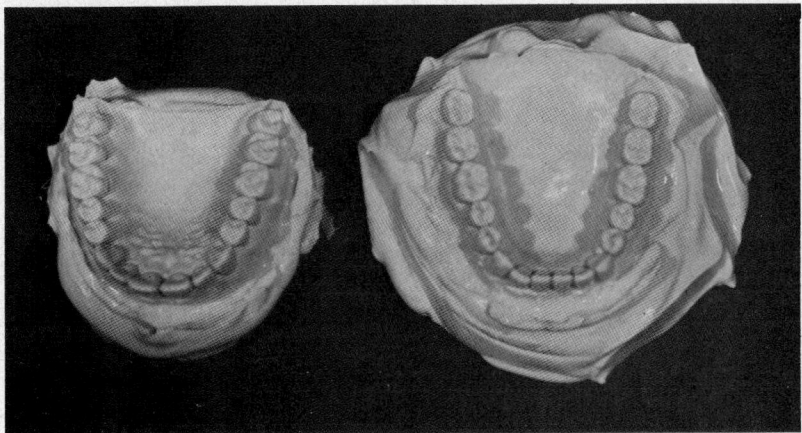

Fig. 16-29. Models removed from alginate impressions and ready to be soaked in water before being trimmed.

illustrated in Fig. 16-28. The following guidelines should be followed when trimming models. Some practitioners recommend very specific guidelines for trimming models, such as those presented by Robson (1973) or Roswick and Simon (1974b). The generally accepted guides recommended by Thurow (1977) are presented and described in the accompanying illustrations. The degree of precision in the shape of the bases depends upon the specific use for which the models are intended. Those used for treatment planning presentations, patient education, and orthodontics records need to be carefully formed. Those to be mounted on an articulator and used for occlusal analysis, ap-

pliance fabrication, and so on may not require an elaborate base form.

The models should be soaked in water before trimming (Fig. 16-29). The maxillary cast is trimmed first; then the mandibular cast is trimmed to match the maxillary cast. As mentioned previously, only the base is trimmed; the anatomic portions are not trimmed. The posterior border of the maxillary cast is trimmed first so that it is flat and perpendicular to the midline of the palate (Fig. 16-30). Ultimately, the models will be able to stand on end without wobbling or moving out of occlusion (Fig. 16-31). Next, the top of the maxillary cast is trimmed so that it is parallel with

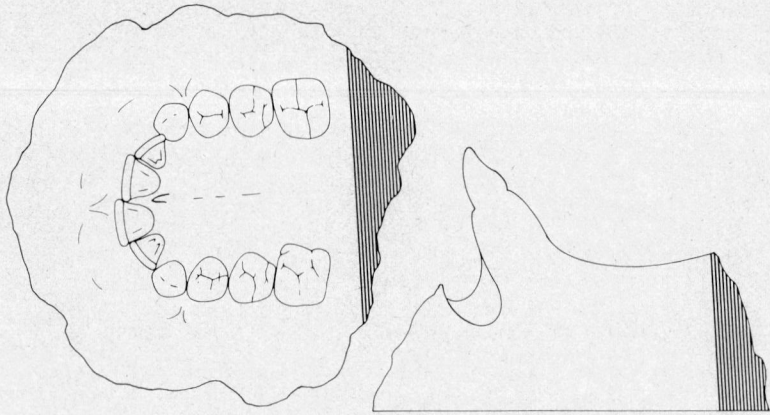

Fig. 16-30. Back surface of maxillary model is trimmed flat.
(From Thurow RC: Atlas of orthodontic principles, ed 2, St Louis, 1977, The CV Mosby Co.)

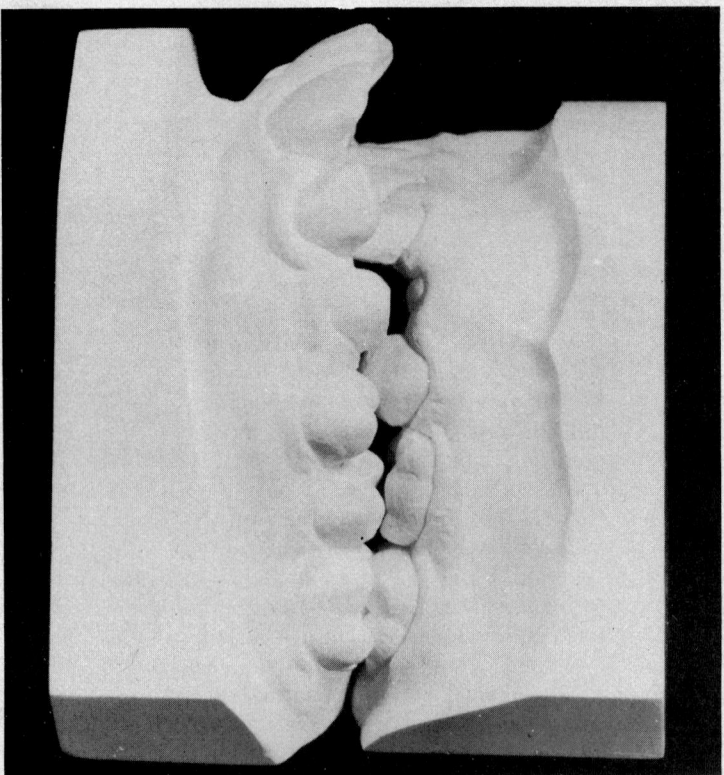

Fig. 16-31. Casts are trimmed so that they will occlude correctly when resting on posterior surfaces.
(From Thurow RC: Atlas of orthodontic principles, ed 2, St Louis, 1977, The CV Mosby Co.)

the occlusal plane (Fig. 16-32). Then the sides of the cast are trimmed to remove the gross excess and to begin the shape of the base (Fig. 16-33). The shapes of the bases of the maxillary and mandibular casts are shown in Figs. 16-1 and 16-28. Note that the posterior borders and the sides of both casts are the same shape—the posterior borders are perpendicular to the midlines; the posterior angles are trimmed to be parallel with the opposite cuspids; and the sides are parallel to a line through the cusps of the cuspids and the central grooves of the posterior teeth. On the maxillary cast the anterior border forms a point over the midline; each side is parallel to a line through the incisal edges of the anterior teeth. The anterior border of the mandibular cast is rounded from cusptip to cusptip of the cuspids. After the rough shape of the maxillary cast is formed, the mandibular cast is trimmed to form the rough outline. The first step is to trim off the excess width of the mandibular cast (Fig. 16-33). Then the posterior border of the mandibular cast is trimmed to be even with the posterior border of the maxillary cast (Fig. 16-34). It is a good idea to keep the interocclusal record between the teeth during this step to prevent damage to the teeth. The wax should be cut back so that it is not touching the

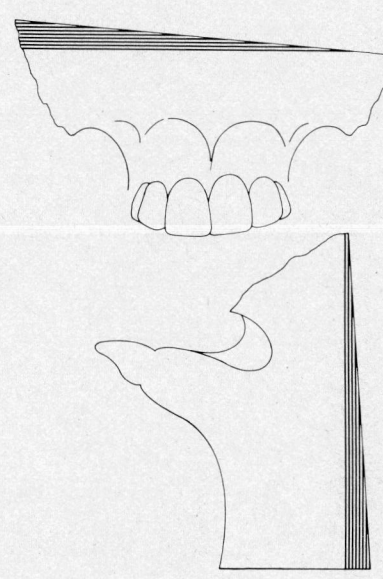

Fig. 16-32. Top of maxillary cast is trimmed to be parallel with occlusal plane.
(From Thurow RC: Atlas of orthodontic principles, ed 2, St Louis, 1977, The CV Mosby Co.)

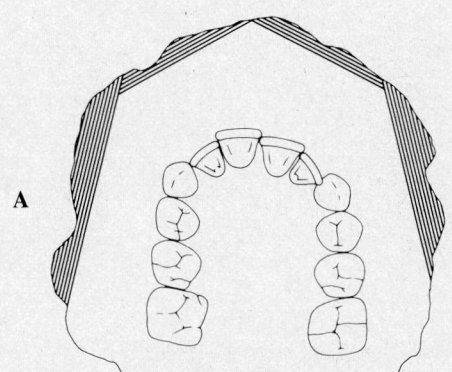

A

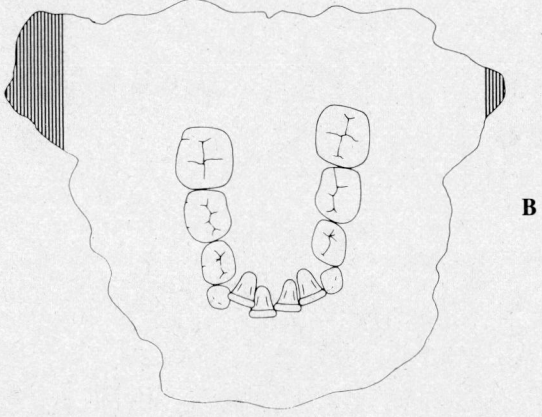

B

Fig. 16-33. Sides of maxillary *(A)* and mandibular *(B)* casts are trimmed.
(From Thurow RC: Atlas of orthodontic principles, ed 2, St Louis, 1977, The CV Mosby Co.)

trimmer wheel. Next, the bottom of the model is trimmed to be parallel with the top of the maxillary cast (Fig. 16-35). As the top of the maxillary cast is parallel to the occlusal plane, the bottom of the mandibular cast also should be parallel to the occlusal plane. The finished product should sit on a flat surface with the bottom of the mandibular cast, the occlusal plane, and the top of the maxillary cast all parallel to the flat surface (Fig. 16-1). The sides of the mandibular cast are trimmed. After forming the approximate shapes, gradually trim each cast to its final shape (Fig. 16-36). Fig. 16-37 shows casts being trimmed with a model trimmer.

Study models can be smoothed and polished with fine sandpaper and then soaked in a soap solution and buffed to make them worthy of display if they are to be used for a professional presentation. Mark each model with an identifying number or the patient's name in case the models become separated. They can be stored in a box labeled with the patient's name and chart number.

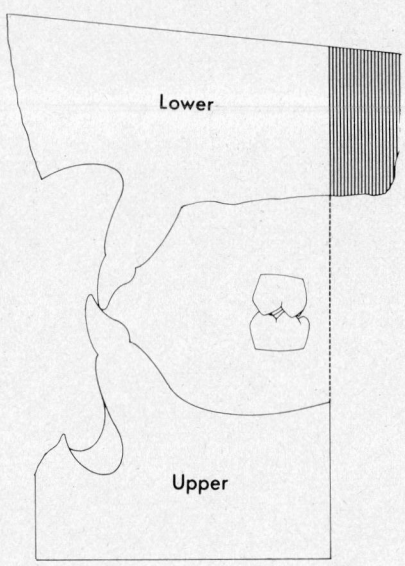

Fig. 16-34. Posterior border of mandibular model is trimmed to match maxillary model.
(From Thurow RC: Atlas of orthodontic principles, ed 2, St Louis, 1977, The CV Mosby Co.)

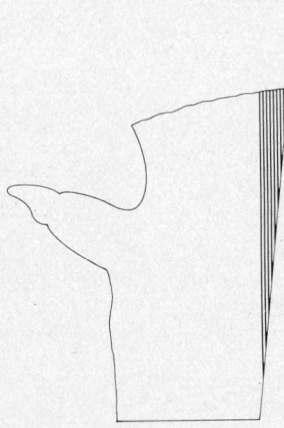

Fig. 16-35. Bottom of mandibular model is trimmed.
(From Thurow RC: Atlas of orthodontic principles, ed 2, St Louis, 1977, The CV Mosby Co.)

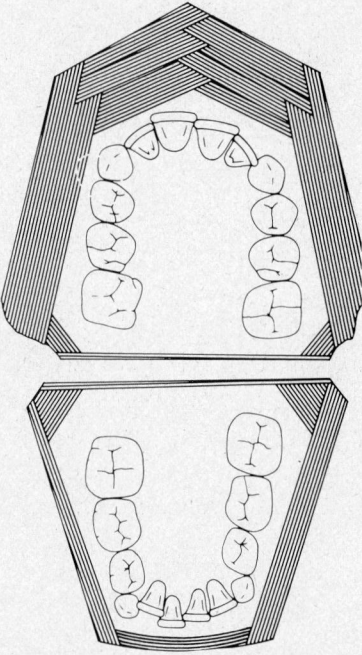

Fig.16-36. Final shapes of both casts are achieved.
(From Thurow RC: Atlas of orthodontic principles, ed 2, St Louis, 1977, The CV Mosby Co.)

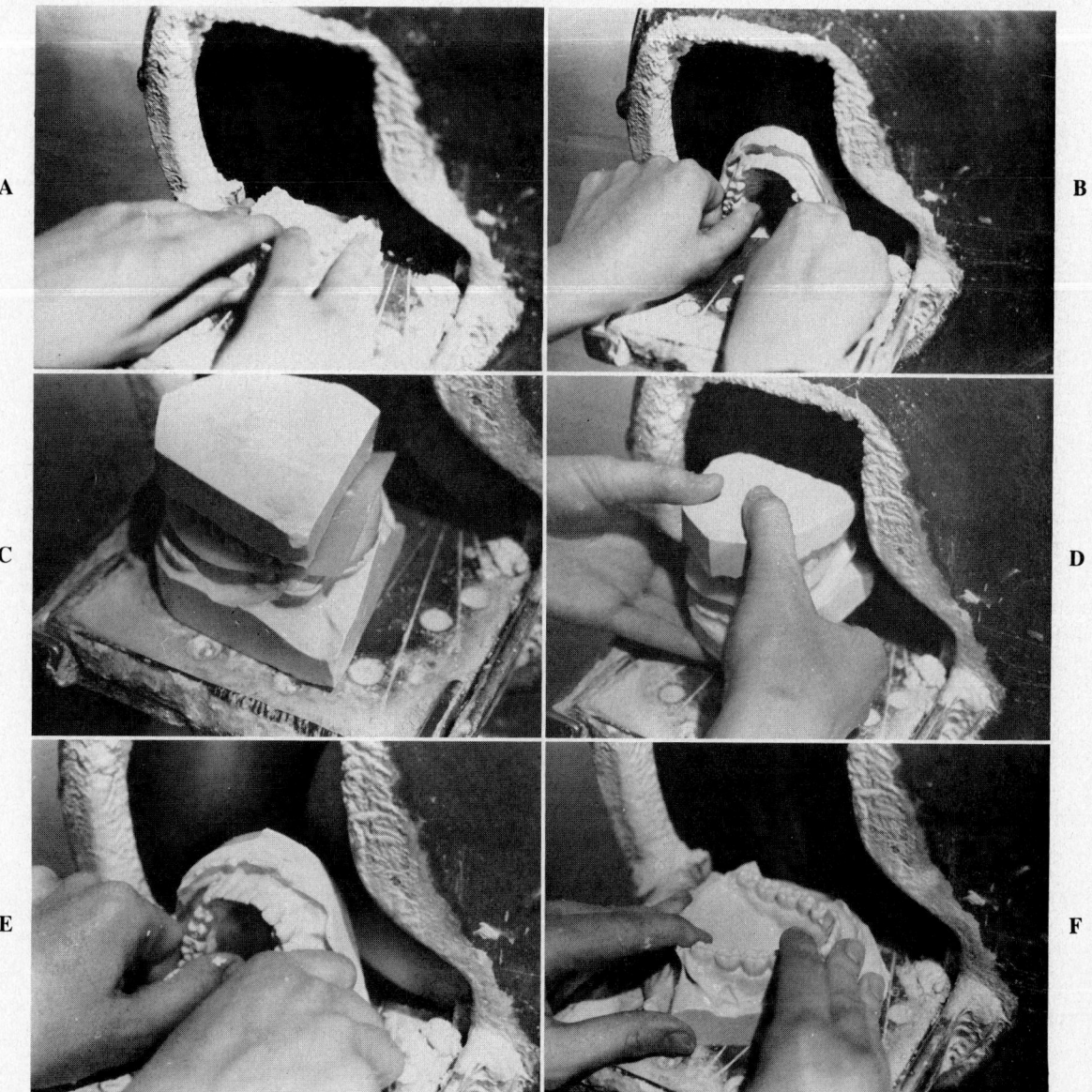

Fig. 16-37. Trimming casts with model's trimmer; note firm grip used to hold cast against blade. **A,** Back surface of maxillary cast is trimmed flat. **B,** Top of maxillary cast is trimmed. **C,** Maxillary and mandibular casts are related with interocclusal record. **D,** After posterior border of wax is removed, casts are trimmed together. **E,** Bottom of mandibular cast is trimmed. **F,** Sides of mandibular cast are trimmed.

Continued.

Fig. 16-37, cont'd. **G,** Mandibular casts are related to each other to see if further trimming is needed. **H,** Basic outline is achieved; top, occlusal plane, and bottom are parallel. **I,** Occlusal blebs are removed with Buffalo knife. **J,** Extensions of gypsum are removed.

ACTIVITIES

1. View videotapes produced by the Quercus Corporation *(Taking an Impression,* 1976; *Trimming a Cast,* 1976).
2. Watch a more experienced clinician prepare study models—making the impressions and pouring and trimming the models.
3. Prepare a set of alginate models for a partner; pour and trim the models (see check-off sheets pp. 311-313).
4. After making impressions for a partner and after being a patient for the procedure, discuss what it was like to be a patient during the procedure. In light of this experience, would either clinician like to modify his or her technique?
5. Secure a set of study models and chart as many findings as possible on the caries or periodontal chartings.
6. Read about health hazards and precautions of alginate material. See the ADA Council report (1981) listed in the references.

REVIEW QUESTIONS

1. What are the four uses of study models?
2. What three factors are important to remember when manipulating alginate and gypsum?
3. What is the criterion for determining if a tray is the proper size?
4. Describe how to place a maxillary tray filled with alginate into a patient's mouth.
5. What is border molding, and why is it performed?
6. What can the clinician do if a patient gags while the impression is being made?
7. What is the problem in removing an alginate impression from the mouth with a slow rocking motion?
8. What is the purpose of an interocclusal record?
9. How should gypsum be flowed into the impression during the pouring procedure?
10. Draw and label the outline forms of the art bases for the maxillary and mandibular casts.

Making an Alginate Impression

Suggested check-off sheet

Mark **S** for satisfactory completion or **U** for unsatisfactory completion of each criterion in the appropriate space

PERFORMANCE CRITERIA:	FACULTY	STUDENT
1. Assemble the armamentarium		
2. Prepare the patient		
3. Select the proper tray		
4. Apply beading wax		
5. Mix alginate properly		

Mandibular impression

	FACULTY	STUDENT
6. Fill the tray to the level of the beading wax		
7. Insert the tray properly by retracting one cheek with the fingers and the other with the side of the tray		
8. Have the patient raise his or her tongue		
9. Muscle mold		
10. Stabilize the tray		
11. Control gagging if necessary		
12. Remove the tray with a quick motion while protecting the opposing teeth		

Maxillary impression

	FACULTY	STUDENT
13. Fill the tray to the level of the beading wax		
14. Insert the tray properly by retracting one cheek with the fingers and the other with the side of the tray		
15. Muscle mold		
16. Stabilize the tray		
17. Control gagging if necessary		
18. Remove the tray with a quick motion while protecting the opposing teeth		
19. Take the interocclusal record		

EVALUATION:

	FACULTY	STUDENT
20. Impressions free of voids and tears		
21. All necessary structures included		

ADDITIONAL COMMENTS:

Pouring the Impressions

Suggested check-off sheet

Mark **S** for satisfactory completion or **U** for unsatisfactory completion of each criterion in the appropriate space.

PERFORMANCE CRITERIA:	FACULTY	STUDENT
1. Assemble the armamentarium		
2. Mix the gypsum properly		
Mandibular impression		
3. Fill in the tongue area		
4. Flow a small increment into the teeth		
5. Gradually flow larger increments into the teeth and impression		
6. Fill the base former		
7. Invert the impression into the base former, and set it away from the vibrator		
Maxillary impression		
8. Flow a small increment into the teeth		
9. Gradually flow larger increments into the teeth and impression		
10. Fill the base former		
11. Invert the impression into the base former, and set it away from the vibrator		
12. Allow the casts to completely harden before separating the impressions from the casts		
EVALUATION:		
13. Impressions free of excessive voids, fractures, and/or air bubbles		
14. Impressions smooth and hard		

ADDITIONAL COMMENTS:

Trimming the Casts

Suggested check-off sheet

Mark **S** for satisfactory completion or **U** for unsatisfactory completion of each criterion in the appropriate space.

PERFORMANCE CRITERIA:	FACULTY	STUDENT
1. Soak the casts in water		
Maxillary cast		
2. Trim the posterior border to be perpendicular to the midline		
3. Trim the top of the cast to be parallel to the occlusal plane		
4. Trim the sides to be parallel to a line from the cuspid to the last molar		
5. Trim the anterior portion from the cuspids to form a point over the central incisors		
Mandibular cast		
6. Trim the excess width		
7. Trim the posterior border to be even with the posterior border of the maxillary cast		
8. Trim the bottom of the cast to be parallel to the occlusal plane and the top of the maxillary cast		
9. Trim the sides to be parallel to a line from the cuspid to the last molar		
10. Trim the anterior portion to be rounded from cuspid to cuspid		
11. Trim the posterior angles of both casts to be even with the opposite cuspid		
EVALUATION:		
12. Proper outline form		
13. Anatomic structures undamaged		
14. Adequate art base—width and thickness		
15. Models remain occluded when positioned on posterior borders		

ADDITIONAL COMMENTS:

REFERENCES

ADA Council on Dental Therapeutics and Council on Pros. Services and Dent. Lab. Relations: Guidelines for infection control in the dental office and the commercial dental laboratory, JADA 110:969, 1985.

ADA Council on Materials, Instruments, and Equipment: Dentist's desk reference, ed 2, Chicago, 1983, American Dental Association.

Alginate impressions and diagnostic models. Haywood, Calif, Quercus Corp, US Department of Health, Education, and Welfare, 1976.

Appelbaum MB: Abused and misused—the alginate impression technique: a timely reminder, Quintessence Int 12:1051, 1981.

Brune D et al: Levels of airborne particles resulting from handling alginate impression materials, Scand J Dent Res 86:206, 1978.

Buchanan S, and Peggie RW: Role of ingredients in alginate impression compounds, J Dent Res 45:1120, 1966.

Carlyle LW: Compatibility of irreversible hydrocolloid impression materials with dental stones, J Prosthet Dent 49:434, 1983.

Chasteen JE: Four-handed dentistry in clinical practice, St Louis, 1988, The CV Mosby Co.

Craig RG, editor: Restorative dental materials, ed 6, St Louis, 1980, The CV Mosby Co.

Craig RG, O'Brien WJ, and Powers JM: Dental materials: properties and manipulation, ed 3, St. Louis, 1983, The CV Mosby Co.

de Freitas JF: Potential toxicants in alginate powders, Aust Dent J 25:224, 1980.

Durr, DP and Novak, EV: Dimensional Stability of alginate impressions immersed in disinfecting solutions, J. Dent. Child. 54(1):45-48, 1987.

Eisner S: Morphodynamics of the human dentition, Philadelphia, 1976, University of Pennsylvania.

Firtell DH et al: Sterilization of impression materials for use in the surgical operation room, J Prosthet Dent 27:419, 1972.

Goldman HM, and Cohen DW: Periodontal therapy, ed 6, St Louis, 1980, The CV Mosby Co.

Graber TM: Orthodontics: principles and practice, ed 3, Philadelphia, 1972, WB Saunders Co.

Greenlee JS: Review of currently recommended aseptic procedures, II. Dental instrument preparation, Dent Hyg 57(12):12, 1983.

Hattab F: Absorption of fluoride following inhalation and ingestion of alginate impression materials, Pharmacol Ther Dent 6:79, 1981.

Hattab F et al: The release of fluoride from alginate impression materials, Comm Dent Oral Epidemiol 6:273, 1978.

Herrera, SP and Merchant, Va: Dimensional stability of dental impressions after immersion disinfection: JADA 113(3): 419-422, 1986

Hill CJ, and Gellin ME: Impression taking for the young child who gags, JADA 81:161, 1970.

Hollenback GM: A study of the physical properties of elastic materials (the linear overall accuracy of reversible and irreversible hydrocolloids), IV, J South Calif Dent Assoc 31:403, 1963.

Knapp JG et al: Syringe application of alginate impression material, J Mich Dent Assoc 63:220, 1981.

Jarvis RG, and Earnshaw R: The effects of alginate impressions on the surface of cast gypsum, I. The physical and chemical structure of the cast, Aust Dent J 25:349, 1980.

Leung RL, and Schonfeld SE: Gypsum casts as a potential source of microbial cross-contamination, J Prosthet Dent 49:210, 1983.

Lorton L: A method to facilitate impressions of orthodontically bonded teeth, J Prosthet Dent 48:356, 1982.

Matyas, J. et al: Effects of disinfectants on dimensional accuracy of impression materials. J. Dent. Res. (Special Issue) 65:764, Abs. A 6. 344, 1986.

Miller JB, and Burch JG: Criteria and procedures for cast trimming, J Prosthet Dent 30:843, 1973.

Morris JC et al: Effect on surface detail of casts when irreversible hydrocolloid was wetted before impression making, J Prosthet Dent 49:328, 1983.

Phillips RW: Skinner's science of dental materials, ed 8, Philadelphia, 1982, WB Saunders Co.

Pouring study casts. Lexington, 1977, Dental Auxiliary Education, Department of Dental Hygiene, University of Kentucky.

Robson E: Preparation of orthodontic study models. Dent Tech 26:50, 1973.

Roswick NA, and Simon WJ: Impression for study models, Dent Assist 43:10 (a), 1974.

Roswick NA, and Simon WJ: The pouring of models. Dent Assist 43:9 (b), 1974.

Rowe AH et al: The probability of contamination and a method of disinfection, Br Dent J 145:184, 1978.

Rudd KD: Making diagnostic casts is not a waste of time, J Prosthet Dent 20:98, 1968.

Sanad ME et al: The repair of gypsum casts, J Prosthet Dent 48:492, 1982.

Selection and preparation of the impression tray for alginate impression. Lexington, 1977, Dental Auxiliary Education, Department of Dental Hygiene, University of Kentucky.

Skinner EW, and Hoblit NE: A study of the accuracy of hydrocolloid impressions, J Prosthet Dent 6:80, 1956.

Stankewitz CG et al: Bacteremia associated with irreversible hydrocolloid dental impressions, J Prosthet Dent 44:251, 1980.

Storer R et al: An investigation of methods available for sterilizing impressions, Br Dent J 151:217, 1981.

Taking an alginate impression. Lexington, 1977, Dental Auxiliary Education, Department of Dental Hygiene, University of Kentucky.

Taking an impression. Haywood Calif, 1976, Quercus Corp.

Thompson EO: Constructing and using diagnostic models, Dent Clin North Am (Mar):67, 1963.

Thurow RC: Atlas of orthodontic principles, St Louis, 1977, The CV Mosby Co.

Trimming a cast. Haywood, Calif, 1976, Quercus Corp.

Trimming study casts. Lexington, 1977, Dental Auxiliary Education, Department of Dental Hygiene, University of Kentucky.

17 INTRAORAL PHOTOGRAPHY

OBJECTIVES: *The reader will be able to*

1. Discuss how intraoral photography can be used in dentistry.
2. List the objectives to be met by a clinical camera system.
3. Describe a camera system that meets the objectives.
4. Identify the parts of a 35 mm camera used for clinical photography.
5. Define the following terms:
   a. Shutter speed
   b. Aperture setting
   c. Depth of field
   d. ASA film speed
6. State the purpose for using cheek retractors and mirrors as intraoral photographic accessories.
7. Load and unload a film cartridge for a 35 mm camera.
8. Describe the composition of the intraoral photographic series consisting of 12 views.
9. State the criteria for evaluating a slide.
10. Insert the cheek retractors with minimal patient discomfort.
11. Select the appropriate mirror for a particular photograph, considering not only the composition but also the differences in patient oral anatomy.
12. Place the mirror for each view to aid retraction, light, and accessibility for the camera operator.
13. Handle photographic equipment properly.
14. Compose the picture through the viewfinder.
15. Compose a picture that is centered vertically and horizontally.
16. Compose a picture free of extraneous objects (fingers, retractors, mirror edges, excess saliva bubbles, mirror fog) to the best of the clinician's and patient's ability.
17. Focus the camera for each view.
18. Display concern for the patient through:
    a. Gentle insertion of mirrors and retractors
    b. Considerate direction and communications
    c. Efficiency in time required to take each view
19. Record the camera use as specified by clinic guidelines.

Clinical photography has become a part of dental practice. Clinicians in both general practice and specialties have found the pictorial representation of the patient's conditions to be an invaluable part of the patient's record (Dahlberg, 1968; Meister et al, 1978; Nuckles, 1975; Rosenfeld, 1976).

The photographic series captures the actual state of the patient as no other diagnostic aid can. Chartings of patient's restorations are useful for patient identification and reference, but these are time-consuming to complete and may be inaccurate because of human error. Chartings of this type are usually done on a diagram, making actual tooth morphology and alignment configuration difficult to illustrate. Study models capture the form of the teeth and adjacent soft tissues but are limited because not all areas of the oral cavity can be subjected to the impression technique. Radiographs are excellent for assessing bony anatomy, caries, and restorations. A look at underlying conditions is provided, but representation of the soft tissue is lost.

Photography captures the color, shape, texture, and characteristics of the oral cavity. The camera objectively records its subject, revealing conditions that may be lost in written notation.

A complete series of intraoral photographs such as that in Plate 3 is useful for treatment planning. The series can be referred to at the clinician's convenience. With the series and the use of other diagnostic aids, the patient's presence may not be necessary for the clinician to assess treatment needs.

With the photographic series and treatment plan in hand, the clinician is ready for the case presentation. The patient studies his or her oral conditions, considers treatment needs, and realizes the scope of dental care. With the help of intraoral photography, the patient is able to see the oral conditions from "the outside." This may encourage the patient to ask questions or discuss therapy from a more objective position. If the clinician has photographic records of other completed treatment, the patient is able to study the before and after photographs of someone who underwent similar care. Although identical results cannot be guaranteed, the photographs help the lay person visualize the proposed treatment. The visual communication of the clinician's work may enhance trust in the clinician's skills.

Photography is part of documenting patient care and makes the patient record more accurate and complete. Images establish the patient's actual oral conditions before treatment. Made during treatment, the color slides record the progress of care (such as improvements in tissue or steps in restoration). At the completion of a phase of therapy, a final series establishes the treatment outcome. The entire series of images, which can be referred to at a future date, provides a record of treatment. Too often, when recall is necessary, the memory is inadequate, and written documentation is sketchy. Should a legal question concerning treatment arise, photographic records may provide invaluable information. Case documentation procedures are described in Chapter 35.

As an educational resource, photography has almost endless possibilities. Tissue changes occur slowly, making day-to-day appreciation of the healing process difficult, but patients are motivated by seeing themselves in photographs before and after treatment. Clinicians may also be motivated as the patient's improvement is monitored.

Kodachrome slides can be made to create an instructional series. Quality color or black and white prints can be made from these slides. In this way educational materials can be developed in the clinic or office to present information suited to the clinical philosophy. Series depicting the use of brushing techniques, flossing principles, or the use of auxiliary aids are examples.

The slide collection rapidly becomes a resource for presenting information to groups of patients or peers for a variety of instructional or educational purposes. As the concept of peer review grows, photography may become even more important as a dimension for assessing quality care. Visual documentation of treatment may be required as third-party payment mechanisms increase.

Intraoral photography has become part of comprehensive oral health care. Photography is useful as an aid in the following:

Patient identification
Diagnosis
Treatment planning
Case presentation
Case documentation
Patient education and/or motivation
Instruction and/or peer review

SELECTING A CAMERA SYSTEM

Daniels and Sherill (1975) have summarized the objectives of a clinical camera system that provides excellent quality and the maximum in flexibility for photographing all aspects of the oral cavity by the following criteria. The camera system is able to do the following:

1. Provide for a simple and repeatable clinical procedure requiring approximately 1 minute for taking a photograph at any image size.
2. Provide for minimum manipulation (that is, does not require changing accessories or components) regardless of the subject area being photographed.
3. Provide for accurate focusing and composing of that subject.
4. Provide a continuous focusing range from very

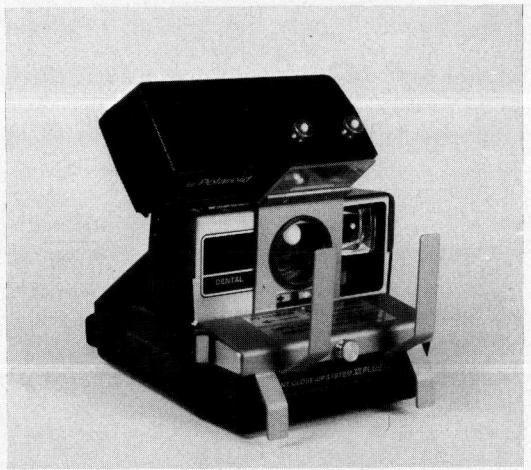

Fig. 17-1. Dental-Pro instant close-up camera.
(Courtesy Trojan Camera, Los Angeles, Ca.)

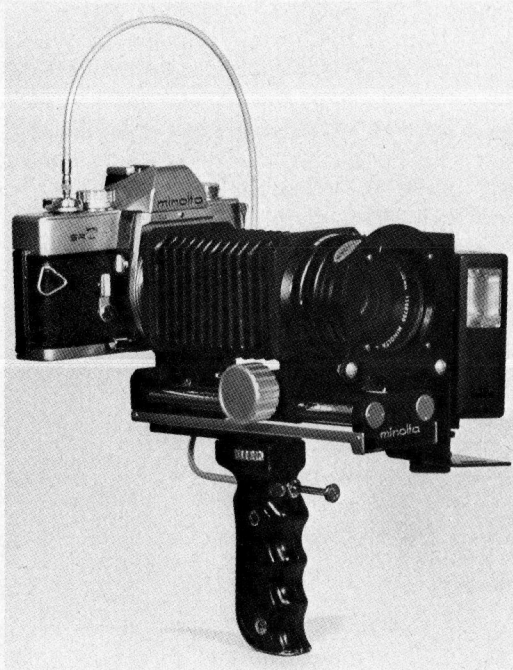

Fig. 17-2. Complete Minolta bellows clinical camera unit.
(Courtesy CL Freehe, Sumner, Wash.)

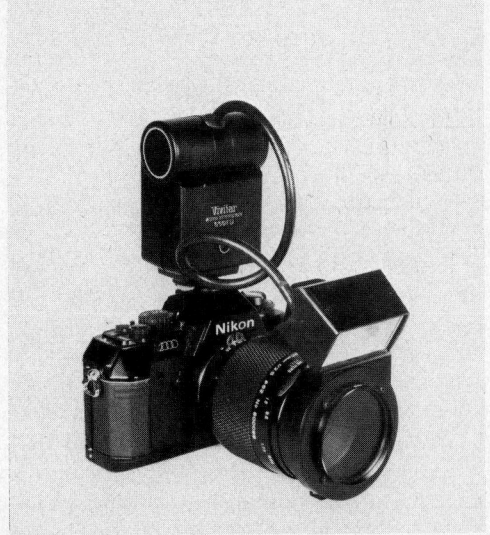

Fig. 17-3. Trojan clinical camera system. Auto system N2000, 90 mm-F/2.5 macro-lens with rotating point source flash unit.
(Courtesy Trojan Camera, Los Angeles, Ca.)

close (1:1) magnification to a "head-to-clavicle" size for maximum convenience and flexibility.

5. Provide for adequate working and lighting distance.

6. Provide for optimum photographic quality in the final result.

In general, three types of clinical camera systems are useful in dentistry. These are (1) an instant close-up camera, (2) a macro-lens camera, and (3) a bellows camera system.

The instant close-up camera system is designed to provide instant pictures for basic patient identification. The advantage is that these photos can be placed in the chart or given to the patient immediately. The camera can make head-and-neck views and general intraoral views such as occlusal, buccal, or direct facial photos. These cameras do not produce finely detailed photographs, very close-up views, or images with lasting color quality. The photos are adequate for basic record keeping or for creating bulletin board displays. Another advantage is that these cameras are very easy to operate (Fig. 17-1).

For documenting treatment with slides that show excellent detail and have professional color, select one of the other clinical camera systems. These systems are made up of component parts that require some manipulation and care but are simple to operate (Figs. 17-2 to 17-4).

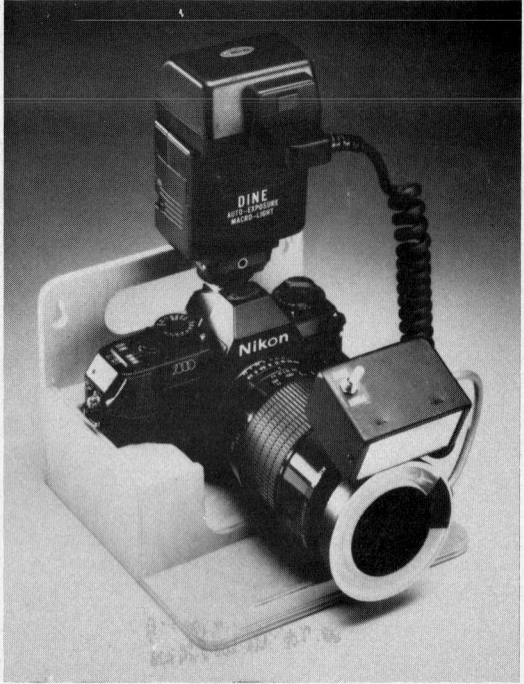

Fig. 17-4. Dine auto exposure system. Nikon N2000, 105 mm-F/32 macro-lens with ring light and point source flash combination lighting units.
(Courtesy Lester A. Dine, Inc., Farmingdale, N.Y.)

The companies listed at the end of the chapter are excellent sources for camera components, complete clinical systems, and a variety of photographic accessories.

Camera body and viewing system

A clinical camera system includes a 35 mm camera body. This number refers to the size of film that the camera holds.

The viewing system of the camera body is very important. A standard 35 mm camera often has a *range finder* viewing system. With this system, the photographer is not able to look directly through the lens to compose the view, because the view window is placed beside the lens. The photographer is able to see the general composition of the view, which is satisfactory for taking a picture of a large scene. It is not accurate when taking close-up views, where a few millimeters of difference could eliminate important details. The discrepancy between what the lens sees and what the photographer sees when using a range finder viewing system is called *parallax.* The viewing system for intraoral photography must be SLR (single-lens-reflex). This means the photographer is able to look directly through the lens with the help of mirrors to compose the actual view the lens sees. Because of the accuracy of this viewing system, it is best suited for intraoral photography.

Lens

Clinical photography requires that the camera lens be between 90 and 135 mm. The standard 35 mm camera usually comes equipped with a 50 mm lens. This lens is good for general, nonclinical photography because it "sees" approximately what normal vision sees. If used clinically for close-up photos, a 50 mm lens has to be placed about 4 inches from the subject. This does not allow enough working space or room for proper lighting of the subject. At best, in a close frontal view, the anterior teeth would appear distorted and wider than normal. Lenses between 90 and 135 mm do not distort the close-up subject. They allow a working distance of approximately 8 inches between the camera lens and the subject. If images are made during a clinical procedure, this distance provides an adequate working field for dental instruments and photographic accessories such as mirrors and retractors. All 35 mm camera lenses between 90 and 135 mm are free of perspective distortion.

The lens can be attached to the camera body or to an automatic bellows. A macro-lens attaches to the camera body and allows focusing from infinity to close-up. Depending on the lens, an adapter extension may be necessary to achieve full life size (1:1) magnification. Some practice is necessary to become comfortable with the size and weight of the macro-lens camera system. This fact and the need to use an adapter occasionally may be important in deciding whether this type of camera system is best suited to the clinician's needs.

Fig. 17-5 shows a complete macro-lens camera system. Components have been separated for display along with a custom storage case.

Another camera system utilizes a 100 mm short-mount lens, attached to an automatic bellows system. The bellows is an adjustable accor-

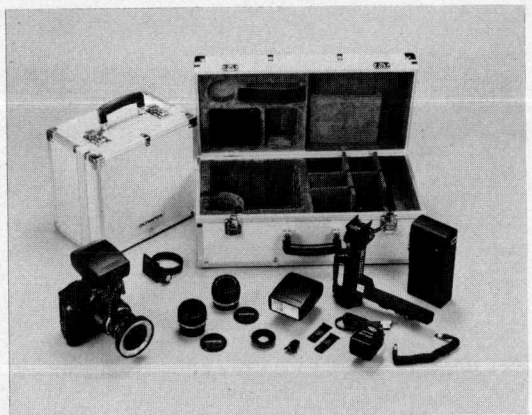

Fig. 17-5. Olympus medical/dental and scientific photography system. Components include: OM-2 Body Black, 135 mm/F4.5, 50 mm/F3.5, 80 mm/4.0 macro-lenses, T10 ring flash, T power control, ring flash filter, electronic flash T32, bounce grip, power pack, TTL auto connector and cord, Macrophoto/Medical Case B.
(Courtesy Olympus Corporation, Woodbury, N.Y.)

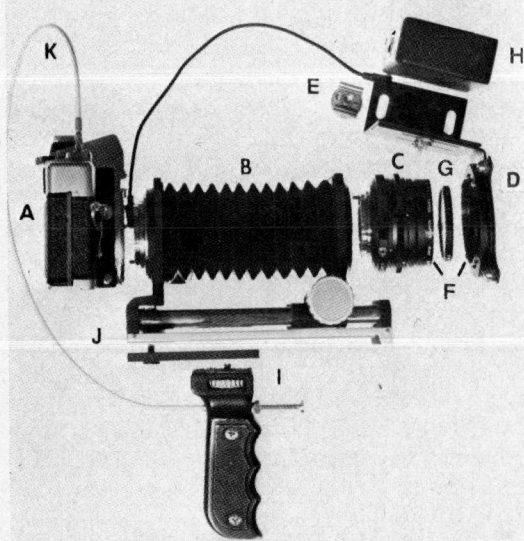

Fig. 17-6. Camera and parts needed for a fully automatic bellows clinical unit. **A,** Single-lens—reflex camera body; **B,** fully automatic bellows; **C,** 100 mm short-mount lens; **D,** Washington Scientific 180-degree rotating flash bracket; **E,** shoe and bolt for flash; **F,** S-7 lens adapter rings; **G,** S-7 color correction filter; **H,** vertical electronic flash unit; **I to K,** pistol grip with 20-inch cable release and balance bar.
(From Freehe CL: Dent Clin North Am 27:3, 1983.)

dion-type apparatus. The main characteristic of the bellows system is that it is continuously adjustable. The short-mount lens and bellows are capable of focusing from 4½ feet to 7 inches, achieving orthodontic views ranging from a head-to-clavicle view to one consisting of four to five anterior teeth. No other parts need to be added or adjusted.

The bellows apparatus attaches to a pistol grip, which is helpful in providing stability when handling the camera. A cable release allows the shutter to be released by activating a trigger in the pistol grip. This enables the free hand to adjust the bellows, aid in focusing the view, assist the patient, or place an instrument in the view. The size of the bellows system may be considered by some to be a disadvantage. The 100 mm short-mount lens and automatic bellows camera system has been specifically designed for intraoral photography. This camera can be recommended for use in other health, natural science, and research fields where quality close-up photography is desired (see Fig. 17-6).

Lighting units

Lighting is the most critical feature in photography. The direction and power of the lighting cre-

ate the image of the subject. Lighting for clinical photography can be achieved by using a single point source flash mounted on a rotating bracket, a ring light flash unit, or a combination ring light and point source flash that can be used selectively.

A point-source flash is mounted on a rotating bracket and adapter rings on the front of the lens. When attached in this manner, the flash unit moves with the lens to provide correct lighting for the view and proper exposure. The light source can be rotated from the 3 o'clock position on one side of the lens to the 12 o'clock position at the top and to the 9 o'clock position on the other side of the lens to provide adequate illumination of the field and cast a shadow for definition.

The position of the flash close to the lens is important, as a horizontal placement too far from the lens will produce too much shadow, creating a poor image.

A ring light attachment encircles the lens. In this way the light source moves with the focusing of the lens to provide adequate lighting for the photographic field. Some ring lights have a rheostatic power control and require adjusting the power up or down, depending on the view for proper exposure. In addition to the time it takes to make the proper adjustments, this can cause a change in slide color. The right light produces an image that may lack definition, contrast texture, and good color. The center of the image has no shadow, whereas a hazy 360-degree shadow is cast around the subject. These images may appear flat when compared with point-source lighting, which provides a more natural, three-dimensional image by the contrast created by lighting the subject from one side. All quality art or scientific images require some directed shadow to capture true form.

The bellows system uses a point-source light unit, and a macro-lens system uses a ring light. With the proper modifications, a ring light and point-source flash could be used together on a camera system. The clinician's preference for lighting control and color and the adaptability of the camera/lens system will determine the best lighting solution.

Electronic flash units may be manual or automatic (TTL, through the lens). An automatic flash is programmed for specific exposures at each camera setting depending on the light sensitivity of the film. The light meter reads the light reflected off the film through the lens and adjusts the flash automatically. Manual systems set the flash for a specific exposure at each camera setting. As long as the film is consistent, the exposure will be reliable. The color output of the flash unit should be as close to 5500° Kelvin (K) as possible. Most flash units have a color output of 5600° to 6400° K, which produce images with blue or purple tissue color. If the color output is below 5500° K, tissue color will be red to yellow. Depending on the flash unit and the type of lighting in the clinical setting, color correction filters over the lens and flash are necessary to achieve ideal color. A light yellow filter is indicated if the films appear blue. A bluish filter will improve a yellow color. The dental light can also affect the color tone of the slides. This light is directed on the cheek, and not on the area to be photographed.

Flash units can be AC or battery operated. Using AC power offers convenience, but access to electrical outlets and maneuverability may be a consideration. Rechargeable batteries are recommended if battery operation is preferred. The flash should recycle within 5.7 seconds to aid in taking a series of pictures at one time. A flash duration of 1/800 to 1/1000 second is also recommended.

Once the camera system is selected, a roll of practice film should be exposed in the clinical setting to determine the necessary corrections in lighting and color filtration.

Camera adjustments

The shutter speed, aperture setting, and film speed work together with the lighting to create high-quality images. Each of these factors requires specific settings on the camera.

The shutter speed is the period of time the shutter remains open, thus determining the amount of light that strikes the film. The shutter speed is usually recorded on the camera in fractions of a second: 1/60, 1/125, 1/250. The higher the shutter speed, the more efficiently it will "stop" the action of the subject.

To set the shutter speed, simply rotate the shutter speed dial until the desired speed is aligned with the indicator on the camera body. For intraoral flash photography, the shutter speed is 60, or 1/60 of a second. This is the speed at which the electronic flash is automatically synchronized with the opening of the shutter. On some makes of cameras, the synchronized flash speed may be as high as 1/125 of a second. The shutter and flash must be synchronized.

The aperture setting refers to the size of the lens opening. It is also called the f-stop. This setting is important because it determines the depth of field, or the area of the image in which all objects are in focus. A great depth of field is desired in intraoral photography to achieve sharpness of all objects in the picture. The smaller the aperture opening, the greater the depth of field. The smallest aperture opening is indicated by the largest f-stop number. The f-stops usually range from 4 (lens wide open) to 32 (very small opening). As the aperture is closed from each f-stop to the next smaller one, the light reaching the film is decreased by 50%.

Cameras with fully automatic lenses allow the photographer to compose the view by looking through the lens at the largest f-stop, 4. This allows enough light to see the view clearly, but the depth of field is very small. Only one tooth may be in focus. The photographer should compose the view by focusing one-third of the way into the scene. For a full direct facial view of the teeth in occlusion on a normally curved arch, this means focusing on the midline of the cuspid. With the automatic lens, when the shutter is tripped, the aperture closes to the preset f-stop. The full direct view would be present at f-19; everything in the final image from the central incisors to the first molars would be in sharp focus.

For a normal head-to-clavicle view taken at a distance of 5 feet, the aperture setting would be f-8, with the focus on the eyes. For most intraoral views consisting of four to six teeth, the f-stop is 22. Intraoral views of dark-skinned or black people should be set one-half more open, at f-19. Conversely, a pure white subject requires less light. For a view of a set of plaster casts, the aperture setting should be f-27 (Freehe, 1983).

Film selection

The principal purpose of the photograph will determine the type of film to be used.

Color film available for slides is called *transparency film;* an example is Kodachrome film. Color print film, such as Kodak Vericolor (VPS-135-type III) Professional film, is called *negative film.*

Color negative film can be used to produce color prints, black and white prints, or fair color slides, but with each generation of processing a small amount of photographic quality is lost. Kodachrome 64 film produces a grainless color transparency. The film exposed in the camera is processed and mounted to make the slide, thereby preserving the greatest resolution of the original quality. When necessary, color or black and white prints can be produced from the original color slide by making an internegative. These copies are of the same quality as those from any negative film, as Kodachrome is grainless. Kodachrome is

the only permanent color film today. Its color can last 100 or more years. Ektachrome slides or negative film will last 4 to 20 years.

The film is given an ASA number that refers to its light sensitivity. This is the amount of time the film needs to be exposed to light to create a quality image. This is also called film speed. A fast film with a high ASA number, such as 400 or 1000, indicates that the film is extremely sensitive to light. Less light is necessary to produce an acceptable image. Although useful in some types of photography, these films are not practical for intraoral photography, where excellent color and detail are the main concerns. As film speed increases, grain size increases and contrast decreases. An intermediate film speed such as Kodachrome 64 is ideal for slide production or color print copy because of its high sharpness and lack of grain. Kodachrome 25 could be used, but it has too much magenta for dental photography unless the proper light filters are used to correct for excessive redness. When an electronic flash is used and color is corrected with a filter for 5500° K, color daylight film should be used. Kodachrome (ASA) 64 with the proper electronic flash is the correct choice for medical and dental photography.

PHOTOGRAPHIC ACCESSORIES

Accessories for intraoral photography include cheek retractors and mirrors.

Cheek retractors

Cheek retractors are used to clear the area to be photographed of the lips and labial and buccal mucosa. This, in turn, improves visibility and allows the maximum amount of light to enter the oral cavity. Cheek retractors are available in clear plastic or metal (Figs. 17-7 and 17-8). Metal retractors are less attractive but can be autoclaved. This is of particular concern when photographing a patient who may transmit infectious pathogens to dental personnel or to the next patient. The main use of the metal retractor is to hold the mirror for a buccal view. Only one wire retractor is necessary, as a plastic retractor is used for retracting the lips on the other side (Fig. 17-9). The transparent plastic retractors are esthetically most acceptable. Natural tissue color shows through

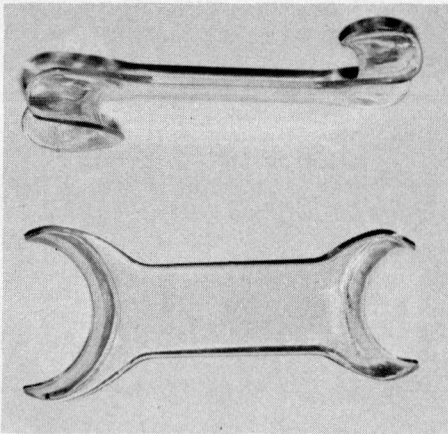

Fig. 17-7. Clear plastic cheek retractors, double ended.

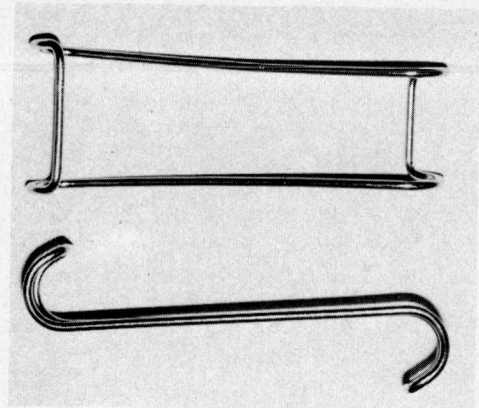

Fig. 17-8. Metal cheek retractors, double ended.

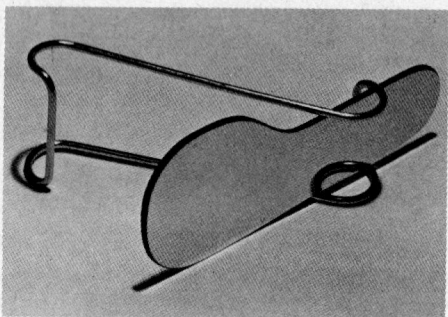

Fig. 17-9. Use of Columbia wire lip retractor with buccal mirror for posterior buccal view. Use one curved plastic lip retractor on opposite side.
(From Freehe CL: Dent Clin North Am 27:3, 1983.)

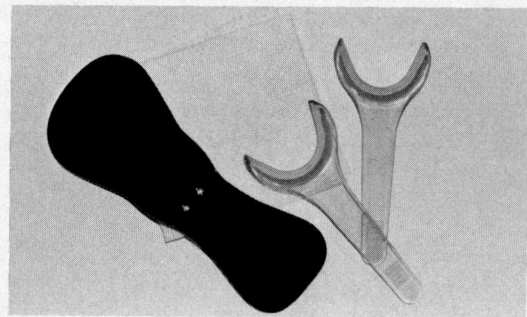

Fig. 17-10. Lester Dine mouth mirror and single-ended plastic cheek retractors.

this retractor, limiting the potential for distraction.

Retractors are either single or double ended. The double-ended retractors provide a small curvature and a larger curvature. This feature allows adaptability to a variety of mouth sizes. The extra retractor end acts as a handle, which also enhances retraction. Single-ended plastic retractors (Fig. 17-10) have longer, tapered handles. The curved end is larger for excellent lip retraction, and these can be cut down or modified to make smaller sizes.

Chemical sterilization procedures are necessary, since plastic retractors cannot be autoclaved. After sterilization, the retractors should be rinsed well to remove all traces of the chemical, which may be irritating to the patient. Directions should be followed for the timing of chemical sterilization because extended time in the solution may damage the plastic.

Technique for inserting retractors (Valentine, 1975)
1. Moisten the retractors in water.
2. Ask the patient to relax the lips and open the mouth slightly.
3. Place the rim of the retractor onto the edge of the lower lip (Fig. 17-11).
4. Rotate the handle of the retractor until it is parallel to the corner of the mouth (Fig. 17-12).

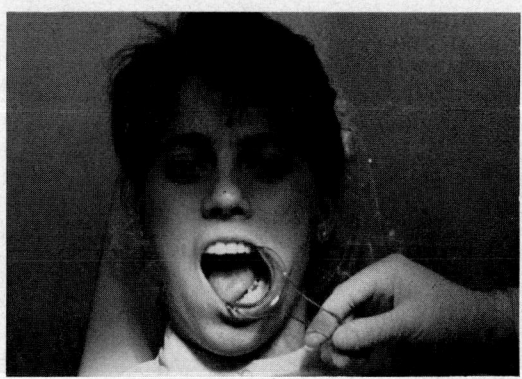

Fig. 17-11. Cheek retractor insertion. With patient's mouth open slightly and lips relaxed, place the rim of the retractor onto the edge of the lower lip. Gently rotate the retractor to the side.

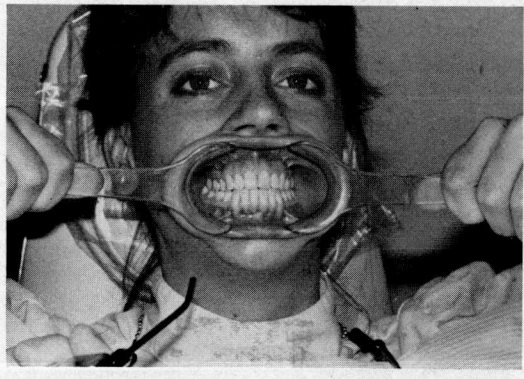

Fig. 17-12. Place the second retractor onto the lower lip and rotate to the opposite side. Pull out laterally and slightly forward.

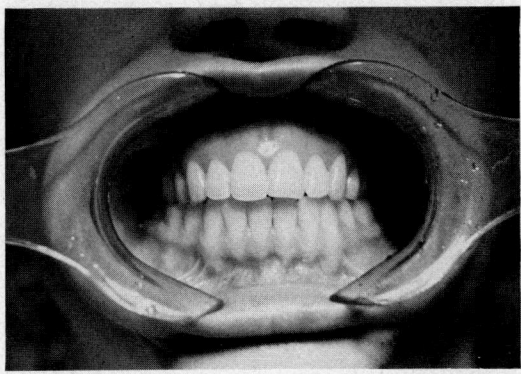

Fig. 17-13. Position for full direct facial views (see Plate 3, *A* and *B*).

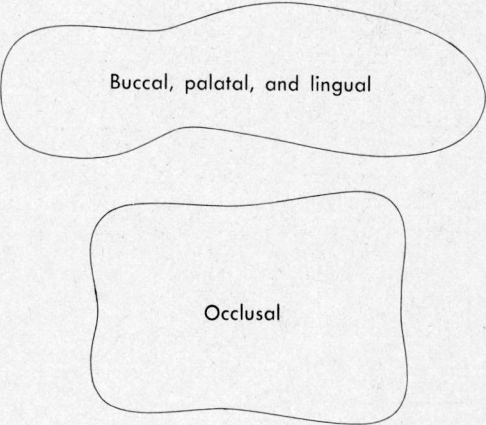

Fig. 17-14. Intraoral mirrors.

5. Repeat this for the other side of the mouth if necessary.
6. Instruct the patient to bite down on the posterior teeth. Pull out the retractors laterally and slightly forward (Figs. 17-12 and 17-13). Avoid pulling the retractor handles toward the ears. This will cause the buccal mucosa to be pressed onto the buccal surfaces of the teeth, as well as causing the patient discomfort when the retractor is pressed against the gingiva and alveolar process.

Intraoral mirrors

Intraoral mirrors are used to provide a reflected image for photographing. It is impossible to obtain a direct view of many of the intraoral structures.

Glass mirrors that have been rhodium plated on both sides create an excellent reflective surface. Intraoral mirrors may be purchased in several sizes. The two mirrors shown in Fig. 17-14 allow flexibility with minimal equipment for general adult photography. For photography of the pedodontic patient, smaller-size mirrors are recommended, especially a child-size occlusal mirror.

Another type of mirror is shown on the tray set-up in Fig. 17-10. The large end of the mirror provides an excellent surface for capturing oc-

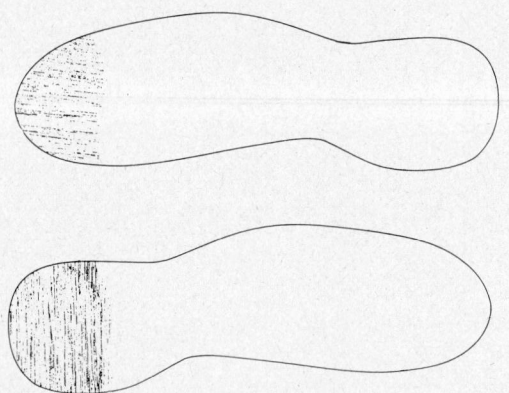

Fig. 17-15. Shaded area indicates portion of mirror that is used for the reflected image in anterior lingual views.

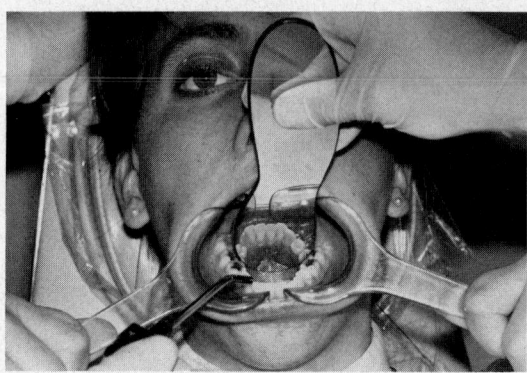

Fig. 17-16. Mirror and retractor placement for mandibular anterior lingual view (see Plate 3, *C*).

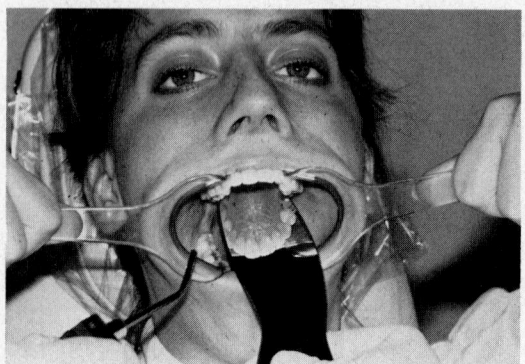

Fig. 17-17. Mirror and retractor placement for anterior palatal view (see Plate 3, *D*).

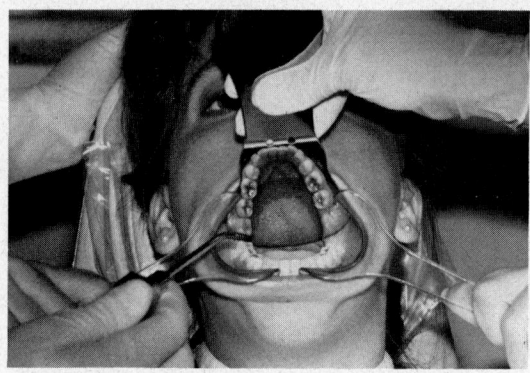

Fig. 17-18. Mirror and retractor placement for mandibular occlusal view (see Plate 3, *E*).

clusal views and the smaller end can be placed for palatal and lingual views. The mirror is easy to hold and keeps fingers from being too close to the scene.

Mirrors are washed with detergent and water and sterilized between patients. They should be rinsed thoroughly with plain water before being used in the patient's mouth. Care must be taken when using the mirrors because they can be easily scratched or broken. They should be wiped with a soft tissue or cloth and wrapped in cloth or felt for safekeeping.

Technique for inserting mirrors

1. Place the mirror in warm water prior to use to prevent fogging. A small heating pad could also be used to keep mirrors warm.

2. Insert the appropriate cheek retractors.
3. Select the mirror and the appropriate end for the desired view.
4. Place the mirror flat into the mouth. As you retract with your fingers, rotate the mirror into position. Take care not to hit the teeth or press into the alveolar process, as this is annoying and uncomfortable for the patient.
5. Hold the mirror securely at the opposite end while maintaining retraction.
6. If fogging occurs, blow a gentle stream of compressed air onto the mirror.

Figs. 17-15 to 17-25 diagram that portion of the mirror used for the reflected image. Additional directions for mirror placement are given in the section on technique for individual views.

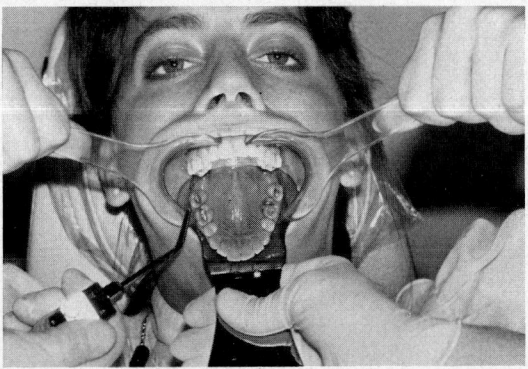

Fig. 17-19. Mirror and retractor placement for maxillary occlusal view (see Plate 3, *F*).

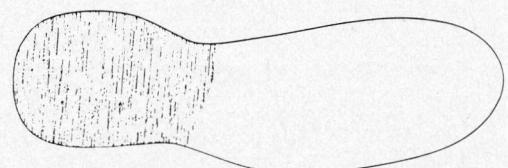

Fig. 17-20. Shaded area indicates portion of mirror used to reflect posterior palatal view.

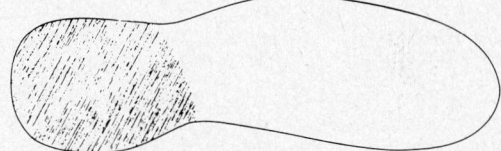

Fig. 17-22. Shaded area indicates portion of mirror used to reflect posterior lingual view.

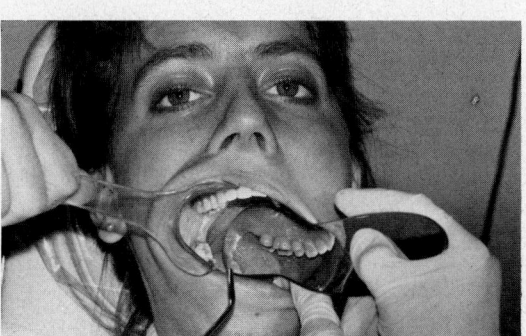

Fig. 17-21. Mirror and retractor placement for right posterior palatal view (see Plate 3, *G*).

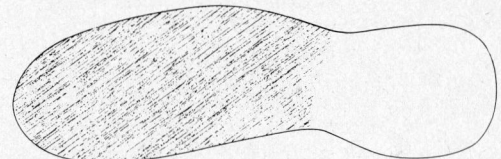

Fig. 17-24. Shaded area indicates portion of mirror used to reflect buccal view.

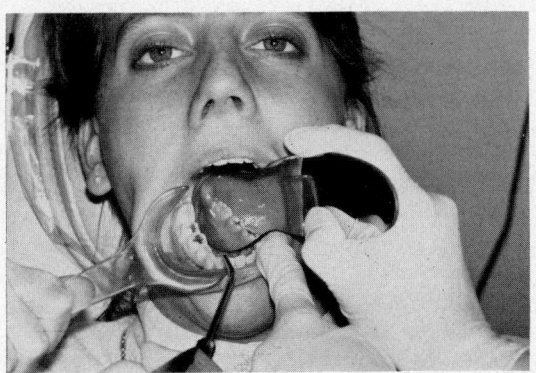

Fig. 17-23. Mirror and retractor placement for right posterior lingual view (see Plate 3, *I*).

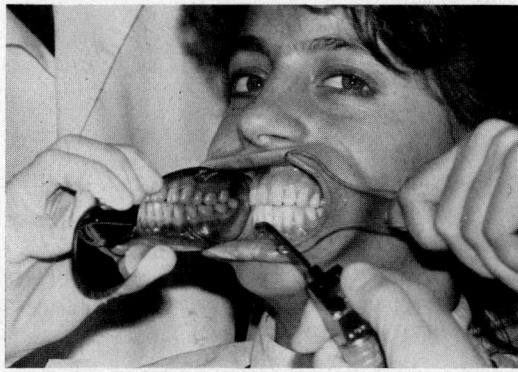

Fig. 17-25. Mirror and retractor placement for left buccal view (see Plate 3, *L*).

RECORD KEEPING AND STORAGE

A record book is placed in the case with the camera. The record book consists of pages with numbers corresponding to the exposures available (such as 24 or 36 exposures). On the line that corresponds to the camera exposure number, record the patient's name and the view that was exposed. Other information may include the date, the photographer's name, or the camera setting if adjustments were made.

Recording the date and the name of the person who loaded and unloaded the camera is helpful in determining the status of the film in the camera. When a film cartridge is unloaded, the camera is reloaded out of courtesy to the next user. This ensures that the camera is ready to be used at a moment's notice.

When the film is processed, the slides are sorted according to the notation in the record book. For identification, each slide is labeled with the patient's name and the view. The clinician's name and the appointment at which the exposure was made are also helpful. The month the slide was processed is generally already imprinted on the slide mount.

Storage

Clear plastic sheets that hold 20 or 36 slides are available to fit three-ring binders. The labeled slides are arranged according to the patient and either stored in a central location or incorporated in the patient's record (Barch, 1972). Slides should be projected or viewed on a color-corrected viewer. The radiographic view box will cause the slides to have poor color. Manual slide viewers that magnify the image are also available. As color slides may fade with time, protection from unnecessary exposure or handling is advised. Kodachrome film has permanent color, so slides need only to be protected from dirt, dust, and finger oils.

GENERAL PHOTOGRAPHIC TECHNIQUE
Camera parts

Proper handling of a camera, as with every other piece of equipment, requires knowledge of its parts and their function. The manufacturer's instruction booklet is most helpful in this regard. In general, it is important to be able to identify the following parts:

Shutter and ASA speed dial
Film advance lever
Shutter release button
Frame counter
Finder eyepiece
Aperture setting, f-stop
Lens and lens cover
Electronic flash unit attachment
Flash plugs connecting at "X" on camera and on flash attachment
Flash "ready" light
Film rewind crank and back-cover release
Film cartridge chamber
Film take-up spool
Film pressure plate
Film rewind button on camera base
Battery cover and switch on camera

Loading the camera

Following are general principles for loading and unloading the film. Consult the manufacturer's directions for specific steps suited to the particular camera.

1. Raise the back-cover release knob and "pop" the back open.
2. Place the film cartridge in the cartridge chamber at the left. Replace the back-cover release knob to hold the cartridge, and feed the film leader onto the take-up spool.
3. Operate the film advance lever. The film will begin to wind around the spool. Watch that the film perforations are engaged on the *upper* and *lower* teeth of the sprocket gears.
4. Press the shutter release button when the advance lever locks. After two shutter releases, the film should be well secured.
5. To make sure the film is flat against the pressure plate, as well as attached to the take-up spool, carefully rotate the film rewind crank in the top of the back-cover release knob to increase the tension slightly. *Always* move the crank in the direction of the arrow. At this point the back of the camera can be closed.
6. Continue to advance the film to the "1" position. As the film advances, look to see if the rewind knob is moving, showing that the film is unwinding.
7. Record your name and the date the camera was loaded.

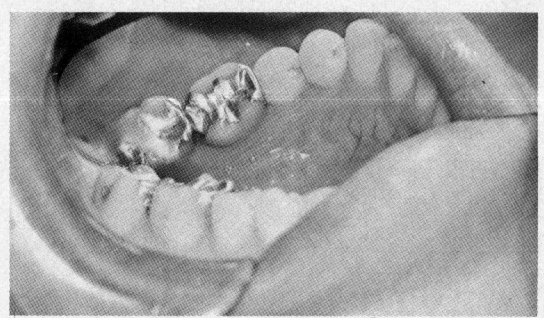

Fig. 17-26. Natural teeth and reflected image create a confusing picture. Capture only the reflected image. Use a stream of air to defog the mirror.

Removing the film

1. Press the rewind button on the bottom of the camera base.
2. Rotate the rewind crank in the top of the back-cover release knob in the direction of the arrow. This winds the film back into the cartridge.
3. As you wind toward the end of the film, you will feel resistance on the crank. Usually after a click that signals the release of the film from the spool, the tension is then released and the crank will move effortlessly. You can then assume that all the film is back in the cartridge.
4. Raise the back-cover release knob, and the back will open.
5. Place the film in its protective canister and send for developing.
6. Record your name and the date of unloading. It is camera courtesy to load the camera for the next person.

Making the photograph

The steps in making a photograph include checking the camera settings, placement of accessories, and composing the view.

1. Check the shutter speed—60 for intraoral photography.
2. Check that the f-stop is set at 22, 19, or 8, depending on the view.
3. Check that the electronic flash "ready" light is on.
4. Check that the film has been advanced.
5. Hold the camera with the pistol grip in the right or left hand. If a macro-lens is used with no pistol grip, place the safety strap from the camera body around your neck.
6. Insert the cheek retractors and mirrors if necessary.
7. When using mirrors and a rotating flash unit, make sure that the flash unit is placed on the same side as the mirror.
8. Dry the field with compressed air as needed.
9. Check the picture composition and the mirror reflection for any adjustments needed at this point.
10. Look through the viewfinder. The bellows is used to obtain the correct composition of the picture. Adjusting the bellows to the most extended position provides the most magnified, close-up view. Change the bellows position for each view as necessary. The bellows does not focus the image; it only provides image ratio or size changes for intraoral views.
11. Correct the mirror placement if necessary. For the best image, position the mirror so that only the reflected image is seen through the viewfinder. Often the natural teeth are observed, which creates a confusing slide (Fig. 17-26). To correct this problem, move the entire mirror further away from the subject. Although it is not always possible to clear the natural teeth from the field, particularly on occlusal or buccal views, attempting to do so is generally beneficial. Often a movement of 1 or 2 mm is all that is necessary.
12. Focus the view. For maximum brightness during focusing, the automatic bellows lens is always at its largest opening (f-4). With the lens aperture set to f-19, for example, it is wide open during focusing but closes down to f-19 as the shutter is triggered. The view is focused by rocking the camera and photographer's body back and forth until the center image in the viewfinder is sharp. Focus on a

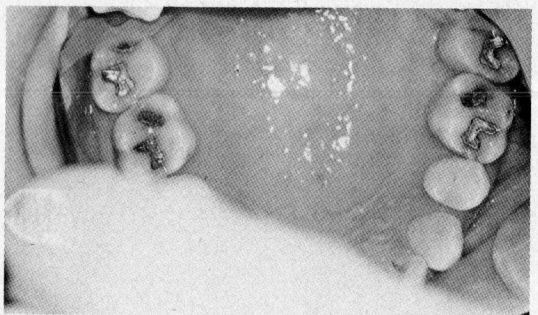

Fig. 17-27. Fingers can be distracting in final picture. As the edge of the view may not be in focus in the viewfinder, check the composition clearly before taking the shot.

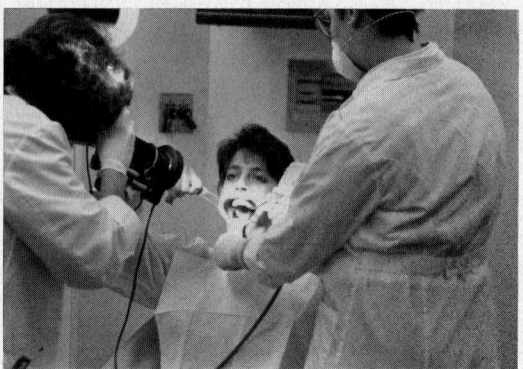

Fig. 17-28. Intraoral photography is a cooperative effort. While looking through camera, the photographer gives directions to the patient holding the retractors and to the person holding the mirror and compressed air.

point one-third of the way into the scene of the subject. For example, use the mesial aspect of the first molar for focus on palatal or mandibular posterior lingual views.

13. Make a final check through the viewfinder for distracting fingers, mirror, or retractor edges, and natural teeth (Fig. 17-27). At this point, the photographer gives the assistant verbal directions for adjusting the accessories without taking his or her eyes away from the viewer. This eliminates additional time spent composing the view and focusing again (Fig. 17-28).

14. While steadying the camera, gently squeeze the shutter release.

15. If correct exposure is uncertain, make the necessary adjustments and take the additional exposure. Film is inexpensive compared with the cost of setting up again or losing the record forever.

16. Record the exposure in the record book.

THE PHOTOGRAPHIC SERIES

A complete series of intraoral photographs is shown in Plate 3. It consists of 12 views of the teeth and adjacent soft tissues. The series does not include a full face or profile view, which may be incorporated depending on the clinician's preference. If the slides identify a person and are going to be used for display or educational purposes, a permission or release form can be developed for the patient to sign (Nuckles et al, 1975). A view of the teeth provides only necessary identification for dental personnel; it does not provide easy recognition of the patient by other observers.

TECHNIQUE FOR INDIVIDUAL VIEWS
Anterior facial views

Composition. Full direct view: The photograph includes all teeth in occlusion as far posteriorly as possible. The incisal and occlusal plane should run in a straight line horizontally across the middle of the slide. The midline is centered (Valentine, 1975) (see Plate 3, A).

Anterior direct view: The photograph includes the area from the distal aspect of the right cuspid to the distal aspect of the left cuspid, as well as an adequate zone of gingiva. The incisal plane should run in a straight line across the middle of the slide. The midline is centered (Valentine, 1975) (see Plate 3, B).

Patient position. The patient sits upright in the chair, with the head resting securely in the headrest. The mandible is parallel to the floor when the teeth are in occlusion. The photographer approaches the subject from a position directly in front of the face. To prevent leaning over the dental chair, the photographer can ask the patient to turn his or her head toward the camera.

Retractors. Both retractors are pulled laterally when composing these pictures (Fig. 17-13).

Mirror. None is required.

Flash. The point-source flash is in the 3 or 9 o'clock position for both the full direct view and the anterior direct view.

Helpful hints. Beware of the upper lip casting a shadow on the maxillary gingiva if the flash is used at the 12 o'clock position. If the cheek retractors are pulled too far posteriorly, the buccal mucosa will press into the buccal surfaces of the teeth.

Anterior lingual views: mandibular

Composition. The photograph contains a lingual view of the mandibular anterior teeth and gingiva from the distal aspect of the right cuspid to the distal aspect of the left cuspid. The incisal plane runs in a line horizontally across the slide, and the midline is centered (Valentine, 1975) (see Plate 3, *C*).

Patient position. The patient is tilted back slightly in the chair with the head resting securely in the headrest. The mouth is opened wide, with the tongue relaxed in the floor of the mouth.

Retractors. Both retractors are used in retracting the lower lip.

Mirror. Either end of the tapered mirror can be used in composing this picture, depending on the width of the patient's mandibular arch (see Fig. 17-15). It is placed one tooth distal to the teeth that are to be photographed and held as parallel as possible to the long axis of the anterior teeth (see Fig. 17-16).

Flash. The point-source flash is in its top position for this view, or if more light contrast is desired, the flash can be placed in the 3 or 9 o'clock position.

Helpful hints. To avoid an excess of saliva in the composition, ask the patient to swallow first.

Anterior lingual views: maxillary anterior palatal

Composition. The photograph contains a palatal view of the maxillary anterior teeth and gingiva from the distal aspect of the right cuspid to the distal aspect of the left cuspid. The incisal plane runs in a line horizontally across the lower edge of the slide, and the midline is centered (Valentine, 1975) (see Plate 3, *D*).

Patient position. The patient should be tilted back slightly in the chair, with the head resting securely in the headrest. The mouth is opened wide, with the tongue resting against the mandibular anterior teeth.

Retractors. Both retractors are used straight out with a slight upward rotation to retract the upper lip.

Mirror. Either end of the mirror can be used in composing this picture, depending on the width of the patient's maxillary arch and the size of the palatal vault. It is placed one tooth distal to the teeth that are to be photographed and held as parallel as possible to the long axis of the teeth (see Fig. 17-17).

Flash. The point-source flash is in the 3 or 9 o'clock position for this view.

Helpful hints. To prevent inclusion of the patient's nostrils in the photograph, make sure that the lower edge of the mirror is depressed as far as possible against the mandibular teeth when the mouth is opened wide.

Occlusal/soft tissue views: mandibular

Composition. The photograph includes the mandibular arch around the perimeter of the mirror (occlusal surfaces) and the floor of the mouth or the tongue (Valentine, 1975) (see Plate 3, *E*).

Patient position. The patient is tilted back in the chair, with the mandible pointed slightly up. The occlusal plane is parallel to the floor when the mouth is opened wide. The tongue may be placed lightly on the soft palate or left to relax in the floor of the mouth.

Retractors. Both retractors are used for this view. Retract the lip downward as necessary.

Mirror. The occlusal mirror is used specifically for this view. Depending on the size of the patient's mouth, either the small or large end of the mirror is inserted posteriorly until the borders of the mirror rest on the retromolar pad. The mirror is then adjusted until it rests at a 45-degree angle to the plane of the occlusion. Blow a stream of compressed air to defog the mirror before taking the photograph (see Fig. 17-18).

Flash. The flash is in the 3 or 9 o'clock position for this view.

Helpful hints. To avoid seeing the fingers or retractors in your composition, hold the mirror at its very edge. Tilt the chair back slightly if necessary. In some cases the cheek retractors do not have to be used if the lips are not obscuring the view. Have the patient swallow to prevent pooling saliva.

Occlusal/soft tissue views: maxillary

Composition. The photograph includes the maxillary arch around the perimeter of the mirror (occlusal surfaces) and the palate (Valentine, 1975) (see Plate 3, *F*).

Patient position. The patient is sitting in the chair with the head resting securely in the headrest. The mouth should be opened wide and the tongue relaxed against the mandibular teeth.

Retractors. Both retractors are used in this view.

Mirror. The occlusal mirror is used specifically for this view. Depending on the size of the patient's mouth, either the small or large end of the mirror is inserted posteriorly until the borders of the mirror rest on the retromolar pad. The mirror is then adjusted until it rests at a 45-degree angle to the plane of the occlusion (see Fig 17-19).

Flash. The flash is in 3 or 9 o'clock position for this view.

Helpful hints. To avoid seeing the fingers or retractors in your composition, hold the mirror at its very edge. If the nostrils are still in view, depress the mirror more toward the mandibular teeth or have the patient open wider. Tilt the chair back slightly if necessary. If some cases the cheek retractors do not have to be used if the lips are not obscuring the view.

Posterior palatal views (right and left)

Composition. The photograph includes a palatal view of the maxillary posterior teeth and gingiva from the distal aspect of the cuspid to the maxillary tuberosity. The occlusal plane runs in a straight line horizontally across the slide (Valentine, 1975) (see Plate 3, *G* and *H*).

Patient position. The patient is tilted back slightly in the chair, with the head resting securely in the headrest and usually turned slightly

to the side being photographed. The patient's head is turned slightly to the side to permit the best view of the mirror.

Retractors. Both retractors are used to retract the lips and provide access for the mirror on the specific side.

Mirror. The rounded end of the buccal mirror is preferred for this view (see Fig. 17-20). It is placed along the midline of the palate until its distal portion is adjacent to the maxillary tuberosity. The anterior end may rest on the incisal surfaces of the lateral incisor of the opposite quadrant. For a direct palatal view, the mirror is maintained as parallel to the long axis of the teeth as possible (see Fig. 17-21).

Flash. The flash is rotated to the same side as the mirror for this view.

Helpful hints. To avoid simulating a gag reflex, do not rest the mirror on the soft palate. If the patient's natural teeth are in the composition, move the entire mirror toward the midline.

Posterior lingual view

Composition. The photograph includes the area from the distal aspect of the cuspid up to and including the retromolar pad. The view is a direct lingual view and shows as little of the occlusal surfaces as possible (Valentine, 1975) (see Plate 3, *I* and *J*).

Patient position. The patient is tilted back slightly in the chair with the head resting securely in the headrest. The mouth is opened wide with the tongue relaxed on the floor of the mouth.

Retractors. Both retractors are used to retract the lips and provide access for the mirror on the specific side.

Mirror. The more rounded end of the mirror is preferred for this view, with the arc toward the floor of the mouth (see Fig. 17-22). The tongue is gently retracted away from the lingual surfaces of the teeth with the mirror as it is positioned just distal to the retromolar pad. The mirror will cross the arch diagonally, and the anterior portion of the mirror will rest as far posteriorly on the bicuspids of the opposite quadrant as possible. The mirror is held as vertically as possible to provide the best view. If the top edge of the mirror is tilted toward the teeth, too much of an occlusal view will be observed. The entire mirror is moved away from the teeth if the natural teeth are in view (see Fig. 17-23).

Flash. The flash is rotated to the same side as the mirror for this view.

Helpful hints. Work quickly with this view, as it is not only uncomfortable but is taken in an extremely wet field. Be careful not to retract the tongue too harshly, stimulating the gag reflex.

Posterior buccal views (right and left)

Composition. The photograph includes the area from the distal aspect of the cuspids to the distal aspect of the most posterior tooth in each arch, as well as a glimpse of the retromolar pad or the maxillary tuberosity. The occlusal plane runs in a straight line horizontally across the midline of the slide. The view is as direct a buccal view as possible, rather than a mesial view (Valentine, 1975) (see Plate 3, *K* and *L*).

Patient position. The patient is sitting upright in the chair, with the head resting securely in the headrest. With the teeth in occlusion, the mandible is parallel to the floor.

Retractors. One wire retractor is used to hold the mirror for the best view. A plastic retractor is used on the opposite side to retract the lip.

Flash. The flash is rotated to the same side as the mirror for this view.

Mirror. The long tapered end of the buccal mirror is preferred for composing this picture (see Fig. 17-24). The mirror is inserted into the frame of the wire retractor and placed between the buccal surfaces of the teeth and the buccal mucosa all the way to the distal aspect of the last tooth in the arch. It should be pulled laterally away from the alveolar process as much as possible (see Fig. 17-9). An alternative technique does not use a wire retractor. The mirror is placed and positioned as described. A secure grip should be kept on the mirror to prevent the buccal musculature from pushing the mirror anteriorly or medially (see Fig. 17-25).

Helpful hints. Retract the tissue firmly and as close to a 45-degree angle as possible from the natural teeth to provide the photographer with the best view.

Summary

These directions are intended as a guide for the beginner. Depending on the camera system and the clinical environment, experience will help each clinician determine the best technique. Slight adjustments in chair position and cheek retractor and mirror placement usually have to be made, depending on the patient's oral conditions.

EVALUATION OF SLIDES

The student is encouraged to evaluate the slides he or she has taken according to clinical criteria. Following are suggested criteria for slides:

Above average
1. Inclusion of all desired oral structures
2. Excellent photographic detail; excellent focus
3. Excellent lighting/color
4. No extraneous material
5. Structures well centered
6. Slide labeled properly

Average
1. Inclusion of desired oral structures
2. Adequate photographic detail
3. Lighting/color improvement needed
4. Extraneous material included, but not to detraction of slide's value
5. Centering improvement needed
6. Slide labeled properly

Unacceptable
1. Omission of desired oral structures
2. Inadequate photographic detail
3. Inadequate lighting/color
4. Obvious extraneous material included
5. Subject completely off-center
6. Slide incorrectly labeled

Following the student evaluation, an instructor meets with the student to discuss the slide evaluation. Discussion focuses on suggestions to improve technique for forthcoming photography sessions. Positive comments and encouragement are helpful, as hours of practice are necessary to reach competence in this psychomotor skill.

The criteria sheet on p. 332 is included for process evaluation of student progress during laboratory or clinic instruction.

Intraoral Photography

STUDENT: _____

DATE:

PERFORMANCE CRITERIA: COMMENTS

1. Prepare all equipment for intraoral photography (camera, sterile mirrors, retractors, film, record book)
2. Make all adjustments on the camera to ensure a successful exposure (1/60 shutter speed, electronic flash "ready", appropriate f-stop)
3. Position the electronic flash according to the area of the mouth to be photographed
4. Insert cheek retractors with a minimum of trauma to the patient
5. Correctly place the intraoral mirrors to obtain the desired composition.
6. Use compressed air to dry the area to be photographed
7. Hold the camera securely
8. Focus the camera by adjusting the bellows and body position, or by adjusting the macro-lens
9. Record all photos in the record book
10. Store the camera without cocking the trigger
11. Rack the bellows to the full "in" position for storage, or correctly position and store the macro-lens
12. Sterilize and store the cheek retractors and mirrors appropriately
13. Care for the photographic equipment in a responsible manner
14. Load and/or unload the camera properly
15. Evaluate the quality of slides and recommend variations in photographic technique to correct inadequate exposure

CONCLUSION

Intraoral photography has become a part of modern dentistry. With this skill the clinician enhances the process of treatment planning and accurate documentation of the patient's care. Basic photographic skills have been presented for handling a clinical camera system and composing a series of intraoral views.

Companies to contact for clinical camera systems and photographic accessories

Washington Scientific
Camera Co.
P.O. Box 88681
Tukwila, WA 98188

Trojan Camera
3540 S. Figueroa
Los Angeles, CA 90007
(800-338-9433)

Lester A. Dine
100 Milbar Blvd.
P.O. Drawer F
Farmingdale, NY
11735-0905
(516-454-6100)

Olympus Corporation
Crossways Park
Woodbury, NY 11797
(516-364-3000)

Competitive Camera
Corporation
157 West 30th Street
New York, NY 10001
(212-868-9175)

U.S. Schizai
5261½ E. Beverly Blvd.
Los Angeles, CA 90022
(213-685-5960)

Evaporated Metals Films
(mirrors only)
701 Spencer Road
Ithaca, NY 14850

ACKNOWLEDGMENT

The author is grateful to the Department of Dental Hygiene at Thomas Jefferson University, College of Allied Health Sciences in Philadelphia, Pennsylvania, and especially to Jaclyn Gleber, R.D.H., M.Ed., and dental hygiene students Kathleen O'Brien and Elizabeth Clark for providing the views of photographic technique presented in this chapter.

ACTIVITIES

1. Identify the parts of a camera. Practice loading and unloading a "test" film cartridge.
2. View slides of the complete intraoral series, identifying the composition of each view. Unacceptable slides may be shown to illustrate common photographic errors.
3. Divide into lab groups of four students: photographer, patient, mirror holder, and an extra to hold retractors, position light, dry field, and other tasks. Rotate being photographer and practice taking the intraoral views (1 hour per session is suggested). One faculty member per group of students is ideal. Eight to ten sessions are suggested for mastering basic skills.
4. When slides are returned from processing, meet as a group to critique the views and plan new technique strategies.
5. Practice photographic skills by taking complete series of intraoral photographs for clinical patients as a part of treatment and case documentation.

REVIEW QUESTIONS

1. State four ways in which intraoral photography can be useful in dentistry.
2. List the components of a clinical camera system.
3. Match the terms in column 1 with those in column 2 that are most closely related. Place the appropriate number in the space provided.

___ a. Single-lens reflex	1. Error in viewing
___ b. Aperture setting	2. 60
___ c. Focus	3. Controls photographic composition
___ d. Shutter speed	4. Produces shadow for definition
___ e. Parallax	5. "Rocking" adjustment with body and camera
___ f. Depth of field	
___ g. Film	6. Lens
___ h. 100 mm	7. ASA 64
___ i. Point-source light	8. Plane of focus
___ j. Bellows position	9. Mirror viewing system
	10. f-22

4. Give the steps for placement of intraoral cheek retractors.
5. Give the composition of the following views:
   a. Mandibular anterior lingual
   b. Buccal of right side
   c. Anterior direct
   d. Maxillary occlusal

REFERENCES

Barch L: Storage and filing of dental color slides, J Acad Gen Dent 20:24, 1972.

Bengel W: Standardization in dental photography, Int Dent J 35(3):210, 1985.

Bernstein ML: The application of photography in forensic dentistry, Dent Clin North Am 27(1):151, 1983.

Brackett WW: Dental photography: getting started, Compend Contin Educ Dent 7(4):297, 1986.

Clinical Research Associates: Camera for clinical photography. Newsletter (Provo, Utah) 7(5):1, 1983.

Cooley RL, and Barkmeier WW: Adapting a flash unit for dental photography, Dent Radiogr Photogr 52(3):62, 1979.

Costello MJ: A simple and standardized approach to clinical photography, Aust Orthod J 7(1):48, 1981.

Dahlberg W: Photography in periodontics, Dent Clin North Am 763, 1968.

Daniels T, and Sherill C: Handbook of dental photography, San Francisco, 1975, University of California School of Dentistry.

Faucher RR: Dental photography in the graduate teaching program, Dent Clin North Am 27:109, 1983.

Freehe CL: Dental retractors and accessories, Dent Clin North Am 731, 1968.

Freehe CL: Clinical dental photography: equipment and technique. In Clark J, editor: vol. 1. New York, 1976, Harper & Row, Inc.

Freehe CL: Photography in dentistry: equipment and technique, Dent Clin North Am 27:3, 1983.

Freehe CL: Dental photography, Funct Orthod 1(4):41, 1984.

Gholston LR: Reliability of an intraoral camera: utility for clinical dentistry and research, Am J Ortho 85(1):89, 1984.

Gordon PD: Principles of close-up photography, Br Dent J 162(6):229, 1987.

Gordon PD: Techniques for dental photography, Br Dent J 162(8):307, 1987.

Gordon PD: Specialized equipment for dental photography, Br Dent J 162(9):346, 1987.

Gregg TA: A modified lighting system for dental photography, J Ir Dental Assoc 30(1):3, 1984.

Hamilton AI: Preparing text, tables, and illustrations for a journal editor, Dent Clin North Am 27:197, 1983.

Hetherington W and Freehe C: Single lens reflex cameras and associated equipment for use in dental photography, Dent Clin North Am 699, 1968.

Jordan R et al. 1983. A clinical lecturer's application of dental photography, Dent Clin North Am. 27:121.

Lund DN: A clinical camera for dental photography, Aust Orthod J 6(3):110, 1980.

McGrannahan W: Clinical camera, J Mo Dent Assoc, 63(5):162, 1983.

Meister F et al: The value of photography in a periodontal survey, Dent Radiogr Photogr 51:8, 1978.

Morgan J et al: Methods of presentation in dental photography, Br Dent J 162(11):429, 1987.

Nelson LC: Photography: its uses in dental practice, lectures, and the home, Dent Clin North Am 27:171, 1983.

Nuckles D et al: Close-up photography in the dental office, JADA 90:152, 1975.

Osborne P et al: An evaluation of a 90 mm lens for use in intraoral photography, Gen Dent 35(3):193, 1987.

Rayman MS and Eilers A: Basic intraoral photography technique, CDA J 13(4):53, 1985.

Rosenfeld L: Periodontics: photos tell the tale, Dent Stud 54:29, 1976.

Stern N: Indexing and storing teaching slides, Dent Radiogr Photogr 46:86, 1973.

Tilly D and Hagen A: Preparing graphics for visual presentation, Dent Clin North Am 27:75, 1983.

Toljanic JA and Groetsema WR: Inexpensive intraoral photography, Ill Dent J 52(4):228, 1983.

Tribe H: Selecting and preparing illustrations for publication and presentation, Dent Clin North Am 27:95, 1983.

Valentine RM: Expanded duties: a self-determined pace laboratory program, Philadelphia, 1975, Department of Dental Hygiene, School of Dental Medicine, University of Pennsylvania.

Walker RS: Guide to dental photography systems, LDA J 43(3):17, 1984.

Wander P: Setting up: equipment, lighting, and accessories, Br Dent J 162(7):268, 1987.

Wander P: Specific applications of dental photography, Br Dent J 162(10):393, 1987.

Wander P and Gordon P: Dental Photography. London, 1987, Professional and Scientific Publications.

Zukerman A: Utilization of instant closeup photography for the esthetic improvement of multiple full coverage restorations, Quintessence 15(5):545, 1984.

PART TWO

PLANNING

Once the site is prepared and assessment data are gathered, it is time for logical *planning* for the patient. This includes (1) developing an action plan to solve the problems that have emerged from the assessment phase and (2) setting goals for the patient's health progress.

Involving the patient in planning is an important key to ensuring active participation and shared ownership of the plan. Therefore, in Chapters 18 to 20, the patient is an integral part of the planning of care.

Some signs of implementation will begin to emerge in these planning chapters, as the line between planning and implementation is often difficult to define. The planning process in many ways triggers the patient's needs to know and to receive care. The dental professional's responsibility is to ensure that planning is adequately defined and that the program moves into implementation at a point when the patient is most receptive.

18

FORMULATING A TREATMENT PLAN, CASE PRESENTATION, AND APPOINTMENT PLAN

OBJECTIVES: *The reader will be able to*

1. Given assessment data from a variety of cases (including medical history, vital signs, intraoral and extraoral examinations and chartings, radiographic surveys, diagnostic casts, and the patient's expectations), do the following:
   a. Design a treatment plan best suited to the specific needs of each patient
   b. Design at least one alternative plan for each case
   c. Design a case presentation format for each patient that meets (1) the legal requirements of *informed consent* and (2) the basic principles of interpersonal communication
   d. Design a logical sequence of planned appointments to fulfill the treatment plan for each case
2. Given a variety of treatment needs, identify priorities for treatment, including:
   a. Emergency needs
   b. Prevention of disease
   c. Restorative and surgical needs
   d. Maintenance needs

NATURE AND ROLE OF TREATMENT PLANNING

Treatment planning saves patients from an automated approach to dental and dental hygiene care. Completing an individualized treatment plan does not allow, for instance, for the assumption that all people need an oral prophylaxis or a fluoride treatment. It guides the health care provider in identifying specific *problems* and specific *health goals* and in identifying treatment or other procedures to solve the problems and to meet the health goals. Careful planning allows these two foci to be accomplished in tandem.

In addition, treatment planning provides an opportunity to specify those problems and goals so that they can be shared with the patient and explained in rational, understandable terms. It provides an opportunity to organize the sequence of care and to plan care so that the patient can identify with and participate in progress as it is made. Such organization maximizes efficiency and reduces frustration.

The written, agreed-on treatment plan is a legal contract that forms the basis of the legal relationship between the health care provider and the patient. It is an invaluable resource in a court of law as well as at the chairside. It provides a medium for discussing wants, needs, and expectations and for promoting a free exchange of perceptions (Clark and Morton, 1977).

PREPARING A TREATMENT PLAN

Once all of the assessment phases of care have been completed, the data from each of these procedures should be analyzed carefully and synthesized into a comprehensive picture of the needs of the individual patient (Clark and Morton, 1977; Fechtner, 1978; Fishman and Ortiz, 1977; Wood, 1978).

The medical history, review of systems, and vital signs should point out precautionary measures to ensure the general well-being of the patient. The need for a physician's clearance or referral to a physician should have been identified clearly before intraoral examination. Be especially aware of general signs of fatigue, unrest, anxiety, or other conditions based on this carefully collected data.

The significant findings from each examination and charting should be identified and compared. Clinical evidence of health and disease should be compared with radiographic evidence. Evaluations of the conditions of the teeth should be compared with soft tissue findings in their respective areas of the dentition. Results of plaque indices should be laid alongside patterns of disease occurrence for the teeth and periodontium. A comprehensive picture of the objective clinical needs of the patient should emerge, or further questions about health status should be raised (Barsh, 1981; Morris, 1983).

A logical way to design a treatment plan is (1) to systematically review each assessment finding in terms of its significance; (2) to identify each significant finding as a problem or goal; and (3) to identify an appropriate course of action. Once these three steps are complete, then (4) a priority should be established for each procedure; from this, (5) a specific sequence in care should be assigned; and (6) estimated time needed should be identified for each step (Wood, 1978).

The treatment planning worksheet shown in Table 18-1 can be modified to meet the individual dental hygienist's approach to planning. Such a worksheet makes it easier to identify critical needs, goals, phases of care, sequencing, and time needs. It minimizes the chance of overlooking specific findings and displays groups of findings so that correlations among data are more apparent.

As objective needs emerge to form a series of preventive or treatment procedures appropriate for the patient, more subjective needs, particularly those expressed by the patient during the self-assessment of needs, contribute to the overall picture of care that should be planned for the patient. The health care provider's attitudes toward these needs and expectations is demonstrated in how they are accounted for in the treatment plan and can have a significant effect on the patient's perception of the health care provider's ability to help the patient meet long-term and short-term health goals (Goldberg, Plume, and Nacman, 1973).

The assignment of priorities reflects the philo-sophic approach of the dental hygienist to providing care. Most clinicians would agree that clinical problems that are causing pain or are likely to cause pain in the near future are *emergency treatment* procedures that should receive top priority. Therefore deep caries, the presence of an apical radiolucency, or a suspicious oral lesion will delay preventive care.

Differences in philosophy are more apparent among health care providers when deciding whether *preventive* procedures or *restorative* and *surgical treatment* are the next highest priorities. Many clinicians believe that ensuring the patient's *control* of his or her dental health supersedes any treatment other than emergency procedures. Others believe that prevention should follow basic treatment procedures. Many combine these priorities by integrating preventive procedures into each treatment appointment. *Maintenance* care, which ensures long-term periodic examinations and preventive procedures, logically follows the completion of therapeutic procedures.

The sequence of treatment does not necessarily follow the priority assignment, as some high-priority elements are more effective if they follow other preliminary procedures. For instance, curettage procedures to reduce chronic inflammatory periodontal disease may have a high priority but may be sequenced after thorough removal of hard deposits and after the patient has mastered brushing and flossing. Another example is the application of sealants, which may have a very high priority for a child with deep pits and grooves but which should follow other treatment needs, such as those prompted by active caries.

Estimating the time needed to complete each procedure is an important step in treatment planning and should be noted while the assessment data are fresh in the clinician's mind. The large, subgingival deposits of calculus noted on the charting and visible on the radiographic survey can prompt more realistic estimates of time needed for debridement than can later recollections.

Once the treatment plan is complete, the dental hygienist should review the patient's wants, needs, and expectations to ensure that they are met, or at least addressed. A useful preliminary step is to imagine oneself as the patient who will soon learn about this plan. A series of questions

Table 18-1. Treatment planning worksheet

Assessment tool	Significant findings	Problem or goal	Indicated course of action	Priority	Sequence in care	Time needed
Medical history						
Review of systems						
Vital signs						
Dental history						
Extraoral examination						
Intraoral examination						
Periodontal examination						
Calculus charting						
Dental charting						
Radiographic charting						
Guided self-assessment						
Plaque index						
Hemorrhage point index						
Nutritional self-assessment						
Patient's expressed wants, needs, and expectations						

339

that may prove helpful in ensuring that the wants, needs, and expectations expressed at earlier appointments are met and in translating the treatment plan into a case presentation are as follows:

Where in the plan are the patient's expressed needs addressed?

Is the *course of action* in meeting those needs and their *priority* likely to be satisfactory to the patient? Why or why not?

What additional phases of care are included in the plan that are related to needs of which the patient may be unaware?

How can those needs be described simply and accurately for the patient? How can self-assessment data substantiate the findings?

Is the patient likely to be alarmed or upset by these additional findings? Is the patient likely to view these plans as a luxury or as unnecessary?

How can the proposed treatment and its likely outcomes be described so that the patient's confidence and trust are maintained? What questions is the patient likely to ask?

What specific goals for health should be emphasized? How can the patient become involved in helping realize those goals?

What alternative plans for care could be followed and with what consequences?

Is the patient likely to be concerned about appearance, pain, cost, and/or time? How does each of those concerns appear justified in terms of the proposed treatment plan?

What would be the likely outcome if the patient refused care or selected a modified plan?

The treatment plan, therefore, requires considerable knowledge of the implications of the assessment data as clinical and radiographic signs are interpreted. It is a critical point in individualizing and personalizing care and in applying knowledgeable professional judgment (Wood, 1978).

DESIGNING A CASE PRESENTATION

After having completed the planning worksheet and answered the aforementioned questions regarding the patient's likely perceptions, the dental hygienist should be prepared to define the treatment plan in an understandable case presentation. The primary purposes of the case presentation are to solidify the understanding of needs and plans and to formalize the contractual relationship between the patient and the dental hygienist for the treatment phase of care. *Informed consent* is the legal reason for the case presentation (Miller, 1979; Rosoff, 1981). *Mutual understanding* and *cooperation* are the more personal reasons for the case presentation.

The guidelines for establishing informed consent form a natural framework for explaining the case to the patient. First, the nature of the patient's condition should be described in understandable terms, with ample opportunity for responding to the patient's concerns and requests for further explanation. It may be helpful to show the patient his or her study models and radiographs and to refer to other data gathered. The suggested plan or treatment should follow, with a discussion of the likely outcomes of the treatment. Risks involved should be described; the likely outcome of not proceeding with care should be described as well. Finally, alternative treatment approaches should be offered, with a discussion of their advantages and disadvantages (Fishman and Ortiz, 1977; Miller, 1979; Rosoff, 1981).

If the patient is involved fully in the case presentation and agrees to proceed with care, informed consent is secured (Miller, 1979; Rosoff, 1981). The costs of care (usually expressed as a close estimate) and the time needed should be discussed also to minimize surprises and to further involve the patient in decision making (Miller, 1979; Rosoff, 1981). The time estimates and sequence identified in the treatment plan should enable the hygienist to identify an order and number of appointments most compatible with the time constraints of the patient.

Although the practice of including the requirements of informed consent in the case presentation is an important preventive approach in avoiding litigation and misunderstanding, two additional points are important in the legal ramifications of the contractual relationship. First, if any additional procedures are to be included in treatment, the patient's informed consent must be obtained for those new elements of care. If this is not done, the dental hygienist is liable for *technical assault* or *battery* (performing a procedure to which the patient did not consent) under tort law. Second, all procedures agreed to in the case presentation must be performed within a reasonable time with a reasonable standard of care. If a procedure is to be omitted or delayed, the patient first must be informed and must agree. If this is not done, the dental hygienist can be subjected to a breach of contract suit (Fechtner, 1978; Miller, 1979; Rosoff, 1981).

More altruistic reasons for the case presentation are to decrease the patient's fear of the unknown, to build trust, and to form a helping relationship that maximizes positive outcomes. The case presentation should be thorough but simple, and it should be presented with a modicum of enthusiasm. Too much intensity can destroy the message (Keltner, 1973). The thorough, thoughtful case presentation should improve the patient's desire to cooperate by appearing for appointments, following preoperative and postoperative instructions, and paying for services. A sense of participation in care promotes this cooperation; the patient develops a sense of ownership of his or her needs and the methods to meet those needs (Cohen, 1975; Keltner, 1973). Likewise, the dental hygienist may derive great satisfaction from having learned about and cared for a person who needed assistance.

The case presentation also helps the patient recognize the significance of the numerous assessment procedures in the beginning phases of care. The patient learns about good dentistry and good health care and experiences shared responsibility in care by having the opportunity to participate in the discussion.

No matter what the quality of the assessments of the patient's needs, the logic of the treatment plan, and the interest of the case presentation, the patient may decline treatment. A health care provider cannot force a patient to accept care (Fishman and Ortiz, 1977; Miller, 1979). While it may be shocking to hear the patient say, "I really don't think I want all this dental work," that kind of honesty is preferable to a nonverbal expression of the refusal to accept care—the broken appointment. It can be risky to ask, "Would you like to proceed with treatment?" It can be difficult to hear the response, "No." However, the direct positive response is usually a strong indicator of the patient's commitment to cooperate in care. It indicates that the patient accepts the described health needs as real and the proposed course of action as

appropriate. A negotiated or compromised treatment plan, although it may not be ideal in the health care provider's view, is usually an even more positive sign of a solid partnership relationship with mutual respect between the patient and the health care provider (Clark and Morton, 1977; Keltner, 1973). With this kind of a relationship the "ideal" plan is more likely to be realized in the long run.

Hesitancy to accept the plan or a simple rejection deserves follow-up discussion (Fishman and Ortiz, 1977). Questioning about the patient's concerns may elicit perceived roadblocks to care (financial problems, fear of discomfort or altered appearance, lack of time) or apparent misunderstandings of the problem or the plan. The health care provider can help reduce or eliminate the roadblocks by further clarifying the specifics of the treatment plan. In any case, if the patient declines treatment, the reasons should be fairly clear, and the health care provider should be able to accept that decision as the patient's right. "Good persuasion endures and allows people to make intelligent choices; it does not take advantage of people's weaknesses" (Keltner, 1973).

With acceptance of the final plan, the development of an appointment plan solidifies the agreement and defines a set of expectations: when and for how long the patient and health care provider agree to receive and provide treatment, respectively. A commitment is made.

APPOINTMENT PLANNING

Translating the treatment plan into specific appointments requires several considerations. Using 15-minute increments (for example) as appointment units simplifies blocking out appointment time. Obviously, the estimated time needed for each procedure and the logic of grouping procedures that are interrelated are the primary determinants in designing appointments.

The patient's tolerance for long sessions in a dental chair (or for frequent trips to the dental office) is an important consideration. Children, for instance, usually should be scheduled for short appointments at a time of day when they are least fatigued. Some patients prefer a series of short appointments; others prefer fewer, longer appointments. For most treatment needs, procedures can be sequenced to accommodate patient preferences.

Tables 18-2 to 18-5 describe the translation of assessment data into treatment plans and then into appointment sequences. These examples reflect the time requirements of a hygienist who has achieved a satisfactory level of time-and-motion management. Beginning clinicians will define their time needs for treatment differently. Time needed to complete various procedures will decrease with greater skill and practice. Another important variable, regardless of the skill and experience of the clinician, is the amount of time spent waiting or participating in discussion with co-workers regarding the case. In health care delivery systems that require patient evaluation in several different clinics or departments, the time requirements in the beginning phases of care may be high. In less complex systems, time requirements for activities such as consultations, preparing release forms, and referral procedures may be less. Therefore, these examples are given primarily to illustrate how individual differences and needs can affect the planning of treatment and appointments and are not intended to reflect ideal time usage.

The case outlined in Table 18-2 describes an adult with chronic, inflammatory periodontal disease (Lynch, 1977). Medical complications are minimal. Assessment findings show a pattern of caries development and high plaque scores despite frequent dental visits. The indicated course of action focuses on monitoring the blood pressure, eliminating the periodontal problem, and instituting a strong preventive program for the patient. The key in motivation, and a factor to be kept in mind in planning, is the patient's concern for cost.

Table 18-3 outlines a case involving a leukemic patient who should be maintained on a solid, albeit low-pressure, preventive program to minimize irritants that could cause gingival problems (Lynch, 1977). Scheduling is based on the medical status of the patient, and traumatic procedures are minimized. The relative significance of good teeth for both this patient and the family should be kept in mind. The primary motivator is that teeth and their surrounding tissues should cause no additional problems. Therefore, an easily followed preventive routine is appropriate.

The third case (Table 18-4) is an outline for a patient with acute necrotizing ulcerative gingivitis (ANUG) (Lynch, 1977). The sequence of care is altered by the history of rheumatic fever. No probing or exploring could be performed until the patient had achieved satisfactory blood levels of antibiotics to counteract any microorganisms entering the blood-stream (bacteremia) through incidental hemorrhage. Once the premedication was ensured, the periodontal examination was completed and debridement was begun (Lynch, 1977).

The fourth, and final case (Table 18-5) describes dental hygiene care planned for a postsurgical cancer patient, for whom the clinician needs to identify individualized needs, to coordinate efforts with other health care providers, and to reinforce oral hygiene procedures to reverse the progress of disease secondary to oral cancer therapy (Rose and Kaye, 1983). The changes in the oral tissues, the rise in the presence of caries and gingivitis, the reduction in oral fluids, and the patient's response to treatment all deserve careful attention and planning before any "routine" care is provided. (See Chapter 33 for further discussion.)

Dental hygiene treatment planning should always question the appropriateness of "routine" care. It seeks out and responds to the individual needs of patients, whether they are startlingly apparent or elusive. Such planning is an essential, professional responsibility of dental hygienists.

The ideal way to develop the ability to translate assessment data into a plan and then into an appointment sequence is to practice with a variety of hypothetical and real cases. Case presentations can then be role played, with students serving as patients and observers who report whether informed consent requirements were met and whether the "dental hygienist" listened to the expressed wants, needs, and expectations of the "patient" and responded to those concerns. Such practice facilitates clinical application of these basic skills in synthesis, planning, and communicating.

TREATMENT PLANNING AND DIAGNOSIS: LEGAL AND PROFESSIONAL RESPONSIBILITIES

In an era when the dental hygienist's role and responsibility are not uniformly defined by law, in

Text continued on p. 351.

Table 18-2. Case 1

Assessment tool	Significant findings	Problem or goal	Indicated course of action	Priority	Sequence in care	Time needed
Medical history	Within normal limits	—	—	—	—	—
Review of systems	Within normal limits	—	—	—	—	—
Vital signs	130/86 right arm sitting (ras) Pulse: 75	Potential high bp	Record bp at each visit	A	First at each appointment	5 min per appointment
Dental history	Regular visits to dentist (every 6 months)	Maintain this habit	Reinforce behavior	—	6—at last appointment; recall system entry	5 min last appointment
Extraoral examination	Crepitus in TMJ	Determine its significance	Refer to dentist for assessment	D	At first treatment appointment	5 min first appointment
Intraoral examination	Within normal limits	—	—	—	—	—
Periodontal examination	Red, edematous tissue—generalized Minimal attached gingivae—3 to 6 mm pockets	Normal gingivae	Plaque control Debridement Review for soft tissue curettage Refer for periodontal consult	C	4	2 hrs (1-hr appointments)
Calculus charting	Generalized ledge and crustaceous calculus	Debride	Ultrasonic scaling	C	3	1 hr
Dental charting	Three suspicious areas of possible caries; one defective restoration (No. 30) Numerous restorations (24 total covering 60 surfaces)	Evaluate for need for restorative treatment	Refer to dentist for assessment Recommend fluoride rinses	C B	At first treatment appointment 2	5 min
Radiographic charting	Within normal limits	—	—	—	—	—
Guided self-assessment	Presence of numerous restorations despite regular dental visits Presence of red tissue	Reduce frequency of caries	Nutritional counseling Review brushing and flossing Consider phosphate fluoride treatment	B	2	15 to 20 min per appointment
Plaque index	Plaque on 60% of surfaces	Reduce plaque	Review brushing and flossing, antiplaque agents	A	1	5 min per appointment

Table 18-2. Case 1 —cont'd.

Assessment tool	Significant findings	Problem or goal	Indicated course of action	Priority	Sequence in care	Time needed
Hemorrhage point index	30 areas of spontaneous hemorrhage	Reduce tissue inflammation	Debridement and improved plaque control; irrigation	—	—	5 min per appointment
Nutritional self-assessment	High intake of refined sugars / Minimal intake of fruits and vegetables	Reduce sugar and add fruits and vegetables	Dietary counseling	B	3	10 to 15 min per appointment
Patient's expressed wants, needs, and expectations	Worried about cost	Minimize time needed and involve patient in self-care program to enhance healing and prevent recurrence	Teach plaque control and dietary counseling early / Use fluoride on suspicious carious lesions	A	1,3 / 5	5 min

Appointment plan

Appointment 1 (postassessment)
1. Record bp — 5 min
2. Request dentist consult for
   Crepitus
   Carious areas (and decision to restore or treat with fluoride) — 10 min
3. Begin plaque/caries control — 30 min
   Brushing/antiplaque agents
   Flossing/irrigation
   Dietary modifications
   Recommend fluoride rinses
4. Ultrasonically scale entire dentition — 60 min
SCHEDULE: 105 min (7 units)*

Appointment 2
1. Record bp — 5 min
2. Review plaque control — 25 min
   Take indices
   Observe techniques of brushing, flossing
   Add oral physiotherapeutic aids (OPTA) as needed
   Review 3-day diet
3. Root plane mandible — 45 min
SCHEDULE: 75 min 5 (units)

Appointment 3
1. Record bp — 5 min
2. Review plaque control (see Appointment 2) — 20 min
3. Root plane maxilla — 45 min
SCHEDULE: 70 min (5 units)

Appointment 4
1. Record bp — 5 min
2. Record indices and discuss plaque control and diet as needed — 15 min
3. Evaluate for curettage — 30 min
   Perform selected areas of curettage as needed
   Polish selected teeth (if curettage is contraindicated) and apply fluoride
   Place on recall or refer for dental treatment
SCHEDULE: 50 min (4 units)

Appointment 5 (if needed)
1. Remove periodontal pack — 5 min
2. Polish selected teeth — 15 min
3. Apply fluoride — 5 min
4. Place on recall or refer for dental treatment — 2 min
SCHEDULE: 27 min (2 units)

*Each unit = 15 minutes.

Table 18-3. Case 2

Assessment tool	Significant findings	Problem or goal	Indicated course of action	Priority	Sequence in care	Time needed
Medical history	Leukemia	Avoid adding to medical problem	Treat during period of remission Seek physician consult and recommended procedures	A	—	—
Review of systems	Blood dyscrasia due to leukemia	Same as above	Same as above	—	—	—
Vital signs	120/84 ras Pulse: 80			—	—	—
Dental history	Pattern of numerous restorations at each visit (4 per year) Currently working with dietician	Reduce caries rate	Identify ways to improve diet—consult with physician and dietician	B	1	30 min
Extraoral examination	Palpable lymph nodes (cervical and submandibular) bilaterally	May be related to leukemia	Consult with physician	B	1	—
Intraoral examination	Within normal limits, but mucosa is generally a pale gray-pink			—	—	—
Periodontal examination	Gingivae are pale gray-pink with hemorrhage areas obvious in sulcus (*prior* to probing)	Characteristic of leukemia	Consult with dentist and physician regarding significance	B	2	30 min
		Attempt to improve gingival health and minimize irritation of tissues	Emphasis on daily, gentle removal of irritants	C	2	30 min
			Scale and polish (depending on physician consult)	D	3	30 min
Calculus charting	None	Minimize recurrence of decay		—	—	—
Dental charting	Numerous restorations (32 surfaces) One new area of caries (D No. 30)	Restore area	Refer to dentist Dietary counseling Recommend fluoride rinses	—	—	—
Radiographic charting	Confirms area of caries (D No. 30)	Same as above	Same as above	—	—	—
Guided self-assessment	See soft tissue findings from intraoral and periodontal examinations	Minimize emphasis on systemic causes; emphasize means of improvement	Plaque control	C	2	—

Continued.

Table 18-3. Case 2—cont'd.

Assessment tool	Significant findings	Problem or goal	Indicated course of action	Priority	Sequence in care	Time needed
Plaque index	Plaque on 30% of surfaces	Redo at each appointment	Plaque control	C	2	5 min per appointment
Hemorrhage point index	Omitted due to generalized passive hemorrhage	Decrease plaque Not necessary	Antiplaque agents	—	—	—
Nutritional self-assessment	Frequent intake of sweets	—		—	—	—
			Nutritional counseling	—	—	—
Patient's expressed wants, needs, and expectations	Dental care becoming an increasingly lower health priority	Keep at least minimal oral health habits easy and attractive as a routine	Keep simple	—	—	—

Appointment plan

Before appointment: Consult with physician, dentist, and dietician   30 min (or more as needed)

Appointment 1 (postassessment)
1. Plaque control and dietary counseling, fluoride usage   30 min
2. Oral prophylaxis (scale, polish as needed)   30 min

SCHEDULE: 60 min (4 units)

Appointment 2
1. Plaque index: review plaque control   15 min
2. Review dietary counseling (3-day diet)   15 min
3. Refer for restorative care

SCHEDULE: 30 min (2 units)

Table 18-4. Case 3

Assessment tool	Significant findings	Problem or goal	Indicated course of action	Priority	Sequence in care	Time needed
Medical history	Rheumatic fever at age 10	Possible subacute bacterial endocarditis from dental care	Prophylactic premedication	A	1	Delay in appointment
Review of systems	Cardiovascular: rheumatic heart; valve damage	Same as above	Same as above	—	—	—
Vital signs	124/82, ras Pulse: 90	—	—	—	—	—
Dental history	Complains of halitosis and bleeding and painful gums	ANUG	Debride and use antibiotic therapy Begin plaque control and nutritional education	B	2	1 hr
Extraoral examination	Within normal limits except for palpable submandibular lymph nodes	—	Consult with physician regarding nodes	A	1	—
Intraoral examination	Halitosis	Improve oral hygiene	Begin plaque control	C	3	30 min
Periodontal examination	Pain with probing; cratered interdental papillae; white membranelike appearance on gingivae; generally red and enlarged (probable ANUG)	Normal gingivae; reduce pain and debris	Use ultrasonic scaler for initial debridement; subsequent fine scaling and root planing	D	4	2 hr
			Refer for periodontal consult regarding gingival form	E	5	15 min
Calculus charting	Moderate amounts of supragingival and subgingival deposits	Debride	Ultrasonic and hand scaling	—	—	—
Dental charting	Caries-free	Maintain	—	—	—	—
Radiographic charting	Minor loss of crestal bone height	Stop loss of bone	Refer for periodontal consult regarding gingival and bone form	—	—	—
Guided self-assessment	Red hemorrhagic gingivae Halifosis, foul taste Sound teeth	Improve soft tissue; maintain teeth	Plaque control Antiplaque agents	—	—	—
Plaque index	Large amounts of visible plaque	Reduce plaque	Plaque control	—	—	—
Hemorrhage point index	Generalized bleeding	Improve gingival condition	Plaque control	—	—	—

Continued.

Table 18-4. Case 3 —cont'd.

Assessment tool	Significant findings	Problem or goal	Indicated course of action	Priority	Sequence in care	Time needed
Nutritional self-assessment	Total lack of green vegetables; minimal fruit and yellow vegetables; other groups adequate	Secure vitamins and minerals from missing foods	Dietary counseling; evaluate at each visit	F	6	30 min
Patient's expressed wants, needs, and expectations	Eliminate bad breath / Stop gums from bleeding	—	Same as above	—	—	—

Appointment plan

Appointment 1*

1. Periodontal evaluation — 15 min
2. Ultrasonically scale entire dentition — 60 min
3. Begin plaque control and dietary counseling; introduce antiplaque agent — 30 min

SCHEDULE: 105 min (7 units)

Appointment 2

1. Review plaque control and dietary modifications — 15 min
2. Scale and root plane mandible — 45 min

SCHEDULE: 60 min (4 units)

Appointment 3

1. Review plaque control and dietary modifications — 15 min
2. Scale and root plane maxilla — 45 min
3. Polish entire dentition — 15 min
4. Repeat periodontal evaluation and arrange periodontal consult — 15 min

SCHEDULE: 90 min (6 units)

*At the initial visit no procedures that could induce a bacteremia were performed. Antibiotic premedication was initiated after consultation with the physician. The patient returned for the periodontal examination, at which time relevant data were added and treatment as outlined commenced.

Table 18-5. Case 4

Assessment tool	Significant findings	Problem or goal	Indicated course of action	Priority	Sequence in care	Time needed
Medical history	Age: 48 yrs Squamous cell carcinoma—hard palate and maxillary alveolus and sinus; chemotherapy and radiation	Watch for recurrence; help patient adjust; prevent secondary oral complications	Modify treatment; focus care to respond to this development and its ramifications	A	2	—
Review of systems	Receiving chemotherapy and radiation therapy Low platelet count due to bone marrow suppression	Possible secondary complications Possible clotting delay	Monitor oral conditions at each appointment; frequent recall Consult with physician re platelet count	—	—	—
Vital signs	128/84 (ras) Pulse: 78	—	—	—	—	—
Dental history	Minimal caries or evidence of periodontal disease Regular visits	Maintain at least historical level of oral health	Compare current with historical status	B	1	15 min
Extraoral examination	Skin on right side of face is red and dry Slight loss of symmetry—right side	Proper care of skin during radiation therapy	Consult with dentist or physician regarding skin preparation recommendations; reinforce instructions for use	D	1	5 min
Intraoral examination	Obturator replaces right side of palate and portion of maxilla Minimal saliva; tongue and mucosa abnormally dry and irritated	Maintain cleanliness of prosthesis and supporting structures Improve oral lubrication and cleansing	Work with patient to establish a routine for oral self-care, with special aids as needed Consult dentist or physician regarding saliva substitute or other measures to reduce dryness	B	1	15-20 min
Periodontal examination	Gingivae are red and tender; general inflammation and presence of irritants	Restore periodontal health and adjust oral care	Dental health education and initial periodontal treatment	D	3	30 min
Calculus charting	Moderate generalized supra- and subgingival deposits; recently formed	Restore periodontal health Enable patient to resume or adjust oral health maintenance	Scale and polish; selective root planing and curettage (*requires consult with physician, dentist given low platelet count*)	E	5	60 min

Continued.

Table 18-5. Case 4—cont'd.

Assessment tool	Significant findings	Problem or goal	Indicated course of action	Priority	Sequence in care	Time needed
Dental charting	Nos. 2, 3, and 4 replaced by obturator Clinical evidence of 10 areas of new or recurrent caries Numerous areas of decalcification, especially near cervical portion of crowns	Recalcify new areas of incipient caries Ensure that caries requiring restoration are treated	Institute fluoride therapy program Alert dentist to evidence of caries	C	4	15 min
Radiographic charting	None currently; complete set is 3 years old	—	Consult dentist and physician regarding need for exposure of diagnostic films	C	2	5 min
Guided self-assessment	Inadequate care of obturator and teeth Decreased mouth moisture and oral hygiene frequency Painful mucosa	Better self-care Increased oral moisture	Involve patient in plans for better oral self-care and procedures for improving moisture	D	3	—
Plaque index	Plaque on 70% of surfaces	Improved gingival health	Plaque control	D	3	—
Hemorrhage point index	15 areas of spontaneous hemorrhage	Improved gingival health	Plaque control	D	3	—
Nutritional self-assessment	Diminished taste; chews sugared lemon drops; eats small amounts of food frequently; loss of appetite; eats soft foods Working with dietician	Minimize sugar intake; continue good dietary habits	Substitute noncariogenic saliva stimulant Consult with dietician Reinforce good habits	C D C	4 3 4	15 min —
Patient's expressed wants, needs, and expectations	Afraid a new lesion will develop; dislikes having a prosthesis and does not like to look at it or postsurgical area	Reduced fear; acceptance of early detection procedures and self-care	Review oral cancer self-exam Show acceptance of patient's state Supportive watchfulness and acceptance	A	3	10 min

Table 18-5. Case 4—cont'd.

Assessment tool	Significant findings	Problem or goal	Indicated course of action	Priority	Sequence in care	Time needed

Appointment plan

Before appointment: Consult with dentist, physician, dietician, and psychologist; compare previous status with current and modify treatment as needed — 30 min (or more as needed); 15 min

SCHEDULE: 45 min (3 units)

Appointment 1 (postassessment)
1. Review of self-care and plaque control; recommend lemon drop substitute — 30 min
2. Review oral cancer self-exam and care of appliance — 10 min
3. Begin fluoride therapy — 15 min
4. Scale (and polish) one quadrant — 15 min

SCHEDULE: 90 min (6 units)

Appointment 2
1. Reassess oral self-care and reinforce plaque control and fluoride regimen — 10 min
2. Scale and polish remaining teeth — 40 min
3. Reinforce nutritional changes — 10 min

SCHEDULE: 60 min (4 units)

Appointment 3
1. Reassess oral self-care, soft tissue health, plaque control, dietary habits, and use of fluorides — 15 min
2. Evaluate for further instrumentation — 15 min
Recall: 2 months (or less depending on recommendations of dentist or physician and on patient's desire to be seen more frequently)

SCHEDULE: 30 min (2 units)

clinical practice settings, or in educational programs, the use of the term *treatment planning* may raise concern among some persons that such a role is "beyond the scope" of the dental hygienist. Most licensing jurisdictions specifically reserve treatment planning and diagnosis for the dentist.

However, many dental hygienists arrange appointment sequencing and scheduling specifically for the dental hygiene care to be provided. For this to be done, assessment data must be gathered and translated into a meaningful summary and conclusions forming a *dental hygiene* diagnosis.

Generally, the dental hygienist prepares this initial synthesis and then discusses and confirms findings requiring a *dental diagnosis* with the dentist responsible for the overall dental needs of the patient. The dentist makes the dental diagnosis and the patient is informed of the results of the assessment. The keys to remaining within the law and to building and maintaining a cooperative team relationship with the dentist are (1) to perform thorough, reliable assessment, (2) to draw preliminary conclusions from the data, (3) to use the dentist as a resource and arbiter of decisions regarding the patient's status and proper treatment, and (4) to follow through with high-quality dental hygiene care, providing status reports for the dentist as the case progresses and ensuring that the patient receives follow-up care related to the dental diagnosis.

In this way the dental hygienist's understanding of basic, behavioral, and dental sciences can be used and expanded with each case while the hygienist remains within the bounds of professional responsibility and maintains an interdependent relationship with the dentist. Maintaining this balance is critical, as the patient's well-being and the profession's credibility depend on it.

ACTIVITIES

1. Assemble assessment data from clinic patients who are receiving care from advanced dental hygiene students. Complete a treatment planning worksheet for three or more patients. Share your worksheets and appointment plans in groups of four or five, and develop composite plans, which then can be shared with the entire class.
2. Role play case presentations derived from the plans generated in the preceding activity. A "dental hygienist" should present the case to a "patient" while

a third student serves as an observer, watching for the elements of informed consent and the presence of sensitivity to the patient's wants, needs, and expectations. Rotate roles to give each student the opportunity to be an observer, patient, and dental hygienist.

3. Read Miller's: "Dental Hygiene Diagnosis" RDH 2(4):46, 1982. As individuals and then as a class, define dental hygiene diagnosis and develop a preliminary diagnostic nomenclature.

REVIEW QUESTIONS

1. What six elements must be included in a case presentation to meet the requirements for informed consent?
2. If a procedure is performed for a patient to which the patient did not give consent, the clinician may be charged with _____.
3. What is a critical reason for integrating the patient's wants, needs, and expectations in the treatment plan?
4. The first priority in the sequence of care is treatment to meet any _____ needs of the patient.
5. How can a dental hygienist function responsibly and legally as part of the dental team when performing treatment planning for dental hygiene care?

REFERENCES

Barsh, LI: Dental treatment planning for the adult patient. Philadelphia, 1981, WB Saunders Co.

Clark JD, and Morton JC: Behavioral assessment: an appraisal of beliefs and behaviors relating to treatment, Dent Clin North Am 21:515, 1977.

Cohen DW: Preventive periodontics, J Indian Dent Assoc (Special Issue), p. 273, 1975.

Fechtner JL: Treatment planning, Dent Clin North Am 22:219, 1978.

Fishman SR and Ortiz E Jr: Effective case presentation, Dent Clin North Am 21:539, 1977.

Goldberg, HJ, Plume M, and Nacman, M: The importance of attitude in the delivery of health services, J Public Health Dent 33:35, 1973.

Kagan AR, and Miles JW: Head and neck oncology: controversies in cancer treatment. Boston, 1981, GK Hall & Co.

Keltner JW: Elements of interpersonal communication. Belmont, Calif, 1973, Wadsworth Publishing Co.

Lynch MA: Burket's oral medicine. Philadelphia, 1977, JB Lippincott Co.

Miller SL: Legal aspects of dentistry. New York, 1979, GP Putnam's Sons.

Miller, SS: Dental hygiene diagnosis. RHD 2(4):46, 1982.

Morris RB: Principles of dental treatment planning. Philadelphia, 1983, Lea & Febiger.

Rose L, and Kaye, D: Internal medicine for dentistry. St. Louis, 1983, The CV Mosby Co.

Rosoff A: Informed consent. Rockville, Md., 1981, Aspen Systems Corp.

Wang, CC: Radiation therapy for head and neck neoplasms: Boston, 1983, John Wright/PSG, Inc.

Wood K: Treatment planning: a pragmatic approach. St. Louis, 1978, The CV Mosby Co.

19 CONTROLLING DENTAL DISEASE

OBJECTIVES: *The reader will be able to*

1. Explain the importance of dental health education as a function of the dental hygienist.
2. List at least five prevention topics that should be included in dental health education in a dental practice or a community health setting.
3. Apply the model of assessment, planning, implementation, and evaluation to dental health education.
4. Individualize prevention programs for a variety of patient needs.
5. Critique prevention programs for the following qualities:
    a. Appropriateness to patient needs
    b. Completeness
    c. Attention to strategies for modifying behavior
    d. Timing and pace of learning
    e. Involvement of the learner
    f. Scope and method of evaluation of success
6. Describe implements used for mechanical control of bacterial plaque, including toothbrushes, floss, stimulators, and other aids.
7. Describe the role of the irrigator in disrupting plaque.
8. Review the characteristics of several prescription agents that can be used to control pathogenic microflora, including metronidazole, tetracyline, stannous fluoride, and chlorhexidine.
9. Review the characteristics of several over-the-counter agents available for the chemical control of microbial plaque, including essential oils, sanguinaria, cetylpyridinium chloride, and surfactants.

If you ask the person on the street what a dental hygienist does, the typical answer will be: "She's the person at the dental office who cleans my teeth." With a little probing, the person will add that the hygienist advises flossing and some different way of brushing, and that there is a lot of discussion about plaque and its evils.

There is no question that subgingival instrumentation is a very important part of treating and preventing disease. It disrupts the microbes that inhabit the periodontal pocket, retarding their ability to infect and inflame tissues and initiate the destruction of the periodontal attachment structures. It removes hard deposits that trap bacterial plaque, and it makes the patient "feel good" to have clean teeth and a fresh start.

But no matter how effective the oral prophylaxis may be in setting back a disease trend, the aspect of dental hygiene care that is most important in controlling and preventing disease is the ability of the dental hygienist to move each patient into a daily routine of good oral hygiene, so that plaque is disrupted supra- and subgingivally and thus does not have an opportunity to proliferate and cause disease. Having outstanding instrumentation skills is important for a hygienist, but in the long run being an outstanding patient educator undoubtedly contributes more.

Patients who have their teeth cleaned every 6 months often end up in the periodontist's office with deep pockets, a diagnosis of periodontitis, and a prescription for corrective surgery. At this point, the patient is introduced to meticulous oral hygiene. The dental hygienist who stops short of introducing that meticulous care while the patient is healthy is practicing supervised neglect (Dunbar, 1976). The patient is lulled into a false sense of security, believing that twice-yearly visits ensure that disease will not strike.

Hygienists who carefully assess each patient's individual needs and then develop a preventive program for each person know that improving a patient's habits is the most challenging part of dental hygiene practice. People change slowly and sometimes not at all. Preventive programs require good planning, persistence, frequent follow-up, a wide array of reinforcement, and interpersonal skills. With many patients, the instrumentation procedures are relatively easy compared with the effort required to launch a workable, effective program of disease prevention.

Although dental health education is addressed in this chapter primarily in terms of working with individual patients, the principles given here also apply in large part to working with groups of people. Even those hygienists who vow to work on a one-to-one basis with patients rather than as community hygienists will have opportunities for working with school groups, senior citizens, birthing classes, patients with special needs, and others. The content of the teaching often is the same. So is the need to focus on the specific needs and characteristics of the persons involved and to evaluate the success of the program.

PREVENTION TOPICS

Plaque control is the most critical aspect of prevention in the control of caries and periodontal disease; thus it will receive the most attention here. Several other topics, however, are of major importance in a prevention program.

The importance of fluoride in controlling caries is a topic that should head the dental health education agenda for persons who (1) have a caries problem, (2) belong to a caries-prone family, (3) are entering caries-prone years, (4) are pregnant or will soon have a new child in the family, or (5) are voters who may someday consider a fluoride referendum in the community. Chapter 28 introduces the importance of fluoride in prevention, so details will not be discussed here. However, it is important to plan to incorporate fluoride education into any prevention plan.

Identifying changes in the normal structures of the mouth is an additional, essential component of dental health education. It is important for people to know what their oral structures look like and then to monitor those structures at least monthly for changes in color, shape, size, tenderness, and tendency toward bleeding. This monitoring includes inspecting the gingival tissues for a tendency toward periodontal problems. It goes beyond the gingivae to include buccal mucosa, tongue, lips, soft palate, alveolar bone, floor of the mouth, and other structures. The oral cancer self-exam is described in Chapter 10. These procedures are especially critical for adults who smoke or chew tobacco, consume alcohol, or have personal or family histories of cancer.

Nutritional education is receiving more attention in dentistry as the public emphasis on fitness and personal responsibility for general health rises. The link between diet and cardiovascular disease and cancer is becoming clearer, and medicine is taking nutritional education more seriously. Dentistry is shifting its emphasis from a narrow discussion of sugar consumption to an understanding that a visit to the dentist may be the ideal time to discuss nutrition and diet from the standpoint of general health and oral health. Chapter 20 provides more detail and strategies on this topic.

Need for specialized dental care is often a health education topic that falls within the purview of a dental hygienist. Patients may have missing teeth, malocclusion, faulty or aged dental work, cosmetic problems, or other dental conditions that will require a dentist's attention. The hygienist can identify conditions that require dental diagnosis and discuss how they affect dental and general health and appearance. The hygienist discusses the fundamentals of the procedures used to correct the problems and provides information about new options for treatment. This area of education is frequently employed after a dental consultation. A dental diagnosis has been provided and procedures recommended; the hygienist then discusses the plan with the patient and addresses questions that may not have been raised in the consultation with the dentist. Some dentists rely upon their hygienists to present proposed treatment plans; others recognize the role of the hygienist in ferreting out patients' reservations and questions about procedures after the dentist has presented the plan to the patient. In any case, providing this kind of information is an important part of dental health education.

INDIVIDUALIZING DENTAL HEALTH EDUCATION

Designing a dental prevention program starts with a careful *assessment* of the patient's needs. This phase of care is based upon the results of the medical and dental history, the intraoral and extraoral examinations, dental radiographs, plaque and gingival indices, and a discussion of the patient's perceived needs and concerns. Using assessment data to plan dental health education makes it less likely that an automated approach to prevention will be followed.

It is easy to fall into the habit of teaching brushing and flossing and imploring the patient to follow those procedures. Brushing, flossing, and motivation are frequently the topics of a plaque control program, but they are not the sum total of prevention. Furthermore, if you follow this automated approach, patients will probably withdraw from the discussion in amazement at the efficiency with which you give instructions, without attending to the fact that they already know, appreciate, and even follow much of the information.

Imagine that you are visiting a dental hygienist who does not know or forgets that you are a dental hygienist. Just before the instrumentation procedures, the hygienist pulls out a new brush, demonstrates the proper methods of brushing, and then goes on to show you how to floss. There you sit, already fully cognizant of these facts. Similarly, many people, even though they are not dental professionals, have memorized brushing and flossing instructions over a long series of dental visits. More important issues, such as slight texture changes in the buccal mucosa, a problem with canker sores, or a nasty crossbite, may go undiscussed.

If the patient has been involved in the assessment procedures, following your moves with a hand mirror and attending to your explanation of each procedure and each finding, the assessment will provide the clues necessary for developing a prevention program. You will be designing that program with the patient during the assessment

phase. For example, after showing the patient his or her crossbite and comparing the position of the teeth to those shown on a typodont or study models, the hygienist can suggest, "We probably ought to discuss the ramifications of having that crossbite, how it affects your dental health. How about if we include that as a topic at our next visit?"Or the patient may want to know about it now, so the hygienist may briefly describe its importance during the assessment of occlusion and make a note to mention it again during subsequent visits.

Fig. 19-1 provides a sample case that is typical of patients frequently encountered in dental practice. Mr. Johnson has restorative problems, periodontal problems, a smoking habit, esthetic problems, and soft tissue changes. He uses an outmoded brushing technique, is sporadic with flossing, and seems unaware of most of his oral conditions. If examination procedures involve the patient, awareness should increase and attitudes should become apparent as the hygienist and the patient discuss each finding and as the patient reveals his attitudes and beliefs. Plaque control will be an important focus of the health education for this patient, but several other topics deserve discussion and inclusion in a health education plan.

Once the assessment data have been gathered, it is time to *plan the goals, steps, priorities, and time* for each component of the prevention program. (See Chapter 18 for a discussion of treatment planning.) Briefly, the best procedure is to list your assessment findings, specify prevention goals and their importance related to each finding, and decide which can and should be handled in what sequence during the provision of dental hygiene care.

Referring to Mr. Johnson's assessment data, what might be appropriate goals for his care? Fig. 19-2 lists several goals for each of his observed conditions. Related to each are action and instruction statements that translate the goals into concrete procedures designed to help achieve those goals. Each goal is given a priority and a sequence; these are then translated into an appointment plan (Fig. 19-3).

Typically, prevention is integrated with other phases of dental hygiene care. At the initial session, the first phases of prevention are introduced; at subsequent appointments, instrumentation pro-

---

Dental health education—home care assessment

DATE: 10/10/88

PATIENT: Mr. John Johnson is a new patient who has not had regular dental care for the past 3 years. Age: 34.

CHIEF COMPLAINT: "Painful back tooth"

CLINICAL FINDINGS:

1. *General:* Tooth No. 30 has a fractured amalgam. Teeth are lightly tobacco stained. Moderate calculus is obvious supragingivally in the mandibular lingual anterior area. Mandibular lingual gingiva in the posterior area appears red and edematous, especially in the interdental areas. Tongue is coated and stained.

2. *Periodontal survey:*
    a. Pocket depth: Highest readings (4 mm) ML and DL of Nos. 18 and 19, also Nos. 28 to 31.

Pocket depth	3					2						3				
Tooth number	1	2	3	4	5	6	7	8	9	10	11	12	13	14	15	16
Bleeding points			X												X	
Bleeding points	X	X		X		X	X		X					X	X	
Tooth number	32	31	30	29	28	27	26	25	24	23	22	21	20	19	18	17
Pocket depth	4					3						4				

    b. Bleeding index: 10 (signified by X)
    c. Plaque index: 48 areas of visible plaque
    d. Problem areas: Interproximal areas: mandibular lingual, posterior and anterior

HOME CARE: Combination roll stroke and scrub brush method. Completes maxillary teeth, then mandibular teeth; does not brush mandibular lingual or tongue. Demonstrates acceptable technique for flossing except in area of the most posterior molars. Brushes twice a day to "keep teeth clean and stop bad breath." Flosses occasionally "because food gets caught sometimes."

AWARENESS: Patient does not worry about gum disease. He believes his teeth will take care of themselves because he's generally a healthy person. Has had few problems in the past. He is unaware of dental plaque and does not know the purpose of a disclosing agent. He cannot remember ever being shown how to clean his teeth.

Fig. 19-1. Sample case on home care assessment.

cedures are integrated as needed with reinforcement of oral hygiene and modification or addition of procedures. To avoid overloading the patient, you can add oral hygiene information in small increments at these subsequent visits.

Most clinicians recommend that dental hygiene education precede any dental care (other than emergency care) to emphasize that the patient can make an observable difference in oral conditions just by instituting changes in the oral hygiene routine. Extensive dental care, including restorative reconstruction such as extensive crown and bridgework, orthodontic care, and periodontal surgery are scheduled after the patient has learned

---

SAMPLE CASE

Dental health education—planning needs and goals

DATE: 10/12/88

PATIENT: Mr. John Johnson

GOALS OF PREVENTIVE EDUCATION

1. Halt current progress of periodontal disease and prevent its recurrence
   a. Describe the nature and source of the disease
   b. Identify several oral hygiene procedures to prevent disease establishment and progress
   c. Correctly demonstrate those procedures
   d. Select an antiplaque rinse for daily use
   e. Integrate procedures into a daily routine
   f. Recognize the signs of the disease in his own mouth
   g. Look for signs of disease recurrence
   h. Report signs of recurrence to the dentist and hygienist
   i. Keep appointments for removal of hard deposits and root planing
   j. Schedule and keep appointment for recall/follow-up visits
2. Reduce or stop tobacco use
   a. Recognize the effects of smoking on his teeth and mucosa
   b. Decide on the relative importance of the perceived benefits of smoking and the need to halt soft tissue changes
   c. Investigate and participate in a smoking cessation program
   d. Cite the health problems associated with other forms of tobacco
3. Reduce the risk of root caries
   a. Recognize the signs of recession in his mouth
   b. Identify the causes of recession
   c. Alter his oral hygiene procedures to minimize recession while cleaning exposed areas adequately
   d. Review the role of fluoride in caries inhibition
   e. Add a fluoride topical supplement (such as low concentration oral rinse or gel) to his daily routine

TREATMENT: Temporize # 30. Scale and root plane. Soft tissue curettage as needed.

PREVENTION: *Instruction*—Discuss plaque, inflammation, progression of periodontal disease. Discuss the effects of smoking upon soft tissue health and upon appearance of the teeth and tongue. Discuss recession and the potential for root caries; the role of fluoride in inhibiting caries; and the importance of the planned treatment and patient participation in reversing and controlling the disease. *Action*—Show the patient the inflammation and bleeding, the tissue changes in the buccal mucosa, and the stain on the teeth and tongue. Disclose the plaque. Show the patient the gingival recession. Show the patient how to look for changes in the gingiva and other oral structures. Ask the patient to demonstrate brushing and flossing; correct the method as necessary. Introduce antiplaque rinses and an additional source of low concentration fluoride.

MOTIVATIONAL APPROACH: Capitalize on the "straight facts"—establishment of good habits to enhance appearance and sociability and to maintain health. Stress prevention of problems as an alternative to ignoring beginning signs and allowing disease to progress. Emphasize patient's decision-making power; provide information to help guide those decisions. Reinforce each small step that indicates patient's acceptance of responsibility and movement toward health. Avoid judging the patient's reluctance to change or his slow progress.

Fig. 19-2. Sample case on planning needs and goals.

SAMPLE CASE

Dental health education — implementation

PATIENT: Mr. John Johnson

Appointment 1
1. Present preventive oral hygiene plan; agree on goals
2. Temporize No. 30 (dentist)
3. Complete guided self-assessment
4. Identify signs of inflammation
5. Explain etiology of inflammatory disease and periodontitis
6. Show patient signs of tissue change on buccal mucosa and stain on tongue and teeth; discuss cause
7. Show patient gingival recession; discuss cause
8. Take pretreatment photographs
9. Ask patient to disclose and identify plaque
10. Discuss patient's usual oral hygiene routine
11. Ask patient to demonstrate current brushing routine
12. Modify brushing routine as necessary to remove plaque and minimize gingival recession problems
13. Suggest an antiplaque agent; ask the patient to use it, evaluating patient response to taste, etc.
14. Discuss what will occur at the next appointment
ESTIMATED TIME NEEDED: 60 minutes

Appointment 2
1. Check tissue color, texture, shape, and bleeding with chartings from previous week and with slides from last visit; share observed changes with the patient
2. Reinforce oral hygiene efforts
3. Ask patient to brush, using technique followed since last visit; disclose and ask patient to identify areas missed
4. Inquire about use of suggested antiplaque agent and fluoride rinse; encourage their use or suggest alternative
5. Ask patient to demonstrate flossing (if he claims knowledge) or introduce its use; improve the technique and add helpful devices such as a floss holder or threader
6. Ask the patient about past efforts to stop smoking; express concern regarding early signs of soft tissue changes in buccal mucosa
7. Scale and root plane a sextant or quadrant
ESTIMATED TIME NEEDED: 90 minutes

Appointment 3
1. Evaluate periodontal tissue and buccal mucosa and tongue
2. Ask patient to brush and floss; disclose plaque and ask patient to look for areas missed
3. Modify brushing and flossing as necessary
4. Inquire about use of antiplaque rinse and fluoride rinse; reinforce their use
5. Teach patient the oral cancer self-examination; explain policy of calling when any change is observed
6. Inquire regarding the patient's willingness to stop smoking
7. Recommend available smoking cessation programs
8. Scale and plane additional sextant or quadrant
ESTIMATED TIME NEEDED: 60 minutes

Appointment 4
1. Evaluate periodontal tissue and buccal mucosa; point out changes in soft tissue for the patient's evaluation and compare instrumented segments with others
2. Ask patient to brush and floss; disclose plaque and ask patient to identify areas missed

Fig. 19-3. Sample case on implementation.

SAMPLE CASE

Dental health education—implementation—cont'd

3. Reinforce good oral hygiene procedures; modify procedures as necessary; introduce other aids, such as supragingival irrigation, perio-aid, and yarn, to enhance efforts
4. Encourage use of rinses as recommended
5. Inquire about intentions to cease smoking
6. Scale and root plane sextant or quadrant

ESTIMATED TIME NEEDED: 60 minutes

Subsequent treatment appointments
1. Reinforce oral hygiene
2. Reinforce efforts to cease smoking
3. Monitor soft tissue health
4. Scale and plane sextants or quadrants as appropriate until completed
5. Photograph dentition and oral tissues during progress of treatment
6. Encourage patient to evaluate his progress

ESTIMATED TIME NEEDED: From 15 to 60 minutes

One-month recall appointment
1. Evaluate soft tissue health; ask patient to evaluate it
2. Ask patient to demonstrate oral hygiene procedures
3. Disclose plaque and ask patient to identify areas missed
4. Inquire about continued use of oral rinses
5. Refer for other restorative needs
6. Replane areas needing instrumentation; curette areas that indicate inadequate tissue response
7. Polish teeth as necessary to improve esthetics; photograph
8. Provide topical fluoride treatment
9. Schedule a 3-month recall appointment

ESTIMATED TIME NEEDED: 60 minutes

Fig. 19-3, cont'd. Sample case on implementation.

---

good oral hygiene procedures and has plaque and soft tissue health under control. These dental procedures will typically fail if the patient is not faithfully following a good oral hygiene program. Caries will recur around the margins of restorations, or supporting bone necessary to maintain a fixed prosthesis will be lost; areas next to orthodontic bonds or bands will decalcify, resulting in caries or an unesthetic result; periodontal pockets will recur. Many dentists will not attempt extensive procedures until the patient follows recommended procedures.

Changing habits, particularly well-established ones, is extremely difficult, as any smoker who has tried to quit can testify. For the educational process to succeed, the learner must demonstrate a change in behavior. To do this, the learner moves through several stages as the commitment to a new behavior is established. These stages are awareness, interest, involvement, action, and fi-

nally habit (Katz, McDonald, and Stookey, 1979).

The preventive educator is a partner in this entire process. Too often, the educator feels that after the initial instruction the remainder of the work is the patient's responsibility. In actuality, the educator's role is only beginning. The individualized approach in a plaque control program characterized by frequent assessment, planning, implementation, and evaluation strategies helps keep the continuing process of communication and education between the patient and the clinician vital, meaningful, and progressive.

When the plan has been determined, it should be shared with the patient. Are the goals acceptable? What goals does the patient have? Is the patient committed to the plan? The patient who has an investment in the preventive program usually offers maximal cooperation. Following are four accepted steps to keep in mind during planning

---

SAMPLE CASE
Dental health education—evaluation summary

DATE: 12/10/88
PATIENT: Mr. John Johnson

Mr. Johnson came for dental treatment 10/10/88 with a broken filling. He was unaware of the potential for severe periodontal disease according to the inflammatory condition of his gingival tissue. Assessment data were obtained and shared with the patient. He agreed to begin a preventive education program.

Although a bit reserved at first, the patient was interested in maintaining his "independence" with good oral health. He responded well to facts about the progression of dental disease, and motivation appeals were directed at his ability to understand and control his own dental conditions. The patient is well coordinated and picked up technique suggestions easily.

During the past 2 months, the patient has reduced his plaque index to the goal level. The bleeding index came close to the goal level, but malposed teeth continue to be a problem (Nos. 22 to 25). The patient recognizes signs of inflammation, readily identifies plaque, and can describe the process of dental disease. Mr. Johnson has practiced home care techniques and reports being much more regular about flossing. He never misses brushing the lingual surfaces any more. Overall, the goals of this initial phase of preventive dental health education were accomplished. The 3-month recall will be important for evaluating maintenance of health.

Fig. 19-4. Sample case on evaluation summary.

(Katz, McDonald, and Stookey, 1979; Pipe et al, 1972):

1. *Small step size.* Provide the theoretical or factual information in increments that the patient can digest at points when the patient has expressed a *need* to know.
2. *Active participation.* Involve the patient in an activity that will enhance the learning and retention of the information.
3. *Immediate feedback.* Let the learner know the evaluation of his or her participation and progress. Positive feedback is supportive and encouraging.
4. *Self-pacing.* Stay in tune with the learner's needs. If the learner cannot or will not handle more information, do not push. If interest is being shown, pursue the patient's signals.

Once dental health education is planned, it is *implemented* using up-to-date, research-based information. The content of the message is of course an essential part of education. Intertwined with the content is the style of the message—the motivational component. This component provides the reinforcement, the encouragement, the support, the challenge, the need for change. Impeccable content will fall on deaf ears if the style of the message is lackluster, negative, demanding, demeaning, overzealous, judgmental, or frightening. Strategies for both information content and sound style are discussed later in this chapter.

At each step in a patient's care, the patient's progress in carrying out good oral hygiene should be evaluated. *Evaluation* means determining whether or not your educational program is working. It is the bottom line of success. As any teacher knows, just because the teacher teaches doesn't mean the student learns. This is certainly true in teaching dental health. Typically, health education programs for individuals or groups succeed or fail because of the second component of the message—the style. But regardless of the reasons for the outcome, the hygienist must evaluate progress, determine what is missing in the message, and try again to (1) help the patient understand his or her needs as the clinician sees them, (2) identify and remove roadblocks to implementing specific procedures, and (3) delineate markers for the patient to see progress (see Fig. 19-4).

Philosophy of prevention

Typically, dental health education is a continuing circuit through the phases of assessment, planning, implementation, and evaluation. The hygienist and the patient improve with each circuit as long as they work together to identify progress and further needs.

Fortunately, today's general population is more attuned to self-care and responsibility for health than was the case several years ago. A trend toward greater health consciousness is seen in the emphasis upon exercise and diet. People are more willing to play a role in maintaining health and to ask questions about proposed treatment. Commercial advertisers have been educating the public about plaque, calculus, and periodontal disease. Therefore, it is easier to capture a patient's attention with a message about home care than it was 10 or 20 years ago. The message is taken more seriously, and reinforcement for teaching good oral hygiene to patients is more frequent.

Research is showing that good oral hygiene can prevent or control dental disease, which makes it easier to specify procedures likely to help patients when they follow recommendations. Research into motivational strategies is providing guidance for inducing patients to change and reinforcing their efforts.

Designing and conducting preventive programs with individuals and groups is both a skill and an art. It may be the most important function a hygienist learns and performs. This chapter provides a basis for learning how to teach prevention; it is a springboard for perfecting the art of working with people who could benefit from change.

It is no longer acceptable for a dental office to skip over or minimize dental health education. Education now is seen as a hallmark of a good dental practice and the primary way to ensure that good dental health and quality care are maintained over a lifetime. Omitting prevention education is coming to be considered grounds for malpractice.

Essential to any prevention program is a sincere commitment to a preventive philosophy. Because the clinician selected a caring profession as a career, he or she is likely dedicated to helping others. Some choose to serve by becoming experts in reconstruction or in maintenance; others provide service by researching or teaching the concepts of prevention. Realistically, the latter course has the potential for the greatest effect. Treatment is essential, but it is a losing battle to try to control dental disease by treatment alone.

Embracing a preventive philosophy and practicing it are two entirely different levels of commitment. Each practitioner must identify his or her own commitment.

On a personal level, this means maintaining one's own oral health status. Being a good example will model the benefits of prevention. In a broader sense, much of what makes an oral health educator is seeing it as a primary career role. Often the clinician is defined by the skills dictated by the employment situation. For example, if scaling and polishing teeth are the sole activities of the day, then seeing oneself as a health educator may be difficult. Ideally, the employment situation will allow the clinician to develop a personal approach to home care with each patient. During the day, time should be devoted to assessing oral conditions, providing educational information, and evaluating patients' efforts in addition to performing a variety of clinical services. These circumstances will permit practicing a preventive philosophy in an environment conducive to providing health education.

While remaining committed to a preventive philosophy, the person responsible for preventive education needs to be sensitive to the individuality of each patient. With this comes the realization that a program of prevention must be flexible and individualized to be effective.

Motivational strategies

Although no particular preventive program is proven to be "best," well-designed programs pay particular attention to identifying individual needs. Instructional formats and motivational appeals are selected for their appropriateness in each case, and long-term reinforcement strategies are included. Closely supervised teaching on a multiple-visit basis with periodic reinforcement can result in a significant, sustained improvement in oral hygiene, but there is a tendency for regression in performance over time after the instruction (Melcer and Feldman, 1979). Boyer and Nikias (1983) surveyed 123 randomly selected adult patients who had participated in a plaque control program. Slightly more than a third of the patients were highly compliant in performing prescribed procedures. Another third was moderately compliant, and the remaining third was poorly compliant. Almost all patients had adopted the preventive dental procedures for some length of time. Keeping the patient motivated about oral health over the long term seems to be a key goal in any plaque control program.

Much has been written about Maslow's hierarchy of human needs in relation to motivation (Katz, McDonald, and Stookey 1979; Maslow, 1970; Pipe et al, 1972). A pyramid model is used to represent the levels of human need from the most basic level—the physiologic need for food, shelter, warmth, rest, and reproduction—to the apex of the pyramid, labeled self-actualization. At this highest need level, a person aspires to be personally fulfilled by reaching his or her potential. The intermediate levels are security needs, social needs, and esteem needs. Except under special circumstances, the physiologic and security need levels of the general population in our society are fairly well satisfied.

Maslow proposes that higher-level needs do not emerge until lower-level needs are satisfied; one has little energy to spend on esteem needs if food or shelter needs are not satisfied. He also states that once a need has been satisfied, it no longer continues to be highly valued or to act as a motivating force.

To a person suffering from a toothache or other painful conditions, pain could be interpreted as a threat to the individual's security. The person has a need to be removed from physical peril. Certainly, at this point the need for help occurs, and one becomes desperate to follow the steps necessary to remove the cause of the threat. Often, preventive education takes this opportunity to make its greatest appeal: "Ah-ha. These teeth are loose and causing you discomfort because of severe periodontal disease. This is caused by the accumulation of plaque, calculus, and the resultant bacterial toxins that have irritated and destroyed the ligaments in the supporting tissues which actually hold the tooth in the bone. If this continues, you will lose all your teeth." The patient gasps, "Can you help me?" "Yes, we can do something about this. First I'll show you a new or better way to care for your teeth to help remove the irritants. Then a thorough prophylaxis and possibly a bit of surgery will be done to remove the tissue that is beyond healing and reattachment." The patient's natural response is "Of course anything." The follow-through with home care and the necessary treatment proceed smoothly.

After the "problem" has been resolved, the clinician may continue to motivate the patient by appealing to the security level. "You remember what happened before, don't you?" It seems to be human nature to forget unpleasant or frightening experiences. The memory of the discomfort, time involved, money spent, and inconvenience may not be vivid. Furthermore, the problem was essentially solved by treatment. The patient naturally assumes that treatment could resolve the problem again.

This example shows how effective the appeal to a security need can be as a motivator over a short period of time. It also points out the pitfalls of this appeal as a motivator over a longer term (Pipe et al, 1972). It is difficult to estimate how many patients who were motivated with short-term threats have become edentulous over the years. The hope that dental treatment (even if it is inconvenient and expensive) will save the patient's teeth in the nick of time eventually is proved false.

The two need-level appeals that do have potential as long-term motivators are those directed at social and esteem levels (Pipe et al, 1972). Throughout life a person generally wishes to remain socially acceptable and feel personally valued. A healthy mouth that projects an attractive smile and is free of disease makes anyone feel more comfortable in a social setting. Physical self-care often reflects the way a person values himself or herself. Because social and esteem needs are lifelong, appeals to these levels are more appropriate long-term motivators to be incorporated in the preventive program.

In describing some sociopsychologic perspectives motivating change in oral hygiene behavior, Evans (1978) stresses the need to avoid a situation wherein the patient is dependent on the health professional for the focus of therapy. Motivating the patient to make new oral hygiene behaviors last means fostering long-term self-determination on the patient's part. A "therapeutic alliance" should exist between the patient and the health professional. Direct patient involvement should occur from the outset of treatment. The patient and clinician must work together to prevent dental disease. The professional role is as a reinforcer of the patient's desire to do something good for himself or herself.

After studying several plaque control programs, Weinstein (1982) identified seven common problems in the way preventive programs are structured and managed. The first three are as follows:

1. Plaque control programs begin too early.
2. Plaque control begins without patient readiness.
3. The motivational appeal is often "canned," not personalized.

Each of these problems is related to plaque control programs beginning before a relationship is established with the patient. The patient has the sense of being plugged into a routine that everyone gets. An assessment of the patient's wants and needs has not taken place, so the patient feels that the program is not really designed for his or her dental condition.

Problems 4 through 6 are as follows:

4. The dental staff's assumptions about the patient's nonperformance are often mistaken.
5. Patient's receive feedback too infrequently.
6. Plaque control programs lack adequate follow-up.

These three issues deal with the way the dental staff follows the patient's progress. The dental health educator often fails to consider the effort it takes to establish and maintain a new habit. The clinician should establish and maintain a new habit. The clinician should recognize that lapses in the patient's skill or motivation do not mean the patient does not know how or does not care. It is necessary to provide regular feedback and to review skills without making the patient feel he or she has failed. Changes in oral health habits seldom last more than 6 months. Everyone has difficulty becoming proficient at and sustaining a new behavior. A positive attitude toward the patient's problems with motivation is essential.

The seventh common problem of plaque control programs is that the time spent on them is not financially rewarding. When the practitioner is

faced with the low probability of patient follow-through and a high likelihood of little financial reward for the dental staff's time, preventive activities are minimized or squeezed into treatment. Financial incentives need to be worked into a successful program. The health professional's time is valuable, whether it is spent observing a home care technique or placing a fluoride tray. The issue is complicated by third-party payers who refuse to promote such preventive programs and by patients who are reluctant to pay for counseling time they feel is not a helpful personal service. By waiting for an indication from the patient that he or she desires to improve his or her oral health status, the clinician can be more assured that the patient is ready to assume both the time and cost of a customized preventive program.

Of course, many aspects of patient education will never be paid for directly. Helpful advice the clinician provides during contact with the patient is a natural part of oral health care. All patients should be exposed to the opportunity to learn about good home care practices during the course of dental care regardless of entry into a specific plan of preventive visits.

A plaque control program that avoids some of the previously mentioned problems combines humanistic application of behavioral strategies in oral hygiene instruction. In such a program the clinician is a skilled listener and provides information in line with the patient's concern for preventive education. When the patient expresses a desire to do something about the dental problem, the clinician is ready to assess the patient's skills and suggest changes. The patient becomes involved by collecting data at home about the new skill. The clinician and patient set goals together and decide on techniques that patient can use to cue the new behavior. This could include such things as making a chart to place on the bathroom mirror, carrying dental floss in the lunch bag, or deciding to perform brushing and flossing at a particular time. Perhaps completing the oral hygiene routine *before* the usual morning shower will assure its place in the day more than if the routine is left to be done "if time permits." These kinds of steps will act as reminders to sustain the new skill long enough for the patient to see a positive change occurring. A written contract can be made, with the patient to set the goals and time to be devoted to the program effort.

Habit formation is reviewed after about 2 weeks to make any modifications and provide positive feedback. The program ends with the patient and clinician planning how to avoid "back-sliding" on the new behavior. The dental professional facilitates the patient's behavior change. The patient remains responsible for establishing better home care that will influence future dental needs.

In another conceptual model for patient motivation and education, Bakdash (1979) emphasizes the assessment of the patient's incoming behavior. Taking time to identify the patient's perceptions of his or her dental problems and recognizing the emotional aspects of the patient's behavior and the socioeconomic factors that contribute to the patient's attitudes will influence the type of information and style of the preventive education program best suited to the patient. Once this is done, a plan including appropriate motivational strategies can be followed. Frequent contact and positive reinforcement to encourage the patient's self-confidence also contribute to a successful result.

Motivation is an important part of patient education on the part of both the learner and the instructor. An unmotivated teacher rarely has motivated students. It is especially important for the preventive educator to stay enthusiastic about preventive goals. Over time, however, treatment of numerous dental problems associated with a variety of patient personalities can be extremely exhausting. In addition, it is often difficult to accept the fact that people do not always do what is good for them or will not learn what seems obvious. Such frustration does nothing to enhance the educator's motivation. The commitment to a preventive philosophy laced with patience and determination is the backbone to sustaining this energy. Staying enthusiastic means keeping the goals of disease prevention in mind. Helping patients achieve a better state of health and a greater degree of independence from dental disease continues to be the best reason to persist.

When patient education is individualized and the clinician and patient share an interest in the preventive plan, changing human behavior is merely difficult—not impossible.

DAILY PLAQUE CONTROL: MECHANICAL DISRUPTION

The goal in plaque control instruction is to help the patient practice a nontraumatic method of disrupting plaque supra- and subgingivally. Disrupting bacterial organization in dental plaque remains a primary way to control periodontal disease. Supragingival disruption helps prevent gingivitis. Regularly disturbing the subgingival flora helps reduce bacterial proliferation associated with periodontitis. Periodontitis is due to a complex interplay of factors attributable to individual immunity and to bacterial toxicity (Listgarten, 1987). Until treatments can be developed that pinpoint enzymes, toxins, and host-mediated factors, the most widely accepted prevention procedure is to reduce the organization and numbers of microorganisms residing on the teeth and particularly in the periodontal pocket. Both the patient and the clinician must be aware of the areas where plaque accumulates. Currently, these areas are assessed by using a disclosing agent supragingivally and by assessing subgingival plaque with a microscope.

Disclosing agents

Dental plaque is not easily identified because of its colorless, or invisible, nature. An agent is therefore necessary to make the plaque obvious to the patient. As described in Chapter 13, a disclosing agent stains plaque so that the patient is able to assess areas where plaque remains on clinical crowns.

Several materials are available that stain plaque. Arnim (1963) discovered the first coloring that could be used routinely and safely as a dental disclosant. The food coloring erythrosine remains the most widely used agent and is dispensed in tablet or solution form. Erythrosine indiscriminately stains plaque, calculus, intraoral tissues, clothing, toothbrush bristles, towels, and skin (Yankell and Emling, 1978). This seems to be its only drawback, making instructions and warnings for its use advisable (see Plate 1, *I,* for plaque stained with erythrosine).

Color combinations such as FD & C red No. 3 and FD & C green No. 3 stain plaque differentially according to thickness of formation and maturation.

Another solution, sodium fluorescein, stains plaque but is only visible under blue light (Plate 1, *J*). This may be particularly useful in a dental practice from which patients may be returning to daily business where pink-stained oral tissues are unacceptable.

All types of disclosing products are useful. The patient's preference is important.

The patient should use disclosing tablets or solution to assess plaque retention areas and to make self-evaluation of home care techniques possible. The routine use of disclosing agents has been shown to decrease periodontal disease as compared with the incidence of periodontal disease in groups who perform routine oral hygiene measures without the aid of a disclosing agent (Squillaro, Cohen, and Laster, 1975).

Disclosing agents may be most helpful at the beginning of a preventive program. As the patient becomes more proficient in assessing gingival status, the disclosing agent may be used less frequently to check the thoroughness of plaque removal (Tan, 1980; Melcer and Feldman, 1979).

Microscopic evaluation

Culturing for specific bacterial species, as well as more sophisticated procedures as immunofluorescence and the DNA probe, can determine specifically the bacterial species located on the teeth and in the pocket. In many instances, such definitive identification is necessary—particularly for recurrent or rapidly progressive periodontitis.

However, simpler techniques can be used in a clinical setting to help patients to understand the bacerial nature of periodontal problems and to monitor their progress in controlling subgingival flora. Phase contrast microscopy can be used to characterize plaque samples as highly motile (where there is a evidence of rapid streaming of bacteria and heavy spirochete activity), moderately active, or minimally active. This broad characterization of what is visible through the microscope can reveal changes in the nature of the plaque sample, which can be monitored at recall visits.

Darkfield microscopy uses a slightly more sophisticated technique. Specific bacterial forms are counted as they move out of the field of vision. Spirochetes, motile rods, cocci, and "other" are counted on a counting machine until 100 organisms have been observed. The counter provides a percentage distribution among the four forms, which can be compared to counts taken on previous visits and to the patient's "normal" distribution. Health is characterized by low percentages of spirochetes and motile rods. A shift to cocci and other forms indicates that a positive change is occurring in the bacterial composition of the plaque (Listgarten and Levin 1981; Listgarten and Schifter, 1982).

The toothbrush

The primary tool in the removal of dental plaque is the toothbrush (Bass, 1948). Because the main areas that harbor plaque are the tongue, the cervical one-third of the tooth, and the gingival sulcus, a brush that is highly adaptable and that will not harm the soft tissue is most desirable. Synthetic or nylon bristles have the advantages of being manufactured in a consistent size. The diameter of the bristle determines its resiliency (Yankell and Emling, 1978). The smaller the diameter, the softer the texture. Soft bristles with polished ends are flexible and gentle on the oral tissues. To adapt the bristles with uniform pressure, the height of the bristles should be the same. Bristles can be clumped together to form a tuft, which may stand isolated, or several tufts can be placed close together (multitufted). The multitufted brush may cover an area more completely than a brush with separated tufts. Either brush style is acceptable.

Brushes are manufactured in a wide variety of sizes and shapes. The most common configuration for brushes for adults is three or four rows of bristles. Most brushes are flat in profile. The individual manufacturer decides on the size of the toothbrush head. The profusion of sizes and shapes results from the lack of evidence as to which is the most effective brush (Figs. 19-5 and 19-6).

In summary, the toothbrush of today has soft synthetic bristles with polished ends of uniform height, in sharp contrast to the hard-textured, natural boar-bristle brushes of the past.

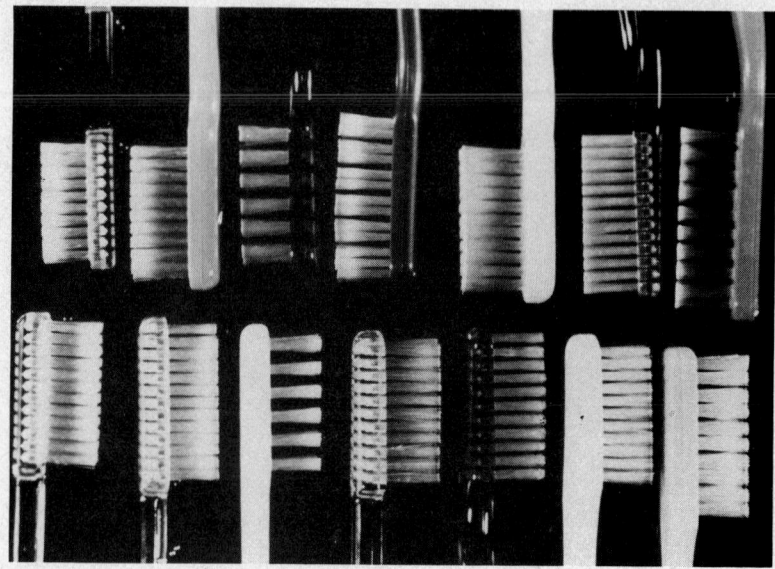

Fig. 19-5. Various acceptable brushing tools.
(From Yankell S and Emling R: Contin Dent Educ 1[76], 1978.)

Brushing methods

A few techniques for brushing the oral tissues are presented here. It is important to emphasize that although knowledge of specific techniques of brushing may be important for the health educator, the most important procedure for the patient to master is thoroughness in reaching all areas of the mouth. One method is not in and of itself better than another. A patient may need to use principles of several techniques to clean adequately. Guiding the patient toward methods that meet individual needs is more important than stressing a particular technique.

Rolling stroke brushing. The roll method is a general cleaning method to remove food and plaque primarily from the crowns of the teeth. This method places little emphasis on cleaning the sulcus and is rarely recommended today.

Method: The patient is instructed to grasp the brush so that the bristles are pointed apically and placed on the gingiva (Fig. 19-7, *A*). With a sweeping motion, the bristles are gently rolled over the gingiva and teeth toward the incisal or occlusal surfaces (Fig. 19-7, *B*). The brush is replaced, and this roll stroke is continued in the

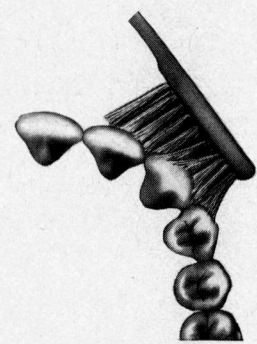

Fig. 19-6. Soft-textured brush adapts well to contours of dentition.
(From Yankell S and Emling R: Contin Dent Educ 1[18], 1978.)

same area five to ten times. Depending on the length of the brush head and the size of the teeth, two to four teeth may be cleaned with one brush placement. When the strokes for one section have been completed, the toothbrush is moved to the next area, with care taken to overlap at least one tooth.

The narrow anterior lingual portion of the arch

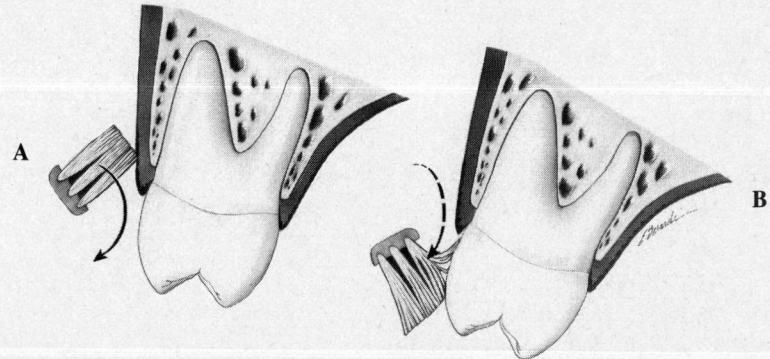

Fig. 19-7. Rolling stroke brushing method. **A,** Place bristles pointing apically on gingiva. **B,** Sweep bristles over teeth from gingiva toward incisal or occlusal surface.

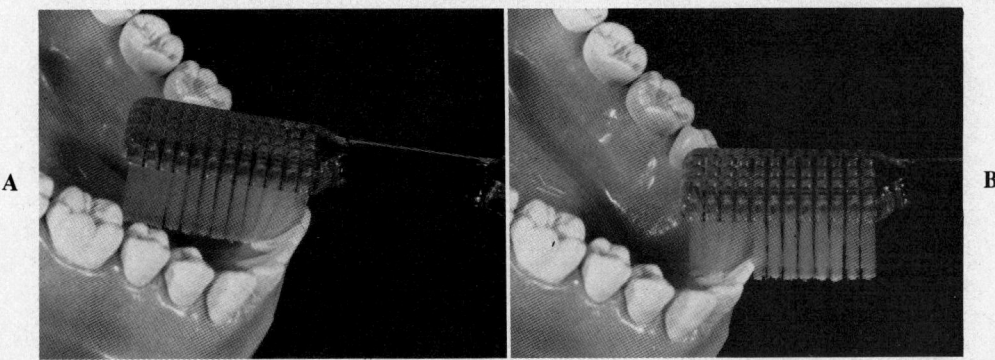

Fig. 19-8. Anterior lingual brushing method. **A,** Place brush vertically into narrow anterior portion of arch. **B,** Sweep brush from gingiva toward incisal edge.

presents a problem because the brush head generally is too large to be placed horizontally. The patient repositions the brush vertically and sweeps from the gingival to the incisal edge (Fig. 19-8).

When both maxilla and mandible are completed on the facial and lingual surfaces, the occlusal surface should be scrubbed by moving the bristles back and forth (Fig. 19-9).

Cleaning the tongue. The surface of the tongue is an ideal location for bacterial plaque and food debris to collect. The papillae of the tongue create a surface similar to a thick-piled carpet. The patient should be instructed to scrape or brush the tongue to clean it. By cleaning the tongue, the patient removes deposits that may be

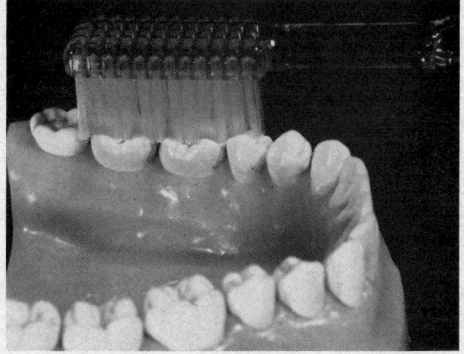

Fig. 19-9. Occlusal cleaning method. Flex, tap, or move bristles back and forth along occlusal surface to clean this portion of dentition.

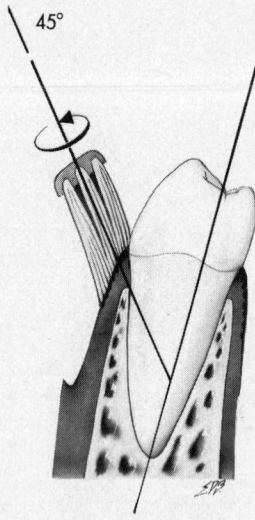

Fig. 19-10. Stillman's brushing method. Place bristles on attached gingiva and gingival margin at 45-degree angle. Activate bristles with a small circular motion to stimulate tissue and clean cervical area. Following this step, place bristles to complete rolling stroke to clean clinical crowns (modified Stillman's).

causing odors or contributing to plaque formation in other areas of the mouth.

Method: while leaning over a sink, the patient extends the tongue. Using plenty of water, the tongue is cleaned by placing the brush as far posteriorly as possible and sweeping the brush anteriorly. After several strokes the patient inspects the tongue for coating.

Gagging may be avoided by displacing the tongue as little as possible. An alternate method is to clean the tongue in its normal resting position with the head erect.

Stillman's method (modified). Stillman's (modified) method is useful for stimulating and cleaning the cervical area. The roll stroke is then included for cleaning the clinical crowns.

Method: The toothbrush is grasped and the bristles, pointing apically at about a 45-degree angle, are placed on the attached gingiva. The bristles should be flexed with enough pressure to cause slight gingival blanching and are activated with a small rotary (circular) motion (Fig. 19-10). The rotation is repeated about eight to ten times. When this is completed, the brush is rolled from the gingiva toward the occlusal surfaces. With a

soft-bristled brush, the bristles adapt to the interproximal areas as the roll is completed. The rotation/roll sequence is performed several times before the brush is placed in the next area, with care taken to overlap at least one tooth to ensure that the brushing sequence cleans all areas. The anterior lingual section is brushed by placing the heel or toe of the brush on the gingiva, rotating, and sweeping toward the incisal edges. In this area only about two teeth at a time will be cleaned by each brush placement.

Bass method

The Bass method of brushing is generally accepted for effectively removing plaque from the sulcus area.

Method: The toothbrush is grasped and the bristles, pointing apically at a 45-degree angle to the long axis of the tooth, are placed at the gingival margin. Generally, only the first row will approximate the sulcus while the adjacent row will touch the gingival margin (Fig. 19-11, *A*).

When the brush is pressed lightly, the soft bristles contour themselves into the sulcus and interproximal area. About ten short back-and-forth vibration strokes are used to disorganize the plaque in the area, without lifting the brush (Fig. 19-11, *B*). If the bristles make a scrubbing sound, the pressure of vibration is too great or the size of the back-and-forth stroke is too large. The pressure is relaxed, and the brush is moved to the next area, with care taken to overlap at least one tooth for each placement in the sequence. The main objective is sulcular cleaning. The buccal and lingual surfaces of the dental arches are completed in this manner. In the anterior lingual area the brush is inserted vertically, and the bristles of the heel or toe of the brush are placed at the sulcular area and vibrated. The lingual surface is cleaned by the bristles being pulled over the tooth surface.

The roll stroke method may be used in conjunction with this brushing method either as a procedure performed prior to the sulcular placement or afterward. This is called the *modified Bass method.*

Scrub brush method. This method is used for general cleaning. The brush is usually placed perpendicular to the long axis of the teeth. Vertical, circular, or horizontal strokes are employed. When a soft toothbrush is used, such a technique

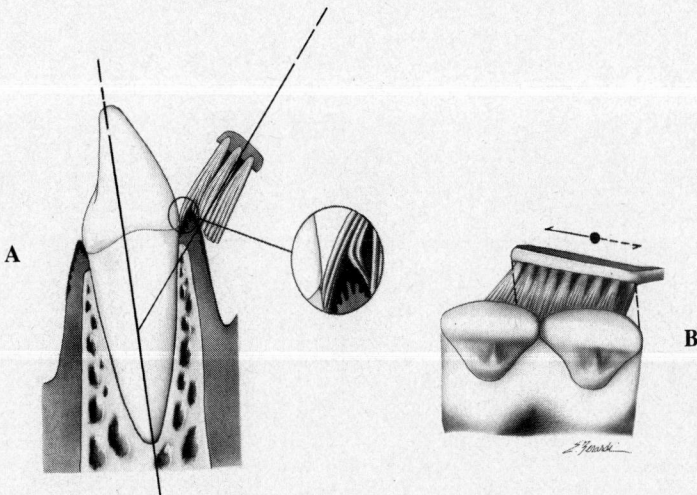

Fig. 19-11. Bass brushing method. **A,** Place bristles pointing apically at 45-degree angle to long axis of tooth. First row of bristles will approximate sulcus, and adjacent row will touch gingival margin. **B,** Activate brush with a short back-and-froth vibration to disorganize plaque in sulcus. Following this step, place bristles to complete rolling stroke to clean clinical crowns (modified Bass).

may adequately remove plaque on the clinical crowns. In general, vigorous brushing in such a random fashion is discouraged, since trauma to the teeth or gingiva may result. A brushing method such as this does not purposefully clean the interproximal or sulcular area, so critical areas may be missed.

However, this technique may work well with some patients. Children, patients with limited dexterity, or patients with specific tooth alignment problems may find this technique useful. Encourage a sequence of brushing, the use of other cleaning tools to complement this brushing method if necessary, and short brushing strokes.

Summary of brushing methods. Brushing in an appropriate and thorough manner removes the food and plaque accumulation on the major portions of the clinical crowns of the teeth. The buccal, lingual, and occlusal areas are cleaned, in addition to a major portion of the sulcus and the gingiva. The tongue, palate, and buccal mucosa can be gently cleaned also. The tissue area that is yet untouched is the tooth surface protected by the interdental papillae in the interproximal area. This area collects plaque as easily as the other areas, but cleaning it with a brush is virtually impossible. The inflammatory and caries processes may occur here without interruption for long peri-

ods of time unless interproximal cleaning is performed.

Before addressing interproximal cleaning, the clinician determines the patient's skill level with brushing. The following questions are suggested for summarizing this aspect of the patient's preventive program:

1. Does the patient use a disclosing solution? Can the patient identify plaque in the mouth?
2. Does the patient realize the relationship of plaque to dental disease?
3. Is the patient's brush tool suited to his or her needs?
4. How effectively does the patient's cleaning method remove bacterial plaque and food from all surfaces?
5. Does the patient use a cleaning sequence?
6. Does the patient care for the oral soft tissues, gingiva, and tongue?
7. Does the patient recognize the limitations of brushing when caring for his or her oral health?

Interproximal cleaning

Dental floss and tape are the primary interproximal plaque removal tools. Basically, a material is needed that can easily fit through the tight contact areas of the teeth to clean the interproximal sulcus

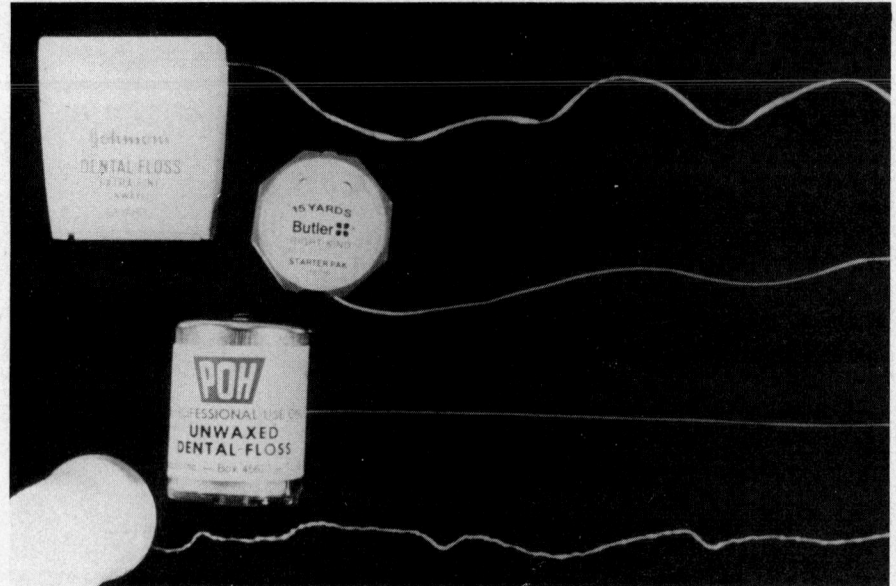

Fig. 19-12. Variation in acceptable interproximal plaque removal tools.
(From Yankell S and Emling R: Contin Dent Educ **1:**[7], 1978.)

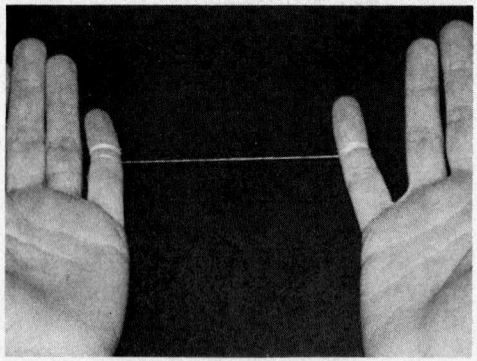

Fig. 19-13. Flossing technique. Wrap length of floss around fourth fingers of each hand.

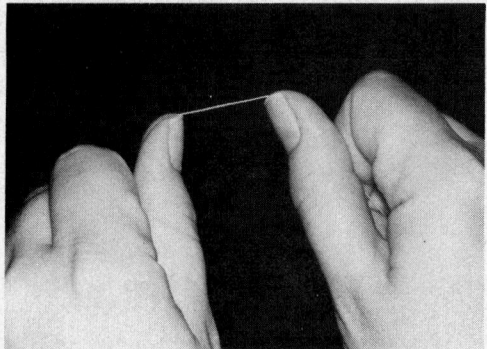

Fig. 19-14. Stretch floss over thumbs to clean maxillary teeth.

and the mesial or distal portion of the tooth untouched by the brush. Not all contact areas are the same. Consequently, several types of floss, from the thin, nonwaxed products to heavier, waxed tapes, have been marketed (Fig. 19-12). Even a variable-diameter floss that combines a stiff end for threading beneath contact areas, a section of regular unwaxed floss, and an area of yarn-type floss is available.

French and Friedman (1975) found that both

waxed and unwaxed products cleaned effectively. Stevens (1980) and Lobene and Soparkar (1982) have reported similar studies, in which variable-diameter and mint-flavored floss removed plaque as well as other floss products. The floss type is selected according to the patient's specific conditions. Someone with normally firm contacts between teeth may need an average-weight unwaxed floss. Someone with crowded teeth, tight contacts, or rough interproximal restorations may be

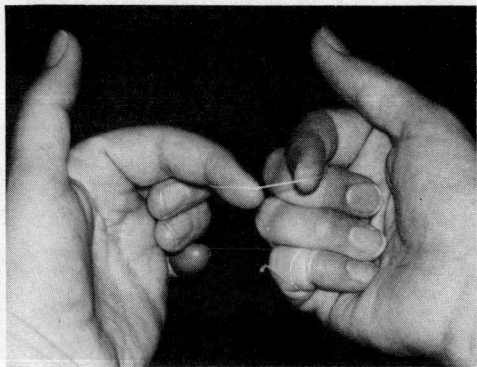

Fig. 19-15. Stretch floss over index fingers to clean mandibular teeth.

thoroughly frustrated by interproximal cleaning unless a waxed floss, which resists fraying, is used. Manual dexterity may determine the appropriate type of floss. A very fine, threadlike floss may be impossible for a person who handles a heavier tape beautifully. The purpose is to remove the plaque in the easiest, safest, and most efficient way; offering instruction for tools that the dental professional prefers may not help the patient if they do not meet the patient's needs and limitations.

Suggested flossing techniques. A piece of floss approximately 18 inches (45 cm) long is taken. Both ends are wound around the second or fourth finger of each hand (Corn and Marks, 1978) (Fig. 19-13). The floss is secured with the index fingers and thumb of each hand with a length of ¾ to 1 inch (1.9 to 2.5 cm) between each hand. This length of floss will be manipulated into the contact area between the teeth. When floss is wrapped around the fourth finger, the excess floss is tucked out of the way, allowing maximum maneuverability for the index fingers and thumbs. In the maxilla, the floss is stretched over the thumbs, and these fingers are used to guide the floss (Fig. 19-14). On the mandible, the floss is stretched over the index fingers, and these are used to guide the floss (Fig. 19-15). One thumb or index finger is placed on the buccal side of the area being flossed, and the thumb or index finger from the other hand is placed on the lingual side (Figs. 19-16 and 19-17). Approximately 1 inch of floss is used to "work" through the contact area of the teeth. The span of floss is inserted into the contact area by sliding it against one of the in-

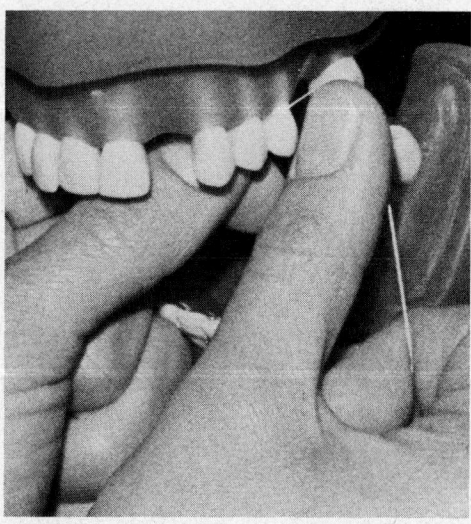

Fig. 19-16. Placement of thumbs and floss for maxillary technique. To clean interproximally, one thumb is placed on lingual side of tooth; other thumb is placed on facial side with approximatley 1 inch (2.5 cm) of floss between the thumbs.

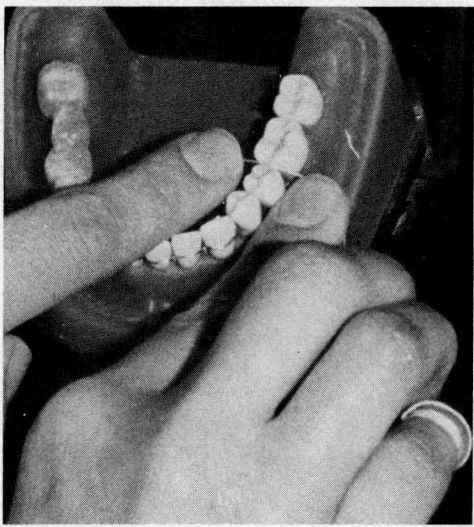

Fig. 19-17. Placement of index fingers for mandibular technique. To clean interproximally, one finger is placed on lingual side of tooth; other finger is placed on facial side with approximately 1 inch (2.5 cm) of floss between fingers.

terproximal surfaces (mesial or distal) of the tooth (Fig. 19-18). The floss is worked along the tooth with a back-and-forth motion at the contact area (Fig. 19-19). With the floss pulled firmly around the tooth surface, this seesaw motion flattens the

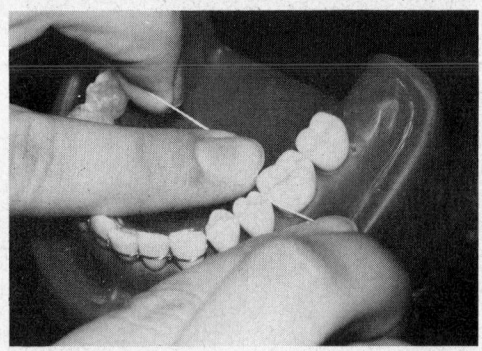

Fig. 19-18. Insert span of floss into contact area. Hold floss around one of the teeth to help ease past contact.

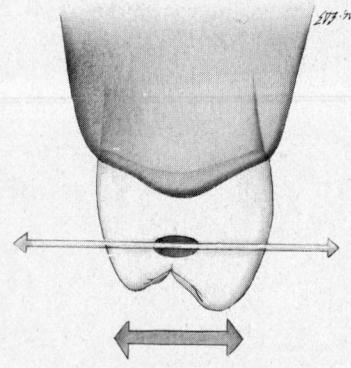

Fig. 19-19. Diagram illustrates back-and-forth, seesaw motion as floss is moved through contact area.
(From Corn H and Marks M: Contin Dent Educ **1**:14, 1978.

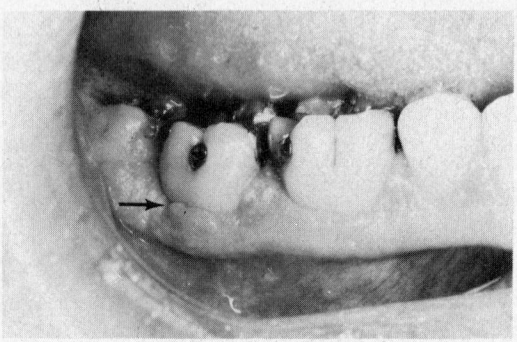

Fig. 19-20. With improper placement, a gingival cleft may result from dental floss being continually forced into sulcus.
(From Corn H and Marks M: Contin Dent Educ **1**;16, 1978.

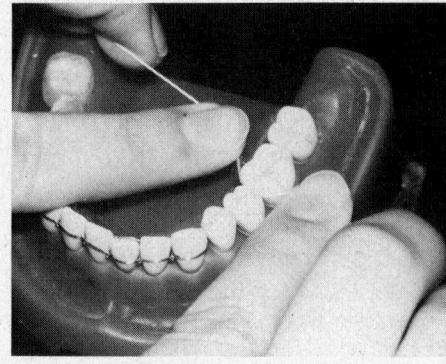

Fig. 19-21. Once past contact area, wrap floss around tooth and move floss up and down on proximal surface.

floss as much as possible to ease it through the contact area. This part of flossing is often the most difficult, as control is needed not to slip through the contact too rapidly and cause trauma to the sulcular gingiva (Fig. 19-20). Once eased gently past the contact point, the floss is wrapped around the tooth and moved up and down against the tooth between the sulcus and the contact area of one tooth (Figs. 19-21 and 19-22). The same cleaning is performed on the adjacent tooth in the interproximal space (Fig. 19-23). The floss is removed by being held against one of the teeth and using the seesaw motion again through the contact area. If the teeth are extremely tight or restoration margins are causing particular problems, one end of the floss is released. The remainder of the floss

is pulled out of the interproximal area without struggling through the contact area and possibly breaking the floss. When moving to the next area, the used floss is wound around the finger to permit access to a clean, fresh span.

Another method for flossing uses the floss tied in a loop (Katz, McDonald, and Stookey, 1979;) (Fig. 19-24). It works the same way, but often the patient does it better than the finger-wrapping technique. This can be especially good for parents flossing the teeth of a child or to allow persons with less nimble hands to maneuver the floss themselves.

Summary of flossing techniques. In general, flossing is best learned in a progressive way. Flossing the anterior teeth is practiced first so the

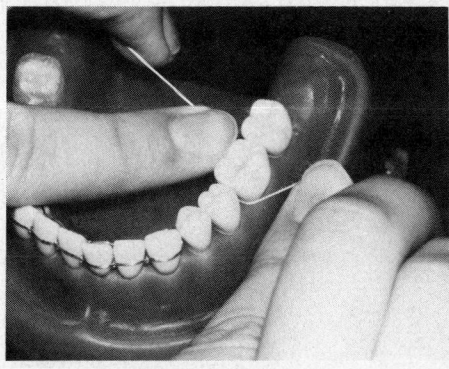

Fig. 19-22. Entire area from contact point to gingival sulcus is cleaned with floss well adapted to tooth.

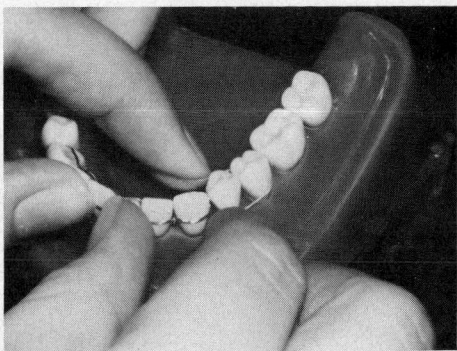

Fig. 19-23. When first proximal surface is completed, wrap floss around adjacent tooth, and use same cleaning stroke on this tooth.

patient can learn to manipulate the floss in an area that is easily viewed and accessible. When the clinician is assured of the patient's safe technique, the posterior areas are tackled.

This aspect of home care may be the newest to the patient. It should be understood that time, practice, and patience are critical to aiding the patient's realization that flossing is important and not impossible to make habitual.

The patient should be assisted with problem areas and allowed to experiment with different wrapping techniques. The emphasis for evaluation is on the success of plaque removal and the safety of the patient's method with whatever product is most comfortable. The following questions are suggested for summarizing this aspect of the patient's preventive program:

1. Does the patient recognize the value of flossing in addition to brushing?
2. Has the patient identified a product that he or she can use effectively?
3. Has flossing been added to the patient's home care procedures on a regular basis? (If not, identify the reason. Chances are that the skill does not need to be retaught. Review planning to identify and remove motivational roadblocks).

Additional cleansing tools

With thorough brushing and flossing, most patients will be on the way to preventing dental disease. However, some patients have conditions that require instruction in the use of special aids.

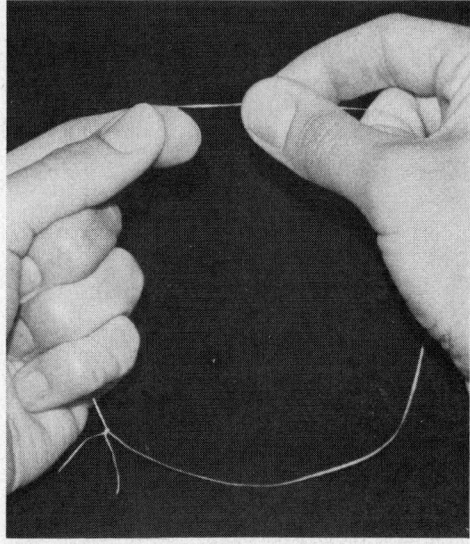

Fig. 19-24. Floss tied in a loop may be maneuvered more easily for some patients. Follow guidelines for finger placement and cleaning stroke as described in previous figures.

Following are some of these conditions with the possible aids listed for each group:

1. Limited dexterity due to age, disability, or coordination
   a. Floss holder
   b. Electric toothbrush
   c. Modified brush
2. Areas of fixed bridges, splints for stabilization, or

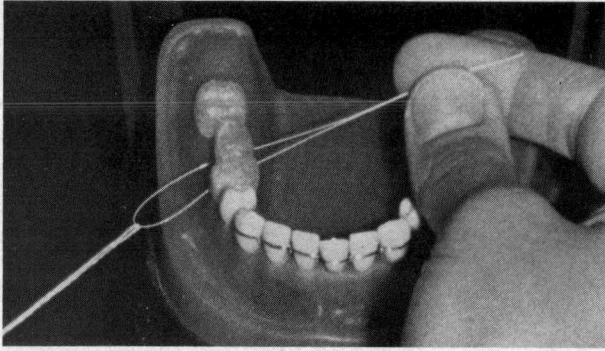

Fig. 19-25. Floss threader. Place floss through loop in threader (Butler), and feed floss under bridge or tight contact area.

orthodontic wires that do not permit flossing as usual
  a. Floss threader
  b. Variable-diameter floss or yarn
  c. Oral irrigation
3. Wide interdental areas where the normal contour of the gingiva has been lost because of resolution of disease or surgery (these areas may be adequately cleaned by brushing and flossing methods, but sometimes the patient needs additional massage or cleaning assistance to maintain the area in a health state)
  a. Yarn
  b. Periodontal aid
  c. Balsa wood wedge
  d. Interproximal brush
  e. Rubber tip stimulator
4. Sulcular areas with a pocket depth greater than 3 mm that cannot be adequately cleaned with the brush and floss but can be maintained indefinitely with an additional aid until surgical correction
  a. Periodontal aid
  b. Toothpick holder
  c. Oral irrigator
5. Teeth that are isolated or are adjacent to edentulous areas
  a. Yarn
  b. Gauze Strip
6. Tooth contours that present difficulty because of access, furcations, or malposed or malformed teeth
  a. Periodontal aid
  b. Rubber tip
  c. Pipe cleaner
  d. Oral irrigator

When advising the use of any of these aids, keep the overall home care armamentarium sim-

ple. Many of these aids can be used for the same problem. Efforts to add a wide variety of oral hygiene measures beyond toothbrushing can meet with poor compliance (Johansson et al, 1984). Select the one that is easiest for the patient and that the patient will enjoy using. Additional instruction or trial-and-error experience may be necessary to find the aid that works best for a particular patient. The more cumbersome home care methods become, the more difficult it is to motivate the patient to perform the skills. When unrealistic demands are made on a patient's performance, the patient will feel guilty and avoid further contact if possible. Following is a brief description of the aforementioned aids.

Floss threader. Several floss threaders are available. They consist of a flexible material through which the floss can be threaded. These are used as a guide to insert the floss into the contact area so that cleaning may take place. Once the floss is threaded under the bridge or under the contact, the flossing technique described previously is used (Figs. 19-25 and 19-26).

Variable-diameter floss. This floss is used with the same technique as regular floss. The variation in the body of this floss allows it to be threaded under fixed bridges or below tight contact areas (Figs. 19-27 and 19-28). It may be used as yarn for wide embrasures or open contacts in addition to its regular flossing function (Figs. 19-29 and 19-30). It cleans effectively, but not better than regular floss (Spindel and Person, 1987).

Floss holder. This device may be especially important for those patients who have limited

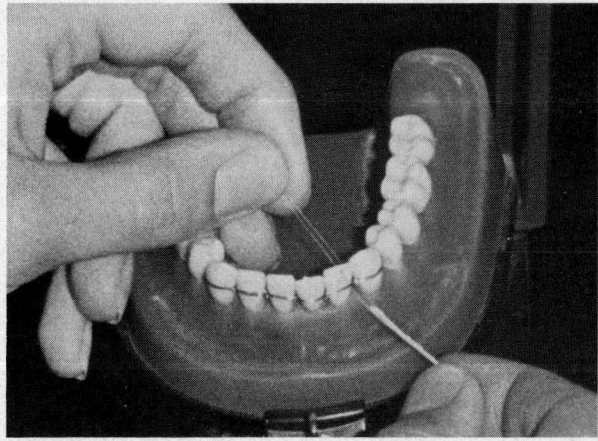

Fig. 19-26. Floss threader. Place floss through eye of clear plastic threader (Zons), and feed floss under appliance, tight contact, or bridge area.

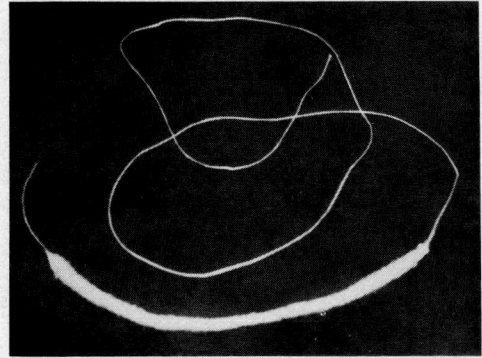

Fig. 19-27. Variable-diameter floss. This product combines a stiff end for threading, an area of yarn-type floss, and a large section of regular floss. This versatility may be well suited to some patients.

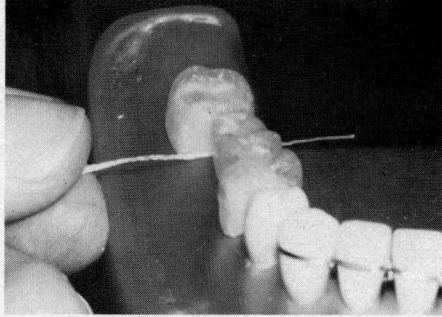

Fig. 19-28. Variable-diameter floss threader section being fed under bridge.

dexterity or the use of only one hand. The holder is a frame that supports a length of floss. It holds the floss taut so that it can be manipulated between the teeth. Enough "play" exists so that by pressure against the tooth, the floss will adapt itself adequately around the interproximal area (Fig. 19-31).

Yarn. This is a thick, soft, and absorbent type of cleaner for wide interproximal areas or abutment teeth. Approximately 14 inches (35 cm) of synthetic yarn should be used. White is the best choice, since some dyes may run when moistened. If access between the teeth allows the yarn

to be used as regular floss, previously mentioned techniques are followed. After the yarn is slid interproximally, a vertical stroke is used to remove plaque and polish the tooth surface. A floss threader may be used to assist in the yarn placement if necessary (Fig. 19-32).

Gauze strip. The cotton is removed from the gauze. The gauze is then folded and used as though shining a shoe; in the wide interdental or abutment area, the gauze is rubbed back and forth to clean and polish the interproximal surface (Figs. 19-33 and 19-34).

Several other types of interdental aids are described below.

Pipe cleaner. Pipe cleaners can be adapted easily to achieve access to furcation areas or mal-

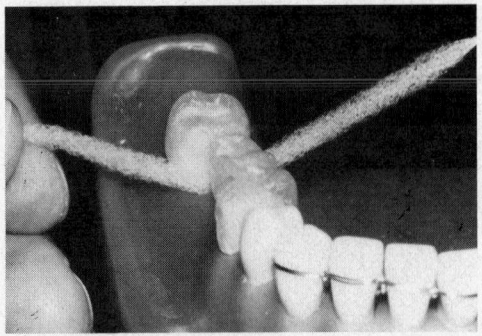

Fig. 19-29. Yarn section of variable-diameter floss for cleaning under bridge or in area where space permits.

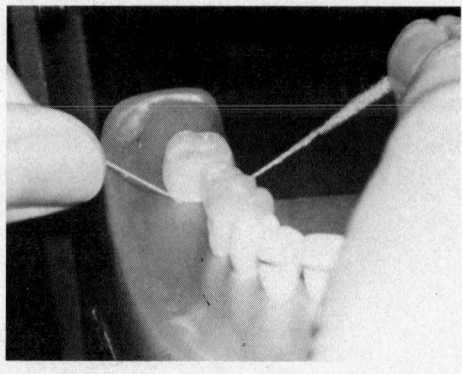

Fig. 19-30. Floss section of variable-diameter floss adapted for standard flossing technique.

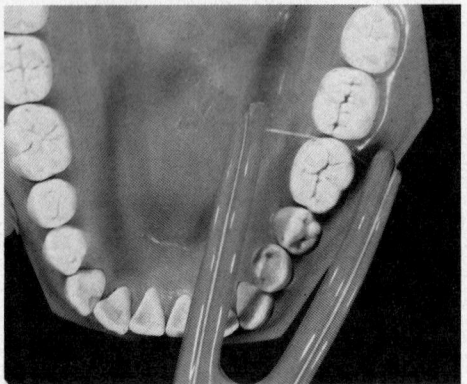

Fig. 19-31. Floss holder. Floss is stretched over frame and can be maneuvered for standard flossing with one hand.

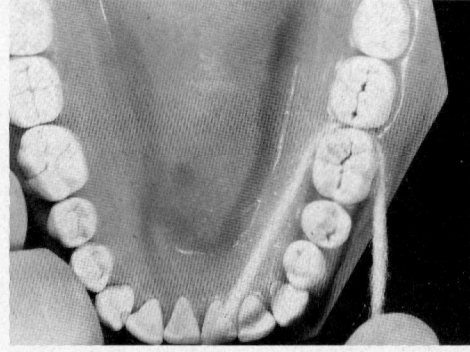

Fig. 19-32. White synthetic yarn makes excellent cleaner for wide interproximal areas.

posed teeth. The pipe cleaner is used to rub the tooth free of plaque and food debris. Care must be taken not to damage the tooth or tissue with the wire of the pipe cleaner. The pipe cleaner is discarded after use (Fig. 19-35).

Periodontal aid. Generally, the periodontal aid consists of a toothpick and plastic holder. The toothpick is softened and applied to the gingival margin. With the tip directed at less than 45 degrees to the long axis of the tooth, it can be used to remove plaque in the sulcus. Another use is for desensitization with the periodontal aid used to massage fluoride or other desensitizing agents into the root of the tooth (Figs. 19-36 and 19-37).

Rubber tip. A cone-shaped rubber tip can be used to clean the tooth surface and massage tis-

sues. The tip is placed on the interdental area, with the tip end directed toward the occlusal surface; a rotation or back-and-forth motion with the side of the tip is used to massage the tissue. The tip can be used in a similar fashion in an exposed furcation area (Fig. 19-38).

Wood wedge. Wedge-shaped toothpicks may be used for cleaning interdental areas and stimulating tissues. The patient should soften the wedge and apply the base of the triangle to the interdental area with the tip directed slightly occlusally. The interproximal area is cleaned by using a vertical or horizontal stroke against the tooth surface. The proximal surface of one tooth should be cleaned and then that of the adjacent tooth. When the wedge begins to fray, it should

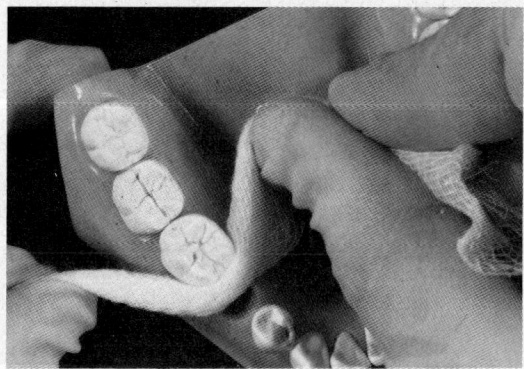

Fig. 19-33. Gauze strip can be folded and adapted to polish a wide interdental area.

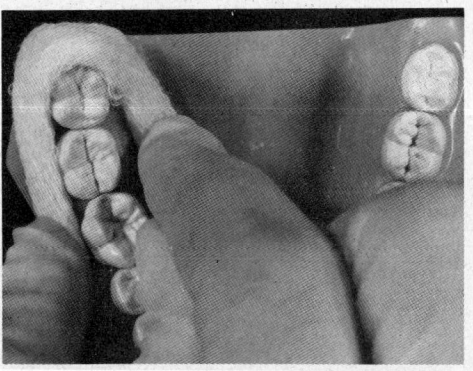

Fig. 19-34. Gauze strip becomes excellent polisher for hard-to-reach areas such as distal surface of last tooth in arch.

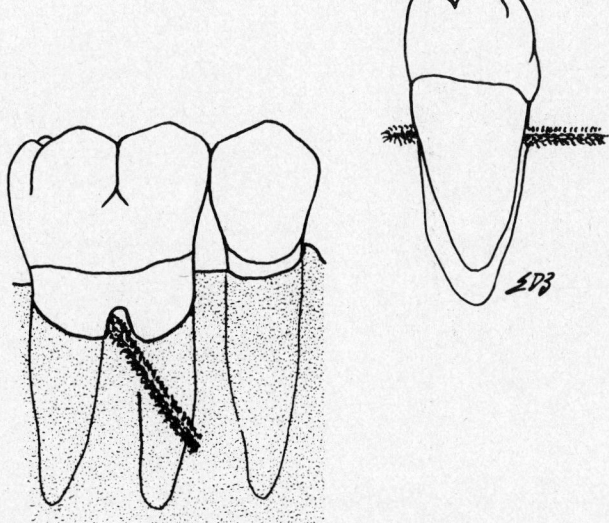

Fig. 19-35. Pipe cleaner can be bent and adapted to area of difficult access or to furcation area to remove plaque and food debris.

be discarded (Fig. 19-39). Wood wedges can also be used help the clinician and the patient determine gingival inflammation through evidence of papillary bleeding. The Eastman Interdental Bleeding Index assesses the presence or absence of bleeding upon stimulation with the wooden pick. Patients can use the picks to clean interdentally and to observe areas where bleeding occurs (Abrams et al, 1984; Caton and Polson, 1985; Amato et al, 1986; Barton and Abelson, 1987).

Interproximal brush. This is a small spiral brush or single tuft of bristles attached to a handle. The bristles are soft and adapt to the interproximal area of a wide embrasure. The brush is manipulated with a slight rotation or scrub motion and may be helpful for patients with appliances that present hard-to-clean areas (Fig. 19-40).

Modified toothbrush. An endless variety of brushes can be created with modified handles, bristle heights, or extensions. These are especially

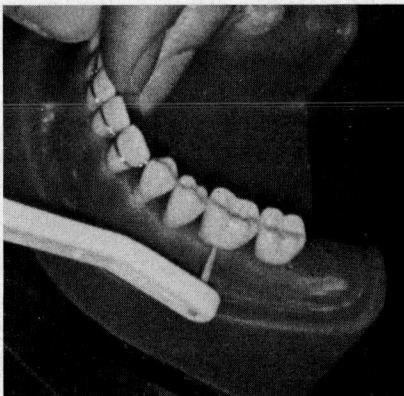

Fig. 19-36. Periodontal aid is toothpick in plastic holder. Toothpick is softened by wetting and applied to gingival margin. Tip can be moved gently in sulcus at less than 45-degree angle to remove plaque or can be adapted on cervical surface to burnish fluoride into the exposed root for desensitization.

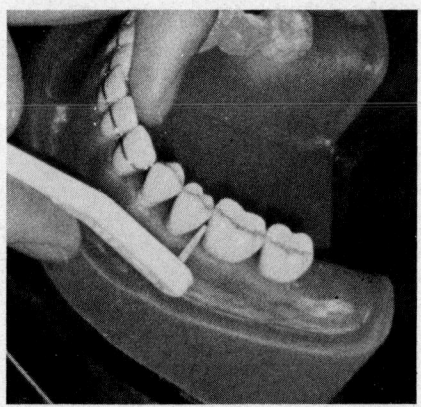

Fig. 19-37. Periodontal aid can be used to clean proximal surface of tooth. Tip is directed occlusally and moved along cervical area.

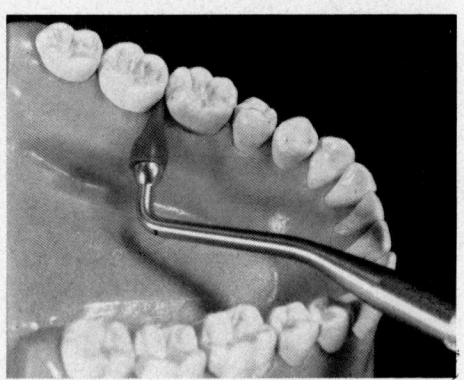

Fig. 19-38. Place rubber tip in interdental area pointed occlusally. Massage tissue by rotating tip against tissue.

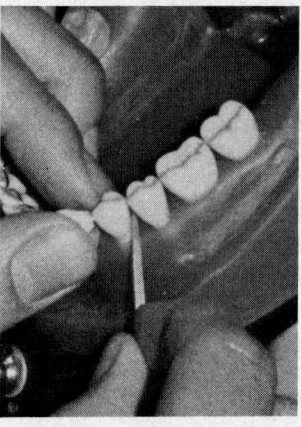

Fig. 19-39. Wood wedge is softened and placed with base of wedge on tissue. Point wedge occlusally and clean proximal surface by sliding wedge against tooth. At the same time, this stroke helps stimulate and recontour tissue.

helpful for patients with a limited grasp, reach, or control in cleaning. Once an appropriate tool is designed, a brushing stroke is applied to meet the patient's needs (Fig. 19-41). (See Chapter 33 for more information on modifying toothbrushes for patients with special needs.)

Automatic toothbrush. An electrically or battery-powered brush offers an alternative for patients unable or unwilling to use a manual toothbrush. Vibratory, reciprocating, and arcuate motion brushes are available with soft bristles. Studies indicate that automatic brushes compare quite

well with manual brushes; the degree of motivation and thoroughness in technique is most important. However, interproximal cleaning with floss or another aid may be necessary (Schifter et al, 1983).

Two new designs in automatic toothbrushes offer interproximal cleaning superior to that achieved with a hand brush. The Rotodent® brush rotates a single rotating tuft, which can be applied to interproximal areas and embrasure spaces. Dif-

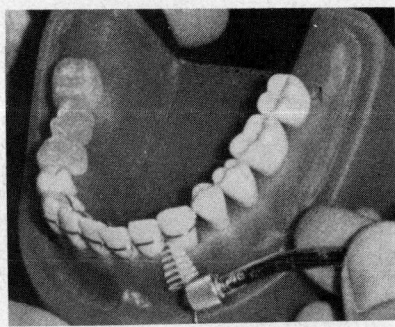

Fig. 19-40. Interproximal brush is spiral-shaped brush that can be placed in wide interdental areas to clean proximal surfaces and stimulate interdental tissue.

ferent brush shapes are interchangeable to fit the patient's individual needs. The Interplak® brush head has several individual tufts that rotate a turn and a half back and forth, providing an individual swirling action to clean the teeth and resulting in increased mechanical action on proximal surfaces.

A recent study showed that the WaterPik® automatic toothbrush with a simulated, modified Bass technique was equivalent to the Interplak brush for plaque removal ability when evaluating all tooth surfaces (Ciancio, 1988). New brushes engineered to improve interdental access will undoubtedly be introduced to provide an array of options.

Oral irrigation: supra- and subgingival plaque control

Nearly all of the devices introduced above are restricted to supragingival plaque control. Brushing and flossing are effective in the mechanical removal of most supragingival plaque, but they are limited in subgingival removal by the physical constraints of the device in conjunction with the gingiva (Plate 1, *K*). Manual brushing can approach 1.5 to 3 mm subgingivally (Waerhaug 1976), and flossing reaches to a depth of 2 to 3 mm (Reitman, 1980). Toothpicks, pipe cleaners, and interdental brushes have minimal effect on subgingival plaque; even in areas where they may be able to move below the margin of the gingiva, size and shape limit their access and usefulness.

One device has access to subgingival areas and can offer patients a way of disrupting the plaque which proliferates in those sites. That device is

the oral irrigator. The first powered oral irrigation device (the Water Pik®) was accepted by the American Dental Association in 1968 for its ability to flush food particles and debris from between teeth and under the gum line. Although the device was widely recommended (especially for orthodontic and prosthodontic patients), early research found no relationship between debris and periodontal disease and no evidence that irrigation could significantly reduce plaque.

As dental researchers expanded their understanding of bacterial plaque, however, they discovered that oral irrigation disrupts the subgingival microbiota. The pulsating action of the water penetrates subgingivally and changes the *quality* of the plaque, detoxifying it. The introduction of antimicrobials (to be discussed in the next section) for the chemical control of dental plaque has further expanded the usefulness of the irrigator. Antimicrobials can be delivered "site specifically" to the sulcus or pocket by an oral irrigator. These two advances in dental research have made oral irrigation an important procedure in planning preventive care, establishing it as much more than a device to flush away debris.

As described in Chapter 13, plaque is a complex organization of bacteria made up of supragingival and subgingival organisms. The supragingival plaque is comprised of attached plaque (AP) that clings to the tooth's surface and an outside layer of loosely attached plaque (LAP) that moves in and out of that attached matrix. Subgingival plaque similarly includes both an attached layer against the root surface and a loosely attached component floating freely between the root and the epithelial lining of the pocket. The subgingival LAP extends beyond the attached component to the epithelial attachment (Plate 1 K and L).

Gingivitis follows the accumulation of supragingival plaque; regular removal of supragingival plaque will prevent gingivitis (Cumming and Löe, 1973). Supragingival plaque influences the establishment and relative proportions of subgingival microorganisms (Loesche and Syed, 1978; Kornman, 1986). Once mature plaque is established, subgingival plaque cannot be controlled by removal of supragingival plaque (Tabita et al, 1981). The loosely attached subgingival plaque directly contacting the epithelial lining is most likely to initiate periodontitis (Carranza, 1979).

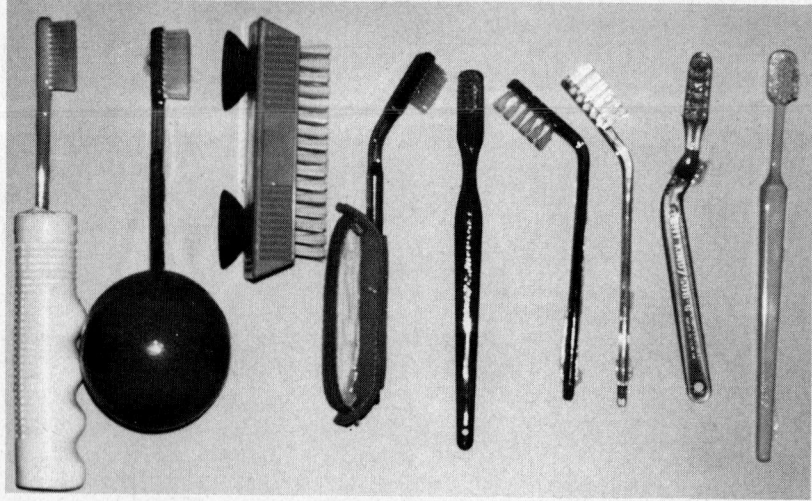

Fig. 19-41. Variety of modified brushes. Some patients have physical limitations that may require creation of a customized tool. Note variety in handles and bristle shapes.

The obvious conclusion is that *supragingival plaque must be controlled to prevent and treat gingivitis, but subgingival plaque, especially the loosely attached component, must be controlled to prevent and treat periodontitis.* Various combinations of professional and home care methods are required for prevention, treatment, and maintenance, depending on the individual patient and disease status.

Most early research on oral irrigation was designed to test its efficacy in removing debris and supragingival plaque. Tempel and colleagues (1975) concluded that water irrigation was significantly more effective than oral rinsing in removing particulate debris and soluble bacterial products, both before and after toothbrushing and flossing. In 1971, Hoover and Robinson found that oral irrigation users had significantly less plaque and calculus accumulation and experienced highly significant reductions in the periodontal index and plaque index in the 3-month test period following prophylaxis.

Lobene (1969) found that oral irrigation, as a supplement to the toothbrush, reduced calculus formation by approximatley 50% and effected a 50% reduction in gingivitis. Lobene suggested that the pulsating water jets might qualitatively have altered the composition of the plaque, which in turn accounted for the reduction in gingivitis. A later study by Brady, Gray, and Bhaskar (1973) used the electron microscope to verify that the pulsating water of the oral irrigator did remove plaque and also produced qualitative changes in the adherent plaque left on irrigated tooth surfaces.

Depth of delivery and chemotherapy

Eakle and others (1985) found that the Water Pik® oral irrigator delivered solution into subgingival pockets of various depths (from 3 to more than 7 mm) and averaged a penetration of approximately half the depth of the pocket.

White and others (1988) verified earlier work by Aday (1982) and West (1982) by evaluating the effect of water irrigation on various bacteria associated with untreated gingivitis and periodontitis at pocket depths up to 6 mm. Irrigated sites improved in both shallow and deep pockets. Results also demonstrated a dramatic reduction of *Bacteroides melaninogenicus* and *Bacteroides intermedius,* with a statistically significant reduction of spirochetes and motile rods in deep pockets.

A recent ultrastructural study using oral irrigation and electron microscopic methods (Cobb,

Using the Oral Irrigator

The heart of the first oral irrigator, as well as today's, is a mechanical pump designed to deliver pulsating bursts of water at a predetermined force. The user is instructed to start with the lowest pressure setting and to hold the delivery tip at the interproximal space, almost touching the tooth at a right angle to the long axis of the tooth. In this position, the pulsating water is dispersed into droplets that emanate in all directions from the original point of contact (Plate 1, *L*). For maximum benefit, the user should pause interproximally for several seconds. The idea behind powered oral irrigation is for water or solution to move with enough energy to flow between the teeth and into the sulcus or pocket. Extensive research has determined optimal pressure settings.

Rogers, and Killoy, 1988) evaluated untreated pockets in patients with advanced, chronic adult periodontitis after a single exposure to pulsating oral irrigation with saline solution. They found qualitative differences in microbial morphotypes at various pocket depths with no injury to soft tissues. When compared with rinsing, oral irrigation has proved superior at distribution of antimicrobial agents (Lang and Raber, 1981; Brownstein et al, 1987).

Boyd and fellow researchers found (1985) that self-administered daily irrigation with 0.02% stannous fluoride resulted in significant improvement in periodontal health when used as an adjunct to brushing and flossing. In 1987, Ciancio and others studied the efficacy of oral irrigation with Listerine as a supplement to normal hygiene. They found that irrigation, with placebo or Listerine, significantly improved probing depth and attachment level measurements. Irrigation with Listerine, furthermore, significantly reduced plaque and bleeding and was shown to be an effective oral hygiene adjunct, both with and without previous dental prophylaxis. Most recently, Brownstein and others (1987) showed that irrigation once daily with 0.06% chlorhexidine was superior in reducing gingival index and bleeding on probing when compared with twice-daily 0.12% chlorhexidine rinsing. Recently M. Newman and colleagues (1988) reported results of a study confirming the Brownstein work. Irrigation with 0.06% chlorhexidine was significantly superior to rinsing twice daily with 0.12% chlorhexidine for gingivitis, bleeding upon probing, and plaque. Water irrigation proved clearly therapeutic in reducing gingivitis, bleeding, without concomitant plaque reduction. In fact, once-daily irrigation with placebo reduced gingival bleeding as well as twice-daily rinsing with chlorhexidine.

Two other studies evaluated the use of sanguinaria (Viadent®) when delivered supragingivally. One study evaluated the effects of irrigation and sanguinaria on established plaque and gingivitis (Parsons et al, 1987). A second evaluated their effects on newly forming plaque and gingivitis (Southard et al, 1987). Both studies used a model in which subjects refrained from brushing for 2 weeks and used either only the irrigator with water or sanguinaria or only a manual oral rinse to control plaque growth. The results showed that irrigation with water or with sanguinaria reduced established gingivitis and inhibited the development of gingivitis in healthy subjects. Adding a dilute solution of Viadent (0.00225% sanguinaria) as an irrigant controlled plaque in both studies.

A number of other studies have compared the efficacy of irrigation with that of rinsing and the benefits of irrigating with one chemical agent over another (Lang and Raber, 1981; Lang and Ramseier-Grossman, 1981; Derdivanis et al, 1978; Alfant et al, 1983; Wolff et al, 1982; Sanders et al, 1986; Aziz-Gandour and Newman, 1986). The consistent conclusion appears to be that delivery with oral irrigation enhances the effect of whatever agent is used. Oral irrigation, because of its proven ability to penetrate gently deep into periodontal pockets, demonstrates benefit even with dilute concentrations. This can be especially important when prescribing chemical agents whose taste and staining are of concern.

Some patients require site-specific subgingival delivery in their home maintenance regime. Subgingival delivery tips designed for patient use are currently being evaluated by researchers both for efficacy and safety. These tips offer promise for

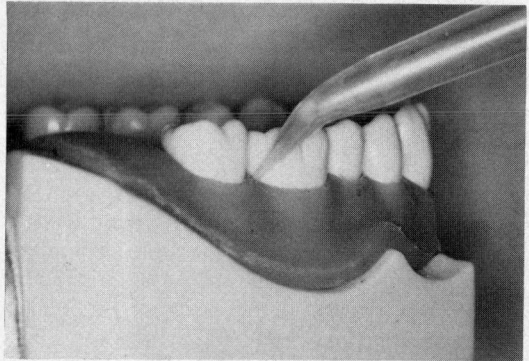

Fig. 19-42. SulcusTip® is designed to carry water or antimicrobial agents to the gingival sulcus or the periodontal pocket.

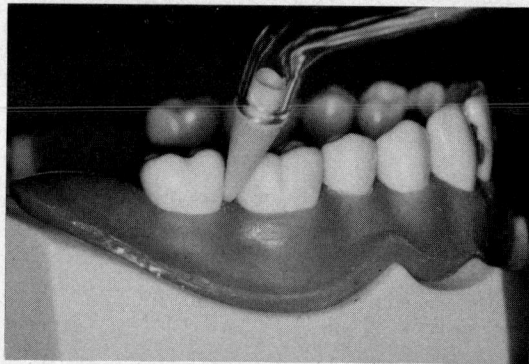

Fig. 19-43. PikPocket® is designed like a rubber tip stimulator and is also used to reach subgingivally with water or antimicrobial agents.

more targeted delivery into deep pockets by patients at home. (Figs. 19-42 through 19-44).

Chemomechanical subgingival irrigation for professional use

In-office subgingival delivery of antimicrobial agents has been used by many professionals for a number of years. Most of the early research centered around the delivery of chemical agents subgingivally with the use of the hand syringe (Hardy, Newman, and Strahan, 1982; Mazza, Newman, and Sims, 1981; Perry et al, 1984).

In recent years, the powered irrigation device has been fitted with a special handpiece and cannula for subgingival delivery in the operatory (Figs. 19-45 and 19-46). The cannula can be placed into the sulcus or pocket to enable professionals to deliver solutions under extremely low pressure directly into periodontal pockets.

Kelly and others (1985) compared delivery pressure of the Water Pik® powered irrigation device to that of the peristaltic pump and the hand syringe. Delivery force was more consistent and physiologically acceptable with the powered irrigator.

More recently, researchers have examined the use of the powered irrigator with specialized subgingival cannulae in the delivery of antimicrobial solutions. Watts and Newman (1986) found subgingival delivery to be clinically effective in reducing inflammation and pocket depth, but saw no significant difference between chlorhexidine

and placebo results. Researchers continue to investigate various antimicrobial concentrations and intervals of administration in addition to alternative methods of subgingival delivery. It is likely that further research will prove the attributes of powered oral irrigation for site-specific subgingival delivery of chemical agents, at a consistent rate and force, as an another adjunctive use of direct irrigation in the dental operatory.

In-office irrigation can be used following routine scaling and root planing to flush away calculus and plaque fragments and to introduce an antimicrobial agent to impede reestablishment of plaque.

Cannulas can deliver the irrigant deeper into the pocket than can a supragingival tip (Fig. 19-47). The cannula is a blunt needle which attaches to a special office-use handpiece. The cannula has either an end-port with the orifice at the end or a side-port with the orifice on the side. The choice is a matter of professional preference.

The cannula is used much like a periodontal probe. It is gently inserted approximately 3 mm into the pocket or sulcus. The footpedal is then activated, starting the gentle stream of liquid into the pocket. (Plate 1, C and D). The liquid should surround the tooth in the moatlike subgingival space and emerge from the pocket. (Plate 1, E). Move the cannula around the tooth and move on to the next site to be irrigated.

The cannula must be discarded after use. Disassemble the handpiece, autoclave it, and allow liq-

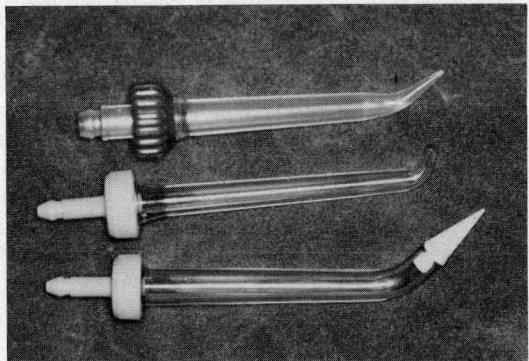

Fig. 19-44. From the top are the SulcusTip®, a standard irrigating tip, and a PickPocket® each of which is safe for home use.

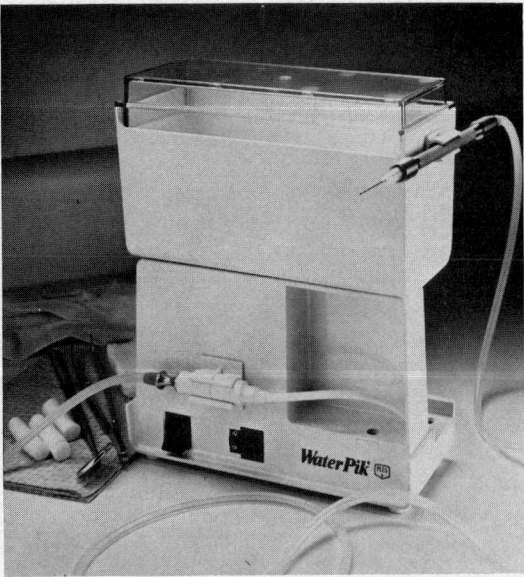

Fig. 19-45. The WaterPik® in-office irrigator with a cannula.

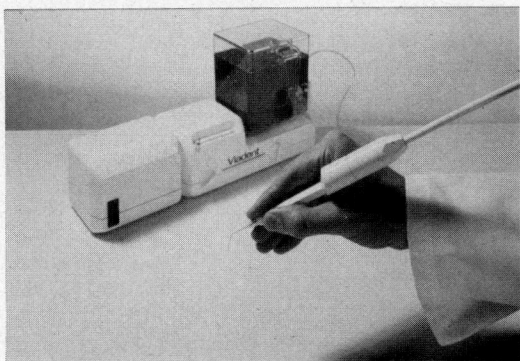

Fig. 19-46. The Viadent Via-Jet® irrigator with a cannula and handpiece with heater.

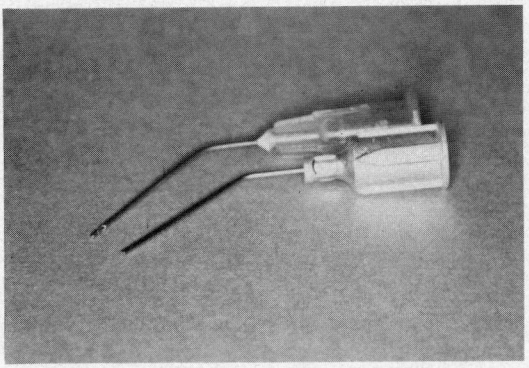

Fig. 19-47. Cannulae with side-port (top) and with end-port.

uid to flow through the tubing before and after use.

Placing an antimicrobial in the pocket after instrumentation can provide an opportunity to discuss how the patient can incorporate at-home irrigation with an antimicrobial agent appropriate for maintenance therapy.

DAILY PLAQUE CONTROL: CHEMICAL INHIBITION

Toothbrushes, floss, wood wedges, and the other implements of plaque disruption focus on *mechanical disruption* of plaque. Even the irrigator has a mechanical effect upon plaque. Dentifrices contain abrasives that remove or disorganize

plaque. This mechanical control has been the focus of daily plaque control for decades. Unfortunately, some people are unable to control their plaque even with conscientious effort. Patients with a low commitment to plaque control will be even less successful. Plaque seems to form readily or to be overlooked in the places where it can do the most harm—interproximally and in difficult-to-reach areas.

The last two decades, in particular the mid- to

Benefits and Applications of Oral Irrigation

Home Irrigaton

- Has potential to irrigate periodontal pockets
- Disrupts and flushes away some supragingival plaque
- Disrupts and flushes away subgingival loosely attached plaque
- Removes microscopic food particles that may contribute to health problems
- May be used with water or recommended antimicrobials
- Convenient and easy to use for daily therapy at home

Applications for Home Irrigation

- Gingivitis
- Gingivitis with coexisting periodontitis
- Poor oral hygiene
- Malpositioned teeth
- Orthodontics
- Prosthodontics
- Implants
- Orthognathic surgery

Professional Irrigation: Subgingival Delivery of Antimicrobials

- Used to augment skilled scaling and root planing
- Efficient
- Used during initial therapy as well as maintenance recall apppointments

Applications for Professional Irrigation

- After deep scaling, during initial and maintenance appointments
- During surgery
- Between visits to control microflora
  Note: In general, patients considered at high risk for bacteremia should be premedicated and carefully instructed before recommendation on oral irrigation is given. Research has demonstrated that oral irrigation poses no greater risk to these patients than brushing and flossing, but the usual precautions should be taken.

late 1980s, have begun a new era in plaque control. There are now several options to consider for the *chemical inhibition* of plaque. Antimicrobial agents reduce plaque proliferation and help control gingivitis. They do not replace mechanical oral hygiene; they augment it.

Various anticalculus dentifrices and oral rinses have appeared on the market since the mid-1980s. It is important to recognize that although these agents contain ingredients (usually pyrophosphates or zinc chloride) that can inhibit calculus formation, they do not exert an antiplaque effect. Their action is to keep calcium and phosphorus from precipitating into the plaque matrix on the teeth. Several other agents, some prescription and others available over the counter, do exert antiplaque effects.

Systemic antibiotics offer one option, although they typically are selected for patients who are experiencing rapid periodontal destruction or who have recurrent bouts with the disease. Patients with recurrent periodontitis seem to benefit from a course of systemic antibiotics in combination with subgingival root planing, monthly recall visits, and a program of daily plaque control (Lundstrom et al, 1984).

Two frequently cited agents are metronidazole and tetracycline. The disadvantages are that they affect the flora of the entire body and thus have undesirable effects. Also, clinicians often chose to reserve systemic antibiotics for general health situations that demand their use. They can be used for one or more short courses of treatment but generally are not selected for long-term maintenance therapy.

Chlorhexidine (0.2%) has been studied and used successfully in Europe for 2 decades as an antiplaque, antigingivitis topical rinse or gel. Research is unequivocal in establishing the agent's effectiveness. Chlorhexidine is known to cause taste alteration, which diminishes after product use ends. One study showed that the ability to taste salt was impaired (Lang et al, 1988). A 0.12% rinse, Peridex, was introduced in the United States in 1986 as a prescription agent. Side effects of reversible tooth-staining and altered taste sensation are reduced with the lower concentration but still occur. The agent can be used to help control plaque and gingivitis, particularly during initial therapy, when patients are mastering mechanical removal techniques and when healing is critical.

Chlorhexidine is toxic to red blood cells and to polymorphonucleated cells at a concentration of 0.02%. Cells are protected by serum (such as flows from the periodontal pocket) but apparently not by saliva (Gabler et al, 1987). Labeling information for the prescription agent does not limit the duration of its use. However, patients should be monitored for staining, taste alteration, tissue response, and patient compliance before suggesting (or assuming) its continued use.

Stannous fluoride also possesses antimicrobial properties. It is active against bacteria because of the stannous ion, which affects the ability of cells to metabolize polysaccharides. It can be administered subgingivally by a clinician at a concentration of 1.64%; bacteria require several weeks to return to baseline values (Mazza et al, 1981). Gel preparations of 0.4% can be used twice daily to help control plaque. The gels are brushed onto the teeth and then swished and expectorated. As with any prescription agent, stannous fluoride should be monitored for adverse effects and patient compliance.

Nonprescription agents are available for controlling plaque and gingivitis, too. Listerine, which contains a combination of essential oils, has demonstrated efficacy against plaque and gingivitis when used as a rinse, full strength, for 30 seconds twice daily (Axelsson and Lindhe, 1987; DePaola et al, 1986; Lamster et al, 1983). The studies used 20 ml of the product. Its major drawback is its strong taste and its 26.8% alcohol content. It is not as effective as chlorhexidine but can be used as a long-term maintenance rinse.

Viadent is available in nonprescription toothpaste and rinse forms. They contain sanguinaria, an alkaloid extract from the bloodroot plant. The cationic sanguinarine molecule combines chemically with dental plaque and remains detectable in the plaque for up to 4 hours after use. It is antimicrobial (Dzink and Socransky, 1985) and it appears to alter the receptor sites in freshly formed pellicle, reducing the ability of bacteria to adhere to it (Babu, 1986). Alcohol content is 10%. Short-term studies (1 month or less) indicate effectiveness for both toothpaste and oral rinse (Klewansky, 1984; Wennstrom and Lindhe 1985, 1986). One 6-month study suggests long-term ef-

ficacy for the toothpaste (Lobene, et al, 1986). Another 6-month study demonstrated statistical differences between Viadent and a placebo for plaque and gingivitis and showed no bacterial overgrowth (Palcanis, et al, 1986). Two longer-term studies with orthodontic subjects, using both the toothpaste and the oral rinse for 9 weeks (Miller et al, 1988) and 6 months (Hannah et al, 1989), suggest good effectiveness for this type of subject, known for problems with plaque and gingivitis.

Scope and Cepacol contain 0.05% cetylpyridinium chloride (CPC) as an antiplaque ingredient; Scope also contains domiphen bromide. Alcohol content ranges from 14% to 16%. CPC shows mild activity at the percentage included in these mouthwashes.

Plax is described as a prebrushing rinse that enables the mechanical action of the brush and floss to remove plaque more easily. Two short-term studies show activity; however, in both trials subjects brushed for only 15 seconds and did not use toothpaste. The effeciveness of this pretoothbrushing mouthrinse, compared with normal toothbrushing with a dentifrice, is undetermined (Emling and Yankell, 1985; Lobene et al, 1986). The active ingredient is not specified; the concentrations of sodium laurel sulfate and sodium borax (soaping agents) suggest that it may be a surfactant action. Sodium content is high in this product, which should not be recommended for people on sodium-restricted diets (Wagner et al, 1988).

Sodium bicarbonate and hydrogen peroxide have a synergistic antimicrobial effect (Miyasaki et al, 1986). However, clinical trials have been unable to demonstrate that using a slurry of these two agents with a toothbrush, oral irrigator, rubber tip, or periodontal aid was more effective than normal oral hygiene (Rosling, et al, 1982; Wolff, et al, 1982; Cerra and Killoy, 1982; West and King, 1983; Greenwell et al, 1983).

A direct comparison of 0.12% chlorhexidine with 1% hydrogen peroxide showed that hydrogen peroxide produced modest reductions in gingivitis and bleeding and no significant reduction in plaque, compared with chlorhexidine's dramatic reduction in all three parameters (Gusberti et al, 1988).

Other agents will undoubtedly emerge as the dental profession and the public look for ways to augment mechanical oral hygiene with chemical control. This area of development is particularly active; research is regularly reported on a wide array of agents. An increased number of options will make it easier for clinicians to suggest alternatives that fit patients' needs and preferences.

CONCLUSION

This chapter has introduced the most important function of a dental hygienist—helping the patient learn to prevent disease. The task is twofold: (1) the information and advice must be accurate and up to date, and (2) a clear understanding of each patient's needs and motivation "windows" must be developed and used to design a prevention program.

Efforts made today may not have an effect for months or years. But today's words may be the ones that result in someone's decision to adopt good health behavior and prevent disease. This is our fundamental objective as dental professionals and the most significant measure of our success.

ACTIVITIES

1. Discuss the need for developing a preventive philosophy. Write down a few of the ideals you value, and share them with other students in small groups. Stress that with such values, right or wrong is not an issue. Working in small groups, develop the components of a preventive philosophy, and present your group's philosophy to the entire class.
2. Investigate alternative methods of brushing. Demonstrate these methods and discuss the merits of all brushing techniques.
3. Make up several trays with samples of the additional tools for cleaning or providing oral physiotherapy. Practice with these aids on a typodont.
4. After sufficient practice with brushing techniques and the use of cleaning aids, form small goups. Each group is given an envelope filled with slips of paper asking for a demonstration of a particular facet of instruction. Select a slip of paper and demonstrate what is called for to the small group.
5. Present sample dental health education assessments. Discuss these and develop individualized education plans to meet the sample patient's needs. This can be done with the entire class or in small groups.
6. The following exercise may take several weeks to complete. It is designed to help each dental hygiene student bring personal oral health to an optimal level. Complete a dental health assessment with a classmate. Plan for this patient's needs. Set

aside one (or several) instruction sessions and a follow-up evaluation session. (As these concepts and instruction methods are new to most students, instructor participation at each step is recommended.)
7. Provide individualized preventive education for a clinical patient. Keep a journal of events documenting the initial assessment, the educational plan, the instruction sequence, and the follow-up evaluation. Share this in a small group for feedback and suggestions.
8. Invite community hygienists, preventive therapists, or dentists to present a seminar on the preventive education format that is used in their practice settings. Share preventive education materials and discuss experiences.
9. Prepare a review of the literature on one or more of the antimicrobial agents. Conduct a panel discussion of the relative merits and indications for the each of the agents.
10. Select a patient who is having difficulty controlling plaque and gingivitis with brushing and flossing. Provide the patient with an irrigator and ask him or her to irrigate twice daily with water. Document the before and after appearance of the soft tissue with photographs. Document the plaque using a plaque index. What effects did you observe with the irrigation?
11. Use a microscope to observe bacterial form and motility in supra- and subgingival plaque samples.
12. Prepare a review of the literature on the relative merits of delivering chemotherapeutic agents subgingivally. What new research suggests that such a procedure may be appropriate before and/or after instrumentation?

REVIEW QUESTIONS

1. Discuss the hygienist's role as educator.
2. How has oral research affected patient education?
3. What is the value of presenting an indivdualized approach to education?
4. State the rationale for using the following methods in patient education:
   a. Small step size
   b. Active participation
   c. Immediate feedback
   d. Self-pacing
5. After three preventive visits the patient demonstrates good brushing techniques, but the plaque index is not improving and inflammation is still obvious. Which of the following responses is appropriate?
   a. Review brushing once again, emphasizing the need to place the brush in an overlapping sequence.
   b. Send the patient for medical consultation.

c. Talk to the patient about what you have observed.

d. Decide that you have tried, "it's his mouth," and finish the prophylaxis.

6. Which of the following are short-term motivators and which are long-term motivators? Also identify the need level appeal to which the statement is directed.

a. You'll have more cavities the next time if you don't brush your teeth.

b. You meet many people in your line of work; keeping your breath fresh with clean teeth and healthy gingiva must be important to you.

c. The bleeding will continue unless you get serious about flossing.

d. You really show you care about yourself by spending the time to clean your teeth after lunch at work.

7. Indicate whether you agree or disagree with the following statement and why: "Following a specific technique for brushing is the most important part of preventing dental disease."

8. Besides a soft brush and dental floss, what additional tools might you suggest for a patient who has wide embrasures after periodontal surgery, a fixed maxillary bridge, and a removable lower partial denture?

9. Why is it important to emphasize the following in patient instruction?

a. Using a disclosing agent

b. Brushing in a sequence

c. Paying particular attention to the anterior lingual area

d. Caring for the tongue and soft tissue

10. List five prevention topics that should be included in dental health education.

11. True or false:

a. The oral irrigator's usefulness is limited to flushing away food debris.

b. The oral irrigator changes the quality if not the quantity of plaque on the teeth.

c. The irrigator (even with a supragingival standard tip) can deliver liquids approximately halfway into the pocket.

d. A cannula is a special cone-shaped plastic tip used by the patient at home to carry antimicrobials to the pocket.

e. Irrigators are ideal for delivering antimicrobials subgingivally.

12. List the active agent in each of the following antimicrobials and indicate which is a prescription agent:

a. Listerine

b. Peridex

c. Viadent

d. Cepacol

e. Plax

f. Stannous fluoride

REFERENCES

Abrams K, Caton JG, and Polson AM: Histologic comparisons of interproximal gingival tissues related to the presence or absence of bleeding, J Periodontal 55:629, 1984.

Aday B: An evaluation of an oral irrigation device's ability to quantitatively reduce the bacterial count of spirochetes, filaments, fusiforms, and motile bacteria from subgingival plaque. Thesis in the Department of Periodontics. University of Missouri at Kansas City, 1982.

Alfant M, Walker CB, and Bhaskar S: Local delivery of tetracycline as a possible adjunct to conventional periodontal therapy, J Dent Res 62(special issue); Abst 1083, 1983.

Amato R et al: Interproximal gingival inflammation related to the conversion of a bleeding to nonbleeding state, J Periodontol 57:63, 1986.

Arnim SS: The use of disclosing agents for measuring tooth cleanliness, J Periodontol 34:227, 1963.

Axelsson and Lindhe J: Efficacy of mouthrinses in inhibiting dental plaque and gingivitis in man, J Clin Periodontol 14:205, 1987.

Aziz-Gandour IA, and Newman HN: The effects of a simplified oral hygiene regime plus supragingival irrigation with chlorhexidine or metronidazole on chronic inflammatory periodontal disease, J Clin Periodontol 13:228, 1986.

Babu JP, et al: Anti-plaque activity of a sanguinaria-containing oral rinse: an *in vitro* study, Compend Contin Educ 7:(supp):S209, 1986.

Barton J and Abelson D: The clinical efficacy of wooden interdental cleaners in gingivitis reduction. Clin Prev Dent 9(6):17, 1987.

Boyd RL, et al: Effect of self-administered daily irrigation with 0.02% SnF_2 on periodontal disease activity. J Clin Perio, 12:420, 1985.

Boyer EM, and Nikias MK: Self-reported compliance with a preventive dental regimen, Clin Prevent Dent 5(1):3, 1983.

Bakdash MB: Patient motivation and education: a conceptual model, Clin Prevent Dent 1(2):10, 1979.

Bass CC: The optimum characteristics of toothbrushes for personal oral hygiene, Dent Items 70:696, 1948.

Brady JM, et al: Electron microscopic study of the effect of water jet devices on dental plaque, J Dent Res 52:1310, 1973.

Brownstein C, et al: Gingival irrigation with chlorhexidine resolves naturally occurring gingivitis. Presented at American Academy of Periodontology annual meeting, 1987, San Antonio, Tex.

Carranza FA Jr: Glickman's clinical periodontology, Philadelphia, 1979, WB Saunders Co.

Caton JG, and Polson AM: The interdental bleeding index: a simplified procedure for monitoring gingival health, Compend Contin Educ 6(2):88, 1985.

Cerra M, and Killoy W: The effect of sodium bicarbonate and hydrogen peroxide on the microbial flora of periodontal pockets, J Periodontol 53:599, 1982.

Ciancio SG, et al: The effect of oral irrigation with Listerine on plaque, gingivitis, and the subgingival microflora, J Dent Res 66 (special issue): Abst 1028, 1987.

Ciancio SG: Free communication presentation, #FC410,

ADA/FDI Joint World Dental Congress, Washington, D.C., 1988.

Cobb CM, Rogers RL, and Killoy WJ: Ultrastructure examination of human periodontal pockets following the use of an oral irrigation device in vivo. J Periodontol 3:155-163, 1988.

Corn H, and Marks M: The integration of a preventive dentistry program into a dental practice. Cont Dent Educ, University of Pennsylvania School of Dental Medicine 1:No. 10, 1978.

Cumming BR, and Löe H: Optimal dosage and method of delivering chlorhexidine solutions for the inhibition of dental plaque, J Periodont Res 8:57, 1973.

DePaola LG, et al: Chemotherapeutic inhibition of supragingival dental plaque and gingivitis development, J Dent Res 65(special issue): Abst 941, 1986.

Derdivanis JP, Bushmaker S, and Dagenais F: Effects of a mouthwash in an irrigating device on accumulation and maturation of dental plaque, J Periodontol 49:81, 1978.

Dunbar S: Term coined for continuing education for dental hygienists.

Dzink JL, and Socransky SS: Comparative in vitro activity of sanguinarine against oral microbial isolates, Antimicrobial Agents and Chemotherapy 27:663, 1985.

Eakle WS, Ford C, and Boyd RL: Depth of penetration in periodontal pockets with oral irrigation, J Clin Periodontol 13:39, 1985.

Emling RC and Yankell SL: First clinical studies of a new prebrushing mouthrinse, Compend Contin Educ 9:636, 1985.

Evans RI: Motivating changes in oral hygiene behavior: some social psychological perspectives, J Prevent Dent 5(4):14, 1978.

French CI and Friedman LA: The plaque removal ability of waxed and unwaxed dental floss, Dent Hyg 49:449, 1975.

Gabler WL, Roberts D, and Harold W: The effect of chlorhexidine on blood cells, J Perio Res 22:150, 1987.

Greenwell, et al: Clinical and microbiologic effectiveness of Keyes' method of oral hygiene on human periodontitis treated with and without surgery, JADA 106:457, 1983.

Gusberti FA, et al: Microbiological and clinical effects of chlorhexidine digluconate and hydrogen peroxide mouthrinses on developing plaque and gingivits, J Clin Periodontol 15:60, 1988.

Hannah J, et al: Long-term clinical evaluation of toothpaste and oral rinse containing sanguinaria extract in controlling plaque, gingival inflammation, and sulcular bleeding during orthodontic treatment. American J Ortho, in press, 1989.

Hardy JH, Newman HN, and Strahan JD: Direct irrigation and subgingival plaque, J Clin Periodontol 9:57, 1982.

Hoover, DR, et al: The comparative effectiveness of a pulsating oral irrigator as an adjunct in maintaining oral health, J Clin Periodontol 42:37, 1971.

Johansson L, Oster B, and Hamp S: Evaluation of cause-related periodontal therapy and compliance with maintenance care recommendations, J Clin Periodontol 11:689, 1984.

Katz S, McDonald J, and Stookey G: Preventive dentistry in action, Upper Montclair, NJ, 1979, DCP Publishing.

Kelly A, et al: Pressures recorded during periodontal pocket irrigation, J Periodontol 56:297, 1985.

Klewansky P, and Vernier D: Sanguinarine and the control of plaque in dental practice, Compend Contin Educ 7(supp):S94, 1984.

Kornman KS: The role of supragingival plaque in the prevention and treatment of periodontal diseases: a review of current concepts, J Perio Res 21:5, 1986.

Lamster, I, et al: The effect of Listerine antiseptic on reduction of existing plaque and gingivitis, Clin Prev Dent 5(6):12, 1983.

Lang N, et al: Quality-specific taste impairment following the application of chlorhexidine digluconate mouthrinses, J Clin Periodontol 15:43, 1988.

Lang NP, and Raber K: Use of oral irrigators as vehicle for the application of antimicrobial agents in chemical plaque control, J Clin Periodontol 8:177, 1981.

Lang NP, and Ramseier-Grossman K: Optimal dosage of chlorhexidine digluconate in chemical plaque control when applied by the oral irrigator, J Clin Periodontol 8:189, 1981.

Listgarten MA: Nature of periodontal diseases: pathogenic mechanisms, J Periodont Res 22:172, 1987.

Listgarten MA, and Levin S: Positive correlation between the proportions of subgingival spirochetes and motile bacteria and the susceptibility of human subjects to periodontal deterioration, J Clin Periodontol 8:122, 1981.

Listgarten M, and Schifter C: Differential darkfield microscopy of sub-gingival bacteria as an aid in selecting recall intervals: results after 18 months, J Clin Periodontol 9:305, 1982.

Lobene RR: The effect of a pulsed water pressure cleansing device on oral health, J Periodontol 40:667, 1969.

Lobene R, and Soparker P: Use of dental floss, effect on plaque and gingivitis, Clin Prevent Dent 4(1):5, 1982.

Lobene RR, et al: Plaque removal with a prebrushing mouthrinse, 65 (special issue):Abst #406 (IADR), 1986.

Lobene RR, Soparkar PM, and Newman MB: The effects of a sanguinaria dentifrice on plaque and gingivitis, Compend Contin Educ 7(Supp):S185, 1986.

Loesche, WJ, and Syed SA: Bacteriology of human experimental gingivitis—effect on plaque and gingivitis scores, Infection and Immunity 21:830, 1978.

Lundstrom A, Johansson L, and Hamp S: Effect of combined systemic antimicrobial therapy and mechanical plaque control in patients with recurrent periodontal disease, J Clin Periodontol 11:321, 1984.

Maslow AH: Motivation and personality, New York, 1970, Harper & Row.

Mauriello SM, et al: Effectiveness of three interproximal cleaning devices, Clin Prev Dent 9(3):18, 1987.

Mazza JE, Newman MG, and Sims TN: Clinical and antimicrobial effect of stannous fluoride on periodontitis, J Clin Periodontol 8:203, 1981.

Melcer S, and Feldman S: Preventive dentistry teaching methods—improving oral hygiene: a summary of research, Clin Prevent Dent 6(1):7, 1979.

Miller RA, McIver JE, and Gunsolley JC: The effects of sanguinaria extract on plaque retention and gingival health in active orthodontic patients, J Clin Orthodontics, 1988 (in press).

Palcanis KG, et al: Longitudinal evalution of sanguinaria: clinical and microbiologic studies, (supp)7:S179, 1986.

Parsons LG, et al: Effect of sanguinaria extract on established plaque and gingivitis when delivered as a manual rinse or under pressure in an oral irrigator, J Clin Periodontol 14:381, 1987.

Perry DA, et al: Stannous fluoride adjunct to root planing, clinical and antimicrobial effects, J Dent Res 63 (special issue): Abst 702, 1984.

Pipe P, et al: Developing a plaque control program: a motivational approach to involving patients in dental care, Berkeley, Calif, 1972, Praxis Publishing Co.

Reitman WB, et al: Proximal surface cleaning by dental floss, Clin Prev Dent 2:7, 1980.

Rosling BG, et al: Topical chemical antimicrobial therapy in the management of the subgingival microflora and periodontal disease, J Periodont Res 17:541, 1982.

Sanders PC, Linden GJ, and Newman HN: The effects of a simplified mechanical oral hygiene regime plus supragingival irrigation with chlorhexidine or metronidazole on subgingival plaque, J Clin Periodontol 13:237, 1986.

Schifter, et al: A comparison of plaque removal effectiveness of an electric versus a manual toothbrush, Clin Prevent Dent 5(5):15, 1983.

Southard GL, et al: Effect of sanguinaria extract on development of plaque and gingivitis when supragingivally delivered as a manual rinse or under pressure in an oral irrigator, J Clin Periodontol 14:377, 1987.

Spindel L, and Person P: Floss design and effectivenss of interproximal plaque removal, Clin Prev Dent 9(3):3, 1987.

Squillaro RC, Cohen DW, and Laster L: A comparison of micirobial plaque disclosants after personal oral hygiene instruction and prophylaxis, J Prevent Dent 2:3, 1975.

Stevens AW Jr: Comparison effectiveness of variable diameter versus unwaxed floss, J Periodontol 51:666, 1980.

Tabita P, et al: Effectiveness of supragingival plaque control on the development of subgingival plaque and gingival inflammation in patients with moderate pocket depth, J Clin Periodontol 52:88, 1981.

Tan AE: The role of visual feedback by a disclosing agent, J Clin Periodontol 7:140, 1980.

Tempel TR, Marcil JFA, and Seibert JS: Comparison of water irrigation and oral rinsing on clearance of soluble and particulate materials from the oral cavity, J Clin Periodontol 46:391, 1975.

Waerhaug J: The interdental brush and its place in operative and crown and bridge dentistry, J Oral Rehabil 33:107, 1976.

Wagner, MJ, et al: Sodium retention from rinsing with commercial mouthwashes, J Dent Res 67 (special issue): Abst 2312, 1988.

Watts EA, and Newman HN: Clinical effects on chronic periodontitis of a simplified system of oral hygiene including subgingival pulsated jet irrigation with chlorhexidine, J Clin Periodontol 13:666, 1986.

Weinstein P: Humanistic application of behavioral strategies in oral hygiene instruction, Clin Prevent Dent 4(3):15, 1982.

Wennstrom J, and Lindhe J: Some effects of a sanguinarine-containing mouthrinse on developing plaque and gingivitis, J Clin Periodontol 12:867, 1985.

Wennstrom J, and Lindhe J: The effect of mouthrinses on parameters characterizing human periodontal disease, J Clin Periodontol 13:86, 1986.

West BL: An evaluation of an oral irrigating device's ability to reduce the microbial count of subgingival plaque at six millimeters in depth. Thesis in the Department of Periodontics, University of Missouri, Kansas City, 1982.

West TL, and King WJ: Toothbrushing with hydrogen peroxide-sodium bicarbonate compared to toothpowder and water in reducing periodontal pocket suppuration darkfield bacterial counts, J Periodontol 54:339, 1983.

White CL, et al: The effect of supervised water irrigation on the subgingival microflora of untreated gingivitis and periodontitis, J Dent Res 67(special issue): Abst 2298, 1988.

Wolff LF, et al: Phase contrast microscopic evaluation of subgingival plaque in combination with either conventional or antimicrobial home treatment of patients with periodontal inflammation, J Periodont Res 17:537, 1982.

Yankell S, and Emling R: Understanding dental products: what you should know and what your patient should know, Contin Dental Educ 1(7), 1978.

20 NUTRITIONAL SELF-ASSESSMENT AND MODIFICATIONS

OBJECTIVES: *The reader will be able to*

1. Describe the role of dietary assessment and planning in dental hygiene care.
2. Briefly describe the ways in which diet can affect the overall health of the body and specifically of the oral cavity.
3. Identify the basic role of each of the following nutrients in the health of the patient:
   a. Carbohydrates
   b. Proteins
   c. Lipids
   d. Vitamins
   e. Minerals
   f. Water
4. Describe the usefulness and limitations of the Recommended Dietary Allowances (RDAs) and the four food groups in assessing a person's diet and in recommending modifications.
5. Describe how carbohydrates and plaque promote caries.
6. Explain how diet has been shown to influence cancer formation.
7. Explain strategies for assessing a patient's diet using a 1-day diet review or a 3-day or 7-day diary.
8. Conduct a dietary assessment for a patient, using the self-assessment strategy.
9. Given a variety of completed dietary assessments, assist each patient in determining which components of the diet could be changed, why they should be modified, and how the modification could be accomplished.
10. Identify several environmental factors that affect whether modifications are likely to occur following the self-assessment session.
11. Conduct a follow-up, reinforcement session as part of dental care to evaluate the progress the patient is making and to assist the patient in identifying alternative approaches to diet modification.

The growing knowledge and awareness of the relationship between good dietary habits and good general health have brought nutritional assessment and dietary counseling into focus as essential components of dental hygiene care. Many of the effects of dietary habits are clearly reflected in the oral cavity, because poor nutrition has negative effects on hard and soft oral tissues as well as on general well-being. Dental hygienists see their patients more frequently and more regularly than do most other health care providers. Thus the hygienist has more opportunity to detect dietary

problems and help the patient adopt changes (Diet, 1984). The hygienist needs to know how to assess a patient's diet, what changes are indicated by the results, and when a patient's nutritional problems require the expertise of a dietitian.

Private dental practices that focus on prevention include nutritional assessment for new patients, with periodic review at recall intervals for established patients in the practice. Other sites, such as hospitals, nursing homes, day care centers, and other community-based settings include nutritional counseling as a significant part of the overall program to improve general and oral health.

Any dental professional who will be assessing patients' diets and helping patients identify changes needs a complete course in nutrition, a good grounding in communication and basic counseling skills, and supervised clinical experience with a range of patient cases. This can be accomplished as part of the educational preparation with clinic patients. This chapter provides only a survey of basic nutrition and an introduction to the philosophy of nutritional assessment and patient-centered dietary counseling.

For clinicians who understand the basics of proper nutrition in general and in oral health in particular and who include a dietary focus in their everyday clinical care, a dietary assessment for every patient is the best way to ensure that the focus is established and maintained.

The assessment can be a routine component of the overall assessment phase of dental hygiene care and be the means for identifying patients for whom simple dietary counseling is necessary and also those who may need referral to a dietitian or physician. It may also identify those patients whose diets are well within normal limits and who do not need modifications. The critical point, as with the gathering of all other assessment data, is that the "assumption" of need no longer determines how dietary or nutritional counseling is planned into care. Assessment information can help both the patient and the dental hygienist arrive at a well-informed decision about the need to proceed with further discussions of diet.

IMPORTANCE OF DIET IN GENERAL AND ORAL HEALTH

"We are what we eat." is a well-worn, yet appropriate, cliche. Dietary patterns dictate how well the body grows and functions. Failure to consume appropriate amounts of carbohydrates, lipids, proteins, vitamins, minerals, and water can result in general fatigue, dysfunction, and disease.

The first three nutrients (carbohydrates, proteins, and lipids) provide calories for the body. Most of the body's energy is derived from carbohydrates. They make up a major portion of most diets, as they are reasonably inexpensive, easily assimilated, and frequently palatable.

Carbon, oxygen, and hydrogen are the three elements that make up *carbohydrates*. The simplest form of a carbohydrate is a *monosaccharide* (or simple sugar), such as glucose, fructose, or galactose. *Disaccharides* are double sugars made up of two of the simple sugars. Sucrose, lactose, and maltose are disaccharides. The most complex carbohydrates, polysaccharides, are made up of several units of one type of monosaccharide. Starch, dextrins, cellulose, pectins, and glycogen are examples of *polysaccharides*. Energy becomes available for use when complex carbohydrates, such as sucrose, lactose, and starch, are broken down to their simplest form (monosaccharides) and then are metabolized in the cells to form carbon dioxide and water; a release of energy accompanies this process.

Metabolism makes energy available for the functioning of the organism and produces, maintains, or breaks down protoplasm, the basic substance of cells.

Carbohydrates serve other functions in the body. They are an essential component of nerve tissue and can facilitate the oxidation of fats. They contribute to the structural elements of the body, such as collagen. Because complex carbohydrates, such as whole grains, contribute to food bulk, they assist normal digestion and elimination. Dietary carbohydrates should constitute from 50% to 65% of the total diet; this is an increase of approximately 10% over levels previously recommended. Increased complex carbohydrates can replace the less desirable fats that have been shown to increase the risk of heart disease and cancer (Good news, 1987). Carbohydrates, particularly whole grains, can help meet the body's need for fiber, generally accepted as an important way to help the body's alimentary canal function correctly (Looking for fiber, 1987). Oats, used in addition to a diet low in cholesterol, can reduce serum cholesterol levels even further (Reducing cholesterol, 1986).

If too much carbohydrate is ingested, the excess is converted to fat and deposited in the body's adipose tissues. Therefore a large intake of carbohydrates can lead to obesity. Because fermentable carbohydrates are essential for the development of dental caries, frequent ingestion, particularly of retentive carbohydrates (such as caramels and hard candies), promotes tooth decay and is unhealthful (Firestone, 1982; Nizel, 1981; Randolph and Dennison, 1981; Diet, 1984).

Proteins supply energy for the body, but their more critical role is as an essential component of body tissues, enzymes, and hormones. Approximately 50% of dry body weight is protein. It plays a major role in the body's chemical reactions in digestion, assimilation, and metabolism. A lack of protein in the diet can have major consequences if protein is lost from the system and not replaced (Nizel, 1981).

Lipids, a term used for fats and fatlike substances, also have important functions in the body. They are integral components of cells and cell membranes. They are necessary for normal growth and skin health, and they carry the fat-soluble vitamins A, D, E, and K. Stored fats help insulate and cushion the body. Additionally, they lend flavor to food, and they are digested slowly, thus reducing hunger sensations. They make up approximately 40% of the American diet, a figure that is too high in light of recent findings linking fats and cancer (to be discussed later in this chapter) and to heart disease. Foods should be selected to minimize fats from meats, margarine, and cooking oils. Fats provide 9 calories per gram, while carbohydrates and proteins provide only 4.

Caloric intake from these three nutrients should balance with calories expended in daily activities. If intake exceeds energy used, the excess will be converted to and stored as fat deposits, and weight gain will occur. Conversely, if intake is lower than output, weight loss will occur. Because of the multiple functions that these three nutrients serve, none of them should be strictly eliminated from the diet. Moderation in all three, with the total calories consumed balanced with energy used, is a healthier approach to weight control.

Vitamins, in contrast to carbohydrates, proteins, and fats, do not supply energy. They function as catalysts or as coenzymes to regulate metabolism and to assist in forming body tissues. As mentioned earlier, vitamins A, D, E, and K are fat-soluble vitamins. Any excess is stored and can cause an adverse effect if this excess reaches critical levels. The other vitamins are water soluble and thus are not readily stored in the body. Excess amounts are largely excreted.

The vitamin B complex consists of 11 different vitamins. All of them are water soluble and are found primarily in liver and yeast. All but three (inositol, choline, and para-aminobenzoic acid) are classified as necessary nutrients for human beings. The complete metabolism of carbohydrates depends on the presence of adequate amounts of each of the six energy-releasing vitamins: niacin, thiamin, riboflavin, pantothenic acid, vitamin B_6, and biotin (Nizel, 1981).

Folic acid and vitamin B_{12} are essential in the formation of red blood cells. Vitamin B_6 (pyridoxine) is an energy-releasing vitamin, and it serves as an antianemic coenzyme (Nizel, 1981). Vitamin B_6 deficiency is often associated with the use of oral contraceptives. High doses of this vitamin are often recommended to help combat premenstrual syndrome; if this malady is suspected, a dietitian should be consulted in order to determine appropriate supplementation, as vitamin B_6 can be toxic (Fahey et al, 1987b; Vitamin B_6 toxicity, 1986).

Because the B-complex vitamins are so interrelated, a discrete deficiency of any one of them probably does not occur; rather there is a deficiency of many. Therefore, for symptoms of Vitamin B deficiency, a supplement that includes the range of B vitamins is indicated.

Ascorbic acid, vitamin C, is also a water-soluble vitamin and is found in citrus fruits, red and green peppers, parsley, turnip greens, and other leafy vegetables. Vitamin C plays an essential role in collagen synthesis, and therefore it is an important component in tissue formation, particularly in wound healing. A person with a vitamin C deficiency often bruises easily because of capillary fragility. Vitamin C is involved in phagocytosis and acts as a detoxifying agent. Its presence can increase the resistance of traumatized tissues to infection. In addition, it influences the formation of hemoglobin. Appropriate amounts of the vitamin (60 to 100 mg daily) are obviously essential for health, including oral health. The soft tissue of the oral cavity, particularly the gingiva, is less susceptible to irritation and bleeding if vitamin C in proper dosages is ingested.

Vitamin C is often mislabeled the "sunshine vitamin," probably because of its association with orange juice and that industry's advertising approaches. However, the real sunshine vitamin is vitamin D, because of its formation in the presence of ultraviolet light. It is absorbed through the digestive tract as it is ingested in food and drink. Less dietary vitamin D is required if there is extensive exposure to sunshine. It is commonly added to milk to ensure a dietary source. As vitamin D is best absorbed in the presence of calcium and phosphorus, milk is an ideal medium.

The primary function of vitamin D relates to the absorption and homeostasis of calcium. It distributes calcium and phosphorus ions within the bony matrix. Therefore it is critical to the proper formation of teeth and their supporting bone.

Vitamin D can be extremely toxic if taken in excess. Large amounts can cause intense calcification of bone, formation of renal calculi, and calcification of blood vessels. This is one instance where megavitamin doses can be extremely harmful (Nizel, 1981; Randolph and Dennison, 1981).

Vitamin A is another vitamin that can result in severe toxicity if it is ingested in large amounts. Yellow skin and oral mucosa (carotenemia), anorexia, hyperirritability, skin lesions, bone decalcification, and increased intracranial pressures are signs of toxicity.

In its proper dosage, vitamin A is essential for proper vision, control of the differentiation of epithelium in mucus-secreting structures, bone remodeling, normal activity of the reproductive system, and the activity of the body's enzymes. Therefore it is important to the oral cavity with its plethora of mucus-secreting structures and as bone is remodeled to adjust to occlusal patterns and orthodontic treatment. Milk is fortified with vitamin A, and the vitamin is found in many vegetables.

Vitamin K is produced by microorganisms in the intestinal tract. It also occurs in green vegetables, egg yolk, and liver. It is essential for the formation of prothrombin and other clotting factors. Blood will not clot without prothrombin, thus vitamin K is important in health and disease. As it is produced in the intestinal tract, it is not given as a supplement except in instances where pregnancy or an imminent surgical procedure indicates the need.

The last of the four fat-soluble vitamins is vitamin E. Its primary functions relate to reproduction and membrane stability, probably because of its role as an antioxidant in reducing the destruction of lipids carrying other fat-soluble vitamins and necessary fatty acids (Nizel, 1981).

Several inorganic elements that are essential for health are found in quantifiable amounts in the human body. Calcium, phosphorus, magnesium, sodium, potassium, sulfur, iron, and chlorine all contribute to the growth, development, and function of the body. Trace amounts of elements, including copper, manganese, zinc, iodine, cobalt, molybdenum, selenium, and fluoride, affect the body's biologic systems. Besides these, several other elements found in the body are not considered essential for health or have not been fully studied.

The most critical elements in terms of dietary intake are calcium and phosphorus for the development and health of bones and teeth, iron for hemoglobin formation, iodine for thyroid regulation, and fluoride for decay-resistant teeth. The others are critical as well, but usually are ingested in adequate amounts if the aforementioned specific elements are found in the diet (Nizel, 1981; Randolph and Dennison, 1982).

Calcium is receiving increased attention because of its link to osteoporosis, a debilitating nutritional disease in which calcium is depleted from the bones, causing skeletal deformities and increasing the likelihood of bone fractures. This problem is most evident in postmenopausal women, who seem to lose calcium from the system more rapidly. Calcium absorption decreases with age. Impaired renal function, decreased intestinal absorption of vitamin D, and low exposure to sunshine seem to contribute to the problem. Fluoride consumption helps retard the loss of calcium; the concentrations found in community water supplies provide a satisfactory amount. The elderly require from 50% to 100% more vitamin D than young adults, and calcium intake should be 700 to 1000 mg per day. Additional research on the effects of dietary supplementation is needed (Schaafsma et al, 1987).

Calcium deficiency is prevalent and should be checked for as a part of routine nutritional assessment and recommendations. Persons susceptible to osteoporosis include young, growing people and adults who do not consume dairy products; elderly, sedentary people living primarily indoors; and patients with anorexia nervosa (Schaafsma et al, 1987). One cup of milk contains approximately 300 mg of calcium; people who cannot or will not consume dairy products can take calcium carbonate supplements. Such a recommendation should be made even for women as young as 20 years of age and certainly for those of 40 or more years (Fahey et al, 1987b). Patients should also learn that exercise and vitamin D help bone strength and that cigarette smoking, caffeine, and alcohol appear to be detrimental to calcium balance (Sutnick, 1987).

Water, which serves as the fluid medium for the body's chemical and physical reactions, is probably the most critical dietary component. Without water, all the other nutrients would be incapable of acitivity. Water carries nutrients and oxygen to all parts of the body through the blood and the lymphatic system. It helps control body temperature and removes metabolic waste in urine and sweat. The average adult consumes and excretes about 2 to 3 quarts of water each day in various forms. People who work in a warm climate and perspire greatly require more. The body needs six to eight 8-ounce glasses of water each day, whether we feel thirsty or not (Getting the most, 1986).

People require different amounts of certain nutrients during times of stress. If an individual is marginally deficient in particular nutrients, stress may make the condition worse. In fact, undernutrition is a form of physical stress (Kipp, 1985). Alcoholics place a special form of stress on the body, frequently have poor diets, and suffer additional nutritional depletion through adverse alcohol-nutrient interactions (Lieber, 1984). Cancer patients have special nutritional needs (Lum et al, 1984). Poor nutrition reduces the probability of survival of victims of head and neck cancer. This may be due, in part, to compromised immune responses (Brookes, 1985; Homsy et al, 1986).

Rapid growth, pregnancy, lactation, and advanced age indicate special nutritional needs (Fahey et al, 1987a, 1987b). Athletes require increased levels of certain nutrients and can improve performance by decreasing certain types of food and drink (American Dietetic Association, 1987a; Wilmore and Freud, 1986). Deuster and colleagues (1986) reported that highly trained women athletes consumed diets that exceeded some of the RDA values and that were substantially below recommendations for some nutrients.

Consuming too much as well as too little of most of the nutrients can increase the body's propensity for disease. Obesity, scurvy, rickets, and dental caries are prime examples of conditions based largely on deleterious dietary habits.

With the mention of dental caries as a nutritional disease, it may become more apparent that nutrition may have a direct effect on oral health as well as on general physical well-being. The oral cavity has been described as a barometer of general health (Randolph and Dennison, 1977; Randolph, 1981). This is particularly true in relation to nutritional problems. The nature of the oral structures allows them to reflect the body's nutritional maladies. The oral mucosa may appear extremely pallid or quite red. The texture of the tissue may indicate edema or friability. Cracks or fissures in the corners of the mouth or a heavily coated tongue may be signs that the general health of the individual is less than ideal. The presence of a large number of carious lesions provides information about the patient's consumption of fermentable carbohydrates (Randolph and Dennison, 1981).

TOXICITY

The preceding section mentions the toxic effects of some vitamins taken in large quantities. This is true for the fat-soluble vitamins (A, D, E, and K), for vitamin C, and for pyridoxine (B_6), which recently was found to produce toxic effects, including severe sensory nervous system dysfunction and ataxia (Schaumberg et al, 1983). Minerals such as zinc, fluoride, and iron, essential in prescribed amounts, produce toxic effects in large doses (Hamilton and Whitney, 1982; Randolph and Dennison, 1981).

In recent years there has been a widespread trend toward taking large doses of vitamin C to prevent or cure infectious diseases and cancer. No well-controlled studies have supported this practice, and several have failed to show significant differences between vitamin C and a placebo. In addition, large doses of vitamin C raise the uric acid level or urine (sometimes triggering gout in susceptible persons); they obscure the results of some medical tests; and they impair the ability of white blood cells to kill bacteria, actually worsening infections. They may cause kidney stones, affect fertility, and induce a deficiency rebound in newborns whose mothers routinely took large doses.

Toxic reactions to large doses of vitamins are becoming more of a problem since the awareness of good nutrition has grown among the general public. Some people have erroneously assumed that more of a good thing is better. Self-prescribed doses may far exceed needed amounts and may be seen as a substitute for eating proper foods. In addition, lay articles advocating the use of megavitamin doses are omnipresent, unwittingly recommending levels of vitamins or minerals that not only exceed what is needed for normal functioning but that actually produce negative effects. In some cases the toxic response is very similar to the deficiency symptoms, which may prompt the person to take even more of the nutrient. It is therefore very important during a nutritional assessment to inquire about what vitamin supplements are being taken, in what doses, and with what frequency (Hamilton and Whitney, 1981).

DENTAL CARIES AND DIET

Most research related to the nutritional effect on caries has centered on systemic fluoride's effect on teeth. Teeth with a high fluoride content are less susceptible to caries. The effects of other dietary components have been less extensively studied (Hefferren, 1981). Still, many findings influence the way patients should be guided.

There is a direct correlation between sugar intake and plaque. The more sugar consumed, especially the disaccharide, sucrose, the thicker and more plentiful the plaque (Carlsson and Egelberg, 1965). When oral hygiene is poor, even low quantities of sugar consumption promote caries (Kleemola-Kujala and Räsänen, 1982).

Binns (1981) and Newbrun (1982b) have summarized the numerous epidemiologic and clinical studies that show that eating high-sugar diets predicts a high caries rate. People living in countries where sucrose is consumed in large quantities have higher caries rates than people living where intake is low. Sreebny (1982) confirms that a diet of manufactured or processed food that contains higher levels of sucrose promotes higher levels of caries activity.

Retentive, sticky sugars (such as caramels or taffy) that are not quickly diluted by saliva and flushed from the oral cavity promote caries to a greater extent than do liquid sugars (such as soda pop). Complex carbohydrates (such as whole grain cereals and breads) are less cariogenic than simple sugars, but even these carbohydrates promote caries if food particles are retained around the teeth. The complex carbohydrates are reduced by the amylase enzyme in saliva to more simple forms, and they can be fermented by the bacteria in plaque.

Plaque can form on teeth even when carbohydrates are not ingested; but it is thin and is not as highly structured as the thick, dense plaque that is associated with a high-sucrose diet. Plaque that is not fed a carbohydrate diet does not promote caries, because acid is not produced; its presence is therefore more associated with periodontal disease resulting from the soft tissue inflammation caused by bacterial toxins, antigens, and enzymes.

Once plaque is present, ingested carbohydrates can diffuse into it. Then the bacteria, especially *Streptococcus mutans*, ferment the simple sugars, producing acid that demineralizes the teeth, initiating a carious lesion (Hefferen, Ayer, and Koehler, 1981).

Plaque is especially important in promoting smooth-surface caries, since it provides the matrix for holding the bacteria and fermenting sugars against a surface that does not otherwise easily retain food. Pit and fissure caries formation relies less on plaque, since the anatomy of the tooth enhances sugar retention and access to acid-forming bacteria.

The longer sucrose is in contact with plaque, the lower the interdental plaque pH (that is, the greater the acidity of the plaque). Therefore all-day suckers or lollipops, chewing gum, or slowly dissolving hard candies and mints pose a major risk in caries formation. So does the slowly sipped drink of cola or other sugared beverage. The passive, continual availability of sucrose keeps the acidity of the plaque high, enhancing ongoing tooth dissolution (Firestone, 1982; Newbrun, 1982a).

This point is especially evident in cases where babies are put to bed with a bottle of formula, milk, juice, or other substance that contains or is easily converted to simple sugars. The liquid, which stays in the infant's mouth with periodic replenishment as the child sucks during sleep, is chemically reduced and fermented, causing rampant tooth destruction, referred to as baby-bottle caries or nursing caries (Randolph and Dennison, 1981).

Thus a major emphasis in dietary counseling is the reduction of the frequency and duration of ingestion of fermentable carbohydrates and the elimination of sticky sweets. Patients who have a high rate of smooth-surface caries (usually on the gingival third of mandibular teeth) are prime candidates for reviewing snacking habits. A patient with this clinical evidence may keep a box of cookies in the desk drawer at work, eat sugared mints or lozenges, chew gum, or frequently consume sugared drinks such as sweetened coffee or tea, soda pop or lemonade.

Sreebny (1982) has concluded, based on epidemiologic data, that the "safe" upper limit of daily sugar consumption may be 50 g. For many individuals even this may be too much. Ingesting more than this raises the risk of caries considerably. This amount takes on more significance when the amounts of sugar in typical portions of commonly ingested foods are known: ketchup, 5 g; fruit yogurt, 18 g; canned fruit, 46 g; milk chocolate bar, 26 g; hot chocolate, 12 g; cola, 32 g (Wykeham-Martin, 1981).

Foods with a sugar content of 15% to 20% or higher are poor snack food choices because they are highly cariogenic. Even items that are 10% to 20% sugar should be restricted from between-meal use (Newbrun, 1982a). Any item that lists sugar or sucrose early in the list of ingredients on the label should be avoided.

A large number of sugar substitutes have been introduced in order to satisfy the public's demand for sweeteners that do not add calories and that do not promote tooth decay. Cyclamates, saccharin, and aspartame have all come under scrutiny for their links with cancer in laboratory animals. Cyclamates were banned in the United States in 1969. Saccharin-containing products are labeled as hazardous in the United States. Saccharin is banned in Canada, but cyclamates are allowed there. Aspartame is now widely used as a sugar substitute, having been reviewed by the FDA and found to have no adverse effects for most people (Safety of aspartame, 1986; American Dietetic Association, 1987b).

In recommending a reduction in sugar intake, the proposed alternatives should be evaluated for their safety in general health as well as for their role in dental health. Every clinician should be aware of what is available, what is "safe," and what foods or snacks it is found in.

Recent research suggests that malnourished children are more likely to harbor the bacteria associated with periodontal disease than are well-nourished children (Sawyer et al, 1986). There is growing evidence that nutritional deficiencies may enhance *Candida* infections (Samaranayake, 1986). Poor nutrition also compromises the integrity of the periodontal tissues, rendering them more susceptible to disease (Diet, 1984; DePaola et al, 1984). Nutrition is not the primary cause of the disease, but it can be considered a contributing factor. Much attention in periodontal disease has focused on altered immunity; the disease becomes active and degenerative when the host is susceptible. It is clear that malnutrition can alter a person's immunity (Homsy et al, 1986). This makes nutritional assessment and recommendation an even more important part of a total periodontal prevention, treatment, and maintenance program. Finally, a major nutritional factor associated with dental health is that tooth loss adversely affects a person's ability to eat correctly. There is a reciprocal relationship between oral health and nutrition (Geissler and Bates, 1984).

DIET AND CANCER: NEW FOCUS IN NUTRITIONAL ASSESSMENT

Dental professionals help promote good general health when they help patients replace high-calorie, caries-promoting food with nutritionally well-balanced choices. This can be accomplished by eliminating or reducing snack foods and high-sugar breakfast choices (doughnuts, sweet rolls, processed cereals), and for the most part dental professionals limit their nutritional guidance to this sphere. They may emphasize the need for vegetables, fruits, and protein sources, but the diet in general has been less of a focus for most. New evidence of the importance of diet in relation to cancer in general raises, however, the consideration of how far a dentist or hygienist should extend advice in counseling patients.

The Committee on Diet, Nutrition, and Cancer of the National Academy of Sciences reviewed hundreds of published research findings to identify those pointing conclusively to the influence of dietary habits on cancer formation.* They reviewed epidemiologic studies of population groups with varying dietary patterns. They linked the findings of those studies with laboratory and case study results. Having identified several series of studies repeatedly pointing to the influence of diet, they released the following interim guidelines that should be followed in reviewing your own diet as well as the diets of patients:

1. Reduce the percentage of both saturated and unsaturated fat to approximately 30% of total calories. This represents a 25% reduction from the typical U.S. diet percentage. An even lower percentage is indicated by the data; the committee saw this reduction as more "moderate and practical."
2. Minimize consumption of salt-preserved, smoked, or salt-pickled food.
3. Drink alcohol in moderation or not at all.

The committee also recommended that carcinogenic and mutagenic contaminants in food be prevented through regulation and continued study of food additives and processing (Palmer and Bakshi, 1983).

Many of the findings relating fat consumption to cancer have come from studies designed to investigate fats and cardiovascular disease. In addition to linking high fat intake, especially of saturated fats, to heart and blood vessel problems, they have found that diets rich in either saturated or unsaturated fats are highly correlated with cancer of the breast, colon, and prostate gland. Cancers of the testis, uterus, ovary, and pancreas have also been associated with high dietary fat levels (Palmer and Bakshi, 1983).

In these studies persons who had a high fat intake but who also consumed large quantities of vegetables had a lower risk of colon cancer. Several other studies have shown that "consumption of vegetables in general, raw vegetables (e.g., lettuce and celery), or cruciferous vegetables in particular (e.g., cabbage, cauliflower, brussels sprouts, and broccoli)" is inversely related to cancer of the alimentary tract (the esophagus, stomach, or colon). It is difficult to determine the mode of their anticarcinogenic activity. Some attribute it to their high fiber content, whereas others cite their vitamin A content or suspect some yet unknown biochemical function (Palmer and Bakshi, 1983).

Fresh fruit consumption or estimated vitamin C intake has also been shown to be inversely related to cancer incidence, especially of the stomach, esophagus, and larynx, and to uterine cervical dysplasia.

Bacon, ham, and other foods preserved with salt, smoke, or salt pickling are now known to be highly carcinogenic. But vitamin C tends to reduce their harmful effect (Palmer and Bakshi, 1983).

Numerous studies have shown a correlation between alcohol and cancer of the esophagus, tongue, pharynx, hypopharynx, larynx, lung, lip, glottis, and the supraglottic region. Studies also have shown "an interactive role between tobacco and alcohol in tumorigenesis of the oral cavity, larynx, lung, and esophagus" (Palmer and Bakshi, 1983).

Given that dental professionals have the most regular and frequent contact with healthy people, and given the convincing evidence of dietary contributions to cancer, hygienists can assume a role of major importance in reviewing individual's diets and moving them toward more healthful choices that are likely to reduce the risk of cancer.

CLINICAL ASSESSMENT: INTRAORAL AND EXTRAORAL EXAMINATION

During the complete intraoral and extraoral examination phases, the appearance of the gingivae, teeth, lips, and oral mucosa, as well as the texture of the hair and the skin, may provide some clue that the patient has nutritional problems that should be carefully assessed (Christakis, 1973). Therefore the dental hygienist is in an ideal position to identify potential nutritional and other general health problems during the complete examination of the patient's head and neck.

*The complete report can be found in National Academy of Sciences. 1982. Diet, nutrition, and cancer. Washington, D.C.: Committee on Diet, Nutrition, and Cancer Assembly of Life Sciences, National Research Council. The Palmer and Bakshi citation in the text is a summary report of the 500-page original document.

When a nutrient is not present in the diet, blood and tissue levels are maintained by reserves in specific tissues. No clinical signs are evident until the reserve stores are depleted and biochemical changes occur. Thus a person with obvious clinical symptoms can be assumed to have a relatively long-term deficiency rather than a poor diet for a day or two (Chipponi et al, 1982). Similarly, rampant caries reflects nutritional patterns that have existed for more than a few days.

However, the examination procedures are only one step in the nutritional assessment component of care. Just as the patient learns to conduct a self-assessment of oral structures and observe healthy structures as well as those that have changed in appearance or texture over time, the patient should learn how to self-assess dietary habits. Leading a patient through the self-assessment procedure is a learning procedure in itself. Additionally, it provides key data for making a decision regarding the need for dietary modifications and/or referral.

NUTRITIONAL SELF-ASSESSMENT

One way to include nutritional self-assessment routinely in dental hygiene care is to develop a simple questionnaire that can be used to determine what a "usual" day's diet is like (Nizel, 1981; Randolph, 1977). This can be done by asking a patient what he or she ate the day before, including the time of day each element was ingested and the approximate amounts eaten. The questionnaire can be given to the patient to complete; after the questionnaire has been completed, a discussion can follow, or the hygienist can ask the questions in an interview format. Twenty-four hour recalls can provide reliable information if they are completed as interviews (Morgan et al, 1987).

Generally, a patient can be expected to recall with reasonable accuracy the previous day's intake. As with any questionnaire that seeks to gather information but not to place any particular values on behavior, the questions should be phrased in such a way that the patient does not begin to be embarrased, angry, or puzzled by a failure to comply with the pattern of activities suggested by the questionnaire (Randolph, 1977). For instance, asking "What did you have for breakfast?" implies that breakfast should have

been eaten. An alternative question is, "What was the first thing you ate or drank yesterday?" Then the following question can be, "What time of the day did you eat (drink) that?" and "How much of it did you consume?" A series of such questions can elicit the approximate kinds of foods and beverages consumed, the times of day they were ingested, and the approximate amounts taken. Keeping cups, spoons, drinking glasses, and plastic containers handy can help the patient identify more precisely the amounts ingested (Christakis, 1973). It is important to ask the patient about between-meal snacks, glasses of water, and any pills or other medications that were consumed. People often feel that snacks do not count in a dietary assessment and may ignore water or vitamin pills as sources of nutrients.

The question regarding pills and other medications may help expose a noncompliance with prescribed dosages of drugs. For instance, if the patient reports during the medical history that a drug to control high blood pressure has been prescribed, the hygienist might assume that the patient takes the medication. However, if during the dietary assessment the patients fails to report having taken the medication during an entire day, this may be a sign that the patient takes the medication sporadically or not at all, regardless of the fact that it has been prescribed. This is also one way to determine if the patient has adopted any other habits related to prescribed drugs or over-the-counter medications. In any case, just as the other phases of patient assessment can yield valuable clues regarding nutritional problems, the dietary assessment can provide valuable information regarding the medical status of the patient.

Once all the suggested questions have been answered and the dietary form completed, the hygienist should ask, "Is this a typical day's eating pattern? Would you normally eat and drink this amount of food at these times of day?" Further questioning should be, "What about on days when you are at work?" (or, "What about on days when you are at home?") A person's eating habits may differ greatly from the weekday to the weekend or from days spent at work to days spent off work (Randolph, 1977; Randolph and Dennison, 1981). If the day described is atypical, the assessment should be repeated at a subsequent visit for a more valid assessment (Christakis, 1973).

According to Randolph (1977), "We tend to choose food and beverage on the basis of where we are, who we are with, the time of day, the next scheduled activity, the way we feel, the money we have and are willing to spend, and what is available." Current peer group norms (particularly among college students or institutionalized persons and certainly in families) affect dietary choices (Porter, 1987).

A homemaker may have a substantially different pattern of eating when the family is home than when he or she is home alone. A question regarding this may ferret out information about the hoard of chocolate bars in the bed stand or the secret supply of beer hidden in the old refrigerator in the attic. With the right questions, the hygienist can learn a great deal about the patient's dietary habits.

Once a full day's inclusions have been identified and verified as representing a pattern in the patient's daily living, the hygienist should ask the patient to circle in red all those solid foods that he or she knows contain sugar. Most patients can identify a large number of foods that contain sugar (Randolph, 1977; Randolph and Dennison, 1981). An orange pencil should then be used to circle liquids that contain sugar. Dairy foods should be identified by the patient and circled in yellow. Meat can be identified and circled in blue, and vegetables and fruits circled in green. Bread and cereals should be circled in brown. Observing the patient circling the items according to each of the food groups and identifying sugar-containing products should let the hygienist assess the patient's knowledge of nutrition.

Once the circling is complete, the hygienist should ask the patient if there is anything he or she would like to change about the diet. In most instances, this too will be a strong indicator of what the patient knows but does not necessarily practice. Nutritional behavior (actual food choices) may not correlate well with knowledge about proper nutrition (Shepherd and Stockley, 1987). Hearing the patient say all the right things about what to increase and what to decrease can be quite an awakening. In most instances, pre-planned lectures on proper diet and nutrition are abandoned. No doubt there also will be considerable evidence regarding the patient's attitude about changes. For instance, if the patient can identify what should be changed but says, "There's no way I'm going to change it, however," the hygienist may need to be reasonably cautious about offering multiple suggestions for change. Not all patients want this kind of help; many may resent it. People will not attend to a message unless there is some need to hear what is being said. A person who has no perceived need to change probably will doze through a lecture on what to change in the diet. The hygienist must awaken the need to know; this may not occur until after several encounters or after several decades (Porter, 1987).

Once the patient has had an opportunity to assess what should (or could) be changed in the diet, the hygienist can begin to provide a few insights into the patient's diet of which the patient may not be aware. For instance, most patients are not aware of the vast number of foods that contain refined sugars. Therefore several additional items on the day's menu may need to be circled in red or orange to reflect their actual contents. Keeping common food items in the dental operatory or counseling room can be helpful in showing the patient that ketchup, many canned vegetables, and crackers, for instance, contain sugar. By pointing out how foods are labeled, the patient can learn about concentrations of sugar and salt in the product. In all instances the approach should be "You might be interested to know that. . . ." rather than "Well, there are several you missed in circling the sugar foods."

In many instances the four foods groups will be marked accurately, although they, too, should be reviewed to ensure reasonable accuracy. Table 20-1 provides an overview of these food groupings.

Two steps that are helpful in determining the effect of the day's diet on the patient's well-being include identifying the amount of time sugar has been active in the oral cavity and identifying how closely the patient's diet adheres to the Recommended Dietary Allowances (RDAs) (Table 20-2) and/or each of the four food groups. The former determination involves counting the number of times sugar was consumed and multiplying by 20. Each time sugar is ingested, it provides 20 minutes of acid production to promote tooth decay and the proliferation of plaque. Therefore calculating the number of minutes (or hours) that acid

Table 20-1. The four food groups

Food group	Recommended servings
Meat Poultry Fish Dried beans and peas Nuts Eggs	One serving of 3 to 4 ounces of cooked meat or fish or 3 to 4 ounces of beans, lentils, or other vegetables high in protein twice daily. It is best to choose lean meat and to limit the intake of egg yolk to three times per week.
Vegetables Fruits	One serving of ½ cup at least four times weekly, including green leafy vegetables, dark yellow vegetables, and fruits or fruit juices. Citrus fruits should be included daily.
Bread Cereals	Whole grain or enriched breads recommended: one serving (slice) four times daily. Muffins, pasta, biscuits, cereal, and rice are included in this group.
Milk products	One serving (usually an 8-ounce glass of milk) three times daily for children to age 12, four or more times daily for teenagers, and twice daily for adults. Cheese, cottage cheese, ice cream, and buttermilk are included in this group.

The four food groups are useful for assessing dietary intake with recommended dietary standards. They are not, however, a recommended mechanism for preparing a detailed dietary analysis with specific amounts of nutrients identified in measurable quantities. Food value charts that identify the specific nutrients present in a wide variety of foods provide a more detailed resource for such an analysis.

has been active in the mouth can provide an interesting summary of the effect of the diet on the teeth. Likewise each of the other items circled in various colors should be tabulated to determine if frequency and amount relate to that suggested by federal standards. The Food and Nutrition Board of the National Research Council of the National Academy of Sciences has the responsibility for recommending a specific optimum quantity, based on sex and age, for each nutrient. Recommendations are issued every 5 years. The quantities suggested provide a margin of safety and are designed for an average person; therefore they do not address individual differences or the nutritional needs of medically compromised people. As a basic reference, the RDAs provide overall useful guidelines in quantifying a diet. If specific amounts of nutrients ingested can be identified, they can be compared with RDA standards to determine if the intake approximates the optimum level (Hamilton and Whitney, 1981; Randolph and Dennison, 1981).

Many nutrition texts include comprehensive listings of food values that make it possible to perform a detailed analysis of a diet. The RDA does not suggest appropriate intakes of fat, carbohydrate, cholesterol, or fiber. It does not describe associations between disease and diet or provide guidance in controlling obesity or in selecting foods (Harper, 1987). Olson describes the RDA as "a suggested level of intake that prevents signs of deficiency, provides a defined adequate reserve and is fully consistent with the health of most members of a healthy population group" (1987). Because the 1985 edition of the RDA was rejected due to differences of opinion on the changes, the 1980 guidelines will stand until a revision is agreed upon (Olson, 1987; Sutnick, 1987).

For purposes of dietary assessment and most dietary counseling in dental hygiene care, qualitative assessments using the four food groups may be more useful than detailed quantitative analyses. In any case, the patient should be able to determine if food selection is reasonably appropriate.

In addition to these two basic assessments, estimates of caloric intake may be made. The texture of the foods should be identified, as a diet of soft, nonfibrous foods can adhere to the teeth and cause problems with digestion and elimination. The distribution of eating during the day should be identified as well. Encouraging the practice of eating a good breakfast should be viewed as more than "mom's advice." A recent study suggests that persons who eat ready-to-eat cereal regularly for breakfast consume less fat and cholesterol during the day; conversely, those who skip breakfast typically consume a diet during the remainder of the day that is lacking in essential nutrients.

Males who do not eat breakfast tend to eat more during the day than do those who eat breakfast (Morgan, Zabik, and Stampley, 1986). Children who eat breakfast tend to perform better on problem-solving skills in late morning than do those who do not (Rapoport and Kruesi, 1984).

Food choices are based on beliefs and attitudes that may be outdated or mistaken. In addition, food choices are a part of daily living and constitute habits that are not easily changed. Research suggests that people select foods and utilize nutrients based on sensory experiences—some positive and some negative. It may be possible to identify these associations of sensory properties with foods and then use or alter them to improve dietary choices (Mattes, 1987). Even if habits are changed, these changes will affect not only the patients but those people around them who share social relationships, most notably families (Martin et al, 1984). Also, the positive results of dietary changes are often delayed, providing little short-term reinforcement for continued behavior (Gillespie, 1987). Change must be incremental and directed to those areas where the patient can identify the need to change and take small, concrete steps to alter behavior.

It is sometimes preferable to draw a line between assessment of need and implementation of dietary counseling. This is especially true if the patient appears to be apprehensive or reluctant to participate. If the assessment shows a need for such counseling, it can be included in a treatment plan and discussed at the case presentation.

In a number of instances, the patient may be able to identify at the time of assessment the kinds of modifications that are important for improved health. The patient may say, "I guess I never realized that I ate so few vegetables." Or the patient may say, "I knew I was a nibbler, but I would never have said that I could be found eating at 10 different times during a given day!" If the patient comes to one of these conclusions about the diet, then it may be appropriate to ask, "Would you like some suggestions for modifica-

tion?" In all likelihood, the patient who has just had a revelation about daily eating patterns will be open to at least a few suggestions for change.

The next question would be, "Where do you think you need guidance?" This question gives the patient the opportunity to say, for example, "Well, I know I can handle adding a few vegetables to my diet, but I really don't know what I'm going to do about all the sugared beverages I drink." This cues the hygienist to ignore the missing vegetables for the moment and turn the patient's attention to substitution foods that will make the decrease and possibly the eventual elimination of sugared beverages from the diet more tolerable. Once this patient-identified priority is addressed, the hygienist may return to the issue of the vegetables and ask, "What kinds of vegetables do you like? How do you usually prepare them?" Even though the patient may believe he or she can resolve a certain dietary problem, the verbal expression of plans for improvement and discussion of potential difficulties and varieties of ways in which to resolve the problem can help clarify the patient's goals and increase the likelihood of change. Another way of bringing the planned change closer to reality is to ask, "What can you do tomorrow to implement the changes you think you need?" The patient may decide to purchase the different foods today to make change possible for tomorrow. In almost all behavior changes, the goals need to be reduced to definable short-range steps that the patient can identify and accomplish, one by one. In any case the patient should be given ample opportunity to think and reply.

Merely giving instructions and information without including incremental behavior change strategies may improve the patient's knowledge and awareness of dietary needs but will have no more than a negligible effect on actual performance (Morasky and Lilly, 1980).

If, after several moments of silence, the patient seems to be at a loss as to how the diet should change, the hygienist can provide missing information. The stock of canned and bottled goods can be brought into view for an assessment of what those foods contain. The hygienist can discuss the retention of food and the frequency of intake of sugar in terms of the total amount of time acid is produced in the mouth. Or he or she may point out the vitamins and minerals that are in-

Table 20-2. Food and Nutrition Board, National Academy of Sciences—National Research Council Recommended Daily Dietary Allowances, a revised 1980: designed for the maintenance of good nutrition of practically all healthy people in the U.S.A.

	Age (yr)	Weight (kg)	Weight (lb)	Height (cm)	Height (in)	Protein (g)	Vitamin A (μg RE)[b]	Vitamin D (μg)[c]	Vitamin E (mg α-TE)[d]	Vitamin C (mg)	Thiamin (mg)
Infants	0.0-0.5	6	13	60	24	kg × 2.2	420	10	3	35	0.3
	0.5-1.0	9	20	71	28	kg × 2.0	400	10	4	35	0.5
Children	1-3	13	29	90	35	23	400	10	5	45	0.7
	4-6	20	44	112	44	30	500	10	6	45	0.9
	7-10	28	62	132	52	34	700	10	7	45	1.2
Males	11-14	45	99	157	62	45	1000	10	8	50	1.4
	15-18	66	145	176	69	56	1000	10	10	60	1.4
	19-22	70	154	177	70	56	1000	7.5	10	60	1.5
	23-50	70	154	178	70	56	1000	5	10	60	1.4
	51 +	70	154	178	70	56	1000	5	10	60	1.2
Females	11-14	46	101	157	62	46	800	10	8	50	1.1
	15-18	55	120	163	64	46	800	10	8	60	1.1
	19-22	55	120	163	64	44	800	7.5	8	60	1.1
	23-50	55	120	163	64	44	800	5	8	60	1.0
	51 +	55	120	163	64	44	800	5	8	60	1.0
Pregnant						+30	+200	+5	+2	+20	+0.4
Lactating						+20	+400	+5	+3	+40	+0.5

From Recommended Dietary Allowances, revised 1980. Washington, D.C.: Food and Nutrition Board, National Academy of
[a]The allowances are intended to provide for individual variations among most normal persons as they live in the United States which human requirements have been less well defined.
[b]Retinol equivalents. 1 retinol equivalent = 1 μg retinol or 6 μg β carotene.
[b]As cholecalciferol. 10 μg cholecalciferol = 400 IU of Vitamin D.
[d]α-tocopherol equivalents. 1 mg d-α tocopherol = 1 α-TE.
[e]1 NE (niacin equivalent) is equal to 1 mg of niacin or 60 mg of dietary tryptophan.
[f]The folacin allowances refer to dietary sources as determined by *Lactobacillus casei* assay after treatment with enzymes
[g]The RDA for vitamin B_{12} in infants is based on average concentation of the vitamin in human milk. The allowances after weaning intestinal absorption.
[h]The increased requirement during pregnancy cannot be met by the iron content of habitual American diets nor by the existing iron substantially different from those of nonpregnant women, but continued supplementation of the mother for 2-3 months after

cluded in the dietary plan, making obvious those that are missing. A brief discussion of how those missing elements affect health and well-being may have an added impact on the patient's perception of the diet. The hygienist may find it appropriate to discuss the effects of an imbalance of caloric intake and utilization. It may be that the patient will decide to expend more calories through exercise as well as decrease the intake if obesity seems to be a problem.

In some instances the patient may inquire about what kinds of foods should be eaten to fulfill a nutritional recommendation. A wise response is to list a number of foods that are appropriate and ask the patient to specify which foods he or she enjoys and are available. It is important to remember that many food choices may not be available to patients because of financial and/or cultural barriers (Hamilton and Whitney, 1981; Nizel, 1981; Randolph and Dennison, 1981). Patients may have allergies to certain foods. And, most important, there are some foods a person simply does not like and will not eat.

As mentioned before, it is important for the pa-

| | Water-soluble vitamins | | | | | Minerals | | | | |
Riboflavin (mg)	Niacin (mg NE)[e]	Vitamin B$_6$ (mg)	Folacin (μg)	Vitamin B$_{12}$ (μg)	Calcium (mg)	Phosphorus (mg)	Magnesium (mg)	Iron (mg)	Zinc (mg)	Iodine (μg)
0.4	6	0.3	30	0.5[g]	360	240	50	10	3	40
0.6	8	0.6	45	1.5	540	360	70	15	5	50
0.8	9	0.9	100	2.0	800	800	150	15	10	70
1.0	11	1.3	200	2.5	800	800	200	10	10	90
1.4	16	1.6	300	3.0	800	800	250	10	10	120
1.6	18	1.8	400	3.0	1200	1200	350	18	15	150
1.7	18	2.0	400	3.0	1200	1200	400	18	15	150
1.7	19	2.2	400	3.0	800	800	350	10	15	150
1.6	18	2.2	400	3.0	800	800	350	10	15	150
1.4	16	2.2	400	3.0	800	800	350	10	15	150
1.3	15	1.8	400	3.0	1200	1200	300	18	15	150
1.3	14	2.0	400	3.0	1200	1200	300	18	15	150
1.3	14	2.0	400	3.0	800	800	300	18	15	150
1.2	13	2.0	400	3.0	800	800	300	18	15	150
1.2	13	2.0	400	3.0	800	800	300	10	15	150
+0.3	+2	+0.6	+400	+1.0	+400	+400	+150	3	+5	+25
+0.5	+5	+0.5	+100	+1.0	+400	+400	+150	3	+10	+50

Sciences—National Research Council.
under usual environmental stresses. Diets should be based on a variety of common foods in order to provide other nutrients for

(conjugases) to make polyglutamyl forms of the vitamin available to the test organism.
are based on energy intake (as recommended by the American Academy of Pediatrics) and consideration of other factors, such as

stores of many women; therefore the use of 30-60 mg of supplemental iron is recommended. Iron needs during lactation are not
parturition are advisable in order to replenish stores depleted by pregnancy.

tient to express what he or she could do the next day to alter the diet in the ways the patient had previously suggested. It is also wise to suggest incremental changes. One small change over a few weeks followed by other small changes may actually result in long-term major changes. A crash program to change the entire structure of a person's diet is often shortlived, as can be verified by the numbers of people who have gained and lost and gained back again hundreds of pounds over the years on fad approaches to weight loss. Ideally, the specific changes can be identified in

writing for the patient and placed in the patient's record. Each change should be identified in a time frame. As each change is implemented, the patient can identify the date and time of day the change was implemented, thus tracking whether or not real change has occurred.

Finally, the hygienist should integrate follow-up assessments of progress into each dental hygiene visit. People do not always do everything they say they will do; a supportive, helpful hygienist will remember to identify the areas in which even minor success has been achieved and reinforce that change. If recommended changes did not occur, the hygienist might ask, "What seemed to be the biggest roadblock to making the change?" Setting out to remove or diminish each roadblock as it appears can be an effective way to facilitate change over an extended period of time.

REFERRALS

Even though the dental hygienist has courses in nutrition and feels confident about proper dietary intake, there will be times when it is essential to refer the patient to a dietitian or a physician for more complete nutritional analysis and counseling (Nizel, 1981; Randolph and Dennison, 1981). In most instances if the patient's health history indicates diabetes, alcoholism, an obvious chronic nutritional debility, or any other complicated combination of disease and nutritional problems, the hygienist should recommend that the patient see a person more qualified to make recommendations and work with the patient. A protocol for these kinds of referrals should be established for the practice site so that co-workers are able to ensure rapid, safe referral for the patient. Subsequent to such referrals, the hygienist should inquire whether the patient was able to obtain assistance from the dietitian or the physician. Just as medication to control high blood pressure can remain in the bottle, appointments with other health care providers to whom the patient is referred may not always occur. A helpful step is to contact the person to whom the patient was referred to ensure that the patient complied with the recommendation and to determine if the hygienist's findings were accurate. This is one way to establish whether assessment skills in patient observation and history preparation are adequate. A dialogue with coprofessionals can be beneficial to the dental hygienist as well as to the patient under discussion.

SUMMARY

With a solid knowledge of basic nutrition and its relationship to health and disease, a dental hygienist can play a valuable role in helping improve the dietary patterns of patients. The use of simple patient self-assessment procedures and the approach of guiding the patient in identifying necessary modifications can result in improvements in health and in patient cooperation in all phases

of care. Perhaps the most essential point is for the hygienist to assume the facilitator role rather than the directive role. Decisions that the patient makes are most likely to lead to actual behavior change. The hygienist's role is to ensure that the decisions are guided properly and that roadblocks to their fulfillment can be identified and reduced.

ACTIVITIES

1. Prepare 1-day, 3-day, and 7-day, dietary assessments with a student partner. Use nutritional texts and articles to prepare a comprehensive evaluation of the records to reveal the following:
   a. Caloric intake and expenditure
   b. Consumption of bulk foods
   c. Consumption of liquids
   d. Degree of compliance with the four food groups and the RDAs
   e. Frequency and form of carbohydrates ingested
   f. Percentage of fat consumed.
2. Videotape the dietary assessment encounter with a student partner to reveal the process of communication, verbal and nonverbal cues, and the approach used by the student dental hygienist.
3. Read Binns's (1981) article listed in the references at the end of this chapter.
4. Critique the General Mills ad on pp. 142-143 of the January 1981 issue of the *Journal of the American Dental Association*. How are research results manipulated to convince readers that they should counsel patients to eat processed cereals, regardless of their sugar content?
5. Form groups of five. Visit a grocery store and review labels on products in each of the following categories for the presence of sugar:
   a. Breakfast cereals
   b. Bread
   c. Juice
   d. Canned fruits, vegetables
   e. Tomato sauce and prepared spaghetti sauces
6. Compare findings, identifying brand names of products high in sugar as well as those that are low in sugar or contain none.
7. Review the literature regarding requirements for athletes. Specify which nutrients should be increased or decreased. Refer to: Position of the American Dietetic Association: nutrition for physical fitness and athletic performance for adults, *Journal of the American Dietetic Association* 87:933, 1987 and to more recent citations.
8. Prepare a report giving the truth or fiction about one or more of the following popular beliefs:
   a. Honey is more wholesome than sugar
   b. Fish is brain food
   c. Eating carrots improves eyesight

d. Garlic lowers blood pressure
e. Brown eggs are superior to white eggs
f. White bread is not as good as whole wheat bread
Refer to the January 1988 issue of the Tufts University *Diet and Nutrition Letter* for information and other topics to research and debate.
9. Search the current literature for the most recent version of the RDA guidelines. Compare those values with the ones in the table 20-2.

REVIEW QUESTIONS
1. Identify the three nutrients that provide calories for the body.
2. Which of the three nutrients given in response to Question 1 can cause weight gain if consumed in excess?
3. Match the following nutrients with their important functions in the health of the human body.

___ a. Protein
___ b. Fat
___ c. Carbohydrate
___ d. Vitamin B complex
___ e. Vitamin D
___ f. Vitamin A
___ g. Vitamin K
___ h. Vitamin E
___ i. Iodine
___ j. Fluoride
___ k. Calcium and phosphorus
___ l. Iron
___ m. Water

1. Contributes to thyroid regulation
2. Serves as fluid medium for the body's chemical and physical reactions
3. Essential for development of healthy bones and teeth
4. Helps teeth become resistant to decay
5. Essential component of nerve tissue
6. Essential component in body tissues, enzymes, and hormones
7. Helps cushion and insulate the body
8. Important in collagen biosynthesis and wound healing
9. Critical for the complete metabolism of carbohydrates and for energy release
10. Formed in the presence of ultraviolet light; important for the absorption and homeostasis of calcium
11. Essential in prothrombin formation
12. Essential in hemoglobin formation
13. Primary functions relate to reproduction and membrane stability
14. Essential for vision and control of differentiation of epithelium in mucus-secreting structures and in bone remodeling

4. Why is it a useful strategy to ask the patient to identify the presence or absence of specific foods in his or her diet?
5. What role do the RDAs and the four food groups play in dietary assessment?
6. How does plaque aid caries formation?
7. What foods have been proved to be highly associated with cancer?
8. What foods tend to reduce the incidence of cancer?

REFERENCES
American Dietetic Association: Nutrition for physical fitness and athletic performance for adults, J Am Diet Assoc 87:933, 1987(a).
American Dietetic Association: Appropriate use of nutritive and non-nutritive sweeteners, J Am Diet Assoc 87:1689, 1987(b).
Binns NM: Caries and carbohydrates—a problem for dentists and nutritionists, Dent Health 20(4):5, 1981.
Brooks GB: Nutritional status—a prognostic indicator in head and neck cancer, Otolaryngol Head Neck Surg 93:69, 1985.
Carlsson J, and Egelberg J: Effect of diet on plaque formation and development of gingivitis in dogs, II: Effect of high carbohydrate versus high protein-fat diets, Odontol Rev 16:42, 1965.
Chipponi JX, et al: Deficiencies of essential and conditionally essential nutrients, Am J Clin Nutr (supp 5) 35:1112, 1982.
Christakis G: Nutritional assessment in health programs. Am J Public Health (supp) 63, 1973.
DePaola DP, Alvares O, and Etzel DR: Nutrition and periodontal disease, TIC 43(6):5, 1984.
Diet, nutrition, and oral health: a rational approach for the dental practice, JADA 109:20, 1984.
Deuster PA, et al: Nutritional survey of highly trained women runners, Am J Clin Nutr 44:954, 1986.
Fahey PJ, Boltri JM, and Monk JS: Key issues in nutrition: from conception through infancy, Postgrad Med 81(1):301, 1987(a).
Fahey PJ, Boltri JM, and Monk JS: Key issues in nutrition: supplementation through adulthood and old age, Postgrad Med 81(6):123, 1987(b).
Firestone AR: Effect of increasing contact time on sucrose solution of powdered sucrose on plaque pH in vivo, J Dent Res 61:1243, 1982.
Geissler CA, and Bates JF: The nutritional effects of tooth loss, Am J Clin Nutr 39:478, 1984.
Getting the most from the most essential nutrient, Tufts University Diet and Nutrition Letter, 4(8):3, 1986.
Gillespie AH: Communication theory as a basis for nutrition education, J Am Diet Assoc 87(9) (supp): S-44, 1987.
The good news about complex carbohydrates, Tufts University Diet and Nutrition Letter, 5(6):3, H, 1987.
Hamilton EMN, and Whitney EN: Nutrition concepts and controversies, St. Paul, Minn, 1982, West Publishing Co.

Harper AE: Evolution of recommended dietary allowances—new directions? Ann Rev Nutr 7:509, 1987.

Hefferren, J.J. 1981. A look ahead: diet and nutrition research, J. Am. Dent. Assoc. 102:624.

Hefferren, J.J., Ayer, W.A., and Koehler, H.M., editors. 1981. Foods, nutrition, and dental health, vols. 1-3, Park Forest South, III.: Pathotox Publishers, Inc.

Homsy J, Morrow WJW, and Levy JA: Nutrition and autoimmunity: a review, Clin Exp Immunol 65:473, 1986.

Kipp D: Stress and nutrition, ASDC J Dent Chil 52:68, 1985.

Kleemola-Kujala E, and Räs'auanen L: Relationship of oral hygiene and sugar consumption to risk of caries in children, Community Dent Oral Epidemiol 10:224, 1982.

Lieber CS: Alcohol-nutrition interaction, ASDC J Dent Chil 51:137, 1984.

Looking for fiber? Start with cereal, Tufts University Diet and Nutrition Letter, 5(1):7, 1987.

Lum LLQ, and Gallagher-Allred CR: Nutrition and the cancer patient: a cooperative effort by nursing and dietetics to overcome problems, Cancer Nurs 7:469, 1984.

Martin BJ, Austin JB, and Stewart JS: Role for the dentist in behavioral intervention: families with poor eating patterns, Oral Health, 74(11):11, 1984.

Mattes RD: Sensory influences of food intake and utilization in humans, Hum Nutr Appl Nutr 41(2):77, 1987.

Morasky RL, and Lilly KP: Nutrition management for dental health: a behavioral approach, Clin Prevent Dent 2(4):7, 1980.

Morgan KJ, et al: Collection of food intake data: an evaluation of methods, J Am Diet Assoc 87:888, 1987.

Morgan KJ, Zabik ME, and Stampley GL: The role of breakfast in diet adequacy in the U.S. adult population, J Am coll Nutr 5:551, 1986.

Newbrun E: Sugar and dental caries, Clin Prevent Dent 4(3):11, 1982(a).

Newbrun E: Sugar and dental caries: a review of human studies, Science 217:418, 1982(b).

Nizel AE: Nutrition in preventive dentistry: science and practice, 1981, Philadelphia, WB Saunders Co.

Olson JA: Recommended nutrient intakes: guidelines for the prevention of deficiency or prescription for total health, J Nutr 116:1581, 1986.

Palmer S, and Bakshi K: Diet, nutrition, and cancer: interim dietary guidelines, JNCI 70:1151, 1983.

Poplin LE: Cautions in nutritional counseling, Dent Hyg 55(2):40, 1981.

Porter SB: Using communication theory: the development of a conceptual framework to map students' thinking about food, J Am Diet Assoc 87(9) (supp): S-53, 1987.

Randolph PM: Dietary counseling. in Boundy SS, and Reynolds NJ, editors: current concepts in dental hygiene, vol 1, St Louis, 1977, The CV Mosby Co.

Randolph PM, and Dennison CI: Diet, nutrition, and dentistry, St Louis, 1981, The CV Mosby Co.

Rapoport JD, and Kruesi MJP: Behavior and nutrition: a mini-review, ASDC J Dent Chil 51:451, 1984.

Reducing your level of cholesterol? Try oats, Tufts University diet and Nutrition Letter 4(9):1, 1986.

Safety of aspartame upheld again, Tufts University Diet and Nutrition Letter 4(4):2, 1986.

Samaranayake LP: Nutritional factors and oral candidosis, J Oral Pathol 15:61, 1986.

Sawyer DR, et al: Comparison of oral microflora between well-nourished and malnourished Nigerian children, ASDC J Dent Chil 53:439, 1986.

Schaafsma G, et al: Nutritional aspects of osteoporosis, Wld Rev Nutr Diet 49:121, 1987.

Schaumberg H, et al; Sensory neuropathy from pyridoxine abuse, N Engl J Med 309:445, 1983.

Shepherd R, and Stockley L: Nutrition knowledge, attitudes, and fat consumption, J Am Diet Assoc 87:615, 1987.

Sreebny LM: Sugar availability, sugar consumption and dental caries, Community Dent Oral Epidemiol 10:1, 1982.

Sutnick MR: Nutrition: calcium, cholesterol, and calories, Med Clin North Am 71(1):123, 1987.

Vitamin B_6 toxicity and premenstrual syndrome, Tufts University Diet and Nutrition Letter 3(12):7, 1986.

Wilmore JH, and Freund BJ: Nutritional enhancement of athletic performance. In Winick M: Nutrition and exercise, New York, 1986, John Wiley & Sons.

Wykeham-Martin J: Hidden sugar, Dent Health 20(3):14, 1981.

PART THREE

IMPLEMENTATION

Implementing care in dental hygiene practice is defined in the following 15 chapters in terms of periodontal care (Chapters 21 to 26), caring for appliances (Chapter 27), using chemical agents for the prevention of dental caries and for the control of tooth hypersensitivity (Chapter 28 to 30), controlling pain (Chapters 31 and 32), modifying dental hygiene care for patients with special needs (Chapter 33), and performing restorative procedures (Chapter 34).

Most of the highly technical skills of dental hygiene practice are further developed and expanded in these chapters, with a firm grounding given in the scientific basis for these procedures. During this phase of development the student may begin to recognize that the cycle of assessing, planning, implementing, and evaluating is not a single large cycle but occurs in a series of minicycles throughout implementation and each of the other phases. Even while a clinical procedure is being implemented, the thinking clinician is assessing the state of the tissue and its response, planning the next move, carrying out each sequence of the procedure, and evaluating the performance of each procedure.

21 REMOVING HEAVY DEPOSITS: HAND SCALING

OBJECTIVES: *The reader will be able to*

1. Use a pen grasp, fulcrum, wrist rock, and a variety of stroking patterns to remove calculus from teeth with the following instruments:
   a. Sickle scalers
   b. Universal curettes
   c. Hoes
   d. Chisels
   e. Files
2. Given a variety of calculus deposits, use exploratory and working strokes to identify deposit location and size and to engage the deposit for removal.
3. Differentiate between exploratory and working strokes.
4. Differentiate among vertical, horizontal, oblique, and circumferential stroking patterns.
5. Identify instances in which the selection of a sickle, universal curette, hoe, chisel, or file for calculus removal is appropriate.
6. Describe the uses and limitations of each of the calculus removal instruments.
7. Describe an order of instrumentation for effective utilization of the calculus removal instruments, based on effective clinician and patient positioning and effective time and motion economy.
8. Demonstrate four alternative fulcrum placements.
9. Identify methods for evaluating complete deposit removal.
10. Explain briefly why removing calculus and ensuring good oral hygiene are not sufficient to stop periodontal disease.

Writings from 1000 years ago include references to calculus deposits and suggestions for their removal (Ring, 1987). The problems of deposit formation and their effective removal have been with us for a long time and have been the subjects of many research articles and treatment plans.

Removing calculus deposits from the teeth is still a large part of what a clinical dental hygienist does in the daily routine. This is an important role in the initial therapy that patients receive, and it is an integral part of maintenance care or prevention. The very term, *prophylaxis,* which is the profession's term for scaling and polishing teeth, means *prevention.* This procedure is viewed as part of a total regimen of professional and self-care that can prevent most instances of dental caries and periodontal disease. Yet, there has been considerable controversy regarding exactly how much the oral prophylaxis is able to prevent. Does oral prophylaxis in itself prevent disease? In most instances, dental hygienists and other health professionals would agree that it does not in itself prevent disease. At least, the periodic recall prophylaxis administered every 6 months is unlikely to do so. Certainly, the single event of a complete oral prophylaxis in initial periodontal therapy does not in itself prevent periodontal disease. However, most practicing dental hygienists can show that in combination with thorough, habitual plaque removal and proper diet, the oral prophylaxis is one contribution to maintaining oral health.

Research findings support this belief. Periodontal patients who receive initial therapy including these procedures show significant decreases in oral disease over a 1-month period (Morrison et al, 1980). Similar results have been reported for maintenance periods of 13 months (Badersten et al, 1981) and 6 years (Axelsson and Lindhe, 1981). Periodontal patients maintained with regular prophylaxes *without* surgical intervention over an 8-year period have shown no significant difference in oral status from patients with comparable conditions for whom surgery was performed (Knowles et al, 1980). Muller and colleagues (1986) showed that a single course of scaling and root planing resulted in shallower pockets, a gain in clinical attachment, and a shift in the subgingival microflora to a healthier picture. Thus scaling, root planing, and soft tissue curettage have been shown to be efficacious modes of treatment when combined with a high degree of oral hygiene.

Taken in its proper perspective as part of a complete program of prevention, the oral prophylaxis is an important service for the patient. It removes irritants from the teeth, smooths surface irregularities that enhance plaque formation and growth, and provides the patient with a clean feeling that he or she is more likely to want to preserve. Also, the teeth may look better as a result of the oral prophylaxis.

If the oral prophylaxis is given too much significance by the patient or the hygienist, however, it may become a flimsy crutch. A preoccupation with the short-term cosmetic effects, an acceptance of the recurrent deposits on the teeth, and the patient's reliance on the dental hygienist as the source of clean teeth all are signs of abuse of the procedure and are a certain pattern for supervised neglect. Teeth that are cleaned every 6 months but that have no regular daily care in the form of plaque removal and that are subject to cariogenic foods will not be safe from caries, slow periodontal destruction, and eventual loss.

The dental hygienist's goal is to be so effective as a health educator and as a motivator that the oral prophylaxis becomes basically nonessential for the patient. Over the course of a few months or years, the patient should become increasingly interested in self-care and in long-term health. As deposits are not allowed to reaccumulate between professional appointments, less and less scaling and polishing will be needed. Maintenance becomes a process of evaluating tissue health (both hard and soft tissues, intraorally and extraorally) and of providing the patient with information and suggestions for maintaining optimal oral health (Parr et al, 1976). The dental hygienist becomes a resource rather than a "tooth cleaner."

In initial care and for those patients who have not yet achieved control of oral health, the dental hygienist needs to have skills in deposit detection and removal. Chapter 6 presents the basic principles of detection.

This chapter presents the principles of deposit removal; in later chapters the principles of root planing and curettage, as well as other procedures that support complete periodontal care, are discussed. The oral prophylaxis procedure and more advanced periodontal instrumentation need to be learned so that they can be performed safely, efficiently, and thoroughly. At this point the dental hygienist begins to develop as a therapist as well as a data gatherer and health educator.

COMMON PRINCIPLES OF INSTRUMENTATION FOR EXPLORING AND REMOVING CALCAREOUS DEPOSITS

The basic principles of instrumentation presented in Chapter 6 will be extremely useful in learning the principles of deposit removal. For nearly all the calculus removal instruments the modified pen grasp, fulcrum placement, wrist rock, and stroking patterns discussed in Chapter 6 are the same as those used in detecting deposits and in probing subgingivally.

Recall that the instrument is held between the thumb and the first *two* fingers (a *modified pen grasp),* with the first two sections of the index finger flat against the instrument for maximum control. The third finger, or ring finger, is used as a *fulcrum,* giving the movements of the instrument control and stability. Usually the fulcrum (also called a finger rest) is on the occlusal or incisal surfaces of the teeth, near the operative site. The *wrist rock* is the unified lateral or vertical hand and arm motion that causes the instrument to move in a prescribed *stroking pattern* on the tooth for detecting calculus or for removing it and other irregularities from the tooth. The stroking pattern can be vertical, oblique or diagonal, or circumferential. *Exploratory strokes* require minimal pressure against the tooth, as nerves in the

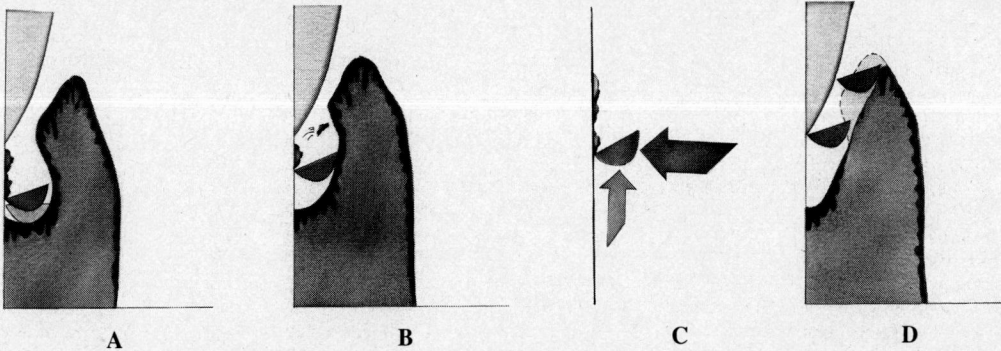

A   B   C   D

Fig. 21-1. **A,** Scaler inserted to base of sulcus and beneath a calculus deposit. **B,** Calculus being removed by properly angulated blade (more than 45 degrees and less than 90 degrees to tooth). Calculus is removed by increased horizontal pressure against tooth as working stroke is activated, **C,** and motion out of sulcus is completed, **D.** Coincidental curettage of sulcus wall occurs in some instances as cutting instrument moves out of sulcus.
(Adapted from Seibert JS: Contin Dent Educ **1**:8, 1978.)

fingers must detect the slight variations in the texture and morphology of the teeth that cannot be seen when working subgingivally, but that can be felt with a fine explorer or probe. The *adaptation* of the instrument tip against the tooth as it moves around the circumference of the tooth is critical in detecting root variations and in preventing accidental piercing of the soft tissue with the point. All of these principles are important in exploring and probing. They also are important in removing deposits. In addition, two new principles of instrumentation require mastery for safe removal of deposits: working stroke and angulation. The principle of a working stroke is described here. Angulation is described after a description of the parts of a scaler and an introduction to the necessary terminology.

Working stroke

One critical difference between probing and removing deposits relates to the type of stroke used. Although the same gentle stroke is used with a scaler in moving into the sulcus, once a deposit is located with the scaler, the motion out of the sulcus becomes a *working stroke*. A working stroke involves increased pressure laterally against the tooth at the edge of the deposit as the instrument is brought out of the sulcus with the wrist rock motion. The increased pressure against the tooth forces the deposit to fracture away from the tooth (Fig. 21-1). The goal is to fracture away the en-

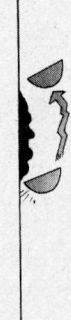

Fig. 21-2. Instrument may merely chatter over or smooth down a calculus deposit if insufficient horizontal pressure is used or if blade is dull.
(Adapted from Seibert JS: Contin Dent Educ **1**:8, 1978.)

tire deposit if possible. It is *not* to chip away or wear down the deposit. If adequate pressure is not maintained against the tooth, the instrument will slide over the deposit, smoothing it down but not removing it from the tooth (Fig. 21-2). Also, the horizontal pressure against the tooth prevents the instrument from being pulled from the sulcus with a jerk. All alternating exploratory and working strokes should remain under solid control and generally be maintained subgingivally until the surface feels smooth with the scaler. As with the probe and explorers, the instrument should not exit completely from the sulcus with each stroke. Rather, the instrument should remain subgingivally until the area being scaled feels smooth. Then the instrument can be used to scoop out any loose calculus or other debris, and the area can be flushed thoroughly with water or air irrigant When an entire sextant or quadrant is scaled and feels smooth to the scaler, the clinician should then reevaluate the areas with a fine explorer or periodontal probe for more definitive detection of deep deposits or residual pieces of deposits.

A critical element in ensuring a light-handed approach to instrumentation is to use working strokes only when calculus or roughness is detected on the tooth. Otherwise it is best to use exploratory strokes with cutting instruments.

The horizontal pressure against the tooth is effective only if the instrument doing the calculus removal has a sharp blade (Parr et al, 1976; Seibert, 1978). The sharp blade on the cutting instruments used in deposit removal distinguishes them from the probe and explorers used thus far in instrumentation. Like the explorers, the cutting instruments must be designed so that they have access to all areas of the mouth and so that they will not damage healthy tooth structure and soft tissue during proper use. A wide variety of instruments meets these criteria, from them an experienced dental hygienist may select his or her instruments of choice.

A solid working knowledge of the types available and their general use in deposit removal makes it possible for each individual to try a wide range of instruments suitable for the variety of cases that challenge the clinician (Parr et al, 1976; Seibert, 1978). Deposit location, size, tenaciousness, and accessibility place limitations on the variety of instruments that may be selected for use.

Sickle scaler

The basic design of the working end of a sickler scaler is shown in Fig. 21-3. The working end is formed by two blades terminating in a point. Each of the two blades is formed by the bevel or facial surface and a lateral surface. The two lateral surfaces join at the bottom of the instrument to form an unused third edge. It should be obvious that two hazards in using the instrument are the potential trauma caused by the point (just as with the point on the explorer) (Fig. 21-4) and by the edge on the bottom of the instrument. Careful adaptation of the sickle scaler can ensure that the point does not wander into soft tissue. Generally,

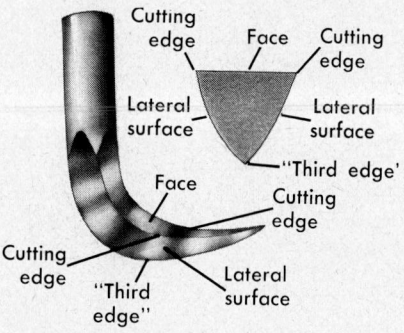

Fig. 21-3. Sickle scaler has two cutting edges. Lateral surfaces join at back of instrument to form a third "edge" that should be dulled to reduce possible tissue trauma. Face (or bevel) of instrument is surface between the two blades converging to form a point.
(Adapted from Seibert JS: Contin Dent Educ 1:8, 1978.)

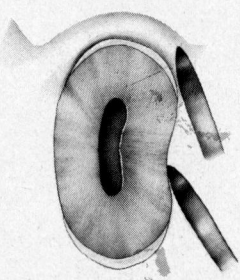

Fig. 21-4. Side of point of sickle must be carefully adapted to tooth to ensure that it does not pierce soft tissue, particularly as it is guided around line angles of tooth.
(Adapted from Seibert JS: Contin Dent Educ 1:8, 1978.)

the "third edge" can be made less of a problem by dulling the underside with a sharpening stone. A few strokes directly over the bottom of the scaler reduce potential difficulty.

The relatively short shank and relatively long straight working end limit the sickle scaler's usefulness (Seibert, 1978). Generally, it is limited to removing supragingival calculus or subgingival calculus that is only 1 to 2 mm beneath the margin of the gingiva. It is not effective for deep deposits and will cause tissue trauma if an attempt is made to use it in deep pockets.

The solid design of the instrument makes it strong enough to remove reasonably heavy deposits as long as it is sharp and is used with adequate pressure against the tooth during the working stroke.

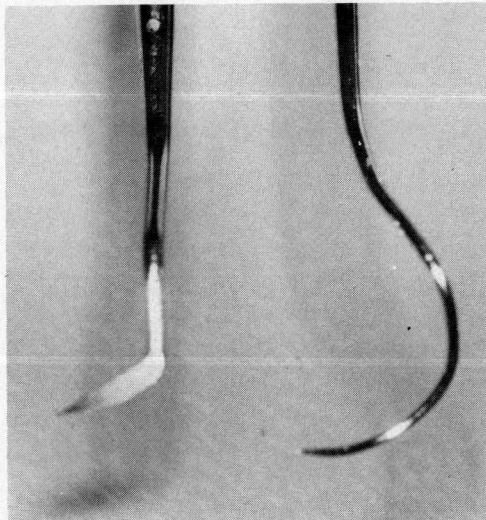

Fig. 21-5. By comparing ends of contra-angled (pigtail or cowhorn) explorer and sickle scaler, it is possible to find matching ends that curve in same direction. Sickle scaler can then be selected for use in areas of dentition by following same principles as for selecting appropriate end of contra-angled explorer.

Selecting the proper end is a reasonably easy task once proper end selection with the cowhorn or pigtail explorer has been mastered (Chapter 6). The best way to determine the proper end is to place the double-ended sickle next to the cowhorn or pigtail and determine which ends match. One end of the cowhorn will curve in the same direction as one end of the sickle scaler (Fig. 21-5). The other ends will match likewise. Careful comparisons will reveal that the terminal shank of the instrument adjoining the working end matches the terminal shank of the explorer. Therefore the process used to establish which end of the explorer to use is also used to select the proper end of the sickle scaler. The end of the explorer used on the mandibular right buccal, for instance, provides a model for the end of the sickle scaler that is appropriate for that area of the mouth. Without referring to the explorer's matching end, it is possible to place either end of the sickle against the mesial surface of a tooth in the mandibular right sextant and determine which end is aimed across the mesial surface and also has a terminal shank in parallel relation to the long axis of the tooth. Its pair should be usable on the lingual surface of the mandibular right sextant, with the shank par-

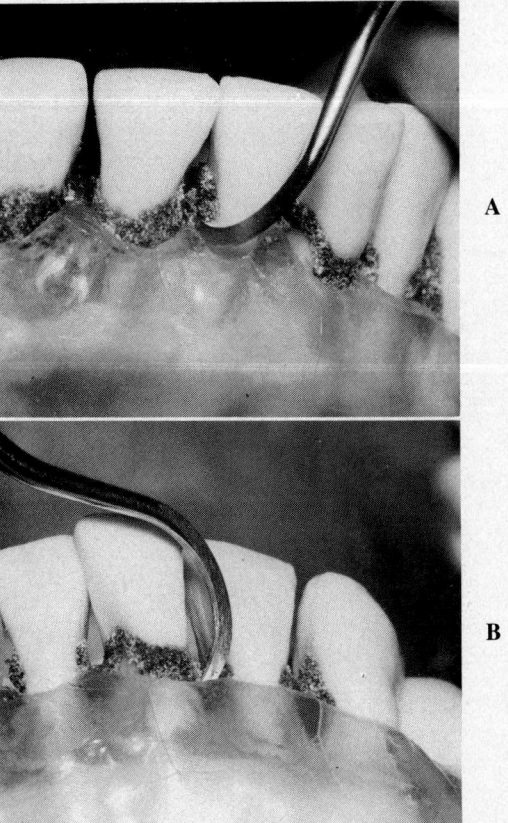

Fig. 21-6. **A,** Anterior sickle with less angular working end in this case is shown adapted to mandibular anterior tooth on proximal surface. Shank is angled in toward midline of tooth to ensure that angle of blade to tooth is less than 90 degrees. Side of tip is carefully adapted to tooth to avoid piercing soft tissue with point of sickle. **B,** Anterior or straight-shanked sickle can be used with circumferential or horizontal stroke on direct facial and lingual surfaces to remove deposits that are otherwise inaccessible. Extreme care is necessary in adapting blade and in ensuring use of short strokes to prevent tissue trauma.

allel to the long axis of the tooth. Thus the basic principles of instrument selection for explorers should be useful in selecting paired contra-angled sickle scalers.

Anterior sickles have a straight shank. *The simpler the shank, the more anterior the intended area of use for the instrument* (Fig. 21-6). Anterior sickles can be adapted on anterior proximal surfaces or on the direct facial and lingual surfaces of teeth using a horizontal or circumferential stroke.

Angulation

While basic principles of end selection, grasp, fulcrum, wrist rock, and stroke are basically the same as for explorers (except for the increased horizontal pressure with the working stroke), *angulation* is a critical difference that is important when using cutting instruments. The blade must be angled to the tooth so that it can engage the deposits optimally and so that the edge that is not placed against the tooth surface is not engaging soft tissue (Parr et al, 1976; Seibert, 1978). To ensure that these two needs are met, the blade should be angled so that it is less than 90 degrees and more than 45 degrees to the tooth. If the angle of the blade is less than 45 degrees to the tooth, the blade is "too closed," and the facial aspect of the working end is almost completely in

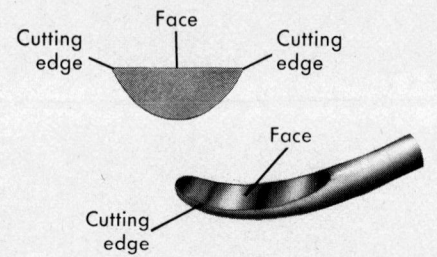

Fig. 21-7. Universal curette has rounded back and rounded toe, which enhance its use in subgingival areas, as this back and toe are less likely to cause inadvertent trauma than are sharp-edged back and pointed toe of sickle scaler.
(Adapted from Seibert JS: Contin Dent Educ **1**:8, 1978.)

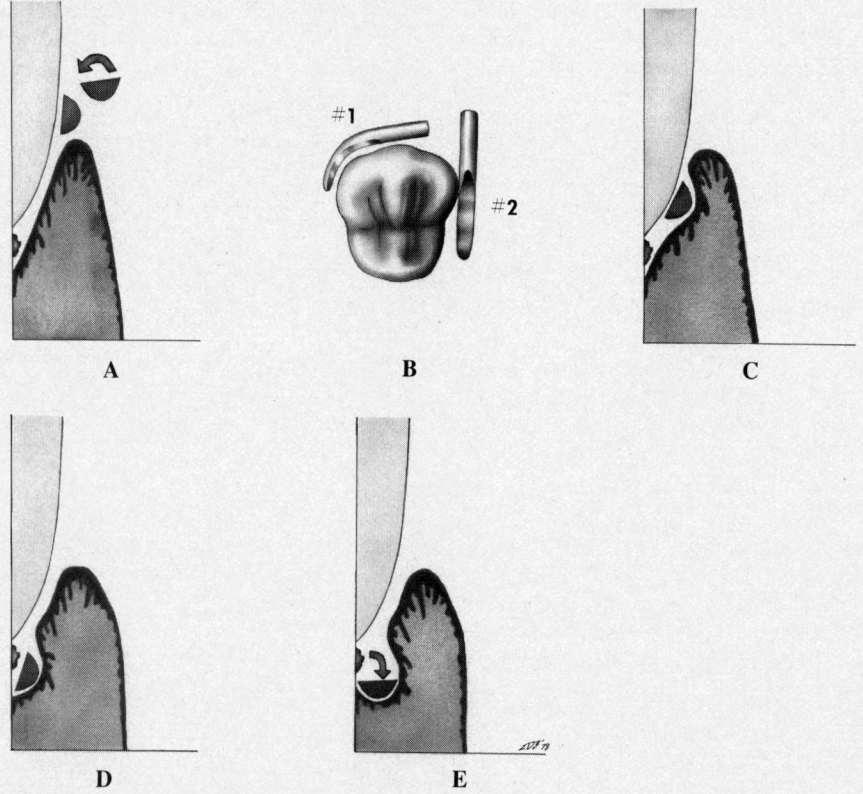

Fig. 21-8. Curette is inserted into sulcus at 0 degrees angulation. **A,** so that is resembles curette No. 1 in **B.** Curette is moved into sulcus and past calculus with exploratory stroke, **C** and **D.** At base of sulcus, blade is opened to between 45 and 90 degrees before beginning working stroke, **E.** If 90-degree angle (as shown here) is used, soft tissue will be removed also. Closing it to 75 to 80 degrees minimizes this hazard.
(Adapted from Seibert JS: Contin Dent Educ **1**:8, 1978.)

contact with the tooth. Instrumentation is therefore ineffective. If the angle of the blade is at 90 degrees or more to the tooth, the angle of the blade is "too open," therefore posing a hazard of tissue damage as well as decreased effectiveness in deposit removal.

Universal curette

A universal curette is shown in Fig. 21-7. It, too, is a paired instrument. Universal curettes come in a variety of sizes and shank lengths for use in heavy calculus removal and in fine scaling (Parr et al, 1976; Seibert, 1978). The shape of the working end of curettes allows them to be used safely in subgingival areas. The universal curette has a rounded toe instead of a point and does not have a third edge on the back. It is generally more spoon-shaped and thus is less hazardous to surrounding soft tissue. Yet is is a relatively strong instrument that can be extremely useful in removing heavy, deep deposits. The curved blade (which extends around the toe to form two useful cutting edges) allows it to be more readily adapted to curved root surfaces.

When inserting the universal curette for subgingival scaling, the blade should be closed against the tooth to 0 degrees and inserted to the base of the sulcus past the deposit with this same closed angle. At the base of the sulcus the angle is opened to between 45 and 90 degrees and prepared for the working stroke to remove the deposit (Seibert, 1978) (Figs. 21-8 and 21-9).

The stroking pattern can be a series of vertical or oblique strokes that overlap (Fig. 21-10) to

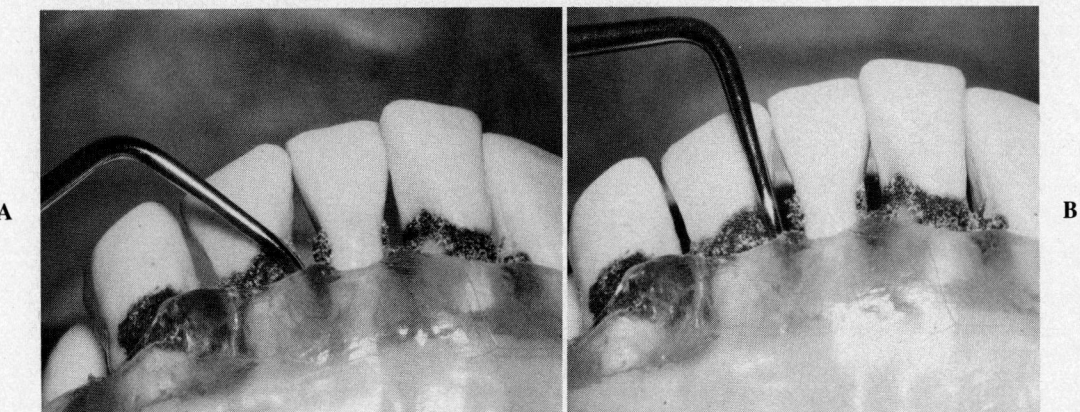

Fig. 21-9. **A,** Curette inserted at 0 degrees and then **B,** opened to approximately 75 degrees in sulcus.

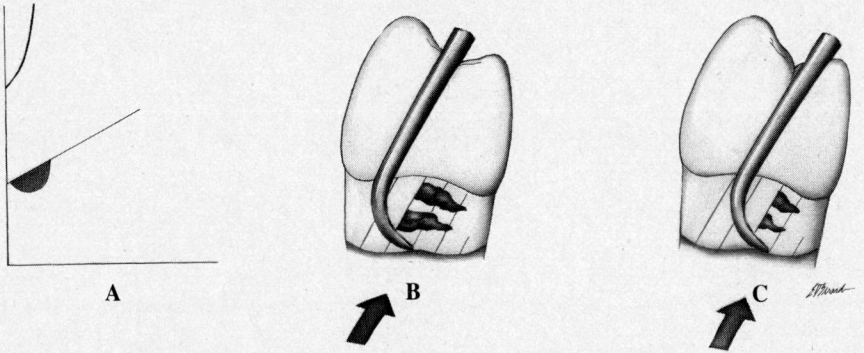

Fig. 21-10. Once blade is engaged at proper angle to tooth, as suggested in **A,** vertical or oblique overlapping working strokes can be used to remove calculus deposits in **B** and **C.**
(Adapted from Seibert JS: Contin Dent Educ **1:**8, 1978.)

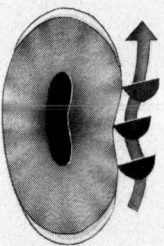

Fig. 21-11. Horizontal or circumferential stroke uses blade with toe aimed more apically so that blade engages lateral side of deposit rather than the most apical aspect of deposit. Horizontal stroking is useful when vertical strokes are not successful and for removing deposits from line angles and from the very base of a pocket. Horizontal stroking also helps obtain adaptation in root furrows and grooves.
(Adapted from Seibert JS: Contin Dent Educ **1:**8, 1978.)

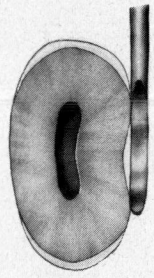

Fig. 21-12. Often a vertical stroke will not be adequate in scaling convoluted roots, especially in furrows and deep grooves. Adaptation is critical, as calculus often forms in these protected areas. Rather than trying to adapt full length of blade to proximal surface as shown, adapt first 2 mm of blade and follow contours of root as shown in Fig. 21-4.
(Adapted from Seibert JS: Contin Dent Educ **1:**8, 1978.)

cover the root or crown surface (Parr et al, 1976; Seibert, 1978). This stroke is used for initial scaling around the tooth and is highly successful in removing most deposits. A second kind of stroke is the circumferential or horizontal stroke (Fig. 21-11). The stroking pattern engages the deposits on the sides and allows another approach to calculus that will not come off with a vertical stroke. It also is a useful stroke for removing small pieces at the line angles of teeth and for gaining access to the very base of the pocket and to furrows and grooves on root surfaces that may be incompletely scaled by vertical strokes (Fig. 21-12).

The same process used in selecting the paired explorer and the paired, contra-angled sickle is used in *selecting the proper end* for the universal curette. Placing the universal curette next to the contra-angled sickle and the explorer allows the clinician to match ends based on direction of curvature and location of the terminal shank. When the universal curette is placed intraorally, the terminal shank should be parallel to the long axis of the tooth as the toe of the instrument is aimed across the proximal surface of the tooth to be scaled (Fig. 21-13). The same principles of grasp, fulcrum, wrist rock, and stroke are used with this type of instrument.

In general, the shank design and working end design of the universal curette allow the instrument to be used with a slightly less restricted pattern of adaptation in the dentition than that allowed by the sickle. Just as with the cowhorn explorer and the paired contra-angled sickle, the instrument can be used in any given sextant from the facial or lingual surfaces, *with one edge adapting against the mesial aspect and the opposite edge on that same end adapting on the distal aspect.* In other words, the same end of the instrument is used for all proximal surfaces in a given sextant from the buccal aspect. And, of course, the opposite end is used in that same sextant from the lingual aspect on all proximal surfaces. The two edges on a given end of the instrument make it possible to scale the mesial surface and then the distal surface and so on by merely changing the edge being used and the orientation of the shank in relation to the long axis of the tooth.

With the universal curette it is possible to use the *opposite end* of the instrument to scale most distal surfaces as well. That is, the end that normally would not be used on a given sextant from a particular aspect can be used on the distal surfaces safely and with the proper angulation. For example, one end can be used on the mandibular right area from the buccal aspect; the other end can be used in that quadrant from the lingual aspect. With the universal curette the end used from the lingual aspect can also be used on distal surfaces from the buccal aspect. The terminal shank, however, will not be parallel to the long axis of the tooth in this case. Return to Fig. 21-13, *A,* which shows the position for using the *opposite*

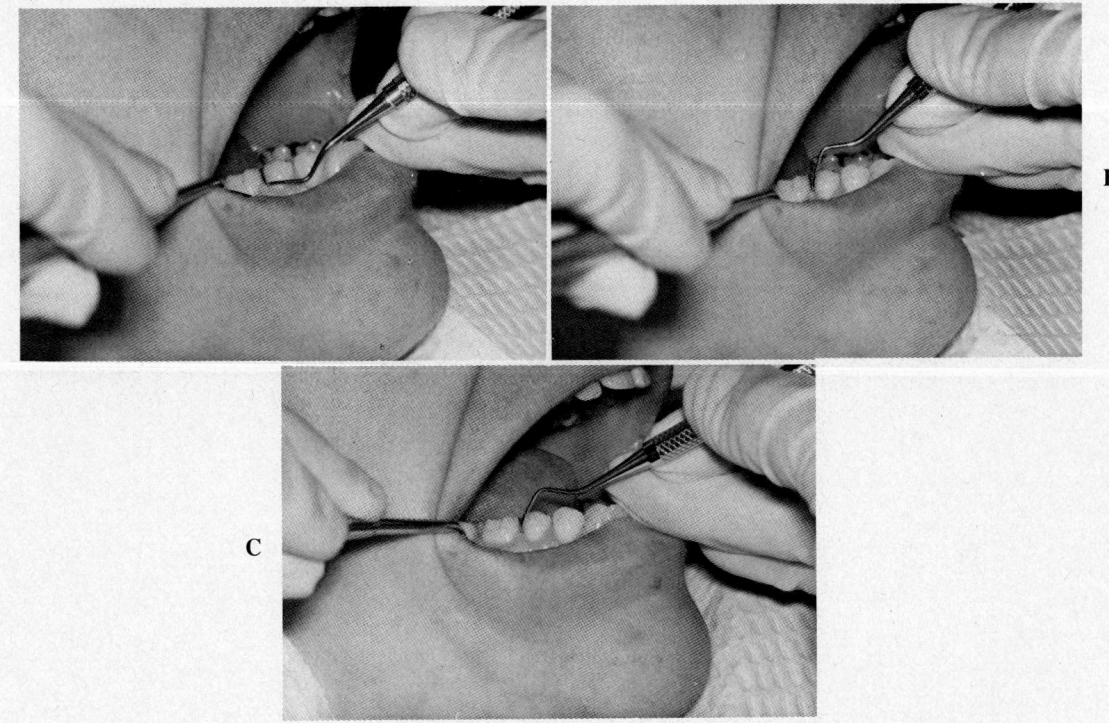

Fig. 21-13. **A,** Universal curette is adapted with toe directed proximally but with terminal shank perpendicular to long axis of tooth. **B,** Universal curette is adapted with terminal shank parallel to long axis of tooth. **C,** Angulation is closed to less than 90 but more than 45 degrees before beginning working stroke.

end. By raising the shank to a 45-degree angle to the long axis of the tooth, the instrument can be adapted on the distal surface safely. Generally, this particular use of the instrument is an adjunct to regular patterns of instrumentation largely because it necessitates an additional change of ends of the instrument, which is not necessary if the opposite edge of the same end is used as usual. It is helpful to know that this adaptation can be safely accomplished, as there are times when a slightly different approach to an area will allow the right adaptation to remove a particularly challenging deposit.

Selecting a curette: design variations

Many varieties of universal curettes are available; therefore considerable opportunity exists for selecting a specific curette for a particular patient's need. Variations in shank angle, shank strength, and shank length allow for use in remote or more anterior areas of the dentition, for heavy tenacious deposits, and for very deep or relatively shallow pockets. Tissue tightness to the tooth often dictates the size of the shank or blade that may be selected. Extremely tight tissue will not allow a heavy, large instrument adequate access to remove subgingival deposits.

The length of the blade is another variable in selecting a universal curette. Longer blades are needed to gain access across the relatively broad proximal surfaces of posterior teeth but may be quite inappropriate for use on the narrow mandibular anterior teeth.

The universal curette is often the instrument of choice for removal of moderate or heavy amounts of calculus and when the width and depth of the pocket can accept the havier shank, but other curettes are more appropriate for use in deep, tight pockets and for removal of fine deposits and root planing. Gracey curettes are examples of instruments with longer, thinner shanks and with more delicate blades. They are characterized by a preangled blade design. The blade and bevel are set at the correct angle to the terminal shank so that the shank can be kept parallel to the long axis of the tooth throughout instrumentation. The universal curettes (and the sickle scalers) require that the blade be angled to between 45 and 90 degrees after it is inserted; the shank is then angled toward the long axis of the tooth during instrumentation. The Gracey curettes are introduced in Chapter 23.

General guidelines for selection of universal curettes include (1) reserving heavy, large curettes for heavy deposits and finer, smaller curettes for finer deposits or for access to tight subgingival areas; (2) using long-shanked instruments for deep pockets; and (3) selecting the blade length according to the size of the tooth surface to be scaled.

Sequence

Whether the universal curette or the sickle scaler is being used for removing moderate to heavy amounts of calculus, the same general sequence is followed as described in detail in Chapter 6.

The mandibular posterior sextant closer to the clinician (mandibular right for right-handed clinicians; mandibular left for left-handed clinicians) is scaled first, moving from the most posterior tooth through the first premolar. The distal, facial, and mesial surfaces are scaled using overlapping exploratory and working strokes as calculus is detected and engaged for removal. The stroking pattern should carry the instrument past the proximal midlines of each tooth to ensure that typically elusive deposits are not left.

The clinician then scales the mandibular sextant on the opposite side of the mouth, approaching it from the lingual surfaces. The lingual surfaces on the side of the mouth nearer the clinician are next, and then the buccal aspect of the opposite side of the mouth is scaled. At this point all the posterior teeth are scaled. If the instrument has reached sufficiently far across the proximal surface under the deposits to engage and remove them with overlapping strokes, few deposits should remain. With either a posterior sickle or a universal curette, this can be accomplished with only one position change (moving to the rear position for the buccal surfaces on the side away

from the clinician) and with only one instrument change (changing ends when moving from the lingual surfaces of the distant sextant to the lingual surfaces of the near sextant).

The anterior teeth can then be scaled either from the rear or front position.

Many clinicians stop and explore the mandibular teeth for remaining deposits before moving to the maxilla. If considerable deposits remain on these teeth, time will be needed to return to these locations and remove the calculus and recheck.

Once no deposits are detected on the mandibular teeth, the clinician moves to the buccal aspect of the maxillary sextant closer to the clinician and then to the lingual aspect of the distant posterior maxillary sextant. The clinician changes ends and positions (to a rear position) and scales the lingual surfaces of the nearer maxillary sextant, followed by the buccal aspect of the distant sextant. The anterior teeth are then scaled from the rear position. The maxilla is explored for residual deposits and rescaled as needed.

Particularly difficult deposits may require the use of adjunct instruments such as hoe or file. Deposits located in areas defying access may need to be approached with an unconventional adaptation or fulcrum placement.

Hoe

The hoe is an instrument that is usually limited to removal of large ledges of calculus (Seibert,

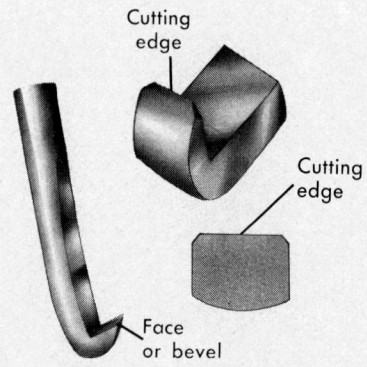

Fig. 21-14. Hoe has one blade and firm shank. When placed beneath a ledge of calculus, a vertical stroke will usually be successful in removing deposit. As shown, corners of blade should be clipped off with sharpening stone. (Adapted from Seibert JS: Contin Dent Educ **1:**8, 1978.)

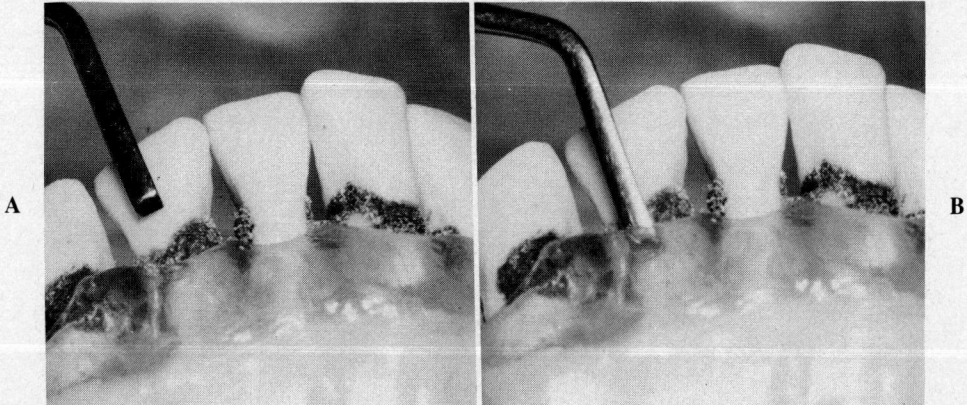

Fig. 21-15. **A,** Hoe with shank parallel to long axis of tooth. **B,** Instrument is moved below edge of calculus with exploratory stroke. Vertical working stroke pattern will engage and remove deposit.

1978). Calculus that rings the tooth, particularly on the facial, lingual, and distal surfaces of teeth that have no posterior tooth adjacent to them, can be removed relatively easy with a hoe.

Fig. 21-14 shows the design of a hoe. It has one blade. The angle of the shank determines the area of use. Generally, the instruments are paired so that one end can be used on the facial surface and its pair can be used on the lingual surface of a given tooth. The companion instrument has one end that can be adapted on the distal surface of a tooth, while its pair can be adapted on the mesial surface of the tooth. The mesial and distal pairs are useful when the adjacent tooth is missing. Thus they are especially helpful in removing ledge calculus from the distal surface of the last tooth in the quadrant and on the direct lingual surface of the lower anterior teeth, especially when a large bridge of calculus is present.

The same modified pen grasp, fulcrum, and wrist rock are used with hoes as with the previously described instruments. However, in implementing the stroking pattern, the instrument is limited to a vertical pattern of strokes (Fig. 21-15). The instrument is placed into the sulcus and moved apically past the deposit of calculus. It is not possible or advisable to force the instrument near the attachment because of its bulk. Once the instrument has moved past the ledge of calculus, it should be held firmly against the tooth with the horizontal pressure of a working stroke and moved coronally out of the sulcus. The blade should engage the deposit and remove it in large

pieces. The instrument can be used to detect any residual pieces of calculus, but it is not known for fine detection potential. It is a heavy working instrument that generally precedes additional scaling with fine curettes.

Most clinicians maintain a sterile set of hoes for those times when a heavy case requires their use. They are not regular inclusions in a standard tray setup for scaling, however, because of their limited use.

Chisel

The chisel is another instrument that is usually maintained as an adjunct instrument. The Zerfing chisel is illustrated in Fig. 21-16. It is used solely to remove large ledges of calculus from the lingual surfaces of the anterior teeth. It is used with a horizontal push stroke with the blade held

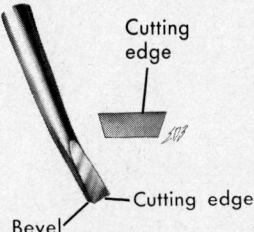

Fig. 21-16. Chisel has single blade and straight shank. Cutting edge is at end of instrument so that when it is pushed against a deposit, leading cutting edge will engage calculus. It is sharpened with flat stone on bevel.

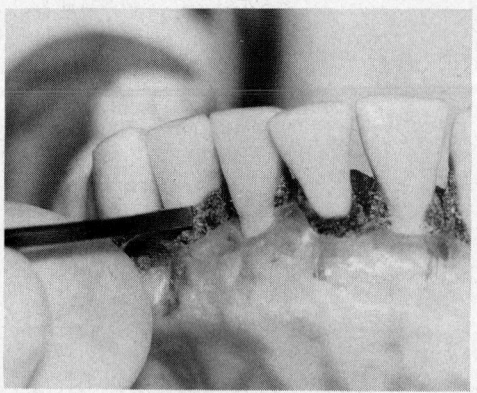

Fig. 21-17. Chisel is used solely to remove lingual calculus on anterior teeth by placing bade against proximal surfaces from labial aspect and pushing toward lingual aspect.

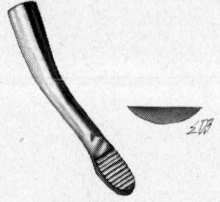

Fig. 21-18. Files are composed of a series of parallel blades on a flat working head. Heavy files have a few large blades, whereas fine files have many small blades.

against the proximal surfaces of the anterior teeth and entering from the labial aspect (Fig. 21-17). The blade is adapted against the distal surface, then against the mesial surface, and so on with a gentle push stroke between the teeth until the large bridge of calculus is adequately loosened and can be removed from the lingual aspect of the teeth. It is never to be pushed down into the gingival sulcus, and it is not designed for a pull stroke out of the sulcus. Its sole function is in the anterior areas, where most instruments would crumble the deposit, and more time would be required to remove a bridge formation of heavy calculus.

File

When an area of subgingival calculus defies removal with universal curettes, sickles, hoes, and other instruments generally used for universal scaling, a file can be used effectively to crush the deposit and roughen it so that other instruments can remove the fine remnants of calculus (Fig. 21-18). The size of files varies, but generally speaking the small fine files that can be readily adapted subgingivally provide the greatest flexibility and accessibility. In design, files are like several small hoe blades placed in a row on a flat head. They are usually paired to allow access on direct facial and lingual surfaces with one pair of instruments and on mesial and distal surfaces with the other pair of instruments. Thus, in basic de-

sign and in areas of access, files are quite similar to hoes. However, the instruments designed for mesial and distal surfaces can be used even in areas where there is an adjacent tooth. Files have a variety of head shapes, ranging from rectangular to oval to oblong. The number of cutting edges or "lips" on the each varies also. Also varying are the size of the lip closest to the shank and the size of the rake farthest from the shank (the heel); these determine how far the instrument will displace soft tissue when used in pockets. The lip closest to the shank should be 90 degrees to the back of the head of the instrument, and the rake angle between lips should be 55 degrees to the back of the head. Ratcliff files are large, thick, working files with four lips. Others, such as the Rhein 31/32 and UW B46, are best used as finishing files, to smooth the roots after calculus has been removed, for smoothing CEJs, and for finishing restorative margins; such files have 10 or more lips. Hirschfeld files remove calculus and root roughness in many otherwise inaccessible areas, such as root furrows, deep pockets, and places where the gingival tissues are tight. They have only three rakes and have small heads (Hoople, 1985).

Files have long been considered as adjunct instruments. However, in some parts of the country they are used extensively in root planing and are often preferred to curettes. They can be an extremely valuable choice depending upon the clinical situation.

Fig. 21-19 illustrates a file approaching the mesial surface of a tooth. The instrument is carefully inserted between the papilla and the tooth, is used to find the tenacious deposit, and is engaged against the deposit with the head of small blades pressed against the deposit and ground into the

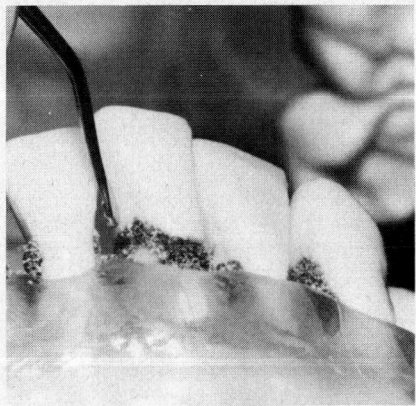

Fig. 21-19. File is adapted to crush calculus and smooth area. Follow-up strokes with a curette are important for removing small fragments and smoothing tooth structure.

deposit, crushing it. Horizontal and vertical strokes can follow this crushing motion. A curette or a finer file can be used to finish the area.

Files are usually placed in the category of adjunct instruments and therefore may not be used routinely in general practice or in a recall program.

Other instruments

Many other kinds of shank designs, working end sizes, and shank strengths are available. However, the basic designs apply to most instruments and can be helpful in selecting instrument ends and in selecting which type of instrument to use for each type of case. Regardless of the type of instrument presented, a careful analysis of the position of the blade(s), shank size and angulation, and size of the head of the instrument will determine its usefulness and limitations. While the student of dental hygiene functions with a limited set of instruments, it is helpful to have a wide variety of instruments available for advanced instrumentation in the later phases of clinical development.

EVALUATING FOR COMPLETE DEPOSIT REMOVAL

The working instruments provide some amount of tactile sense in determining the presence of deposits in the mouth, but all scaling procedures should be carefully evaluated with instruments that provide maximum tactile sensitivity. The explorer or probe should be used at the completion of scaling in each quadrant or arch to determine whether deposits are completely removed. These finer instruments may uncover deposits located just apical to the contact area, a location difficult to reach with heavy instruments, or the explorer may detect a small portion of a deposit at the corner of the tooth or just above the attachment, both of which easily can be missed with a heavier instrument.

During the scaling procedure itself, it is wise to use exploratory strokes with the working instruments to detect relative smoothness of the tooth surface before moving on to another area. However, it is essential that all areas be thoroughly evaluated with explorers or a probe before an area is declared complete.

As mentioned in Chapter 12 it is sometimes possible to detect calculus in subgingival areas by directing a stream of compressed air into the sulcus. The tissue, particularly if not tight to the tooth, can be deflected from the tooth, allowing the clinician to look into the sulcus. Also, after a period of healing, the tissue can be evaluated to identify any particular areas of continued inflammation. Often, isolated areas of poor healing identify the location of residual calculus deposits. Sometimes those deposits will be visible as a dark shadow at the margin of the gingiva. A stream of air can confirm that finding, along with thorough follow-up exploring.

Supragingival calculus is best detected with air and with a well-directed beam of light. The calculus will appear as a chalky white layer across the tooth surface. It will feel crusty and soft to the explorer rather than smooth and hard, as enamel is. Disclosing solution will usually stain this crustaceous calculus. Even the fine grains that cannot be seen clearly with air and light will be visible with a disclosant. It is important to differentiate calculus deposits from plaque, as even repeated polishing will not remove them from the teeth. A sharpened curette or sickle is necessary to remove the fine, residual grains of calculus. If they remain on the teeth, they provide an opportunity for new plaque to adhere, and they can be felt by the patient's tongue.

Whether the deposits are visible or not, it is essential to remove all deposits from the teeth and use thorough evaluation procedures to ensure their complete removal. The time-honored goal in the profession is 100% removal of all deposits—sub-gingival as well as supragingival.

Researchers use two ways of determining instrumentation effectiveness. In the first, teeth are treated in the mouth (in vivo), extracted, and evaluated under the microscope (stero, light, or scanning electron). In the second, teeth are treated and the soft tissue surrounding the teeth is examined at intervals to measure healing and continued health (O'Leary, 1986). The practicing hygienist will typically rely upon the second approach, as the objective of care is to ensure that the teeth stay in the mouth. However, clinicians can learn a great deal about the effectiveness of their instrumentation if they scale teeth that are designated for extraction and then carefully observe the efficiency of their scaling under the microscope. Typically, areas will be visible without aid of magnification; magnification reveals calculus fragments, stainable plaque, scratches, gouges and other irregularities, instilling a deep sense of humility in the clinician.

Surgical access, by laying back the gingiva from the teeth and bone, improves the ability of the clinician to remove calculus and other deposits and irregularities, but even after surgical access fragments can be detected microscopically, particularly in furcation areas (Eaton et al, 1985; Matia et al, 1986; Buchanan and Robertson, 1987).

At some point in a clinician's career, particularly when he or she is at the point of believing that clinical skills are quite well developed, it may be useful to observe a periodontal surgery being performed for one of the patients the clinician has had the opportunity to scale. A great deal can be learned about adequacy and thoroughness as a clinician by seeing a flap laid in the area of scaling and seeing if areas of calculus remain despite even the most careful efforts. Research shows that it is extremely difficult to remove all calculus, especially when it is embedded in irregularities and when it is in deep pockets (Nishimine and O'Leary, 1979; Rabbani et al, 1981; Eaton, et al, 1985). Complete scaling and evaluation is a skill that develops with time; 100% removal for all patients may be a goal to be striven for rather than a valid measure of day-to-day success.

ALTERNATIVE FULCRUM PLACEMENT

As described in Chapter 6 and earlier in this chapter, the usual location for a fulcrum or finger rest is on the occlusal surfaces of teeth. The tooth surface should be dry so that the clinician's finger is less likely to slip, particularly during a working stroke, when control is absolutely essential. If the finger rest is lost, the instrument may accidentally traumatize the patient's palate, lip, gingiva, or the clinician's hand. The first choice for a finger rest or fulcrum is on a dry, stable tooth. Slippery mucosa or no finger rest are unsafe choices.

There are instances when an alternative fulcrum is needed (1) in order to reach inaccessible areas, (2) when even slight pressure against the lip or stretching of the lips is not easily tolerated, (3) when there are not enough teeth in the sextant to provide a fulcrum, or (4) when removing a particularly tenacious calculus deposit demands the greater leverage available from having a more distant fulcrum.

Figure 21-20 shows an alternative rest for the lingual aspect of the maxillary left quadrant for a right-handed clinician. The left index finger is laid across the mandibular arch in the area of the premolars, and the fulcrum finger of the right hand rests stably on it. This is a useful approach for patients with small mouths or in instances when there are few teeth in that sextant to provide a fulcrum.

Figure 21-21 shows the fulcrum finger placed on the left index finger, which is resting securely in the labial vestibule, retracting the lip. This alternative is useful when using circumferential strokes on the facial surfaces or when there are too few teeth to provide a ready fulcrum site. It is the fulcrum of choice when using a horizontal, facial-to-lingual push stroke with a chisel.

Chapter 6 contains considerable discussion regarding access to the buccal aspect of the maxillary teeth in the sextant closest to the clinician. Two rests are described: one posterior to the operative site and one anterior to the site. The two approaches require different wrist rocks (see Fig. 6-21 for a right-handed clinician or 6-33 for a left-handed clinician). The finger rest posterior to the operative site is described as using the orbicularis oris muscle at the corner of the mouth to provide much of the stability, particularly for extreme

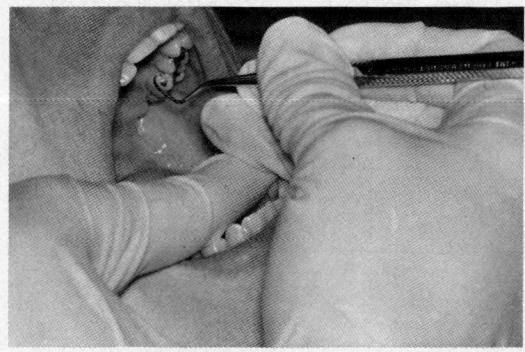

Fig. 21-20. Alternative fulcrum placement for maxillary left lingual sextant uses left index finger resting on mandibular arch.

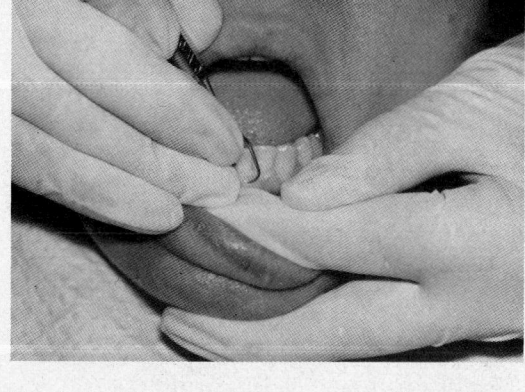

Fig. 21-21. Fulcrum finger rests on index finger placed in mandibular anterior vestibule.

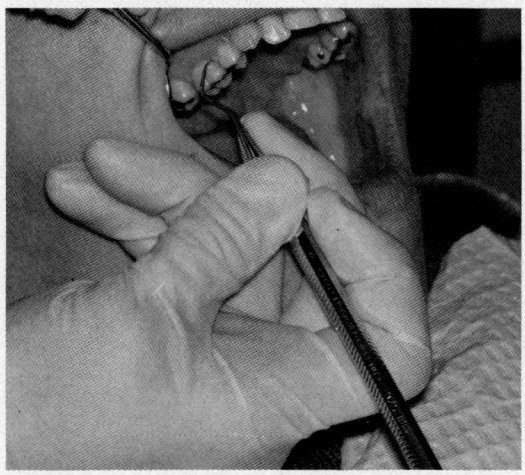

Fig. 21-22. Backs of third and fourth fingers are pressed extraorally against cheek for fulcrum for access to maxillary right buccal area.

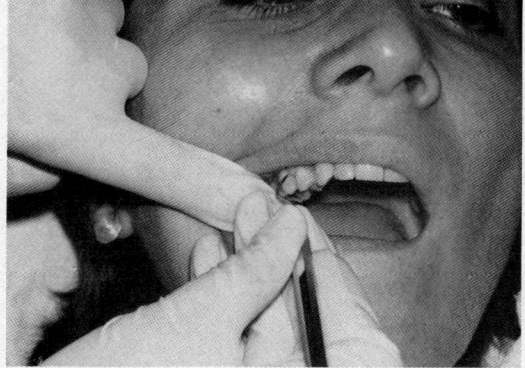

Fig. 21-23. Left index finger retracts cheek; right fulcrum finger rests on it for access to maxillary right buccal area.

posterior instrumentation sites. When the last tooth in the quadrant is being explored or scaled, all fulcrum support is localized on the elastic resistance of the corner of the mouth.

There are two other alternatives for access to this area. Fig. 21-22 shows a rest where the backs of the third and fourth fingers are pressed firmly against the cheek, serving as an extraoral fulcrum. Or the left index finger can be used to retract the cheek, with the right fulcrum finger resting on it (Fig. 21-23).

Although it was once considered heresy to teach many alternative hand placements for establishing a fulcrum, there is currently a movement to encourage creative approaches in order to gain access to areas of the mouth that are remote or provide no ready conventional fulcrum. These approaches include establishing a fulcrum on the mandible while scaling the maxilla and on the opposite side of the arch, causing the fulcrum finger and the grasp of the instrument to separate. Virtually any approach to an area now receives a fair hearing, but it is important to have a firm grasp and stable fulcrum or rest on something to ensure both safe use of the instrument and sufficient leverage to enable deposits to be removed efficiently.

BEYOND CALCULUS REMOVAL

This chapter has focused on removing calculus deposits with hand instruments. As noted in Chapter 12, calculus must be removed in order to create an environment less conducive to the accumulation of plaque. However, initial and maintenance therapy for patients with periodontal involvement requires more than just calculus removal. It requires that all plaque and the endotoxin byproducts of plaque be removed from the root surfaces so that the surrounding soft tissues can repair and generate reattachment. It requires that surrounding soft tissue be prepared for healing, which may necessitate soft tissue curettage.

Simply removing calculus and polishing teeth, even when combined with good patient oral hygiene, are not adequate to halt disease. The subgingival plaque front can progress apically, and cementum-bound endotoxin will continue to irritate soft tissues, causing continued subclinical destruction despite the deceivingly healthy appearance of the gingivae (Daly et al, 1982; Aleo et al, 1974; Waerhaug, 1978a, 1978b).

In the next few chapters other instrumentation procedures are introduced for removing calculus, for debriding the root surfaces, and for performing curettage. Given our growing understanding of the progress and prevention of periodontal disease, these functions are essential components of the scope of practice of a dental hygienist.

ACTIVITIES

1. Compare the contra-angled sickle and the universal curette with the cowhorn or pigtail explorer. Identify which ends match in terms of the direction of the shanks. Given either end of the contra-angled sickle or universal curette, identify all areas in the dentition where that end may be used so that the point aims across the intended proximal surface, the terminal shank is parallel to the long axis of the tooth, and the handle exits the mouth from the front.
2. Use the suggested sequence of positions to adapt the contra-angled sickle, straight sickle, and universal curette in each sextant of the dentition. Be certain to do the following:
   a. Use a modified pen grasp
   b. Establish a firm fulcrum
   c. Use all fingers as a unit to generate a wrist rock, pivoting on the fulcrum finger
   d. Adapt the side of the tip to the tooth to avoid piercing the tissue with the point or toe of the instrument
   e. Angulate the face of the instrument at greater than 45 degrees and less than 90 degrees to the tooth
   f. Execute exploratory stroke around the tooth with the scaler or curette, using horizontal pressure against the tooth when engaging a deposit (working stroke)
   g. For the universal curette, use the *opposite end* on distal surfaces and analyze its usefulness
3. Adapt the hoe, chisel, and file on a typodont and on calculus-laden teeth set in plaster. Explore apically with the hoe and file to detect calculus and engage horizontal pressure apically to remove it. Use a push stroke from labial to lingual surfaces to loosen a bridge of calculus by engaging the blade of the chisel on the proximal surfaces.
4. Scale a quadrant for a more advanced student's patient. Have the advanced student watch the procedure and offer suggestions. Observe as the student uses air, light, explorer, probe, and/or disclosant to evaluate for residual calculus.
5. Role-play ways of responding to hypothetical patients, employers, and peers who describe the dental hygienist as a person who cleans teeth.
6. Develop a role definition of dental hygiene that adequately describes the class's perception of how the oral prophylaxis fits into the scope of practice.
7. Compare the effects of a dull blade and a sharp blade for calculus removal from plaster-mounted calculus-laden teeth.
8. Compare the shank sizes and shapes and the sizes of the working ends for a variety of the following instruments:
   a. Universal curettes
   b. Hoes
   c. Files
9. Given descriptions of clinical conditions, such as amounts and locations of calculus, sulcus or pocket depth, and gingival tissue conditions, practice selecting appropriate scalers for removing the deposits.
10. Review the radiographs in Chapter 11 that show supra- and subgingival calculus. Select scalers and/or curettes that would most efficiently remove the deposits.

REVIEW QUESTIONS

1. What are two major differences between scaling with a cutting instrument and exploring?

2. True or false (correct the false statements):
   a. A chisel is useful for removing large bridges of calculus from the lingual surface of the mandibular anterior teeth.
   b. The chisel is used with a pull stroke.
   c. The hoe is useful for removing ledge calculus that is readily accessible to a heavy instrument.
   d. The file is used to crush calculus.
   e. The universal curette is used primarily for deep calculus removal.
   f. The sickle scaler is the most versatile instrument, as it is effective for deep scaling as well as supragingival scaling.
   g. As long as calculus is removed from the teeth, the soft tissues will be able to heal with time.
3. What are three methods for clinically evaluating complete calculus removal?

REFERENCES

Aleo JJ, et al: The presence and biological activity of cementum-bound endotoxin, J Periodontol 45:672, 1974.

Axelsson P, and Lindhe J: The significance of maintenance care in the treatment of periodontal disease, J Clin Periodontal 8:281, 1981.

Badersten A, et al: Effect of nonsurgical periodontal therapy, J Clin Periodontol 8:57, 1981.

Buchanan SA, and Robertson PB: Calculus removal by scaling/root planing with and without surgical access, J Periodontol 58:159, 1987.

Daly C, et al: Histological assessment of periodontally involved cementum, J Clin Periodontol 9:266, 1982.

Eaton KA, Kieser JB, and Davies RM: The removal of root surface deposits, J Clin Periodontol 12:141, 1985.

Hoople S: Files provide desirable results in patient treatment procedures, RDH Mag 5(10):22, 1985.

Knowles J, et al: Comparison of results following three modalities of periodontal therapy related to tooth type and initial pocket depth, J Clin Periodontol 7:32, 1980.

Matia, J. et al: Efficiency of scaling of the molar furcation area with and without surgical access, Int J Periodont Restorative Dent 6:25, 1986.

Morrison E, et al: Short-term effects of initial, nonsurgical periodontal treatment (hygienic phase), J Clin Periodontol 7:199, 1980.

Muller H-P, Hartmann J, and Flores-de-Jacoby L: Clinical alterations in relation to the morphological composition of the subgingival microflora following scaling and root planing, J Clin Periodontol 13:825, 1986.

Nishimini D, and O'Leary TJ: Hand instrumention versus ultrasonics in the removal of endotoxins from root surfaces, J Periodontol 50:345, 1979.

O'Leary T: The impact of research on scaling and root planing, J Periodontol 57:69, 1986.

Parr RW, et al: Subgingival scaling and root planing. San Francisco, 1976, University of California School of Dentistry.

Rabbani GM, et al: The effectiveness of subgingival scaling and root planing in calculus removal, J Periodontol 52:119, 1981.

Ring ME: A brief history of dental prophylaxis, Compend Contin Educ 8:470, 1987.

Seibert JS: Incorporating root planing and gingival curettage into a clinical practice, Contin Dent Educ, 1:8, 1978.

Waerhaug J: Healing of the dento-epithelial junction following subgingival plaque control, I: As observed in human biopsy material, J Periodontol 49:1, 1978(a).

Waerhaug J: Healing of the dento-epithelial junction following subgingival plaque control, II: As observed on extracted teeth, J Periodontol 49:119, 1978(b).

22 REMOVING HEAVY DEPOSITS: ULTRASONIC AND SONIC INSTRUMENTS

OBJECTIVES: *The reader will be able to*

1. Given information about oral conditions and general health status, determine whether ultrasonic scaling is or is not an appropriate choice for particular patients.
2. Describe the advantages and disadvantages of ultrasonic scaling.
3. Briefly describe how ultrasonic and sonic scalers remove deposits.
4. Identify precautions that must be taken to minimize cross-contamination during ultrasonic scaling.
5. Given a patient for whom ultrasonic scaling is indicated, describe the procedure for ensuring patient confidence, obtaining informed consent, and providing the patient with sufficient information to enable the patient to decide whether or not to proceed.
6. Identify four important measures for helping the patient cope with water flow.
7. Given an ultrasonic unit, prepare it for operation by connecting the following:
   a. Electrical outlet
   b. Foot control
   c. Water supply
   d. Handpiece
8. Describe the procedure for preparing an instrument tip for use in a manual tune unit.
9. Identify the design and usefulness of each of the following tips:
   a. Chisel
   b. Beaver-tail
   c. Universal curette style
   d. Periodontal probe style
10. Describe the best sequence and stroking pattern to produce a smooth tooth surface with an ultrasonic or sonic scalers.
11. Describe the length and speed of the stroke used with an ultrasonic or sonic instrument.
12. Contrast ultrasonic and sonic instrumentation principles with those employed with hand instruments.
13. List three functions of the water lavage in ultrasonic scaling.
14. Describe the procedure for adjusting temperature of the water lavage.
15. Given a series of patients for whom ultrasonic scaling is indicated, do the following:
    a. Prepare the patient for maximum comfort and provide him or her sufficient information for informed consent.
    b. Prepare the equipment and take precautions to prevent microbial cross-contamination.
    c. Select an appropriate area for completion.
    d. Use appropriate tips in a sequence that removes stain and calculus both supragingivally and subgingivally.
    e. Explore all areas for removal of deposits.
    f. Root plane all areas to completion, obtaining a hard, smooth surface.
    g. Ensure that plaque control measures are being learned and employed by the patient to ensure the best possible tissue resolution.
16. Briefly describe research findings related to effectiveness, tissue response, tooth structure smoothness, and safety precautions when ultrasonic instruments are used.

A complete intraoral assessment of a patient may reveal large amounts of calculus. Some patients have calculus that bridges the teeth, especially in the mandibular anterior and maxillary posterior areas. Large, tenacious deposits may prevent the patient from adequately flossing interdental areas, and if they are visible, their presence may be of major concern to the patient, as they are an esthetic problem.

From a treatment-planning point of view, many clinicians feel it is advantageous to remove calculus early in treatment so that the patient is able to begin a new routine of self-care and to feel better about his or her mouth immediately. Additionally, thorough early removal of the heavy deposits makes it possible to assess pocket depth more accurately and establish a prognosis.

An ultrasonic scaling device can be used to remove heavy deposits with minimal trauma to soft tissues in a relatively short amount of time. These devices and their functions were reviewed by the ADA (1985). Although hand instruments designed for heavy deposits such as chisels, hoes, and heavy universal curettes can be used, the ultrasonic scaler requires less time and results in less clinician and patient fatigue and discomfort (Green and Sanderson, 1965). Depending on the type of deposit and the expertise of the clinician, scaling with ultrasonic instruments may require only 20% to 60% of the time required to complete the procedure with hand instruments alone.

Less chair time for the patient is valuable to both the patient and the clinician. The patient who has accumulated large amounts of calculus has usually had a long sabbatical from dental care and is pleased to have preliminary appointments that are brief and maximally productive.

Likewise, the clinician who is confronted with several years' accumulation of calculus can anticipate a proportionate amount of hand fatigue when using hand scalers. The ultrasonic scaler results in almost no hand fatigue, as it requires only a light grasp and virtually no pressure against the tooth. Two arches of supragingival and subgingival scaling can be accomplished by the experienced clinician in a 45-minute to 1-hour appointment. Less experienced operators may select one arch to complete during an appointment, with re-evaluation of the scaled arch and scaling of the remaining arch reserved for a later appointment.

One major advantage of ultrasonic scaling is its positive influence on tissue responses. The water lavage that accompanies the calculus removal is apparently largely responsible, along with a coagulation of the necrotic soft tissue wall adjacent to the tooth surface (Ewen, 1961). The lavage flushes most small calculus fragments and dislodges necrotic tissue from the sulcus so that the site has few if any local irritants remaining to retard healing. It is frequently described as the instrument of choice for patients with acute necrotizing ulcerative gingivitis (ANUG), a painful, inflammatory disease. Symptoms disappear more rapidly when ultrasonic scaling is used, and patients report less discomfort immediately following treatment (Fitch et al, 1963). One study has reported that after 8 weeks there was no statistically significant difference between tissue healing after hand scaling and tissue healing after ultrasonic scaling (Torfason et al, 1979).

Ultrasonic scaling is, however, not without controversy. For the 35 years that it has been used in dentistry, research into its effect on the teeth and surrounding tissues has resulted in mixed reports (Green and Sanderson, 1965; Benfenati et al, 1987). Most of the studies that question its long-term merit focus on the changes the instrument makes on root structure, particularly in contrast to the results obtained from using hand instruments in root-planing procedures. A more complete discussion of these controversies is given at the end of this chapter.

ORIGINS AND MECHANISM

Ultrasonic instrumentation was first used in dentistry in the 1950s. An ultrasonic drill was used to prepare teeth for restorations, but it relied on an abrasive slurry to cut the tooth and therefore reduced visibility considerably. High-speed turbine drills were developed about that time as well. As the turbine drill was found to be quite effective, the ultrasonic drill was phased out (Ewen and Glickstein, 1968; Green and Sanderson, 1965).

An ultrasonic instrument reappeared in 1955 for periodontal instrumentation and was first described by Zinner (1955). It has undergone many changes in design and usefulness since that time. The bulky, complex units are now compact and easy to adjust. The variety of tips has increased, and many tips carry the needed water supply through an internal tube rather than by means of an external tube, which can easily bend out of alignment with the tip. Several manufacturers have developed units, each with unique features. Air-driven units that generate less heat are available for direct connection to air turbine hoses, competing with the ultrasonic devices largely because of their ease of operation, lower cost, and simple storage (Woodruff, Levin, and Brady, 1975).

Ultrasonic instruments use high-frequency sound waves to fracture deposits from teeth and to cavitate the accompanying water supply to mechanically flush the area. The instrument tip vibrates approximately 25,000 cycles per second, with the water spray creating a halo of tiny bubbles surrounding the tip in a fine mist (Green and Sanderson, 1965).

Whereas ultrasonic scalers oscillate at 25,000 or more cycles per second, "sonic" scalers follow an elliptical pattern of between 16,000 and 18,000 cycles per second. These are air-driven devices rather than electrical. A sonic scaler consists of an autoclavable handpiece and a set of tips. The handpiece attaches to the tubing of the air turbine handpieces used for caries removal or polishing. These are the most portable scalers. They typically operate with a water spray, which remains an important aspect of the therapeutic benefit of this type of scaling, even though the air-driven sonic scaler does not require water as a coolant. One evaluation of the sonic scaler demonstrated that increased load against the scaler will alter the oscillation and then stop it without a noticeable change in detectable sound. Perpendicular application to the tooth structure can damage the tooth, as can the misapplication of the ultrasonic tips. Thus it is important not to apply excessive pressure against the tooth and to apply the side of the tip rather than the end of the instrument to the tooth during scaling (Gankerseer and Walmsley, 1987).

Because the "vibrating" tip and cavitating water cleanse the tooth, there is no need for sharp instruments. In fact, for purposes of scaling and curettage, the tips must be dull. There is no need to engage a sharp blade against the deposit or tissue; the vibrations merely from placing the activated tip on the operative area cause the deposits to fracture away and necrotic tissue to coagulate.

Placing the tip against the deposit and then moving it over the surface results in a calculus-free area and a smoother tooth surface. No pressure against the tooth is necessary. Usually the instrument will simply stop if pressed against the tooth, although damage to the tooth can sometimes occur.

INDICATIONS, CONTRAINDICATIONS, AND PRECAUTIONS

When the ultrasonic scaler was first introduced, overly zealous users employed it for all prophylaxis procedures, as it was much easier than hand scaling. However, indiscriminate use of the ultrasonic scaler is a mistake. It is best reserved for patients with large amounts of calculus. As hand planing should, according to most investigators, follow ultrasonic instrumentation, use of the ultrasonic scaler for the patient with almost no calculus will result in more chair time than necessary. And, of course, there are instances in which the medical history or certain oral conditions preclude its use.

Generally, the ultrasonic scaler should be used for those patients who have large, tenacious deposits and stains on their teeth. It can be used to remove deposits from teeth that will be extracted, minimizing the possibility that calculus will lodge in the extraction site. But its greatest usefulness is in preparing teeth for definitive periodontal therapy. Teeth with heavy deposits can be cleansed so that only the final stages of root planing are necessary. As mentioned previously, patients with ANUG frequently commence treatment with ultrasonic debridement (Ewen and Glickstein, 1968; Fitch et al, 1963).

Ultrasonic scaling is extremely useful for clearing local irritants in pericoronitis and gingival and periodontal abscesses. It can be used to clear deposits in cases of chronic marginal gingivitis, periodontitis, idiopathic fibrous hyperplasia, drug-induced hyperplasia, and hormonal gingivitis such as that associated with pregnancy, puberty, or menopause (Ewen and Glickstein, 1968).

Ultrasonic instrumentation with a water lavage appears to have an antimicrobial effect. The cavitation activity, heat, and acoustic streaming are the probable causes for the decrease in numbers of bacteria at sites that have been ultrasonically debrided. The mechanical effects of cavitation (shock and stress waves) can disrupt and lyse bacterial cell walls (Clarke and Hill, 1970; Rooney, 1972; Cunningham, 1982). One study suggests that the active motile rods typically associated with periodontal disease are the most sensitive to ultrasonics and that the gram positive bacteria characteristic of healthy sites are resistant to sonication (Olsen et al, 1981). Another study demonstrates that ultrasonically debriding root canals will be more likely to sterilize the site than hand instrumentation (Sjogren and Sundqvist, 1987). This antimicrobial property makes ultrasonic scaling an appropriate choice for dental conditions where bacteria need to be reduced in numbers, such as periodontal disease and endodontic therapy.

A study comparing the amount of residual bacterial plaque following hand and ultrasonic scaling indicates that remarkably little plaque and few bacterial colonies remain after instrumentation. Fourteen of the 17 teeth determined to have no bacteria under SEM evaluation had been treated with ultrasonics. Hand instruments tended to leave plaque near the apical border of the pockets and in areas near residual calculus (Breininger et al, 1987). Another study showed similar effects for hand and ultrasonic methods (Oosterwaal et al, 1987).

Going a step further, Leon and Vogel (1987) demonstrated that ultrasonic instruments were about the same as hand curettes when treating Class I furcation involvements but more effective when compared in the treatment of Class II and III furca. Darkfield counts of motile rods and spirochetes were significantly lower in these sites where ultrasonic scaling was used than where hand curettes were used.

Hunter and others (1984) showed no significant differences between ultrasonic scaling and hand scaling for purposes of calculus removal except on the mesial surfaces of anterior teeth, where the hand instruments left 4.51% residual deposits, compared with 7.17% left by ultrasonic instruments. The resulting statistical difference probably would not be clinically apparent to most observers.

Composite resins, especially Class IV and V restorations, should be avoided when scaling ultrasonically, as the action of the instrument tends to cause margin leakage leading to marginal staining and loss of retention (Pollack and Kronenberg, 1981). Similarly, ultrasonic instrumentation tends to damage amalgam restorations widening or chipping the margin between the tooth structure and the alloy (Rajstein and Tal, 1984) or roughening the surface (Blanchard, 1984). Ultrasonic scaling is contraindicated for any patient with a pacemaker, because the sound frequencies of the scaler may disrupt the electronic mechanism with electromagnetic interference. (Adams et al, 1983). Although most newer models of pacemakers have shielding to prevent such interference, it is unwise to subject the patient to such a risk. It is also not to be used for patients with local osteomyelitis, chronic cyclical gingival infections, gingivosis of menopause, nutritional deficiencies of a chronic debilitating nature, severe uncontrolled diabetes, and local neoplasms of metastic nature. It should not be used on young, growing tissues or for patients undergoing immunosuppressive or prolonged antibiotic and/or corticosteroid therapy (Ewen and Glickstein, 1968; Gross, Divine, and Cutright, 1976).

The majority of research into the safety of ultrasound has been associated with the heat generated, particularly during diagnostic procedures for pregnant women. Less information has been generated regarding the effects of acoustic cavitation on tissues. More research on the shockwaves from expanding and collapsing bubbles within tissues should be forthcoming. (Carsten, 1986).

The ultrasonic scaler generates heat, which is cooled by water. However, if insufficient water is used to reduce heat or if the instrument is held against one area of a tooth for more than a few seconds, the temperature in the pulp chamber can rise to hazardous levels. The thermal conductivity of restorations and the thickness of tooth structure separating the instrument from the pulp affect the likelihood of a rise in pulp temperature. Usually the patient will feel discomfort and alert the clinician, preventing continued trauma. But if the operative site is anesthetized, damage could be considerable (Abrams et al, 1979). Walmsley and colleagues (1986) measured the rise of temperature in the pulp due to the transference of acoustic energy from the tip through the water coolant to the tooth. The observed increase in temperature suggests that only 3.6% of the energy being expended was absorbed by the tooth causing a temperature increase, indicating that pulp trauma is highly unlikely. However, water flow must be maintained and the instrument must be kept moving at all times in order to reduce the possibility of pulp trauma. Walmsley (1984) demonstrated that cavitating water has a cleansing effect that contributes significantly to the overall effectiveness of the ultrasonically vibrating tip. This helps emphasize the importance of an adequate flow of water to the tip during ultrasonic procedures.

Because the water spray that accompanies the procedure creates an aerosol of water and microorganisms that contacts the clinician and settles on adjacent equipment surfaces, it is *essential* that the clinician wear protective lenses and a face mask. The entire area should be disinfected thoroughly after each use. It is also recommended that the air in the operatory be continually flushed with a laminar airflow system, which circulates and filters the air of microorganisms (Williams, 1970). When the ultrasonic device is being used, there is a thirty-fold increase of airborne microorganisms, most of which are known to be normal flora of the mouth (Holbrook et al, 1978). Of the airborne contaminants that could cause infection of the clinician or subsequent patients, 97% can be removed with laminar airflow (Williams, 1970). Obviously, it would be unwise to use the ultrasonic device for patient known to have hepatitis or tuberculosis, when the aerosol of pathogens would be extremely dangerous, but precautions should be taken to ensure that even the less virulent organisms are contained.

Another potential hazard of the ultrasonic device is the microbial contamination that can be carried to the surgical site by the water lavage itself (Gross, Devine, and Cutright, 1976). Public water supplies with high counts of microorganisms inoculate the surgical area. Also, the narrow tubing in the unit provides an ideal site for bacterial growth. Water valve connections in the unit may be a site of growth of microbes and of the accumulation of mucin and debris. The results of one study suggest that sterile water should be used (Ballinger, Brasher, and Maupin, 1976). A more recent study has shown that there are no statistical differences in postoperative infections between patients treated with ultrasonic scaling using sterile water and those treated with ultrasonic scaling using regular tap water (Reinhardt et al,

1982). With or without separate water supplies, it is important to assess for backwash of bacteria into the unit and subsequent contamination of the water.

One early study suggested that ultrasonic scaling could cause temporary tinnitus (ringing in the ears) and hearing shifts. It is therefore probably wise to avoid extremely prolonged, repeated use for any patient (Möller, Grevstad, and Kristofferson. 1976). However, a 1987 study contradicts those findings (Walmsley et al, 1987). In any case, ultrasonic scaling is typically of short duration. If a hearing shift does occur, it should be of short duration, as found in the 1976 study.

Once the patient's conditions have been established and it is apparent that the ultrasonic scaler is the instrument of choice, several specific procedures should be followed if the patient is to be comfortable, if the procedure is to be efficient, safe, and effective, and if the equipment is to be properly maintained.

PREPARATION OF THE PATIENT

Perhaps the most important phase of preparation is readying the patient for the procedure. Most patients look warily at humming machines that are rolled into view. Therefore the first step is briefly to explain to the patient the condition that warrants a scaling procedure, why scaling should be done, the consequences of not having complete scaling, the likely aftereffects of the procedure, and the time and cost involved. Included with this explanation should be an introduction to the machine itself.

Following is a typical case presentation in preparing the patient for ultrasonic scaling:

Presentation: I'd like you to take a look in the mirror while I show you something. (Patient grasps mirror; clinician retracts lips to expose gingivae and heavy calculus, using a mouth mirror.) These dark, crusty deposits are hard, chalklike pieces of calculus that are firmly attached to the teeth. They usually go hand in hand with disease of the gum tissue (or gingiva) and bone. Their presence makes it difficult for you to use floss and to adequately cleanse your teeth. (Pause to answer any questions and to follow up on the patient's nonverbal responses.)

One of the first things that needs to be done is to remove these deposits. Once they are gone, your tissue should begin to feel better, and it should be easier to keep up your home care routine. Besides, your teeth will look better.

Sometimes right after the deposits are removed, your teeth will be sensitive to cold. You've had all that crusty insulation for a few years, and once it is gone, the teeth will need to generate their own internal insulation. Other than the sensitivity and a couple of days of tender gingiva, the properly performed procedure has no known harmful effects.

There are two ways in which we can complete the procedure. One is with hand instruments, which you may have had used on your teeth some time ago. Have you ever had your teeth cleaned with metal instruments? (Pause for response and discussion.) The other way is to use the ultrasonic scaler. This latter method should take a good deal less time, because sound waves from this tip remove the deposits (rather than hand pressure) and it is constantly flushing the area to clear away the loosened debris. Usually it feels a good deal better both during and after the procedure, because there isn't extensive pressure and the instrument is gentler on the soft tissues. Healing time may be less also, because the soft tissue is disturbed less and because the water lavage creates a clean site for the tissues to respond.

One problem you may encounter is tooth sensitivity during the procedure. Some patients do experience this sensation—although many feel it with hand instruments as well. (Pause for questions and discussion.)

If we use hand instruments, it may take up to three or four 1-hour appointments to remove all deposits and smooth the roots. If we use the ultrasonic instruments, the first appointment should result in removal of almost all deposits. Two more appointments will involve fine smoothing of the roots of the teeth to ensure that all irritants are removed and to produce a hard root surface. The cost per visit, as mentioned earlier, is $ _____.

Do you have any questions about your condition or the procedure? (Most patients will ask how the ultrasonic device works. It is usually helpful to let the patient see the tip work with the water spraying around it and to let them feel a tip that is kept handy for demonstration purposes. However, you do not want the patient to contaminate sterile equipment with his or her fingers. Also, you can try the sterile tip on a readily visible area while the patient observes in the mirror as the deposits are removed. Usually, after ultrasonic scaling has been contrasted with one or two areas of hand scaling, the patient will choose ultrasonic scaling.)

It is a maxim that fully informed, consenting patients are more cooperative and generally more relaxed. Participation in their own care seems to make the difference. Many patients feel uncomfortable when they feel they are the *objects* of care, *to whom* instead of *for* or *with whom* care is being provided.

Other preparations for patient comfort include placing a plastic drape and an absorbent napkin, giving the patient a wipe to catch any stray trickles of water, and placing the patient in a full supine position. The "halfway" position usually stimulates considerable gagging. *In all cases,* be certain to have *adequate suction.* The passive suction of the saliva ejector is inadequate. High-volume suction manipulated by an assistant or linked to a saliva ejector is essential.

Also, it is important to explain to the patient that the water can be adjusted if it is too warm or too cold. Sensitivity associated with the procedure often can be reduced by means of a simple adjustment of water temperature or by lowering the power setting used with the tip that is selected.

PREPARATION OF THE EQUIPMENT

The equipment for most units includes a control box, foot control, water connector, and handpiece. Insert tips for the handpieces are separate.

The control unit should be moved close to the chair for easy access for adjustments. It should be plugged into the electrical outlet. If the foot control is separate, it usually plugs into the back of the unit. Matching the shape of the plug prongs with the shape of the holes in the unit determines the correct outlet. Next the water hose is attached to the unit. Usually it is either a "quick disconnect" clip-on junction or a junction with threads for screwing the hose endpiece into the unit. It is important that all connections be secure. If the handpiece is separate, matching the prongs with the outlet (usually found on the front of the control box) is again important.

When starting an ultrasonic unit after several hours or more of nonuse, turn the unit on the high setting and activate the foot pedal, allowing water to flow through the system for at least 2 minutes to clear stagnant water and associated contaminants. Bleed air from the handpiece by holding the handpiece up so that the water flows back over the edge of the handpiece, allowing air bubbles to rise and dissipate (Fig. 22-1). This is necessary to prevent overheating. This procedure

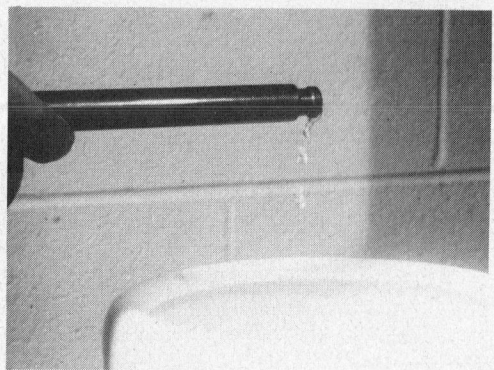

Fig. 22-1. Before placing tip insert, activated handpiece should be held upright until water emerges from opening. It should then be turned to the side and water flow adjusted until water trails from edge in steady flow of nearly contiguous drips.

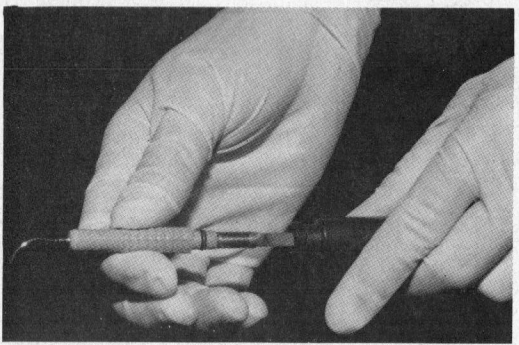

Fig. 22-2. After water has run freely from handpiece for at least 2 minutes, first tip to be used may be inserted into handpiece. Many different methods of insertion are used by different manufacturers. In this case, insert slides into handpiece.

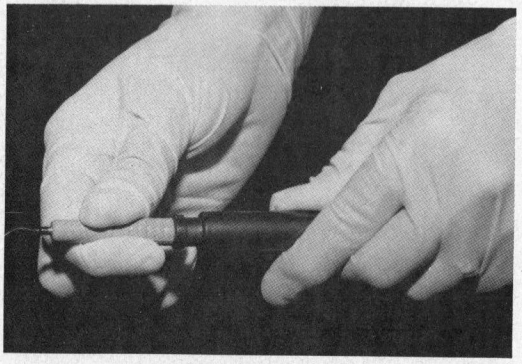

Fig. 22-3. Insert is locked firmly in place before tuning.

should be repeated each time an insert is changed. Once the water flows upward from the handpiece without spurting, an insert can be placed in the handpiece. (Fig. 22-2). Select the proper power setting for the tip.

Most units tune automatically. Simply lock in the handpiece (Fig. 22-3) and activate the footpedal, and the tip will be tuned in a few seconds. Manual tune units require turning the tune control to its highest position and backing it downward while activating the footpedal. When the tip is in tune the water will bursts from the tip in a halo of fine mist (Figs. 22-4 and 22-5). The water flow can be adjusted so that it cools properly and produces a manageable spray in the mouth.

Because a wide variety of ultrasonic and sonic units is available, read and follow the manufacturer's instructions for each unit you encounter.

INSTRUMENT SELECTION

The selection of an appropriate tip is an important component of ultrasonic scaling. It is just as essential as the selection of appropriate hand instruments for scaling and root planing.

The tip should be heavy enough to adequately remove the deposits but not heavier than necessary. The tip should readily adapt to tooth surfaces.

Just as in hand scaling, the heaviest instruments are used to remove the heaviest deposits. For a patient who has bridges of calculus linking the teeth together, the tip shaped like a Zerfing chisel can be employed to loosen the bridge in one or two pieces (Fig. 22-6). The chisel is applied horizontally with a push stroke, flat against the proximal surfaces, and moved from labial to lingual aspects (Fig. 22-7). Once the heavy bridges are removed, the flat-tipped instrument, often referred to as a *beaver-tail* tip, can be used on all surfaces to remove large deposits (Fig. 22-8). This tip should be used until the heaviest and most tenacious chunks are dislodged. Because of its size and shape, it is not the tip of choice for deep or small deposits.

After using the beaver-tail tip, clinicians often use the universal tip, which is most commonly used in practice. Its shape is similar to that of a Gracey 7/8 curette, except, of course, for the fact that it has no cutting edge. This tip can be in-

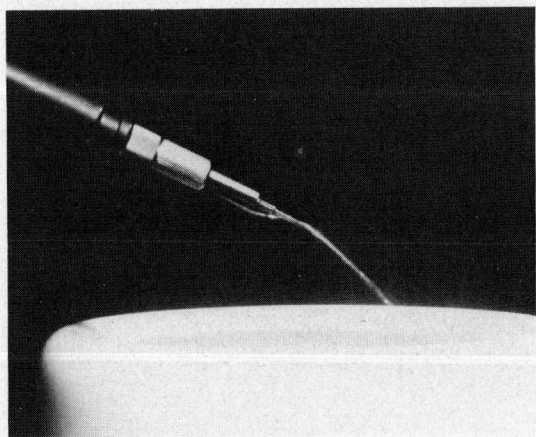

Fig. 22-4. Before proper tuning, water runs or sprays off end in a stream.

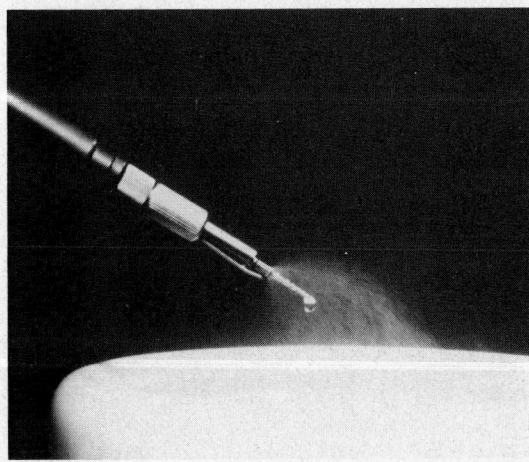

Fig. 22-5. When tip is in tune, water should spray around tip in a "halo." High-pitched squeal is heard at this point. One or two shakes of handpiece will eliminate drop from tip.

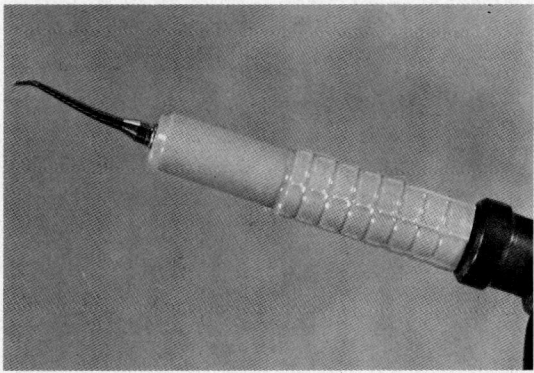

Fig. 22-6. Tip shaped like a Zerfing chisel can be used to loosen and remove lingual bridges of calculus. Water flows through instrument and strikes working end at correct angle to create cavitation.

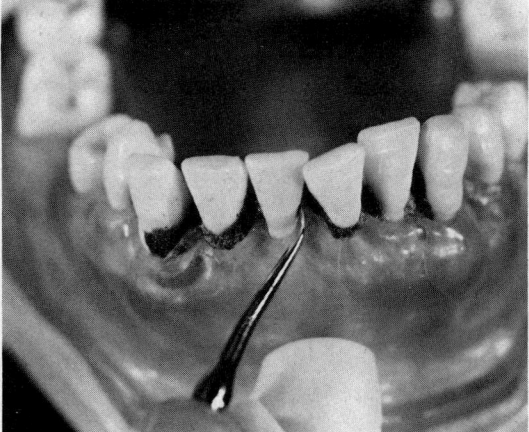

Fig. 22-7. Chisel-shaped tip is used with "blade" against proximal surfaces from labial aspect with horizontal push stroke. As it is applied to each surface, bridge of calculus on lingual surfaces is gradually loosened and can be lifted out in one or two pieces.

serted into 3 or 4 mm pockets, adapts more readily to curves, and still can remove relatively heavy deposits (Fig. 22-9).

Once the quadrant, arch, or other designated segment of the mouth has been thoroughly scaled with the beaver-tail and universal tips, it is appropriate to move on to the tip with a shape similar to that of the periodontal probe (Fig. 22-10).

This tip removes fine deposits and helps smooth clinically detectable root roughness. It is used to remove small residual irritants and is extremely useful in furcations, root furrows, and other anatomic depressions. It is, however, basically ineffective in the removal of heavy deposits.

Other tips are useful adjuncts and may meet the individual preferences of experienced clinicians. There are, for instance, contra-angled versions of

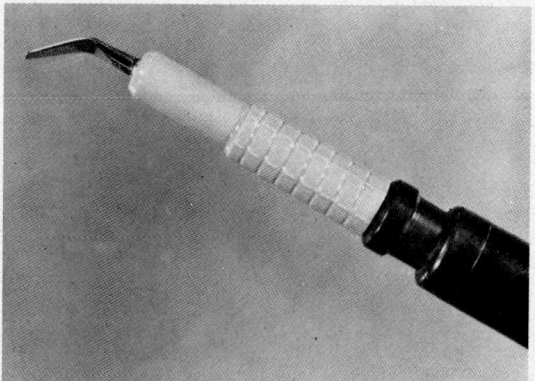

Fig. 22-8. Flat-tipped beaver-tail tip is used to remove large, tenacious deposits throughout mouth.

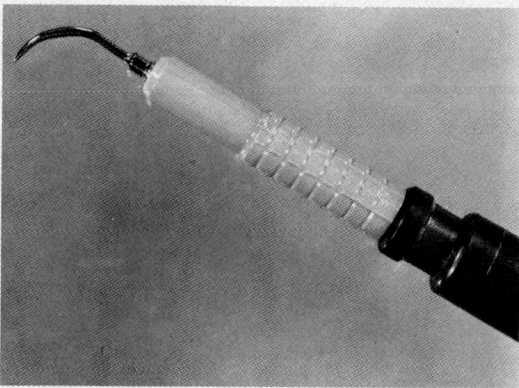

Fig. 22-9. Universal curette tip is probably most commonly used in practice. This tip has access to 3 to 4 mm pockets and adapts readily to curved tooth surfaces.

the universal tip that are useful on proximal surfaces of posterior teeth. Each manufacturer has a selection of tips. It is important to assess the variety of available tips before purchasing a unit, as poorly designed tips will not result in a thorough scaling. Watch for very fine tips that can be placed into deep pockets as they are brought to market.

TREATMENT PLANNING AND ORDER OF INSTRUMENTATION

A patient for whom ultrasonic instrumentation is indicated can usually have the entire mouth scaled by an experienced clinician in 1 hour, unless the deposits are particularly firmly attached. A beginning clinician should plan to complete one quadrant or, at most, one arch.

As each tip is used, the entire designated area to be completed in the appointment should be scaled before tips are changed. A common error is to scale all areas and then change to a finer tip before the area has been evaluated for deposits remaining and before all heavy deposits have been removed. The unactivated tip can be used to detect the presence of deposits in each area as it is scaled. However, detection with an explorer or periodontal probe will provide a more accurate and thorough evaluation.

Therefore, once the chisel and beaver-tail tips have been used both supragingivally and subgingivally, the areas should be explored and air should be used to deflect the tissue to examine the

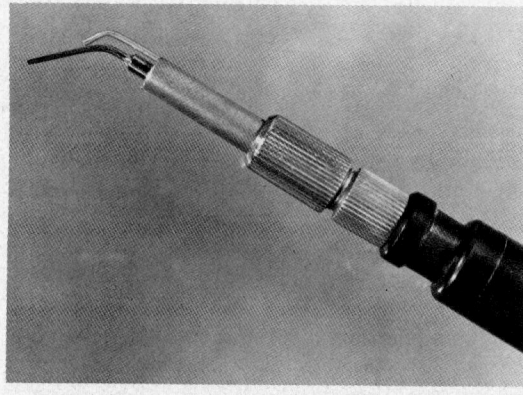

Fig. 22-10. Tip shaped like periodontal probe removes fine deposits. It has best access to deep pockets and furcation areas. This tip has external tube water source targeting working end. All tips shown are now available with only internal or external tubing.

areas. If deposits remain, it is wise to leave the heavy tip in place and remove them. Then the tip can be changed.

Another error is to use one tip to remove "gross deposits" throughout the mouth, with no single area brought to completion at the appointment. This can lead to difficulty in future scaling appointments if the tissues close down over deep deposits. Also, there may be an added danger of periodontal abscesses forming. The best rule is to complete the predetermined areas. At subsequent appointments the areas can be rechecked to ensure completion.

Ewen and Glickstein (1968) have described a stroking pattern that ensures the smoothest surface. It involves a series of vertical, horizontal, and cross-hatching strokes on each area. If the instrumentation moves from the heaviest to the lightest tips, following the suggested stroking pattern, the first set of strokes on an area (excluding the infrequently used chisel) are made with the beaver-tail tip, the second set of strokes is done at a right angle to the first set with the universal tip, and the final cross-hatching strokes are done with the probe tip.

Regardless of the tip selected, the terminal end of the blade (or point) should never be applied at a perpendicular angle to the tooth. The cycle and direction of motion would hammer at the tooth, causing pain and structural damage to the tooth. The terminal end should be maintained at an angle between 10 and 30 degrees to the tooth to ensure that the direction of motion is working tangentially to the tooth rather than hammering at it (Clark, 1969; Stapff, 1975).

If this sequence is followed, it is possible to follow a logical order of instrumentation that minimizes tip changes and maximizes the cleansing of the tooth structure. Such an order is the following:

1. Use the *chisel* tip to break out bridges of calculus.
2. Use the *beaver-tail* tip with horizontal strokes on proximal surfaces and with vertical strokes on direct facial and lingual surfaces (Fig. 22-11). The sequence is as follows:

Horizontal on distobuccal No. 32
Vertical on buccal No. 32
Horizontal on mesiobuccal No. 32
Horizontal on distobuccal No. 31
Vertical on buccal No. 31
Horizontal on mesiobuccal No. 31

3. Use the *Universal curette-style* tip with vertical strokes on proximal surfaces and with horizontal strokes on facial and lingual surfaces (Fig. 22-12). The sequence is as follows:

Vertical on distobuccal No. 32
Horizontal on buccal No. 32
Vertical on mesiobuccal No. 32
Vertical on distobuccal No. 31

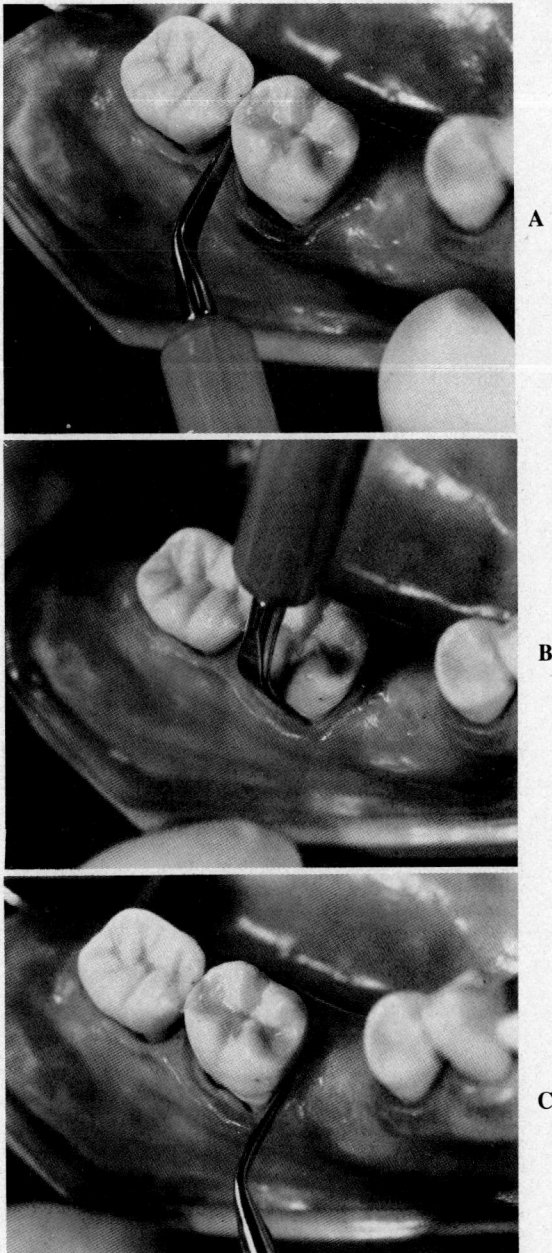

A

B

C

Fig. 22-11. In beginning a pattern of strokes, beaver-tail tip is used **A,** on distal surface on tooth No. 31 from buccal aspect with horizontal stroke; **B,** on facial surface with vertical stroke; and **C,** on mesial surface from buccal aspect with horizontal stroke.

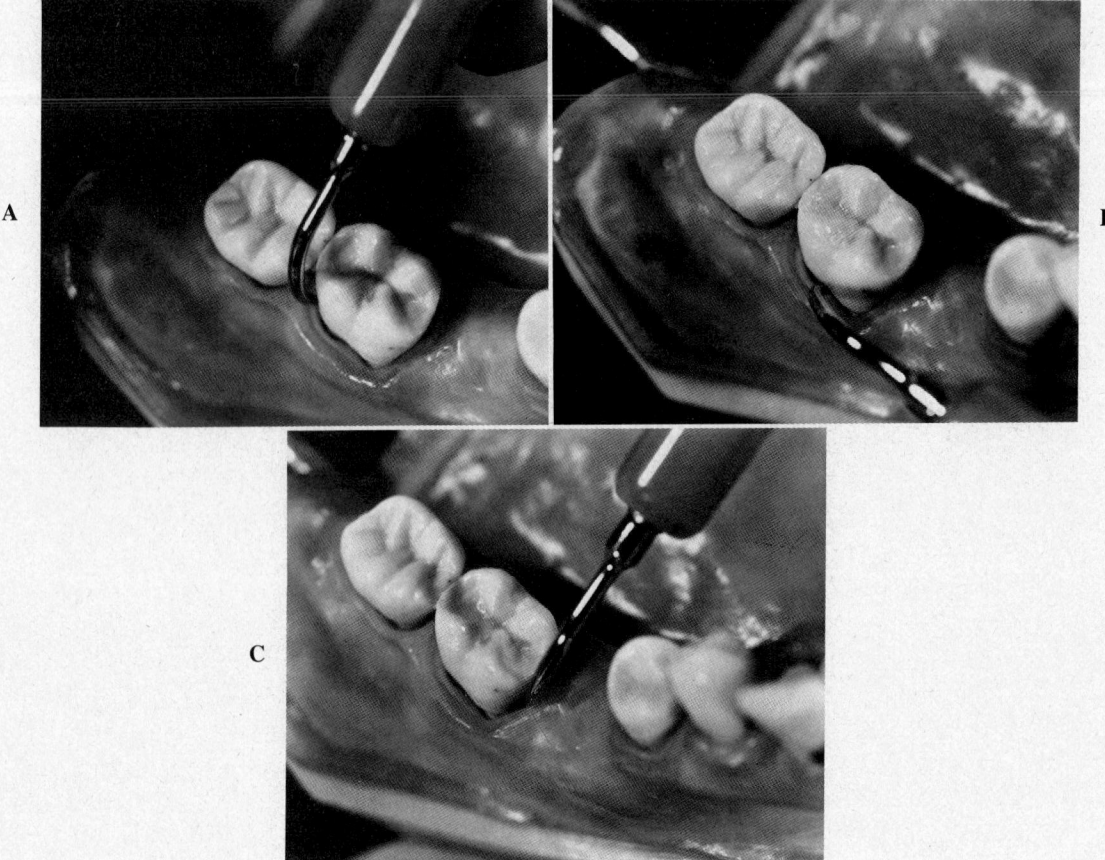

Fig. 22-12. Second pattern of strokes is **A,** vertical on distal surface with universal curette-style tip; **B,** horizontal on facial surface; and **C,** vertical on mesial surface.

Horizontal on buccal No. 31
Vertical on mesiobuccal No. 31

4. Use the *periodontal probe* tip with diagonal cross-hatching strokes in the following sequence (Fig. 22-13):

Diagonal toward lingual on distobuccal No. 32*
Diagonal toward mesial on buccal No. 32
Diagonal toward distal on buccal No. 32
Diagonal toward lingual on mesiobuccal No. 32*

Rapid short strokes should be used. The tip should be constantly moving, as some units generate heat that can damage soft tissue and heat the

---

*Diagonal strokes on proximal surfaces angled toward the buccal aspect are completed from the lingual side of the tooth.

pulp if it contacts the tooth for longer than 1 or 2 seconds. The wrist rock used for most hand scaling is replaced by finger motion to generate the strokes. The speed of the stroke is approximately two sets of back-and-forth strokes across a surface per second. Short strokes enable the tip to fracture away deposits at their most vulnerable point—their edges. As the edges break away, the stroke moves further across the surface to engage more of the deposit.

WATER LAVAGE/TEMPERATURE REGULATION

Because most units generate heat and because water is essential to adequately flush away debris, a water spray must accompany ultrasonic scaling.

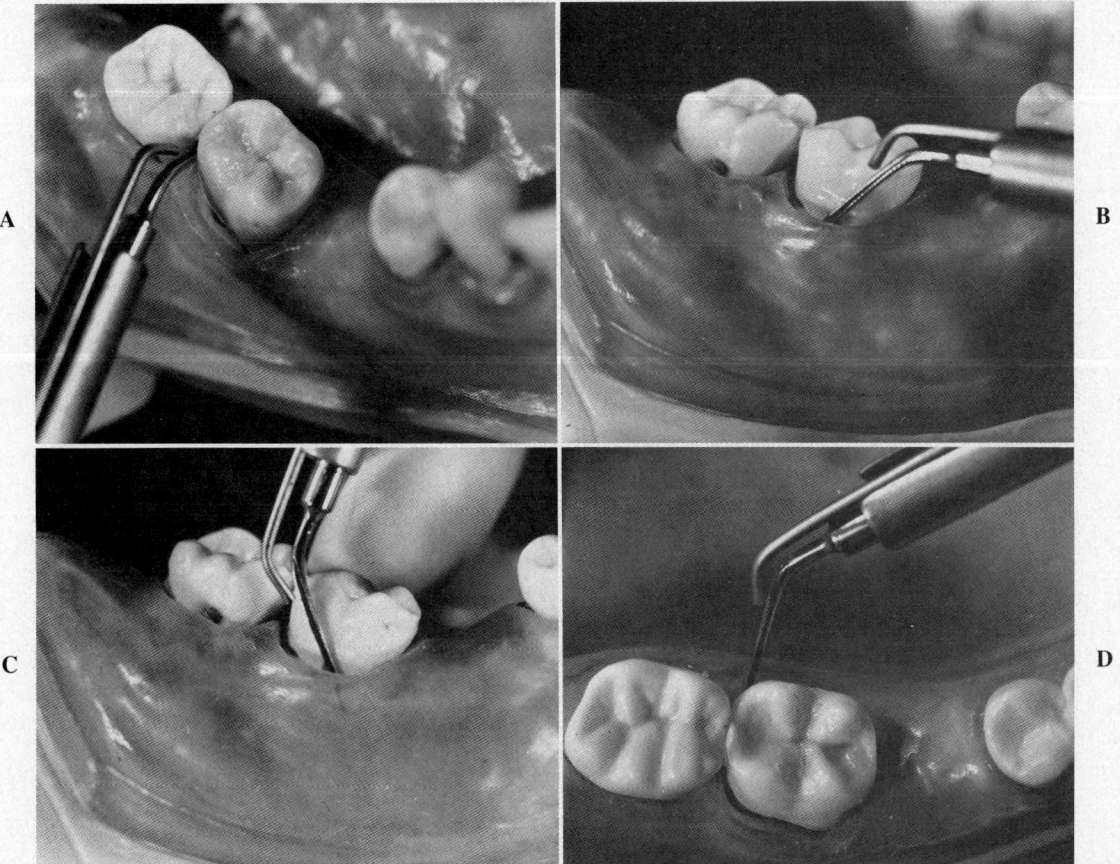

Fig. 22-13. Periodontal probe tip is used **A,** in diagonal pattern on distal aspect; **B** and **C,** in cross-hatched diagonal pattern on facial aspect; and **D,** in diagonal pattern from lingual surfaces on distal aspect. Mesial and lingual surfaces are scaled similarly.

With many types of units it can be harmful to use a tip on the tooth without a flow of water. Water serves as a coolant, lubricant, and cleansing agent. When it is cold, it reduces hemorrhage. When it is warm, it aids in dissolving debris and in floating out fatty substances.

As the water meets the vibrating tip, it cavitates into a spray of bubbles that collapse inward. This is what causes the halolike appearance of the water at the tip.

If the patient complains about cold water, the recommended procedure is to *reduce* the flow of water past the tip to allow more time for the working tip to warm the water. Conversely, if the water is too warm, the water flow should be increased (Ewen and Glickstein, 1968). If the teeth are hypersensitive even though the water temperature is moderate, the power setting on the unit should be reduced so that sensitivity is also reduced, but so that the tip is still effective. Consider anesthetising the area if the patient still experiences discomfort. Most manufacturers recommend power settings for various tips, but often these tips can and should be operated at the lowest effective power setting. It is not wise to operate the tips at power settings higher than those recommended by the manufacturer because they may be damaged.

FINISHING PROCEDURES

When the designated area is completed, each surface should be evaluated for remaining deposits. Definitive exploration should follow any ultrasonic scaling to ensure that remaining fine particles or especially deep deposits are detected and removed. A universal curette is usually the instrument of choice for such needs.

The results of one study suggest that intentional curettage of the wall of the pockets should be done immediately after ultrasonic (and hand) scaling to remove loose calculus that is embedded in the wall of the sulcus. The study showed that some of the wall is removed unintentionally; therefore it was suggested that the curettage procedure be performed. The study concluded that water lavage and exploring procedures alone do not ensure removal of loosened calculus, and remaining calculus combined with a partially curetted sulcus wall may hamper healing (Schaeffer, Stende, and King, 1964).

If curettage is indicated after ultrasonic scaling, it may be easily accomplished with the ultrasonic tip, as the instrument has been demonstrated to be highly effective for this purpose (Sanderson, 1966).

When all areas have been completed, the patient should receive postoperative instructions to brush all areas with a soft brush several times a day and to rinse with warm saline solution or an antimicrobial rinse. Flossing may be recommended depending on the case.

The equipment should be stored, with water flushed and then drained from the hoses and the tips sterilized for future use.

The surrounding area should be swabbed thoroughly with a disinfectant after the visit.

The areas that were scaled should be thoroughly reevaluated at a subsequent appointment, and the roots should be planed to ensure that no roughness remains. The objective is to create the smoothest, hardest surface possible to prevent continued disease.

CONTROVERSY: THE IMPLICATIONS OF RESEARCH FINDINGS

Early investigations demonstrated that ultrasonic scaling devices did not harm soft tissues of the periodontium (McCall, and Szmyd, 1960; Zinner, 1955). Many subsequent studies have shown that considerable benefit in terms of improved healing of gingivae is derived from the use of ultrasonic instrumentation. It has been established that the instrument should not be used *on* bone (Ewen, 1961). However, in a study on cats, there was no greater postsurgical bone loss when the ultrasonic scaler was used to scale the teeth (*adjacent* to bone) than when hand instruments were used (Glick and Freeman, 1980).

Controversy is focused on the effect of ultrasonic scaling on tooth structure, particularly that of the root. Early investigations relied on histologic sections of teeth and on the profilometer, a mechanical device used to measure tooth roughness. Later the scanning electron microscope (SEM) allowed researchers to photograph tooth surfaces at extremely high power so that minute structures and defects could be seen for purposes of contrasting ultrasonically prepared teeth with teeth prepared by a variety of other techniques.

Researchers generally agree that ultrasonic devices remove calculus, subgingival plaque, and endotoxin as well as do hand instruments (Lie and Meyer, 1977; McCall and Szmyd, 1960; Moskow and Bressman, 1964; Nishimine and O'Leary, 1979; Stende and Schaffer, 1961; Thornton and Garnick, 1982; Wilkinson and Maybury, 1973; Vosterwaal, 1987). Disagreement centers on how smoothly roots can be prepared with ultrasonic instrumentation and whether it is effective in root planing.

Many studies using one or more of the three basic techniques of investigation have shown that curettes result in a smoother planed surface (Kerry, 1967; Van Volkinburg, Green, and Armitage, 1976; Wilkinson and Maybury, 1973). A few report actual root "damage" that can be improved only with subsequent thorough root planing. Others report undamaged surfaces but do not advocate ultrasonic root planing. A few report that surfaces as smooth as curetted ones are attainable with ultrasonic instrumentation (Moskow and Bressman, 1964; Pameijer, Stallard, and Hiep, 1972).

One study suggests that a surface as smooth as one curetted with a new, sharp blade can be achieved if the ultrasonically cleaned surface is polished with an abrasive (Benfenati et al, 1987). A similar study evaluated the benefit of using an air powder polish following ultrasonic instrumentation on root surfaces. The study found no benefit or detriment from using the follow-up polishing procedure (Madden et al, 1987). Unfortunately, even if polishing does provide a benefit, only exposed root surfaces can benefit from this follow-up procedure; subgingival areas require a different finishing. Most of the recent articles concur that variance in the methods of assessing root structure as well as in pressure, power, tip selection, and strokes may account for the mixed results (Clark, Grupe, and Mahler, 1968; Wilkinson and Maybury, 1973; Woodruff, Levin, and Brady, 1975; Benfenati et al, 1987). Holbrook advocates reshaping ultrasonic tips so that they will fit the root anatomy and reach the base of deep pockets (Low and Holbrook, 1987). Because the cavitational activity of the tips varies greatly with the acoustic power output, the power settings vary greatly, and instrument designs react differently to the same setting, future research probably should measure and report the displacement amplitude so that results across studies can be compared (Walmsley et al, 1986).

A thorough review of the literature can lead to any number of conclusions. The most logical seem to be that the benefits of the instrument warrant its use in *selected cases* as described earlier; that the instrument can be safely and effectively used subgingivally on root surfaces; that the instrument can approximate root planing, depending on the skill of the clinician, and because clinicians are limited in most instances to clinical evaluation of success, that each such procedure should be followed with hand root planing with a curette. The skilled clinician should have to perform less hand instrumentation following ultrasonic scaling than the less experienced clinician.

The research clearly demonstrates that using the lowest effective power for a given tip and a limited number of light strokes (Ewen et al, 1976) will result in less tissue trauma (Clark, 1969; Clark, Grupe, and Mahler, 1968). Research comparing commercial brands of equipment reveals few significant differences in their effectiveness (Pearlman, 1982; Van Volkinburg, Green, and Armitage, 1976; Woodruff, Levin, and Brady, 1975). Tip design does limit access to various tooth surfaces. Two studies have shown that the sonic air-driven turbine blade causes less surface damage to teeth than ultrasonic instrumentation

(Allen and Rhoads, 1963; Lie and Meyer, 1977). A more recent study compares brands of sonic devices with ultrasonic instrumentation. It supports use of some of the air turbine devices, but it relied upon a unidirectional stroking pattern and upon visual (rather than tactile) cleanliness of extracted teeth (Lie and Leknes, 1985).

Loos et al (1987) used either a sonic scaler or an ultrasonic scaler in a single episode of scaling for periodontally involved teeth. They found no significant differences between the two methods when measuring dental plaque, bleeding on probing, probing depths, or probing attachment levels every 3 months for 12 months. No hand scaling was used in this trial.

Gellin and colleagues (1986) suggest that better results are obtained with the sonic scaler if hand instruments are used following initial debridement with sonics. Using only the sonic scaler resulted in 31.9% surfaces with residual calculus, compared with 26.8% surfaces with hand instrumentation and 16.9% with sonic and hand instrumentation.

With the advent of antimicrobial agents in the treatment and prevention of periodontal disease, it is likely that there will be increased investigation of the effects of the simultaneous delivery of such agents during ultrasonic or sonic instrumentation. It would appear that the antimicirobial effects of the instrument's activity could be enhanced by the chemical activity of agents such as chlorhexidine, tetracycline, sanguinaria, and others. One trial was reported in 1986 (Blumenthal and Ewen) in which .03% sanguinaria produced lower mean gingival index scores compared to water and to baking soda/hydrogen peroxide when delivered during ultrasonic debridement. One manufacturer has introduced an ultrasonic unit which delivers antimicrobial solutions during instrumentation (Fig. 22-14).

Regardless of the type of instrument, experience and careful attention to precautions and protocols will increase positive results.

OTHER USES

In addition to removing deposits, ultrasonic tips can be used for soft tissue curettage (Sanderson, 1966), periodontal surgery, irrigating periodontal abscesses, recontouring restorations, removing orthodontic cement (Shaver, Siefel, and Nicholls,

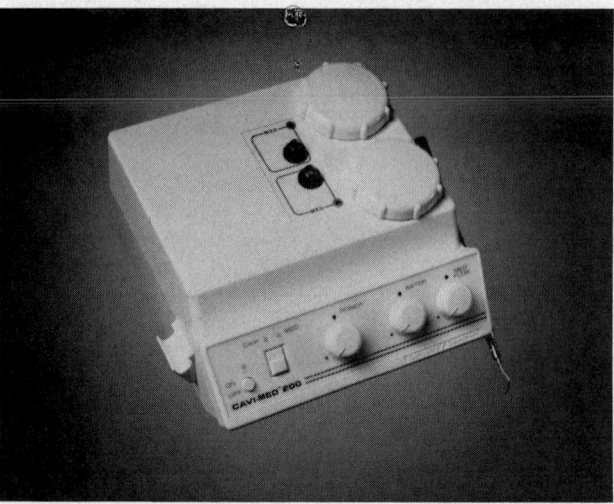

Fig. 22-14. The Cavi-Med® enables the clinician to deliver antimicrobical solutions while instrumentating.
Courtesy Dentsply.

1975), administering drugs, cleansing root canals (Martin et al, 1980), and stripping contact areas of crowded teeth (Clark, 1969).

Endodontic procedures require a thorough debridement of pulp canals, often difficult with hand instrumentation. The ultrasonic endodontic tips seem to enable the clinician to reach areas otherwise often missed. The antimicrobial properties of ultrasonic instrumentation, particularly in combination with a sodium hypochlorite lavage, make it an important adjunct to conventional treatment (Johnson and Zelikow, 1987). It also has proven useful in the removal of silver points and fractured posts (Glick & Frank, 1986).

The most frequent use of ultrasonic instrumentation is in periodontal procedures. It can be a valuable adjunct to therapy when the patient and clinician understand its usefulness as well as it limitations (Forrest, 1967; Green and Sanderson, 1965).

ACTIVITIES

1. Debride extracted teeth with an ultrasonic scaler using the sequence of tips and the stroking pattern suggested. If possible, submit the teeth for scanning electron microscopy (SEM) evaluation.
2. Role-play the process of informing the patient about his or her periodontal conditions and the relative merits of ultrasonic or sonic scaling to remove hard and soft deposits.
3. Conduct a clinical evaluation of the usefulness and efficacy of ultrasonic scaling for one or more patients by preparing one-half of the mouth with ultrasonic scaling and the other half with hand scaling alone. Document immediate preoperative and postoperative results with intraoral photographs. Rephotograph the areas after 3, 7, 10, and 15 days of healing time.
4. Investigate the variety of ultrasonic and sonic scaling devices, comparing the following qualities
   a. Ease of operation
   b. Variety of tips available
   c. Cost and maintenance needs
5. Select two or more of the recent articles evaluating ultrasonic instrumentation. Review the study design and findings and identify how the results could have been different with an altered study design.

REVIEW QUESTIONS

1. Ultrasonic scaling should be limited to patients (select the best answer):
   a. With large deposits of calculus and stain
   b. Who have basically healthy oral tissues
   c. Who show signs of tooth sensitivity
   d. Who have limited time for treatment
   e. Who have extremely resilient teeth
2. A patient who has generalized subgingival ledge calculus, chronic marginal gingivitis, severe diabetes, and oral tori is *not* an appropriate case for ultrasonic scaling. Which of the above factors contraindicates ultrasonic scaling?
3. A 10-year-old patient has drug-induced hyperplasia

with large amounts of hard and soft deposits. Is this patient appropriately treated if ultrasonic scaling is performed? Why or why not?

4. What are four safety precautions that should be followed to minimize the danger of cross-contamination from the microbial aerosol created by the ultrasonic scaler?

5. How does the ultrasonic scaler remove deposits?

6. If the water is too cold, the water flow should be _____ ; if it is too hot, the water flow should be _____ .

7. List the four most commonly used tips in the sequence of their use (first to last).

8. Mark those statements *true* that accurately summarize reasearch findings related to ultrasonic scaling:

   a. Ultrasonic scaling is very effective in removing hard and soft deposits.

   b. Some studies have shown that roots planed ultrasonically are as smooth as hand-curetted roots, but most have concluded that hand planing must follow ultrasonic scaling.

   c. Some minor temporary tinnitus and hearing shifts have been detected in patients who were treated with an ultrasonic scaler.

   d. Using the lowest effective power and a limited number of light strokes minimizes root trauma.

   e. Ultrasonic debridement yields excellent results in treating patients with ANUG.

REFERENCES

Abrams H, et al: Temperature changes in the pulp chamber produced by ultrasonic instrumentation, Gen Dent 27(5):62, 1979.

Adams D, et al: The cardiac pacemaker and ultrasonic scalers, Dent Health 22:6, 1983.

Allen EF, and Rhoads RH: Effects of high speed periodontal instruments on tooth surface, J Periodontol 34:352, 1963.

American Dental Association, Council on Dental Materials, Instruments, and Equipment: Status report on professional sealing and stain-removing devices, JADA 111:801, 1985.

Ballinger ME, Brasher WJ, and Maupin CC: Water contamination and the ultrasonic scaler, Va Dent J 53:10, 1976.

Benfenati MP, et al: Scanning electron microscope: an SEM study of periodontally instrumented root surfaces, comparing sharp, dull, and damaged curettes and ultrasonic instruments, Inter J Perio Restor Dent 7(20):51, 1987.

Blanchard JS: The periodontal curet and the ultrasonic scaler: their effectiveness in removing overhangs from amalgam restorations, Dent Hyg 58:450, 1984.

Blumenthal NM, and Ewen SJ: A short term evaluation of ultrasonically delivered medications in the treatment of moderate periodontal disease, Ill Dent J 55(1):12, 1986.

Breininger DR, O'Leary TJ, and Blumenshine RVH: Comparative effectiveness of ultrasonic and hand scaling for the removal of subgingival plaque and calculus, J Periodontol 58:9, 1987.

Carstensen EL: Biological effects of acoustic cavitation, Ultrasound Med Biol. 12:703, 1986.

Chandler HH, Rupp NW, and Paffenbarger GC: Poor mercury hygiene from ultrasonic amalgam condensation, JADA 82:553, 1971.

Clark SM: The ultrasonic dental unit: a guide for the clinical application of ultrasonics in dentistry and in dental hygiene, J Periodontol 40:621, 1969.

Clark SM, Grupe HE, and Mahler DB: The effect of ultrasonic instrumentation on root surfaces, J Periodontol 39:135, 1968.

Clarke P, and Hill C: Physical and chemical aspects of ultrasonic disruption of cells, J Acoust Soc Am 57:649, 1970.

Cunningham WT, et al: A comparison of antimicrobial effectiveness of endosonic and hand root canal therapy, Oral Surg 54:238, 1982.

Ewen SJ: The ultrasonic wound—some microscopic observation, J Periodontol 32:315, 1961.

Ewen SJ, and Glickstein C: Ultrasonic therapy in periodontics. Springfield, Ill, 1968, Charles C Thomas.

Ewen SJ, et al: A comparative study of ultrasonic generators and hand instruments, J Periodontol 47:82, 1976.

Fitch HB, et al: Acute necrotizing ulcerative gingivitis, J Periodontol 34:422, 1963.

Forrest JO: Ultrasonic scaling: a five-year assessment, Br Dent J 122:9, 1967.

Gankerseer EJ, and Walmsley AD: Preliminary investigation into the performance of a sonic scaler, J Periodontol 58:780, 1987.

Gellin RG, et al: The effectiveness of the Titan-S sonic scaler versus curettes in the removal of subgingival calculus, J Periodontol 57:672, 1986.

Glick DH and Frank AL: Removal of silver points and fractured posts by ultrasonics, J Prosth Dent 55:212, 1986.

Glick DH, and Freeman E: Postsurgical bone loss following root planing by ultrasonic and hand instruments, J Periodontol 51:510, 1980.

Green GH, and Sanderson AD: Ultrasonics and periodontal therapy—a review of clinical and biologic effects, J Periodontol 36:232, 1965.

Gross A, Divine M, and Cutright DE: Microbial contamination of dental units and ultrasonic scalers J Periodontol 47:670, 1976.

Holbrook WP, et al: Bacteriological investigation of aerosol from ultrasonic scalers, Br Dent J 144:245, 1978.

Hunter RK, O'Leary TJ, and Kafrawy AH: The effectiveness of hand versus ultrasonic instrumentation in open flap root planing, J Periodontol 55:697, 1984.

Johnson TA, and Zelikow R: Ultrasonic endodontics: a clinical review, JADA 114:655, 1987.

Kerry GJ: Roughness of root surfaces after use of ultrasonic instruments and hand curettes, J Periodontol 38:340, 1967.

Krupa CM, et al: *In vitro* evaluation of air-powder polishing as an adjunct to ultrasonic scaling on periodontally involved root surfaces. Iowa City, Iowa, 1987, University of Iowa, Second National Dental Hygiene Research Conference Abstracts.

Leon LE, and Vogel RI: A comparison of the effectiveness of hand scaling and ultrasonic debridement in furcations as evaluated by differential dark-field microscopy, J Periodontol 58:86, 1987.

Lie T, and Leknes KN: Evaluation of the effect on root surfaces of air turbine scales and ultrasonic instrumentation, J Periodontol 56:522, 1985.

Lie T, and Meyer K: Calculus removal and loss of tooth substance in response to different periodontal instruments, J Clin Periodontol 4:250, 1977.

Loos B, Kiger R, and Egelberg J: An evaluation of basic periodontal therapy using sonic and ultrasonic scalers, J Clin Periodontol 14:29, 1987.

Low S, and Holbrook T: Ultrasonic instrumentation in periodontal therapy. Denver, 1987, American Academy of Periodontology Annual Meeting.

Martin H, et al: Ultrasonic versus hand filing of dentin: a quantitative study, Oral Surg 49:79, 1980.

McCall CM, and Szmyd L: Clinical evaluation of ultrasonic scaling, JADA 61:559, 1960.

Möller P, Grevstad AO, and Kristoffersen T: Ultrasonic scaling of teeth causing tinnitus and temporary hearing shifts, J Clin Periodontol 3:123, 1976.

Moskow BS, and Bressman E: Cemental response to ultrasonic and hand instrumentation, JADA 68:699, 1964.

Nishimine D, and O'Leary TJ: Hand instrumentation versus ultrasonics in the removal of endotoxins from root surfaces, J Periodontol 50:345, 1979.

Olsen I, and Socransky SS: Ultrasonic dispersion of pure cultures of plaque bacteria and plaque, Scand J Dent Res 89:307, 1981.

Oosterwaal PJM, et al: The effect of subgingival debridement with hand and ultrasonic instruments on the subgingival microflora, J Clin Periodontol 14:528, 1987.

Pameijer CH, Stallard RD and Hiep N: Surface characteristics of teeth following periodontal instrumentation: a scanning electron microscope study, J Periodontol 43:628, 1972.

Pearlman BA: Ultrasonic root planing, Aust Dent J 27:109, 1982.

Pollack BF, and Kronenberg EB: A pilot study on the effects of ultrasonic instrumentation on composite resins, NY J Dent 51:151, 1981.

Rajstein J, and Tal M: The effect of ultrasonic scaling on the surface of Class V amalgam restorations—a scanning electron microscopy study, J Oral Rehab 11:299, 1984.

Reinhardt RA, et al: Effect of nonsterile versus sterile water irrigation with ultrasonic scaling in postoperative bacteremias, J Periodontol 53:96, 1982.

Rooney J: Shear as a mechanism for sonically induced biological effects, J Acoust Soc Am 52:1718, 1972.

Sanderson AD: Gingival curettage by hand and ultrasonic instruments: a histologic comparison, J Periodontol 37:279, 1966.

Schaeffer EM, Stende G, and King D: Healing of periodontal pocket tissues following ultrasonic scaling and hand planing, J Periodontol 35:140, 1964.

Shaver RL, Siefel IA, and Nicholls JI: Effect of ultrasonic $ZnPO_4$ cement removal on band adhesion and cement solubility under orthodontic bands, J Dent Res 54:206, 1975.

Sjogren U, and Sundqvist G: Bacteriologic evaluation of ultrasonic root canal instrumentation, Oral Surg Oral Med Oral pathol 63:366, 1987.

Stamps JT, and Muth ER: Reducing accidents and injuries in the dental environment, Dent Clin North Am 22:389, 1978.

Stapff KH: Debridement with ultrasonics, I. Quintessence Int, 6:57, 1975.

Stende GW, and Schaffer EM: A comparison of ultrasonic and hand scaling, J Periodontol 32:312, 1961.

Thorton S, et al: Comparison of ultrasonic to hand instruments in the removal of subgingival plaque, J Periodontol 53:35, 1982.

Torfason T, et al: Clinical improvement of gingival conditions following ultrasonic versus hand instrumentation or periodontal pockets, J Clin Periodontol 6:165, 1979.

Van Volkinburg JW, Green E, and Armitage GC: The nature of root surfaces after curette, Cavitron and Alphasonic instrumentation, J Periodont Res 11:374, 1976.

Walmsley AD, et al: Investigation into patients' hearing following ultrasonic scaling, Br Dent J 162:221, 1987.

Walmsley AD, Laird WRE, and Williams AR: A model system to demonstrate the role of cavitational activity in ultrasonic scaling, J Dent Res 63:1162, 1984.

Walmsley AD, Laird WRE, and Williams AR: Displacement amplitude as a measure of the acoustic output of ultrasonic scalers, Dent Mater 2:97, 1986.

Walmsley AD, Williams AR, and Laird WRE: Acoustic absorption within human teeth during ultrasonic descaling, J Dent 14:2, 1986.

Wilkinson RF, and Maybury JE: Scanning electron microscopy of the root surface following instrumentation, J Periodontol 44:559, 1973.

Williams GH III: Laminar air purge of microorganisms in dental aerosols: prophylactic procedures with the ultrasonic scaler, J Dent Res 49:1498, 1970.

Woodruff HC, Levin MP, and Brady JM: The effects of two ultrasonic instruments on root surfaces, J Periodontol 46:119, 1975.

Zinner DD: Recent ultrasonic dental studies, including periodontia, without the use of an abrasive, J Dent Res 34:748, 1955.

23 REMOVING FINE DEPOSITS AND ROOT PLANING

OBJECTIVES: *The reader will be able to*

1. Define root planing.
2. Identify the objectives for performing root planing.
3. Contrast root planing techniques with scaling of heavy deposits in terms of instrument selection and the number, length, direction, and pressure of working strokes.
4. Describe design differences between Gracey curettes and universal curettes.
5. Discuss the importance of irrigation as part of root planing.
6. Describe adaptation of Gracey curettes to the teeth.
7. Discuss the criteria used to evaluate the root planing procedure and their application.
8. List the factors that may complicate implementation of root planing and suggest ways of eliminating or responding to them.
9. Discuss five contraindications for performing definitive root planing for a patient.
10. Discuss the limitations of nonsurgical treatment of periodontal disease.
11. Discuss the importance of establishing a frequent and regular maintenance program following periodontal treatment.
12. Define "supervised neglect" in the context of periodontal maintenance therapy.

The use of hand instruments for fine scaling and root planing is an effective method of treatment for patients with gingival and periodontal inflammation. The two procedures, scaling and root planing, complement each other in treating the hard tissue side of the sulcus or pocket by removing the foreign and diseased substances that are attached to the tooth and that cause inflammation and destruction of the adjacent soft tissues and supporting bone. *Fine scaling* involves the use of hand instruments and ultrasonic devices (see Chapters 21 and 22) to detect and remove deposits of plaque and calculus from the surface of the enamel or cementum. During scaling, the emphasis is on removal of soft and hard deposits and smoothing plaque-retentive surfaces (such as overhanging amalgam restorations), but no intentional attempt is made to remove the surface cementum completely. *Root planing* extends the treatment of the root surface that has been exposed to the oral environment of the periodontal pocket as a result of the loss of previously attached gingival fibers. This exposed cementum,

which has been altered by the disease process, is carefully and completely planed, or shaved away, from the root surface during root planing to ensure the removal of all embedded calculus, plaque, and its toxic byproducts (endotoxins), as well as any surface cementum that may still harbor inflammatory substances.

It is important to have a clear understanding of the inflammatory process of periodontal disease when considering its treatment. Many studies have underscored the importance of plaque as the primary etiologic agent in periodontal disease. Chief among these studies is the one by Loë and colleagues (1965) in which it was demonstrated that normal healthy tissues became inflamed after 21 days when plaque removal procedures are not employed. The inflammation was reversed when plaque control was reinstituted in these same subjects. Later studies confirmed the role of plaque as the etiologic agent in gingival inflammation and periodontal disease (Theilade et al, 1966; Waerhaug, 1977, 1978a).

Supragingival plaque control measures such as

brushing, flossing, and the use of auxiliary plaque control aids have been emphasized as effective means of preventing inflammatory disease. In the patient who has not experienced any prior irreversible inflammatory disease, these measures can be effective in preventing its onset.

The situation is different, however, for the patient who has already suffered the loss of gingival attachment and bone as a result of inflammation. When plaque has formed submarginally, it is no longer accessible to removal by routine home care procedures such as those mentioned above. It is unlikely that the bristles of a toothbrush will clean more than 1 mm below the gingival margin (Waerhaug, 1981). Waerhaug (1976) reported an effective cleaning depth of no more than 2.5 mm for the small interdental brush. Once plaque has migrated along the tooth surface to a submarginal depth of 2 to 3 mm, it becomes inaccessible to these methods of removal. Several studies have described the effect of subgingival plaque on the dentogingival junction and indicated that it is the presence of this subgingival plaque that leads to the inflammatory tissue reactions that result in loss of gingival attachment and periodontal destruction. Supragingival plaque that had not been removed completely gave rise to an advancing plaque front that moved apically into the sulcus area. This plaque front was estimated to move at a speed of about 1 to 2 μm a day toward the dentogingival junction. When it reached the level of the gingival attachment, it began to destroy the attachment apparatus. The loss of attachment kept speed with the advancing plaque front.

Waerhaug emphasized the need for complete subgingival plaque removal through scaling and root planing in order to reestablish a healthy dentoepithelial junction and to prevent further destruction. In addition to being formed from available supramarginal plaque, submarginal plaque can also reform from remnants that are left behind following ineffective subgingival scaling and root planing. It was noted that the speed of reformation of subgingival plaque from these sources will occur just as rapidly as from supragingival sources. These studies stressed the necessity of performing complete submarginal plaque control in addition to daily, effective supramarginal plaque control (Waerhaug, 1978a, 1978b).

It now appears that the most important determinant of the pathogenicity of plaque, or its ability to cause disease, is the quality of the plaque rather than its quantity. Older, more mature plaque, which is associated with the initiation of gingival and periodontal disease, has been found to contain a higher proportion of spirochetes and motile organisms, whereas younger plaque, which is found in mouths with healthy periodontal tissues, contains predominantly coccoid and nonmotile organisms. It has been determined that shifts in these bacterial proportions are associated with clinical changes in the gingival tissues. Inflammation occurs when the proportion of spirochetes and motile forms increases and it subsides as the number of these organisms is reduced as a proportion of total plaque organisms. Monitoring of subgingival microbes following scaling and root planing has shown that subgingival instrumentation results in a significant decrease in the numbers of pathogenic plaque organisms for a period of time (Listgarten et al, 1978). Within weeks or months, however, these pathogenic organisms tend to repopulate the subgingival areas. Performance of supragingival plaque control by the patient, no matter how thorough, is not sufficient to prevent the subgingival plaque composition from maturing and shifting towards more pathogenic forms, especially in the presence of deep (6 mm or more) pockets (West and King, 1983; Kho, 1985). Therefore, the patient's plaque control measures cannot be counted on to prevent further periodontal destruction in the absence of frequent professional plaque control measures, including supra- and subgingival instrumentation (Listgarten et al, 1978; Greenwell et al, 1983; Greenwell and Bissada, 1984; Hinricks et al, 1984).

Aleo and others (1974) demonstrated the presence of plaque endotoxin or endotoxinlike substance on the cemental surfaces of periodontally involved teeth. This substance was toxic for gingival fibroblasts and prevented their growth and proliferation (Aleo et al, 1975). These studies generated interest in the role of plaque endotoxins as the major etiologic factor in periodontal disease. Thorough root planing of the cemental surfaces of periodontally involved teeth has been found to be effective in removing most of the cementum-bound endotoxin and restoring the root surface to endotoxin levels comparable to those of healthy teeth with no periodontal disease (Jones and O'Leary, 1978; McCoy et al, 1987). Thus, it would seem that root planing is an effective means of treating the root surfaces of periodontally involved teeth through its ability to produce a clean, endotoxin-free environment that is conducive to the repair and regeneration of the adjacent soft tissues.

The role of calculus as an etiologic agent in periodontal disease has been studied over the years. One theory stated that the calculus acted as a mechanical irritant to the soft tissues, producing an inflammatory response. Later studies demonstrated, however, that the mere presence of calculus alone was not a primary factor in the incidence of gingival inflammation. Rather, it was the plaque that covered the calculus deposits that induced the inflammation. Baumhammers and others (1973) performed a scanning electron microscopic study of calculus and described how the rough and porous nature of calculus makes it suitable for plaque accumulation and permeable to penetration by endotoxins. It is these plaque-retentive characteristics of calculus, then, that make it incompatible with the achievement of a healthy gingival sulcus. In order to restore periodontally affected tissues to health, all such plaque retentive surfaces, including calculus and improperly contoured restorations, must be removed from the environment. They not only harbor plaque and its endotoxins but also make it difficult, if not impossible, for the patient to practice effective supragingival plaque control measures.

Although it is now known that calculus is not responsible for initiating gingivitis and periodontal disease, there is no doubt that it does contribute significantly to the maintenance and/or progression of disease. Calculus contributes to the disease process by acting as a porous reservoir for bacteria and associated toxins so that its presence increases the potential for destruction over that of bacterial plaque alone (Schroeder, 1969; Mandel and Gaffar, 1986). In a review of the literature on this topic, Mandel further stated that clinical studies conducted over the last 15 years have clearly established the effects of subgingival calculus in promoting periodontal disease. These studies have also underscored the importance of the frequent removal of calculus in order to prevent the progression of this disease. Lindhe and others (1984) noted that the critical factor that would determine

the success of periodontal therapy was the effectiveness of root planing in treating the root surface rather than the type of technique (that is, surgical or nonsurgical) used to eliminate the periodontal infection.

Calculus removal by scaling alone is not always possible because of the ways in which calculus can attach to the root surface (Chapter 12). Canis and colleagues (1979) reviewed the nature of this attachment and identified three ways in which it could occur. One method involved attachment of calculus into cemental irregularities in such a way that a mechanical locking of the deposits and the cementum occurred. Another method of attachment was by direct contact of the intracellular matrix and the root surface. Either of these two methods of attachment would require removal of the cementum in order to guarantee complete calculus removal. This finding is significant because it indicates that even if the clinician scales the root surface until it feels smooth, remnants of undetectable calculus can still remain embedded in the surface itself. Root planing of the cementum surface is necessary to remove the remnants of calculus that remain after fine scaling has been accomplished. There have been many reports of the ineffectiveness of scaling in removing all calculus from the root surface (Kerry, 1967; Jones et al, 1972; Wilkinson and Maybury, 1973; Volkinbrug et al, 1976; Rabbani et al, 1981). Many reasons for this ineffectiveness have been proposed, including, the impossibility of detecting calculus that lies embedded in depressions and resorption lacunae in the cemental surface, or calculus that has been smoothed or burnished during scaling. Even the finest tactile sense and sensitive exploration cannot discriminate between calculus and cementum under these circumstances. The only guarantee that these root surfaces are clean of toxic substances is removal of the cementum itself.

It should be clear by now that no matter how well the patient performs self-care and even if scaling and polishing are accomplished, the affected root surface will remain an irritant to the soft tissue wall of the pocket unless the diseased cementum, which contains active endotoxins is removed and all plaque-retentive qualities of that surface have been eliminated (Jones and O'Leary, 1978). In summary, the problems that exist here are: (1) an inflammatory process that is causing destruction of tissues; (2) a root surface environment that favors the inflammation; and (3) an inability by the patient to affect these conditions by regular home care methods. What is needed is a means of removing the irritants from the root surface so that the tissues can heal and a method for preventing this situation from recurring.

Fine scaling followed by root planing can be successful in treating periodontally involved root surfaces, but it must be accompanied by the ability and willingness on the part of the patient to perform daily, effective plaque control and a commitment to a regular and frequent professional maintenance program. Both procedures must occur in order to produce long-term improvements in the oral health of the periodontal tissues. Root planing can create an environment that favors healing in the soft tissues, but lack of effective sub- and supramarginal plaque control will undermine these efforts in only a short period of time by allowing the plaque and associated endotoxins to reform again in the pocket area. The objectives of root planing are as follows:

1. To eliminate plaque and associated endotoxins or endotoxinlike substances from the root surface
2. To remove all calculus and other plaque-retentive surfaces from the root
3. To produce a smooth, hard root surface that may be less likely to attract and retain plaque and calculus deposits, and one that enhances the patient's ability to remove accessible plaque
4. To promote gingival healing and the resultant shrinkage and reduction in pocket depth
5. To provide an environment that favors the new attachment of epithelial and gingival tissues to the surface of the tooth

COMPARISON OF FINE SCALING AND ROOT PLANING

To accomplish the goals of scaling, the clinician must detect and recognize the presence of plaque, calculus, and plaque-retentive surfaces both supramarginally and submarginally. Then, with the aid of hand instruments or the ultrasonic scaler, these deposits and/or surfaces can be removed so that the tooth and root feel smooth to an explorer and the deposits can no longer be detected visu-

ally. To accomplish the goals of root planing, the entire root surface must be thoroughly cleaned of affected cementum by shaving away the root surface until it feels "polished" (that is, exceptionally smooth, hard, and homogeneous). Scaling should always precede root planing. The more obvious deposits must be removed before the clinician can evaluate the nature of the root surface itself. The clinician may choose to use the same or different instruments for scaling and root planing, depending on the type and amount of deposits that are present initially. Scaling procedures can be accomplished with the use of ultrasonic devices, curettes, sickle scalers, hoes, files, or a combination of any of these instruments. Root planing is best accomplished with instruments designed for optimal adaptation to deep submarginal areas and for delivery of sensitive tactile transmissions to the clinician.

The instrumentation skills that are employed for fine scaling must become highly developed and refined to facilitate effective root planing. The clinician must have mastered the principles of adaptation, insertion, and angulation and must be able to direct working strokes effectively to avoid injuring the inflamed soft tissues. Although this is certainly important for all submarginal instrumentation, it is especially crucial during root planing because of the large number of strokes that are employed to treat every portion of the root surface during this procedure. The ability of the clinician to control the amount of pressure applied to each working stroke must also be developed so that the root surface is not gouged or overplaned, resulting in unnecessary loss of cementum. The clinician must be able to apply the instrument to the cementum with a constant pressure and effective angulation. In addition, the clinician is required to evaluate the progress of the procedure continuously and to determine if adjustments in pressure or angulation are needed either to accelerate or to minimize the removal of cementum depending on the quality of the surface.

The most important skill required for root planing is the clinician's ability to receive a wide variety of delicate tactile sensations, to discriminate among them, and to interpret them accurately. The clinician must detect roughness, graininess, or subtle abnormalities of the root surface that indicate the presence of fine or burnished calculus deposits, diseased cementum, or ridges and gouges created by earlier instrumentation. Because of the nature of these surface irregularities, they will be less obvious to the tactile sense than were the larger deposits and plaque-retentive surfaces that were encountered during the preceding scaling procedures. At other times the clinician may be unable to detect any surface roughness at all, but must still perform some root planing of the surface cementum in order to remove plaque and its associated endotoxins from the root surface. It has not been established exactly what type of attachment exists between endotoxins or endotoxin-like substances and the cementum surface, so it is difficult to determine how deeply these substances have penetrated into the affected cementum. Clinicians should avoid unnecessary removal of the cementum during root planing and must monitor the gingival response to determine if the root surface has been made biologically acceptable to the adjacent soft tissues.

Because most root planing occurs submarginally, unless there has been gingival recession, the clinician must have a reliable mental picture of root morphology to assist the tactile sensations in guiding the adaptation of the instruments. It should be added, however, that no matter how well the clinician knows "normal" root morphology, there is no guarantee that all teeth will fit the "normal" mold. This awareness of root morphology, coupled with a keenly developed tactile sense, will allow the clinician to detect and navigate the contour of root surfaces, including depressions, grooves, line angles, and furcation entrances. The curette blade and explorer must follow the irregular contour of root surfaces exactly, delivering both exploratory and working strokes that cover every square millimeter of the root surface. In addition, this task must be accomplished without traumatizing the inflamed soft tissues with which the instruments are in close contact.

It is often difficult to achieve effective adaptation of curettes to the proximal surfaces of teeth for complete root planing due to the presence of concavities that lie within 5mm apical to the CEJ on most teeth (Fox and Bosworth, 1987). These concavities are likely to become exposed to the pocket environment after even minimal loss of periodontal tissues and may be too deep to be reached either by a curette or by flossing. As a re-

sult, calculus that forms in these conca often be burnished or smoothed over du ment and remain undetected. Clinicians aware of the presence of concavities on surfaces so that instrumentation in those ꞏ ꞏꞏ will be as thorough as possible. In addition, patients must be taught alternative measures of plaque control for these surfaces (such as an interproximal brush, rubber tip stimulator, or perio-aid), as flossing is more likely to bridge these areas than to clean them.

Another critical area for instrumentation during root planing is the apical extent of the pocket at the dentogingival junction. Waerhaug (1978a) studied the effect of subgingival plaque removal on this dentogingival junction and reported that the proximity of the plaque front to this junction could be as close as 0.5 mm. This means that the instrument must be located at the very base of the pocket and in some cases must compress the apical soft tissues in order to remove effectively plaque and calculus that have formed there. Because this plaque results in destruction of the gingival fiber apparatus, it is crucial that it be removed during instrumentation. Effective plaque and calculus removal at the base of pockets is a challenge for all clinicians, because it is precisely in this part of the pocket that calculus deposits are often missed. Waerhaug (1978b) issued the ultimate challenge to clinicians when he stated that "removal of 99% of subgingival plaque is likely to be just as bad as no plaque control at all in the long run." It should be clear that definitive root planing is an exacting and time-consuming procedure that demands a great deal of skill, diligence, and patience on the part of the clinician.

ROOT PLANING
Armamentarium

The instruments and supplies used for root planing are much the same as those that might be used for scaling heavier deposits. Instruments that may be used are curettes, hoes, and files. Any of these instruments can successfully remove light deposits and cementum in accessible areas. Several studies comparing the three have shown that curettes produce the smoothest root surface and inflict the least amount of damage to the cementum and the surrounding soft tissues (Kerry, 1967; Wilkinson and Maybury, 1973). In light of these studies, curettes are recommended for use in root planing. Hoes and files may be used as supplemental instruments for heavy and fine scaling in preparation for root planing by the curette. Clinicians who are skilled in the use of hoes and files can adapt them submarginally with good results. The size of the working ends of these instruments has decreased over the years, improving their accessibility to submarginal areas. Although the use of these instruments may speed the scaling and smoothing process, it should always be followed by the use of a curette to achieve the smoothest surface possible. Not only does the curette design faciliate optimal adaptation to the root surface, but the rounded toe and back also protect the soft tissues from trauma during the procedure.

In choosing the best type of curette for the root-planing procedure, several factors must be considered. The clinician needs an instrument that will adapt to a wide variety of pocket depths and shapes. The curette must be versatile enough to be used in any part of the mouth and to reach apically into deep pockets. It must have a blade design that facilitates its use in small, confined areas such as furcations (Bower, 1979). The curette must also be designed with maximum ability to transmit minute vibrations from light calculus deposits and rough cementum and yet be rigid enough to remove these deposits effectively. A narrow blade is necessary because in many cases the deepest pockets are also very tight and allow only limited access to instruments. The Gracey curette designs meet all of the criteria mentioned and are preferred for root planing by many clinicians. Examples of the various area-specific Gracey curette designs are shown in Fig. 23-1.

There are several differences between the design of a Gracey curette blade and that of a universal curette blade. One major difference is that the two cutting edges are not parallel to each other. Instead, the Gracey curette has offset cutting edges so that one edge appears to be lower than the other. In the universal curette design, both cutting edges can be correctly adapted for use on a tooth (as discussed in Chapter 21), but only the lower cutting edge of the Gracey curette should be adapted to the tooth for working strokes. The Gracey curette also has a characteristic beveled surface adjacent to one of its cutting edges, which universal curettes do not have. The different blade design of the Gracey curette gives

it what is called a *self-angulating* capability. This term means that when the Gracey curette is correctly adapted to the tooth so that the terminal shank or last bend in the shank nearest the blade is parallel to the long axis of the tooth, the blade is already aligned at the optimal working angulation and further adjustments are unnecessary.

Gracey curettes also differ from universal curettes in that there are a variety of shank designs available for them. Each shank design permits optimal access of that instrument to a specific area of the mouth or to specific tooth surfaces. This means that more than one of these instruments is needed in order to fine scale and root plane the entire mouth thoroughly. In contrast, each universal curette is designed so that it can be used "universally" throughout the mouth. The following list gives the design numbers of the Gracey curettes shown in Fig. 23-1 and the areas for which optimal adaptation can be obtained:

Gracey ½ and ¾: anterior teeth
Gracey ⅚: anterior and premolar teeth
Gracey ⅞ and ⁹⁄₁₀: posterior teeth, buccal and lingual surfaces
Gracey ¹¹⁄₁₂: posterior teeth, mesial surfaces
Gracey ¹³⁄₁₄: posterior teeth, distal surfaces

Gracey curettes designed for use in anterior segments of the mouth have a rather straight and simple shank design, whereas those designed for harder-to-reach areas in the posterior segments of the mouth have shanks with more complex and convoluted designs. Although each of these curettes is useful in its own way, the efficient clinician will limit the choice of instruments for the root-planing tray setup to only those designs that are absolutely required to get the job done. Too much time can be wasted hunting for essential instruments among a tray cluttered with extras. A good "starter set" of Gracey curettes that will provide accessibility to any area of the mouth includes the ½, ⅞, ¹¹⁄₁₂, and ¹³⁄₁₄.

Other instruments or supplies that are necessary for the root-planing procedure include a mouth mirror, explorer, probe, sharpening supplies, and anesthesia setup. The clinician should carefully choose the explorer to be used for evaluating root planing. A fine, long-shanked explorer should be included because this procedure requires optimal tactile sensitivity for detection of fine deposits and root irregularities. The design of the explorer should allow the clinician access to even the

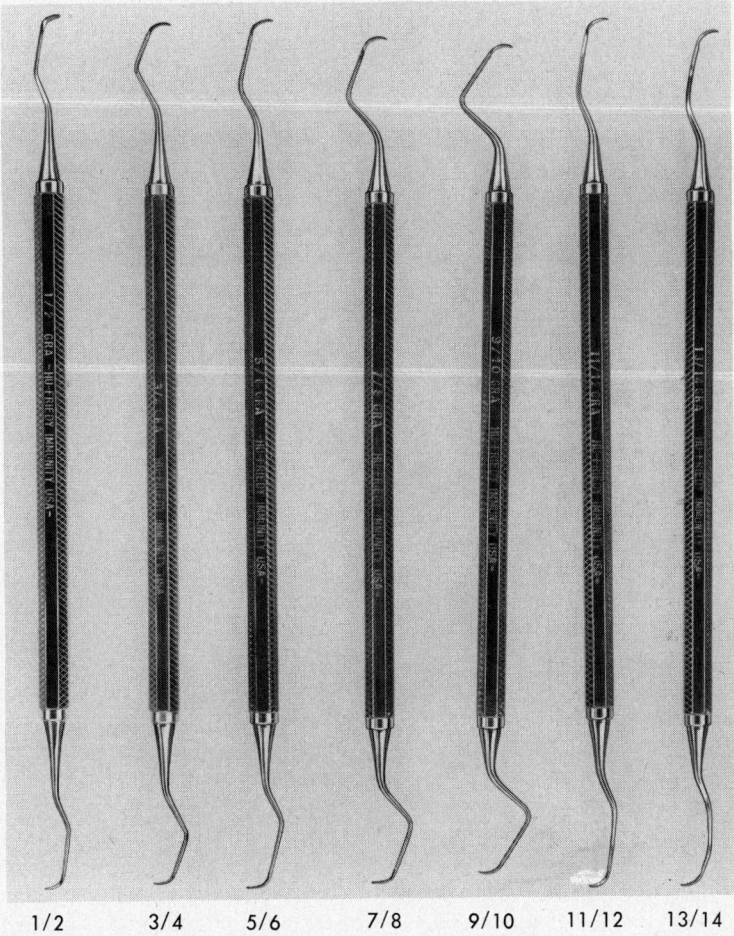

1/2   3/4   5/6   7/8   9/10   11/12   13/14

Fig. 23-1. Gracey curettes provide a variety of shank designs to facilitate access to all areas of dentition. Working-end design is well suited to root planing and removal of fine deposits.

deepest pockets. Curved explorers (such as the pigtail or cowhorn) cannot reach the apical extent of all pockets. The length of the explorer's working end, its ability to be maneuvered in deep pockets, and its ability to transmit subtle vibrations (that is, diameter of the working end) all must be considered. Some explorers that fit these criteria, such as the fine No. 17 or No. 20 design shown in Chapter 6 (see Fig. 6-1), may not adapt easily to the distal surfaces of posterior teeth because of their straight design. For these surfaces, the clinician may elect to use a periodontal probe or another instrument for exploration. An explorer introduced by Hu-Friedy in 1988 is designed with a shank similar to the Gracey $^{11}/_{12}$ making it a good choice for subgingival exploration.

The experienced clinician can also use a sharp curette blade to accomplish much of the detection. There are many advantages to developing tactile sensitivity with the curette blade for definitive exploration. According to basic instrumentation principles, this ability is necessary as a prelude to each working stroke performed with the instrument. The student should take time to practice and develop skill in using the curette for exploration because it will increase operating efficiency. This skill will facilitate deposit removal, because the clinician will have a more accurate idea of location and type of deposit, and it will also require less time and motion than continually switching from curette to explorer and back. Beginning students should depend on an explorer to evaluate the tooth surface until they have developed their tactile sensitivity with the curette. In addition, the final check or evaluation of the procedure always should be performed with an explorer, even though earlier evaluations with the curette blade indicated completion. This instrument allows the clinician to perform a definitive evaluation of all areas of the root surface for optimal results.

The importance of frequent sharpening of curettes during root-planing procedures was reinforced by a study that evaluated the amount of wear (dulling) that the cutting edges of curettes underwent during prescribed numbers of root-planing strokes. Curettes that had been used for only 15 strokes showed signs of dulling, as evidenced by the presence of a slight bevel, when observed under a scanning electron microscope. Even wider bevels were observed after 45 strokes. Jones and O'Leary (1978) suggested that as many as 45 strokes might be necessary for root-planing only one tooth. Therefore, considering that 15 to 45 root-planing strokes might include treatment of only one or two teeth, it is apparent that instruments become dull very quickly when used for this purpose and must be resharpened frequently to maximize the effectiveness and efficiency of the root-planing procedure.

Use of topical or local anesthesia, or nitrous oxide and oxygen conscious sedation during root planing is dependent on individual patient needs. Many patients find any kind of instrumentation performed in inflamed areas somewhat uncomfortable, and because of the exacting requirements of this procedure it may be necessary and advisable to administer some type of pain control. Pain control should not be a cover-up for poor instrumentation technique but should be introduced only in consideration of patient comfort when even safe and effective techniques produce symptoms of pain.

Technique

Root planing employs and builds on many of the principles of basic instrumentation already described for scaling. Some comparisons between fine scaling and root-planing techniques are discussed on pp 446-447. In addition, some of the specific modifications of the scaling technique as presented in Chapter 21 are discussed below as they pertain to root planing. These modifications include the number of strokes, the direction of the strokes, tactile sensitivity, pressure, the length of the strokes, and time required.

Strokes for root planing usually require less pressure against the wall of the tooth than those for scaling. Because cementum is significantly softer than enamel, there is more chance of gouging the root surface if too much pressure is used. Root planing is essentially a shaving process that removes diseased cementum, attached calculus, and endotoxins layer by layer. The desired root surface is one that feels smooth and free of root irregularities, which would attract and retain plaque and calculus. Lateral pressure of the blade against the root surface should be moderate at first until the surface debris of nonvital cementum and calculus is removed. These strokes should be followed by lighter strokes that remove less cementum while continuing to smooth the root surface. The clinician should be careful not to apply heavy pressure at the onset of the stroke; instead, the same amount of pressure should be applied through the entire stroke. This will prevent ditching of the cementum at those areas where the strokes begin. Strokes used for root planing may also be longer than the ones required for scaling. In scaling the objective is to fracture calculus away from the tooth, and the working stroke can end as soon as the deposit is dislodged. In root planing the initial strokes should be relatively short, overlapping, and controlled until the area is smooth. As more and more of the tooth surface has been planed and the root is approaching smoothness, the planing strokes can be lengthened to blend the completed areas into each other. Short strokes are used initially because they are somewhat easier to control and adapt. Adaptation and control of instruments is especially important during root planing because of the wide variations in root morphology that may be encountered and the close proximity of soft tissues to the cutting edges of instruments.

The application of different types of stroking patterns over a given area is likely to produce a smoother surface than the use of only one stroke

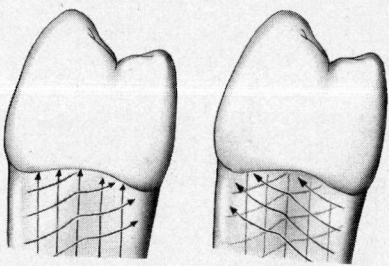

Fig. 23-2. Representation of overall smoothing effect that is produced during root planing through use of a wide variety of overlapping strokes. Result of this cross-hatching pattern of strokes is a surface that is completely planed and polished.

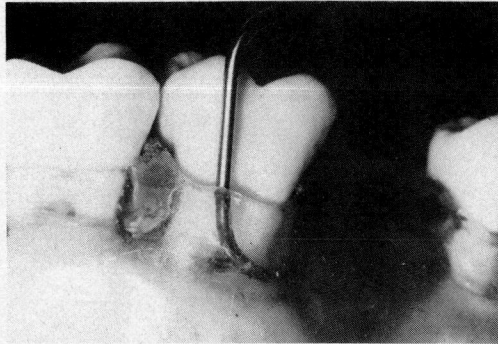

Fig. 23-3. Gracey ⅞ curette is properly adapted for implementation of vertical stroke on mesiobuccal line angle of tooth No. 30. Note that terminal shank is parallel to long axis of tooth for this stroking pattern. This adaptation ensures proper working angulation of lower cutting edge against tooth surface.

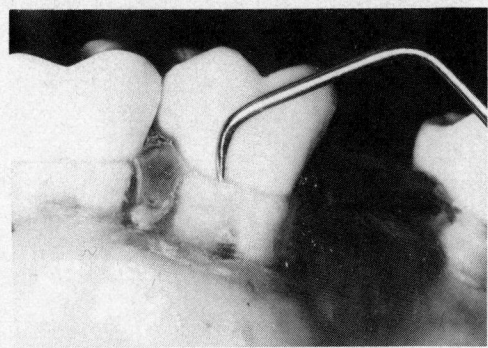

Fig. 23-4. Gracey ⅞ curette is being inserted in preparation for horizontal stroke. Note that toe will be along base of pocket and that terminal shank is not parallel to long axis of tooth.

direction. For instance, if initial root planing is done with vertical strokes, an even smoother surface will be produced by also applying a series of overlapping oblique and horizontal strokes over the same area (Fig. 23-2). Instrument adaptation for vertical and horizontal strokes is shown in Figs. 23-3 and 23-4. This pattern of strokes is identical to the pattern recommended for ultrasonic scaling (see Chapter 22).

One major difference between scaling and root planing is the time required for each. Hand scaling a tooth usually requires only a few well-executed strokes in given areas, whereas root planing requires complete coverage of the entire root surface of the pocket with short, overlapping, continuous, and repeated strokes. Therefore, it takes much longer to root plane a tooth than to scale a tooth. While a whole mouth may be scaled in 1 hour, it may take the same amount of time to root plane only a few teeth carefully and completely. Complete scaling and root planing of periodontally involved roots require much more time and effort than the typical 45-minute recall appointment. In studies comparing the effectiveness of surgical and nonsurgical approaches to periodontal treatment, clinicians involved in nonsurgical treatment of patients, spent from 5 to 8 hours on scaling and root planing alone. Total time spent on these procedures was spread over from three to eight appointments. These time estimates are based on the clinical proficiency of skilled clinicians who have mastered instrumentation and sharpening skills. It is apparent that these procedures are exacting and time-consuming if successful results are to be achieved. Less experienced

clinicians and students should expect to spend even more time to achieve acceptable results. Greenwell and others (1987) noted that "it is questionable whether procedures involving lesser amounts of time should actually be classified as 'non-surgical therapy'." Obviously, root planing is much more exacting and definitive than fine scaling and requires a great deal of precision. It cannot be mastered after a few experiences, and many clinicians will admit that it is the most difficult treatment procedure to perfect. Students will increase their appreciation of this fact as they perform some of the activities recommended at the

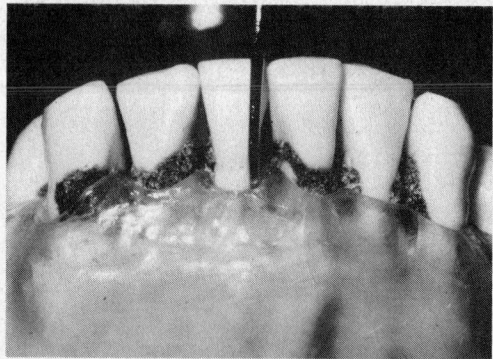

Fig. 23-5. Gracey ½ curette is being adapted to mesial surface of lower right incisor. Again note that terminal shank is adapted parallel to long axis of tooth. Deviation from this orientation will result in working angulation being too open or too closed.

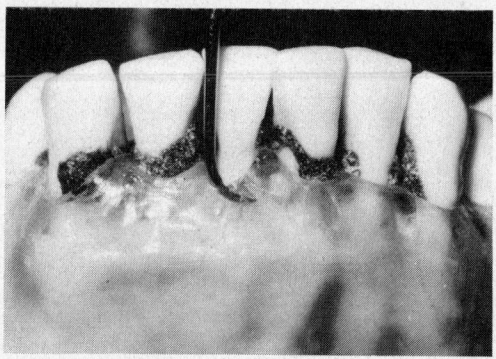

Fig. 23-6. Adaptation of curette blade along narrow labial surface of mandibular incisors is difficult and must be done with a great deal of tactile sensitivity to ensure that toe does not gouge into soft tissues.

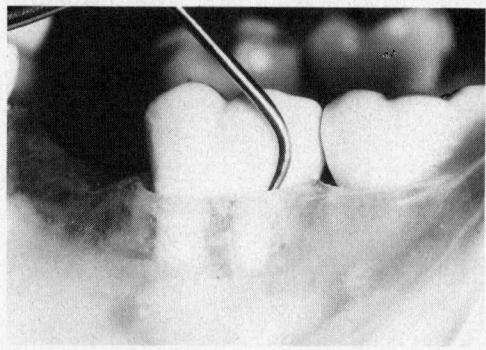

Fig. 23-7. First in a series of photographs demonstrating a variety of approaches to scaling and root planing buccal surface of mandibular left molar tooth in which furcation opening poses additional work. One approach is to use Gracey ⅞ curette on all surfaces except distal surface of mesial root, where it will not adapt. Starting at distal line angle and using vertical and oblique strokes, Gracey ⅞ curette can be used easily in this illustrated buccal area.

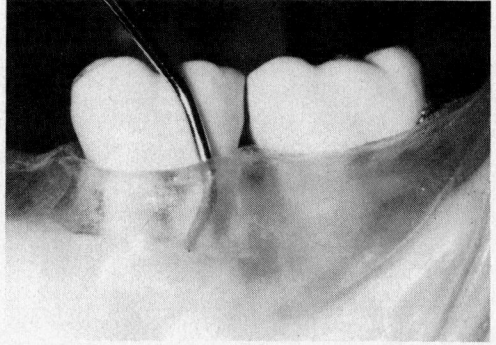

Fig. 23-8. Gracey ¹¹/₁₂ curette is adapted to mesial surface of distal root and into furcation area. This instrument can also be adapted on buccal surfaces of tooth and root with success. As with Gracey ⅞ curette, this instrument will not adapt to distal surfaces of either root.

end of this chapter. A variety of approaches to root planing are shown in Figs. 23-5 to 23-11.

Evaluation

How does the clinician determine when to *stop* root planing? The best evaluation of the success of root planing lies in the response of the soft tissue side of the pocket. If, after a healing period, the clinical signs of inflammation subside and reduction of the pocket depths has occurred, then some of the objectives have been met. Waerhaug (1978a, 1978b) warned that if a patient's *supragingival* plaque control is effective, gingival conditions may appear normal even though subgingival plaque is still present. Therefore, the external appearance of the soft tissues can be misleading regarding the disease process, which is still occurring subgingivally. A more reliable test for the presence of inflammation is gingival sulcus bleeding. When the patient returns for reevaluation, if there is no bleeding on probing in the areas that were root planed and if home care has been optimally maintained, it can be assumed that the

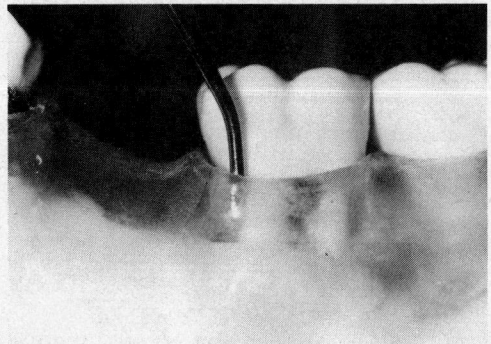

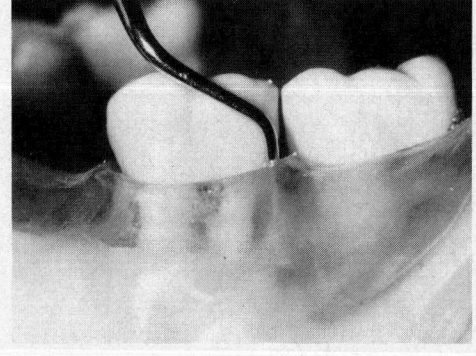

Fig. 23-9. Gracey ¹¹/₁₂ curette is used to continue root planing on mesial surface of tooth and mesial root. It is optimally designed to serve this surface. Note that terminal shank is always parallel to long axis of tooth when this instrument is correctly adapted.

Fig. 23-10. Correct adaptation of Gracey ¹³/₁₄ curette. Again, terminal shank, which is somewhat buried submarginally, is oriented as much parallel to long axis of tooth as possible to facilitate adaptation and angulation.

newly prepared root surface is now *biologically acceptable* to the adjacent soft tissues. Soft tissue evaluation cannot be reached until after several days of healing.

The clinician must be able to provide an ongoing evaluation of the root-planing procedure to identify whether treatment objectives are being reached. How, then, can it be determined that the tooth is *clinically acceptable* and that root planing should cease? In making this determination the clinician can rely on several visual, audio, and tactile clues.

Visual. There are many more visual clues when part of the root surface to be planed is exposed to the oral cavity as a result of gingival recession than when it is submarginal. The clinician can see the color and texture of the exposed root surface and determine whether or not pieces of calculus or diseased cementum are still visible. The use of an air syringe to dry the tooth will aid in this evaluation. If drying reveals white flecks of calculus, diseased cementum, or extrinsic stains, more root planing is indicated. A root surface with a smooth, shiny appearance and homogeneous color indicates effective root planing. The clinician should also evaluate the root surface for signs of ditching or overplaning from previous instrumentation. This was a common result of root planing in the 1950s, when it was thought that the only way to prepare the root surface adequately was to cut well into the healthy dentin,

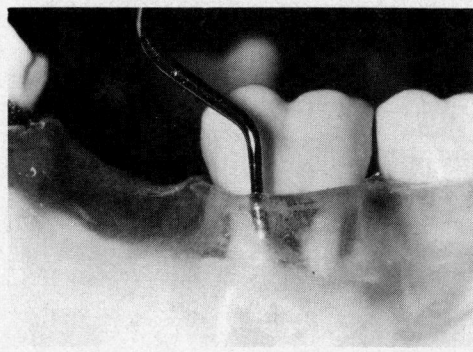

Fig. 23-11. Gracey ¹³/₁₄ curette allows adaptation of blade into furcation area so that distal surface of mesial root can be treated. This is instrument of choice for this area on tooth.

leaving the teeth with roots that were narrow and had an hourglass appearance (Riffle, 1956). (see Fig. 26-6)(In cases where substantial root planing from previous treatment has removed a great deal of hard tissue, the clinician must evaluate whether additional removal of cementum and dentin will be beneficial or detrimental to the patient in the long term.) That practice has become outdated, but a controversy still remains as to how much of the cementum and dentin must be removed to ensure that the root surface is biologically acceptable to the soft tissue wall of the pocket. Before this controversy can be resolved, more research is necessary to determine exactly how the toxic substances that are thought to provoke the inflammatory response (endotoxins) attach to the root surface and how deeply they penetrate into cementum and dentin. One study suggests that laying a surgical flap and polishing the root may be sufficient (Nyman, et al, 1988).

Another way of visually assessing the root surface is to disclose the exposed portions and identify those areas that still attract the disclosant because of surface deposits or root irregularities. The use of disclosing solution may not be a valid measure of the true extent of plaque microorganisms and their byproducts. Organic material and instrumentation debris may also retain the stain immediately after instrumentation, so that not all visibly stained surfaces may represent potential microbial threats to the periodontal tissues (Breininger, 1987). The clinician must also remember that the toxic by-products of plaque are not clinically visible and are frequently located submarginally. Therefore the only reliable method for evaluating the removal of these substances is by observing the gingival response to treatment.

Audio. A rough root surface produces a scratchy, coarse sound when it is being root planed. As the root gets smoother, the sound of the curette blade against the root begins to diminish or take on a higher, squeaky pitch. By listening to the sound produced by the curette, the clinician will receive some clues as to whether or not a smooth, hard surface is being achieved. This sound can be amplified for the beginning student by placing the handle end of a single-ended curette in the rubber tube of a stethoscope from which the bulb has been removed. With the stethoscope the student should hear the change of pitch as the root goes from rough and irregular to smooth (Seibert, 1978). After hearing the amplified sound changes, it may be easier for the student to detect these same audio changes without the aid of the stethoscope.

Tactile. The most frequently used and most important of all clues for evaluating the clinical acceptability of root planing is the tactile sense of the clinician. Most root planing occurs submarginally, where visual and audio clues are not available. Therefore, the clinician must rely on an acute sensitivity to vibrations transmitted through the instruments to the fingers to recognize surface changes that are occurring as a result of the root planing procedure. The tactile sense also must guide the clinician carefully around the root mor-

phology during all working and exploring strokes to ensure optimal adaptation and angulation of the instrument against the root surface. It takes a great deal of time and experience to distinguish between the rough, bumpy, irregular, somewhat sticky feel of the diseased root surface embedded with calculus and plaque and a thoroughly prepared root surface.

The beginning clinician must develop an acute tactile sense by learning to concentrate on tactile sensations and to interpret accurately the vibrations that are transmitted through the instruments to the fingers. Reception of tactile vibrations is easiest when a light grasp is maintained on the instrument for all exploration of the root surface. Another aid in developing and maximizing the tactile sense is the use of fine instruments; these include explorers with small-diameter working ends, as described in Chapter 6, and curettes with fine blades and thin, light shanks, such as the Gracey finishing curettes. Many clinicians also find that instruments with hollow handles transmit more vibrations than those with solid handles. The fingers can detect more subtle vibrations with a sharp curette than with a dull one. Sharpening skills are of utmost importance in root planing for optimum efficiency of the procedure. Much time can be wasted by root planing with dull curettes; the procedure can be performed much more quickly and easily if the instruments are kept optimally sharp.

Exploring exercises on extracted teeth will help the beginning student develop and improve detection skills for root planing as well as calculus detection. One such exercise, described at the end of Chapter 12, p 230, is to explore an extracted tooth with the eyes closed, concentrating on the different textures and curves of the root surface. Comparisons also can be made using different instruments and a variety of root surfaces irregularities. After the surface is explored and a mental image formed of its appearance, the eyes can be used to evaluate the accuracy of the tactile impression. Students should continue to test their tactile sense while working with clinic patients by comparing the feel of different root morphologies, deposits, and restorations and analyzing what makes them feel different from each other. With continual practice a fine, discriminatory tactile sense will eventually develop.

Clinicians frequently evaluate the effectiveness

of root planing on the basis of tactile information, because this is often the only source of information available during the procedure. The "finished" root surface has been described as velvety smooth, glasslike, or hard to an explorer, because these clinical characteristics seem to accompany the removal of calculus and diseased cementum. The concepts of smoothness and hardness, however, should be examined more closely as to their validity and reliability for predicting that a root surface is biologically acceptable and that an optimal healing response will occur. Both of these qualities can be measured only subjectively, because they are evaluated according to the tactile skills, clinical experience, and interpretation of each clinician. It is difficult, therefore, to explain to the beginning clinician exactly what is meant by a smooth or a hard root surface. The following discussion should help the reader review the significance and limitations of each of these clinical parameters.

The effect of periodontal disease on the surface cementum that is exposed because of apical migration of the dentogingival junction is variable. Cementum that is adjacent to the inflamed soft tissues of the pocket undergoes demineralization, reducing the microhardness of the cementum. Cementum that has been exposed to the oral cavity, however, by means of gingival recession may become remineralized to the extent that its microhardness approaches normal levels (Ruben and Shapiro, 1978). The exposed cementum has the apparent ability to absorb minerals such as calcium, phosphorus, and fluoride from the pocket environment and saliva. Unfortunately, this tendency to absorb also extends to the toxic substances within the pocket environment, which inflame the adjacent soft tissues. This information would lead the clinician to believe that the resistance of pocket cementum to planing might be less than that of normal cementum. Rautiola and Craig (1961), however, measured the microhardness of cementum and dentin in extracted teeth that had never been scaled. Their results indicated that there is no significant difference between the hardness of cementum that has been exposed to periodontal inflammation versus cementum that is unexposed. The study also indicated that there are no significant differences in the hardness of inner and outer layers of cementum and that outer layers of dentin that interface with cementum have

hardness values similar to that of the cementum. Several important questions remain to be answered in light of these conflicting reports. If there is a difference in the hardness of periodontally affected cementum as compared with healthy cementum, is it a large enough difference to be clinically detectable to the extent that the clinician can determine exactly when intact, healthy cementum or dentin has been reached and root planing should cease? Is root hardness a reliable measure of the extent to which toxic substances have penetrated the root surface? Until answers to these questions are available, the clinician should use tactile information regarding root hardness only as supplemental feedback regarding the progress of the root-planing process.

What is the risk of overplaning the cementum surface and removing excessive amounts of acellular cementum in the quest for a hard surface? Stahl (1977) studied the mechanisms of repair of the soft tissues to the treated root surface and concluded that by removing the acellular cementum, which is unlikely to regenerate, the clinician is more likely to achieve a repair involving the close adherence of the new junctional epithelium to the root surface rather than actual new attachment of connective tissue fibers—the preferred method of repair. The results of this study imply that excessive removal of cementum can reduce the chances of gaining this type of new attachment during the healing process. A dilemma is created for clinicians, because all diseased cementum must be removed to make the root surface biologically acceptable, yet the actual removal also reduces the chances of gaining new attachment.

If there is no clinically detectable difference between cementum and dentin, as reported by Rautiola and Craig, then it is impossible to determine when all cementum has been removed and dentin is encountered. It is difficult to decide how much to plane away from the tooth. Although it is necessary to remove all the endotoxin-bearing hard tissues, most clinicians try to proceed no further into dentin than necessary, to avoid distortion of the root surface or unnecessary hypersensitivity of the root surface caused by overplaning. It is apparent, however, that because of the need to prepare the root surface thoroughly, it is likely that the patient may experience some sensitivity from the root-planing procedure. When this occurs, the patient should be referred to special home care techniques designed to diminish the sensitivity. Chapter 30 deals with the treatment of hypersensitivity in greater detail. The cementum is especially thin near the cementoenamel junction, and extensive root planing in this area is likely to result in sensitivity.

The degree of root smoothness should be used only as a clinical indicator of the presence of calculus and cannot be depended on as a valid measure of the effectiveness of the root-planing procedure. Clinicians should be wary of relying too heavily on this criterion alone as a predictor of the success of root planing. Although the relative smoothness of the root can provide tactile feedback to the clinician regarding the progress of the root-planing process and the presence of remaining calculus deposits, it cannot provide any assurance that the root surface is free of the toxic byproducts of plaque or that the root is biologically acceptable to the soft tissues. Several studies have demonstrated that root surfaces that feel smooth to an explorer still harbor calculus deposits that can be detected visually (Moskow and Bressman, 1964; Jones et al, 1972; Walker, 1976; Jones and O'Leary, 1978; Nishimine and O'Leary, 1979; Rabbani et al, 1981). The remaining deposits may be either burnished or simply too small to be detected tactilely.

It is frequently assumed that one of the reasons for producing a smooth root surface is that it will be less plaque-retentive, more easily maintained by the patient, and therefore less susceptible to gingival inflammation. Rosenberg and Ash (1974) tested this assumption by comparing the plaque accumulation and gingival inflammation scores for roots that had been root planed with hand instruments and roots that had been ultrasonically scaled. They found that although there was a statistically significant difference in the roughness values of the two groups of teeth, there was not a significant difference in the amount of plaque accumulation or gingival inflammation scores for the two treatment groups. This study has caused researchers to question the validity of promoting root smoothness as a means of preventing future plaque accumulation and gingival inflammation.

Interest in the significance of root roughness to periodontal repair has generated investigations of the role of root roughness in promoting the reattachment of connective tissue fibers. Results indicate that in some cases areas of root roughness

appear to facilitate this reattachment (Khatiblou and Ghodssi, 1983). More research is necessary to clarify this relationship.

It is important that clinicians understand the limitations regarding the use of root smoothness as an indicator of the completion of root planing. Although it is the best clinical indicator available for determining the presence of calculus, it can be unreliable. If a surface that feels smooth can still harbor calculus, then it certainly can harbor plaque and its byproducts. Clinical smoothness of a root surface cannot be relied on as a means of preventing plaque accumulation or gingival inflammation, nor can it or any other clinical clue be relied on as a final test of the effectiveness of the root planing procedure. In fact, some research indicates that a rough root surface that is biologically clean may be preferred as a means of gaining clinical attachment. Although clinical indicators or clues provide helpful feedback regarding the progress of root planing, the only valid and reliable measure of the success of root planing is the response of the soft tissues to the treatment when supported by effective mechanical and chemical supragingival plaque control by the patient.

Complicating factors

A number of factors complicate the root planing process: limited access to the root surface, bleeding, sensitivity, and root texture. In many situations, access to the affected area is difficult, if not impossible.

Exposed furcation entrances and the complex anatomy of root surfaces not only play a significant role in the pathogenesis of periodontal disease but also pose a difficult clinical challenge in the treatment of that disease (Bower, 1979b; Gher and Vernino, 1980; Goldman et al, 1985; Ramfjord et al, 1987). Furcation involvements may be large enough to permit the accumulation of plaque and its endotoxins but too small and too confined an area for access with a curette. Bower (1979a) compared the width of several commonly used curettes and determined that 58% of the furcation entrances that he studied had entrance widths that were smaller than the width of most curette blades. He concluded that it was unlikely that curettes would be able to clean the entrance area to furcations in a clinical situation. Access to furcations in maxillary molars and premolars is especially limited. Unlike the buccal and lingual furcations of mandibular teeth, these maxillary teeth have furcations opening on mesial and distal surfaces adjacent to other teeth. In addition, there may be trifurcation involvements rather than bifurcation involvements. Certainly, the clinician must be well aware of the root morphologies of these teeth to treat these difficult areas (Fig. 23-12).

Another access problem is that of maneuvering even a small curette blade to the bottom of a deep, tight pocket. To ensure the removal of subgingival plaque and calculus, the curette must be inserted all the way to the dentoepithelial junction at the base of the pocket. Since most pockets become narrower at their apical extent, the pressure of the sulcular tissues against the instrument blade as it is inserted may fool the clinician into thinking prematurely that the base has been reached. Not only must the curette reach the base of the pocket, but slight compression of these tissues may also be necessary to locate the cutting edge near the pocket base and below the plaque and calculus that has formed there (Waerhaug, 1978b). This does not mean, however, that instrumentation should go on at the base of the pocket without consideration for the soft tissues. Excessive damage to the gingival fibers underlying the junctional epithelium and damage to the deeper periodontal ligament could result in the formation of an even deeper pocket after healing. The clinician must walk the fine line between damaging underlying soft tissues and allowing calculus and plaque deposits to remain subgingivally. The goal is the removal of the plaque and calculus with as little soft tissue damage as possible. An almost certain result of the root planning procedure will be some *coincidental curettage*. This is the unintentional removal of soft tissue from the pocket wall adjacent to the treated root surface. It is impossible for the opposite cutting edge of the curette to avoid contact with the pocket wall. In many cases coincidental curettage is considered to be more beneficial than detrimental to the patient because it assists in the removal of inflamed soft tissues and aids the wound-healing process. The clinician should be aware that any manipulation of inflamed soft tissues may be painful for the patient.

Another access problem is posed by the close proximity of roots, as in the lower anterior areas,

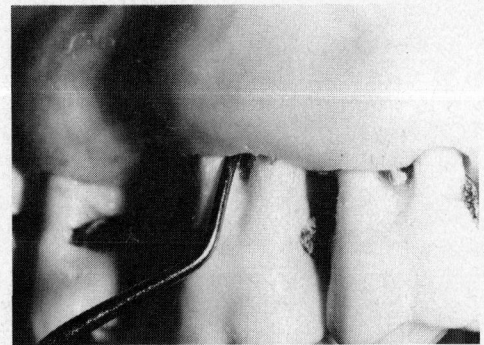

Fig. 23-12. With transparent gingiva removed, it can be seen that access to furcation areas is limited and that there is little room for maneuverability even with narrow blade of Gracey curette. Add to this the fact that normally this area is not visible during instrumentation, and it is easy to see why these areas complicate root-planing procedures.

making instrumentation in these confined areas difficult. Additional access problems may be experienced in distal pockets of posterior teeth where there is not much room for manipulation of an instrument to gain leverage for working strokes.

Bleeding is another complicating factor during root planing. Bleeding can be expected whenever instrumentation is done in an inflamed area. It serves a useful purpose during scaling and root planing by clearing loosened calculus, plaque, and other debris from the pocket, thereby promoting healing. The disadvantage of bleeding is that it hampers visibility and fulcrum stability. For optimal working conditions the area should be kept as free of blood as possible. This can be accomplished easily with water irrigation and suctioning devices. Slight bleeding can be controlled by blotting and light pressure to the wound site with a sterile gauze sponge. More profuse bleeding can be controlled through the use of irrigation and suctioning during the procedure. A stream of water from the water syringe may be directed at the area, followed by suction evacuation of the fluids. Do not use a forced spray of water and air combined to rinse the area because it increases the production of blood-contaminated aerosols, which then are propelled at the operating team and can serve as sources of cross-contamination (see discussion of aerosols in Chapter 3). For patients who need anesthesia, the vasoconstrictor in the anesthetic solution will provide some hemostasis or control of bleeding to the area where it is injected. Control of bleeding will make the patient more comfortable and increase tolerance of the procedure. Patients may not realize that bleeding is a normal response to instrumentation in inflamed areas, and they should be assured in advance that it is expected and beneficial to the healing process. This explanation may help avoid a misunderstanding about the cause of bleeding.

Patient sensitivity often accompanies the root-planing procedure. This sensitivity may arise from the inflamed soft tissues or from the root surface. Because patient cooperation and comfort are important, this sensitivity should be reduced as much as possible. Optimal instrumentation skills will minimize the pain and trauma for the patient but often are not sufficient to eliminate all sensitivity. Nitrous oxide and oxygen conscious sedation and/or a local anesthetic should be available to reduce the patient's discomfort during root planing if requested. Tolerance of pain varies greatly among patients; while some may tolerate the procedure well without anesthesia, others may need anesthesia. The use of any type of anesthesia must not be a cover-up for poor instrumentation technique; all treatment should be performed with concern and respect for the soft tissues whether or not anesthesia is used. Damage caused by inappropriate instrumentation not only will hinder wound healing and repair of the gingiva, but also will destroy patient trust and confidence in the clinician.

As a result of root planing, the patient may also experience increased root sensitivity to stimuli such as hot or cold temperatures, resulting from the removal of cementum or dentin on the root surface. The patient should be informed that this might be a complication of treatment and why it may occur. In many cases this is only a temporary discomfort for the patient, and with proper desensitization procedures and home care it should diminish.

Contraindications

Contraindications for root planing include (1) lack of motivation to perform home care procedures; (2) teeth with severe periodontal disease and mobility; (3) severe pocket depth requiring some form of surgery or osseous recontouring; (4) extreme hypersensitivity; and (5) acute periodontal infections.

Root planing is a time-consuming and exacting effort to provide an environment in the periodontal pocket that will promote healing. If the patient will not maintain home care, the results of root planing will be short-lived, and the pocket will soon return to a diseased condition. No matter how clean and plaque-free the pocket may be at any one time, it will reverse itself in the presence of plaque and its endotoxins. A patient who does not make any effort to maintain supramarginal plaque control will soon have the plaque front again migrating apically into the pocket, and the disease process will recur. Patients must be informed that the success of the treatment is dependent on their ability and willingness to perform effective daily plaque removal.

Patients exhibiting severe periodontal destruction, such as deep infrabony pockets, mucogingival involvement, and mobility, require more definitive periodontal treatment than root planing alone can provide. Fine scaling and root planing should be part of initial therapy for these patients because removal of the etiologic factors will provide some reduction in pocket depth and reduction of inflammation in the soft tissues. In less severe cases root planing may produce significant healing before surgery so that the indications for surgery no longer exist. In more severe cases the initial therapy, which includes root planing, can improve the tissue condition so that there is less bleeding and less damage to tissues during surgical manipulation. Occasionally, cases of severe periodontal destruction may be treated by conservative measures such as root planing and curettage because other surgical procedures are contraindicated due to medical complications, economic limitations, or stress factors.

When root planing is part of initial therapy preceding other surgical interventions, it is often accomplished under *open-flap* conditions. This means that a flap is raised so that the soft tissues can be retracted away from the root surfaces. In this way the clinician can see the root morphology and calculus deposits, increasing the effectiveness and efficiency of the root-planing procedure.

Dentinal hypersensitivity may exist in some patients, especially those who have undergone previous root-planing treatment. Although the root planing itself can be accomplished with these patients under local anesthesia, the clinician should realize that the patient's sensitivity may be increased following treatment. The pain and discomfort of extreme hypersensitivity is likely to override any benefits that the patient perceives as the result of root planing and also may interfere with effective home care procedures. Root planing should be postponed until this situation can be brought under control (see Chapter 30).

Patients with acute periodontal inflammation, such as acute necrotizing ulcerative gingivitis (ANUG), should be treated for the acute condition before the tissue is extensively manipulated, as in root planing. When acute infections occur, the tissue is friable and prone to traumatic injury until the condition subsides. There is also increased chance of bacteremia because of the number of bacteria and other infective microorganisms present at the site. Extensive instrumentation will increase the patient's discomfort and pain. These procedures should be postponed until the acute condition of the tissues is relieved.

Soft tissue response to root planing

The primary goal of root planing is to provide a biologically clean root surface on the hard tissue side of a periodontal pocket that will encourage healing and repair of the inflamed soft tissues. After removal of irritants both within the pocket and on the tooth surface, the body can work to reverse the inflammatory process and repair the damaged gingival tissues. The coincidental curettage that occurs as an indirect result of root planing assists in the healing process. In most cases some amount of coincidental curettage cannot be avoided and results in the partial removal of the ulcerated sulcular epithelium, the junctional epithelium, and superficial layers of the underlying inflamed connective tissues. The inadvertent removal of these diseased tissues facilitates wound healing. Coincidental curettage should not be confused, however, with intentional curettage, which is described in Chapter 24.

The clinician should be aware that incomplete calculus removal in patients with chronic periodontal disease can, in some cases, result in an acute periodontal abscess. A periodontal abscess can occur when a foreign substance such as calculus or food particles occludes the pocket opening, preventing drainage of inflammatory exudate. A chronic periodontal pocket usually can provide its own drainage, but if it becomes blocked the inflammation will spread in other directions and intensify into an acute periodontal abscess, resulting in rapid destruction of tissues.

It is not unusual for a periodontal abscess to occur following scaling procedures, especially if not all subgingival calculus deposits were removed. After the initial scaling, the superficial tissues heal and the pocket orifice tightens and shrinks so that it becomes more adapted to the tooth. If a foreign object such as calculus is still embedded deep in the pocket, the bacteria can proliferate into an abscess. A similar result might occur if the patient initiates sudden and vigorous toothbrushing in an area of periodontitis and subgingival calculus. Clinicians should be aware that incomplete scaling, either by intent (e.g., "gross scale") or by omission (e.g., failure to detect and remove calculus), can have this result. Periodontal abscesses are treated by removal of the irritant, drainage of the exudate, and treatment of the pocket area (Harvey, 1974; Dello Russo, 1985).

Another result of the root-planing process that is not beneficial to tissue healing is the entrapment of calculus, bacteria, and debris in the pocket and adjacent soft tissues following their removal from the root surface. These foreign particles are irritating to the soft tissues and will hinder healing if allowed to remain. Although bleeding and the curette may bring out much of the debris, the pocket should still be thoroughly irrigated with a stream of water to cleanse the area further (Moskow, 1962). Because water with high bacterial counts could result in bacteremia when applied to wounded areas, the water supply to the dental unit should be tested for microbial contamination. To minimize the risk of infection, all surgical wounds should be irrigated with a sterile normal saline solution rather than tap water. Oxygenating rinses may also help cleanse and debride these areas. Following irrigation, healing is further enhanced by the application of gentle compression and readaptation of the tissues to the teeth. This procedure will assist in stopping the bleeding and in forming a thin blood clot against the tissues. Healing is enhanced by the formation of a thin, rather than a thick, blood clot. Performing these procedures immediately after root planing will help accelerate tissue healing and achieve an optimal tissue response.

Root planing has been shown to produce periodontal improvement in the treatment of slight, moderate, and severe periodontitis. Although the ideal result of periodontal treatment would be the creation of new attachment of connective tissue fibers along the root surface, this does not normally occur as a result of root planing. Following root planing, pocket reduction occurs largely as a result of gingival recession (shrinkage) and a secondary gain in the clinical attachment level. The gain in clinical attachment should not be misinterpreted as the creation of a new attachment of connective tissue fibers to the root surface at a more coronal level. This gain in the clinical attachment level is caused by the creation of a new, longer junctional epithelium and the healing of the connective tissue fibers. The repaired gingival fibers consist of healthy, intact tissues that have the ability to provide resistance against the probe tip so that it cannot penetrate as far apically as it could when the tissues were inflamed.

In the presence of inflammation the connective tissue fibers that are located apical to the junctional epithelium are destroyed and replaced by inflammatory cells. Several studies have shown that this destruction allows the tip of a periodontal probe to pass through the junctional epithelium and come to rest only when it encounters intact gingival fibers, at an approximate depth of 0.25 to 0.4 mm beyond the apical extent of the junctional epithelium (Silvertson and Burgett, 1976; Listgarten et al, 1976; Powell and Garnick, 1978; Spray et al, 1978; Listgarten, 1980). When these tissues are permitted to heal, they offer increased resistance to the probe, so that the tip of the probe comes to rest at a point coronal to the junctional epithelium. The clinical probing depth will therefore reflect an apparent gain in attachment levels, although the histologic pocket depth remains the same.

In addition to the secondary gain in clinical attachment, healing also results in shrinkage of the gingiva caused by the reduction of tissue edema. When these two factors are evaluated following treatment, the clinical result is a decrease in the depth of the clinical pocket. The amount of pocket depth reduction seems to be related to the initial severity of the periodontal destruction. Deeper pockets show more depth reduction following root planing than do shallow pockets

(Tagge et al, 1975; Listgarten et al, 1978; Hellden et al, 1979; Cercek et al, 1983).

Histologically, the healed pocket is characterized by the presence of a long junctional epithelium (Caton and Zander, 1979). The ability of a long junctional epithelium to provide effective protection against subsequent inflammatory attacks has been questioned in the literature (Barrington, 1981). This issue was studied by Magnusson and others (1983), who concluded that the presence of a long junctional epithelium offers the same resistance to plaque infection as an epithelial junction of normal length.

Root planing in shallow pockets (1 to 3 mm) can result in an actual loss of connective tissue attachment, followed by a corresponding loss of bone (Knowles et al, 1980; Badersten et al., 1981; Pihlstrom et al, 1981; Lindhe et al, 1982a, 1982b). One reason proposed for this loss of attachment is that it is a result of mechanical wounding and detachment of attached gingival fibers caused by repeated instrumentation (Lindhe, 1982b).

CHEMICAL TREATMENT OF PERIODONTALLY INVOLVED ROOTS

Interest has grown in the possibility of gaining new soft tissue attachment to periodontally exposed roots through the use of chemical agents as an adjunct to mechanical root planing. The best known chemical treatment of planed root surfaces is application of citric acid. Application of citric acid to a planed root surface removes minerals from dentin or cementum and exposes collagen fibers in the cementum; these exposed fibers may connect with collagen fibers from the gingival connective tissue or regenerating periodontal ligament during healing. Some of the surface changes that have been attributed to citric acid as a root conditioner include widening of dentinal tubules, formation of cemental pins, removal of smear layer of cementum, accelerated healing, inhibition of epithelial migration, and formation of a new connective tissue attachment (Register and Burdick, 1976; Cole et al, 1980; Selvig et al, 1981; Albair et al, 1982; Frank et al, 1983; Common and McFall, 1983). Other studies have failed to produce these changes, resulting in a controversy surrounding the effectiveness of chemical root conditioning for the purpose of gaining new attachment (Stahl and Froum, 1977; Otomo and Sims, 1979; Froum et al, 1983).

Several objections have been raised to the use of citric acid as a chemical treatment of root surfaces, including potential damage to pulp, soft tissues, and bone. Studies on animals and humans, however have failed to confirm any harmful effects (Nilveus, 1983). Phosphoric acid has also been investigated for application to planed root surfaces and has been found to have the same potential for enhancing connective tissue reattachment as citric acid (Nilveus, 1983; Heritier, 1984; Rawlinson, 1986). Other chemicals that have been investigated for their potential as adjuncts to mechanical root planing include ethylenediamine tetra-acetic acid (EDTA), sodium hypochlorite, sodium deoxycholate, and Cohn's fraction IV of human plasma (Rawlinson, 1986). Enzymes (elastase and hyaluronidase) and fibronectin (found in plasma and on the surface of fibroblasts) are also being tested for their potential to enhance reattachment following use of citric acid on prepared root surfaces (Caffesse et al, 1987; Smith et al, 1987).

Miller (1982, 1983, 1985, 1987) described a technique using the free tissue autograft procedure following citric acid application to root surfaces in which he achieved "complete root coverage" of areas of recession. "Complete root coverage" has been defined as achievement of the following clinical goals: (1) the soft tissue margin lies at the cementoenamel junction; (2) there is clinical attachment to the root surface; (3) the sulcus is 2 mm deep or less; and (4) there is no bleeding on probing. The technique includes application of saturated citric acid to the root-planed surface for 5 minutes per root. The acid is "burnished" into the root surface with a cotton pledget which is changed every minute to prevent contamination. The area is flushed with water every 5 minutes during the treatment, and the surfaces are isolated from salivary contamination. Chemical root conditioning with citric acid is then followed by placement of a free gingival graft over the treated root surface. Miller reported a success rate of almost 90% in achieving complete root coverage in patients treated with this method and concluded that this technique was currently the most predictable procedure for achieving complete root coverage.

Preparation of the root by mechanical root planing is vital to the success of this procedure. Inadequate root planing is one factor that has been cited for the failure of the free tissue autograft procedure to establish complete root coverage. The purpose of the root planing is not only to prepare the root surface biologically by removing deposits and endotoxins, but also to flatten out the root both at the cementoenamel junction and from the mesiodistal dimension, so that the margin of the graft can be "butted" up against the cementoenamel junction and the graft can be placed in intimate contact with the root surface. This goal is achieved more readily if the convexity of the root surface has been reduced in the area of the graft (Holbrook and Ochsenbein, 1983; Miller, 1985; Miller, 1987). Thus, regardless of the future success of chemical means of treating the root surface, it is still not a substitute for thorough and meticulous root planing. It is more likely that these new procedures, as they are perfected for human treatment, will provide yet another rationale for the complete treatment of the root as an initial step in the preparation for chemical conditioning and surgical procedures.

NONSURGICAL VERSUS SURGICAL THERAPY

A number of long-term clinical studies have led to the current knowledge of the effectiveness of nonsurgical therapy in the treatment of periodontal disease. Nonsurgical therapy includes the procedures of closed root planing and curettage, which are implemented without surgical exposure of the root surfaces. These studies have challenged the long-held belief that surgical techniques are the only route through which gain of clinical attachment, reduction of probing depth, and maintenance of periodontal health can be attained. Ramfjord and colleagues at the University of Michigan compared the effects of surgical techniques with those of meticulous scaling and root planing and found that both approaches to treatment achieved the same objectives and that nonsurgical therapy was indeed an effective treatment for periodontitis. Four treatments (scaling and root planing, subgingival curettage, modified Widman surgery, and pocket elimination surgery) were compared within the same mouth by random assignment to different quadrants. Following treatment, patients were given meticulous professional tooth cleaning on a 3-month basis and followed for more than 8 years. It was noted that regardless of the patients' oral hygiene (as reflected in the plaque scores), clinical probing depth and attachment level averages were not significantly different over the long term. These findings indicated further that strict compliance in the removal of supragingival plaque by the patient is not required for the success of treatment and the maintenance of periodontal health if a professional program of plaque removal is followed on a 2- to 3-month basis. The professional removal of all supra- and subgingival plaque at that interval affected a qualitative change in the plaque flora that was sufficient to prevent further periodontal destruction (Ramfjord et al, 1968; Hill et al, 1981; Ramfjord et al, 1982; Ramfjord et al, 1987).

Another research group (Lindhe and others) confirmed Ramfjord's findings that both surgical and nonsurgical treatment methods were effective in the treatment and maintenance of patients with periodontal disease. One significant difference between the two experimental methods, however, was that the patients in Lindhe's group were recalled for professional prophylaxis every 2 weeks for the 6-month postoperative period and then every 3 months thereafter. These individuals were also required to maintain high levels of plaque control, making this a much more controlled study than the one conducted by Ramjford. Lindhe found that the plaque-free sites maintained shallow probing depths and posttreatment attachment levels more often than sites in which personal plaque control was not maintained (Lindhe, 1982a, 1982b, 1984). When comparing the effects of personal plaque control on the success of nonsurgical or surgical treatment, these studies suggest that successful results do not require perfect plaque control, but that better plaque control measures are more likely to result in better treatment results.

Pihlstrom and colleagues also reported a 6½-year study that compared the results of scaling and root planing with those of modified Widman surgery and supported the conclusions of Ramjford and Lindhe. They also found that both surgical and nonsurgical approaches were able to maintain attachment levels on molar and nonmolar teeth and confirmed Ramjford's finding that

perfect plaque control on the part of the patient did not affect long-term maintenance of health if a strict 3-month recall program of professional removal of sub- and supragingival plaque was followed.

Egelberg and coworkers have provided information about the technical aspects of nonsurgical periodontal treatment. Their findings disclosed that the treatment of scaling and root planing was effective in cases of both moderate and severe periodontitis; that treatment with both hand instruments and ultrasonic devices could be equally as effective; and that repeated instrumentation of teeth was no better than a single episode of instrumentation. Experienced clinicians spent an average of 10 minutes per nonmolar tooth to prepare the root surface so that it would be biologically acceptable, thus requiring several appointments to complete an entire mouth. Studies comparing the effectiveness of home care procedures (supragingival plaque control) to scaling and root planing (subgingival plaque control) indicated that while scaling and root planing resulted in significant clinical improvement, oral hygiene procedures alone did not. These results emphasize that patient home care in the absence of a professional prophylaxis cannot be depended upon to yield improvements in periodontal status.

LIMITATIONS OF SCALING AND ROOT PLANING

A review of the clinical trials comparing surgical and nonsurgical approaches to periodontal therapy seems to indicate that achievement of biologically acceptable root surfaces is all that is necessary for successful periodontal therapy (Greenwell, 1987). Because this goal often can be accomplished through closed scaling and root planing, this approach should be the first one attempted. Nonsurgical therapy may not be successful in resolving the problem, however, and must be followed by surgical interventions. It is crucial that a careful reevaluation of the clinical condition of the soft tissues be made after scaling and root planing. The clinician should also be aware that the likelihood of achieving optimal results with closed scaling and root planing decreases as pocket depth increases.

Stambaugh and others (1981) described some

of the limitations of the scaling and root planing procedure through an analysis of the maximum depth at which a plaque and calculus-free pocket could be achieved through instrumentation with a curette (i.e., curette efficiency) and the maximum depth that an instrument tip could be verified to reach (i.e., instrument limit). They found that the average curette efficiency was 3.73 mm (with a range from 1 to 6 mm) and the average instrument limit was 5.52 mm (with a range from 2 to 10 mm.). Therefore, complete calculus removal was rarely achieved at depths of over 5 mm despite an instrumentation time of approximately 30 minutes for each tooth. A number of factors were associated with technique difficulty, including inability to achieve proper adaptation and angulation, tissue tone, tooth and root morphology, and the presence of furcations. These findings of the limitations of scaling and root planing in pockets greater than 5 mm confirm those of other researchers (Frumker and Gardner, 1956; Jones et al, 1972; Waerhaug, 1978; Jones and O'Leary, 1978; Nishimine and O'Leary, 1979; Tabita et al, 1981; Rabbani et al, 1981; Lindhe and Nyman, 1985; Matia et al, 1986).

The success of nonsurgical treatment should be evaluated carefully in terms of clinical signs of inflammation. These signs should determine whether or not surgery is indicated. If bleeding or other signs of inflammation are still present, then repeated instrumentation or instrumentation with the aid of surgical exposure of the surface in question (i.e., open root planing) is required. Caffesse and others (1986) reported that scaling and root planing in conjunction with flap surgery (open scaling and root planing) increased the probability of removing all plaque and calculus in deep pockets, compared with closed scaling and root planing. Buchanan and Robertson (1987) found that open and closed root planing could be accomplished with equal effectiveness in pockets with depths up to 6 mm, but that open root planing was more effective in deeper pockets, especially on facial and lingual surfaces of anterior and premolar teeth. Residual calculus remained on some tooth surfaces, regardless of whether open or closed root planing was performed and regardless of pocket depth. Complete and thorough treatment of the entire root surface is needed in order to make it biologically acceptable for

healing and new attachment levels. Any site that does not respond to scaling and root planing, regardless of the pocket depth, should be reevaluated for the need for surgical therapy. If the root surface cannot be properly treated by scaling and root planing alone, then surgical approaches that allow visibility and greater access to the root surface are indicated (Greenwell et al, 1987).

THE IMPORTANCE OF MAINTENANCE CARE FOLLOWING PERIODONTAL THERAPY
Objectives of periodontal maintenance
According to Ramfjord (1987), the prime objective of maintenance care is to achieve control of both supra- and subgingival plaque through the combined efforts of the patient and the professionals. Professional plaque control should include removal of all supra- and subgingival deposits with curette and possibly polishing with rubber cups and toothpaste or fine prophylaxis paste, the use of the EVA polishing contra-angle interproximally, and topical application of fluoride. Topical fluoride is helpful in the treatment of hypersensitivity and the prevention of root caries, and it produces a harder root surface due to uptake of fluoride. Tightly adapted gingival walls without evidence of spread of plaque and inflammation should be treated with light scaling or simply polished if no calculus is present. Maintenance therapy should not include routine root planing; only problem areas with bleeding or pus should be planed at recall visits. While the patient's plaque control is of critical importance during the healing phase of therapy (the first 6 months), it is less important after that time. After the first year, the oral hygiene of the patient does not seem to be a factor in the rate of attachment loss or gain following therapy when professional maintenance is performed every 3 months (Ramfjord et al, 1982).

Scheduling maintenance intervals
Once periodontal treatment has been completed and the healing phase of therapy is underway, what is the professional's responsibility in terms of maintenance care in order to maintain the gains that therapy has produced? It has been established that the results of periodontal treatment can be improved and maintained by professional tooth

cleaning every 2 weeks for the first 6 months after treatment, compared with once a month or once every 3 months after treatment (Nyman et al, 1975; Westfelt et al, 1983). In studies conducted at the University of Michigan, professional removal of both supra- and subgingival plaque once a week for the first 4 weeks after treatment and once every 3 months thereafter also was effective in maintaining the health of treated tissues. No studies have compared the effectiveness of these two regimes to determine which is better, but evidence certainly shows that the absence of maintenance care and oral hygiene in treated patients results in further destruction. Nyman and colleagues (1977) also demonstrated that deepening of periodontal pockets and loss of attachment occurred with inadequate plaque control and a 6-month recall interval, so the traditional semiannual recall appointments can no longer be considered adequate for maintenance of periodontal patients.

In the Michigan studies, a recall interval of 3 months has been found to maintain the clinical attachment levels in most individuals, regardless of their own plaque control (Knowles et al, 1979; Ramfjord et al, 1987b). Within the study population, however, some individuals lost teeth in spite of this maintenance program. All teeth that could not be saved were found to have residual calculus deposits that had been missed during the recall appointment. In some of these patients, the ineffective root planing was attributed to furcations and other anatomical factors that restricted access during root planing of the deposits.

Retreatment

One important aspect of the maintenance appointment is to identify teeth that need retreatment of the root surfaces. A tendency of soft tissues to bleed at a 3-month recall is not unusual, but bleeding 2 to 3 weeks after a maintenance appointment indicates the presence of residual calculus and points to the need for retreatment (Ramfjord, 1987). Although surgical exposure of root surfaces can improve visibility and removal of calculus, especially in pockets deeper than 4 to 5 mm, studies have also shown that, regardless of whether the root planing is accomplished under open or closed conditions, residual calculus can remain. Therefore, if there is evidence of bleed-

ing on gentle probing or exudate, the root surface should be retreated even if no calculus is detected. Pockets that bleed or contain exudate should be scaled at the maintenance appointment and the patient recalled in 2 to 3 weeks for further evaluation.

The importance of a frequent recall for maintenance of periodontal patients cannot be overemphasized. A number of reports have indicated that, regardless of the skill and thoroughness of the operator in accomplishing complete scaling and root planing and in educating the patient in plaque control procedures, any benefits that are achieved will become diminished over time if the patient does not receive adequate periodontal maintenance (e.g., frequent recall appointments) and if effective plaque-control measures are not instituted. A lack of routine periodontal maintenance care and plaque control have been found to contribute to progressive bone loss and worsening periodontal conditions (Schei et al, 1959; Nyman et al, 1977; Lindhe et al, 1982; Becker et al, 1984; Devore et al, 1985). In contrast, if optimal oral hygiene is maintained by both professional and individual means, periodontal health can be maintained with no further destruction of supporting tissues (Lindhe and Nyman, 1984).

LEGAL RAMIFICATIONS

Dental care providers who are responsible for the delivery of periodontal treatment are responsible for documenting the diagnosis of disease, informing the patient of the condition, treating the condition according to the current standards of care, documenting disease progression or improvement, and providing maintenance care. Pockets that remain after treatment and inability of patients to perform adequate plaque control require that a recall interval of 3 months be established for professional removal of supra- and subgingival plaque. Patients should be advised of the need for this treatment and their responses to this recommendation should be noted on their charts. Once nonsurgical treatment has been performed, it is incumbent on the clinician to recognize those areas that still are not controlled and to recognize recurrent periodontitis. Failure to recognize these conditions while providing maintenance care or failure to inform the patient of such findings is called "supervised neglect" (Greenwell et al, 1987); it can result in legal liability on the part of the practitioner.

Periodontal treatment that is not followed by supervised maintenance and reevaluation may result in accelerated loss of attachment levels and is certainly ineffective as a means of controlling or preventing disease. It is the responsibility of the practitioner to inform the patient of the need for such a program and to provide the needed services or, in some cases, referral to another practitioner who specializes in periodontal therapy. The patient, having been fully informed, must then decide which course to take. The practitioner cannot be held responsible if the informed patient chooses not to seek the recommended care, but is accountable if diagnosable conditions exist for which treatment is available and the patient is not so informed.

INDICATIONS FOR REFERRAL

As dental hygienists and general dentists are trained more diligently in the methods of treating periodontal disease, they will be able to assume an increasing proportion of the responsibility for treating these conditions. A decision must be made in each case, however, whether nonsurgical therapy will yield a successful result. In general, cases of mild periodontitis characterized by horizontal bone loss and pockets in the 4- to 5-mm range can be treated successfully and maintained. Cases that involve more complex treatment needs, or those which do not respond to nonsurgical treatment, should be referred to specialists. Conditions such as deep pockets, vertical bony defects, and exposed furcations may require the expertise of a specialist to determine whether nonsurgical or surgical approaches to treatment are indicated.

EMERGING CONTROVERSIES

As this text goes to press, research is challenging the fundamental premises of the necessity to definitively remove cementum from periodontally involved roots in order to achieve healing. Emphasis has shifted from being satisfied with maintaining attachment level to creating an environment where periodontal fibers can reattach to the tooth. Nyman and colleagues recently published an article that suggests that laying a flap, remov-

ing calculus, and polishing the remaining cementum may remove the endotoxin and be adequate and perhaps preferrable to the definitive root planing to which that procedure was compared (1988). Cleaning root surfaces with two detergents (in vitro) promoted more attachment of periodontal cells than root planing with either hand curettes or ultrasonic instruments (Blomlöf et al, 1987). There appear to be factors found in the bone and cementum that enhance reattachment. These factors may not be found in dentin; thus reattachment may actually be impaired by removing cementum (Somerman, et al, 1987).

This "new direction" in periodontal research introduces a serious challenge for students, faculty, and practitioners as they determine the "best" way to treat patients. Review the literature for further research developments.

CONCLUSION

Root planing is definitely one of the most exacting tasks that a hygienist must perform. It is extremely valuable in the treatment of patients with periodontal disease and resultant bone loss. It does have limitations, however, and is not the treatment of choice for all periodontally involved cases. The hygienist and dentist must carefully assess each patient's needs to determine whether or not root planing will assist in the restoration of periodontal health and in the provision of long-term benefits.

ACTIVITIES

1. Practice root planing on extracted molar teeth. Use disclosant and a light microscope to help evaluate changes in the root surface as a result of the planing.
2. Remove the end from a stethoscope and insert the handle end of a single-ended curette. Root plane the teeth of clinic patients while listening for changes through the stethoscope.
3. Discuss which teeth would be the hardest to treat because of their root morphology. Discuss approaches to treating various grooves and furcations.
4. If the facilities and personnel are available, root plane a tooth to completion for a patient who will be undergoing periodontal surgery. Observe the surgery to see the effectiveness of the root planing when the tissues are lifted away from the tooth.
5. Have someone in class bring in a piece of wood and a wood-planing tool. Demonstrate some of the con-

cepts involved in the root-planing technique using these tools (e.g., sharpness, constant pressure, smoothing versus gouging, light versus heavy pressure.

6. Review the most recent literature to determine which of these factors is considered most crucial in reversing periodontal disease:
   a. calculus
   b. endotoxin
   c. microbial flora

7. Examine/compare Gracey curettes and their new variations (longer terminal shank, less flex, thinner blade) for ease of use.

REVIEW QUESTIONS

1. Compare scaling and root planing in terms of the following:
   a. Instrument selection
   b. Number of strokes
   c. Direction of strokes
   d. Pressure of strokes

2. Compare Gracey curettes and universal curettes in terms of the following:
   a. Blade size
   b. Cutting edges
   c. Shank design

3. Name four criteria that aid the clinician in determining when root planing is complete.

4. Write a brief response to the following statements, indicating whether or not you agree and your rationale:
   a. You should always root plane a surface until it is hard and glassy smooth.
   b. A skilled clinician never removes healthy cementum during root planing.

REFERENCES

Albair W, et al: Connective tissue attachment to periodontally diseased roots after citric acid demineralization, J Periodontol 53:515, 1982.

Aleo, JA, et al: The presence and biologic activity of cementum-bound endotoxin, J Periodontol 45:672, 1974.

Aleo JA, et al: In vitro attachment of human fibroblasts to root surfaces, J Periodontol 46:639, 1975.

Axelsson P, and Lindhe J: The significance of maintenance care in the treatment of periodontal disease, J Clin Periodontol 8:281, 1981.

Baderstten A, et al: Effect of nonsurgical periodontal therapy, I: moderately advanced periodontitis, J Clin Periodontol 8:45, 1981.

Baderstten A, et al: Effect of nonsurgical periodontal therapy: severely advanced periodontitis. II. Severely advanced periodontitis, J Clin Periodontol 11:63, 1984(a).

Baderstten A, et al: Effect of nonsurgical periodontal therapy, III: single versus repeated instrumentation, J Clin Periodontol 11:114, 1984(b).

Baderstten A, et al: Effect of nonsurgical periodontal therapy, IV: Operator variability, J Clin Periodontal 12:190, 1985.

Barrington EP: An overview of periodontal surgical procedures, J Periodontol 52:518, 1981.

Baumhammers A, et al: Scanning electron microscopy of supragingival calculus, J Periodontal 44:92, 1973.

Becker W et al: Periodontal treatment without maintenance, J Periodontol 55:505, 1984.

Blomlöf, L. et al: New attachment in monkeys with experimental periodontitis with and without removal of cementum, J Clin Periodontol 14:136, 1987.

Bower RC: Furcation morphology relative to periodontal treatment: furcation entrance architecture, J Periodontol 50:23, 1979(a).

Bower RC: Furcation morphology relative to periodontal treatment: furcation root surface anatomy, J Periodontol 50:366, 1979 (b).

Breininger DR: Comparative effectiveness of ultrasonic and hand scaling for the removal of subgingival plaque and calculus, J Periodontol 58:9, 1987.

Buchanan SA, and Robertson PB: Calculus removal by scaling/root planing with and without surgical access, J Periodontol 58:159, 1987.

Caffesse RG, et al: Scaling and root planing with and without periodontal flap surgery, J Clin Periodontol 13:205, 1986.

Caffesse RG, et al: Cell proliferation after flap surgery, root conditioning and fibronectic application, J Periodontol 58:661, 1987.

Canis MF, et al: Calculus attachment, J Periodontol 50:406, 1979.

Caton J, and Zander H: The attachment between tooth and gingival tissues after periodic root planing and soft tissue curettage J Periodontol 50:462, 1979.

Caton J, et al: Maintenance of healed periodontal pockets after a single episode of root planing, J Periodontol 53:420, 1982.

Cercek JF, et al: Relative effects of plaque control and instrumentation on the clinical parameters of human periodontal disease, J Clin Periodontol 10:46, 1983.

Cogen RB, et al: Effect of various root surface treatments on the viability and attachment of human gingival fibroblasts, J Periodontal 54:277, 1983.

Cole RT, et al: Connective tissue regeneration to peridontally diseased teeth—a histological study, J Periodont Res 15:1, 1980.

Common J, and McFall WT: The effects of citric acid on attachment of laterally positioned flaps, J Periodontol 54:9, 1983.

Dello Russo NM: The post-prophylaxis periodontal abscess: etiology and treatment, Int J Perio Rest Dent 5:29, 1985.

DeVore CH, et al: Bone loss following periodontal therapy in subjects without frequent periodontal maintenance, J Periodontol 57:354, 1985.

Eaton KA, et al: The removal of root surface deposits, J Clin Periodontol 12:141, 1985.

Fox SC, and Bosworth BL: A morphological survey of proximal root concavities: a consideraton in periodontal therapy, J Periodontol 57:811, 1987.

Frank RM, et al: Cementogenesis and soft tissue attachment after citric treatment in a human, J Periodontol 54:389, 1983.

Froum SM, et al: Healing responses of human intraosseous lesions following the use of debridement, grafting and citric acid root treatment, I. clinical and histological observations six months postsurgery, J Periodontol 54:67, 1983.

Frumker S, and Gardner W: The relation of the topography of the root surface to the removal of calculus, J Periodontol 27:292, 1956.

Garrett JS: Effects of nonsurgical periodontal therapy on periodontitis in humans: a review, J Clin Periodontol 10:515, 1983.

Garrett JS, et al: Effects of citric acid on diseased root surfaces, J Periodont Res 13:155, 1978.

Gher ME, and Vernino AR: Root morphology—clinical significance in pathogenesis and treatment of periodontal disease, JADA 101:627, 1980.

Glick DH, and Freeman E: Postsurgical bone loss following root planing by ultrasonic and hand instruments, J Periodontol 51:510, 1980.

Goldman MJ, et al: Effect of periodontal therapy on patient maintained for 15 years or longer: a retrospective study, J Periodontol 57:347, 1985.

Greenwell H, and Bissade NF: Variations in subgingival microflora from healthy and intervention sites using probing depth and bacteriologic identification criteria, J Periodontol 55:391, 1984.

Greenwell H, et al: Clinical and microbiologic effectiveness of Keyes' method of oral hygiene on human periodontitis treated with and without surgery, JADA 106:457, 1983.

Greenwell H, et al: Periodontics in general practice: perspectives on nonsurgical therapy, JADA 115:591, 1987.

Harvey RF: Single appointment therapy for periodontal abscesses, J Can Dent Assn 40(5):372, 1974.

Hellden LB, et al: The effect of tetracycline and/or scaling on human periodontal disease, J Clin Periodontol 6:222, 1979.

Heritier M: Effects of phosphoric acid on root dentine surface, J Perio Res 19:168, 1984.

Hill RW, et al: Four types of periodontal treatment compared over two years, J Periodontol 52:655, 1981.

Hinrichs JE: Effects of scaling and root planing on subgingival microbial proportions standardized in terms of their naturally occurring distribution, J Periodontol 56:187, 1984.

Holbrook T, and Ochsenbein C: Complete coverage of denuded root surface with a one stage gingival graft, Int J Periodont Rest Dent 3:8, 1983.

Isidor F, et al: The effect of root planing as compared to that of surgical treatment, J Clin Periodontol 11:669, 1984.

Jones S, et al: Tooth surfaces treated in situ with periodontal instruments, Br Dent J 132:57, 1972.

Jones WA, and O'Leary TJ: The effectiveness of in vivo root planing in removing bacterial endotoxin from the roots of periodontally involved teeth, J Periodontol 49:337, 1978.

Kerry GJ: Roughness of root surfaces after use of ultrasonic instruments and hand curettes, J Periodontol 38:340, 1967.

Khatiblou FA, and Ghodssi A: Root surface smoothness or roughness in periodontal treatment: a clinical study, J Periodontol 54:356, 1983.

Kho D, et al: The effect of supragingival plaque control on the subgingival microflora, J Clin Periodontol 12:676, 1985.

Knowles J, et al: Comparison of results following three modalities of periodontal therapy related to tooth type and initial pocket depth, J Clin Periodontol 7:32, 1980.

Knowles JW, et al: Results of periodontal treatment related to pocket depth and attachment level. Eight years, J Periodontol 50:225, 1979.

Kolinski MK: Use of scaling and root planing in the conservative management of periodontal disease, CDS Review 77(10):30, 1984.

Lasho DJ, et al: A scanning electron microscope study of the effects of various agents on instrumented periodontally involved root surfaces, J Periodontol 54:210, 1983.

Lavanchy DL, et al: The effect of plaque control after scaling and root planing on the subgingival microflora in human periodontitis, J Clin Periodontol 14:295, 1987.

Lindhe J, and Nyman S: Long term maintenance of patients treated for advanced periodontal disease, J Clin Periodontol 11:504, 1984.

Lindhe J, and Nyman S: Scaling and granulation tissue removal in periodontal therapy, J Clin Periodontol 12:374, 1985.

Lindhe J, et al: "Critical probing depths" in periodontal therapy, J Clin Periodontol 9:323, 1982.

Lindhe J, et al: Healing following surgical/non-surgical treatment of periodontal disease, J Clin Periodontol 9:115, 1982 (a).

Lindhe J, et al: Scaling and root planing in shallow pockets, J Clin Periodontal 9:415, 1982 (b).

Lindhe J, et al: Long-term effects of surgical/nonsurgical treatment of periodontal disease, J Clin Periodontol 11:448, 1984.

Listgarten MA: Periodontal probing: what does it mean? J Clin Periodontol 7:165, 1980.

Listgarten MA, and Ellegaard B: Electron microscopic evidence of a cellular attachment between junctional epithelium and dental calculus, J Periodontol 44:143, 1973.

Listgarten MA, et al: Periodontal probing and the relationship of the probe tip to periodontal tissues, J Periodontol 47:511, 1976.

Listgarten MA, et al: Effect of tetracycline and/or scaling on human periodontal disease, J Clin Periodontol 5:246, 1978.

Loe H, et al: Experimental gingivitis in man, J Periodontol 49:337, 1965.

Lopez NJ, and Belvederessi M: Subgingival scaling with root planing and curettage: effects upon gingival inflammation: a comparative study, J Periodontol 48:354, 1977.

Magnusson I, et al: A long junctional epithelium—a locus minoris resistentiae in plaque infection? J Clin Periodontol 10:333, 1983.

Mandel ID, and Gaffar A: Calculus revisited: a review, J Clin Periodontol 13:249, 1986.

Matia J, et al: Efficiency of scaling of the molar furcation area with and without surgical access, Int J Periodontics Restorative Dent 6:25, 1986.

McCoy SA, et al: The concentration of lipopolysaccharide on individual root surfaces at varying times following in vivo root planing, J Periodontol 58:393, 1987.

Miller PD: Root coverage using a free soft tissue autograft following citric acid application, I: technique, Int J Periodont Rest Dent 2:65, 1982.

Miller PD: Root coverage using a free soft tissue autograft following citric acid application. Part II. Treatment of the carious root, Int J Periodont Rest Dent 3:38, 1983.

Miller PD: Root coverage using the free soft tissue autograft following citric acid application, III: a successful and predictable procedure in areas of deep-wide recession, Int J Periodont Rest Dent 5:15, 1985.

Miller PD: Root coverage with the free gingival graft: factors associated with incomplete coverage, J Periodontol 58:674, 1987.

Morrison EC, et al: Short-term effects of initial, nonsurgical periodontal treatment (hygienic phase), J Clin Periodontol 7:199, 1980.

Moskow BS:The response of the gingival sulcus to instrumentation: a histological investigation, I: the scaling procedure, J Periodontal 33:282, 1962.

Moskow BS, and Bressman E: Cemental response to ultrasonic and hand instrumentation, JADA 68:698, 1964.

Nakib NM, et al: Endotoxin penetration into root cementum of periodontally healthy and diseased human teeth, J periodontol 53:368, 1982.

Nightingale SH, and Sheridan PJ: Root surface demineralization in periodontal therapy: subject review, J Periodontol 53:611, 1982.

Nilveus R, and Selvig KA: Pulpal reactions to the application of citric acid to root planed dentine in beagles, J Periodont Res 18:420, 1983.

Nishimine D, and O'Leary TJ: Hand instrumentation versus ultrasonics in the removal of endotoxins from root surfaces, J Periodontol 50:345, 1979.

Nordland SG, et al: The effect of plaque control and root debridement in molar teeth, J Clin Periodontol 14:231, 1987.

Nyman S, et al: Effect of professional tooth cleaning on healing after periodontal surgery, J Clin Periodontol 2:80, 1975.

Nyman S, et al: Periodontal surgery in plaque-infected dentitions, J Clin Periodontol 4:240, 1977.

Nyman, S. et al: Role of "diseased" root cementum in healing following treatment of periodontal disease: a clinical study. J Clin Perio 15:464, 1988.

O'Leary TJ: The impact of research on scaling and root planing, J Periodontol 57:69, 1986.

Otomo JA, and Sims TN: Effects of citric acid demineralization on coronally repositioned flaps, J Dent Res 58 (special issue A, abst 1021): 347, 1979.

Pihlstrom BI, et al: A randomized four-year study of periodontal therapy, J Periodontol 52:227, 1981.

Pihlstom BL, et al: Comparison of surgical and nonsurgical treatment of periodontal disease: a review of current studies and additional results after 6½ years, J Clin Periodontol 10:524, 1983.

Pihlstrom BL, et al: Molar and nonmolar teeth compared over 6½ years following two methods of periodontal therapy. J Periodontol 55:499, 1984.

Polson AM, et al: The production of a root surface smear layer by instrumentation and its removal by citric acid, J Periodontol 55:443, 1984.

Polson AM: The root surface and regeneration: present therapeutic limitations and future biologic potentials, J Clin Periodontol 13:995, 1986.

Powell B, and Garnick JJ: The use of extracted teeth to evaluate clinical measurements of periodontal disease, J Periodontol 49:621, 1978.

Proye MP, and Polson AM: Effect of root surface alterations on periodontal healing, I: surface denudation, J Clin Periodontol 9:428, 1982.

Proye M, et al: Initial healing of periodontal pockets after a single episode of root planing monitored by controlled probing forces, J Periodontol 53:296, 1982.

Rabbani GM, et al: The effectiveness of subgingival scaling and root planing in calculus removal, J Periodontol 52:119, 1981.

Ramfjord SP: Surgical periodontal pocket elimination: still a justifiable objective? JADA 114:37, 1987.

Ramfjord SP: Maintenance for treated periodontitis patients, J Clin Periodontol 14:437, 1987b.

Ramfjord SP, et al: Subgingival curettage versus surgical elimination of periodontal pockets, J Periodontol 39:167, 1968.

Ramfjord SP, et al: Oral hygiene and maintenance of periodontal support, J Periodontol 53:26, 1982.

Ramfjord SP, et al: Four modalities of periodontal treatment compared over 5 years, J Clin Periodontol 14:445, 1987a.

Rautiola CA, and Craig RG: The microhardness of cementum and underlying dentin of normal teeth and teeth exposed to periodontal disease, J Periodontol 32:113, 1961.

Rawlinson A: Periodontally involved cementum: some aspects of its management, old and new, Dental Health 25(4):6, 1986.

Register AA, and Burdick RA: Accelerated reattachment with cementogenesis to dentin, demineralized in situ, II: defect repair, J Periodontol 47:497, 1976.

Riffle, AB: Radical subgingival curettage, J Periodontol 27:102, 1956.

Rosenberg RM, and Ash MM: The effect of root roughness on plaque accumulation and gingival inflammation, J Periodontol 45:146, 1974.

Ruben MP, and Shapiro A: An analysis of root surface changes in periodontal disease—a review, J Periodontol 49:89, 1978.

Sarbinoff JA, et al: The comparative effectiveness of various agents in detoxifying diseased root surfaces, J Periodontol 54:77, 1983.

Schaffer E: Histological results of root curettage of human teeth, J Periodontol 27:296, 1956.

Schei O, et al: Alveolar bone loss as related to oral hygiene and age, J Periodontol 30:7, 1959.

Schroeder HE: Formation and inhibition of dental calculus, Vienna, 1969, Hams Huber.

Seibert J: Incorporating root planing and gingival curettage into a clinical practice. Contin Dent Educ 1:8, 1978.

Selvig KA, et al: Fine structure of new connective tissue attachment following acid treatment of experimental furcation pockets in dogs, J Perio Res 16:123, 1981.

Silvertson JF, and Burgett FG: Probing of pockets related to the attachment level, J Periodontol 47:281, 1976.

Smith BA, et al: Effect of citric acid and various concentrations of fibronectin on healing following periodontal flap surgery in dogs, J Periodontol 58:667, 1987.

Somerman, MJ, et al: *In vitro* evaluation of extracts of mineralized tissues for their application in attachment of fibrous tissue, J Periodontol, 58:349, 1987.

Spray JR, et al: Microscopic demonstration of the position of periodontal probes, J Periodontol 49:148, 1978.

Stahl SS: Repair potential of the soft tissue-root interface, J Periodontol 48:545, 1977.

Stahl SS, et al: Soft tissue healing following curettage and root planing, J Periodontol 42:678, 1971.

Stahl SS, and Froum SJ: Human clinical and histologic repair responses following the use of citric acid in periodontal therapy, J Periodontol 48:261, 1977.

Stambaugh RV, et al: The limits of subgingival scaling, Int J Periodont Rest Dent 1:30, 1981.

Tabita PV, et al: Effectiveness of supragingival plaque control on the development of subgingival plaque and gingival inflammation in patients with moderate pocket depth, J Periodontal 52:88, 1981.

Tagge DL, et al: The clinical and histological response of periodontal pockets to root planing and oral hygiene, J Periodontol 46:527, 1975.

Tal H, et al: Scanning electron microscope evaluation of wear of dental curettes during standardized root planing, J Periodontol 56:532, 1985.

Theilade E, et al: Experimental gingivitis in man, II: a longitudinal clinical and bacteriological investigation, J Periodont Res 1:1, 1966.

Volkinburg JW, et al: The nature of root surfaces after curette, cavitron and alpha-sonic instrumentation, J Periodont Res 11:374, 1976.

Waerhaug J: The interdental brush and its place in operative crown and bridge dentistry, J Oral Rehabil 3:107, 1976.

Waerhaug J: Subgingival plaque and loss of attachment in periodontosis as evaluated on extracted teeth, J Periodontol 48:125, 1977.

Waerhaug J: Healing of the dento-epithelial junction following subgingival plaque control, I: as observed in human biopsy material, J Periodontol 49:1, 1978 (a).

Waerhaug J: Healing of the dento-epithelial junction following subgingival plaque control, II: as observed on extracted teeth, J Periodontol 49:119, 1978 (b).

Waerhaug J: Effect of toothbrushing on subgingival plaque formation, J Periodontol 52:30, 1981.

Walker SL: A study of root planing by scanning electron microscopy, Dent Hyg 50(Mar):109, 1976.

West TL, and King WJ: Toothbrushing with hydrogen peroxide–sodium bicarbonate compared to toothpowder and water in reducing periodontal pocket suppuration and darkfield bacterial counts, J Periodontol 54:339, 1983.

Westfelt E, et al: Significance of frequency of professional tooth cleaning for healing following periodontal surgery, J Clin Periodontol 10:148, 1983.

Wilkinson RF, and Maybury JE: Scanning electron microscopy of the root surface following instrumentation, J Periodontol 42:559, 1973.

24 SOFT TISSUE CURETTAGE

Soft tissue curettage is the process of converting a chronic inflammatory wound to a surgical wound by removing the diseased soft tissue lining of a periodontal pocket (Goldman and Cohen, 1980). Whereas root planing is used to treat the hard tissue wall of the pocket, soft tissue curettage is used to treat the adjacent soft tissue wall. When indications for soft tissue curettage are present, a sharp curette is applied against the soft tissue to remove the inflamed sulcular epithelium and underlying diseased connective tissue. The goal of this procedure is to reduce inflammation and improve healing so that there is reduction of the clinical pocket depth, resulting in tissues that can be maintained in a healthy state by the patient.

The pocket depth can be reduced in one of four ways: (1) shrinkage of the marginal gingiva due to reduction of edema; (2) healing of apical soft tissues resulting in increased resistance to probing (see Chapter 14); (3) formation of a new long junctional epithelium that attaches to the tooth surface; and (4) new attachment of connective tissue fibers. Reduction of edema in the marginal gingiva and interdental papillae will result in shrinkage of these tissues following treatment.

Healing within the pocket restores the soft tissues at the pocket base to their normal firm consistency. When these tissues are inflamed, the periodontal probe can pass easily through the inflamed connective tissue fibers until it reaches intact, noninflamed tissues. Even though the actual attachment of these inflamed fibers is not severed, the clinical measurement indicates that their attachment to the tooth has been destroyed. Following healing, the probe can no longer penetrate through the restored tissue fibers. An apparent gain in attachment is observed, although there is never an actual alteration in the histologic attachment of the tissues.

Caton and Zander (1979) studied tissue healing following root planing and curettage and found that the most frequent means of attachment is the formation of a long junctional epithelium. Listgarten and Rosenberg (1979) reported that the length of this new long junctional epithelium ranged from 1.0 to 4.5 mm in patients who were studied, with an average length of 2.8 mm. This epithelium is impenetrable to a periodontal probe under healthy conditions, and its presence would be likely to produce an apparent gain in clinical attachment and a decrease in the clinical probing depth. A long junctional epithelium forms as effective a barrier against further destruction by bacterial plaque as a normal-length junctional epithelium (Magnusson et al, 1983).

The most desired way to achieve clinical probing reduction would be attainment of a new attachment of connective tissue at a more coronal level of the root surface. Unfortunately this type of reattachment is not likely to occur with current treatment approaches and is unpredictable when it does occur. The events of soft tissue healing are such that epithelial coverage of a wound occurs very quickly, with the result that the new connective tissue does not have an opportunity to reestablish its attachment to the root surface before being obstructed by the new epithelial layer. Therefore, the removal of all epithelial tissue within the pocket, including the junctional epithelium, would be required in order to impede the rapid regeneration of new epithelium from existing remnants of that tissue within the pocket. Many investigators have found that complete removal of all pocket epithelium, including the junctional epithelium, sulcular epithelium, and marginal epithelium, is difficult if not impossible to achieve (Morris, 1954; Stahl et al, 1971; Lopez and Belvederessi, 1977).

The curettage procedure described in this chapter should not be confused with "coincidental curettage," which is described in earlier chapters. Soft tissue curettage refers to a definitive procedure designed for the intentional removal of soft tissues. The term *curettage* can be used in a number of different ways. Some clinicians use curettage to refer to the use of a curette against both hard tissues (i.e., scaling, root planing) and soft tissues. Others use the term to describe the removal of soft tissues that occurs simultaneously with root planing. In this chapter soft tissue curettage is considered a procedure that is performed separately from root planing.

Hall (1983) has provided additional definitions to distinguish between *gingival curettage,* removal of the gingival lining of a shallow true pocket or pseudopocket with gingival shrinkage as the goal, and *subgingival curettage,* removal of the epithelial lining and some subjacent connective tissue in deep pockets with new connective tissue attachment as the goal. Although both gingival and subgingival curettage are discussed in

this chapter, the emphasis is on gingival curettage.

The sequencing of soft tissue curettage as a part of the periodontal treatment may occur in different ways, depending on the preferences of the clinician. Some clinicians prefer to perform soft tissue curettage at the same appointment in which they do root planing, as part of a final effort to create an environment within the pocket that is conducive to optimal wound healing. Their rationale is that much coincidental curettage has already occurred during the root-planing procedure, and healing will be facilitated if the remaining diseased tissue is removed. Advantages to this approach are that the patient is already prepared (i.e., anesthesia and root planing have been accomplished), so that less time is needed to perform curettage during this appointment (Ainslee and Caffesse, 1981; Barrington, 1981).

Other clinicians take a more conservative approach, stating that because soft tissue curettage is a type of surgical procedure, the indications for performing it must be evaluated after other methods of treatment, including plaque control, scaling, and root planing, have been performed. These clinicians prefer to evaluate the need for curettage only after these other treatments and the subsequent healing can be studied. With this approach the indications and need for soft tissue curettage may have been resolved by one or all of the previous treatment modes (Goldman and Cohen, 1980; Wirthlin, 1981). An advantage of this approach is that the patient need not undergo the procedure unless it is necessary, and thus additional manipulation of the tissues is avoided. The decision of which approach to take depends on the preferences and attitudes that prevail in a given practice. Both approaches have been shown to improve the health of the periodontal tissues.

EFFECTIVENESS OF CURETTAGE

There is no doubt that scaling, root planing, and curettage are effective means for reducing gingival inflammation due to chronic gingivitis and periodontitis. An interesting controversy exists, however, as to whether or not curettage is a necessary component of initial therapy. It has been described as the oldest therapeutic procedure in the practice of periodontics and as indispensable for the maintenance of all treated cases (Chace,

1983). Ramfjord and others (1968) compared curettage with other surgical techniques during a longitudinal study that began in 1963. Their conclusions, after 5 years, were that curettage was able to produce more favorable results in pocket depth reduction than surgical elimination of pockets, and that the surgical techniques resulted in a slight loss of attachment that was not seen following curettage. Ten years after treatment, however, results indicated that both experimental groups (surgical pocket elimination and curettage) showed a significant loss of attachment and that pocket reduction was greater and better sustained in the patients who had undergone pocket elimination surgery (Ramfjord et al, 1973). Another report of this longitudinal study included those patients who had completed 8 years of recall treatment and scoring. Those findings demonstrated that soft tissue curettage had resulted in sustained pocket reduction and gains of attachment levels for both moderately deep pockets (4 to 6 mm) and deep pockets (7 to 12 mm). The differences between the treatment results obtained by soft tissue curettage as compared with the two surgical techniques used were not statistically significant. These data indicate that not only is soft tissue curettage an effective method for treatment of moderate to severe cases of periodontitis but also that during the length of this study, soft tissue curettage was just as effective as pocket elimination surgery or modified Widman flap surgery in most cases (Knowles et al, 1979).

Zamet (1975) compared the clinical results after curettage, replaced flap, and apically repositioned flap procedures. After 4 months, results in all three treatment groups were similar for plaque, gingival inflammation, pocket depth, attachment, and contour, with no significant differences between groups, and all procedures reduced pocket depths. This study would seem to confirm the value of curettage as a method of producing pocket depth reduction. Kuren and colleagues (1986) found that root planing followed by gingival curettage was more effective in establishing periodontal health after 6 months than either treatment alone.

Several other investigators, however, have attempted to determine whether curettage following scaling and root planing is any more effective in treating inflamed tissues than scaling and root planing alone. Ainslie and Caffesse (1981) evaluated this question by comparing scaling and root planing in one treatment group with scaling, root planing, and immediate soft tissue curettage in another group. Although both treatment combinations were successful in reducing inflammation, the researchers concluded that there was not a statistical difference in the results obtained by the two treatment groups. They stated further that scaling and root planing alone resulted in a tendency for greater clinical gain of attachment than if curettage was performed. The implications of this study are that soft tissue curettage requires extra effort on the part of both the patient and the clinician without demonstrating additional benefits.

Echeverria and Caffesse (1983) performed a similar evaluation, but they instituted curettage 4 weeks after scaling and root planing rather than performing it concurrently with scaling and root planing. Their findings indicate that although the combination of scaling, root planing, and curettage is an effective treatment to reduce gingival inflammation and pocket depth, it was no more effective than scaling and root planing alone. They concluded that gingival curettage is not necessary in routine treatment of shallow, suprabony pockets.

Many clinicians have discussed the value of soft tissue curettage as a means of treating and maintaining patients suffering from chronic inflammation of periodontal tissues (Hirschfeld, 1952; Deasy and Vogel, 1978; Barrington, 1981; Chace, 1974, 1983; Bradley, 1984; Greenberg, 1985). Gingival curettage also has been advocated for treatment of isolated sites of inflammation that remain unresponsive to scaling and root planing (Buethe et al, 1986). The combination of chemical and mechanical curettage has been found to be an effective means of eliminating microorganisms from deep within periodontal pockets and for achieving control of the quantity and quality of subgingival flora for periods up to 90 days (Adcock et al, 1983; Buethe et al, 1986). Frequent gingival curettage also has been proposed as an approach for provoking regeneration of interdental papillae following their destruction by acute necrotizing ulcerative gingivitis (Shapiro, 1985). Current research, however, casts some doubt on the necessity of performing curettage as a separate procedure in addition to scaling and root planing and suggests that there is no biologic rationale for doing so (Hill et al, 1981; Ainslie, 1981; Escheverria, 1983; Greenstein, 1985; Buethe et al, 1986; Forgas, 1986).

Because of the inclusion of this procedure in clinical practice and in light of the controversy surrounding its effectiveness, the remainder of this chapter will describe a technique for performing gingival curettage as well as explaining the rationale behind each step. In addition to understanding the procedure itself, the clinician must face the bigger challenge of determining how and when it should be used in the control of periodontal disease.

INDICATIONS AND CONTRAINDICATIONS

The *indications* for soft tissue curettage include the following:
1. Soft, boggy, edematous gingiva associated with chronically inflamed tissues
2. Gingival or suprabony pockets
3. Inflammation that persists in spite of plaque control or scaling and root planing
   Contraindications include the following:
1. Deep infrabony pockets
2. Insufficient attached gingiva and mucogingival involvement
3. Systemic complications
4. Acute gingival infections such as acute necrotizing ulcerative gingivitis (ANUG)
5. Gingiva that is more fibrotic than edematous: areas where shrinkage is difficult to achieve, such as the palatal areas of maxillary anterior teeth and retromolar areas (Goldman and Cohen, 1980; Chace, 1974, 1983)

Soft tissue curettage is most effective on edematous tissues because shrinkage of the treated tissues resulting from a resolution of the inflammation is the desired goal. Shrinkage is unlikely in fibrotic gingiva because the bulk of the tissue is due to excess collagen fibers rather than to edema produced by the inflammatory process. The same problem may exist on the palatal surfaces of maxillary anterior teeth and in retromolar areas. Although the clinician should be aware of the considerations, inflammatory conditions may exist within these areas. Curettage may still be considered in these cases if it is felt that there might be some tissue resolution.

The success of soft tissue curettage depends greatly on the ability of the clinician to remove as much as possible of the soft tissues that are inflamed and beyond repair. Adaptation of instruments in deep, narrow pockets without causing traumatic injury to the soft tissues is difficult. Removal of all the inflamed soft tissues without traumatizing the intact tissues is especially difficult in these areas. In these situations curettage may be completed more effectively in an open-flap procedure that is discussed later in this chapter. Probably the most important reason why soft tissue curettage is not the best treatment for deep infrabony pockets associated with moderate to severe periodontitis is that it cannot eliminate the need for surgical treatment of the pocket wall and underlying bone. Pockets displaying these characteristics would not be reduced to a maintainable level by soft tissue curettage alone, and the bone contours would still be nonphysiologic, resulting in a continuation of the disease.

A similar problem exists in cases of inadequate attached gingiva and mucogingival involvement. Not only are these tissues much more delicate and likely to be perforated during curettage, but surgical intervention is required to solve the existing problems so that the patient can resume normal home care and maintenance procedures. Curettage alone often will not meet the patients' needs in these cases. A modification of soft tissue curettage called aggressive curettage has been described as an effective method for treating patients with infrabony pockets. This technique removes the entire col area, so that interproximal tooth surfaces are accessible for cleaning (Green and Green, 1979).

Patients with systemic complications, such as diabetes, or with gingivitis caused by hormonal imbalances or nutritional deficiencies may not be good candidates for soft tissue curettage. Healing is hindered in patients with diabetes, and any tissue manipulation will be more traumatic in these patients. When the inflammatory response is complicated by systemic disturbances, curettage is less likely to effect an acceptable clinical result. Patients who are suffering from medical disorders that limit their ability to withstand the physical or emotional stress of periodontal treatment may not

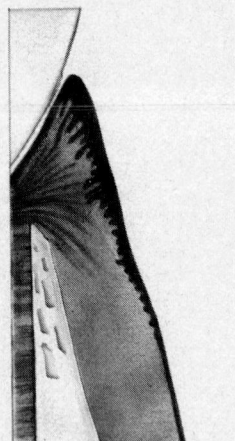

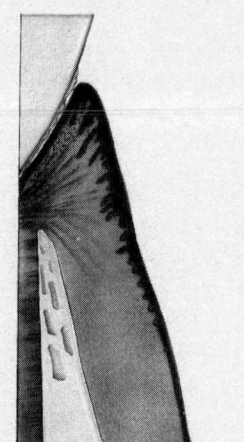

Fig. 24-1. Cross-sectional diagram of normal healthy sulcus. Appearance of sulcular epithelium and underlying connective tissues is normal. There is a slight inflammatory infiltration in subsulcular areas.
(Adapted from Seibert JS: Contin Dent Educ **1**:8, 1978.)

Fig. 24-2. Number of inflammatory cells increases significantly with presence of plaque and calculus in sulcus.
(Adapted from Seibert JS: Contin Dent Educ **1**:8, 1978.)

be good candidates for soft tissue curettage. In some situations, however, curettage for these patients may be the treatment of choice in lieu of more demanding surgical interventions.

Acute periodontal infections such as ANUG or gingivostomatitis are also contraindications for soft tissue curettage. Manipulation of these very delicate tissues not only will be painful for the patient, but also might create unnecessary trauma in the tissues. Periodontal treatment for these patients should be postponed until the acute conditions have been resolved.

Patients who will not or cannot maintain optimal home care procedures to prevent the recurrence of periodontal disease are not good candidates for the curettage procedure. This treatment is aimed at elimination of the inflammation and at reduction of clinical pocket depths so that patients can maintain their mouths in a healthy state. If the patient will not or cannot maintain optimal plaque control, the purpose for performing this procedure is undermined and the curettage will have only short-term value to the patient.

A closer look at the disease process of gingival inflammation shows how soft tissue curettage contributes to the reduction of inflammation. A review of the incipient lesion of gingivitis shows that there is loss of integrity of the sulcular epithelium resulting from inflammation. Ulceration

of these tissues provides access for the inflammatory process into the underlying connective tissues, and the result is bleeding and breakdown of these subsulcular fibers. As the connective tissue fibers become involved in the battle of inflammation, they are destroyed and lose their firm consistency. This allows the sulcular epithelium to proliferate in fingerlike projections (*rete peg)* deeper and deeper into the connective tissues because there is no longer sufficient "contact inhibition" to prevent over-growth of epithelium. As the inflammation persists, there is continuing destruction of gingival fiber groups of the subsulcular connective tissue extending into the major fiber groups and down into the periodontal ligament, junctional epithelium, and bone. The goal of the curettage procedure is to remove the soft, mushy, diseased connective tissue and the affected sulcular epithelium so that the remaining tissues have a healthier environment in which to repair themselves during wound healing. This diseased tissue is often granular in nature and is called *granulomatous tissue.* It is connective tissue that has tried to repair itself but has failed in the unfavorable environment produced by the chronic inflammation. Proponents of curettage believe that the chronic wound is converted to a surgical wound as a result of removal of granulation tissue during curettage and that a more acceptable environment

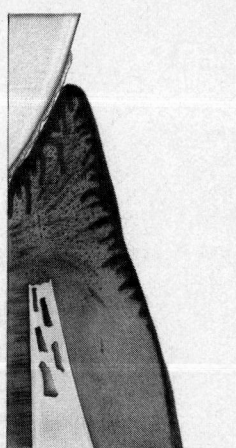

Fig. 24-3. As inflammatory process continues to affect tissues, there is weakening of subsulcular connective tissues, which allows epithelium to proliferate into connective tissue spaces, producing rete peg appearance of these tissues. There is further breakdown of gingival fiber groups, allowing apical migration of junctional epithelium along root surface. Loss of crestal bone is also apparent.
(Adapted from Seibert JS: Contin Dent Educ **1:**8, 1978.)

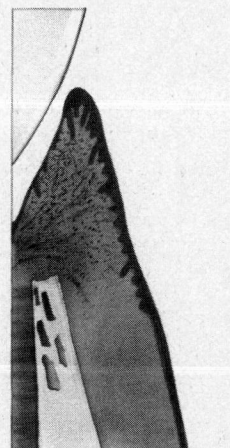

Fig. 24-4. It is difficult to remove all rete peg extensions of epithelium into connective tissue. Coincidental curettage or light curettage might produce a wound site similar to this in tissues.
(Adapted from Seibert JS: Cont Dent Educ **1:**8, 1978.)

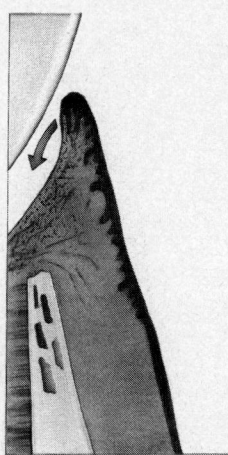

Fig. 24-5. Complete curettage involves removal of all sulcular epithelium and junctional epithelium as is shown here.
(Adapted from Seibert JS: Contin Dent Educ **1:**8, 1978.)

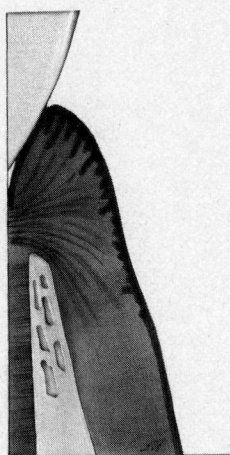

Fig. 24-6. Healing following soft tissue curettage reveals that healthy epithelium has again been restored to sulcus and that subsulcular connective tissues have regenerated to their normal form and function. Although attachment is now slightly apical to where it existed normally, adherence of gingival tissues to tooth is favorable.
(Adapted from Seibert JS: Contin Dent Educ **1:**8, 1978.)

for healing is provided for periodontal tissues (Figs. 24-1 to 24-6). Lindhe and Nyman (1985) reported, however, that the intentional removal of granulation tissue as part of periodontal therapy did not seem to be a critical factor for achieving healing of periodontal tissues and a return to health.

Bacterial invasion of soft tissues

A number of investigators have confirmed that Gram-negative bacteria do penetrate the apical and lateral epithelial walls of deep pockets in cases of advanced chronic periodontitis. Evidence of bacterial invasion into the adjacent connective tissues, into the cementum, and as far inward as the alveolar crest of bone has been observed. These observations have prompted a significant amount of discussion in the literature regarding the role of these invading bacteria in the pathogenesis of periodontal disease. Although there was early skepticism regarding the possibility that bacterial invasion actually takes place, findings obtained using light, electron, and scanning electron microscopes have confirmed that bacteria do invade the periodontal tissues of patients with advanced adult periodontitis, acute necrotizing ulcerative gingivitis, and localized juvenile periodontitis. Organisms have been observed 400 micrometers beyond the epithelium, within connective tissue, as well as in cementum and alveolar bone. Connective tissue of active periodontal lesions was found to contain more organisms than that of sites with no active disease.

The organisms identified have been mainly Gram-negative, including fusiform and spirochetes. Experimental observations suggest that only some of the periodontal organisms gain access to soft tissues and that there are differences in the invasive capacities of certain plaque bacteria and differences in virulence among different strains of bacterial species such as *Bacteroides gingivalis*.

Bacterial invasion by oral pathogens appears to be secondary to the tissue changes of periodontal disease, although there is evidence that some pathogens do create their own entryway into the tissues. Disruptions in the gingival basement membrane and in the sulcular epithelium as a result of the inflammatory process would faciliate bacterial invasion into the deeper tissues, although some organisms are able to pass through gingival epithelium in the absence of ulcerated opening (Saglie et al, 1982; Frank, 1980; Saglie et al, 1985; Nisengard and Basiones, 1987).

The implication of these findings for the treatment of periodontal disease is that the presence of invasive pathogenic bacteria may indicate a source of infection other than the subgingival plaque, which lies within the pocket and the toxic root surface adjacent to it. Although scaling and root planing can successfully remove these etiological factors successfully, these procedures do not remove pathogens that lie embedded within the soft tis-

sues. If these bacteria prove to be sources of reinfection following periodontal treatment, other methods for their removal may be indicated. Soft tissue curettage may be indicated under these circumstances, especially when mechanical and chemical curettage are employed together (Buethe, 1986). These observations do not alter the fact that there is no current clinical evidence of a clinical benefit provided by curettage over that of root planing alone. Clinicians should be aware, however, that much remains to be learned about periodontal disease, its causes, and its treatment. It is incumbent on dental professionals to remain up to date on periodontal literature and to provide treatment that has demonstrated its effectiveness in controlling and preventing disease. At the same time, we must remain openminded regarding the possible implications of new findings.

PATIENT PREPARATION

For the goals of treatment to be realized, the new surgical wound must be able to repair itself in an environment favorable for healing. Several requirements in patient preparation for curettage should be completed before the curettage is performed. First, the patient should be educated and motivated to practice optimal plaque control procedures. Effective plaque control will accomplish two things: (1) the tissue will undergo some healing and improvement from the plaque control alone, so that the indications for curettage can be more carefully evaluated; and (2) the increased health of the tissue and decreased inflammation brought on by plaque control will improve conditions for performing the soft tissue curettage procedure. A reduction in inflammation will result in a reduction in tissue sensitivity and bleeding and in better tissue tonus, or firmness. The firmer the soft tissues are, the easier they will be to manipulate during curettage. Conversely, tissues that are friable and spongy require more careful instrumentation technique and tissue support in order to prevent excessive tissue trauma during curettage. The second reason for the patient to establish good plaque control habits before the curettage is to ensure that the treated areas will be maintained after the procedure. If the patient's home care is less than adequate, it may be advisable to postpone the curettage until there is evidence of the patient's ability to maintain plaque control.

Another prerequisite for the success of curettage is the complete preparation of adjacent root surfaces. This preparation should include removal of all plaque, its associated endotoxins, plaque-retentive surfaces, and calculus. The soft tissue wall of the pocket cannot heal if it constantly encounters the diseased hard tissue wall that was a source of inflammation from the start (Aleo et al, 1974, 1975). Therefore, complete, definitive root planing is needed to prepare the root surface and provide submarginal plaque control before the curettage procedure can be performed (Jones and O'Leary, 1978). If root planing was done at a previous appointment, the results should be re-evaluated and the root retreated as necessary immediately before the curettage.

The patient's assessment data for periodontal treatment should be reviewed before treatment begins. These data should include an updated medical history and periodontal chart so that information regarding pocket morphologies and the degree of periodontal involvement can be examined. This information, in conjunction with clinical signs and symptoms, will help the clinician determine current indications and contraindications for performing soft tissue curettage. The patient must be informed of the purpose of this treatment procedure and provided with a description of what the treatment involves. Patient consent and cooperation are as important for the success of curettage as for any dental procedure. The patient should be encouraged to ask questions, and potential results should be discussed. This dialogue reinforces the importance of the patient's role as a partner in care and encourages self-evaluation of progress through treatment.

Anesthesia is recommended for the soft tissue curettage procedure. Even though there are some patients who feel that they could tolerate the curettage without anesthesia, most patients will be more comfortable if they are anesthetized. An exception to this recommendation may be a case in which only one papilla or other localized area is being treated rather than a whole segment of the mouth. In such an instance, administering appropriate anesthetic may be just as painful for the patient as performing the curettage procedure. Another exception is the patient who is allergic to anesthetic solutions or who refuses anesthesia for reasons that cannot be negotiated. In many cases,

however, the patient already may have been anesthetized for root planing and thus is prepared for soft tissue curettage.

Infiltration anesthesia supplemented with interpapillary injections is best for this procedure (see Plate 4, *D*). A long-lasting injection such as a block is unnecessary for curettage because the procedure can be performed in a relatively short period of time and certainly does not require the same extent of anesthesia as root planing. Interpapillary injections are especially helpful for curettage because, in addition to providing local anesthesia to the area, the solution improves tissue tones, which makes handling of the tissue easier during the curettage. The vasoconstrictor available in most anesthetic solutions will also provide local hemostasis or control of bleeding to the area, which makes the procedure easier for the clinician and the patient. Patients for whom the use of a vasoconstrictor is contraindicated should be given an anesthetic agent that does not contain a vasoconstrictor, even though this will diminish the hemostatic effect.

ARMAMENTARIUM

The instruments and supplies needed for the curettage procedure are essentially the same as those used for root planing. An explorer is used to evaluate the root surfaces for any deposits that are still remaining. The curettes must be extremely sharp so that they will cut the soft tissue easily. Dull curettes will tear and pull on the tissues rather than cut out the inflamed tissues smoothly. The wound created during curettage will heal much faster if the surface is smooth and free of tears, cuts, or tissue tags. Much of the technique for curettage that will be described is aimed at producing a wound that will heal easily and quickly. For this reason, the clinician is advised to keep a separate set of curettes for curettage so that the blades can be maintained in a surgically sharp condition. Curettes used for root planing should not be used for the curettage procedure. Any sharp curette can be used for this procedure as long as it has adequate access to all areas that need to be treated. Gracey curettes are illustrated because they have excellent access to any area or pocket morphology due to their varied shank designs and small blade size. When Gracey curettes are selected, any combination of designs that will serve all areas may be used. A suggested combination is ½, ⅞, ¹¹⁄₁₂, and ¹³⁄₁₄. The basic instrumentation principles are the same in soft tissue curettage as in scaling and root planing, except that the cutting edge is directed toward the soft tissue rather than toward the tooth. When Gracey curettes are used, the lower cutting edge should be turned toward the soft tissue. The working angulation will vary between 45 and 90 degrees to the soft tissue.

Other supplies needed for the curettage procedure include an anesthesia setup, a periodontal probe to record pretreatment pocket depths, a mouth mirror, and gauze sponges. In addition, normal saline and an aspirating syringe should be used for cleansing the area during the procedure to reduce the chances of introducing microorganisms into the surgical site.

The information in Chapter 3 reminds the clinician that the potential exists for large numbers of bacterial colonies to grow in the water supply of the dental unit. The water syringe must be thoroughly flushed before daily use. This procedure is especially important if the unit water supply will be used for a procedure such as curettage. Irrigation of the surgical site is an important factor in providing optimal conditions for wound healing. Inflamed tissue, plaque, calculus, and other debris that the curette may not have carried out of the pocket should be flushed out of the pocket area to cleanse the wound. (See Chapter 19 for a discussion of post-treatment irrigation.) An oxygenating agent may also be included on the tray setup to cleanse the postoperative site further of remaining debris and to facilitate healing.

CURETTAGE PROCEDURE

When the patient has been prepared and the tray setups are ready, the curettage procedure can begin. Five basic steps should be followed to ensure that all the inflamed granulomatous tissue is removed from the site and to obtain a clean wound. These steps are described in detail.

1. *Buccal and lingual pocket walls* should be curetted by placing the instrument with the cutting edge against the soft tissues at a 45- to 90-degree angle and positioning the blade for a horizontal or circumferential stroke (Fig. 24-7; see also Plate 4, *E*). The toe should be positioned near the base of the pocket and moved gently across the bottom

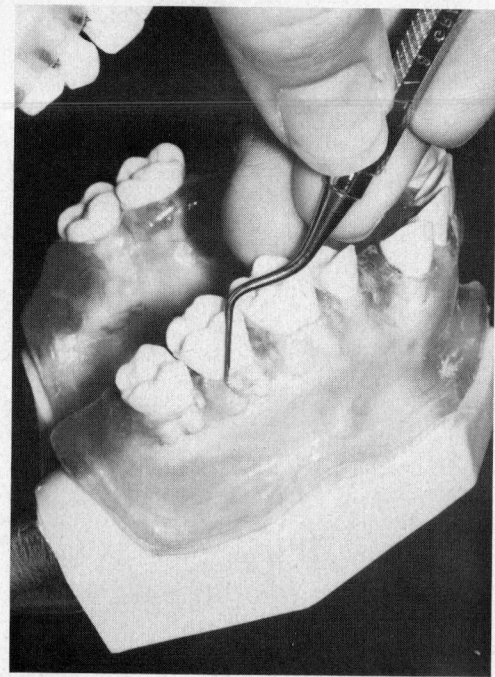

Fig. 24-7. Adaptation of Gracey ⅞ curette is shown on typodont, demonstrating proper adaptation and angulation for soft tissue curettage of buccal wall of this tooth. Transparent "gingiva" allows visibility of curette blade so that reader can see that lower cutting edge is being adapted to soft tissue rather than to root surface.

part of the pocket. The geography of the pocket bases already should have been plotted on the periodontal chart so that the clinician can estimate the location of the junctional epithelium and avoid tearing the underlying gingival connective fibers. The stroke should move in a horizontal direction across the buccal or lingual wall of the pocket from distal line angle to mesial line angle. A smoother incision will be made if the strokes are long and light rather than short and irregular. It is like the difference between cutting a piece of paper with scissors using a long stroke or a series of shorter strokes; the more often the hand stops and starts, the more jagged the edge of the paper will appear. The same is true in curettage along the soft tissue wall. Because tissue tags or even minute tears will hinder the healing of the pocket wall, they should be avoided as much as possible.

The length of the stroke must be guided by the

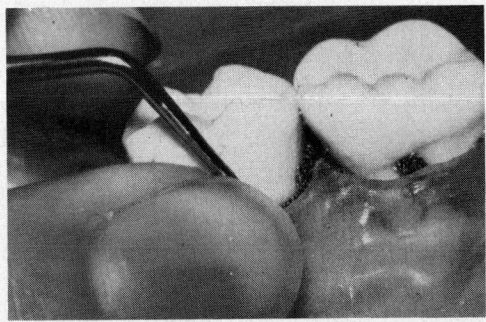

Fig. 24-8. When curettage stroke is initiated against buccal or lingual walls, it is important that soft tissue wall be supported against cutting edge with index finger as shown. Finger should follow strokes as they move across buccal or lingual surfaces.

ability of the clinician to control the adaptation and angulation of the curette. Neither of these two factors should be compromised by the length of the stroke, because they will affect the quality of the wound that is created. It is important to support the soft tissue with a finger of the other hand during each stroke (Fig. 24-8; see also Plate 4, *G*). Unless gentle external pressure is supplied against the tissue being treated, the curette will simply displace the soft tissue rather than cut it. The finger support should be directly opposite the cutting edge at all times. It is therefore necessary to rely on tactile sensations through the curette and the supporting finger and on visualization of the proper orientation of the shank of the curette to monitor instrument application. If the angulation is optimal, the clinician will feel the resistance of the tissues to the sharp cutting edge and the sensation of peeling away diseased tissue from healthy tissue. Another evaluation of angulation is whether or not the clinician is actually removing the granulomatous tissue from the pocket. If not, angulation may be at fault, as may be the amount of pressure being applied against the tissue from either the curette or the supporting finger. Incorrect adaptation of the toe of the curette may be felt by the supporting finger if the toe is directed into the soft tissue or by the operating hand if the toe is being directed against adjacent tooth surface. A light and perceptive operating grasp is as necessary for this procedure as for any other instrumentation technique.

The buccal or lingual pocket walls may require several well-executed strokes over the same area

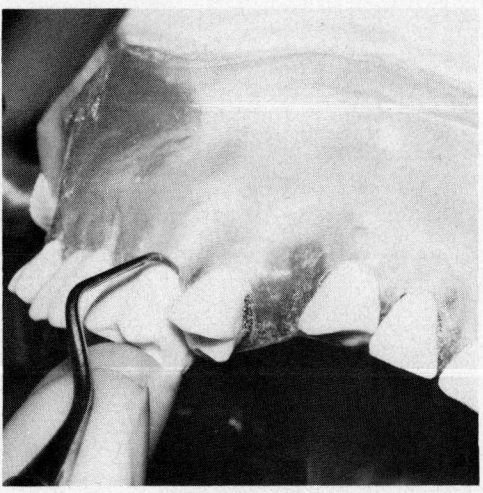

Fig. 24-9. Gracey ⅞ curette is shown being inserted into sulcus for interproximal strokes. Lower cutting edge is directed against soft tissue, and terminal shank of instrument is maintained nearly parallel to long axis of tooth.

to remove all inflamed tissue (see Plate 4, *H*). When the base portion of the wall is curetted, the blade should be moved somewhat coronally. If the length of the curette blade cannot accommodate the entire pocket wall, several strokes may be performed at different levels to complete the curettage of this area. The curettage is complete when the inner pocket wall feels firm to the curette blade, indicating that the inflamed mushy tissue has been removed, and when no more granulomatous tissue is being brought out of the area by the curette.

2. *Interdental papillae* are curetted by placing the curette so that the cutting edge is against one or the other of the papilla walls. A series of short, vertical strokes extends from the base of the interdental pocket area up to the free margin of the papilla (Fig. 24-9). These strokes should extend from the buccal or lingual angles of the tooth and into its midline. While the papilla is being curetted, a finger and thumb of the opposite hand should support both of its sides. The clinician will not be able to see the curettage in these areas because of the finger support (Fig. 24-10 and Plate 4*F*). Tactile information must be used.

3. *Marginal gingiva,* specifically the free gingival margin, is one area that is often curetted inadequately during the procedure. A special stroke

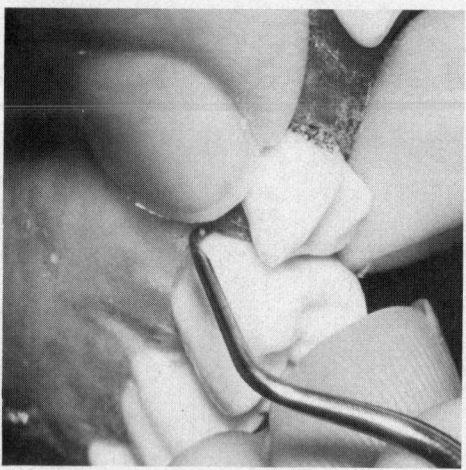

Fig. 24-10. Close-up view of curettage being simulated on interdental papilla, showing that tissue support should come from both sides of papilla with thumb and index finger of other hand. Blade of instrument often will be completely covered from view while these strokes are being implemented.

is warranted to overcome this problem. The curette blade should be placed about 80 degrees from the free margin of the gingiva and moved circumferentially along the margin so that the free gingival crest is retracted away from the tooth. This stroke should remove epithelium and inflamed tissue that still remains at the crest of the gingiva. The presence of any remaining tissue tags that might have been produced by earlier strokes should be detected. These tissue tags will be removed in step 5.

4. *Junctional epithelium* does not usually require a separate step because the other steps of the procedure will have removed all or most of this tissue already. Submarginal scaling and root-planing procedures often will remove epithelium at the pocket base. When shrinkage of the tissue is the goal, total removal of this epithelium is unnecessary. If, however, the goal is for a more coronal reattachment of tissues after healing, then it is necessary to perform a separate step that will guarantee that all sulcular epithelium is removed. This removal can be accomplished by placing the toe of the curette along the base of the pocket and performing light, circumferential strokes along the pocket base. The clinician must consider that a definitive, cutting stroke at the base of the pocket might also cut into the 1 to 2 mm of gin-

gival attachment fibers that exist below the junctional epithelium. There is a chance that a deeper pocket may be produced in this manner as evidenced by a loss of clinical attachment.

5. *Tissue tags* should be removed as a final step in the curettage procedure so that the free gingival margin is smooth and clear of tears or excess pieces of tissue that will hinder the healing process. These tissue tags should be detected during the stroke involving the marginal free gingiva or by close inspection of the margin. They are excised by placing the cutting edge against the tissue and pressing it laterally against the tooth surface. When all steps have been accomplished, the wound should be free of all inflamed tissues, and the gingival margins should be smooth and free of tags, tears, or gouges.

POSTTREATMENT TISSUE MANAGEMENT

After the tissues have been inspected, the pockets should be irrigated thoroughly to remove any tissue remnants (Moskow, 1962). A wound that is clean and smooth will heal more quickly. After irrigation of the pocket, the tissues should be readapted to the teeth by applying gentle lateral pressure for several minutes with a sterile gauze square that has been soaked in warm normal saline. The pressure will stop bleeding, readapt tissue, and help in the formation of a thin blood clot. If this compression is sufficient to control bleeding and the tissue remains in close contact with the tooth, no other postoperative treatment is necessary. If, instead, there is incessant bleeding and/or the tissues tend to stand away from the tooth, placement of a periodontal dressing is indicated. The pressure of the dressing against the wound site will help control the bleeding and assist in the formation of the blood clot. The protective coverage provided by the dressing will also help keep the wound site free of food debris, plaque, and other material that would retard healing. A periodontal dressing is recommended for best results if the goal of the curettage is for reattachment instead of shrinkage. If this is the case, the pack should remain on the wound site for 7 to 10 days. When only shrinkage is expected, the pack can be removed in 3 or 4 days (Chace, 1974). More detailed information regarding periodontal dressings is given in Chapter 25.

The patient should be instructed to perform gentle home care of the curettage site on the first day. This includes rinsing with mild salt water and plaque control with a soft brush or gauze. The patient should be warned not to rinse vigorously for 1 to 2 hours after the procedure to avoid dislodging blood clots. Extreme temperatures and spicy foods should be avoided to minimize sensitivity in the area. Usually, regular home care procedures can be instituted on the day following the procedure. When a periodontal dressing is placed, special instructions regarding its care should be given (see Chapter 25).

WOUND HEALING

Immediately after curettage is performed, the gingiva will show evidence of bleeding and blood clots and will appear red or blue-red in color (see Plate 4, *I*). A day later, the gingiva will show signs of edema and a red or blue-red color. There may still be evidence of sloughing tissue and clotted blood. By the fourth day, the intensity of red in the gingiva will have diminished, as well as the edema and swelling. By the sixth day, the gingiva may appear light red with a further reduction of edema, and marginal gingiva may show constriction and some recession. Healing should be complete in 7 to 10 days unless it has been interrupted by incomplete curettage or root planing, poor plaque control, or systemic complications (Goldman and Cohen, 1980) (see Plate 4, *J*).

EVALUATION OF CURETTAGE

After a week or more of healing, the patient should be recalled for an evaluation of the tissue response to curettage. This examination should include evaluation of tissue color, contour, and consistency, reduction of pocket depth, and status of the sulcular epithelial lining. The appearance of the gingiva should be compared with its precurettage characteristics and expectatons of normal, healthy gingiva. Reexamination and comparison with precurettage periodontal charts will indicate the areas and extent of pocket reduction. Probing will also indicate the status of the pocket lining according to the presence or absence of bleeding.

Any area where signs of inflammation still exist should be carefully reexplored for the presence of plaque or calculus. The possibility of incomplete curettage or residual debris should also be considered. If local factors are at fault, they should be eliminated, and additional curettage should be performed if necessary.

Soft tissue curettage is a procedure that can be performed successfully by the clinician who develops an appreciation for its indications and limitations. Many of the principles of instrumentation are similar to those already used during scaling and root planing procedures, and those skills are transferred easily to the treatment of diseased soft tissue lining of the pocket. A thorough background in the nature of healthy and diseased periodontal tissue will enhance the clinical skills of the clinician in assessment, planning, implementation, and evaluation of soft tissue curettage.

CHEMICAL CURETTAGE

Chemical solutions have been studied as a means of accomplishing the effective removal of inflamed soft tissues within a chronically inflamed pocket. Kalkwarf and others (1982) described a technique for using sodium hypochlorite solution for this purpose and described its effect on the soft tissues. Sodium hypochlorite solution was applied to the soft tissue lining of the treated pockets for 1 minute, with care taken not to spill it on any of the adajcent tissues. Several drops of 5% citric acid were then introduced into the pocket to neutralize the environment. The area was thoroughly irrigated with water prior to instrumentation against the soft tissue wall with a sharp curette. The chemical treatment of the pocket produced chemolysis of the inflamed epithelium and connective tissue, so that it was removed from the pocket with fewer strokes and more completely than by hand curettage alone. Chemical curettage had the additional advantages of not requiring anesthesia, of producing a more predictable and uniform removal of the pocket lining, and of reducing hemorrhage. Healing was similar to that which follows hand instrumentation for curettage. Both root planing and effective plaque control are prerequisites for the chemical treatment, as they are for traditional soft tissue curettage techniques. Vieira and others (1982), in a study done on beagle dogs, confirmed that the effects of chemical curettage using sodium hypochlorite and citric acid (antiformin) were similar to those found after soft tissue curettage. They concluded that healing following chemical curettage involved the formation of a long junctional epithelium, and that the healing response to chemical curettage was similar to, although not improved over, healing following soft tissue curettage.

ACTIVITIES

1. Practice the adaptation of instruments and steps in tissue removal in a laboratory situation using the jaws of freshly killed hogs. Make arrangements with a local slaughterhouse to secure one-half jaw per student. Wearing disposable gloves, create pockets or sulci around each tooth by cutting the tissues away from the teeth using the toe of a large curette. Experiment with the curettage technique, simulating all steps as closely as possible. At the conclusion of the lab, cut a flap at either end of the area worked on and retract the tissue down to check for remaining tissue tags or gouges. This is a useful way to practice curettage on something other than another human being.

2. An analogy between a bruised apple and the principles of curettage is helpful in planning an inquiry approach to learning. All that is needed is a bruised apple floating in a pan of water and a spoon.

    Pose the situation of an apple-bobbing contest with a huge bruise visible on the only available apple. What is wrong with the apple? How can you tell? What could be done about the problem? What kind of tool would be most helpful in removing the bruised area? What technique would you use to implement the tool? How could you tell that all of the bruise was removed? How would you keep the apple from bobbing away from you as you tried to remove the bruise?

    Use answers to illustrate the indication, armamentarium, technique, and evaluation of the soft tissue curettage procedure. It is important that all answers be valued and that their implications and consequences be discussed to help the students develop skills in critical problem solving.

3. Observe a faculty member or more advanced student performing soft tissue curettage for a clinic patient.

4. Observe an open-flap curettage in progress.

5. View a videotaped close-up demonstration of soft tissue curettage being performed for a patient.

6. Investigate equipment designed to deliver sterile water, saline, or antimicrobial solutions to the surgical site for lavage, avoiding contaminated water supplies.

REVIEW QUESTIONS

1. Define the following terms:
    a. Soft tissue curettage
    b. Coincidental curettage

2. Of the two methods of achieving pocket elimination—shrinkage and reattachment—which is most likely to occur as a result of soft tissue curettage?

3. True or false: The only tissue that is likely to be removed during the curettage procedure is the epithelial lining of the sulcus or pocket wall.

4. You performed curettage for a patient 2 weeks ago, and when he returns, you find that the tissue has not healed completely and there is still bleeding on examination, edema, and redness of the treated areas. Plaque control has been maintained, and no systemic disturbances are present. List three possible causes of this failure of the tissues to heal that could be traced to poor clinician technique.

5. Identify each of the following as an indication or contraindication for you to begin soft tissue curettage:
    a. Area has primarily gingival pockets or pseudopockets
    b. Presence of bony defects in the underlying bone
    c. Bleeding on probing
    d. Recent history of cardiac disease and valve damage
    e. Boggy, edematous tissues
    f. Rough root surfaces
    g. Ineffective plaque control
    h. Mucogingival or frenum involvement

6. Which of the following situations would indicate the necessity of placing a periodontal dressing following the soft tissue curettage procedure?
    a. Profuse bleeding follows curettage
    b. Free gingiva adheres closely to the tooth surfaces
    c. Free gingiva stands away from the tooth surfaces
    d. Goal of the procedure is reattachment

REFERENCES

Adcock JE, et al: Effect of sodium hypochlorite solution on thesubgingival microflora of juvenile periodontitis lesions, Pediatr Dent 5:190, 1983.

Ainslie PT, and Caffesse RG: A biometric evaluation of gingival curettage, Quintessence Int 12:519, 1981.

Aleo JJ, et al: The presence and biologic activity of cementum-bound endotoxin, J Periodontol 45:672, 1974.

Aleo JJ, et al: In vitro attachment of human gingival fibroblasts to root surfaces, J Periodontol 46:639, 1975.

Barrington EP: An overview of periodontal surgical procedures, J Periodontol 52:518, 1981.

Bradley RE: The rationale and technique of subgingival curettage in the treatment of periodontal disease, Texas Dent J 101:14, 1984.

Buethe CG, et al: Gingival curettage. Is it a viable therapy alternative? Dent Hyg 60:24, 1986.

Caton JG, and Zander HA: The attachment between tooth and gingival tissues after periodic root planing and soft tissue curettage, J Periodontol 50:462, 1979.

Chace R: Subgingival curettage in periodontal therapy, J Periodontol 45:107, 1974.

Chace R: Subgingival curettage. In Clark JW, editor: Clinical dentistry, New York, 1983, Harper & Row.

Deasy MJ, and Vogel RI: The relevance of curettage in periodontal therapy, Ann Dent 37:70, 1978.

Echeverria JJ, and Caffesse RG: Effects of gingival curettage when performed 1 month after root instrumentation, J Clin Periodontol 10:277, 1983.

Forgas L: Soft tissue curettage. Literature review, Dent Hyg 60:42, 1986.

Frank RM: Bacterial penetration in the apical pocket wall of advanced human periodontitis, J Periodont Res 15:563, 1980.

Goldman H, and Cohen DW: Periodontal therapy, ed 6, St Louis, 1980, The CV Mosby Co

Green ML, and Green BL: Aggressive curettage, Dent Hyg 53:409, 1979.

Greenberg J: Conservative periodontics NY J Dent 55:297, 1985.

Greenstein G: Changing periodontal concepts, II: treatment approaches, Compend Contin Educ 6:253, 1985.

Hall WB: Procedure code 452: eliminating the confusion, CDA J 11:33, 1983.

Hill RW, et al: Four types of periodontal treatment compared over two years, J Periodontol 52:655, 1981.

Hirschfeld L: Subgingival curettage in periodontal treatment, JADA 44:301, 1952.

Hirschfeld L: The role of subgingival curettage in periodontal therapy, Alpha Omegan 55:115, 1962.

Jones WA, and O'Leary TJ: The effectiveness of *in vivo* root planing in removing bacterial endotoxin from the roots of periodontally involved teeth, J Periodontol 49:337, 1978.

Kalkwarf KL, et al: Longitudinal study of periodontal therapy, J Periodontol 44:66, 1973.

Kalwarf KL, et al: Histologic evaluation of gingival curettage facilitated by sodium hypochlorite solution, J Periodontol 53:63, 1982.

Knowles JW, et al: Results of periodontal treatment related to pocket depth and attachment level: eight years, J Periodontol 50:225, 1979.

Kon S, et al: Visualization of microvascularization of the healing periodontal wound, II: curettage, J Periodontol 40:96, 1969.

Kuren S, et al: Comparative effectiveness of gingival curettage with and without root planing on periodontal health, J Dent Res 65:270 (abst 912), 1986.

Lindhe J, and Nyman S: Scaling and granulation tissue removal in periodontal therapy, J Clin Periodont 12:374, 1985.

Listgarten MA, and Rosenberg MM: Histological study of repair following new attachment procedures in human periodontal lesions, J Periodontol 50:333, 1979.

Lopez NJ, and Belvederessi M: Subgingival scaling with root planing and curettage: effects upon gingival inflammation—a comparative study, J Periodontol 48:354, 1977.

Magnusson I, et al: A long junctional epithelium—a locus minoris resistentiae in plaque infection? J Clin Periodontol 10:333, 1983.

Morris M: The removal of pocket and attachment epithelium in humans: a histological study, J Periodontol 25:7, 1954.

Moskow B: The response of the gingival sulcus to instrumentation: a histological investigation, J Periodontol 33:282, 1962.

Nisengard R, and Basiones A: Bacterial invasion in periodontal disease: abstracts from a workshop to consider bacterial invasion in periodontal disease, J Periodontol 58:331, 1987.

Ramfjord SP, et al: Longitudinal study of peridontal therapy, J Periodontol 44:66, 1973.

Ramfjord SP, et al: Subgingival curettage versus surgical elimination of periodontal pockets, J Periodontol 39:167, 1968.

Saglie R, et al: Bacterial invasion of gingiva in advanced periodontitis in humans, J Periodontol 53:217, 1982.

Saglie FR, et al: The presence of bacteria within the oral epithelium in periodontal disease, I: a scanning and transmission electron microscopic study, J Periodontol 56:618, 1985.

Seibert J: Incorporating root planing and gingival curettage into a clinical practice, Contin Dent Educ, 1:8, 1978.

Shapiro A: Regeneration of interdental papillae using periodic curettage, Int J Perio Rest Dent 5:27, 1985.

Stahl SS, et al: Soft tissue healing following curettage and root planing, J Periodontol 42:678, 1971.

Valentine R: Periodontal documentation and therapy: a laboratory program for dental students and expanded duty auxiliaries, ed 3. Philadelphia, 1977, University of Pennsylvania School of Dental Medicine.

Vieira EM, et al: The effect of sodium hypochlorite and citric acid solutions on healing of periodontal pockets, J Periodontol 53:71, 1982.

Wirthlin MR: The current status of new attachment therapy J Periodontol 52:529, 1981.

Zamet JS: A comparative clinical study of three periodontal surgical techniques J Clin Periodontol 2:87, 1975.

25 PERIODONTAL DRESSINGS AND SUTURE REMOVAL

OBJECTIVES *The reader will be able to*

1. List and explain the functions of a periodontal pack.
2. Compare and contrast the properties of a pack that contains eugenol with those of a pack that does not contain eugenol.
3. Describe the placement of a periodontal pack on a surgical area with no missing teeth and on an area with several missing teeth.
4. Describe the removal of sutures and of a periodontal pack.
5. Place and remove a periodontal pack on a typodont and/or partner.
6. Remove sutures.
7. Instruct a patient in caring for a periodontal pack.

Dental hygienists are assuming an ever-expanding role in the treatment of periodontal disease, especially with respect to procedures such as root planing and curettage. More and more dentists and periodontists are using the skills of dental hygienists in the treatment of periodontal disease to provide a team approach that makes maximum use of the training and skills of both types of professionals for the effective and efficient delivery of services to dental consumers. Among the periodontal treatment procedures that the dental hygienist is qualified to perform are placing and removing periodontal dressings after surgical treatment and removing sutures following soft tissue healing. This chapter describes each of these procedures.

PURPOSE OF PERIODONTAL DRESSINGS

Periodontal dressings are mixtures of special materials that are initially soft and puttylike in consistency so that they easily can be placed over and adapted to oral tissues that have been surgically treated. After the dressings are properly placed, they harden in the mouth to form a rigid and protective covering for these tissues while they heal. Periodontal dressings have two primary functions: (1) to protect the surgical area and thus promote healing; and (2) to increase postsurgical patient comfort. The dressing itself does not contain sub-stances that directly stimulate healing, but it does protect the healing surgical area from irritants such as hot or spicy foods, sharp pieces of food, and mechanical trauma during chewing. Periodontal dressings also protect newly exposed root surfaces from temperature changes, stabilize mobile teeth, protect sutures, help maintain the position of repositioned soft tissues, help control bleeding, and act as a template to prevent formation of excessive granulation tissue (Baer et al, 1969; Blanque, 1962; Carranza and Perry, 1986; Goldman and Cohen, 1980; Levin, 1980; Valentine, 1976; Watts and Combe, 1979, Grant et al, 1988). Periodontal dressings have been used after most types of periodontal surgery, including flap procedures, gingivectomy, gingivoplasty, mucogingival surgery, and occasionally soft tissue curettage procedures (Valentine, 1976; Watts and Combe, 1979; Goldman and Cohen, 1980; Carranza, 1984).

PRESENT STATUS AND VALUE OF A PERIODONTAL DRESSING

A great deal of debate has occurred regarding the value and usefulness of periodontal dressings for routine use following all surgical procedures. This controversy has not yet been fully resolved on the basis of experimental evidence. A number of reports have indicated that the routine use of periodontal dressings may not achieve either of the two goals for which a dressing is placed—improved healing and increased patient comfort. Probably the biggest concern is that the presence of a periodontal dressing promotes the accumulation of plaque in and around the wound site. The dressing itself is a plaque-retentive surface that favors the accumulation of plaque. In addition, the presence of the dressing prevents the patient from adequately removing plaque and debris from the area and prevents antibacterial rinses (e.g., chlorhexidine) from contacting the healing surfaces. As a result, inflammation is more likely to occur and healing may be retarded. Studies of the healing process of surgically treated areas found that the tissues without periodontal dressings healed just as well as tissues that had been covered by periodontal dressings (Stahl et al, 1969; Greensmith and Wade, 1974; Jones and Cassingham, 1979; Allen and Caffesse, 1983). Heaney and Appleton (1976) found that the presence of a dressing was associated with more inflammation than in areas that were uncovered and suggested that dressings should be removed within 1 week of surgery. Wampole and colleagues (1978) found an incidence of bacteremia in 24% of patients at the time that the postsurgical dressing change took place. They noted that these findings could have serious implications for patients who were already medically compromised and susceptible to systemic infection. Several of these studies asked patients who had experienced surgery both with and without periodontal dressings which approach they preferred. Many patients reported a preference for no dressing and some even said that they experienced more pain as a result of wearing a periodontal dressing (Greensmith and Wade, 1974; Jones and Cassingham, 1979; Allen and Caffesse, 1983). It would seem from these reports that if the surgical procedure is completed in such a way that the flap is well adapted, the flap serves as a sufficient barrier to infection. Open access to the area also allows the individual to cleanse and rinse it thoroughly to keep the area clean. In many cases, depending on the type of surgery, the patient will be no more uncomfortable without a dressing than with a dressing (Sachs et al, 1984).

Although these reports question the need for routine use of periodontal dressings, there will always be circumstances in which a periodontal dressing is indicated. Dressings may be indicated for retention of an apically positioned flap so that it is not displaced coronally, for additional support to stabilize a free gingival graft, to protect exposed bone from injury during the early stages of healing and thereby reduce patient discomfort, or to act as a guide for healing to prevent overgrowth of granulation tissue (Sachs et al, 1984). The choice to use or not to use a dressing depends on the nature of the surgery and the preferences of the dentist or periodontist. The routine use of periodontal dressings following surgery may decrease as a result of better surgical techniques and increased use of antibacterial mouthrinses (Sachs et al, 1984).

TYPES OF PERIODONTAL DRESSINGS

Several different materials are used in the formulation of periodontal dressings. The two most widely used types of dressing materials are zinc oxide–eugenol dressings and zinc oxide–noneugenol dressings. In addition to these two types, cyanoacrylates and modified methacrylic gels have also been studied for their use as periodontal dressings.

The inclusion of eugenol in periodontal dressings is somewhat controversial and its safety and value as an ingredient in periodontal dressings have been investigated and analyzed by many researchers and clinicians (Frisch and Bhaskar, 1967; Baer et al, 1969; Haugen and Gjermo, 1978; Haugen and Mjor, 1979; Goldman and Cohen, 1980; Haugen, 1980; Levin, 1980; Carranza and Perry, 1986). Eugenol is the main chemical constituent of clove oil; this explains its clovelike odor. It is combined with vegetable oils as the liquid component of zinc oxide–eugenol. As an antiseptic and an anodyne, eugenol is considered to be an *obtundent* material, meaning that it is soothing to living tissues. Some investigators believe that eugenol is an obtundent to all tissues, including bone, and that it should be used in all dressings to promote healing and patient comfort. Other investigators believe that eugenol is irritating to bone and might even stimulate its destruction, and, therefore, that it should not be included in periodontal dressing materials. Reports of animal studies in which zinc oxide–eugenol dressings were placed against exposed bone indicate that there is incomplete healing, or destruction, of the bone due to these substances (Haugen and Mjor, 1979; Goldman and Cohen, 1980; Levin, 1980; Carranza and Perry, 1986). Studies done with animals and humans to compare wound healing with zinc oxide–eugenol and zinc oxide–noneugenol dressings have shown there is no difference in epithelialization and wound healing in spite of the previously mentioned reports of bone destruction (Frisch and Bhaskar, 1967; Haugen and Gjermo, 1978; Haugen, 1980; Levin, 1980). *There is no conclusive research to direct the clinician to choose one type over another using the criterion of compatibility with oral tissues, especially bone.*

Many clinicians select the type of periodontal dressing on the basis of factors other than the absence or presence of eugenol, such as ease of manipulation, consistency of the dressing, and storage factors. Another important criterion for selection of dressing materials is the potential of patient sensitivity to ingredients in the dressing. The dental literature contains several reports of allergic reactions to the eugenol component of some dressing materials (Poulson, 1974; Barkin et al, 1984). In addition, an allergic response to rosin has been described (Lysell, 1976). It is important to assess the patient's history of allergic reactions and relate the allergens to the ingredients in dressing materials, to decrease the probability that allergic reactions will develop as a result of the presence of periodontal dressings.

Because many brand-names of dressing materials are copyrighted, determining the ingredients of a periodontal dressing can sometimes be a challenge. If the material being used is accepted by the American Dental Association, its ingredients will be listed in the most recent *Accepted Dental Therapeutics* (ADA, 1984). If the material is not listed, consult the manufacturer or the research literature. Research articles usually list the ingredients of the materials studied.

In general, the antimicrobial qualities of a dressing seem to have only minor effects on wound healing, and the addition of antimicrobial agents to dressings is of questionable merit. The benefits of the antimicrobial substances must be weighed against their potential for causing allergic responses or sensitivity or for altering the normal oral flora (Sachs et al, 1984).

The use of chlorhexidine as an intraoral antibacterial rinse following surgical procedures has shown merit. Although the effect of the rinse is apparently blocked if a dressing is used, it is quite effective in reducing plaque formation and associated inflammation when the surgical site remains exposed to the oral cavity (Pluss et al, 1975; Addy and Douglas, 1975; Addy and Dolby, 1976). The ability of chlorhexidine to inhibit plaque growth makes it a valuable asset in post-surgical care (Sachs et al, 1984).

Zinc oxide–eugenol dressings

Dressings containing eugenol are prepared by mixing a powder and a liquid. The powder is composed of zinc oxide, tannic acid, and rosin. Some powders also contain ingredients such as kaolin, zinc stearate, or asbestos. Asbestos fibers have been associated with lung disease and are considered a health hazard to dental personnel who prepare the dressings containing asbestos (Bakdash, 1976). Although there is no apparent danger from asbestos to patients after the dressing has been mixed, most products no longer contain asbestos. Tannic acid has also been omitted by some manufacturers because its absorption has been associated with liver disease (Baer et al, 1969; Watts and Combe, 1979; ADA, 1984). The liquid contains eugenol and an oil such as mineral or peanut oil. Ingredients to modify or improve the color and flavor of the dressing may also be included (ADA, 1984; Carranza and Perry, 1986; Watts and Combe, 1979). Table 25-1 lists the ingredients in one commonly used eugenol dressing and the function of each ingredient.

When the components of the zinc oxide–eugenol dressing are mixed together, setting (hardening) occurs due to the chemical interaction between the zinc oxide and the eugenol, which forms zinc eugenolate. This reaction is a slow one, allowing sufficient time to form, place, adapt, and trim the dressing to fit the wound site before the dressing hardens and becomes brittle. Not all of the eugenol is converted to zinc eugenolate during the reaction, with the result that a certain amount of free, unreacted eugenol is present in the dressing mixture. Because the presence of this free eugenol has been associated with harmful effects on oral tissues in some cases, the use of this type of dressing has been controversial.

Table 25-1. Ingredients and some of the functions of a zinc oxide–eugenol dressing*

Ingredient	Amount	Function
Powder (each 100 g)		
Zinc oxide	40 g	Setting reaction; slightly antiseptic and astringent
Rosin	40 g	Filler to increase strength
Tannic acid	20 g	Slightly hemostatic
Liquid (each 100 ml)		
Eugenol	46.5 ml	Setting reaction; slightly anesthetic; obtundent
Peanut oil	46.5 ml	Regulates setting time
Rosin	7.5 ml	Filler to increase strength

From ADA Council on Dental Therapeutics: Accepted dental therapeutics, ed 40. Chicago, 1984, American Dental Association.
*Kirkland Pack, Pulpdent Corporation of America, Brookline, Mass.

Table 25-2. Ingredients and some of the functions of a zinc oxide–noneugenol dressing*

Ingredient	Percentage	Function
Paste 1 (pink)		
Zinc oxide	45	Slightly antiseptic and astringent
Magnesium oxide	32	Setting reaction
Peanut oil	11	
Mineral oil	6	Regulate setting time
Rosin oil	3	
Other formulating and bacteriostatic agents	3	Bacteriostatic
Paste 2 (amber)		
Polymerized rosin	53	Increases strength
Coconut fatty acid	30	Setting reaction
Chlorothymol	3	Bacteriostatic
Peruvian balsam	3	Unspecified
Other formulating agents	3	Unspecified

From ADA Council on Dental Therapeutics: Accepted dental therapeutics, ed 40. Chicago, 1984, American Dental Association.

One reason that zinc oxide–eugenol dressings are preferred by clinicians is that the material can be mixed in a large quantity, divided into smaller amounts, wrapped tightly, and frozen. After dressing material has been frozen, it must be defrosted to room temperature before it can be used. The ability to mix this dressing material in advance is an advantage because the initial mixing is time consuming. Another advantage of eugenol-containing dressings is that they have a consistency that is firm, heavy, and easy to manipulate. These dressing materials do not stick to the clinician's fingers as readily as the noneugenol materials. A related disadvantage, however, is that the firmness of the material makes it necessary for the clinician to use more pressure to manipulate and adapt the dressing against the soft tissues. Because excessive pressure can displace newly repositioned flaps, a softer dressing material is preferred for these situations.

Zinc oxide–noneugenol dressings

The most common noneugenol periodontal dressing (Coe-Pack*) is supplied as two pastes. One paste contains zinc oxide, magnesium oxide, and hexachlorophene; the other paste contains hydrogenated rosin, chlorothymol, and benzyl alcohol (ADA, 1984; Carranza and Perry, 1986; Goldman and Cohen, 1980; Watts and Combe, 1979). Table 25-2 lists the ingredients and functions of each paste. When the two pastes are mixed together a setting reaction, which causes the material to harden, occurs between a metallic ion and fatty acids.

The noneugenol dressing should be mixed at the time of placement. When first mixed it has a very pliable consistency, making it the ideal choice for placement over a repositioned flap or over other fragile tissues. The noneugenol dressing can be made firmer by adding zinc oxide powder, which is usually mixed with a eugenol liquid; the addition of the powder gives the final dressing material more body and makes it less sticky (Valentine, 1976). Placement of a noneugenol dressing in a cup of cold water for several minutes after it is mixed also will have this effect. Noneugenol dressings usually have a more pleasant taste than dressings containing eugenol. Periodontal dressing products are constantly being improved in terms of strength, setting time, handling characteristics, and patient acceptance characteristics.

Premixed zinc oxide–noneugenol dressings are also available. One such dressing, Peripac*, con-

*Coe-Pack, Coe Laboratories, Inc.

*Peripac®, de Trey Frères, S.A., Zurich, Switzerland.

tains calcium phosphate, zinc oxide, acrylate, organic solvent, and flavoring and coloring agents (Haugen and Gjermo, 1978). When this material is exposed to air or moisture, it sets by the loss of organic solvent (Watts and Combe, 1979). After it is set, this dressing becomes quite brittle. The Peripac is not as popular as the zinc oxide–noneugenol dressing. Use of these materials has been associated with greater patient pain and swelling than found with other dressings (Haugen and Gjermo, 1978). A review of the literature on the physical properties of periodontal dressings indicated that none of the currently used dressings have ideal properties for clinical use and that further research is needed to improve these properties (Sachs et al, 1984).

Cyanoacrylate dressings

A number of researchers have investigated the use of cyanoacrylate as an alternative to suturing and as a surface adhesive and periodontal dressing (Frisch and Bhaskar, 1967; Ochstein et al, 1969; Forrest, 1974; Levin et al, 1975). This material has the unique ability to cement together moist, living tissue surfaces. Cyanoacrylate is either applied in drops or sprayed on the tissue. This method of application is time saving and relatively easy to perform. The characteristics of cyanoacrylate make it a near-ideal periodontal dressing in comparison with other dressing materials. The material is much less bulky than that of the other dressings. Other advantages include no apparent side effects; easy adherence to living tissues; immediate hemostasis; no evidence of systemic toxicity or sensitivity; excellent healing results; precision placement of flaps; decreased suturing time; ease of application; reapplication over existing material; patient preference over bulky dressings. Cyanoacrylates have been used for surface application only; adhesive that becomes trapped under the soft tissue flap will delay wound healing (Forrest, 1974; Levin et al, 1975; McGraw and Caffesse, 1978; Watts and Combe, 1979; Levin, 1980). Cyanoacrylate dressings have not yet been approved for use in the United States other than for research.

Methacrylic gel dressings

Methacrylic gels are used primarily in dentistry as tissue conditioners or denture liners. They have an elasticlike consistency that is soft and resilient and will flow under pressure, making them ideal for use in dentures. These gels adapt closely to the tissues and are very compatible with the wound site. Tissue conditioners cannot be used alone as dressings because of their poor retention, but they have been used in conjunction with a zinc oxide–noneugenol dressing (Addy et al, 1975; Watts and Combe, 1979; Levin, 1980). Addy and others (1975) reported the application of an antibacterial agent (such as chlorhexidine) by means of a methacrylic gel and zinc oxide–noneugenol dressing. The major advantage of this material is its ability to carry and release medicaments to the soft tissues. Other properties of this material cause it to have adhesion and retention characteristics that are less favorable than those of other types of dressing material. Methacrylic gel dressings are not widely used.

Addition of antibacterial agents

Antibiotics and other antibacterial agents have been added to periodontal dressings to reduce infection and to promote healing of surgically treated tissues. The effectiveness of adding antibacterial agents to dressings for this purpose, however, has not been proven conclusively (O'Neill, 1975; Haugen et al, 1977). Several concerns exist regarding the addition of antibiotic agents to periodontal dressings. One is that exposure to antibiotics can sensitize a patient to the agent, thereby limiting its application for controlling later infections in these patients. A second concern is that the ingredients in the dressing preparations inactivate the antibiotic. Therefore, the risks of antibiotic use may outweigh its intended benefits (Watts and Combe, 1979; Levin, 1980). The addition of chlorhexidine gluconate to methacrylic gel dressings has already been discussed as an effective means of promoting healing (Addy et al, 1975).

MIXING AND APPLICATION OF A PERIODONTAL DRESSING

The materials used for mixing and placing a periodontal dressing are shown in Fig. 25-1. Petroleum jelly is used to lubricate the patient's lips, and the tongue blade is used to mix the dressing components together. The curette and/or the college pliers are used to adapt the dressing into the

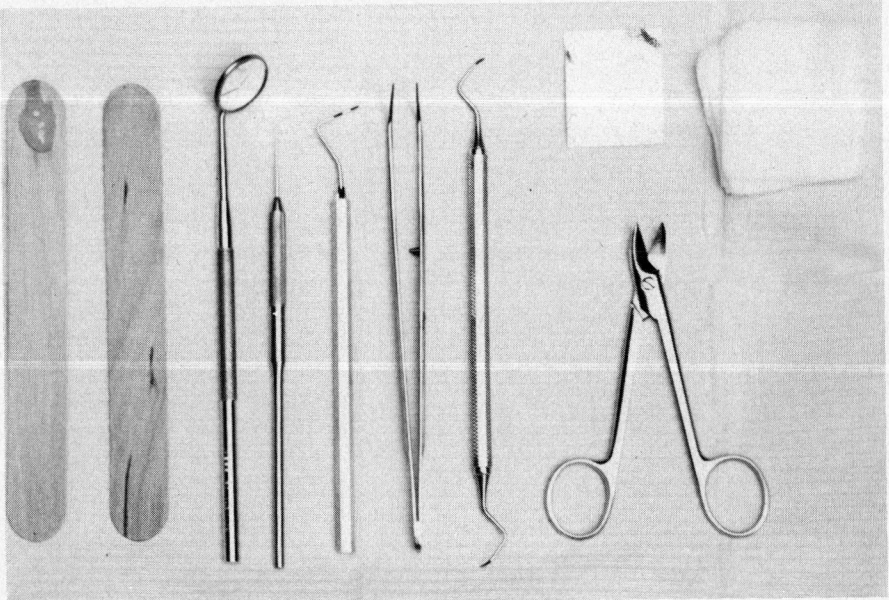

Fig. 25-1. Tray setup for placement of periodontal dressing: petroleum jelly, tongue blade, mirror, explorer, probe, college pliers, curette, dry foil, scissors, and gauze.

interproximal areas of the wound site. The dry foil is used to protect the dressing until it hardens.

Preparing the patient

The hygienist should discuss the purpose of the periodontal dressing with the patient and describe how it will be placed. Patients should also be told how the dressing will taste, feel, and look in the mouth. When the patient and clinician are ready to begin, the patient's lips should be lubricated with a light coating of petroleum jelly to prevent the moist and sticky dressing material from adhering to the lips while it is being placed. Because the noneugenol dressing is commonly used in clinical practice, the technique for mixing and adapting this type of dressing will be discussed first. Later sections will supply additional information necessary for the handling of other types of dressing materials.

Mixing a noneugenol dressing

The following steps are used when mixing a noneugenol dressing. First, mix the dressing according to the manufacturer's directions. For the product shown in the figures, equal lengths of each

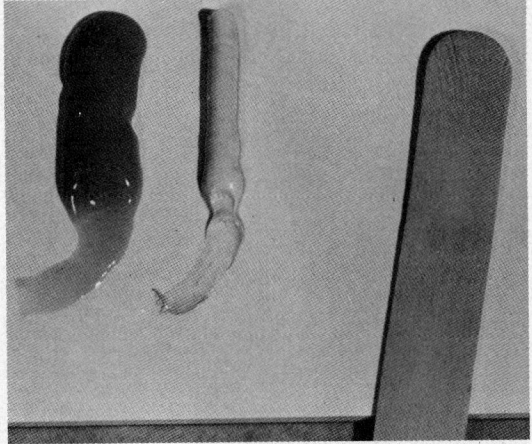

Fig. 25-2. Equal lengths of noneugenol pastes expressed onto pad.

component paste are expressed from the tubes and mixed until they are well blended and the color is homogeneous (Figs. 25-2 and 25-3). The particular stroke used for mixing is not an important consideration, as it is with some dental materials. Zinc

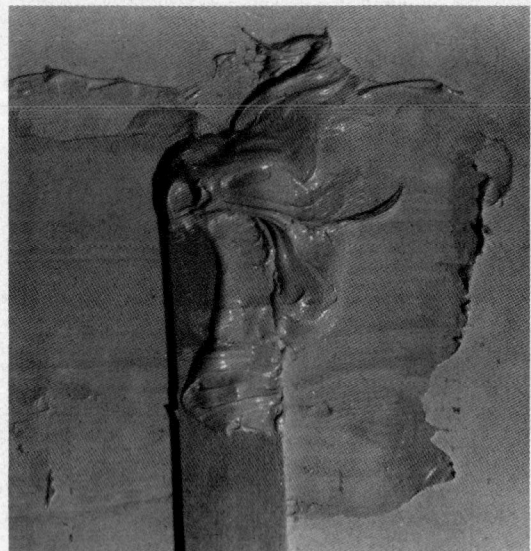

Fig. 25-3. Pastes are mixed until color is homogeneous.

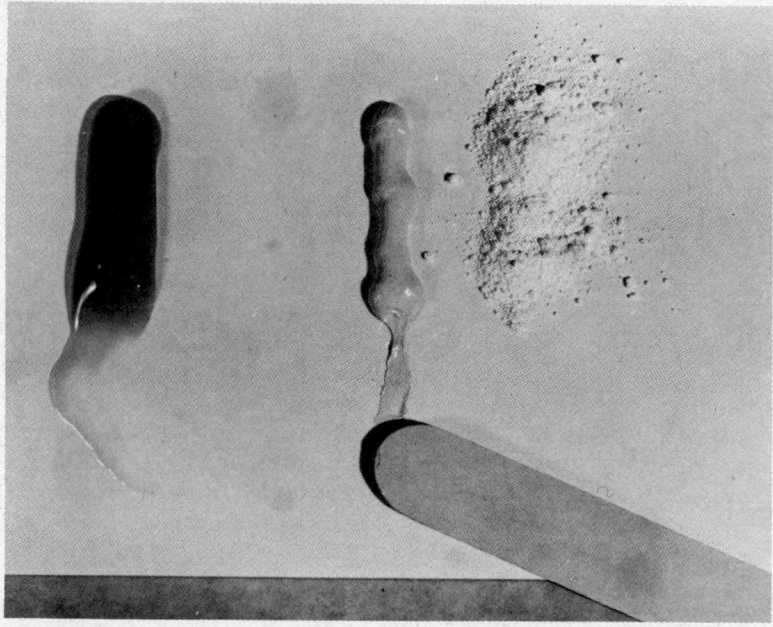

Fig. 25-4. To improve strength and workability, zinc oxide powder is incorporated into paste 1 and then mixed with paste 2.

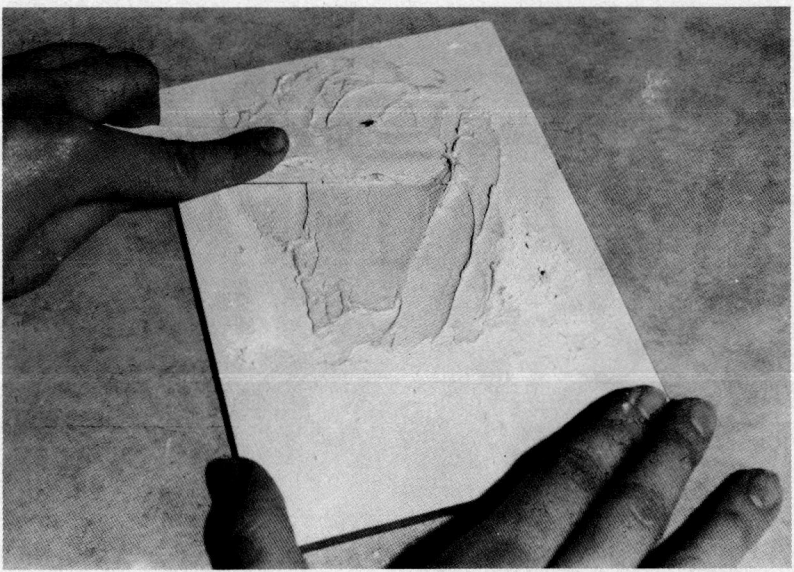

Fig. 25-5. Paste 1, with zinc oxide powder, is being mixed with paste 2 until color is homogeneous.

oxide powder may be added to the mix to make the material stronger and less sticky (Figs. 25-4 and 25-5). After the material is mixed, roll it between the palms of the hands (gloves should always be worn) to form it into cylinders about two-thirds the diameter of a pencil (Fig. 25-6). The length of the roll should correspond to the length of the area to be covered by the dressing.

Placing the dressing

Using sterile gauze, gently dry the area to be covered. Bleeding should be controlled before the dressing is placed. Although the dressing will help control bleeding, it should not be considered the primary means of control. If slight bleeding is present, apply pressure to the area with a sterile gauze sponge until it subsides. If this approach does not stop the bleeding, or if profuse bleeding occurs, the use of hemostatic agents or other measures of control may be required (Carranza and Perry, 1986). After the bleeding has been controlled and the area has been dried, place the roll of dressing material so that it wraps around the most distal tooth in the area to be covered. Adapt the dressing to the area by pressing it gently

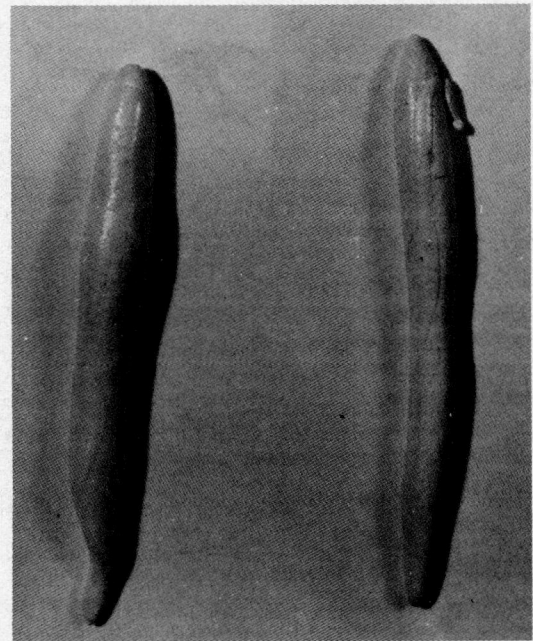

Fig. 25-6. After complete and proper mixing, two rolls, approximating length of wound, are formed.

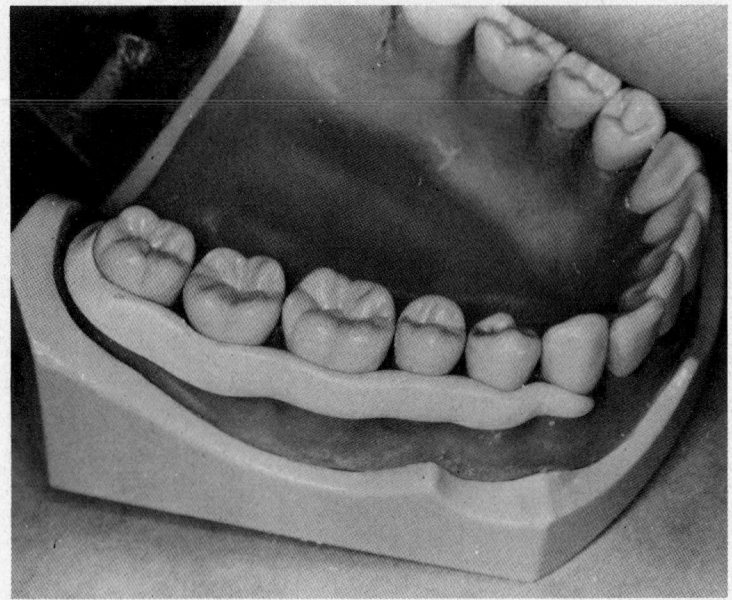

Fig. 25-7. One roll is applied to buccal surface, being wrapped around distal-most tooth and extending to most anterior tooth.

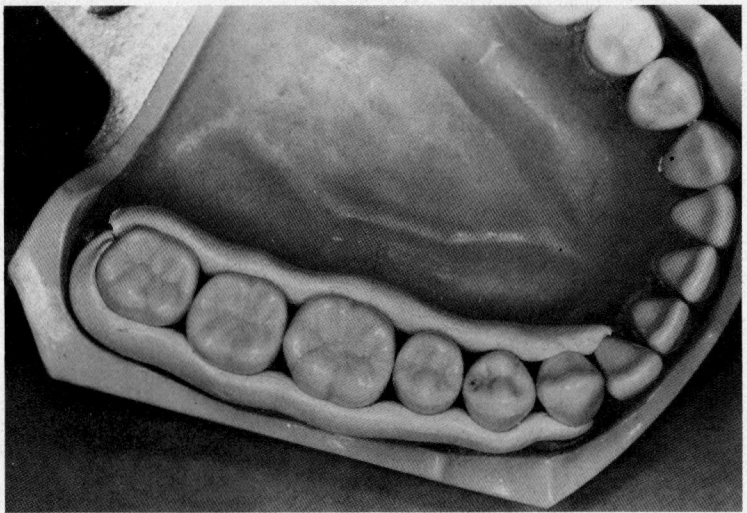

Fig. 25-8. Other roll is applied to lingual surface but is not yet adapted into interproximal areas.

against the wound site and flattening it against the teeth and the soft tissues. The dressing should be extended over the entire wound site up to the most anterior tooth that is involved (Fig. 25-7). Apply a separate roll of material to the opposite side of the involved area (Fig. 25-8). After placing the rolls of material so that they extend the entire length of the wound site, adapt the material to the teeth and gingiva, using a finger which has been wrapped with damp gauze (Fig. 25-9). Gen-

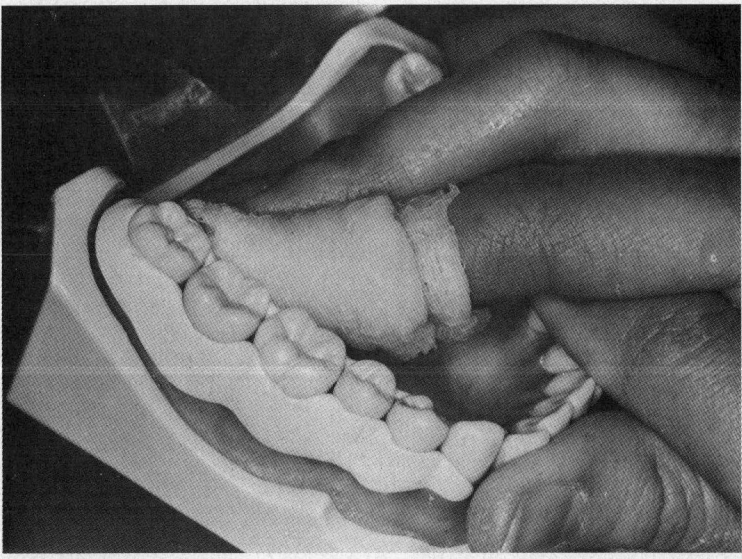

Fig. 25-9. Dressing is being adapted with damp gauze wrapped around clinician's finger. (Note: Under normal clinical circumstances gloves should always be worn.)

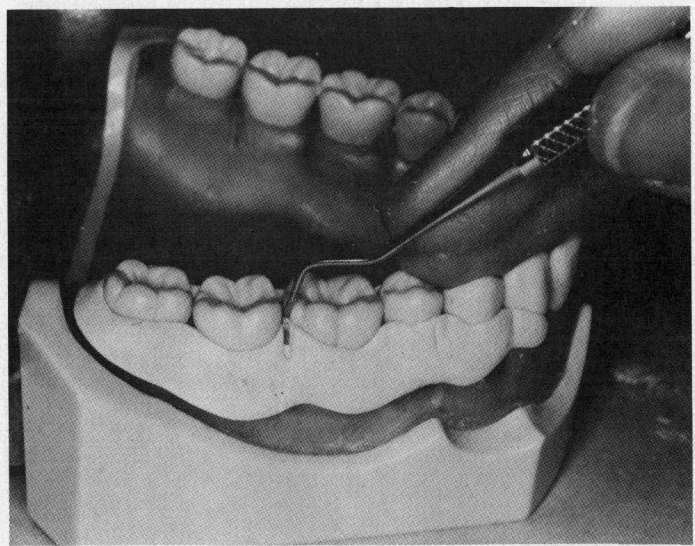

Fig. 25-10. Dressing is being pressed into interproximal areas with back of a curette.

tly compress and flatten the dressing against the teeth and periodontal tissues. Adapt the dressing further into the interproximal areas using the back of a curette or cotton pliers (Fig. 25-10). Adapt the dressing far enough into the interprox-imal areas so that the facial and lingual surfaces of the dressing are joined together, forming a mechanical lock between the dressing and the teeth. Even if the facial and lingual dressings do not join, the dressing still will form a mechan-

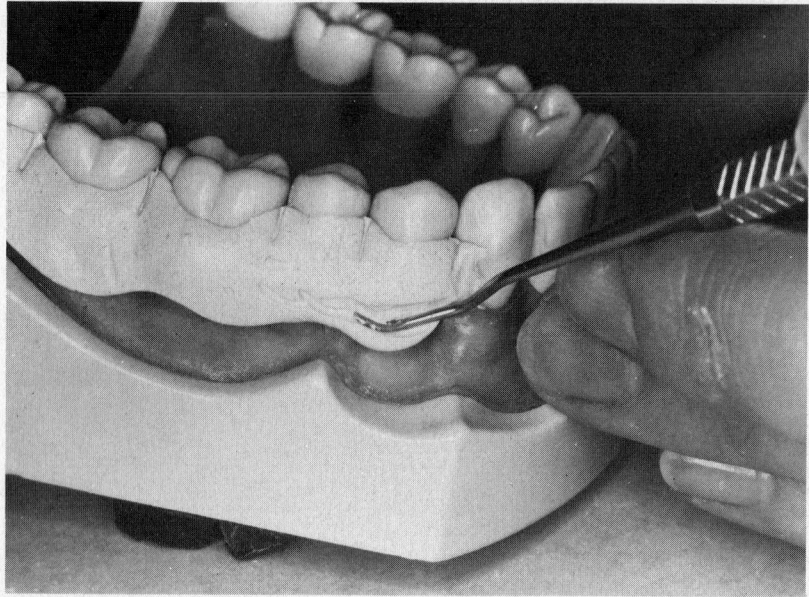

Fig. 25-11. Apical portion of pack is being trimmed by gently and firmly pressing curette into material and peeling away excess material.

ical lock in the embrasure areas between the teeth. This lock is important for retention of the dressing.

Muscle trimming and removing excess material

Careful molding of the periodontal dressing to the shape of the oral structures will permit the patient to perform normal activities without unnecessary interference or discomfort. Once the dressing material has hardened, it should not impinge on the oral musculature. One way of ensuring that this does not occur is to "muscle trim" the dressing by extending the patient's lips and cheeks over the dressing while it is still soft to identify where the dressing may interfere with muscle attachments. When the tissues are pulled against the apical margins of the dressing, the pressure of the soft tissues will cause the margin to fold occlusally in areas where the dressing interferes with muscle attachments or frenula. The clinician can see where this occurs and trim away the excess material until the interference is eliminated. Curettes can be used to trim excess dressing carefully away from soft tissues. The finished dressing

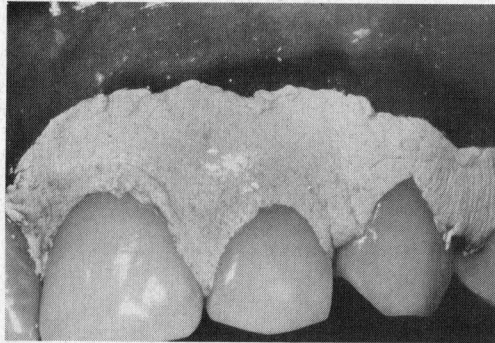

Fig. 25-12. Properly placed, adapted, and smoothed periodontal dressing. It has been muscle molded and trimmed so that none of the material impinges on soft tissue.

should extend occlusally no more than the middle third of the teeth and should not interfere with normal occlusion. Dressing material that is present on occlusal surfaces or is contacted by opposing teeth when occluded must be removed (Fig. 25-11). The clinician must remember that after the dressing hardens it will be very brittle and may irritate soft tissue or break apart if it has

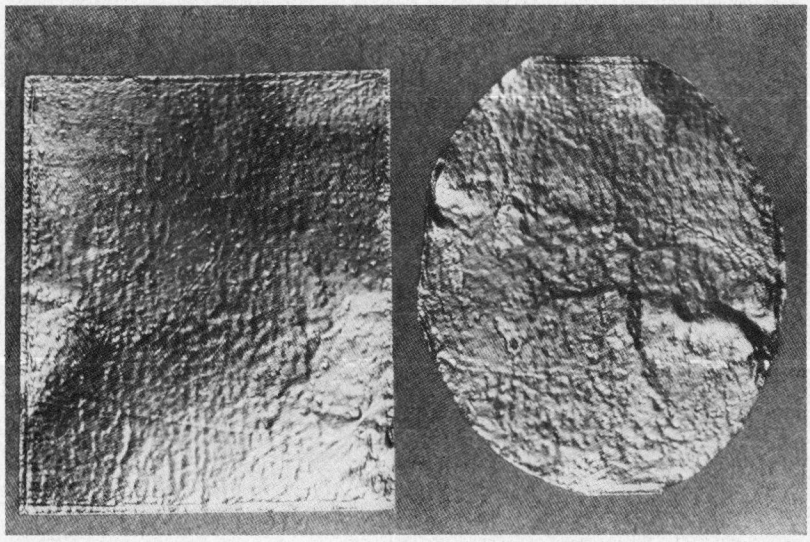

Fig. 25-13. Dry foil on left is as manufacturer supplies it. The foil on right is trimmed and ready to be applied.

not been properly adapted and trimmed. Every effort must be made to provide the patient with a well-contoured, smooth periodontal dressing that is as unobtrusive as possible (Fig. 25-12).

Applying dry foil

Dry foil is a specially treated paper that looks like a small rectangle of aluminum foil (Fig. 25-13). On its nonshiny side, it has an adhesive that can adhere to the periodontal dressing and teeth. The dry foil protects the outer surface of the dressing while it hardens by preventing food and other debris from becoming impregnated into the soft periodontal dressing material, and it helps hold the dressing in place (Fig. 25-14) (Valentine, 1976; Nelson et al, 1977; Grant et al, 1988). Dry foil also can be placed between composite restorations of teeth and dressings to protect the restorations from deterioration (softening) caused by the components of dressing materials (Watts and Combe, 1981). The dry foil can be removed from the dressing several hours after it has been placed; the clinician can instruct the patient how to remove the foil by peeling it away from the hardened dressing. Placing dry foil over the soft dressing is not essential or crucial to the success of the dressing. A dressing will usually harden and remain on

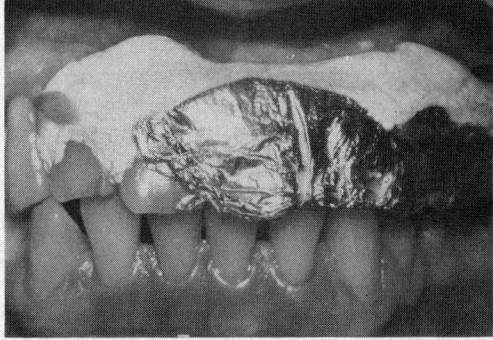

Fig. 25-14. This dry foil had been properly applied; use of foil in anterior is unusual, since it is not esthetically pleasing.

the teeth as long as necessary without the application of dry foil to protect it.

Evaluating the dressing

Evaluate the placement and adaptation of the dressing according to the criteria presented and summarized on page 504 at the end of this chapter. If any of the criteria is not met, the clinician should modify the dressing to meet these criteria. In most instances there is ample working time to modify or add to the dressing as needed. Some types of dressings, however, set very quickly after being exposed to air and moisture; they must be adapted very quickly before they become hard and brittle. Consult the manufacturer's directions for the exact amount of working time for each type of dressing material.

Patient instructions

After placing the dressing, instruct the patient about care of the dressing and oral hygiene procedures. Also provide complete written instructions that can be referred to at home (Fig. 25-15). The patient should be cautioned that the dressing will gradually harden and that care should be taken not to dislodge it within the first few hours. The patient should be advised to avoid eating or drinking within the first hour or until the dressing has hardened. Tart or spicy foods should be avoided immediately after surgery. If the dressing is brushed, it should be done very gently and only with a soft toothbrush. The patient should rinse the mouth thoroughly after eating and can brush and floss the other areas of the mouth, including careful brushing of the occlusal surfaces, which are not covered by the dressing.

Provide the office phone number and tell the

Date: _____ March 1, 1988 _____

Dear: _____ Mr. Philips _____

A periodontal dressing has been placed to protect your gums while they heal. The dressing should remain in place until your next appointment. A few instructions are listed below to help you care for your mouth while the dressing is in place.

1. Avoid eating, drinking or rinsing for the next hour. Avoid the following foods until the dressing has hardened completely (next 3 hours): hard foods (e.g., pretzels), sharp foods (e.g., potato chips), sticky foods (e.g., toffee), or spicy foods (e.g., pizza).
2. Avoid rinsing for the rest of the day. After that you may rinse your mouth with warm water or warm saltwater four or more times a day.
3. You may notice some bloodstains in your saliva for 4 to 5 hours. This is not unusual and will correct itself. If there is considerable bleeding, however, it can usually be stopped by applying pressure against both sides of the dressing with a gauze square in the area where the bleeding is originating. Apply firm pressure for 20 minutes. If the bleeding has not stopped after 20 minutes or if it becomes worse, please call the office for instructions. **Do not try to stop the bleeding by rinsing.**
4. Swelling is not unusual and will usually subside in 3 to 4 days. If it does become painful, however, or appears to worsen, please call the office.
5. To keep the dressing clean you can wipe it with moist gauze or cotton or brush it **gently** with a soft toothbrush. The rest of the areas of your mouth can be brushed and flossed as usual. **BE CAREFUL NOT TO DISLODGE THE DRESSING WHILE CLEANING THE MOUTH.**
6. Do not be concerned if pieces of the pack break off. It is not necessary to call us unless sharp edges are left to irritate your tongue or cheeks.
7. If the pack becomes dislodged from the area during the first 2 days after your surgery, please call the office. If it has been more than 2 days, there is probably no need to replace it unless you are experiencing significant discomfort. Simply rinse all fragments of the pack from your mouth and clean the tissues gently until your next appointment. Do not try to replace a dislodged dressing yourself.
8. Avoid smoking. The heat and smoke will irritate your gums and interfere with healing.
9. Be sure to return to the office for your follow-up appointment on _____.
   If you have any questions, please call the office at _____.

Fig. 25-15. Sample patient instruction sheet.

patient to call if an emergency arises. There may be some slight oozing of blood from the surgical area. Oozing is considered normal, but profuse bleeding should be reported. The patient should be given an appointment to return to the office in 3 to 5 days to have the dressing removed and the tissue evaluated. In some instances, depending on the type of surgery and the progress of healing, the dressing may be replaced for an additional period of time.

Alternative dressing procedures

A modification of the technique for placing the dressing is necessary for edentulous areas between teeth and for isolated or widely separated teeth. If only a few teeth are missing in an area and the dressing cannot be retained there, tie a loop of dental floss around the existing teeth to bridge the open space. The dressing can then be applied against the floss and retained more easily. When single isolated teeth are present in the arch or groups of teeth are widely separated, place a strip of dressing material around each tooth or group of teeth rather than trying to bridge a wide area with floss. If dressing material will not ad-

here around an isolated tooth, tie a small strip of gauze around the cervical area of the tooth and then apply the dressing to the area (Carranza and Perry, 1986).

Mixing a zinc oxide–eugenol dressing

The technique for mixing a zinc oxide–eugenol dressing is shown in Figs. 25–16 and 25–17. The material is usually mixed on a waxed pad with a tongue blade, but if a large amount of material is to be mixed, a piece of waxed paper taped to a counter can be used. Follow the manufacturer's directions, which usually require that the powder be gradually incorporated into the liquid to form a thick paste. The consistency must be very thick; if additional powder is needed, it is added by kneading it into the paste. When the mix has been completed, the dressing is placed as previously described.

Manipulation of a premixed dressing

Manipulation of a premixed dressing should be done according to the manufacturer's directions. Usually, the desired amount of material is removed from the container with a sterile tongue

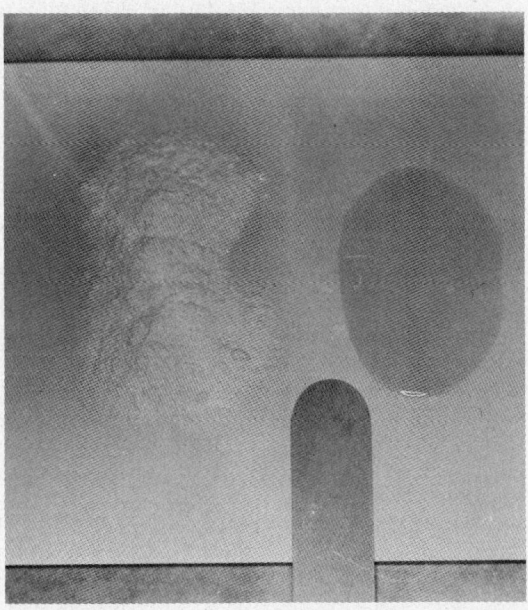

Fig. 25-16. Zinc oxide–eugenol powder and liquid placed on pad before mixing.

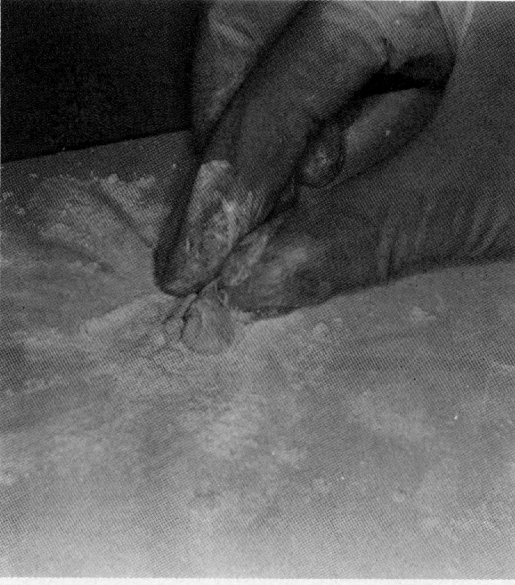

Fig. 25-17. After being mixed with tongue blade, material is being kneaded to incorporate more powder.

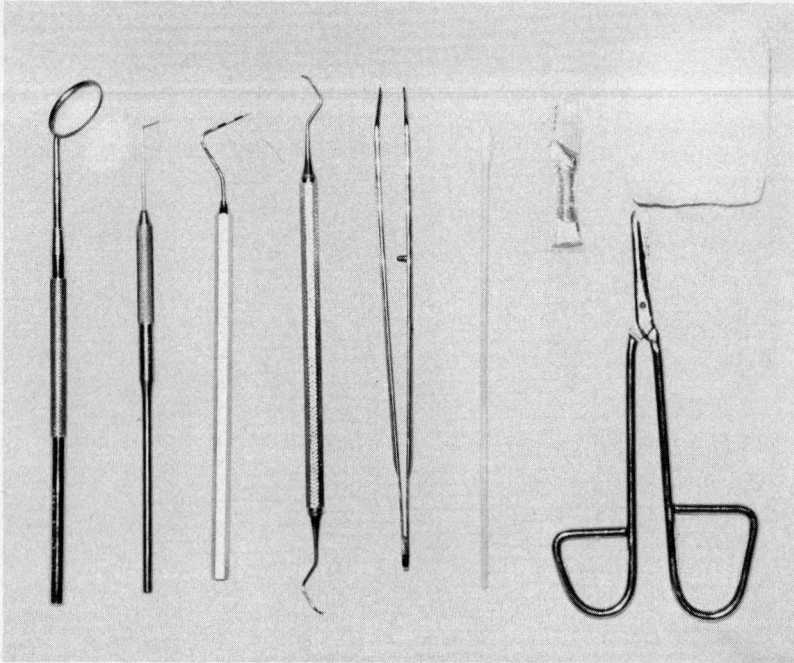

Fig. 25-18. Tray setup for removal of periodontal pack and sutures. Note that suture scissors have a curved blade to reach suture without harming tissue.

blade and placed on a waxed mixing pad. The material can be formed into two strips of the desired diameter and length and applied as described previously.

REMOVAL OF A PERIODONTAL DRESSING (FIG. 25-18)
Loosening the dressing

If foil is present, loosen and remove it with an explorer (Fig. 25-19). Then gently loosen the dressing from the soft tissues with a pair of college pliers and a curette (Figs. 25-20 and 25-21). After the dressing has been loosened sufficiently, lift it away from the wound site (Fig. 25-22). The dressing often can be removed as one solid strip (Fig. 25-23). Remove large pieces of excess dressing from the teeth using a curette, being careful not to traumatize tender soft tissues and newly exposed root surfaces (Fig. 25-24). Rinse the area gently with sterile saline or with an oxygenating solution (e.g., Glyoxide*) to cleanse it

*Marian Labs, Inc., Kansas City, MO.

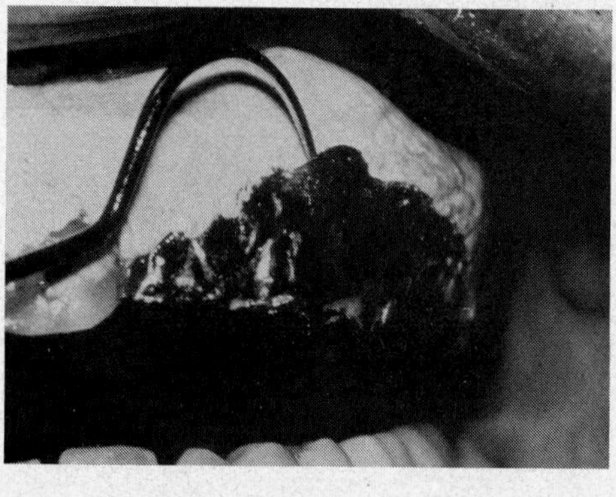

Fig. 25-19. Dry foil is loosened with an explorer and removed.

of surface debris (Figs. 25-25 and 25-26). Special care is needed to remove a dressing placed over a sutured area. Instructions for this procedure are discussed in the following section.

After the dressing has been removed, inspect the wound site to evaluate the healing that has taken place. Gently rinse away plaque and other

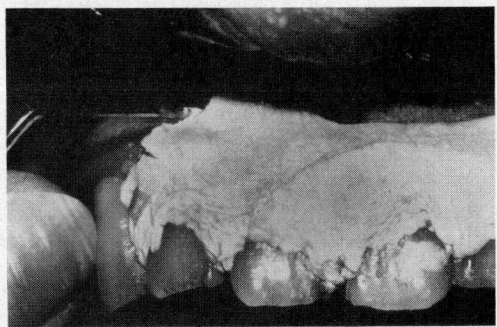

Fig. 25-20. Pack is loosened with a curette.

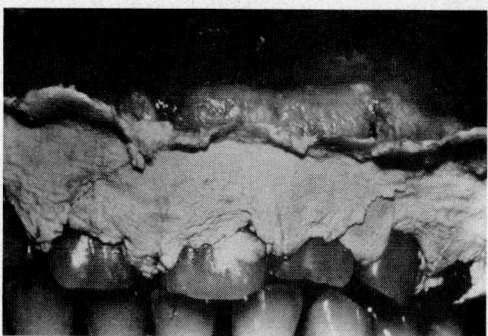

Fig. 25-21. Loosened dressing.

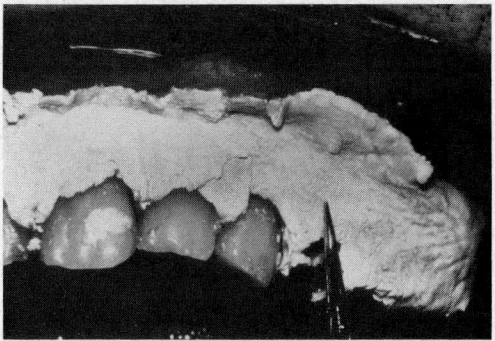

Fig. 25-22. Pack is lifted off wound with college pliers.

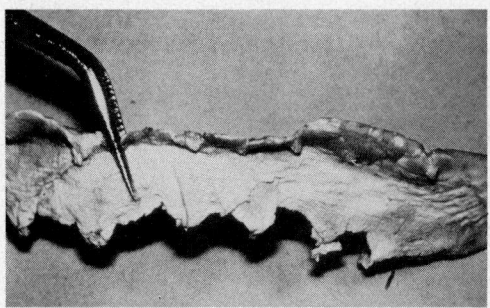

Fig. 25-23. Pack in one piece after removal.

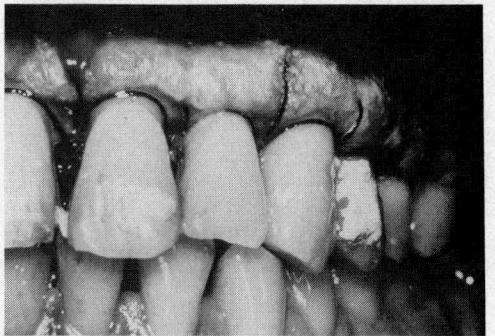

Fig. 25-24. Some large pieces of dressing remain on teeth. Pieces should be removed gently with a curette.

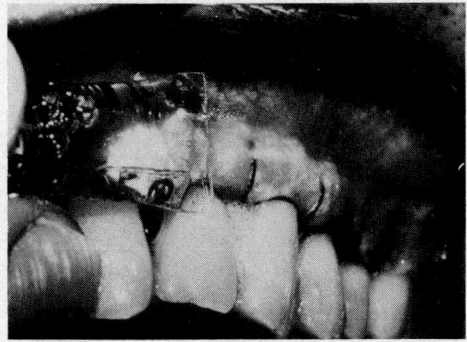

Fig. 25-25. Area is rinsed with oxygenating agent.

debris that is present so the tissue can be viewed carefully. After a period of 5 to 7 days, the tissues should show evidence of epithelialization and healing. If the tissues appear unusually red or inflamed or if exudate is present, examine and ex-

plore the teeth for the presence of plaque and calculus. Remove calculus with a curette. Based on the dentist's evaluation, another dressing may be needed until satisfactory wound healing has occurred. Root surfaces that have been newly ex-

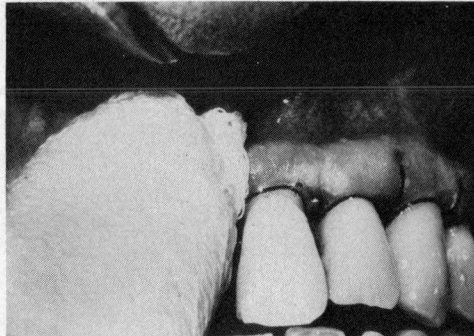

Fig. 25-26. Damp gauze can be used to cleanse area gently of small pieces of dressing and debris.

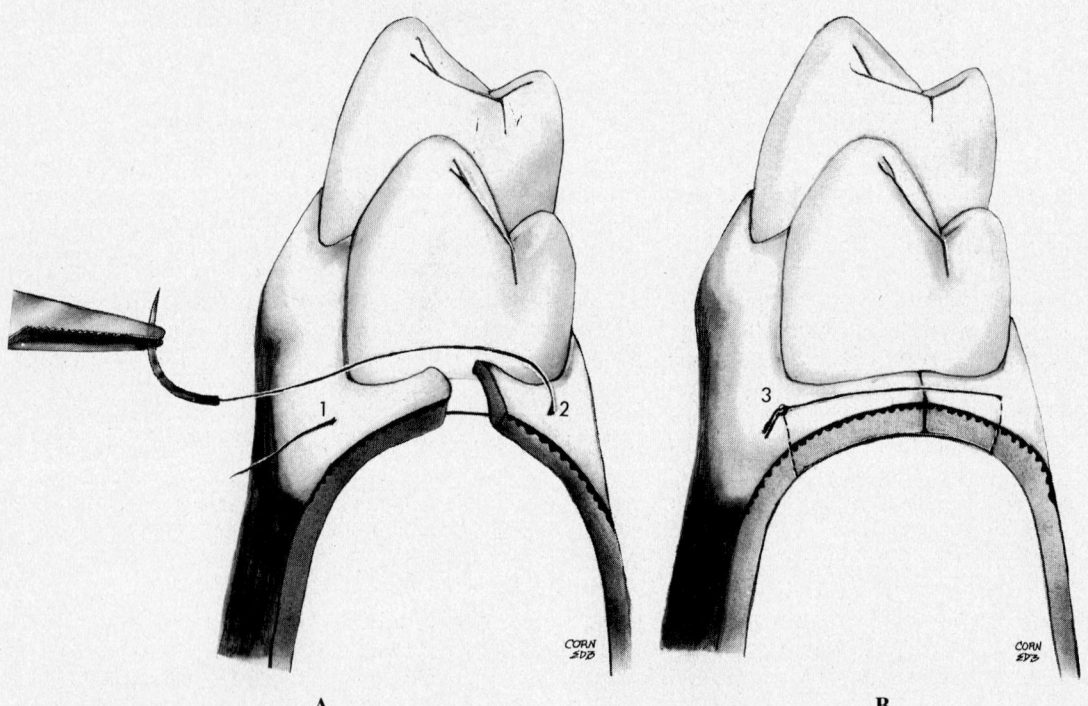

A   B

Fig. 25-27. Placement of interrupted suture with a curved, swaged needle, **A,** Suture penetrates *(1)* facial aspect of buccal flap, enters connective tissue of lingual flap, and *(2)* exits lingual flap. **B,** Suture is carried to facial aspect and tied *(3)*.
(From Goldman HC and Cohen DW: Periodontal therapy, ed 6. St. Louis, 1980, The CV Mosby Co.)

posed due to shrinkage of soft tissues may be sensitive to tactile or thermal stimuli. Therefore, use compressed air on these surfaces with great care (Carranza and Perry, 1986; Goldman and Cohen, 1980).

REMOVAL OF SUTURES

Sutures are used after most surgical procedures to reapproximate (secure together) the soft tissues and to promote healing. A variety of absorbable and nonabsorbable suture materials are available.

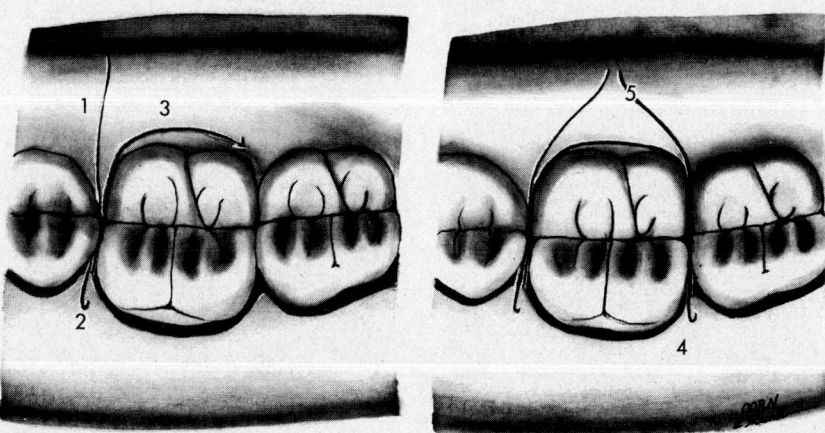

Fig. 25-28. Placement of continuous sling suture to reapproximate buccal tissue. *1,* Needle passes through interdental space from lingual aspect without penetrating tissue and leaves a tail of suture; *2,* buccal tissue is penetrated, and needle passes under contact without entering lingual tissue; *3,* suture is carried around lingual aspect of tooth; *4,* needle penetrates buccal tissue; *5,* suture is knotted on lingual aspect.
(From Goldman HC and Cohen DW: Periodontal therapy, ed 6. St. Louis, 1980, The CV Mosby Co.)

The absorbable sutures include surgical gut, collagen, polyglycolic acid, and polyglactin acid; the nonabsorbable materials are silk, nylon, polypropylene, silver wire and mersilene (Chung and Weinberg, 1978; Goldman and Cohen, 1980). Black silk suture material is the most popular for periodontal surgery because of its easy manipulation, durability, and strength.

The suture material can be threaded through a needle by the clinician, or it may come already attached (swaged) to the needle by the manufacturer (Fig. 25-27). Swaged needles are more popular among dentists and dental specialists. Most of the needles used in dentistry are curved to allow safe, easy manipulation.

Types of sutures

A variety of suture patterns, including interrupted, sling, continuous sling, and simple mattress patterns, are used to reapproximate tissues following surgical procedures. The surgeon selects the type of suture based on the type of surgical procedure, healing considerations, and the desired goal of treatment. It is important for the person who is to remove the sutures to know the type of suture placed, the suturing pattern, the number

of knots, and the location of the knots. Thus it is helpful if the clinician who places the sutures indicates this information in the chart. Figs. 25-27 through 25-29 illustrate and describe three types of commonly used sutures: interrupted, sling, and continuous sling. Note the pattern of the sutures and the location of the knot. Additional suture patterns are shown in a number of textbooks of periodontology.

Principles for removing sutures

Removing sutures is a relatively simple procedure, but a few basic principles must be observed. The knot must *never* be pulled through the tissue. Instead, cut the suture so that the knot is pulled *away* from the tissue (Fig. 25-31). When removing the suture, avoid passing through soft tissues suture material that has been exposed to the oral cavity and may be contaminated by plaque or other oral bacteria and oral debris. Be certain that all of the suture material and knots are accounted for after the removal procedure. Figs. 25-30 through 25-32 illustrate and describe the correct technique for removal of interrupted and sling sutures.

When removing a dressing that has been placed

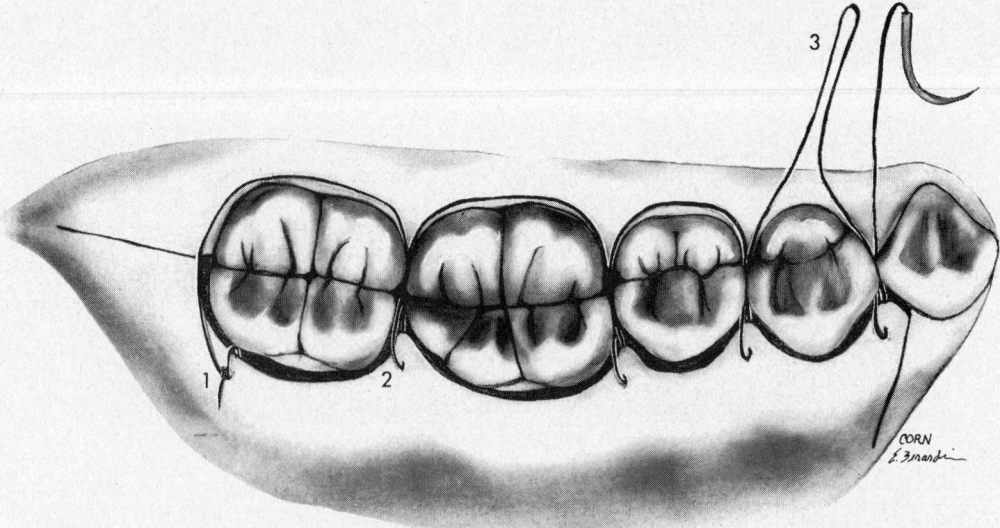

Fig. 25-29. Placement of continuous sling suture to reapproximate lingual tissue. *1,* Loose loop of suture material is tied to ease suture removal; *2,* sling sutures are placed as in Fig. 25-28; *3,* final knot is tied with loop of lingual suture material.
(From Goldman HC and Cohen DW: Periodontal therapy, ed 6. St. Louis, 1980, The CV Mosby Co.)

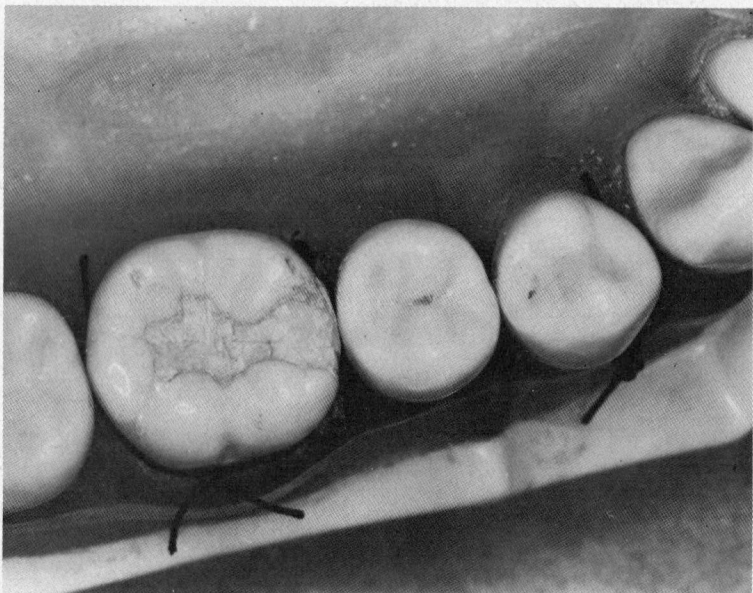

Fig. 25-30. Sling suture to reapproximate lingual tissue around molar and interrupted suture mesial to premolar are ready to be removed.

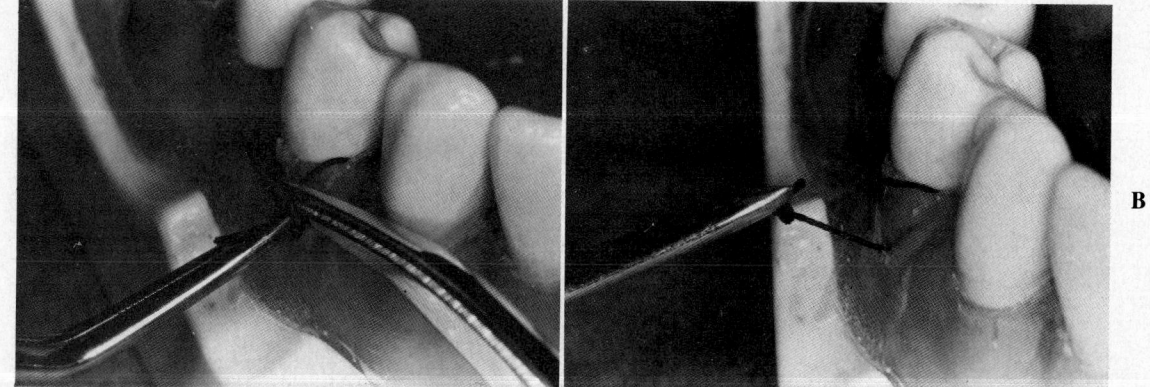

Fig. 25-31. Removal of interrupted suture. **A,** Knot is grasped with cotton pliers, pulled away from tissue, and cut with scissors. **B,** Suture is pulled out of tissue.

Fig. 25-32. Removal of sling suture. Buccal knot was cut first. **A,** Lingual portions of suture entering tissue are cut. **B,** Loose interproximal suture is removed. **C,** Lingual loop is removed.

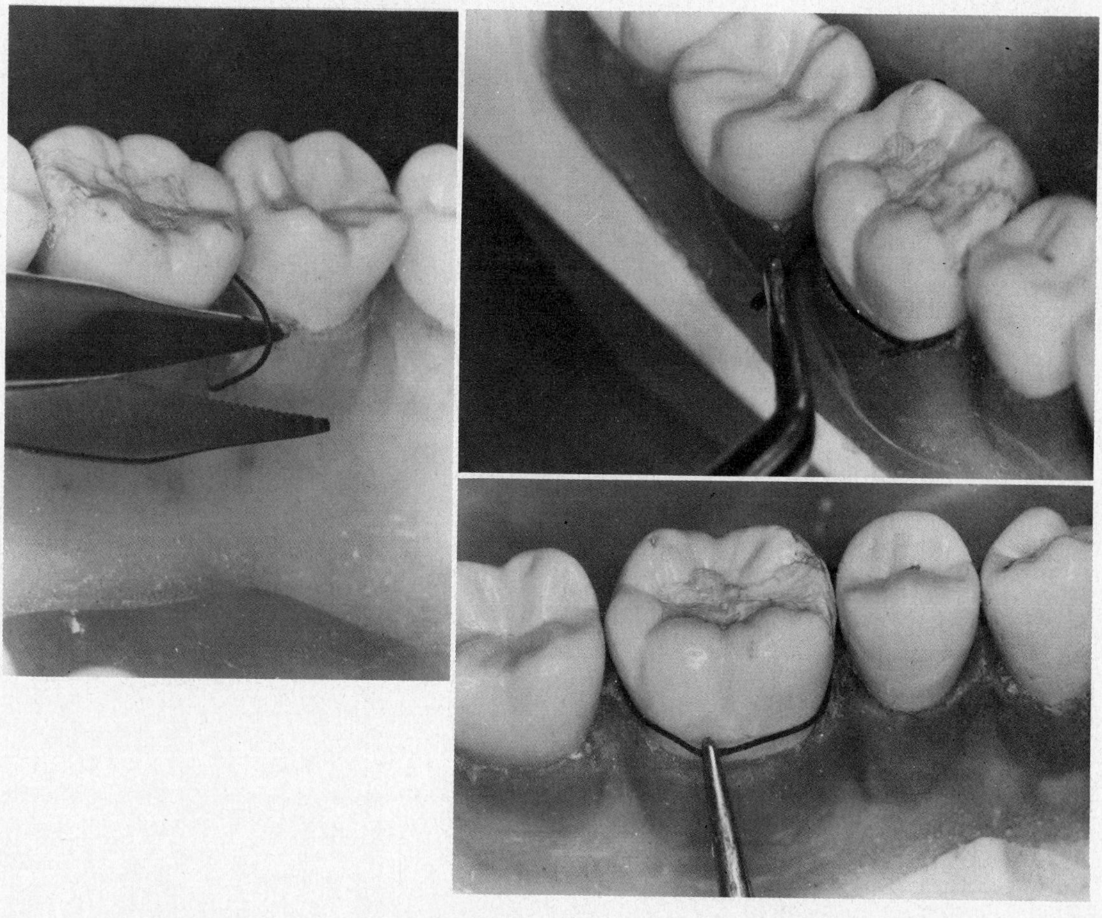

Placement and removal of periodontal packs

Suggested check-off sheet

Mark S for satisfactory completion or U for unsatisfactory completion of each criterion in the appropriate space.

PERFORMANCE CRITERIA	FACULTY	STUDENT
1. Assemble the necessary armamentarium		
2. Mix the pack according to the manufacturer's directions		
3. Shape the pack into two rolls, each the length of the site and two-thirds the diameter of a pencil		
Placement of the pack		
4. Gently adapt the pack to the area with gloved fingers and damp gauze		
5. Adapt the pack interproximally with a curette or cotton pliers		
6. Muscle mold and trim the pack		
7. Smooth the pack		
8. Produce a pack that		
a. Extends to the middle third of the tooth but not onto the occluding surfaces		
b. Extends beyond all margins of the wound		
c. Does not interfere with normal function		
Removing the pack		
9. Remove the dry foil if still present		
10. Loosen the lingual and buccal packs		
11. Remove the lingual pack		
12. Cut sutures from the lingual portion if necessary		
13. Remove the buccal pack		
14. Cleanse the area with an oxygenating agent		
15. Remove remaining sutures if necessary		
16. Recleanse the area		
17. Gently remove any calculus or granulation tissue		
18. Evaluate healing of the wound site		

---

over sutures, the clinician should be aware of the possibility that the suture material may have become incorporated into the hardened dressing. Under these circumstances, remove the lingual portion of the dressing first. This recommendation is due to the fact that sutures are usually knotted on the facial surfaces of the wound site rather than on the lingual surfaces. If the knots have become incorporated within the hardened dressing, the suture should then be cut from the exposed lingual surfaces and the suture material and knots can be removed along with the facial aspect of the pack. After the dressing and sutures are removed, cleanse the area and evaluate the tissue as described previously.

Hygienists may be called upon to place and remove periodontal dressings following procedures that they perform (e.g., curettage) or as an expanded periodontal function in the dental or periodontal practice. Removing sutures is another procedure that the hygienist can perform competently as a member of the dental team. A knowledge of the skills required to perform these functions will help the dental hygienist assume additional responsibilities related to the treatment of periodontal disease (see box on page 504).

ACTIVITIES

1. Place and remove a periodontal dressing in one or more of the following situations:
   a. For a partner
   b. On a typodont with missing teeth
   c. On a typodont with sutures placed
2. Conduct a panel discussion with periodontists and/or dentists from your area on the subject "The need for periodontal dressings."
3. Prepare a table clinic on how to place and remove a periodontal pack.
4. Prepare a review of the literature for any of the types of periodontal dressings.
5. Prepare a presentation about the various suture techniques and the techniques for removing each type.
6. Observe periodontal surgery, suturing, and postsurgical care in a periodontist's office.
7. After having a periodontal dressing placed in your mouth by a fellow student, leave it on until the next day and keep a diary of how it affected your comfort and your ability to eat, talk, and perform oral hygiene procedures.
8. Compile a list of characteristics of an "ideal" periodontal dressing.

REVIEW QUESTIONS

1. List the purposes of periodontal dressings.
2. Which type of periodontal dressing, eugenol or non-eugenol, would most likely be placed after a soft tissue curettage procedure?
3. After a pack has been placed on a surgical site, the patient asks how to care for the pack. Briefly outline the directions to be given to the patient.
4. Describe how to remove sutures that have become embedded in the pack.
5. What reasons have been cited for not placing a periodontal dressing as a routine postsurgical procedure?

REFERENCES

ADA Council on Dental Therapeutics: Accepted dental therapeutics, ed 40. Chicago, 1984, American Dental Association.

Addy M, and Dolby AE: The use of chlorhexidine mouthwash compared with a periodontal dressing following the gingivectomy procedure, J Clin Periodontol 3:59, 1976.

Addy M, et al: A chlorhexidine-containing methacrylic gel as a periodontal dressing, J Periodontol 46:465, 1975.

Allen DR, and Caffesse RG: Comparison of results following modified Widman flap surgery with and without surgical dressing, J Periodontol 54:470, 1983.

Baer PN, et al: Periodontal dressings, Dent Clin North Am 13:181, 1969.

Bakdash MB: Asbestos in periodontal dressings, a possible health hazard, Quintessence Int 7:61, 1976.

Barkin ME: Acute allergic reaction to eugenol, Oral Surg 57:441, 1984.

Blanque RH: Fundamentals and technique of surgical periodontal packing, J Periodontol 33:346, 1962.

Carranza FE: Glickman's clinical periodontology, ed. 6. Philadelphia, 1984, WB Saunders Co.

Carranza FE, and Perry DA: Clinical periodontology for the dental hygienist. Philadelphia, 1986, WB Saunders.

Chung H, and Weinberg S: Suture materials in oral surgery: a review, Oral Health 68(10):31, 1978.

Dahlberg WH: Incisions and suturing: some basic considerations about each in periodontal flap surgery, Dent Clin North Am 13:149, 1969.

Forrest JO: The use of cyanoacrylates in periodontal surgery, J Periodontol 45:225, 1974.

Frisch L, and Bhaskar SN: Tissue response to eugenol-containing periodontal dressings, J Periodontol 38:402, 1967.

Geiger B, et al: Periodontal dressings: rationale and procedures, Dent Hyg 55(9):21, 1981.

Goldman HC, and Cohen DW: Periodontal therapy, ed 6, St Louis, 1980, The CV Mosby Co.

Grant DA, Stern IV, and Everett FG: Periodontics in the tradition of Orban and Gottlieb, St Louis, 1988, The CV Mosby Co.

Greensmith AL, and Wade AB: Dressing after reverse bevel flap procedures, J Clin Periodontol 1:97, 1974.

Haugen E: The effect of periodontal dressings on intact mucous membrane and on wound healing, Acta Odontol Scand 38:363, 1980.

Haugen E, and Gjermo P: Clinical assessment of periodontal dressings, J Clin Periodontol 5:50, 1978.

Haugen E, and Mjor I: Bone tissue reactions to periodontal dressings, J Periodont Res 14:76, 1979.

Haugen E, et al: Some antibacterial properties of periodontal dressings, J Clin Periodontol 4:62, 1977.

Haugen E, et al: The sensitizing potential of periodontal dressings, J Dent Res 57:950, 1978.

Heaney FG, and Appleton J: The effect of periodontal dressings on the healthy periodontium, J Clin Periodontol 3:66, 1976.

Jones TM, and Cassingham RJ: Comparison of healing following periodontal surgery with and without dressings in humans, J Periodontol 50:387, 1979.

Levin MP: Periodontal suture materials and surgical dressings, Dent Clin North Am 24:767, 1980.

Levin MP, et al: Cyanoacrylate as a periodontal dressing, J Oral Med 30:40, 1975.

Lysell L: Contact allergy to rosin in a periodontal dressing, J Oral Med 31:24, 1976.

McGraw VA, and Caffesse RG: Cyanoacrylates in periodontics, Periodont Abstr 26(1):4, 1978.

Macht SD, and Krizek TJ: Sutures and suturing—current concepts, J Oral Surg 36:710, 1978.

Manor A, et al: Unusual foreign body reaction to a braided silk suture: a case report, J Periodontol 53:868, 1982.

Nelson EH, et al: A comparison of the continuous and interrupted suturing techniques, J Periodontol 48:273, 1977.

Ochstein AJ, et al: A comparative study of cyanoacrylate and other periodontal dressings on gingival surgical wound healing, J Periodontol 40:515, 1969.

O'Neill TC: Antibacterial properties of periodontal dressings, J Periodontol 46:469, 1975.

Pihlstrom BL, et al: The effect of periodontal dressing on supragingival microorganisms, J Periodontol 48:440, 1977.

Pluss EM, et al: Effect of chlorhexidine on dental plaque formation under periodontal pack, J Clin Periodontol 2:136, 1975.

Poulson RC: An anaphylactoid reaction to periodontal surgical dressing: report of case, JADA 89:895, 1974.

Sachs HA, et al: Current status of periodontal dressings, J Periodontol 55:689, 1984.

Stahl SS, et al: The effects of periodontal dressings on gingival repair, J Periodontol 40:34, 1969.

Stroh C, and Chinn SA: Periodontal dressings. Seattle, 1976, University of Washington.

Valentine RM: Expanded duties: a self-determined pace laboratory program, Philadelphia, 1976, University of Pennsylvania.

Wampole HS, et al: The incidence of transient bacteremia during periodontal dressing change, J Periodontol 49:462, 1978.

Watts TLP, and Combe EC: Periodontal dressing materials, J Clin Periodontol 6:3, 1979.

Watts TLP, and Combe EC: Effects of noneugenol periodontal dressing materials upon the surface hardness of anterior restorative materials in vitro, Br Dent J 151:423, 1981.

26 POLISHING THE TEETH

OBJECTIVES: *The reader will be able to*

1. Recognize the categories of tooth discolorations or stains.
2. Given a dental stain, identify whether it is intrinsic or extrinsic.
3. Explain to a patient the role of polishing in esthetics and in disease prevention.
4. Explain the function of abrasives in toothpaste and in professional polishing pastes.
5. Describe the advantages and disadvantages of the following:
   a. Porte polishing
   b. Engine polishing
   c. Air-powder polishing
6. Describe ways to minimize frictional heat during engine polishing.
7. Polish stains from teeth using a porte polisher, engine polishing, and air-powder polishing.

Following scaling, root planing, and other necessary periodontal procedures, the teeth should be evaluated for stain. If the dental hygienist involves the patient in removing plaque and food debris with a brush and floss at the beginning of each appointment, it should not be necessary to polish the teeth to remove plaque. Stain that cannot be removed by the patient is the primary factor that determines the need for polishing.

In deciding which teeth to polish and the necessary materials for the polishing procedure, it is important to evaluate the stains present on the teeth and the abrasives and mechanical devices available for optimal use.

The important aspect of dental staining to the patient is the appearance of the teeth. While the patient tends to focus on the color and appearance of the teeth, the dental professional is more concerned with the health of the tissues and teeth as affected by stains and deposits. Dental stains may be associated with deposits that are related to caries and gingival problems, but typically they are a relatively harmless nuisance. They can, however, be used to help motivate patients to improve their oral hygiene if the patients are more concerned about esthetics than disease. In an attempt to achieve a whiter and brighter appearance of the teeth, the patient may practice better toothbrushing and, with this, the cleaning of critical gingival areas.

Most dental hygienists have learned to polish all tooth surfaces after a scaling procedure, regardless of the presence of plaque or stain. It has traditionally been viewed as the finishing procedure of the oral prophylaxis, receiving good acceptance among patients because it makes the teeth feel uniformly smooth and clean (Hunter et al, 1981).

Over the past several years the concept of "selective polishing" has been discussed as a logical alternative to polishing all teeth (Primosch, 1980; Rohleder and Slim, 1981). The rationale is partly to ensure that the patient realizes his or her role in maintaining oral cleanliness and partly to minimize polishing away the fluoride-rich outer layer of enamel (Mellberg, 1977; Retief et al, 1980; Shern et al, 1977). As studies have shown that polishing does not improve the uptake of professionally applied fluoride in enamel, the prime clinical reason for polishing all surfaces has been cast in doubt (Tinanoff et al, 1974; Steele et al, 1982). In addition, polishing and hand planing over years of routine care changes the morphology of the teeth (Swan, 1970). This makes the assumption of a complete polish of all teeth at every recall even more questionable.

Polishing procedures create minute scratches that typically are not visible at 25X power but are noticeable at 200X. The deepest scratches appear to be caused by the edge of the rubber cup as it contacts prominences in the tooth and strikes the dentin at the necks of the teeth. However, the scratches appear to resolve themselves within 21 to 39 days; the mechanism of this resolution is unknown. The scratches tend not to accumulate more stain or calculus. The thin layer of enamel that is lost does not remove all the fluoride-rich surface, but a depth of at least 3 to 4 micrometers is disturbed. The clinical significance of this, in terms of increased caries susceptibility and vulnerability of the enamel, is not known (Christensen and Bangerter, 1987). Russ and colleagues reported a SEM stereoscopic technique to map surface contours that may help assess the effects of polishing on tooth structure (1986).

Polishing can have limited positive effects beyond creating a stain-free smile. One study showed that plaque reaccumulation after polishing was less than on teeth that had been polished when the subjects were not allowed to brush or floss for 3 days after a prophylaxis (Waring et al, 1982). Also, in one trial, orthodontic subjects whose teeth were polished monthly for 10 months and who received oral hygiene instructions experienced dramatic decreases in plaque and gingivitis (Huber et al, 1987). However, Walsh and others (1985b) determined that professional polishing after scaling, as would typically occur in a dental hygiene recall appointment, provides minimal additional benefit beyond scaling and cannot be considered as having great therapeutic benefit.

Ironically, although the relative wisdom of polishing has been debated extensively since the early 1980s, hygienists have tended to select coarse or medium abrasive polishing pastes, typically using pumice as the abrasive (Christensen, 1984). This may be due to a perceived need to remove stains thoroughly and quickly due to time constraints. To minimize such scratches, it may be wise to use a dentifrice rather than an abrasive paste and to use a moderate rather than light pressure so as to polish away the scratches (Tilliss and Hicks, 1987).

The clinical rationale for polishing or not polishing is being investigated, but the trend among hygienists is to turn to selective polishing to remove obvious stains and polish areas that "still feel fuzzy." The larger concern seems to be how to move the profession and the patient population away from expecting that all surfaces will be polished after every scaling or planing. Among hygienists, skepticism is high, partly because the change is a radical departure from how they learned to practice hygiene and have practiced it for years. This general attitude is clear among hygienists who attend continuing education courses where selective polishing is discussed. A second contributing factor is the reluctance of hygienists to introduce the change to their patients. After explaining how polishing causes no harm for years or decades, it is difficult now to explain that polishing is probably not very helpful and may be harmful.

One questionnaire showed that 83% of respondents preferred to have their teeth polished as a part of cleaning. However, these subjects apparently were not informed of the relative merits and demerits of polishing, and their preferences did not correlate strongly with their perceptions of how the polished or unpolished sides of their mouths felt after the procedure (Walsh et al, 1985a). Cross and Carr (1983) found that if the rationale was presented, patients readily accepted selective polishing. Patients should be given a choice regarding polishing once the rationale is explained. They can be moved gradually from a complete polishing to polishing only those areas that warrant use of an abrasive.

The following information about deposits should aid in assessing whether polishing should be selective or universal for a patient and what procedures should be followed.

DENTAL STAINS
Definitions and classifications

Staining or discoloration can occur in three ways: (1) it can adhere directly to tooth surfaces; (2) it can be contained within calculus and soft deposits; and (3) it can be incorporated in the tooth structure.

Discolorations are classified as either endogenous or exogenous (Carranza, 1979; Shaw and Murray, 1977; Vogel, 1975; Winter, Murray, and Shaw, 1978). *Endogenous* is the term used for stains that develop within the tooth. Usually these are dentin discolorations showing through enamel. *Exogenous* stains originate outside the tooth or the oral cavity. Within this classification, exogenous stains are further categorized on the basis of their ability to be removed. *Extrinsic* stains are on the exterior of the tooth and are removable by the individual or the dental professional. *Intrinsic* stains are of exogenous origin but become incorporated into the tooth structure and are not removable by the patient or by polishing and scaling.

Hereditary or genetic factors can affect both the primary and permanent dentitions. Genetic inheritance affects the size of the teeth, their shape, and their color. Therefore, some people have endogenously stained yellow or gray teeth because of family traits passed through generations. A clinician can do little to improve this situation; polishing is of no help. Dental procedures such as bonding of tooth-colored materials to the facial aspects of the teeth can improve an unesthetic appearance.

Endogenous stains can form as the tooth is developing due to medications that the mother takes during fetal growth or that the child takes. Tetracycline is one medication known to cause developmental stains. Excessive repeated intake of fluoride can discolor or mottle the teeth as they develop. Again, polishing has no effect; bonding can improve the problem.

Environmental endogenous stains can be caused by pathological incursions into the tooth, such as dental caries or pulp death due to trauma. Metallic stains from dental restorations or prolonged exposure to metals in the air or water are also possible. Stains caused by dental procedures (usually due to restorative materials, exposure of the dentin to bleeding, and other problems) are *iatrogenic stains*.

Environmental stains can also be exogenous— and therefore more likely to be removable. The stain is on the surface of the tooth. Typical *environmental exogenous* stains are from food, tobacco, tea, coffee, and airborne particles. Chlorhexidine, an agent sometimes recommended to help control plaque and gingivitis, causes brown staining interproximally and at the gingival margin within a few days' use for many people. See Table 26-1 for a list of extrinsic stains. Although many of these stains may be difficult to remove, polishing or scaling is usually effective.

Developmental or *congenital defects* are associated with several disease processes wherein the dental professional can be of value in consulting with the physician; however, little can be done by members of either profession to alleviate these dental defects. Another phase of problems in the developmental or congenital area deals with medications that are delivered to the mother and that affect the developing teeth in utero, or that are given to children during the formation of their primary or permanent dentition. Here the dental professional can be of much value when consulted for information, especially about compounds such as tetracyclines and fluorides.

Individuals vary widely in the rate and amount

Table 26-1. Extrinsic stains

Stain category	Primary tooth sites	Composition	Associated with
Green	Cervical one-third to one-half of labial surfaces of maxillary anterior teeth	Inorganic elements, chromogenic bacteria	Poor oral hygiene; surface irregularities; highest in children
Black-line	Thin band along gingival margin of lingual and buccal surfaces	Ferric sulfide	Iron in saliva, gingival fluid; plaque or bacteria; all ages
Orange	Thin line; cervical one-third of incisors	Chromogenic bacteria	Poor oral hygiene; highest in children
Tobacco	Cervical one-third to one-half of lingual surfaces; pits and fissures	Tars, pigments	Smoking; chewing tobacco
Food	Same as above	Food colors	Consumption of tea, coffee, cola drinks, berries, spices, colored candies
Metallic	Cervical one-third; random surfaces	Associated with particular metals	Environmental, food, water
Drug, therapeutic	Plaque-associated areas	Plaque bacteria; tin; reactions with food colors	Extended antibiotic use, stannous fluoride, chlorhexidine

of *extrinsic* stain accumulation. Certain factors predispose a person to the accumulation of both dental deposits and stains; these include enamel roughness, salivary composition, salivary flow rates, and poor oral hygiene.

Extrinsic stains can be identified by color, distribution, and tenaciousness and by age, sex, home care, and other factors in which the preventive classification and the standard classification agree (Reid, Beeley, and MacDonald, 1977). The major colored stains are as follows:

Green stain. This occurs primarily in the cervical areas of the maxillary anterior teeth and is associated with the primary dental cuticle. It usually is crescent shaped, close to the gingiva, and colored light green to yellow-green to dark green. Usually green stain occurs when an individual practices poor oral hygiene, and it tends to recur after removal.

Black-line stain. This usually occurs as a continuous thin band along the gingival margin and follows the crestal contour on lingual or proximal surfaces. It occurs at all ages and is found more often in females. The primary cause of this deposit is iron compounds in saliva or gingival fluid that become embedded in plaque and/or plaque bacteria. This stain is a ferric sulfide compound (Reid, Beeley, and MacDonald, 1977).

Orange stain. This is fairly rare, occurring in approximately 3% of the population. It occurs usually at the cervical third of incisor teeth and is attributed to chromogenic bacteria.

All of the aforementioned colored stains occur more extensively if home care is inadequate. Professional scaling and prophylaxis will remove these stains easily, but there is a tendency for recurrence.

Tobacco stain. This tooth discoloration ranges in appearance from tan to dark brown or black and covers approximately the cervical one-third to one-half of most teeth. It occurs mostly on lingual surfaces. It is also commonly found in pits and fissures and other irregularities of enamel. Tobacco staining is directly proportional to the number of cigarettes smoked per day (Ness, Rosekrans, and Welford, 1977) (Table 26-2). Staining is also high in individuals who chew tobacco. Tobacco stains may penetrate enamel and become intrinsic.

Food stain. This is a common stain in individuals who consume large quantities of coffee and tea. Other categories of colored food that may contribute to stain include cola drinks, berries such as raspberries and blueberries, spices, and licorice and other colored candies. Stains resulting from ingestion of these

Table 26-2. Effect of smoking on extrinsic stain

Number of cigarettes per day	Percent with moderate to severe stain
0	18
1 to 10	35
11 to 20	51
>20	78

Modified from Ness L, Rosekrans DdeL, and Welford JF: Community Dent Oral Epidemiol **5:**55, 1977.

foods range from tan to dark brown in color and occur over broad tooth surfaces and in pits and fissures.

Metallic stains. These vary in color depending on the metal or metallic salt ingested. Green or blue-green colors result from copper or brass, whereas brown colors may result from an ingestion of materials or dust particles containing iron. While the majority of these stains have been attributed to industrial dust, it is possible to ingest high quantities of metals in various foods and/or water.

Stains due to drug and/or therapeutic agents. These stains can originate from many sources, only a few of which are described here. After extended topical or systemic antibiotic use, or in studies of antibacterial agents with antiplaque activity, surface discolorations and staining have occurred (Moffit et al, 1974; Solheim, Erikson, and Nordbo, 1980). These have been attributed to direct effects of the agents on plaque bacteria, as well as an enhanced affinity for food colorants. A brown to black pigmented stain in plaque-associated areas has also been reported in several clinical studies and is attributed to dentifrices containing stannous fluoride (Yankell and Emling, 1978).

Chlorhexidine causes a dark brown stain that may appear within a few weeks to a year.

Two other tooth discolorations are discussed here from the professional's point of view. The first of these is caries. Initial or incipient carious lesions will appear slightly whiter, chalky, and dull in comparison with unaffected enamel. Often these are not observed by the patient but should be pointed out at a dental examination. Recurring caries will appear as a gray area adjacent to the margin of a defective restoration. With increased caries development or lesion size, the decalcified areas will become stained with food and bacterial debris, and the amount of discoloration will depend on the length of the active decay process. The second discoloration includes stains due to defective restorations. These stains occur around

Table 26-3. Toothpaste composition

Ingredient	Approximate composition (%)	Function
Abrasive(s)	10 to 60	Clean; polish
Water	20 to 50	Provides a vehicle
Humectant(s)	10 to 60	Prevent caking or hardening; retain moisture
Binding agent(s)	1 to 5	Prevent separation; add thickness
Surface active agent(s), detergent(s)	1 to 2	Remove surface deposits, debris; provide foam
Flavor(s), sweetening agent(s)	1 to 3	Add taste
Therapeutic agent(s)	0.01 to 10	Prevent and/or reduce caries, sensitivity, plaque formation, etc.
Miscellaneous	0.1 to 5	Color; preserve; stabilize

Modified from Yankell S and Emling RC: Contin Dent Educ **1:**7, 1978.

the restoration usually because of leakage at the site. The restoration should be replaced.

Prevention (home care)

Toothbrushing is the most common means of home care in this country. Although proper toothbrushing with a toothbrush alone or with water can remove all dental deposits, the pellicle may stain (Manly, 1943). Toothpastes are formulated to aid in the removal of debris and discoloration from tooth surfaces and to impart a gloss or luster (polish). Toothpastes are composed of many ingredients, each with a specific function (Gershon and Pader, 1972; Goldstein, 1976; Yankell and Emling, 1978) (Table 26-3). Following is a summary of abrasives in toothpastes:

Calcium carbonate ($CaCO_3$ [Macleans, Phillips, Aquafresh]). Precipitated calcium carbonate (chalk) was widely used in dentifrice products until the mid 1950s. This material is decomposed in an acid pH.

Dibasic calcium phosphate ($CaHPO_4$ [Colgate, Viadent regular, Pearl Drops]). The anhydrous or the dihydrate form of dibasic calcium phosphate is used. The anhydrous form is much more abrasive than the dihydrate form. Although dicalcium phosphate dihydrate is not compatible with sodium fluoride or stannous fluoride, sodium monofluorophosphate can be maintained in soluble form in the presence of this agent for relatively long periods of time.

Calcium pyrophosphate ($Ca_2P_2O_7$ [Gleem]). Calcium pyrophosphate is more abrasive than dicalcium phosphate dihydrate and more compatible with fluoride compounds because it is one of the most inert calcium phosphate salts.

Tetrasodium pyrophosphate (tartar control toothpastes). This agent has abrasive properties and helps prevent precipitation of salivary salts into dental plaque.

Alumina compounds (Ultra-Brite). Hydrated alumina compounds are available in various particle sizes and thus various degrees of abrasiveness. These compounds do not contain calcium and do not appear to react with fluorides.

Hydrated silicas and silicas (Colgate Winterfresh Gel, Viadent fluoride, Sensodyne, Close-up, Crest, Macleans, Aim, Aquafresh). Silica compounds are available in various grades. When coupled with the proper humectant systems, silicas can be used to produce translucent or transparent clear gel products.

With scanning electron microscopy, changes on the tooth surface have been studied after the use of toothpastes that varied considerably in abrasive composition. Pellicle was present within 24 hours after cleaning the tooth completely, and pellicle thickness increased with time. Thicker pellicles formed during the use of nonabrasive toothpastes. It was concluded that abrasives were necessary to control pellicle thickness and prevent stain buildup. If pellicle was allowed to remain undisturbed, it became more difficult to remove because of changes in physical properties (Saxton, 1976). This study suggests one reason for recommending dentifrices with mild abrasives to be used properly on a consistent basis. A more important reason is to ensure regular, low doses of fluoride for enamel remineralization. For patients with exposed dentin or cementum, it is imperative to stress proper brushing procedures. Because these tooth structures are softer than enamel, they are more susceptible to the abrasives in dentifrices if improperly used. Unfortunately, no standards have been established as to the optimal amount of abrasiveness in toothpastes (ADA Council, 1982).

Professional treatment

Extrinsic stains. After scaling and root planing, areas of stain may be polished professionally. Although many prophylaxis pastes are available, these vary considerably in abrasiveness. The abrasives contained in these products essentially are similar to those in dentifrice products (Craig, O'Brien, and Powers, 1983; Davis, 1978; O'Brien and Ryge, 1978); the major difference is that the levels in professional products are much higher.

Abrasive agents are incorporated into professional products for the purpose of cleaning and polishing (Fig. 26-1). A dental abrasive changes the surface of the tooth by frictional grinding, rubbing, scraping, scratching, and the like to remove irregularities. As this process proceeds from coarse abrasion (cleaning) to polishing, the surface of the tooth passes through various stages; from an irregular surface, to a grooved surface, to a finely scratched surface, which is increased in smoothness and light reflectance. The last stage is regarded as the polished surface.

Factors determining the abrasiveness or polishing potential of an agent include hardness, shape, size, and concentration. Abrasives vary markedly in inherent hardness and shape. Within the same abrasive, sizes are graded from fine to coarse. With abrasive compounds that are harder, of rougher shape, increased particle size, or high concentration, abrasiveness is maximized. As each of these factors decreases, surface abrasion decreases and the surface becomes smooth, or polished.

Additional factors related to the method(s) of applying the prophylaxis product must be considered in the polishing and cleaning procedure. These include the pressure and speed used to apply the product and the surface (enamel, restor-ative material, or other) being treated.

Two abrasive agents used in prophylaxis products or available as chemical compounds are pumice and calcium carbonate (chalk, whiting). Pumice is manufactured in a wide variety of particle sizes, and its use ranges from an abrasive stain removal agent to fine polishing of acrylic dentures. Calcium carbonate is also manufactured in several particle shapes and sizes. This compound has more of a polishing action, as it produces minimal scratching and results in a smooth surface that reflects light.

Although professional products have been categorized as fine, medium, or coarse, there are no standards to define exactly what these terms mean. One manufacturer's fine prophylaxis paste may be more abrasive than another manufacturer's medium paste, as they may contain different abrasives. No attempt should be made to match one manufacturer's fine abrasive product with another manufacturer's product labeled in the same category even if they contain the same abrasive(s). The dental professional must learn how to use each manufacturer's products in his or her own practice. It is important to evaluate different manufacturers' products to become familiar with the polishing and abrasive characteristics in laboratory experiments, if possible, before using them for patients.

Because prophylaxis pastes are more abrasive than toothpastes, it is important to be selective in the teeth that are polished. With a professional prophylaxis and the use of highly abrasive materials, a thin surface of enamel is removed. This is reformed fairly quickly and mineralized in the mouth as a result of the high calcium phosphate content of saliva. It is also recommended that abrasive procedures be followed by professional fluoride treatments, as discussed in Chapter 28.

Professional methods for improving intrinsic stain appearance include such procedures as bleaching the teeth (Heringer, 1976), using composite restoration materials bonded as overlays, and, less frequently using crown(s) to cover completely the affected tooth or teeth. Although bleaching often has been attempted and is satisfactory for relatively minor intrinsic stain(s), a number of concerns have arisen (Cooley, 1976). These include the need to know more about the histologic effects after bleaching and the chemical reactions during the application of concentrated

ABRASION		POLISHING
Large	Particle size	Small
Irregular	Shape	Regular
High	Concentration	Low
Increased	Hardness	Decreased
Firm	Pressure	Mild
Rapid	Speed	Slow
Soft (dentin and cementum)	Tooth surface texture	Hard (enamel)

Fig. 26-1. Factors influencing tooth cleaning.

peroxides. Effects on the pulp after bleaching are unknown, as are potential dehydration effects on the enamel.

Several researchers have used resin veneers or composite materials in 6- to 12-month evaluations (Spencer, 1972; Stuart, 1975; Cooley, 1976). Results have been encouraging, particularly in matching color with other teeth in the mouth, in the relatively short time required to do individual teeth (ranging from 15 to 30 minutes per tooth), and in the excellent patient acceptance after completion of treatments. Difficulties with these materials include flaking or cracking, especially when fibrous or hard-consistency foods are eaten. Tooth capping or full porcelain or acrylic crowns are used when major intrinsic staining has occurred; however, this should not be done on deciduous or young permanent dentition. It is desirable to have complete development of the pulp prior to crowning. A second drawback of this treatment is the expense and time incurred in having the procedure performed. A third difficulty is the creation of an artificial margin between the tooth crown and root, which can be a primary site for plaque adherence. Many dental professionals are reluctant to sacrifice large areas of healthy tooth structure for purely cosmetic purposes.

Stain evaluation

Attempts have been made to develop scoring procedures to evaluate intrinsic and extrinsic staining. One of the first attempts to evaluate stain clinically was the categorization of both the inten-

sity and severity of the stain and the tooth area covered (Lobene, 1968). This scoring system is shown in Table 26-4. This scoring procedure was used to study the effects of dentifrices on tooth stains after controlled brushing times. The products evaluated differed significantly in their ability to remove stains. Another approach to quantitation of tooth stain has been the use of chips of various colors combined with a tooth surface scoring area to evaluate new antiplaque materials (Yankell et al, 1982). A stain index has been proposed to detect small changes in staining levels between different groups. In this procedure, stained areas are drawn on a reproduced grid system to determine the area of the tooth covered. No attempt has been made in this system to quantitate the intensity of tooth stain; rather, staining is graded on a stain, no stain basis (Shaw and Murray, 1977).

What is recommended for the professional office? Staining records should be maintained for individuals who present this problem, whether this symptom is recognized by the patient or evaluated by the professional. The scoring system shown in Table 26-4 offers criteria for analyzing intensity and tooth area and for recording the maximum amount of information to be used for planning treatment and for review of conditions at recall.

MECHANICAL DEVICES FOR POLISHING

The simplest device for polishing stains from the teeth is a *porte polisher* (Fig. 26-2). This hand instrument is designed to hold wooden points, which can be thoroughly adapted to the various aspects of the teeth to rub the abrasive against the tooth surface. Each stroke generated by the wrist rock moves the wedge-shaped, tapered, or pointed wooden point over the tooth surface (Fig. 26-3). This procedure requires considerable hand strength and control and is a slow, tedious process. It does, however, have several advantages, including (1) its portability (as it can be used when electricity is not available, at the bedside, or in other settings where engine-driven equipment cannot be used); (2) the gentle massage provided to the soft tissues as long as strokes are carefully controlled and approximate the gingival margins; (3) ready access to selected tooth surfaces that are obscured by tooth malpositions; (4) generation of minimal frictional heat; (5) lack of

Table 26-4. Scoring tooth stains*

Stain characteristic	Score	Description of stain
Intensity	0	None
	1	Light
	2	Moderate
	3	Heavy
Extent	0	None detected
	1	One third of region
	2	Two thirds of region
	3	>Two thirds of region

Modified from Lobene RR: JADA **77**:844, 1968.
*The facial surfaces of the eight incisors are scored. Each incisor is divided into the gingival and body regions. Each region is scored for both intensity and extent.

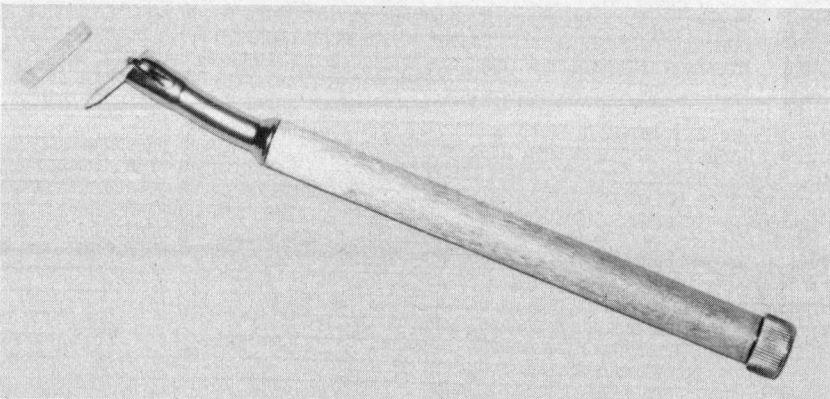

Fig. 26-2. Porte polisher is a hand instrument into which variously shaped orangewood points may be inserted and used to polish teeth with an abrasive.

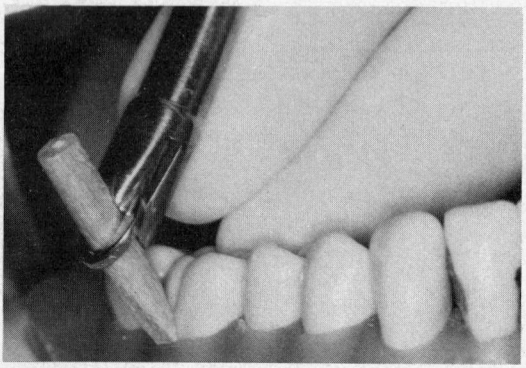

Fig. 26-3. Wooden point is closely adapted to tooth to rub the abrasive against stained areas. Short strokes are used in gingival, middle, and incisal or occlusal thirds of tooth to ensure a clean, well-polished surface.

engine noise (and thus greater acceptance by patients); (6) minimal bacterial aerosol; and (7) simple procedures for cleaning and sterilizing as compared with those required for cleaning and sterilizing engine-driven handpieces and prophylaxis angles.

In the early days of dental hygiene, porte polishing was one of the first procedures learned in educational programs because it developed hand strength, control, and a functional wrist rock. Motor-driven polishing has become more common in educational programs in recent decades, as it requires less time to complete and is the method of choice in clinical practice. Despite the predominant use of motor-driven polishing, however, the porte polisher is a valuable adjunct instrument that should be the method of choice for some patients and in some clinical settings. An activity at the conclusion of this chapter provides students with an opportunity to use the porte polisher.

Engine-driven polishing is more widely used in clinical practice because of its efficiency and the lesser amount of effort required to polish a complete dentition. The power is derived in most instances from (1) an electric motor, which drives a belt over a series of pulleys to turn the handpiece gears (the familiar slow-speed "drill"); (2) a small electric motor that attaches to the base of the handpiece and to electric supply hosing; or (3) compressed air supplied by hosing to an air turbine handpiece. Whatever mechanism or power source is used in any given clinical setting, it is extremely important for the dental hygienist to become familiar with (1) the kind of system used, (2) the specific procedures necessary for operating and maintaining the system, and (3) the checklist of what to inspect if the system fails to rotate the polishing instrument.

The handpiece and the prophylaxis angle (which holds the rubber cup and brush attachments that polish the teeth) require proper care and maintenance. A nonfunctional handpiece, prophylaxis angle, or power line makes motor-driven polishing impossible. Identifying and correcting the reason for the malfunction require the hygienist's mechanical abilities. A sterile porte

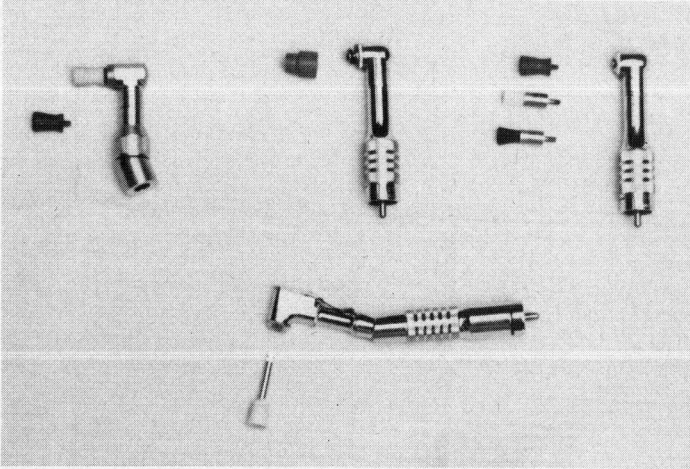

Fig. 26-4. Prophylaxis angles vary in design to accommodate handpiece systems and vary in mechanism used to attach polishing cups or brushes. Attachment may screw in, snap on over a knob, or fit into angle with a mandrel and latching mechanism.

polisher should be kept close at hand for those times when basic cleaning and oiling do not restore function to the modern convenience.

The handpiece selected for use should be specifically designed for the system being used. The handpiece may screw, snap, lock, or clip onto the power source. Attached to the handpiece is the prophylaxis angle, which, as mentioned before, holds the rubber cup or brush (Fig. 26-4). The cup or brush may attach by means of a metal mandrel that is latched into place. The metal mandrel slides through the head of the angle to the latch at the back of the angle head. Other styles of cups and angles enable the rubber cup to screw into the head of the angle. Reverse threads are used so that the rubber cup will not unscrew while running in a clockwise rotation against the tooth. Yet another style allows the cup or brush to snap over a knob on the face of the angle head. The cup and knob must be dry and oil-free, or the cup will slip against the knob instead of gripping it firmly.

Some cups are impregnated with fluoride. They have been shown to increase enamel fluoride content by 400 to 700 ppm and to reduce enamel solubility by 20% to 28%. They also remove stained pellicle more efficiently and with less abrasion of the enamel than the other cups tested. The cups are made of thermoplastic resins and a 6% mix-

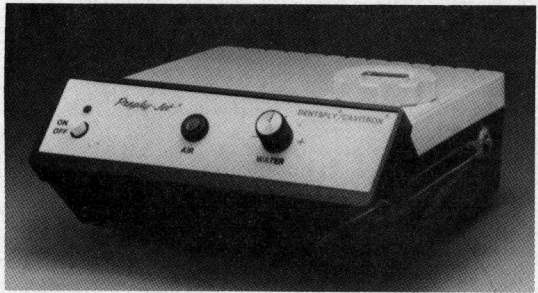

Fig. 26-5. Dentsply/Cavitron Prophy-Jet uses a slurry of sodium bicarbonate and water under air pressure to clean stain and polish teeth.

ture of sodium fluoride and stannous fluoride. In instances where stains require polishing, the use of fluoride-impregnated cups is indicated (Stookey and Schemehorn, 1976; Stookey and Stahlman, 1976).

Air-powder polishing

A third method for polishing the teeth requires no hand pressure against the tooth. The Dentsply/Cavitron Prophy-Jet (Fig. 26-5) projects a slurry of water and sodium bicarbonate against the tooth surface, cleaning away the stain and polishing the teeth. It uses air pressure of 50 to 100 pounds per square inch (psi) and water pressure of 10 to 50

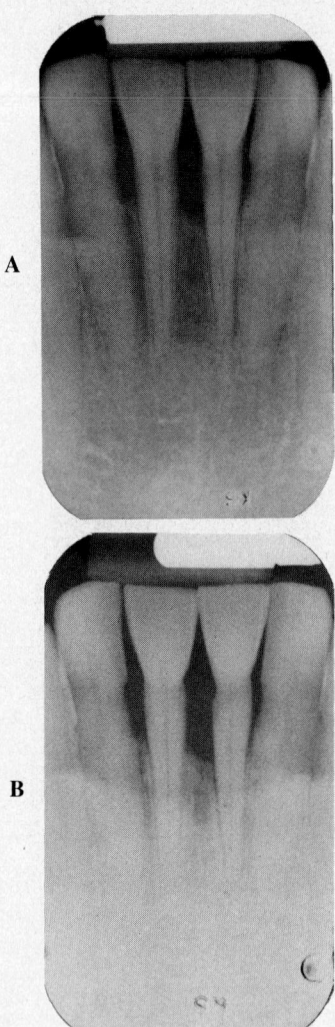

Fig. 26-6. **A,** Radiograph of anterior teeth in 1978. **B,** Radiograph of the same teeth in 1988 after quarterly scaling and polishing, partly to remove tobacco tar from exposed root surfaces. Note the altered root shape.

psi. The water temperature is thermostatically controlled at approximately 37.7° C (100° F). The handpiece has a nozzle through which the slurry is propelled when a foot control is activated. The nozzle should be held 1 cm from the tooth and be angled diagonally toward the tooth and not at right angles to it. The stream should not be aimed at the soft tissue. An air-propelled jet of sodium

bicarbonate powder is surrounded by a concentric water jet.

The air-powder polisher removes plaque and stain as well as a rubber cup and does so in less time (Weeks et al, 1984; DeSpain et al, 1988). However, it may not prevent plaque reaccumulation as effectively as a rubber cup (Baker, 1988). It has little effect on enamel, but can erode cementum and dentin (Boyde, 1984; Kee and Allen, 1988). One study showed that it removed 636.6 micrometers of root structure in 30 seconds, but resulted in a smooth surface free of fibers and debris (Atkinson et al, 1984). Another study showed it to remove approximately 25 microns of cementum when exposed to a root surface for 30 seconds and to result in a slightly rougher surface than that found in untreated control surfaces (Petersson et al, 1985). Study methods probably account for the differences.

Some patients require extensive instrumentation on root structure in order to remove coffee or tobacco stains, particularly at the cementoenamel junction or on areas with extensive recession. If this stain is removed with a curette, which is the accepted procedure when a rubber cup or porte polisher cannot adequately reach the areas in question, the root structure will be pared down over the years, particularly if those patients are on a short recall interval (see Fig. 26-6). The air-powder polisher is preferable to the curette in these instances. The air-powder polisher removes approximately 10.68 micrometers, while the curette removes an average of 27.09 micrometers in a simulated 3-month recall over 3 years. In addition, stain was removed more than three times as fast with the air-powder polisher (Berkstein et al, 1987).

The air-powder polisher also works well in removing plaque and stain from root concavities and furca as an adjunct to periodontal surgery (Horning et al, 1987), but may offer no measurable benefit beyond ultrasonic debridement (Krupa et al, 1988).

One in vitro study suggests that using an ultrasonic scaler followed by air-powder polishing creates an environment where fibroblast growth and vitality is greater than for either ultrasonic scaling alone or control teeth with remaining calculus (Gilman and Maxey, 1986). Another study showed that although there were signs of small

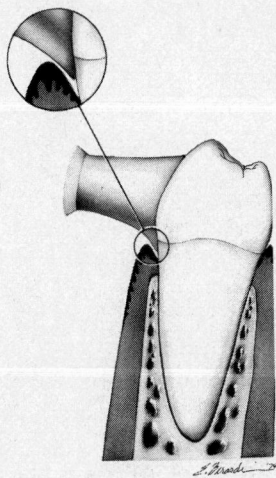

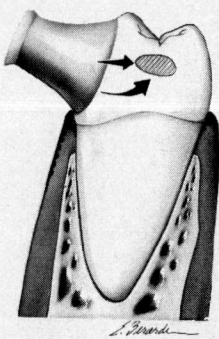

Fig. 26-8. Rubber cup should be adapted so that it has as much access to proximal surface as possible and so that it slides up under contact point.

Fig. 26-7. Rubber cup should be adapted so that it slides slightly subgingivally in cervical area.

blood clots at the margin of the gingiva immediately after use, there were no signs of abrasion or long-term irritation (Mishkin et al, 1986). Soft tissue abrasion of a transient nature can be expected. The air-powder polisher should not be applied on composite restorations. Even a 5-second exposure results in surface changes in several composite materials (Patterson and McLundie, 1984; Lubow and Cooley, 1986). Moreover, using the air-powder polisher generates an aerosol of microorganisms that contaminates surfaces several feet from the operative site (Glenwright et al, 1985; Logothetis et al, 1988). Gloves, mask, protective lenses for patient, operator, and assistant, and a laminar airflow to reduce airborne bacteria are important to minimize this problem. Surface areas require thorough disinfection after this procedure.

Blood sample analysis of one patient before and after treatment with an air-powder polisher demonstrated that serum pH rose to a marginally alkaline state. This condition should be normalized within a day or two in persons whose systems are functioning normally. It is a potential problem for persons with chronic diarrhea or who abuse laxatives or use diuretics extensively (Rawson et al, 1985).

ENGINE POLISHING PROCEDURE

All parts of the handpiece and angle must ensure that adequate torque is maintained to move the abrasive against the tooth for polishing. The abrasive is carried to the tooth by dipping the rubber cup or brush into the abrasive, placing the cup or brush against the tooth, and activating the rheostat so that the applicator rotates, thus polishing the tooth with the abrasive.

The abrasive can be held in a dappen dish or in a small cup held by a finger on the mirror-holding hand for ready access. Or the chairside assistant can apply the abrasive directly to the teeth with a plastic syringe just ahead of the path of the rubber cup or brush. Regardless of how the abrasive is to be placed on the tooth, it is important that adequate amounts be used. Usually a full rubber cup of abrasive will be sufficient for one or two teeth. A bare or saliva-laden cup devoid of polishing agent does not polish the teeth and generates heat (Spierings et al, 1985). Cups are available with internal webbing to retain the agent more readily.

The rubber cup can be adapted to all exposed tooth surfaces. It can and should be slipped slightly subgingivally so that the lip of the cup cleans the most coronal aspects of the sulcus (Fig. 26-7). It should be applied to proximal surfaces by sliding the lip of the cup as far proximally as possible and slightly under the contact point area (Fig. 26-8). Adapting the lip of the cup into the occlusal grooves will often suffice for stain removal from those difficult areas.

When the rubber cup does not remove occlusal stain adequately, a small brush may be attached for use on the occlusal surfaces. Brushes *should not* be used on any other tooth surfaces, as they are highly abrasive (Thompson and Way, 1981), are difficult to control, and easily may abrade the soft tissues. Brushes are available with soft or firm bristles. The softer bristles are usually adequate for stain removal, and they hold abrasive more readily.

Whether a cup or brush is being used, the attachment and abrasive should be used with *moderate intermittent pressure* (Tillis and Hicks, 1987). On-and-off application on the tooth allows the heat that is generated by the process to dissipate between each stroke. Constant pressure of the rubber cup or brush on the tooth builds up frictional heat, causing first discomfort, then pain, and finally possible pulp damage. The rule is to apply the cup on and off the tooth with moderate pressure. This is especially critical for anterior teeth, which provide minimal insulation for the pulp because of the comparative lack of bulk of dentin and enamel.

A study of speed, duration, and load on the rubber cup demonstrated that the clinicians in the trial used consistent speed (approximately 2751 rpms), spent more time on molars than on other teeth, and used greater load (pressure) depending upon the area of the mouth, the surface being polished, and the amount of stain present (Christensen and Bangerter, 1984).

Clinicians should observe the patient's facial expression carefully to detect signs of discomfort from heat. If the clinician suspects that the patient is in pain, the patient should be asked if he or she feels heat, and if so, the polishing procedure should be altered to reduce heat, usually by lessening the duration of each application of the cup or brush to the tooth.

The speed of the cup is critical in both minimizing frictional heat and in ensuring effective polishing., A speeding cup is both harmful and ineffective (Spierings et al, 1985). As it is rarely possible to determine the exact revolutions per minute (rpm) at which the handpiece is operating, most clinicians operate the handpiece at the *lowest possible speed* that moves the cup or brush against the tooth without stalling. Sound also provides a clue for determining whether the cup is rotating too rapidly. A high whine or whistle in the handpiece usually indicates excessive speed. To achieve the lowest possible speed, the rheostat may need to be activated to a high or medium speed and then backed down to a low

speed before the tooth is touched with the attachment.

The order or sequence of polishing can follow the one outlined for instrumentation in Chapter 6. Positioning of the patient, clinician, and assistant is basically unchanged. The procedure will require adequate evacuation, as the polishing agent and the mechanical stimulation usually increase salivary secretions. The tri-syringe can be used to flush the areas with a water stream as each arch segment is completed. At the completion of the procedure, the patient should be encouraged to rinse thoroughly to remove all residual polishing agent. Proximal areas should be flossed.

Inspection for remaining stain should be performed with good intraoral light, compressed air, and the mouth mirror. Final inspection for plaque should be accomplished with a disclosant as described in previous chapters.

Any remaining stain should be removed by the clinician, and plaque should be removed by the patient.

One area that tends to cause frustration is the mandibular anterior lingual area. Frequently a light pink staining will reappear with each disclosing and will not disappear with repeated polishing and brushing. In almost all cases the disclosant is adherent to a thin sheet of calculus, otherwise not visible on the lingual surfaces. Instrumentation with a scaler or curette is necessary to remove it. Then the area can be repolished.

THE ROLE OF POLISHING IN DENTAL HYGIENE CARE

Polishing for stain removal rather than for removing all soft deposits may be a new experience for some patients. Many patients may have learned to treat the professional oral prophylaxis as a cosmetic procedure or as the key to "healthy gums." Accepting a portion of the responsibility may be an unfamiliar role for the patient. Therefore, it is wise to share with the patient the purpose of polishing, the effect of repeated polishing on the teeth, the rate of reformation of plaque on the teeth after polishing, and how the patient can participate in ongoing "prophylaxis" (i.e., *prevention*). This explanation may make it easier for the patient to accept the change and to reinforce the concomitant plaque control messages offered throughout care.

ACTIVITIES

1. Omit brushing your teeth one morning. Rinse your mouth with grape juice (swallow or spit out), and describe how your mouth feels and the appearance of your teeth and deposits. Which deposits do you think are "colored"? How do you think this relates to not brushing after meals and eating colored foods? How can you "feel" the grape juice remaining in your mouth? What do you think is happening with the grape juice and the dental deposits allowed to form overnight? Evaluate the ease of removal of the colored deposits.
2. Examine a series of student partners. If intrinsic stains are found, can you relate them to childhood diseases, medications (antibiotics), fluorides, restorative materials, or other sources? If extrinsic stains are found, can you relate them to tea, coffee, and/or tobacco consumption?
3. Polish stain from a partner's teeth using a porte polisher and engine polishing. Compare the results, the effort involved, and your partner's preference.
4. Examine the variety of tips available for use in the porte polisher.
5. Perform routine maintenance on the handpiece and contra-angle to be used for engine polishing.
6. Given a variety of nonfunctioning engine polishers, determine why each is not working and correct the problem.
7. Change a belt on a belt-driven engine.
8. Use the Prophy-Jet to polish a quadrant of teeth heavily laden with stain. Polish a second quadrant with an engine-driven rubber cup. Compare results regarding (1) cleanliness of the teeth, (2) time, (3) patient acceptance, and (4) amount of recurrent stain at the recall visit.
9. Role-play an encounter with a patient who wishes to have all of his or her teeth polished regardless of the presence of stain.

REVIEW QUESTIONS

1. Define the following stain classifications:
   a. Exogenous
   b. Endogenous
   c. Extrinsic
   d. Intrinsic
2. What is the primary importance of the abrasive in toothpaste?
3. Compare abrasives in toothpastes and professional products.
4. What factors affect abrasiveness and polishing?
5. How can frictional heat be minimized during engine polishing?
6. What are seven advantages of a porte polisher?
7. What is the primary disadvantage of a porte polisher?
8. What is the primary indication for polishing teeth?
9. How does the Prophy-Jet polish teeth?

REFERENCES

ADA Council on Dental Theraupeutics: Accepted dental therapeutics, ed 39, Chicago, 1982, American Dental Association.

Atkinson DR, Cobb CM, and Killoy WJ: The effect of an air-powder abrasive system on in vitro root surfaces, J Periodontol 55:13, 1984.

Baker DJ: Effects of rubber cup polishing and an air abrasive system on plaque accumulation, Dent Hyg 62:55 (abst), 1988.

Berkstein S, et al: Supragingival root surface removal during maintenance procedures utilizing an air-powder abrasive system or hand scaling: an in vitro study, J Periodontol 58:327,

Boyde, A: Airpolishing effects on enamel, dentine, cement and bone, Brit Dent J 156:287, 1984.

Carranza FA Jr: Glickman's clinical periodontology, ed 5, Philadelphia, 1979, WB Saunders Co.

Christensen RP: Brand names and characteristics of polishing products used by dental hygienists in the US: results of a survey, Dent Hyg 58:222, 1984.

Christensen RP, and Bangerter VW: Determination of rpm, time, and load used in oral prophylaxis polishing in vivo, J Dent Res 63:1376, 1984.

Christensen RP, and Bangerter VW: Immediate and long-term in vivo effects of polishing on enamel and dentin, J Pros Dent 57:150, 1987.

Cooley RL, Lubow RM and Patrissi GA: The effect of an air-powder abrasive instrument on composite resin, JADA 112:362, 1986.

Cooley RO: Resin veneer ends discoloration problem, Dent Stud 54:28, 1976.

Craig RG, O'Brien WJ, and Powers JM: Dental materials; properties and manipulation, ed 3, St Louis, 1983, The CV Mosby Co.

Cross GN, and Carr EH: Patients' acceptance of selective polishing, Dent Hyg 57(12):20, 1983.

Davis WR: Cleaning, polishing and abrasion of teeth by dental products, Cosmet Sci 1:38, 1978.

DeSpain B, and Nobis R: Comparison of rubber cup polishing and air polishing on stain, plaque, calculus, and gingiva, Dent Hyg 62:55 (abst), 1988.

Gershon SD, and Pader M: Dentifrices. In Balsam, MS, and Sangarin E, editors: Cosmetics: sciences and technology, vol 1, New York, 1972, Wiley-Interscience.

Gilman RS, and Maxey BR: The effect of root detoxification on human gingival fibroblasts, J Periodontol 57:436, 1986.

Glenwright HD, Knibbs PJ, and Burdon DW: Atmospheric contamination during use of an air polisher, Brit Dent J 159:294, 1985.

Goldstein RE: Esthetics in dentistry, Philadelphia, 1976, JB Lippincott Co.

Heringer E: Bleaching removes some discoloration, Dent Stud 54:31, 1976.

Horning GM, Cobb CM, and Killoy WJ: Effect of an air-powder abrasive system on root surfaces in periodontal surgery, J Clin Periodontol 14:213, 1987.

Huber SJ, Vernino AR, and Nanca RS: Professional prophylaxis and its effect on the periodontium of full-banded orthodontic patients, Am J Orthod Dentofac Orthop 91:321, 1987.

Hunter EL, et al: The prophylaxis polish—a review of the literature, Dent Hyg 55(9):36, 1981.

Kee A, and Allen DS: Effects of air and rubber cup polishing on enamel abrasion, Dent Hyg 62:55 (abst), 1988.

Krupa CM, et al: In vitro evaluation of air-powder polishing as an adjunct to ultrasonic scaling on periodontally involved root surfaces, Dent Hyg 62:55 (abst), 1988.

Lobene RR: Effect of dentifrices on tooth stains with controlled brushing, JADA 77:849, 1968.

Logothetis R, Gross K, and Eberhart A: Bacterial aerosol contamination using an air polishing device, Dent Hyg 62:55 (abst), 1988.

Lubow RM, and Cooley RL: Effect of air-powder abrasive instrument on restorative materials, J Prosth Dent 55:462, 1986.

Manly RS: A structureless recurrent deposit on teeth, J Dent Res 22:479, 1943.

Mellberg JR: Enamel fluoride and its anti-caries effects, J Prevent Dent 4:8, 1977.

Mishkin DJ, et al: A clinical comparison of the effect on the gingiva of the Prophy-Jet and the rubber cup and paste techniques, J Periodontol 53:151, 1986.

Moffitt JM, et al: Prediction of tetracycline-induced tooth discoloration, JADA 88:547, 1974.

Ness L, Rosekrans DdeL, and Welford JF: An epidemiologic study of factors affecting extrinsic staining of teeth in an English population, Comm Dent Oral Epidemiol 5:55, 1977.

O'Brien W, and Ryge G: An outline of dental materials and their selection. Philadelphia, 1978, WB Saunders Co.

Patterson CJW, and McLundie AC: A comparison of the effects of two different prophylaxis regimes in vitro on some restorative dental materials, Br Dent J 157:166, 1984.

Petersson LG, et al: The effect of a jet abrasive instrument (Prophy-Jet) on root surfaces, Swed Dent J 9:193, 1985.

Primosch RE: Rubber cup prophylaxis: a reevaluation of its use in pediatric dental patients, Dent Hyg 54:525, 1980.

Rall D: From the NIH: research findings of potential value to the practitioner, JAMA 237:635, 1977.

Rawson RD, et al: Alkalosis as a potential complication of air polishing systems, Dent Hyg 59:500, 1985.

Reid JS, Beeley JA, and MacDonald DG: Investigations into black extrinsic tooth stain, J Dent Res 56:895, 1977.

Retief DH, et al: In vitro fluoride uptake distribution and retention by human enamel after 1- and 24-hour application of various topical fluoride agents, J Dent Res 59:573, 1980.

Rohleder PV, and Slim LH: Alternatives to rubber cup polishing, Dent Hyg 55(9):16, 1981.

Russ JC, et al: SEM low magnification stereoscopic technique for mapping surface contours: application to measurement of volume differences in human teeth due to polishing, J Microscopy 144:339, 1986.

Saxton CA: The effects of dentifrices on the appearance of the tooth surface observed with the scanning electron microscope, J Periodont Res 11:74, 1976.

Shaw L, and Murray JJ: A new index for measuring extrinsic stain in clinical trials, Comm Dent Epidemiol 5:116, 1977.

Shern RJ, et al: Enamel biopsy results of children receiving fluoride tablets, JADA 95:310, 1977.

Solheim H, Eriksen HM, and Nordbo H: Chemical plaque control and extrinsic discoloration of teeth, Acta Odontol Scand 38:303, 1980.

Spierings TAM, Peters MCRB, and Plasschaert AJM: Thermal trauma to teeth, Endod Dent Traumatol 1:123, 1985.

Steele RC, et al: The effect of tooth cleaning procedures on fluoride uptake in enamel, Pediatr Dent 4:228, 1982.

Stookey, GK, and Schemehorn BR: Studies evaluating a fluoride-containing prophylactic cup, Dent Hyg 50:253, 1976.

Stookey GK, and Stahlman DB: Enhanced fluoride uptake in enamel with a fluoride-impregnated prophylactic cup, J Dent Res 55:333, 1976.

Swan RW: Dimensional changes in a tooth root incident to various polishing and root planing procedures, Dent Hyg 53(1):17, 1979.

Thompson RE, and Way DC: Enamel loss due to prophylaxis and multiple bonding/debonding of orthodontic attachments, Am J Orthod 79:282, 1981.

Tilliss TSI, and Hicks MJ: Enamel surface morphology comparison: polishing with a toothpaste and a prophylaxis paste, Dent Hyg 61:112, 1987.

Tinanoff N, et al: Effect of a pumice prophylaxis on fluoride uptake in tooth enamel, JADA 88:384, 1974.

Vogel RI: Intrinsic and extrinsic discoloration of the dentition; (a literature review), J Oral Med 30(4):99, 1975.

Walsh MM, Heckman BH, and Moreau-Diettinger R: Polished and unpolished teeth: patient responses after an oral prophylaxis, Dent Hyg 59:306, 1985(a).

Walsh MM, et al: Effect of a rubber cup polish after scaling, Dent Hyg 59:484, 1985(b).

Waring MB, et al: A comparison of engine polishing and toothbrushing in minimizing dental plaque reaccumulation, Dent Hyg 56(12):25, 1982.

Weaks LM, et al: Clinical evaluation of the Prophy-Jet as an instrument for routine removal of tooth stain and plaque, J Periodontol 55:486, 1984.

Winter GB, Murray JJ, and Shaw L: Cosmetics and dental history, Cosmet Sci 1:1, 1978.

Yankell S, and Emling RC: Understanding dental products: What you should know and what your patient should know, Contin Dent Educ 1:7, 1978.

Yankell SL, et al: Effects of chlorhexidine and four antimicrobial compounds on plaque, gingivitis, and staining in beagle dogs, J Dent Res 61:1089, 1982.

27 CARE OF REMOVABLE APPLIANCES

OBJECTIVES: *The reader will be able to*

1. List five types of removable appliances and their uses.
2. State a rationale for cleaning dental appliances.
3. Describe the advantages and disadvantages of different denture cleansing agents and methods.
4. Discuss important considerations in the care of soft tissues and abutment teeth of patients with removable appliances.
5. Describe an aseptic technique for professional ultrasonic cleaning of dentures.
6. State criteria for evaluating denture identification methods.
7. Describe and compare three basic methods for marking dentures.
8. Discuss the importance of mouth protectors for prevention of oral injuries.
9. Compare the advantages and disadvantages of the three types of mouth protectors discussed.

Although the number of edentulous individuals is declining, there are still nearly 20 million of them in the United States. More than 90% of these people have some form of prosthodontic replacement, and an estimated one third of these need replacement or refitting of existing dentures. In spite of this need, more than half of the edentulous people questioned in one study reported in 1983 that they had not visited a dentist in the past 5 years (Waldman, 1987). A number of attitudinal and other barriers may be implicated in the failure to use dental services by this population group. Many people may not be aware of the importance of regular dental care for evaluating soft tissues for pathology, for examining existing dentures for fit and function, and for preventive education. The dental hygienist can fulfill an important role by informing edentulous consumers of the importance and need for regular oral examinations and of the professional and preventive services that can be provided for them. The hygienist must also be well prepared to educate all dental consumers regarding the care and cleaning of removable dental appliances of all types.

An understanding of the concepts of oral hygiene maintenance and the motivation to apply these concepts are as critical for dental consumers who have dentures and other types of removable appliances as to those with full sets of natural teeth. Edentulous individuals need to be instructed on the proper care and cleaning of the appliances, as well as on preserving and maintaining the health of remaining teeth and existing soft tissues. Removable dental appliances to be discussed include complete dentures, partial dentures, overdentures, removable orthodontic appliances (retainers), and mouth protectors.

TYPES OF REMOVABLE APPLIANCES

Complete dentures are appliances designed to replace all teeth in an entire arch. The parts of a complete denture are as follows: the denture base; the tissue surface; and the occlusal surface. The *denture base* is the part of the denture that rests on the oral mucosa and to which the denture teeth are attached. It usually is constructed of plastic resin or metal. The surface that is in direct contact with the alveolar ridge is called the *impression, tissue,* or *inner surface*. The external surface is called the *polished surface* because of its highly polished appearance. The *occlusal surface* of the denture is formed by the occlusal surfaces of the denture teeth. Denture teeth may be made

A   B

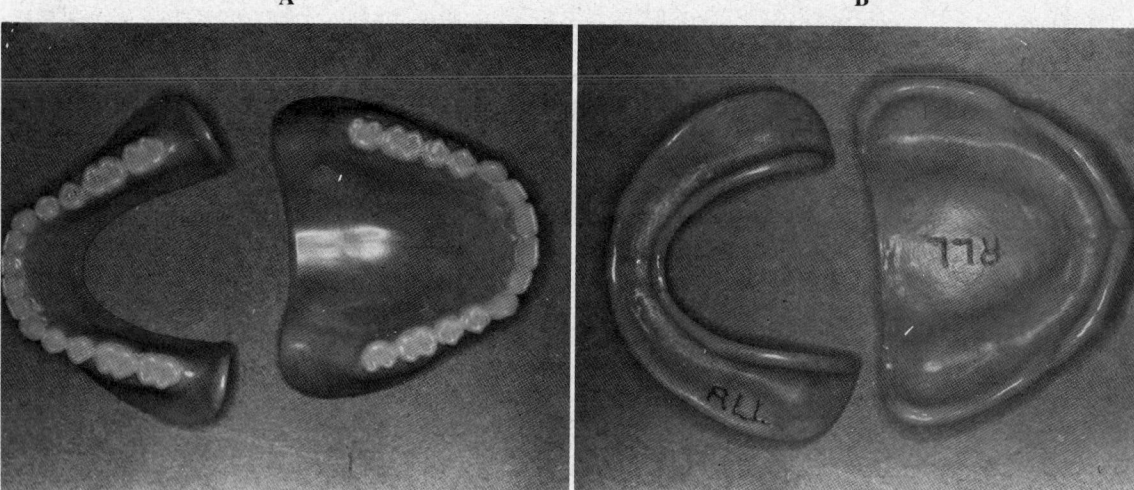

Fig. 27-1. Full dentures. **A,** Polished surfaces and occlusal surfaces. **B,** Tissue or inner surfaces.

of either plastic resin or porcelain materials (Fig. 27-1).

Removable partial dentures replace one or more but not all teeth in a given arch. The denture base is usually made of a metal alloy or plastic resin. Teeth in partial dentures may be made of porcelain, plastic resin, or metal. Partial dentures also have bars of rigid metal called *major connectors* that may span the palate in maxillary dentures or the lingual surfaces of the teeth in mandibular dentures. Partial dentures are anchored or supported by natural teeth (abutment teeth) by means of metal clasps or occlusal rests (Fig. 27-2).

An *overdenture* is a complete denture supported by both retained natural teeth and the alveolar ridge (Fig. 27-3). The presence of natural teeth is an advantage over a completely edentulous arch in that the presence of the teeth helps to preserve surrounding bone, to reduce occlusal stresses on the edentulous ridge, and to stabilize and retain the denture. Overdentures are indicated for situations in which existing teeth can no longer support a removable fixed or partial denture. They are used more frequently for replacement of teeth on the mandibular arch (Johnson and Sivers, 1987).

Removable *orthodontic appliances* (such as the Hawley retainer) are made of lightweight plastic materials that anchor the retaining wire and clasps used to maintain and stabilize the positions of the teeth following removal of fixed orthodontic appliances (Fig. 27-4). *Mouth protectors* or mouth guards are plastic or vinyl forms that are worn over maxillary teeth to prevent injuries to dentition, the temporomandibular joint, and other oral tissues during contact sports or other recreational activities in which blows to the head, face, or mouth might occur (Fig. 27-8).

IMPORTANCE OF ORAL HYGIENE MAINTENANCE

All patients who wear removable appliances must be instructed on their proper care, handling, and cleaning. Daily cleaning is necessary to prevent the build-up of plaque, calculus, and stain on oral appliances. These deposits not only may be problems in terms of esthetics and mouth odor, but can also contribute to irritation and infections, such as candidiasis or denture stomatitis, in the adjacent mucosa. *Denture stomatitis* is the term used to describe pathological changes that occur in the mucosa of denture-bearing tissues. In its mild forms it may appear as a localized inflammation or pinpoint hyperemia. Less mild forms appear as diffuse redness in a pattern that correlates directly with the tissue surface of the denture. In its most severe form, denture stomatitis appears as inflammatory papillary hyperplasia (overgrowth) of soft tissue that lies beneath and adja-

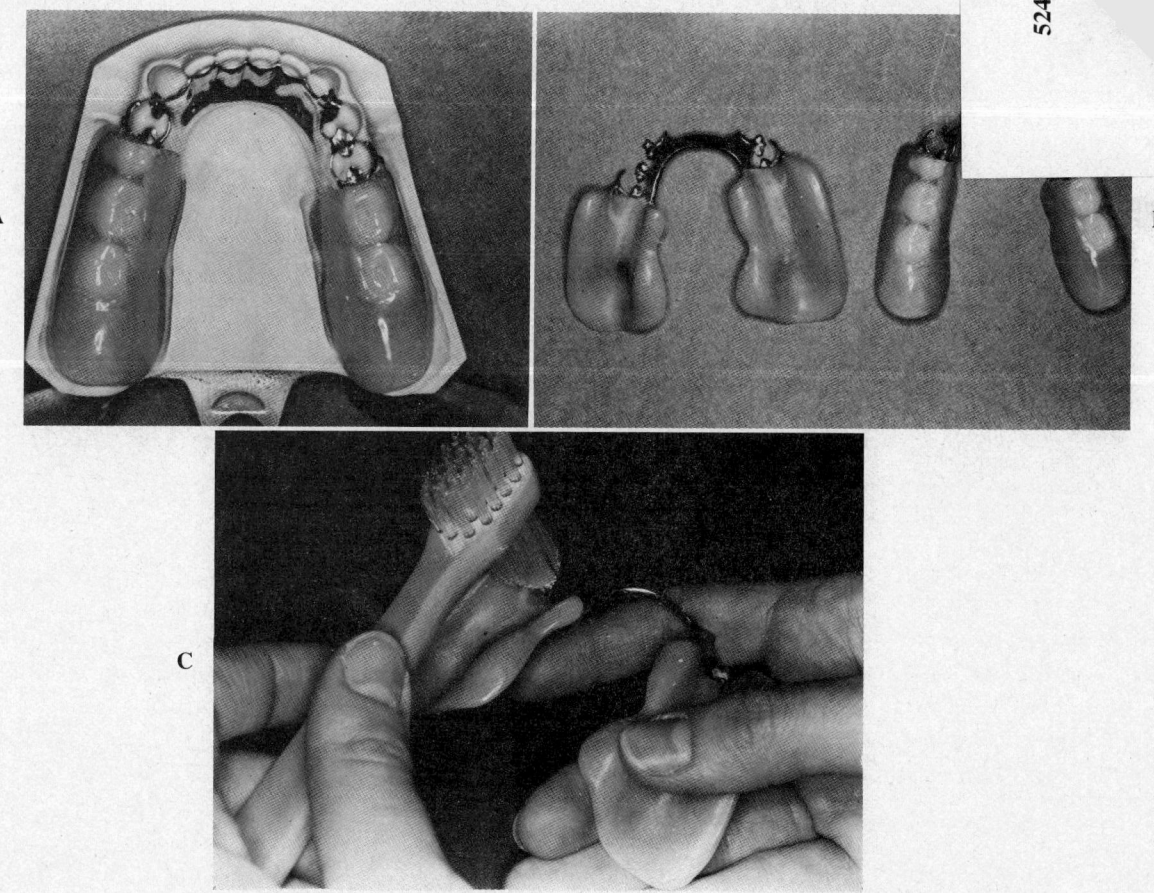

A

B

C

Fig. 27-2. Partial denture. **A,** Partial denture on typodont model. **B,** Partial denture, teeth and soft tissue sides. **C,** Cleaning soft tissue side with a denture brush.

cent to the denture base (Budtz-Jorgensen, 1978).

Irritation of soft tissues underlying dentures can be attributed to a number of possible causes. A major etiological factor is poor oral hygiene, resulting in the formation of mature plaque, which contains not only microorganisms that cause periodontal inflammation but also an abundance of pathogenic yeast microorganisms, primarily *Candida albicans* (Budtz-Jorgensen, 1983; Catalan et al, 1987). This microorganism, although part of the normal oral flora, can cause an inflammatory condition known as candidiasis in susceptible tissues. In a relatively healthy individual, candidiasis can be satisfactorily treated as localized infection through use of antifungal preparations (e.g., Nystatin) and improved hygiene of dentures and soft tissue surfaces. However, in oral cancer pa-

tients whose immune response has been suppressed due to drug therapy and a generally weakened physical condition, the localized infection can become systemic and life-threatening. Optimal control of pathogens related to denture-wearing is imperative for these patients as well as anyone undergoing prolonged therapy with immunosuppressive drugs, antibiotics, or corticosteroids who may be susceptible to yeast infection (Budtz-Jorgensen, 1978).

Irritation of soft tissues underlying dentures also may be attributed to an uneven distribution of stresses on soft tissues resulting from an improper fit of the denture to the supporting structures. In this case the dentist is responsible for evaluating the appliance and adjusting, relining, or replacing it. Patients should be warned

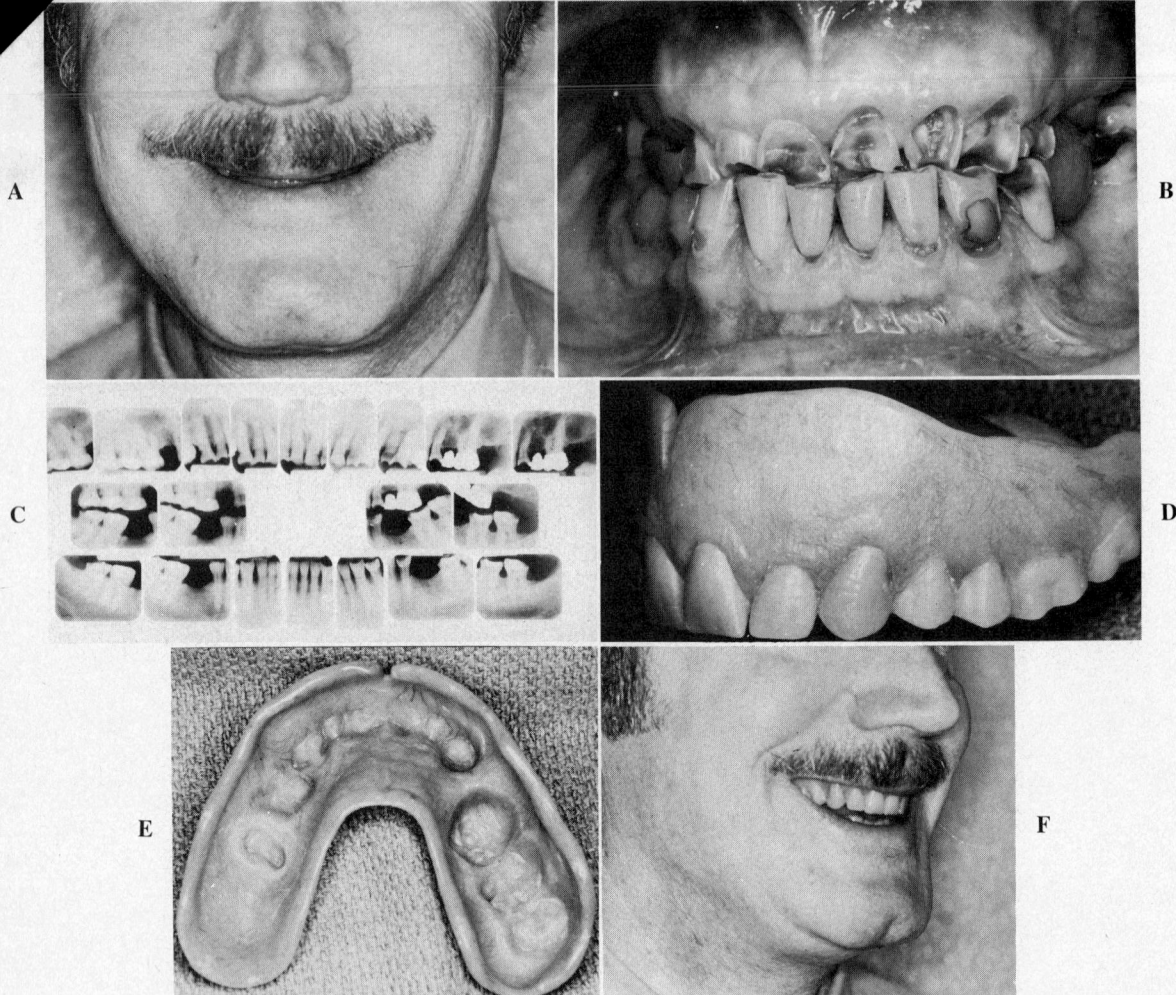

Fig. 27-3. Overdenture. **A,** Patient is shown. **B,** Patient's teeth are eroded. **C,** Radiographic series of the patient's teeth. **D,** View of tooth surface of overdenture. **E,** Inner surface of denture with indentations for natural teeth. **F,** Patient with denture inserted.

(From Brewer, AA, and Morrow RM: Overdentures, St Louis, 1980, The CV Mosby Co.)

against repairing or relining their own dentures to improve retention because this can cause additional problems to oral tissues and usually will not solve the existing problem. Patients with removable appliances should be encouraged to seek professional help for all denture problems.

Build-up of plaque on and under dentures also contributes to bad breath and the adherence and formation of stains and calculus that are estheti-cally unpleasing and can affect not only the self-confidence of the wearer but the impressions of others. Complete oral hygiene for patients who wear dentures and other removable appliances involves procedures to clean both the appliance and the oral tissues. Procedures for cleaning the removable appliance will be discussed first. Information discussed for care of complete dentures is also applicable for partial dentures and overdentures unless otherwise noted.

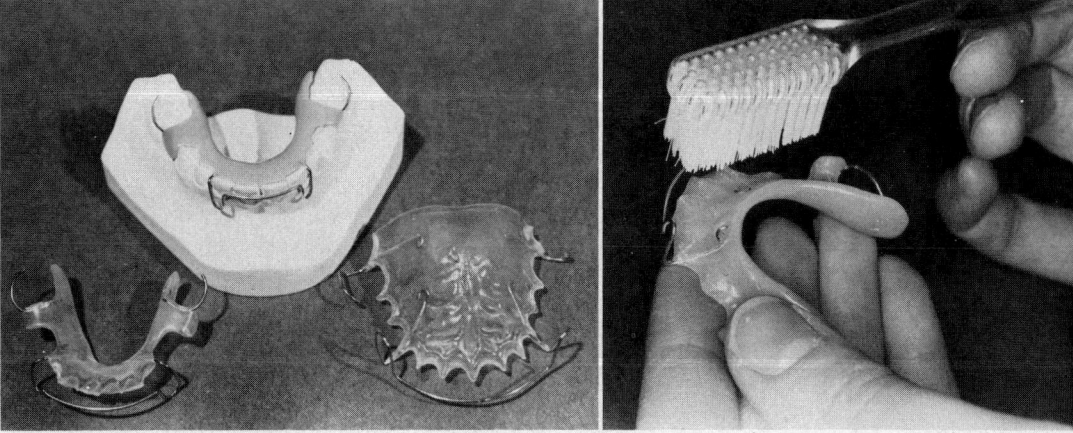

Fig. 27-4. Orthodontic Hawley appliance. **A,** Appliance placed on model and on table surface. **B,** Brushing appliance with a toothbrush.

DENTURE-CLEANING AGENTS
Brushing with soap, adhesive powders, or dentifrices

Dentures may be cleaned either by mechanical action, such as the use of a brush and an abrasive substance, or by chemical action. Although rinsing with water alone is important after eating and during cleaning procedures in order to remove food particles and loosened plaque and debris from dentures and oral tissues, it is not sufficient for removal of plaque and other adherent materials.

Mechanical removal of plaque using a brush alone or in combination with chemical soaking is probably the most effective way of removing denture plaque. A study comparing brushing with a dentifrice formulated for denture use and two popular chemical-soak cleansers found brushing with an abrasive to be superior to soaking for removal of accumulated plaque from all denture surfaces (Tarbet et al, 1984). Dentures should be brushed after each meal, if possible, or at least once daily, preferably before retiring. A soft denture brush is recommended because its two-head design facilitates contact of the bristles with all surfaces of the denture. The longer, rounded tuft of bristles is used to clean the tissue surface of the denture. The flat rectangular portion should be used to clean the polished and occlusal surfaces (Fig. 27-5). A regular soft toothbrush can be used

for cleaning dentures as long as its design permits access to all denture surfaces. It is sometimes difficult to adapt a regular toothbrush thoroughly into the recesses and curves of the tissue surface, resulting in inadequately cleaned dentures. It is important to stress that only a soft-bristled brush should be used on denture materials. Any other type of bristle can abrade and damage the soft denture acrylic. Excessive pressure during overzealous brushing can also result in a damaged surface to the extent that the fit of the denture may be compromised.

Delicate metal clasps on partial dentures should be brushed using a small tapered brush designed specifically for that purpose. Plaque control of these surfaces is especially important because plaque accumulation around abutment teeth and under clasps not only is common but also has significant potential for damaging the gingival and periodontal tissues surrounding these teeth. Use of denture brushes or regular toothbrushes can cause damage and distortion to these clasps, affecting their ability to anchor the partial denture properly. This part of the partial denture must be handled with special care.

Modifications in the choice of brush may be useful for handicapped patients. One modification is to attach rubber suction cups to the bottom of a soft-bristled fingernail or vegetable-brush so that it will adhere to the inside of the sink. The den-

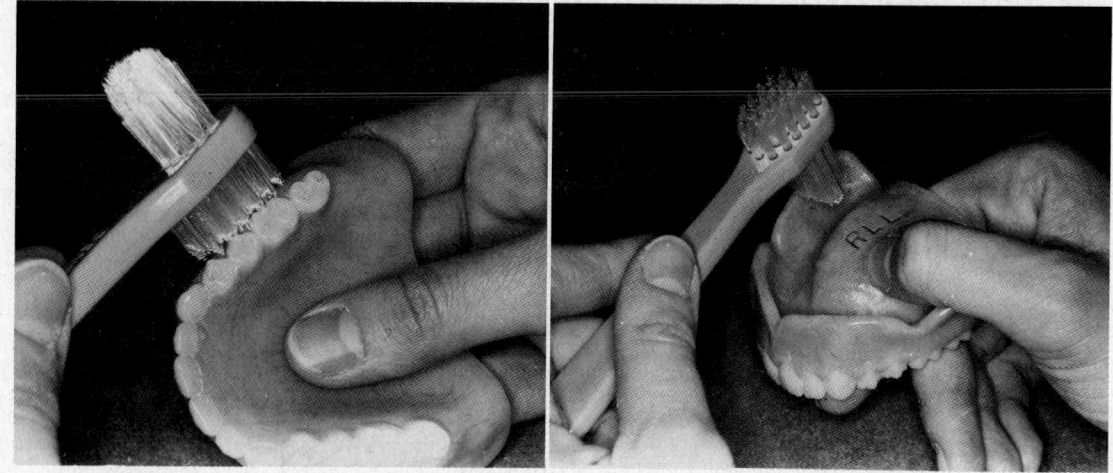

Fig. 27-5. Mechanical brushing of full denture. **A,** Teeth are brushed with flat, rectangular side of a denture brush, and **B,** inner surface is brushed with small rounded brush. It is suggested that this be done over a sink partially filled with water to cushion impact if denture is dropped.

ture can then be brushed by holding it with both hands and moving all surfaces over the bristles of the brush. Fingernail brushes with plastic handles that curve over and around the side of the hand may also be helpful for individuals who cannot grasp a brush with a regular handle.

A number of abrasive powders and dentifrices are commercially available to aid in denture cleaning with a brush. They are manufactured with a mild abrasive such as calcium carbonate, which will not damage denture acrylic as readily as the abrasives in dentifrices used to clean natural teeth. One disadvantage of cream dentifrices is that they are not as easily rinsed off after cleaning. If the patient chooses to use a commercial powder abrasive or dentifrice, recommendations can be made from the list of accepted products published annually by the ADA. Many individuals find that dentures can be cleaned satisfactorily with facial soap or sodium bicarbonate and water. Both of these agents can be used safely and effectively, but patients should be warned never to use other household cleansers on dentures because these preparations are often dangerously abrasive and may be toxic if ingested. Instead, advise patients to have dentures professionally cleaned by dental professionals to remove stain and calculus that cannot be removed by recommended mechanical or chemical cleaning methods.

Dentures should be rinsed thoroughly under cool running water after any cleaning to remove loosened plaque and debris and to clear the denture of the cleaning agent. Brushes should also be rinsed thoroughly under a running stream of water until they are clean of debris and paste and allowed to air-dry. Patients who have both dentures and natural teeth should have a separate brush for cleaning natural teeth so that the brush used on teeth and gums is in good condition. Patients can check the effectiveness of any method of plaque removal with liquid disclosing agents. These solutions allow the patient to see surfaces that have not been thoroughly cleaned.

Patients should be instructed how to handle dentures during cleaning procedures to avoid accidents. Wet dentures are extremely slippery and should be held firmly to avoid dropping them— but not too tightly, because they can be broken if stressed too much. Dentures should be held over the sink with one hand while they are cleaned with the other hand. The bottom of the sink should be lined with a rubber mat or a towel and partially filled with water as protection against breakage if they accidentally slip and fall. Dentures should never be rinsed or soaked in hot water, because high temperatures can damage the acrylic resin. After cleaning at night, dentures should be held in a clean container of either water or one of the commercial soaking agents discussed below. Rinse again before returning them to the mouth. Containers used to store dentures should be rinsed out and cleaned after each use to prevent microbial build-up.

Soft lining materials in dentures should be cleaned with care to avoid damaging the lining and thereby compromising the fit of the denture. Opinions differ regarding the effects of denture cleansers and brushing on these materials. Mäkilä and Honka (1979) reported significant wear of lining materials resulting from brushing over a 30-month period and recommended that dentures with soft liners should be cleaned by immersion rather than brushing. Others, however, found no evidence of abrasion after normal brushing (Wright, 1976; Schmidt and Smith, 1983). Abrasion also can be minimized by cleaning the liners with soft cotton under cool running water. Goll and others (1983) reported that denture cleansers can negatively affect the properties of certain temporary soft tissue liners, such as porosity, shape, size, solubility, and water absorption; they suggested that manufacturers' recommendations for cleaning these materials should be followed. A more recent study, however, subjected soft lining materials to 100 treatments by alkaline hypochlorite, alkaline peroxide, and acidic types of denture cleansers and found that these products did not affect the properties of softness or elastic recovery of the liners tested (Davenport et al, 1986). Dentures with soft linings should be stored in plain water rather than in a commercial soaking solution and should be placed in the storage container with the occlusal surfaces down so that the weight of the denture will not distort the lining material.

Using sonic or ultrasonic units

Although thorough brushing of dentures is probably the most effective way of removing denture plaque, some denture wearers may not have the motivation, time, or perseverance required to perform this task regularly and effectively. Other denture wearers who suffer from debilitating arthritis or other physical limitations, including paralysis, mental incompetence, or blindness, may not be able to perform thorough plaque removal by brushing. For these individuals the use of a sonic or ultrasonic cleaner or a chemical solution may be a more acceptable alternative. Both sonic and ultrasonic units are available for use in cleaning dentures. Sonic cleaners operate through the generation of audible electrosonic energy waves; ultrasonic cleaners operate by means of high-frequency sound waves. Most units available to the general public are the sonic type, which produce less mechanical agitation of solutions than do the ultrasonic units available in most dental offices. The cleaning ability of sonic cleaners has been likened to that of chemical immersion cleansers (Muenchinger, 1975). Although no ultrasonic cleaner has been shown to remove *all* plaque, it has been reported that ultrasonic cleaning is more efficient in plaque removal than either a commercial chemical immersion cleanser or a sonic cleaner (Palenik and Miller, 1984).

There is disagreement as to the effectiveness of these mechanical cleaners in reducing denture plaque. Abelson (1981) found that use of an ultrasonic cleaner and water was effective in removing plaque accumulations and that it was more effective than 15-minute soaks in commercial denture solutions. Myers and Krol (1974) reported that sonic cleaners helped in the removal of calculus and stain from dentures. Nicholson and coworkers (1968) reported that sonic cleaning with a hypochlorite (bleach) solution was more effective in plaque removal than use of that solution alone. The American Dental Association reported that the cleaning ability of ultrasonic devices was related more to the chemical solution in which the denture was immersed than to the ultrasonic action of the device. Budtz-Jorgensen (1979) reported that although ultrasonic treatment by itself did not reduce the number of microorganisms that could be cultured from dentures, it did enhance the effectiveness of disinfecting solutions in which dentures were immersed during the ultrasonic treatment.

Chemicals used for immersion

The use of chemical solutions for soaking dentures is a popular alternative to mechanical cleansing. The advantages of these cleansers are that they require less effort and compliance on the part of the individual and that the solution can reach surfaces on the denture that may be inaccessible to the denture brush. There are several different types of chemical denture cleansers, including alkaline hypochlorites, commercially prepared alkaline peroxides, dilute acids, enzymes, and antibacterials.

Alkaline hypochlorites (e.g., household bleach) are effective as denture cleansers because of their ability to dissolve mucin and other organic substances, thus destroying the plaque matrix so that it can be rinsed or brushed away. These solutions are also bactericidal and fungicidal, making them useful in treating denture stomatitis and for disinfecting dentures. Destruction of the plaque matrix also inhibits calculus formation, and the bleaching action of the solution removes stains from denture acrylic. Alkaline hypochlorites are available as commercial products (e.g., Mersene) or as a homemade preparation in which 1 teaspoon of household bleach and 2 teaspoons of Calgon are combined in 4 ounces of warm water. A number of research studies have found alkaline hypochlorite (Mersene) to be more effective in removing alkaline peroxide products (Hutchins and Parker, 1973; Shannon and Starcke, 1978; Rustogi et al, 1979; Ghalichebaf et al, 1982).

Although they are effective denture cleansers, these solutions have a number of disadvantages. They corrode metal, which restricts their use to appliances that have no metal parts. Kastner and others (1983) also found that the bleach/Calgon solution significantly increased the flexibility of the metal clasps of partial dentures, resulting in poor retention of these appliances. Dentures should be soaked in these solutions for only 10 to 15 minutes for maximum effectiveness; dentures should not soak in these solutions overnight. Hypochlorite solutions have an unpleasant taste and odor, and dentures treated by this method should be brushed and thoroughly rinsed under cool running water afterward. Patients may want to soak dentures in commercial alkaline peroxide rinses after treatment with hypochlorites to minimize taste and odor aftereffects.

Alkaline peroxide preparations are commonly available in tablet or powder form. They consist of an alkaline detergent combined with sodium perborate or percarbonate, which when dissolved in warm water forms an alkaline solution of hydrogen peroxide. The release of oxygen by the hydrogen peroxide causes a bubbling or effervescent action that has a mechanical cleaning effect on the dentures. This mechanical action occurs only during the 10- to 15-minute period during

which the solution is bubbling; additional cleaning usually is not achieved after that period of time.

Use of these agents on a regular basis may help prevent the formation of stain and calculus if followed by brushing and rinsing. Many of these preparations are now formulated with enzymes that enhance their antibacterial action. These products have been found to be safe and effective for treatment of all types of dentures and are the agents of choice for dentures that contain metal parts. Dentures should never be soaked using hot or boiling water, because high temperatures may result in bleaching or distortion of the acrylic resin (Crawford et al, 1986, 1987; Robinson et al, 1985). There are no serious disadvantages to using these products except for the caution needed in storing them so that they cannot be ingested by accident. Tablets can be mistaken by elderly or visually impaired persons for antacid tablets and accidentally ingested. These products should also be stored out of the reach of small children.

Denture soaking as a potential source of infection. Proper care of denture-soaking containers is especially critical for myelosuppressed cancer patients. Chemical soaking solutions can serve as growth media for pathogenic microorganisms that form on the dentures. Contaminated solutions and their holding containers could therefore serve as reservoirs of microorganisms in which clean dentures might be placed. Thus, after storage in these containers, dentures can become a source of infection for the patient. Because of the extreme sensitivity of cancer patients to infection, disposable denture containers should be used and discarded daily. Dentures should be cleaned with a disinfecting detergent (see Chapter 3) and rinsed before being returned to the mouth (DePaola and Minah, 1983; DePaola et al, 1984a and 1984b).

Dilute acids are also used to assist in the cleaning of dentures. They include 3% to 5% hydrochloric acids with or without phosphoric acid, white household vinegar, and more concentrated commercial preparations that are used in ultrasonic units only by dental professionals. Acid solutions dissolve the inorganic components that form on dentures and are good for the removal of persistent stains not removed by regular cleaning methods. Because of their properties as acids, these chemicals should be used with care. A major disadvantage is their ability to corrode metals, limiting their use to appliances with no metal parts. An effective solution for the removal of stain can be made by combining 1 to 2 teaspoons of *white* household vinegar in 4 ounces of warm water. When the formation of calculus on dentures is first noticed, they can be soaked in this solution overnight. Undiluted vinegar can be used to dissolve and loosen heavier calculus deposits by overnight soaking, but this method should be reserved for occasional use and should *never* be used on partial dentures or other metal-containing surfaces.

Enzymes have been incorporated into many commercially available denture-soak products. They have shown effectiveness in destroying the plaque matrix so that plaque can be more easily brushed or rinsed away. Antibacterial agents such as chlorhexidine gluconate have also been suggested for denture cleansing. Although these agents have both antibacterial and antifungal properties, they also are capable of creating stains on denture teeth after repeated use, making them unacceptable for routine treatment of dentures.

COMPARING THE EFFICACY OF DENTURE CLEANSERS

It is difficult to compare the efficacy of the various denture-cleaning products due to the lack of research studies comparing a variety of products used on actual dentures in vivo. Available research results are difficult to compare because of the wide variations in materials and methods, as well as in the quantification of results. In addition to documenting the presence or absence of plaque after use of denture cleansers, studies are also needed to document the pathogenicity of remaining plaque. Dental consumers should be told how to care properly for their dentures and should be informed of the advantages and disadvantages of available products. Consumers should be aware that not all manufacturers' claims for product effectiveness have been documented in published professional research studies. Dental professionals should know the names of products that have been accepted and approved by the ADA Council on Dental Therapeutics. Lists are updated annually identifying products, including denture cleansers, that have been evaluated and accepted for safety, efficacy, quality, and accuracy in advertising claims (Council on Dental Materials, Instruments, and Equipment and Council on Dental Therapeutics, 1988).

CARE OF EDENTULOUS AREAS, SOFT TISSUES, AND ABUTMENT TEETH

In addition to cleaning the removable appliance, individuals also must be instructed about the need to maintain the health of edentulous areas and other soft tissues, as well as that of the abutment teeth and surrounding periodontal tissues. Unless the patient is instructed otherwise by the dentist, dentures should be removed at night and stored in water or in alkaline peroxide cleaning solutions. The acrylic resin materials of which dentures are formed can dry, resulting in distortion, which in turn will compromise the fit of the appliance in the mouth.

The rationale behind removing dentures at night is that this gives the soft tissues beneath the denture an opportunity to rest and recover from the constant compression they undergo between the denture and the bone. Failure to alleviate this stress can result in soreness and irritation of the soft tissues. Removal of dentures at night is preferred by most people because it is less embarrassing and less inconvenient to be without them when one is in the privacy of one's own home. Removal of dentures at night may also be advised for individuals who are known to clench or brux while they sleep, causing additional stress on the soft tissues. In some individuals, however, being without dentures even at night is considered unacceptable. These individuals should understand the importance of maintaining tissue health and should be encouraged to find some time during the day or night when dentures can be removed. It has been recommended that dentures be left out of the mouth for 6 to 8 hours during each 24-hour period (Boucher and Renner, 1982).

After removing, rinsing, and cleaning dentures, the individual also should clean the intraoral tissues using a soft toothbrush or a washcloth. This cleansing not only removes adherent plaque and debris from tissues but also massages and stimulates circulation and keratinization of tissues. Gums and palate also may be massaged after cleaning by applying pressure and stimulation with the fingers. The tongue should also be brushed lightly with a soft toothbrush to remove plaque and to freshen breath. Instructions for the care of remaining teeth are the same as those discussed in Chapter 19. In addition, patients should be instructed regarding the importance of diligent plaque control and caries prevention for abutment teeth. The ability of these teeth to serve as anchors for partial dentures or overdentures depends on the integrity of the supporting periodontal tissues and on the strength of the intact tooth. Periodontal disease and/or dental caries can undermine the ability of these teeth to function properly in retaining the denture. Comprehensive supramarginal and submarginal plaque control, as well as the appropriate use of fluorides for decay prevention, are mandatory for these abutment teeth and paramount to the success of partial or overdentures. Patients should receive detailed instructions regarding appropriate plaque control measures for both abutment teeth and denture materials. Use of fluoride dentifrices as well as topical application of fluoride gels is recommended for control of dental decay. Fluoride gels may be brushed onto the teeth or placed on the inner surfaces of an overdenture that overlies the teeth before inserting the overdenture into the mouth (Johnson and Sivers, 1987; Bergman, 1987).

Care of removable orthodontic appliances involves many of the principles already discussed. Appliances should be worn as directed by the dentist or orthodontist. They should be removed after each meal and rinsed along with the mouth and cleaned with a regular toothbrush and soap or mild abrasive (Fig. 27-5). These appliances should be stored in water when not in the mouth.

Professional denture cleaning usually includes immersion of the denture in professional strength denture cleanser during ultrasonic cleaning. The clinician should receive the denture in a disposable paper towel or napkin and transfer it into a sealable "zip-lock" plastic bag. Protective barrier coverings including mask, gloves, and glasses should be worn while handling and cleaning dentures. The appropriate chemical solution should be selected according to the deposits present on the denture and the materials of which the denture is made. The solution then should be added to the contents of the bag so that the denture is completely immersed. This bag can be placed in a beaker of water in the ultrasonic cleaner (Fig. 27-6). Thus the solution contaminated by the denture can be discarded after cleaning, and other liquids,

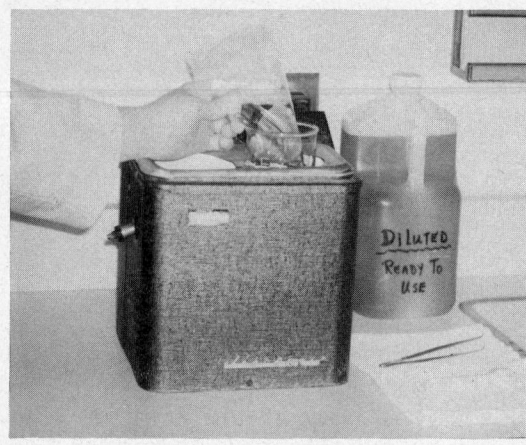

Fig. 27-6. "Zip-lock" sealed plastic bag containing denture and cleaning solution is placed into beaker of water for ultrasonic cleaning.

containers, and surfaces are protected from cross-contamination.

After ultrasonic treatment, the denture should be rinsed thoroughly and brushed with a sterile or disposable denture brush under running water. The original plastic bag should be rinsed before replacing the denture. The denture should be stored in the bag with a small quantity of clean water until returned to the patient. The addition of a small amount of mouthwash to the water in which the clean denture is being held will make the denture taste better when it is replaced in the mouth. Stains and deposits that cannot be removed using the ultrasonic cleaner and brushing may require additional cleansing and/or removal by hand scaling instruments followed by laboratory polishing. Great care must be taken when using these methods in order to avoid scratching or other damage to the acrylic resin material, which might make the denture even more susceptible to build-up of plaque, stain, or calculus deposits.

Denture identification

Dental professionals have recognized the need to mark dentures for identification. Benefits of marking include (1) postmortem identification; (2) identification of persons who are unconscious or who have a loss of memory; (3) identification of dentures in commercial laboratories; and (4) identification of dentures in institutional situations, such as nursing homes (Seals and Seals, 1985).

Minimum critera for dental identification are permanence and full legibility to the patient. American Dental Association guidelines further specify that identification must (1) not jeopardize prosthesis strength; (2) be easy, efficient, and inexpensive; (3) be visible and durable; (4) withstand humidity and fire; (5) be cosmetically acceptable to the wearer; and (6) be in the location least likely to receive damage in an accident (Johanson and Ekman, 1984; Seals and Seals, 1985; Chalian et al, 1986). Opinions vary on what information should be included in the marking because names, identification numbers, dentist's name, and other elements either rely on systems of perpetual and centralized record keeping or are not sufficiently individual-specific.

A variety of techniques has been used for marking dentures. These techniques can be divided into three general types: engraving or scribing into the denture surface; surface marking or writing over the denture base; and inclusion of paper, plastic, or metal markers in the denture's construction (Council on Prosthetic Services, 1982; Johanson and Ekman, 1984; Seals and Seals, 1985).

The engraving method uses an etching or engraving tool to engrave the identifying name or number into the denture. The grooves are then filled with contrasting self-curing acrylic resin or are highlighted with a fine-point, felt-tip pen. Markings are then sealed with clear acrylic resin.

The surface marking method involves using an abrasive pad or emery board to roughen a small area, usually at the back of the denture. The identifying name or number is then written over the roughened surface with a felt-tip pen or a pencil and subsequently covered with clear, self-curing acrylic resin. Surface marking, scribing, and engraving do not provide permanent marks; therefore, dentures identified by these methods must be remarked after a year or more (Johanson and Ekman, 1984).

The inclusion method provides permanent identification. Strips of paper, plastic, or metal are embedded and sealed into the denture (Fig. 27-7). In one approach, the identifying name or number is typed on a small strip of thin white paper. A groove is created in the denture with a dental handpiece, to correspond with the size of the paper strip. After being placed in the groove, the

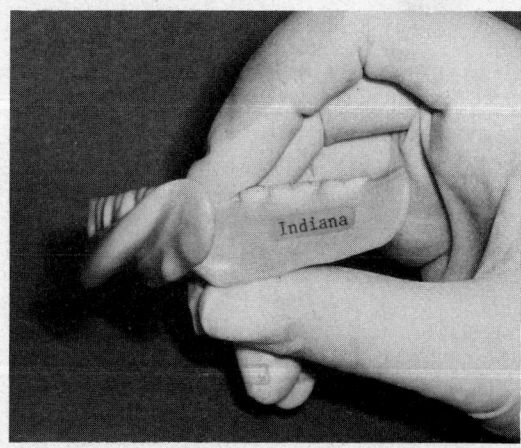

Fig. 27-7. Example of denture marked by inclusion method.

strip is covered with clear acrylic resin and the area is polished, if needed (Council on Prosthetic Services, 1982). Another technique is typing the name or number on a special plastic strip, which is then heated for 1 to 3 minutes in an oven until it shrinks to a hard durable chip. The denture is grooved as described above, and the chip is inserted and sealed with clear acrylic resin. Other inclusion techniques using metal disks or metal strips have also been described (Johanson and Elkman, 1984).

Marking all new dentures for permanent identification is required by law in some states. These statutes do not, however, solve the problems of denture identification for individuals who already have dentures that are unmarked. Denture identification requires minimal time, materials, and effort and can be accomplished in conjunction with regular dental appointments and through community-based dental health programs, such as health fairs or in retirement centers or nursing homes (Williams et al, 1982; Ames, 1985.).

USE, SELECTION, AND CARE OF MOUTH PROTECTORS

The use of mouth protectors in sports has steadily increased over the past 3 decades. First introduced in the direct contact sports of boxing and football, mouth protectors are now being used widely in any sport where there is a risk of falling or being struck in the mouth. The introduction of faceguards in football halved football injuries involving oral trauma, and mouth protectors have nearly eliminated these remaining injuries (Seals and Dorrough, 1984). Unfortunately, oral sports injuries that could be prevented with properly fitted mouth protectors still occur due to a failure to promote the use of protectors for young athletes of both sexes and to the occasional lack of strong endorsement by coaches.

Mouth protectors are usually fitted only over the maxillary teeth, which are the most prone to damage, in order to avoid bulkiness. These devices prevent oral trauma in several ways. They minimize lacerations by holding the soft tissues away from the teeth. They prevent teeth from being damaged by hitting together when subjected to a blow, and they absorb the impact of a direct blow by spreading its force away from individual teeth. This absorption of impact decreases shock to the temporomandibular joint and mandibular condyle, thus protecting against concussions, neck injuries, and more severe central nervous system damage (Seals and Dorrough, 1984).

Several critera must be met for mouth protectors to be accepted into sports programs (Bishop et al, 1985). They must be nontoxic, tasteless, and tissue compatible. They must be comfortable, with a fit that allows retention in the mouth without jaw clenching, and must not interfere with speech. Durability of more than one season, ease of processing and repair, and resistance during sterilization are important. Low cost and easy attainability also improve acceptance of mouth protectors.

Four general types of mouth protectors are available for sports (Fig. 27-8): ready-made or stock; mouth-formed (two types), and custom-fitted (CAL, 1983; Bureau of Health Education, 1984, 1985). Although any type of mouth protector will reduce oral injury, the better it is tolerated by the athlete, the more likely it is that it will be worn and that injuries will be prevented.

Ready-made or stock mouth protectors are commonly available and are the most inexpensive type. They cannot be fitted to the individual, with the result that they are uncomfortable to wear, difficult to retain, bulky, and they interfere with talking and breathing.

There are two types of mouth-formed protectors. The shell-liner type consists of a hard

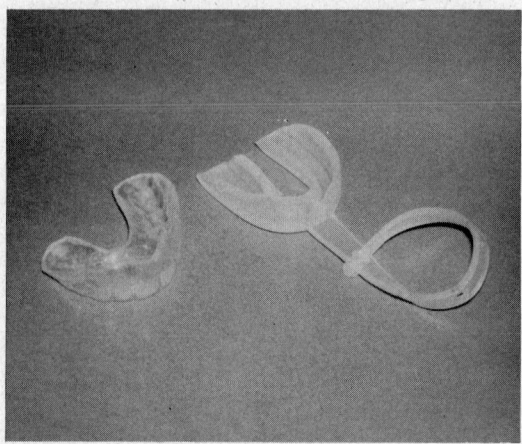

Fig. 27-8. Two types of mouth protectors are shown: custom-fitted mouthgard (left), and thermoplastic mouth-formed type (right).

outer shell of polyvinyl chloride that provides physical strength. A soft liner made of plasticized acrylic gel or silicone rubber is placed in the mouth, molded to the teeth, and then set by thermal or chemical means. A disadvantage of this type is that repeated biting and exposure to saliva cause distortion of the shape and physical properties of the materials. This type is not recommended for athletes with fixed orthodontic appliances.

Thermoplasic mouth-formed protectors are made by immersing the preformed plastic shell in boiling water for 10 to 45 seconds, dipping it in cold water for one second, and then transferring it immediately to the mouth where it is adapted to the teeth. Adaptation can be performed by the individual using finger pressure, tongue pressure, and gentle biting. For best results, however, these protectors should be placed and checked by a dentist. Advantages of this type of mouth-formed protector include comfortable fit, less bulk, reasonable cost, and the ability to reform the plastic if it becomes loose or distorted. These protectors also can be used safely by individuals with fixed orthodontic appliances if they are fitted by dentists. An added advantage of these mouth protectors is that many styles include a strap attachment to anchor the protector to helmet faceguards if desired.

Optimal fit, comfort, and protection are offered

by custom-made mouth guards. They are made of square sheets of a thermoplastic material (e.g., polyvinyl acetate–polyethylene), which are custom-formed to a cast of the individual's maxillary teeth and surrounding tissues and then trimmed for fit and comfort. This procedure should be performed by a dentist to ensure proper fit and function of the final product. Formation of the protector involves heating the thermoplastic material and then vacuum forming it over the cast of the person's teeth for about 2 minutes. After the material cools for a minute, it is then placed in cold water to harden before it is finished. The hardened form is removed from the cast and excess material is trimmed so that it does not impinge on frena, muscle, or soft tissue attachments. Finally, the protector is replaced on the cast and edges are flamed with an alcohol torch for softening and then smoothed with wet fingers. The final product should be evaluated for fit and comfort in the individual's mouth and adjusted as needed by the dentist.

Custom-fitted mouth protectors are usually made to cover all existing teeth in the maxillary arch except for erupting third molars. The protector may be formed instead for the mandibular arch of an individual with a prognathic (protruding, Cl III) mandible because its prominence places that arch at higher risk for injury than the maxilla in these cases. Mouth protectors also can be constructed for edentulous athletes and for those wearing fixed orthodontic appliances.

The individual should be instructed how to care for the mouth protector to preserve its life and function. It should be rinsed under cold tap water after each use and cleaned occasionally in cool soapy water. When not in use, the protector should be stored and transported in a rigid container so that it is not crushed or damaged. Mouth protectors should be inspected regularly for damage or distortion that may affect their fit or ability to prevent injuries (CAL, 1983; Bureau of Health Education, 1985).

Dental professionals should play a role in preparing mouth protectors for athletes or at least in helping the athletes make wise selections. They should be advocates for the use of mouth protectors in all dangerous sports and for all ages and both sexes, not just where mandated by legislation. Athletic coaches, in particular, should be encouraged to support the use of mouth protectors for their athletes in every sport.

ACTIVITIES

1. Get samples of different types of dentures, made of different types of materials from dental offices, laboratories, or dental schools. Discuss the cleaning measures that would most effectively care for each type of appliance, based on its component parts and materials.
2. As a class, plan and implement a community service project for individuals who wear dentures. These projects could include performing an oral cancer screening, providing denture cleaning services, implementing a denture marking service, or making custom-fitted mouth guards for young athletes in conjunction with local dentists. These activities could take place during health fairs or in schools, nursing homes, senior citizen centers, or retirement centers.
3. Survey friends and family members who wear dentures and collect a list of all the methods of cleaning and caring for dentures that they or others they know have used, including "home remedies"; compile all the lists into one master list, noting which techniques are most commonly used and critiquing nonrecommended methods.
4. Practice denture-marking methods using old dentures secured from family members, or ones which have been discarded in nursing homes or institutions.
5. Invite a dentist specializing in denture construction to address the class regarding how dentures are made, the importance of a properly fitting denture, problems in patient adjustment to dentures, and acceptable procedures for relining dentures.
6. Go to a variety of drugstores and grocery stores in the area and compile a list of dental products marketed for use by denture wearers. Compare the list to accepted product lists in *Accepted Dental Therapeutics*. Write manufacturers for more information regarding product use and effectiveness. Critique the products in terms of safety, efficacy, cost, and acceptability.

REVIEW QUESTIONS

1. Which of the following types of denture cleansers should not be used on dentures containing metal parts?
   a. Alkaline peroxide
   b. Dentifrices formulated for denture use
   c. Alkaline hypochlorite solutions
   d. Dilute white vinegar

2. Which method of marking dentures is considered to be the most permanent?
   a. Engraving
   b. Surface marking
   c. Inclusion
3. For which arch are mouth protectors usually fitted?
   a. Mandibular
   b. Maxillary
   c. Both arches
4. True or false: Most people with full dentures seek regular dental care.
5. What is the microorganism which seems to be related to denture stomatitis?
6. What suggestions should be made to patients who complain that calculus forms on their dentures?
7. What precautions should the dental professional take to avoid cross-contamination during denture cleaning procedures?
8. What precautions should individuals take to avoid dropping and breaking dentures during cleaning?

REFERENCES

Abelson DC: Denture plaque and denture cleansers, J Prosthet Dent 45:376, 1981.

Abelson DC: Denture plaque and denture cleansers: review of the literature, Gerodontics 1:202, 1985.

American Dental Association: Guide to dental materials and devices, ed 6. Chicago, 1974, ADA.

Ames RK: Operation IDENT/Nursing home screening project, Broward County, Florida, Flor Dent J 56:42, 1985.

Bergman B: Periodontal reactions related to removable partial dentures: a literature review, J Prosthet Dent 58:454, 1987.

Bishop BM, et al: Materials for mouth protectors, J Prosthetic Dent 53:256, 1985.

Boucher LJ, and Renner RP: Treatment of partially edentulous patients, St Louis, 1982, CV Mosby Co.

Budtz-Jorgensen E: Clinical aspects of *Candida* infection in denture wearers, JADA 96:474, 1978.

Budtz-Jorgensen E: Materials and methods for cleaning dentures, J Prosthet Dent 42:619, 1979.

Budtz-Jorgensen E, et al: Quantitative relationship between yeast and bacteria in denture induced stomatitis, Scand J Dent Res 91:134, 1983.

Bureau of Health Education and Audiovisual Services and Council on Dental Materials, Instruments, and Equipment: Mouth protectors and sports team dentists, JADA 109:84, 1984.

Bureau of Health Education and Audiovisual Services: Mouth protectors: give your teeth a sporting chance. Chicago, 1985, ADA.

Catalan A: Denture plaque and palatal mucosa in *denture stomatitis:* scanning electron microscopic and microbiologic study, J Prosthet Dent 57:582, 1987.

Chalian VA, et al: Identification of removable dental prosthesis, J Prosthet Dent 56:254, 1986.

Council on Dental Materials, Instruments, and Equipment: Denture cleansers, JADA 106:77, 1983.

Council on Dental Materials, Instruments, and Equipment: Accepted dental products, JADA 116:249, 1988.

Council on Prosthetic Services and Dental Laboratory Relations: Operation IDENT. Chicago, 1982, American Dental Association.

Crawford CA, et al: Denture bleaching: a laboratory simulation of patients' cleaning procedures, J Dent 14:258, 1986.

Crawford CA, et al: Bleached dentures: misuse of a denture-cleaning agent, Dent Update (Jan-Feb):29, 1987.

Davenport JC, et al: The compatibility of soft lining materials and denture cleansers, Br Dent J 161:31, 1986.

DePaola LG, and Minah GE: Isolation of pathogenic microorganisms from dentures and denture-soaking containers of myelosuppressed cancer patients, J Prosthet Dent 49:20, 1983.

DePaola LG, et al: Evaluation of agents to reduce microbial growth on dental prostheses of myelosuppressed cancer patients, Clin Prev Dent 6:9, 1984(a).

DePaola LG, et al: Growth of potential pathogens in denture-soaking solution of myelosuppressed cancer patients, J Prosthet Dent 51:554, 1984(b).

Ghalichebaf M, et al: The efficacy of denture cleansing agents, J Pros Dent 48:515, 1982.

Goll G, et al: The effect of denture cleansers on temporary soft liners, J Prosthet Dent 50:466, 1983.

Harrison A: A simple denture marking system, Br Dent J 160:89, 1986.

Hutchins DW, and Parker WA: A clinical evaluation of the ability of denture cleaning solutions to remove dental plaque from prosthetic devices, NY State Dent J 39:363, 1973.

Johanson GK, and Ekman B: Denture marking, JADA 108:347, 1984.

Johanson GK, and Sivers JE: Periodontal considerations for overdentures, JADA 114:468, 1987.

Kastner C, et al: Effects of chemical denture cleaners on the flexibility of cast clasps, J Prosthet Dent 50:473, 1983.

Kempler D, et al: The efficacy of sodium hypochlorite as a denture cleanser, Special Care in Dentistry 2:112, 1982.

Mäkilä E, and Honka O: Clinical study of a heat-cured silicone soft lining material, J Oral Rehabil 6:199, 1979.

Mouth protectors for contact sports, CAL 47:18, 1983.

Muenchinger FS: Evaluation of an electrosonic denture cleaner, J Prosthet Dent 33:610, 1975.

Myers HM, and Kroll AJ: Effectiveness of a sonic-action denture cleaning program, J Prosthet Dent 32:613, 1974.

Nicholson RJ, et al: Calculus and stain removal from acrylic resin dentures, J Prosthet Dent 20:326, 1968.

Ortman LF: Patient education and complete denture maintenance. In Winkler S, editor: Essentials of complete denture prosthodontics, ed 2, Littleton, Mass, 1987, PSG Publishing.

Palenik CJ, and Miller CH: In vitro testing of three denture-cleaning systems, J Prosthet Dent 51:751, 1984.

Rudd RW, et al: Sterilization of complete dentures with sodium hypochlorite, J Prosthet Dent 51:318, 1984.

Rustogi KN, et al: The clinical efficacy of denture cleansers, Quart NDA 37:100, 1979.

Robinson JG, et al: Br Dent J 159:247, 1985.

Schmidt WF, and Smith DE: A six year retrospective study of Molloplast-B-lined dentures. Part II: liner serviceability, J Prosthet Dent 50:459, 1983.

Seals RR, and Dorrough BC: Custom mouth protectors: a review of their applications, J Prosthet Dent 51:238, 1984.

Seals RR, and Seals DJ: The importance of denture identification, Special Care in Dentistry (July-Aug):164, 1985.

Seals RR, et al: An evaluation of mouthguard programs in Texas high school football, JADA 110:904, 1985.

Shannon IL, and Starcke EN: Higher performance denture cleansers, NYJD 48:246, 1978.

Sharp EW, et al: Denture cleansers and in vitro plaque, J Prosthet Dent 53:584, 1985.

Tarbet WJ, et al: Denture cleansing: a comparison of two methods, J Prosthet Dent 51:322, 1984.

Waldman HB: The edentulous population: its use and need of dental services, J Prosthet Dent 58:643, 1987.

Williams JE, et al: A denture identification program for nursing home residents, Special Care in Dentistry 2:76, 1982.

Wright PS: Soft lining materials: their status and prospects, J Dent 4:247, 1976.

28 FLUORIDE THERAPY

OBJECTIVES: The reader will be able to

1. Describe what causes dental caries.
2. Describe how fluoride inhibits dental caries, including the following factors:
   a. The formation of fluorapatite
   b. Its effect on microorganisms and plaque
   c. Its function in the outermost layer of enamel
   d. Its role in calcium and phosphorus remineralization
3. Distinguish between the benefits of systemic and topical fluoride in preventing caries.
4. Specify the optimal level of fluoride in communal water supplies.
5. Describe dental fluorosis and how it is caused.
6. Define posteruption maturation.
7. Describe the logic and results of the Grand Rapids/Muskegon and Kingston/Newburgh studies.
8. Administer a professional topical fluoride treatment using the following:
   a. Sodium fluoride
   b. Stannous fluoride
   c. Acidulated phosphate fluoride
9. Describe the recommended regimen for fluoride rinses containing 0.025%, 0.05%, and 0.20% sodium fluoride.
10. Outline and follow procedures designed to minimize toxic reactions to fluoride during the following:
    a. Daily use of fluoride supplements
    b. In-office topical fluoride treatments
11. Outline the current controversies and trends relating to the following:
    a. Using high concentration topical fluorides
    b. Excessive exposure to fluorides from dietary and professional sources
    c. Polishing teeth before topical fluoride application
    d. Using frequent, low-dose fluorides
    e. Higher-concentration fluorides in dentifrices
    f. Water fluoridation
12. Outline a fluoride therapy program for caries-prone patients.

FLUORIDE AND DENTAL CARIES

Until the last decade, more teeth were lost to dental decay than to any other dental problem. In the past several years, caries incidence has dropped dramatically (U.S. Public Health Service, 1981; Burt, 1983; Downer, 1983). Fluoride is cited as one of the primary reasons for this decline (Granath and McHugh, 1986). Fluoride is found in many public water supplies, in toothpastes, in oral rinses, in lozenge form, in concentrated topical gels, and even in foods. Frequent exposure to multiple forms of fluoride undoubtedly has had a positive effect on tooth enamel's resistance to dental decay. Most dentists and hygienists consider fluoride to be the most reliable preventive agent for caries (Isman, 1984).

Dental plaque, as pointed out in earlier chapters, is rich in microorganisms. *Streptococcus mu-*

tans is believed to be the principal bacterium in caries formation, even for root caries (Keltjens et al, 1987). When *S. mutans* is exposed to simple carbohydrates, such as sucrose, glucose, or fructose, it metabolizes those sugars and produces acid. The acid is held against the enamel, resulting in a loss of mineral content from the tooth. A carious lesion results from numerous pH drops in the plaque that covers enamel if there is no intervening remineralization from salivary or dietary sources.

Fluoride itself remineralizes the tooth, but it also assists calcium and phosphorus in repairing the enamel (Fehr et al, 1970). The beginning carious lesion is usually detected clinically as a white, chalky spot on the tooth. Scanning electron microscopy of the white spot lesion shows eroded focal holes (Driessens et al, 1985) that allow bacteria and acids to enter to deeper layers. If this process persists without an opportunity for the area to remineralize, the lesion progresses inward toward the dentin, from where it can advance rapidly toward the pulp.

FLUORIDE'S MECHANISMS OF ACTION

Fluoride works in several ways to prevent caries. It converts the enamel constituent, hydroxyapatite, to fluorapatite. Fluorapatite resists demineralization. However, fluoride's action at the surface of the enamel is probably the most important function (Newbrun, 1986).

Also, fluoride is antibacterial, and, if highly concentrated in a plaque layer, may inhibit the growth of *S. mutans*. Fluoride is largely chemically bound in the plaque, but becomes available as free fluoride ion as the pH drops (due to acid production by bacteria), at which point it may inhibit harmful enzyme formation or the acid-producing bacteria (Newbrun, 1986). Fluoride may actually inhibit the formation of acid (antiglycolytic activity) as it is gradually released from enamel into the potentially harmful plaque layer (Harper and Loesche, 1986); also, it may, at high concentrations, prevent salivary pellicle formation or the adherence of bacteria on teeth (Newbrun, 1986).

If fluoride is consumed in drinking water, in fluoride lozenges or tablets, or through the inadvertent swallowing of fluoride toothpaste, the fluoride ions travel through the bloodstream and surround the developing teeth before eruption. The fluoride bathes the forming enamel, making it relatively impervious to acid attack from plaque once the tooth is erupted and exposed to dietary sugars. Ingesting water with approximately 1 part per million (ppm) fluoride results in higher amounts of fluoride in deeper enamel (Iijima & Katayama, 1985). Children who live in fluoridated communities for at least 3 years during tooth development show 26.8% fewer carious lesions in their permanent teeth than cohorts who have not lived in fluoridated communities, showing the effects of ingested fluorides on developing enamel (Burt et al, 1986).

Removing the fluoride from a water supply caused the incidence of decayed, missing, and filled surfaces to increase 39.6% over a 5-year period even during a period of nationwide decline in caries incidence (Stephen et al, 1987b).

If the concentration of fluoride in the water is too high (usually more than 5 ppm), the teeth may develop white or even brown mottling. This *dental fluorosis* is disfiguring if it is severe. Therefore, dietary sources of fluoride must be monitored to ensure that children are not overexposed (Heifetz and Horowitz, 1984).

Once the teeth are erupted, exposure to fluorides in the mouth becomes important. The newly erupted tooth goes through a maturation process in which the enamel hardens as it is exposed to salivary minerals, especially fluoride (Driessens et al, 1985). It is more difficult to acid-etch teeth for sealant adherence that have been exposed to oral fluids for an extended period than it is to etch newly erupted ones because of this posteruption maturation.

After teeth erupt, even very low doses of fluoride (.024 ppm) can remineralize tooth structure and help protect the enamel from demineralization (Margolis et al, 1986). The higher concentrations used in professional fluoride treatments (12,300 ppm), which contact the enamel for 4 minutes, are intended to penetrate further into the enamel, converting it to fluorapatite.

The outermost enamel layer is the most impervious to acid attack and the richest in fluoride. Nakagaki and colleagues showed that there was an exponential decrease in fluoride in the enamel as it moved away from the outermost layer toward the middle third of the enamel (1987).

There appears to be a pumping mechanism of inorganic material from inner enamel to the oral cavity and back, continuously regenerating the outer layer (Driessens et al, 1985; Hattab, 1986). The plaque itself provides a reservoir for fluoride that has penetrated the bacterial mass (Charleton et al, 1974; Schamschula et al, 1982), but this fluoride is derived in part from the enamel (Holloway et al, 1981; Klimek et al, 1983).

There is no strong, mathematical correlation between fluoride in enamel and dental caries (Mellberg et al, 1985; Retief et al, 1987), probably because of the many other factors that affect caries, including most notably dietary habits. Frequency of sugar intake and the form in which it is ingested, salivary flow and composition, tooth alignment, brushing and flossing habits, and the microbial population of plaque on the teeth each affect the caries rate in any given individual's teeth. However, even though no correlation has been found between enamel fluoride content and caries, fluoride is well recognized as a major contributing force in preventing decay based on carefully controlled laboratory and clinical experiments. The levels required to prevent decay in one person may not be the same as those required in other individuals. Susceptibility differs from person to person.

COMMUNAL WATER FLUORIDATION

The addition of fluoride to communal water supplies is a relatively new method of controlling dental decay. Dr. S.S. McKay noted among his patients in the Rocky Mountain area of the United States that patients who had intrinsic brown stains (mottling) had less dental decay than those without stain. Dr. H. Trendly Dean conducted investigations in the 1930s linking this brown stain and a lower caries incidence with the presence of fluoride in the drinking water. The next step was to compare towns with varying levels of natural fluoride in the water with towns having minimal fluoride in order to determine what concentration could effectively inhibit decay without enamel mottling. From these results researchers determined the optimum concentration of 1 ppm.

In 1945, Grand Rapids, Michigan, added fluoride to its water supply; the caries incidence over the next several years was compared with that observed in nearby Muskegon, Michigan, which had a very low fluoride level. Likewise, Newburgh, New York, was fluoridated and compared with its neighbor, Kingston, New York. The results of these and subsequent studies showed significant reduction in caries as well as unequivocal safety (ADA Council, 1984; McClure, 1970; Stallard, 1983; Wei, 1974).

After these initial studies, efforts to fluoridate communities throughout the country were launched. Most major cities are fluoridated; however, there are continuing efforts to fluoridate additional communities and to ward off the efforts of antifluoridationists, who typically cite potentially harmful effects and the issue of mass medication in their efforts to remove fluoride from the public drinking supply. Despite 40 years of safety data that reveal no trends in increased disease among populations drinking fluoridated water, these groups persist in presenting to legislative bodies information that would suggest there are harmful effects. Most dentists and hygienists agree that water fluoridation is desirable, and they are willing to work in community campaigns to ensure that the public votes in favor of adding the ion to their water (Isman, 1984). The most effective way to lobby in favor of this public health measure may be to include a discussion of water fluoridation in one-on-one patient education in the dental office. In this way, those people seeking dental care will already be educated to the benefits of fluoridation and be ready to speak and vote in favor of adding fluoride or retaining such a program in the community.

FLUORIDE FORMULATIONS AVAILABLE FOR CONTROL OF CARIES

If the water supply used by your patients is not fluoridated, *sodium fluoride* drops should be prescribed for infants for daily use. Lozenges, which are sucked or chewed, then swished and swallowed, are prescribed for older children. Table 28-1 shows the recommended doses of daily fluoride tablets or drops (ADA Council, 1984). It is important to coordinate with the child's pediatrician or family physician to ensure that the proper amounts are recommended (Levy, 1986).

Sodium fluoride was one of the first forms of fluoride to be applied topically to the teeth. The original protocol called for applying a 2.0% solu-

Table 28-1. Recommended doses of daily fluoride tablets or drops

Patient's age	Fluoride concentration of drinking water (ppm)			Suggested product
	Less than 0.3	0.3 to 0.7	More than 0.7	
	Recommended mg. of fluoride per day			
Birth to 2 years	0.25	0	0	Drops
2 to 3 years	0.50	0.25	0	Tablets or drops
3 to 13 years	1.00	0.50	0	Tablets

Modified from ADA Council on Dental Therapeutics: Accepted dental therapeutics, ed 40, Chicago, 1984, American Dental Association.

tion to clean, dry teeth for 3 to 4 minutes at ages 3, 7, 11, and 13, the ages when newly erupted teeth are present in the mouth. Four applications are given 1 week apart. Caries reductions of 30% to 40% have been measured among children living in low-fluoride areas. Sodium fluoride is chemically stable, has an acceptable taste, is non-irritating, and causes no tooth discoloration. Its major disadvantage is the need to see the patients for 4 consecutive weeks (Horowitz and Heifetz, 1986).

Sodium fluoride is included in some toothpastes in a 0.10% concentration. It is stable, provides good re-mineralization, and is readily taken up into the enamel (Reintsema et al, 1985). Sodium fluoride is also the active ingredient in most fluoride oral rinses sold over the counter (0.05% or 0.025%) or by prescription (0.20%). The formulation's stability in solution makes it ideal for delivering fluoride in a ready-made rinse that may be stored for several months. The 0.025% solution is intended for twice-daily use; the 0.05% solution is for once-daily use; the 0.20% prescription solution is for once-weekly use. Daily rinsing results in approximately 50% reduction in caries; the weekly rinses produced a 44% reduction. Even a 0.01% sodium fluoride rinse (not currently marketed) used for 60 seconds twice daily was found to produce a layer of acid-resistant mineralization at the outer layer of cementum in an in vitro/in vivo study with subjects wearing slabs of demineralized tooth in a prosthetic device while rinsing and during daily activities (Terenaka and Koulourides, 1987).

The famous Three Village Program studies showed that after 7 years the 0.2% rinses produced a 47.2% reduction in caries overall and a 78.9% reduction in caries on proximal surfaces (Ripa et al, 1983b, 1983c; Leske et al, 1984, 1985). The Nelson County, Virginia, study showed a 90% reduction in proximal caries after 11 years of weekly rinsing (0.20%) combined with ingesting 1 mg fluoride tablet daily and using a fluoride dentifrice (Horowitz et al, 1986). Overall, the weekly and daily rinses are considered to decrease caries by 35% (Leske et al, 1984; Horowitz and Heifetz, 1986). In a head-to-head trial 0.05% and 0.20% were shown to be equivalent (Driscoll et al, 1981). Because they are less costly, most school-based programs use the 0.2% rinses weekly (Horowitz and Heifetz, 1986.)

Rinse container sizes are specified by the Food and Drug Administration in order to minimize the possibility of an accidental consumption of a toxic or lethal dose. No more than 264 mg of sodium fluoride or 120 mg of fluoride ion should be prescribed at one time (ADA Council, 1984). Fluoride rinses should be stored out of the reach of children, and their use should be supervised by an adult. The rinses must be expectorated after use and not swallowed. Typically children over 5 years of age can manage thorough expectoration, but even they should be evaluated for their ability to control the swallow reflex. Ask the child to swish with a premeasured 10 milliliters of water and then empty it back into the cup. The amount that is returned should exceed the amount that was premeasured, as the saliva will contribute to the volume of what is returned to the measuring cup. This gauge of ability can help identify subjects who automatically consume whatever is placed in the mouth.

Stannous fluoride (SnF_2) also can be applied topically. A freshly mixed 8.0% solution is applied to dry teeth for 4 minutes, during which the teeth are continually painted with the solution. The treatment requires a single visit and can result in reductions in caries of 48% to 78%. Stannous fluoride is unstable in solution, tastes bad, stains demineralized enamel a yellowish brown, and can irritate the soft tissues (Horowitz and Heifetz, 1986).

Stannous fluoride was included in the first fluoride dentifrice, but its instability rendered it inactive a few months after manufacture. The inactivity results from the binding of the stannous fluoride molecule with abrasives in toothpastes.

Stannous fluoride is now available by prescription in a nonabrasive gel system at a 0.4% concentration, providing 1000 ppm fluoride. It can be used at home and should be brushed on the teeth twice daily after brushing with a dentifrice and rinsing thoroughly to remove all traces of abrasive from the mouth. As it is brushed on the teeth, the gel quickly becomes a liquid, which is swished among the teeth before expectorating. The stannous fluoride not only aids in the prevention of caries, but also has antihypersensitivity properties (see Chapter 30). Several studies indicate that it has antiplaque and antigingivitis effects as well (McDonald et al, 1978; Hock and Tinanoff, 1979; Mazza et al, 1981; Boyd et al, 1988). The disadvantages are its taste (although the gel preparations are more palatable than the 8.0% solutions), the staining of teeth, and its potential toxicity.

Acidulated phosphate fluoride (APF) was introduced in the early 1960s when it was determined that fluoride uptake is better in an acidic environment (Benediktsson et al, 1982). The fluoride gel is either painted on the teeth or applied in preformed trays on both arches simultaneously. It is applied for 4 minutes, during which uptake is very rapid (Newbrun, 1986). The patient should chew lightly on the trays to move the fluoride around the teeth. Also, it is important that the fluoride gel be thixotropic—a gel that becomes fluid when applied to the teeth and agitated by occlusal movements or by movement of an applicator.

APF contains 1.23% fluoride ion derived from sodium fluoride and hydrogen fluoride in 2 moles of orthophosphoric acid at a pH of 3.0. Studies show up to 70% reduction in caries, but the average reduction is 28% (Horowitz and Heifetz, 1986). APF is available in a variety of flavors and is generally believed to be more acceptable than sodium or stannous fluorides. APF gels are available for brushing on the teeth and then swishing between the teeth followed by expectoration.

At least three manufacturers market a *sequential or combined rinse of APF and SnF_2* for use in professional fluoride treatments. These rinses are much higher in total fluoride concentration (0.31% APF and 1.64% SnF_2) and, for obvious safety reasons, should not be recommended for home use. Three studies with extracted teeth show that enamel is less soluble after using a sequential rinse (Shannon et al, 1974a, 1974b; Crall et al, 1983), but most caries researchers agree that demonstration of efficacy is insufficient to recommend the use of sequential rinses even under professional supervision. They are easier to use than 4-minute applications of the other agents, but are not supportable as a choice in place of agents proven to be effective in short- and long-term clinical trials (Horowitz and Heifetz, 1986).

Gels for home use on a daily basis can be recommended. They contain 1.1% NaF, approximately half the concentration of those used in professional treatment. Applied in custom-made trays, they can be a helpful adjunct for patients with rampant dental decay. Only 5 drops per tray should be used to minimize accidental swallowing. They can be used daily for 3½ weeks; their use then should be reevaluated by a dental professional. School-aged children should be carefully supervised during use; children under 3 should NEVER be given these products (Horowitz and Heifetz, 1986).

In addition, *sodium monofluorophosphate* (Na_2MFP) is used to deliver fluoride in some dentifrices. The average benefit, whether in fluoridated or nonfluoridated communities, is a reduction in caries incidence of 25%, with a range of 15% to 40% (DePaola, 1983). Its uptake into enamel and its ability to remineralize white spot lesions are good, but not as rapid as those of sodium fluoride (Reintsema et al, 1985; White and Faller, 1987). However, MFP seems to produce a more thorough remineralization of the early carious lesion, perhaps because it acts more slowly (Mellberg and Mallon, 1984). These differences may have little clinical relevance when fluoride is available from drinking water, fluoride rinses, and professional treatments.

Fluoride varnishes are available in Europe. They are painted on the teeth and deliver fluoride in a controlled release system, improving upon delivery systems that are quickly washed away by saliva and eating. As of 1988, they are not available in the United States. A 2-year study in Finland comparing twice-yearly applications of a varnish with rinsing with 0.20% NaF every 2 weeks showed significant superiority with the varnishes, suggesting a cost-effective alternative to fortnightly rinsing (Seppa and Pollanen, 1987). Varnishes show a mean caries incidence reduction of 48% and a significantly higher concentration of enamel fluoride at 1 and 5 weeks posttreatment than that achieved with an APF treatment (Clark, 1982).

CONTROVERSIES AND CHANGING PROTOCOLS

Historically, dentists and hygienists have used two primary ways to deliver fluoride: (1) in dietary sources, such as communal water supplies and (2) topical fluoride treatments, where a high concentration of fluoride is applied directly to the teeth for up to 4 minutes (ASDC Forum, 1984). The former modality is still universally accepted as an important prevention measure. The latter, however, while still widely accepted and practiced, is being reevaluated.

Professionally applied topical fluorides deliver between 9000 and 19,400 ppm fluoride to the enamel surface. If the presence of .024 ppm fluoride can remineralize tooth structure as noted above, the concentration in professional treatments may be overkill. Likewise, uptake for both sodium fluoride (NaF) and acidulated phosphate fluoride (APF) is linearly dependent upon exposure time (Benediktsson et al, 1982; Arends et al, 1985). One in vitro study noted that a 6-hour application time was optimal for deep penetration of enamel and the formation of fluorapatite (Arends et al, 1985). This is, of course, not a result that is easily adopted in dental hygiene practice.

In addition, high concentrations of fluoride are not necessarily optimal for deep penetration in enamel. These higher concentrations form CaF_2 rather than fluorapatite, blocking the diffusion pathways to the deeper enamel and inhibiting ion penetration into the body of a carious lesion (Benediktsson et al, 1982). However, a 1983 study (Bruun et al) showed that carious areas on extracted teeth retained CaF_2 at measurable levels at the surface at 8 weeks after treatment with APF even when subjected to continuous washing. The release of CaF_2 from the enamel over a number of weeks after the concentrated treatment may be of benefit in helping prevent or remineralize caries (Fejerskov et al, 1981) or in affecting accumulating dental plaque for the short-term. In 1988 Lagerlof and colleagues discovered that a coating of pyrophosphate (found in many toothpastes) may enhance the slow release of CaF_2. These findings provide a rationale for the continued use of high-dose, biannual treatments, particularly if patient access to or compliance of with usage low-dose fluoride rinses and dentifrices is questionable.

Concentration of fluoride treatment is also a topic of discussion. In vitro tests show that there is no difference is enamel fluoride uptake whether an APF concentration is 1100 ppm, 2300 ppm, 2500 ppm, or 12,300 ppm fluoride ion (Dijkman et al, 1982). A 2-year clinical trial comparing 1.23% APF with 0.6% APF demonstrated no significant differences between the two concentrations in the control of smooth surface caries, with the higher concentration more effective on pits and fissures (Hagan et al, 1985). Even drinking fluoridated water has a topical effect on teeth beyond that achieved by the bathing of the unerupted teeth (Mirth et al, 1985). Larsen and Jensen's research (1986) suggest that fluoride activity and pH have a greater impact on CaF_2 than does concentration. Therefore the fluoride concentration in topical treatments may be altered as continued research evaluates fluoride uptake, remineralization, resistance to demineralization, and long-term clinical caries effects.

The *increased incidence of mild fluorosis* among teenagers compared with teens examined 10 years ago suggests that children may be exposed to too much total dietary fluoride (Heifetz et al, 1987; Narendran et al, 1987). Drinking water, most dentifrices, fluoride rinses, and professionally applied treatments provide cumulative effects. The profession has viewed fluoride as incapable of doing harm. However, dental hygienists and dentists are now being urged to assess the levels of fluoride that their patients may be ingesting in order to minimize the likelihood of fluorosis. Patients should be assessed for all sources of fluoride and the frequency of their ingestion. For instance, persons living in dry climates or who engage in heavy physical activity may consume more water each day to replenish fluids than persons living in a humid environment or who have minimal physical activity.

Children should be supervised when using fluoride toothpaste so that they do not eat or inadvertently swallow it. Toothpaste should be treated like a drug and placed out of children's reach when not being used under supervision. Consuming large amounts of fluoride toothpaste can cause nausea and vomiting and create a sufficient spike in blood levels of fluoride to cause fluorosis. Even a single elevated systemic dose of fluoride increases the ion concentration in the bone surrounding the developing tooth, where it may be slowly released in sufficient concentrations to cause fluorosis (Angmar-Mansson and Whitford, 1985).

Recently introduced higher-concentration (2500 ppm) fluoride toothpastes have shown only minimal decrements in caries and should not be selected for small children unless the children have serious caries problems. Again, supervision is imperative.

Until 1984, the accepted protocol regarding *preparation of teeth for a topical fluoride treatment* required all plaque and stain be polished from the teeth in order to ensure optimal contact of fluoride with enamel. Research results with APF gels have changed that standard procedure. A change was first considered when it was discovered that polishing can abrade a thin but significant fluoride-rich layer of outer enamel from the teeth (Vrbic et al, 1967) and was further considered when it was discovered that fluoride uptake into enamel was greater when existing plaque remained on the teeth (Bruun and Stoltz, 1976; Klimek et al, 1982). However, these combined findings did not immediately translate into an altered protocol.

The first finding occurred when researchers were learning about the importance of the fluoride in the outermost layer of enamel. The second finding was tempered by the discovery that plaque-enhanced uptake was due to the demineralization the plaque had caused in the underlying enamel; the demineralized structures acquire fluoride more readily than does intact enamel. This latter finding, however, stimulated a series of clinical studies that established that it makes no difference in uptake or in caries incidence whether plaque is removed with a rubber cup and abrasive, with a toothbrush and floss, or simply left on the teeth before applying topical APF (Steele, 1982; Seppa, 1983; Ripa, 1983a; Leverett and Curzon, 1983; Houpt et al, 1983; Bijella et al, 1985).

Ripa recommends the following revised protocol:

Although the prophylaxis/topical fluoride treatment has been a time-honored sequence in clinical dentistry, enough recent laboratory and clinical evidence exists to recommend the elimination of the prior prophylaxis as a routine procedure when professional topical fluoride applications are performed (Ripa, 1984).

This suggested revision and the growing body of information suggesting that polishing has limited therapeutic value make the inclusion of polishing as a standard procedure in dental hygiene care questionable (see Chapter 26).

In light of this evidence regarding the necessity of a complete prophylaxis before topical fluoride treatments, dental professionals should begin to investigate other options for patient preparation. Within the dental practice, tooth cleaning is one of the priorities of treatment. The patient should be instructed and reinforced regarding the necessity of effective supramarginal plaque control. In addition, the professional bears the responsibility of removing those soft and hard deposits both supramarginally and submarginally that the patient cannot remove. During a preventive appointment, then, tooth cleaning (i.e., scaling, root planing, and prophylaxis) are important. There are a number of ways that the clinician can accomplish coronal cleaning other than with a rubber cup prophylaxis. One alternative might be to have the patient perform supervised brushing and flossing either with a fluoride paste or without one. In this way the professional could instruct and reinforce effective behaviors in the patient while simultaneously accomplishing the tooth cleaning. If a fluoride paste or gel is used during the brushing, the fluoride treatment or application is also accomplished in the same step. If no paste or gel is used, the brushing and flossing can be followed by a topical fluoride treatment if needed.

Another alternative to the traditional prophylaxis is selective polishing of only those teeth with stains that the patient cannot remove. The patient can then brush and floss to remove remaining plaque under professional supervision, and the topical fluoride can be applied. Both of these approaches open up new treatment alternatives that allow the clinician to spend more time with patients, instructing them on home care methods, and less time polishing plaque from the coronal surfaces. They also demonstrate to patients that the primary responsibility for supragingival plaque removal lies with them—rather than with the professional.

In addition to using high-concentration professional topical fluoride treatments, clinicians are *recommending the use of daily, low-concentration fluoride rinses* to prevent caries. This pattern is a response to the growing body of information suggesting that frequency of exposure is more critical than concentration. Patients may be asked to rinse daily with the 0.05% sodium fluoride rinses or weekly with the 0.20% sodium fluoride rinses. Twice-daily rinsing can be recommended with a .025% sodium fluoride rinse. The selection should be made primarily with regard to the ability of the patient to expectorate all the rinse from the mouth and to his or her habit patterns. Some people remember to use a rinse if they use it after each brushing (twice daily 0.025% is best in this case); others are more likely to comply if the regimen is a weekly one (for instance, every Saturday morning, rinse with the 0.20% solution). School programs often opt for the weekly rinses or institute a daily brushing program followed by rinsing with the 0.05% solution.

Another controversy concerns the use of *higher-concentration fluoride in dentifrices*. Typically the concentration of fluoride ion in dentifrices has been from 800 to 1150 ppm. In 1987 the FDA approved a new drug application for a dentifrice containing 1500 ppm. One toothpaste was immediately introduced with the higher level of fluoride ion; its packaging carries a specific warning regarding the need to supervise children using the product. The debate centers on whether a higher-concentration toothpaste is necessary given the decline in the caries rate and the increased emphasis upon limiting ingested fluoride. Clinical trials to demonstrate an incremental benefit from the higher level of fluoride have reported minimal improvement, usually between 10% and 15%, over lower-concentration dentifrices (Stephan et al, 1987a) or no difference (Ripa, 1987). This is due partly to the difficulty of securing a test group with a high caries rate. Opponents contend that if little additional benefit is achieved, the risk of ingesting larger quantities of fluoride outweighs the potential good. Proponents contend that certain populations still have a high caries rate and that the dentifrice should be available for them.

FLUORIDE THERAPY

Dental hygienists confronted with individuals who have a propensity for caries should design a fluoride therapy program that fits the individual's lifestyle and willingness to cooperate. Adding fluoride to the daily regimen of brushing and flossing requires careful planning and a full assessment of the sources of fluoride already present in the patient's daily activities.

First, assess the family, communal or school water supply for fluoride. Assay it if necessary. Many sources have natural fluoride; others sources may not be optimally fluoridated. Determine the need for systemic supplements following the guidelines in Table 28-1. For children under 13, provide the proper prescription for the supplements to the parents, monitor the filling of the prescription (to determine patient compliance), and monitor the use of the supplement by following up with the patient. Remember to adjust the supplement dosage when necessary (as the child ages or as fluoride availability in the drinking supply changes) (Levy, 1987). Following these steps is an important, but frequently ignored, part of the protocol for providing fluoride supplementation (Levy, 1987).

After determining and prescribing the supplement, add a fluoride dentifrice and a fluoride rinse or low-dose home-use gel, giving careful instructions regarding the use of each. In-office topical treatments can be given more frequently than twice yearly depending upon the needs of the patient (Horowitz and Heifetz, 1986). Usually, logic must prevail in how many additional steps can be required of a patient in order to minimize caries. It will be more effective to add one new source of fluoride that the patient can easily adopt than to add several sources that weigh heavily on the pa-

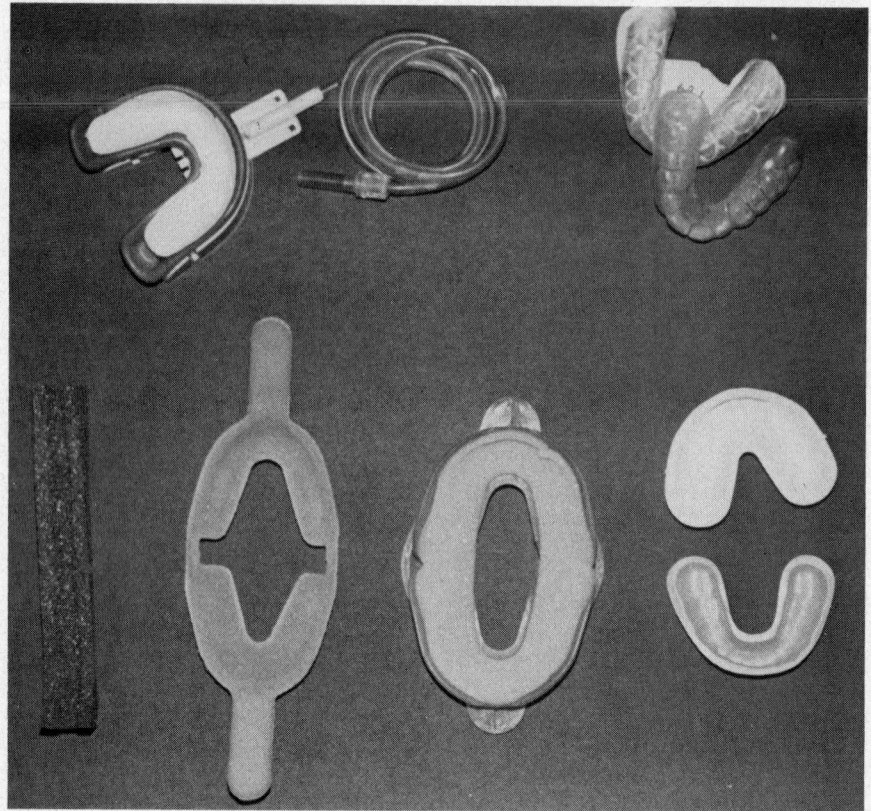

Fig. 28-1. A variety of fluoride trays is available for application of fluoride gels. *Clockwise from upper left:* Reusable tray with hard plastic base, rubber membrane liner, and paper inserts (note also saliva ejector attachment on tray); pliable plastic tray made by forming plastic material directly from patient's arch impressions; styrofoam trays; plastic disposable tray with foam insert; tray in which plastic and foam are fused; foam tray that can be cut and adapted to arch length at time of treatment.

tient's time, financial resources, and commitment.

Fluoride gel application

Professional fluoride applications can be delivered by two different methods. The first method of fluoride application to be discussed is the tray technique, which is used to apply fluoride gels to the teeth. The second involves the application of fluoride solution. Fluoride solution cannot be applied in trays because it would spill out into the mouth, and thus it must be "painted" onto the individual tooth surfaces with cotton-tipped applicators. This technique for applying fluoride solution is described later in the chapter.

The widespread use of fluoride gels for professional fluoride applications has significantly in-creased the ease and simplicity of applying topical fluorides. The gels are inserted into a tray that is designed to fit over all the teeth of one arch, thereby eliminating the need to apply fluoride to individual teeth. The gel is more viscous or thick than the fluoride solutions and is transferred easily into the mouth, where it adheres to the tray and teeth with minimal or no leakage.

Tray selection. A wide variety of fluoride trays is commercially available for use in professional fluoride applications (Fig. 28-1). Although most trays are made of disposable materials, some use disposable liners in a reusable, arch-fitting base (Fig. 28-1, *top left, bottom middle left*). The clinician should consider several factors carefully to determine which type of tray design to pur-

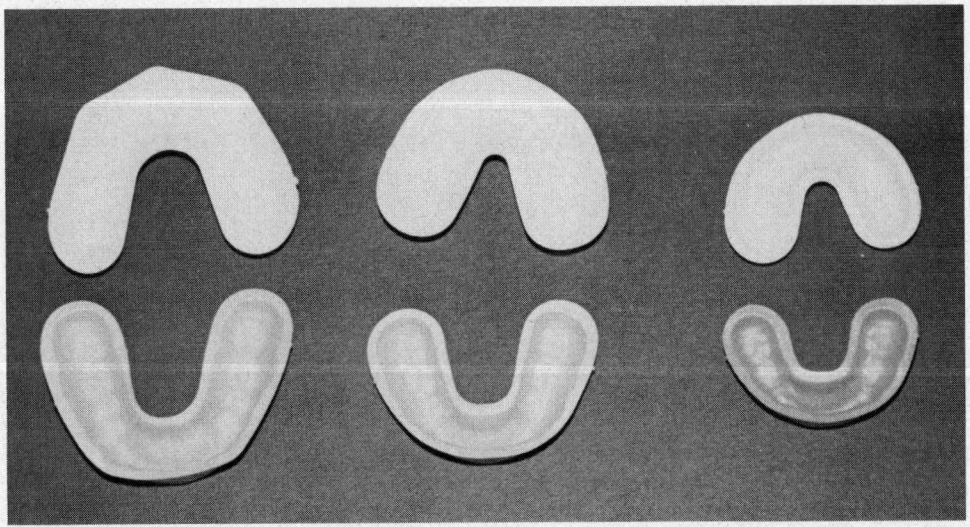

Fig. 28-2. Many disposable fluoride trays come in a selection of arch sizes to ensure optimal fit for each patient.

chase. The tray should be available in a variety of sizes to fit primary, mixed, and adult dentitions (Fig. 28-2). The length of the tray should provide complete coverage of all erupted teeth without extending beyond the most distal tooth's surfaces. The width and depth should provide both effective isolation of teeth and intimate contact of the fluoride gel and the tooth surfaces when it is in place. The ends of the tray should be closed so that fluoride gel is not spilled into the mouth during the procedure. Trays that are custom fitted to the patient's mouth will provide the best fit, because they conform exactly to the teeth and arch (Fig. 28-1, *top right*). A custom-made fit improves the amount of contact between the teeth and the fluoride gel and promotes compression of the gel against the teeth and into interproximal areas. Another advantage of custom-fitted trays is the they require less gel to cover all surfaces of the teeth. Larger amounts of gel may be needed in mass-produced trays to ensure that all tooth surfaces are thoroughly coated during the treatment procedure. A technique that minimizes the amount of gel that will be needed is preferred because it reduces the chances that excess gel will be swallowed by the patient as a result of the treatment. In addition to vacuum-molded custom-fitted trays, those with foam or air-filled liners

also may enhance the adaptation of the fluoride to the teeth.

When standard, disposable trays are used, no more than 2 g of gel should be dispensed into each tray (about 40% of tray capacity). Even smaller amounts should be dispensed into trays for small children. When custom-fitted trays are used by patients who require daily or weekly fluoride application using high-concentration gels, only 5 to 10 drops of the product are needed per tray (LeCompte, 1987).

The trays should be made of a material that is comfortable for the patient and will not interfere with the contact of fluoride with the tooth. Use of custom-made wax trays is not recommended, because the waxy material can adhere to tooth surfaces and can interfere with fluoride uptake. Trays should be easy to handle and to insert into the mouth when filled. Flexible sponge trays and trays that use paper inserts require slightly more handling than do other types of trays, increasing the procedure time (Fig. 28-1, *top left, bottom far left*). The use of disposable trays reduces the chances of cross-contamination and eliminates additional time and handling required to sterilize reusable trays. As most reusable fluoride trays are made of heat-sensitive materials, chemical sterilization must be used to decontaminate them.

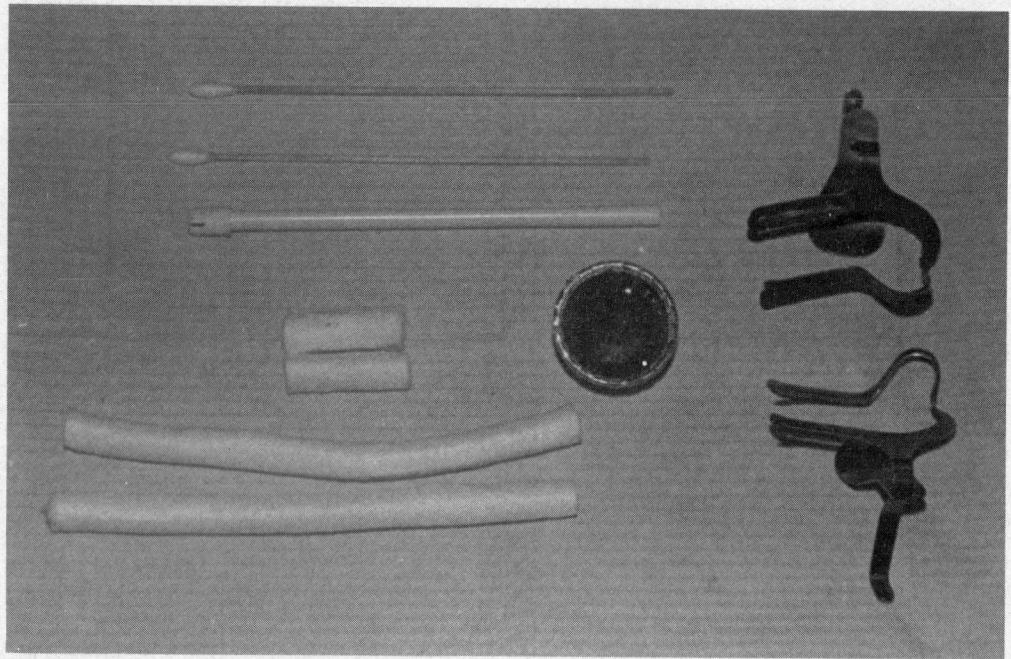

Fig. 28-3. Suggested tray setup for application of fluoride solutions includes cotton roll holders, cotton rolls in two lengths, saliva ejector tip, disposable applicators, and fluoride solution.

Application procedure. The same major steps are followed for the application of both fluoride solution and gel. Tray setups for solution application and gel application are shown in Figs. 28-3 and 28-4 respectively. The patient should be positioned in an upright position to facilitate evacuation of saliva and fluoride and also to reduce the possibility of gagging. All necessary supplies and materials for the procedure should be assembled, and the procedure be explained to the patient. Patient consent should already have been obtained during the treatment-planning stage. It is important to reinforce the patient's knowledge regarding the benefits of the topical fluoride application at this time and to solicit any questions that the patient may have. After the best tray size has been selected for the patient's mouth (Figs. 28-4, and 28-5), both trays should be filled by placing a narrow strip (2 g) of fluoride gel along the bottom of the tray. This amount is sufficient to wet all tooth surfaces thoroughly when the tray is in place but not so much that it overflows the tray boundaries into the mouth where it can be swallowed.

After all materials have been assembled and the patient has been adequately prepared, the first step is to dry all the teeth that will be treated (Fig. 28-6). This should be done slowly and thoroughly to ensure that all tooth surfaces are free of saliva, which might dilute the fluoride concentration and reduce fluoride uptake. The patient should be informed that cooperation is needed to maintain the dry field until the trays are in place. Best results are obtained if the areas least likely to become rewetted are dried first, such as palatal surfaces. Areas near saliva ducts, such as maxillary buccal and mandibular lingual surfaces, should be dried immediately before the fluoride is applied. Dry the teeth with an air syringe using the following pattern:

Mandibular arch. Dry buccal surfaces; then occlusal surfaces; finish on lingual surfaces.
Maxillary arch. Dry palatal surfaces; then occlusal surfaces; finish on buccal surfaces.

Retract the buccal mucosa and labial mucosa away from the dried teeth with either plastic retractors or the fingers of one hand until the tray is

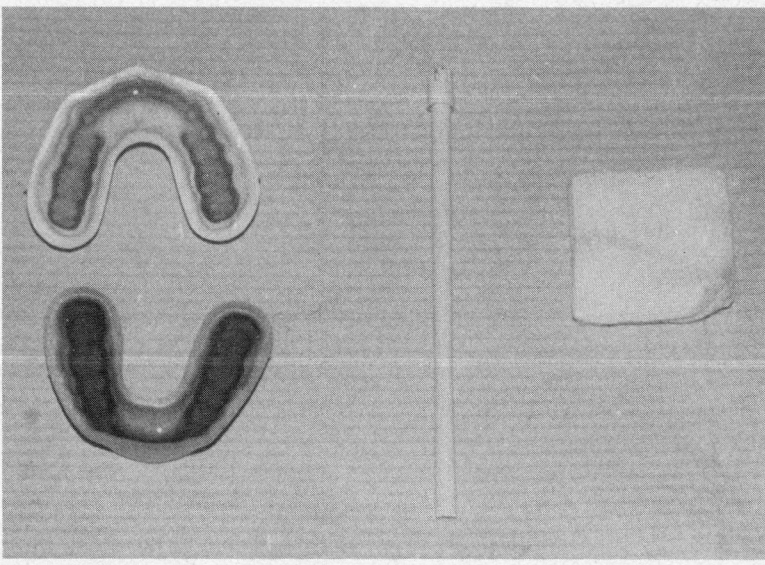

Fig. 28-4. Suggested tray setup for application of fluoride gels.

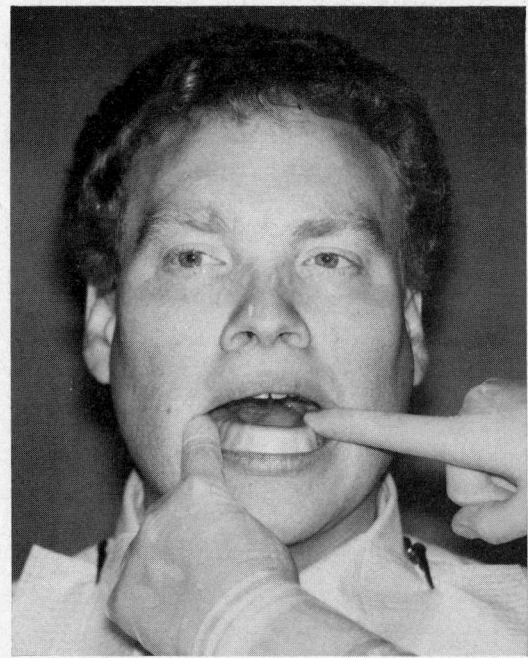

Fig. 28-5. Tray size is selected and tried in patient's mouth to make sure that all teeth will be contacted by fluoride gel.

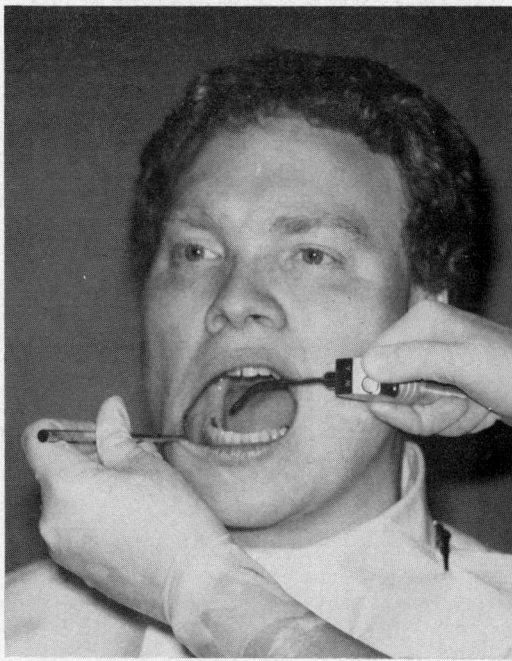

Fig. 28-6. Teeth should be carefully dried and kept as dry as possible until trays are placed. Each arch is dried separately immediately before tray is placed.

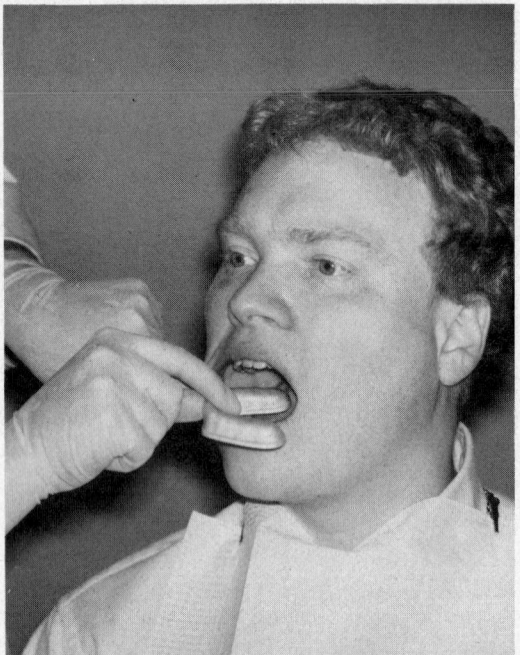

Fig. 28-7. One end of filled mandibular tray is inserted from side of patient's mouth rather than directly from front. This is similar to technique described for insertion of impression trays.

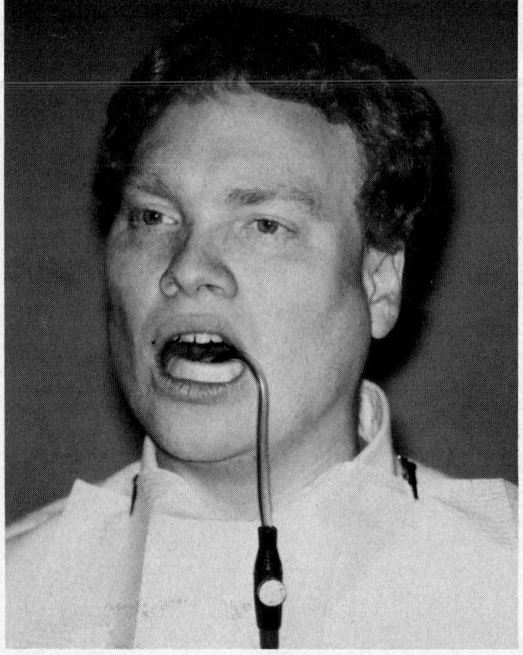

Fig. 28-8. Saliva ejector is inserted *before* maxillary tray is placed.

placed into position on the teeth with the other hand.

If both arches are to be treated simultaneously, position the mandibular tray first, then place the saliva ejector over the tray, and finally insert the maxillary tray. Ask the patient to close the mouth and to bite gently on the trays. The slight pressure from biting will help force the fluoride gel around and between all the teeth that are being treated. Begin timing the procedure after the tray(s) are in position and all the teeth to be treated are thoroughly wetted with the fluoride. Supervise or monitor the patient for the entire 4-minute period. Place the patient in a fully upright position with the chin tilted down to allow fluids to run to the anterior area of the mouth, where the saliva ejector is placed, so that it is maximally effective. All patients, and especially children, should be discouraged from swallowing excess fluoride during the treatment and should be encouraged to rely on the saliva ejector. Patients usually appreciate having disposable tissues on hand to assist in the re-

moval of excess saliva around their mouths during and after the procedure. These steps are shown in Figs. 28-7 to 28-9.

With some trays, such as the ion-fluoridation tray shown in Fig. 28-1, *top left,* only one tray is put in place at a time. This is because the saliva ejector is attached directly to the tray and because simultaneous use of both trays would be too bulky and uncomfortable for the patient. When using only one tray at a time, dry the arch to be treated. Then place the tray, add the saliva ejector, and ask the patient to close the teeth together gently.

At the end of 4 minutes, remove the trays from the mouth and remove excess fluoride and saliva by means of the saliva ejector or high-speed evacuation. Instruct the patient to expectorate any remaining fluids from the mouth, repeating the process for 30 to 60 seconds. Expectoration is the most effective way to reduce orally retained fluoride so that it is not swallowed (LeCompte, 1987). The patient should not be allowed to rinse

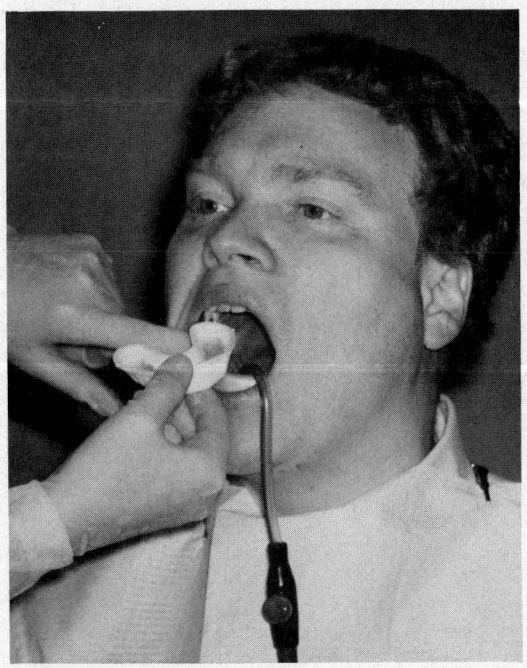

Fig. 28-9. Insertion of maxillary tray.

and should be instructed not to eat, rinse, drink, or smoke for at least 30 minutes following the fluoride application procedure. Stookey and coworkers (1986) reported evidence that rinsing immediately after fluoride application resulted in less fluoride deposition in incipient caries lesions. Therefore, rinsing after a fluoride treatment may reduce the maximum cariostatic potential of the treatment and should not be permitted.

The advantages of the tray application methods are as follows:
1. Ease of application
2. The whole mouth can be treated during a single 4-minute period
3. Trays are used only once, eliminating sterilization procedures
4. Improved patient comfort

The disadvantages of the tray application methods are as follows:
1. Poorly designed or fitted trays may hinder fluoride uptake or allow leakage of gel into the mouth
2. Cost of disposable supplies

Controlling gagging. The fluoride treatment may elicit a gag response in some individuals. Mild gagging can usually be controlled through distraction strategies that focus the patient's attention on something other than the fluoride treatment. Such strategies may include rapidly paced nasal breathing, toe wiggling, or simply talking to the patient about an interesting topic to divert his or her attention.

Patients with more serious gagging problems can be helped by allowing them to practice the procedure in advance (i.e., with empty trays), by giving them some control over the procedure (i.e., holding the saliva ejector), by providing distracting imagery ("imagine walking on the beach in the sunshine"), or by listening to and acknowledging their concerns (i.e., about choking, suffocating, and the like), discussing them, and providing assurance that the procedure poses no risk (Ramsay et al, 1987).

Fluoride solution application

Use of cotton roll holders. Fluoride in solution form requires the painting technique of application because it must be applied in small quantities and would flow easily out of trays and be swallowed. When solutions are used, the teeth are isolated and kept dry by means of cotton rolls, which are held in place adjacent to the teeth that will be treated so that the tongue, cheeks, and saliva do not touch them during the procedure. Cotton roll holders called Garmer clamps are used to stabilize the cotton rolls in the mouth. Garmer clamps can be obtained in two sizes for adults and children. The cotton rolls are inserted onto metal prongs with a short roll on the lingual side of the clamp and a 6-inch roll on the buccal side (Fig. 28-10). The cotton roll holder is placed gently in the mouth so that the lingual cotton roll isolates the lingual surface of the teeth from the tongue and the lowest half of the buccal roll is lying in the mandibular buccal and labial vestibule with the rest extending out of the mouth (Fig. 28-11). The holder should then be stabilized in the mouth by anchoring the clamp snugly under the patient's chin. The rest of the buccal cotton roll should then be securely positioned so that the free end curves up along the maxillary vestibule and returns labially to the central incisors. A slight twist on the end of the cotton roll

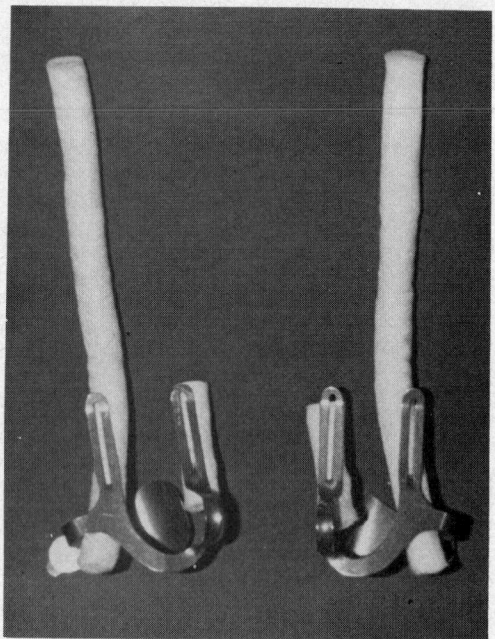

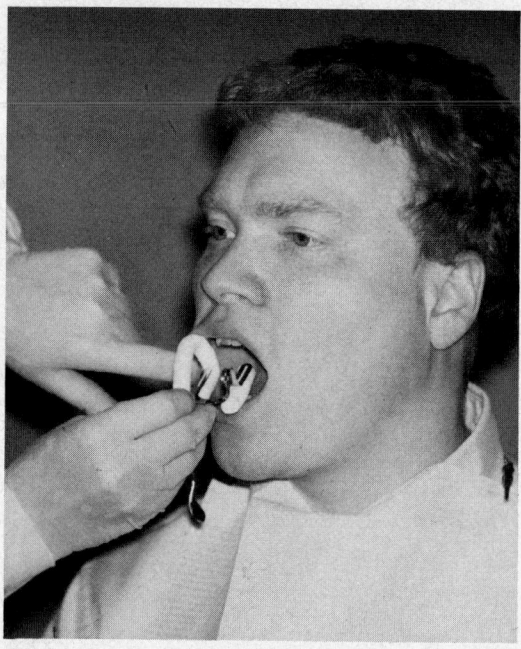

Fig. 28-10. Set of cotton roll holders known as Garmer clamps. Each holder secures two cotton rolls to isolate one half of mouth at a time. Short roll lies against lingual surfaces of mandibular arch, and longer roll isolates buccal surfaces of maxillary and mandibular teeth from mucosa.

Fig. 28-11. Garmer clamp and cotton rolls are placed with short roll side against lingual surfaces of mandibular teeth and long roll side against buccal surfaces. Note that maxillary extension of buccal cotton roll is folded forward and held until clamps are inserted and stabilized.

before placing the lip over it will hold the anterior end in place. A final check should be made to ensure that the cotton rolls are effectively isolating the teeth from the cheeks, lips, and tongue but are not touching the tooth surfaces to be treated.

The lingual roll should not extend beyond the distal surface of the last molar, where it might elicit gagging from the patient. When the cotton roll holder is in place, the saliva ejector should be positioned and the teeth on the side to be treated should be dried thoroughly following the same pattern suggested earlier in the chapter.

Application procedure. Ask the patient to hold the fluoride solution container close to the mouth, or place it on the bracket table near the mouth (Fig. 28-12). Apply the solution first to the mandibular lingual surfaces using an application pattern that moves systematically around the quadrant as follows: posterior on the lingual surfaces, anterior on the occlusal surfaces, and pos-

terior on the buccal surfaces. Apply solution to the surfaces of the maxillary arch by starting on the buccal aspect of the molars and moving forward; then wet the occlusal surfaces and finally the lingual or palatal surfaces. Apply the solution to each tooth liberally with a cotton-tipped applicator, taking care that all accessible tooth surfaces are thoroughly wetted. After all isolated teeth are covered with solution, begin timing the application. During the application period continue to apply solution to the teeth using the same pattern as before to ensure that they are continuously bathed in fluoride. At the end of the recommended application time, remove the saliva ejector and then the cotton rolls and clamps. Suction all remaining fluoride solution and excess saliva from the mouth, and allow the patient to empty the mouth into a cuspidor or funnel-suction device (depending on the equipment available).

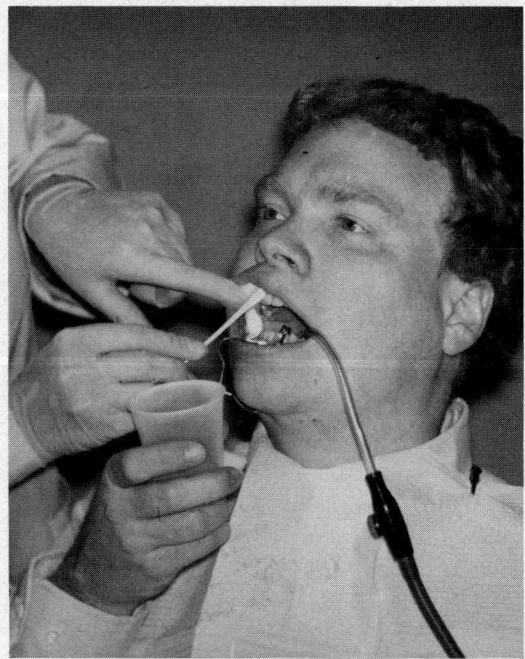

Fig. 28-12. With clamp fastened snugly under the chin and cotton rolls in place, teeth are dried and solution is placed using suggested pattern of application.

The entire procedure (isolation, drying, application) is then repeated on the opposite side of the mouth.

The advantages of this method of isolation are as follows:

1. It provides effective isolation when fluoride solutions are used
2. Garmer clamps can be autoclaved and are reusable, thereby reducing the cost of supplies

The disadvantages of this method of isolation are as follows:

1. The procedure is more time consuming and complicated than tray techniques
2. Only half the mouth can be treated at one time
3. Bulkiness of clamps and cotton rolls may be uncomfortable for the patient

Controlling fluoride ingestion during professional applications

The goal of fluoride therapy is to maximize the benefit provided by topical or systemic fluoride preparation while minimizing the known risks of using the agent. Fluorides, including high-concentration gels and solutions used in the dental office, have been proven time and time again to be safe and effective for prevention of decay when used as recommended. Recently, however, there has been some concern among members of the professional community that the availability of fluoride from multiple sources, including water, food, diet supplements, school fluoride programs, dentifrices, over-the-counter rinses, and professional application treatments, might lead to increased prevalence and severity of dental fluorosis.

A number of investigations have indicated that substantial amounts of fluoride are retained in the mouth after a professional fluoride treatment and subsequently ingested (Owen et al, 1979; Ekstrand and Koch, 1980; Ekstrand et al, 1981; LeCompte and Whitford, 1981, 1982; LeCompte and Doyle, 1982; More et al, 1983; LeCompte and Doyle, 1985). The high amounts of retained fluoride have been reported to result in elevation of fluoride concentrations in body fluids, including plasma concentrations, causing concern that these elevated levels may result in dental fluorosis when they occur in young children with developing teeth (Ekstrand and Koch, 1980; Ekstrand et al, 1981; LeCompte and Whitford, 1981, 1982). Because fluorosis is most likely to occur in young children, efforts to reduce amounts of ingested fluoride in that group are especially important. Although dental fluorosis does not in itself pose a major public health threat, it is a minor side effect that can be controlled effectively through proper application technique.

The possibility that a young child might accidently ingest high doses of fluoride during the professional application procedures is a more serious concern. In order for this to happen, abuses of accepted fluoride application procedures would be necessary, but, unfortunately, the death of one child has been reported due to such abuses (Church, 1976; Horowitz, 1977). Although topical fluoride treatments have been consistently shown to be safe and effective ways of preventing dental decay, this occurrence emphasized the need to ensure that the risks, however minor, are minimized. Although each of the following recommendations has been included when describing the technique for application of fluoride gels or solutions, additional emphasis is warranted. The following recommendations are intended for all professional applications of fluoride, but they are especially important when treating young children, for whom the potential risks of chronic or acute fluoride overdose are greater. Children under the age of 6 with developing teeth are especially susceptible to the effects of dental fluorosis as a result of ingestion of high-fluoride-concentration gels or solutions. Recommendations for controlling the ingestion of high-concentration-fluoride gels and solutions include the following (LeCompte, 1987).

Patient instruction. Patients should be instructed that the purpose of the procedure is to apply fluoride only to the surfaces of the teeth and that fluoride should not be swallowed. They should be shown how to use the saliva ejector effectively and should be placed in a fully upright position with their chins tilted down. It should be explained that maintaining this position will improve the effectiveness of the saliva ejector in removing saliva and excess fluoride.

Tray selection. A tray should be selected that will allow coverage of all teeth in the arch, promote intimate contact of the fluoride to the teeth, and minimize loss of fluoride from the tray and into the mouth. Descriptions of trays and criteria for selection were discussed earlier in this chapter.

Amount of fluoride dispensed. It has been recommended that only about 2 grams of fluoride be dispensed into each tray. This is equal to about 40% of the tray capacity. Even smaller amounts should be dispensed into trays for small children. Studies of the amount of fluoride retained in the mouth or swallowed following fluoride treatments indicate that substantial amounts are retained following all application techniques, both before and after the patient has expectorated. Furthermore, there is a wide variation in the amount of fluoride that may be placed within a tray, depending on the discretion of the individual. In studies investigating how much fluoride gel is dispensed, the average amount dispensed per tray, depending on the type of tray system, ranged from 2.0 to 3.6 g. (i.e., 14.8 to 44.3 mg F per tray) (LeCompte, 1987). These amounts are averages, indicating that some individuals were dispensing even greater amounts into each tray. Most manufacturers of high-concentration fluoride gels are now recommending that only enough gel should be dispensed to fill a third of the tray. The result of overdispensing fluoride gel is that fluoride is ingested by the patient unnecessarily and the product is wasted by the professional.

Use of suction equipment. The use of saliva ejectors and high-speed suction will reduce the amount of fluoride that can be ingested during a professional treatment. Saliva ejectors can be used both during and after the procedure, and high-speed suction devices can be used to clear the mouth further after the trays have been removed. Although these devices are effective in removing significant amounts of retained fluoride, data indicate that there is still substantial oral retention of fluoride in both children and adults even when suctioning is used (More et al, 1983; Eisen and LeCompte, 1985; LeCompte and Doyle, 1985).

Expectoration. Instructing the patients to empty their mouths repeatedly for 30 to 60 seconds following a fluoride treatment is the single most effective way to reduce orally retained fluoride (LeCompte, 1987). Eisen and LeCompte (1985) reported that suctioning procedures with patient expectoration were found to be more beneficial than suction alone.

Patient monitoring. Patients, especially small children, should be monitored during the entire procedure to ensure that they are following instructions and that they are not swallowing the fluoride inadvertently or intentionally. The hygienist should never leave the operatory or be in a position where the patient cannot be seen or heard while the fluoride treatment is in progress. Bottles containing fluoride gel or solution should never be kept within reach of young children. Relatively low concentrations of fluoride can cause gastrointestinal irritation. Complaints of nausea, vomiting, or abdominal pain are not uncommon in patients following topical APF gel applications (Whitford et al, 1987). Children who complain of gastrointestinal upset should be given milk and monitored closely for other symptoms. Never give a fluoride treatment to a fasting child; provide a snack before the appointment if the child hasn't eaten for several hours.

One way to reduce fluoride ingestion would be to develop a product that produces the same cariostatic effect on tooth surfaces as existing fluoride gels but requires a shorter contact time (i.e., 1 minute versus 4 minutes). Although 1.23% APF gels have been formulated and marketed with this goal in mind, there has not yet been sufficient evidence generated by independent researchers (researchers other than the manufacturer) to determine whether these products can be considered as effective as approved APF products applied for 4 minutes (LeCompte, 1987).

Recommended dosages for daily or weekly applications using custom-fitted trays. Certain patients may require frequent use of high-concentration fluoride gel for prevention of rampant caries, especially those undergoing cancer therapy or suffering from xerostomia. The recommended application procedures for these patients involves use of a custom-fitted acrylic tray for delivery of the fluoride. Because of the close fit of these trays to the teeth, less fluoride gel is required and excessive amounts of gel are likely to be forced out of the tray when it is placed. Current recommendations are that only 5 to 10 drops (1 to 2 mg) of the fluoride preparation should be dispensed into trays used for frequent fluoride application. If patients perform this procedure at home, they should be shown the amount of fluoride to be dispensed and instructed regarding the importance of expectorating after the treatment is completed.

Awareness of fluoride dosages in professional applications

In addition to compliance with recommendations regarding fluoride application technique, the hygienist must always be aware of the amount of fluoride being given to the patient and understand the relation of this quantity (expressed as mg F/ml) to toxic dose levels. Chronic overexposure to fluoride even at low concentrations can result in dental fluorosis in children under the age of 6 who have developing teeth. Acute overdosage resulting in poisoning or even death can occur if high-concentration gels or solutions are abused. Lyon (1985) stated that "it is the legal as well as moral responsibility of every hygienist to be able to determine how much fluoride is being administered to a patient."

Only trained dental professionals who are legally permitted to apply topical fluoride preparations should be allowed to perform office fluoride treatments. Each dentist and hygienist must know how much fluoride is being given to patients and how that quantity compares to the Certainly Lethal Dose (CLD) and the Safely Tolerated Dose (STD) guidelines presented in Table 28-2. Table 28-3 provides estimates of the amount of fluoride that is commonly used for professional fluoride treatments and the associated dosages for each of the three common fluoride preparations. It can be seen that if recommended amounts of fluoride are used according to the suggestions in this chapter, the total fluoride dose is well below the suggested CLD for any age level. It should be noted, however, that if the stated amounts of an 8% SnF_2 solution, for instance, were to be ingested by a 2-year-old child, the ingested dose would exceed the STD for that age/weight level. Close monitoring of the fluoride application procedure and care to ensure that containers of fluoride gel or solution are kept out of the reach of children can prevent accidental ingestion of these products.

If a toxic overdose of fluoride is known or suspected, the hygienist must be able to calculate quickly the total amount of topical fluoride gel or solution that may have been ingested and use that information to make appropriate recommendations regarding treatment for fluoride overdose. These quantities can be estimated by using the information in Table 28-3, or they can be calculated more exactly using the simple equations in Table 28-4. More detailed explanations of how to calculate the concentration of any type of topical fluoride product are available so that dental professionals can ascertain acceptable dosages of other fluoride products or combinations of products (Heifetz and Horowitz, 1984; Lyon, 1985; Bayless and Tinanoff, 1985).

After calculating the amount of the overdose, the hygienist can determine which emergency measures to implement. Table 28-5 suggests emergency treatment measures for acute fluoride overdose based on the quantity of fluoride ingested. Whitford (1987) suggested that an oral dose of 5.0 mg F/kg body weight should be regarded as the "Possibly Toxic Dose" (PTD)—that is, the minimum dose that could cause toxic signs and symptoms. He further recommended that an emergency should be assumed to exist if it is even suspected that 5.0 mg F/kg or more has been ingested and that immediate emergency treatment

Table 28-2. Estimated safe, toxic, and lethal dosage levels of fluoride

Certainly Lethal Dose (CLD) = an estimated dosage range with the potential for causing death when consumed
Safely Tolerated Dose (STD) = an estimated dosage that can be consumed without producing symptoms of serious acute
toxicity
Probably Toxic Dose (PTD) = the estimated minimum dosage that could cause toxic signs and symptoms

For a 70-kg adult:
Certainly Lethal Dose (CLD) = 5-10 gm NaF or 32-64 mg F/kg†
Safely Tolerated Dose (STD = (1/4 CLD) 1.25-2.5 gm NaF or 8-16 mg F/kg†
Probably Toxic Dose (PTD) = 5.0 mg F/kg‡

CLDs and STDs and PTDs of fluoride for children of selected ages:

Age	Weight (lb)*	CLD (mg)†	STD (mg)†	PTD (mg)‡
2	22	320	80	50
4	29	422	106	66
6	37	538	135	84
8	45	655	164	102
10	53	771	193	120
12	64	931	233	145
14	83	1206	301	189
16	92	1338	334	209
18	95	1382	346	216

*3rd percentile of the normal age-specific weight distribution.
†Adapted from Heifetz SB, and Horowitz HS: The amounts of fluoride in current fluoride therapies: safety considerations for children, ASDC J Dent Children **51**:257, 1984.
‡Adapted from Whitford GM: Fluoride in dental products: safety considerations, J Dent Res **66**:1056, 1987.

Table 28-3. Amounts of fluoride in professionally administered topical fluoride treatments

Agent	Frequency	F concentration	Volume	Total amount of F
2% NaF	series of 4 every 3 yr	0.91%	2.5 ml	22.8 mg
8% SnF$_2$	1 or 2/yr	1.95%	5 ml	97.5 mg
10% SnF$_2$	1 or 2/yr	2.44%	5 ml	122 mg
APF	1 or 2/yr	1.23%	5 ml	61.5 mg

Adapted from Heifetz SB, and Horowitz HS: The amount of fluoride in current fluoride therapies: Safety considerations for children, ASDC J Dent Children **51**:257, 1984.

Table 28-4. Rapid method of calculating amount of fluoride ingested

Form	Formula
NaF	(4.5) × (no. ml swallowed) × (NaF concentration) = mg F$^-$ (e.g., 0.05%, 1.1%)
SnF$_2$	(2.4) × (no. ml swallowed) × (SnF$_2$ concentration) = mg F$^-$ (e.g., 0.4%, 8%, 10%)
APF	(10) × (no. ml swallowed) × (F$^-$ concentration) = mg F$^-$ (e.g., 1.23%)

Adapted from Bayless JM, and Tinanoff N: Diagnosis and treatment of acute fluoride toxicity, JADA **110**:209, 1985.

Table 28-5. Emergency treatment for fluoride overdose

Milligram fluoride ion per kilogram body weight*	Treatment
Less than 5.0 mg/kg	1. Give calcium orally (milk) to relieve GI symptoms; observe for a few hours 2. Induced vomiting not necessary
More than 5 mg/kg	1. Empty stomach by induced vomiting with emetic; for patients with depressed gag reflex caused by age (<6 months old), Down's syndrome, or severe mental retardation, induced vomiting is contraindicated and endotracheal intubation should be performed before gastric lavage 2. Give orally soluble calcium in any form (e.g., milk, 5% calcium gluconate, or calcium lactate solution) 3. Admit to hospital and observe for a few hours
More than 15 mg/kg	1. Admit to hospital immediately 2. Induce vomiting 3. Begin cardiac monitoring and be prepared for cardiac arrhythmias; observe for peaking T-waves and prolonged Q-T intervals 4. Slowly administer 10 ml of 10% calcium gluconate solution intravenously; additional doses may be given if clinical signs of tetany, or Q-T interval prolongation develops; electrolytes, especially calcium and potassium, should be monitored and corrected as necessary 5. Adequate urine output should be maintained using diuretics if necessary 6. General supportive measures for shocks

*Average weight/age: 1-2 years = 10 kg; 2-4 years = 15 kg; 4-6 years = 20 kg; 6-8 years = 23 kg.
Adapted from Bayless JM and Tinanoff N: Diagnosis and Treatment of acute fluoride toxicity, JADA **110:**209, 1985.

Table 28-6. Basic conversion factors

1 kilogram (kg)	= 2.2 lbs
1 gram (gm)	= 1000 mgs
1 ounce (oz)	= 30 ml (volume)
1 ounce	= 28.3 gm (weight)
1 gm/100 ml	= 1% (% = parts/hundred)
% × 10,000	= parts/million (ppm)
1 mg/ml or 1 mg/gm	= 1000 ppm

Adapted from Lyon TC: Topical fluorides; how much are you using? Dent Hyg **59:**58, 1985.

and hospitalization should occur. This information should be kept where it can be used immediately in case of an emergency. The conversion units listed in Table 28-6 will help the dental professional translate into useful data the information found on labels and in advertisements and research articles that describe fluoride concentration levels and dosages.

SELECTING EFFECTIVE FLUORIDE PRODUCTS

As with many other consumer items, a myriad of fluoride products are being promoted by dental sales representatives, at professional meetings, in advertisements in both lay and professional publications, by other professionals, and by patients themselves. Proponents of each product indicate that theirs is the best, the cheapest, the most efficient, the safest, or the most popular product of its kind on the market. How do dental professionals sort out all of these claims to ensure that they are using or recommending the best product for their patients? A number of suggestions can help professionals make these important choices.

Products that claim to have therapeutic value must have their safety proved to government bodies such as the Food and Drug Administration before they can be marketed for public consumption. Simply knowing that a product is safe, however, is not enough to indicate its choice over other similar products. The professional literature should be consulted regarding research conducted to document is efficacy (ability of the product to produce the desired benefit under controlled conditions), its effectiveness (ability of the product to produce the stated benefit under normal-use conditions), and its comparative efficacy or effectiveness (how it compares to other similar products of an established reputation). A product such as a topical fluoride preparation must go through a number of stages of research before it can be recommended safely. First, laboratory studies must be done to determine the properties and effects of the product using models or extracted teeth, and then the product may be used in live animal studies to establish its safety and effectiveness. These studies are followed by controlled use of the substance in vivo; that is, in the mouths of live human beings. Finally, the product must be tested under realistic circumstances of actual use on large population samples. This entire process can take years or even decades to complete, but the final evidence obtained from long-term clinical studies on humans is an important requirement in order for a product to be professionally recognized as an effective fluoride product.

As a service to the profession and as an aid to practitioners, the American Dental Association has councils (e.g., the Council on Dental Therapeutics and the Council on Dental Materials, Instruments, and Equipment) whose task it is to evaluate the claims of safety and effectiveness of therapeutic and preventive products, materials, instruments, and equipment used in dentistry. These councils evaluate data regarding the safety, efficacy, composition, and quality of products, and they review all labels, package inserts, and advertising to ensure the use of scientifically accurate statements. In addition, these councils encourage, establish, and support research on the therapeutic value of agents used in dentistry. The results and discussion of their findings, as well as lists of accepted products, are compiled for easy reference in a publication entitled *Accepted Dental Therapeutics*. In addition, the councils provide more current updates of the status of new products and of newly accepted products in reports published frequently in the *Journal of the American Dental Association*. Dental professionals should consult these reports and recommendations before adopting any new forms of fluoride treatment. Products that have been approved and accepted by these councils can be used and recommended with confidence. For the most current information on the status of new therapeutic agents or products, the professional can also contact the secretaries of these councils by phone at the offices of the American Dental Assocation.

Dental researchers and faculty members at dental schools may also be consulted for accurate and up-to-date information on new techniques, concepts, or products. Dentists and hygienists should participate in continuing education programs, which will keep them updated in the latest methods and approaches to dental care. Finally, all professionals have a responsibility to keep up to date with professional literature by reading journals published by their professional associations and other related sources. Dental professional also should be aware of information that is being disseminated to the general public through magazines, newspapers, and television so that they can respond with accurate information when consulted about claims transmitted by these media. Finally, dental professionals need to review the information supplied to them by manufacturers of dental materials, instruments, equipment, and products, because many important details can be ascertained from it. Dental professionals also should consider the reputation of a manufacturer within the dental profession when evaluating products. In summary, dental professionals are responsible to their consumers to use accepted and approved methods and products and to be informed regarding the products that are available to the general public. In order to fulfill this responsibility, they must be assertive in their search for reliable information and develop their skills as critical evaluators of new information and new products.

ACTIVITIES

1. Visit the local pharmacy and grocery store and identify all the products available for oral hygiene that include fluoride. Note the type of fluoride included, the concentration, and the directions for use.
2. Calculate the total fluoride available to a person who consumes four 8-ounce glasses of fluoridated water, rinses with a 0.05% sodium fluoride rinse according to manufacturer's instructions, and brushes three times daily with a 2500 ppm fluoride dentifrice using 1 gram of paste at each brushing.
3. Review antifluoridationist literature and prepare a list of their arguments. Locate the sources of their references and review the articles that are available.
4. Review the results of the Grand Rapids/Muskegon and Kingston/Newburgh clinical trials.
5. Conduct a seminar for parents of young children and discuss the ways in which their children use toothpaste.

Fluoride Application Procedure

Suggested check-off sheet

Mark **S** for satisfactory completion or **U** for unsatisfactory completion of each criterion in the appropriate space.

PERFORMANCE CRITERIA:	FACULTY	STUDENT
1. Assess the need for topical fluoride therapy		
2. Explain the benefits of fluoride, describe the application procedure, and obtain the consent of the patient		
3. Evaluate the teeth for removal of calculus, stain, and plaque		
4. Assemble all necessary supplies		
5. Seat the patient in an upright position		

Tray technique

6. Select the appropriate-size tray and check the fit in the patient's mouth		
7. Dispense the proper amount of gel into each tray		
8. Dry the mandibular teeth and isolate them		
9. Insert the mandibular tray		
10. Insert the saliva ejector		
11. Dry the maxillary teeth and isolate them		
12. Insert the maxillary tray		
13. Ask the patient to close the mouth and bite the teeth together gently		
14. Begin timing the procedure		
15. Monitor patient comfort		
16. Remove the trays after the full 4 minutes have elapsed		
17. Remove excess fluoride with a saliva ejector or high-speed evacuation		
18. Allow the patient to expectorate for 30 to 60 seconds		
19. Instruct the patient not to eat, rinse, or drink for 30 minutes following the procedure		

Solution technique

6. Attach cotton rolls to holders properly for maximum effectiveness and patient comfort		
7. Insert cotton roll holders and stabilize them in the mouth		
8. Check the placement of the cotton rolls in relation to the soft and hard tissues		
9. Dry the teeth using the prescribed pattern		
10. Insert a saliva ejector		
11. Apply the solution, using the prescribed pattern, to all tooth surfaces on the isolated side of the mouth		
12. Begin timing the procedure after all surfaces have been covered		
13. Repeat the application pattern throughout the 4-minute period to keep surfaces continuously wet with fluoride		
14. Remove the cotton rolls and holder after the full 4-minute period has elapsed		
15. Evacuate excess saliva and fluoride from the mouth, and allow the patient to expectorate		
16. Repeat steps 6 through 15 for the other side of the mouth		
17. Instruct the patient not to eat, rinse, or drink for 30 minutes following the procedure		

6. Review the literature for epidemiological studies that describe trends in the following areas:
   a. Caries incidence
   b. Fluorosis
   c. Water fluoridation
   d. Use of low-concentration fluorides
   Prepare a panel discussion of one or more of these issues, presenting the data and the controversies generated.

7. Conduct a survey of local family physicians and pediatricians to determine whether they prescribe fluoride drops or lozenges for their patients and in what concentrations.

8. Survey the local town or city and surrounding areas for the presence of fluoride in the drinking water. Take a sample of water from the public supply, from several wells, and from neighboring cities to the health department to assess the level of fluoride in the water.

9. Interview local dentists and hygienists regarding the historical efforts to fluoridate the local community.

10. Assign to groups of five the task of reviewing the literature describing the percentage reductions achieved with (1) each of the topical fluoride agents, including high-concentration professionally applied gels and solutions; (2) home use rinses; (3) dentifrices; (4) home use gels; and (5) sequential rinses of acidulated phosphate fluoride and stannous fluoride. Each group should prepare a report describing the research design, the number of subjects, the age of the subjects, the duration of the trial, the agent(s) tested, the method of evaluation, whether the water supply was fluoridated, whether other fluoride sources were available to the study subjects, and the results.

11. Tour a local water plant and find out how community water fluoridation is implemented and monitored.

12. Determine which students come from areas where the water supplies were fluoridated (optimum level), and relate this to the number of caries for each student. Can any trend be determined?

13. Plan and discuss setting up a clinical study to investigate a new anticariogenic agent in your (or a hypothetical) town. Would you participate, or would you let your child, brother, sister, or other family member participate if you knew you might receive the placebo product?

14. Invite representatives of dental manufacturing companies to discuss their fluoride products and supplies. Collect a wide variety of fluoride trays, and discuss advantages and disadvantages of each tray design.

15. Perform a topical fluoride treatment for a partner in your class (see p. 557).

16. Construct scenarios in which the clinician made errors during the topical fluoride procedure, then have the class critique the procedures and discuss the possible results of the errors.

17. Demonstrate fluoride effectiveness by soaking an egg in a high-concentration fluoride solution overnight. Then take the test egg and a control egg and soak them in household vinegar. Compare the results.

18. Select several members of the class and have each dispense fluoride gel into similar or different tray designs. Weigh each set of trays to determine how much gel was dispensed. Compare results and compute the total fluoride dosage that would be delivered to each patient. Are there differences? How much variation is there? Discuss ways to determine how much fluoride gel is actually needed for the topical procedure.

19. Check the most current edition of *Accepted Dental Therapeutics* for a list of fluoride products that have proven effectiveness. Identify products available to the public that are not on the list. Perform a literature search on these items to determine what claims have been made regarding their effectiveness or lack of effectiveness.

REVIEW QUESTIONS

1. The microorganism most closely associated with dental caries is:

2. True or false:
   a. Fluorapatite is formed in the deep layers of enamel.
   b. Calcium fluoride is formed at the surface of the enamel when exposed to topical fluoride.
   c. Calcium fluoride may serve as a reservoir, releasing fluoride over a number of weeks.
   d. Surface layer fluoride may be more important in preventing dental decay than a high concentration of fluorapatite.
   e. Topical fluoride, even in low concentrations, helps enable calcium and phosphorus to remineralize enamel.
   f. The optimal level of fluoride in communal water supplies is 10 ppm.

3. What is dental fluorosis?

4. What is posteruption maturation?

5. What is the recommended regimen for each of these rinses:
   a. 0.05% NaF
   b. 0.025% NaF
   c. 0.20% NaF

6. Is it necessary to polish the teeth prior to applying topical fluoride or a fluoride mouthrinse?

7. What was the purpose of the Grand Rapids/ Muskegon and Kingston/Newburg caries trials?
8. Describe, in order, the steps involved in performing the following procedures:
   a. A tray application of fluoride gel
   b. The application of fluoride solution
9. When should the 4-minute timing of the fluoride application begin?
   a. After the teeth are dried
   b. As soon as the first tray is in place, or solution has been applied to the first treated teeth
   c. When all teeth to be treated have been thoroughly wetted with the fluoride gel or solution
10. State the lethal dose of fluoride for adults; for children. Compare these amounts with the amounts that are normally dispensed in a topical fluoride treatment.
11. Which of the following are effective antidotes for accidental fluoride poisoning?
    a. Milk
    b. Lime water
    c. Preparations containing large amounts of magnesium
    d. All of the above
12. If a 2-year-old child ingests an entire 10 ml solution of 8% SnF_2 while the dental professional is not watching, how many mg of fluoride would be ingested?
13. In the case above, would the total fluoride dose be over the CLD for a 2-year-old child?
14. Should hospitalization be recommended for the above child in addition to such measures as giving milk or inducing vomiting?

REFERENCES

Aasenden R, et al: Effects of daily rinsing and ingestion of fluoride solutions upon dental caries and enamel fluoride, Arch Oral Biol 17:1705, 1972.

American Dental Association Council on Dental Therapeutics: Accepted dental therapeutics, ed 40. Chicago, 1984, American Dental Association.

American Dental Association Council on Dental Therapeutics: A guide to the use of fluorides for the prevention of dental caries, JADA 113:506, 1986.

American Dental Association Council on Dental Materials, Instruments, and Equipment and Council on Dental Therapeutics: Accepted dental products, JADA 116:249, 1988.

Angmar-Mansson B, and Whiford GM: Single fluoride doses and enamel fluorosis in the rat, Caries Res 19:145, 1985.

Arends J, et al: Time dependence of F uptake in demineralizing enamel from 1000 ppm fluoride, Caries Res 19:450, 1985.

ASCD Forum: The topical fluorides—how should they be used? ASCD J Dent Children 51:150, 1984.

Bayless JM, and Tinanoff N: Diagnosis and treatment of acute fluoride toxicity, JADA 110:209, 1985.

Benediktsson S, et al: The effect of contact time of acidulated phosphate fluoride on fluoride concentration in human enamel, Arch Oral Biol 27:567, 1982.

Bijella MFB, et al: Comparison of dental prophylaxis and toothbrushing prior to topical APF applications, Comm Dent Oral Epidemiol 13:208, 1985.

Boyd RL, Leggott PJ, and Robertson PB: Effects on gingivitis of two different 0.4%SnF_2 gels, J Dent Res 67:503, 1988.

Bruun C, Thylstrup A, and Uribe E: Loosely bound fluoride extracted from natural carious lesions after topical application of APF in vitro, Caries Res 17:458, 1983.

Brunn C, and Stoltze K: In vivo uptake of fluoride by surface enamel of cleaned and plaque-covered teeth, Scand J Dent Res 84:268, 1976.

Burt BA: The epidemiology of oral diseases, In Striffler DF, Young WO, and Burt BA, editors: Dentistry, dental practice, and the community, Philadelphia, 1983, WB Saunders.

Burt BA, Eklund SA, and Loesche WJ: Dental benefits of limited exposure to fluoridated water in childhood, J Dent Res 61:1322, 1986.

Carlos JP: Topical fluorides: optimizing safety and efficacy—introduction, J Dent Res 66:1055, 1987.

Charleton G, et al: Associations between dental plaque and fluoride in human surface enamel, Arch Oral Biol 19:139, 1974.

Church LE: Fluorides—use with caution, J Maryland Dent Assoc 19(Aug):106, 1976.

Clark DC: A review of fluoride varnishes: an alternative topical fluoride treatment, Comm Dent Oral Epidemiol 10:117, 1982.

Crall JJ, et al: SEM and electron microprobe analysis of enamel treated with two-step topical fluorides in vitro, Caries Res 17:481, 1983.

DePaola PF: Clinical studies of monofluorophosphate dentifrices, Caries Res 17(supp 1):119, 1983.

Dijkman AG, Tak J, and Arends J: Comparison of fluoride uptake by human enamel from acidulated phosphate fluoride gels with different fluoride concentrations. Caries Res 16:197, 1982.

Downer MD: Changing patterns of disease in the western world. In Guggenheim B, editor: Cariology Today. Basel, 1983, Karger.

Driessens FC, et al: Posteruptive maturation of the tooth enamel studied with the electron microprobe. Caries Res 19:390, 1985.

Driscoll WS, et al: Caries preventive effects of daily and weekly fluoride mouth rinsing in an optimally fluoridated community: findings after eighteen months. Pediatr Dent 3:316, 1981.

Driscoll WS, et al: Prevalence of dental caries and dental fluoride in areas with optimal and above-optimal water fluoride concentrations, JADA 197:42, 1983.

Duxbury AJ, et al: Accute fluoride toxicity, Br Dent J 153:64, 1982.

Eisen JJ, and LeComple EJ: A comparison of oral fluoride retention following topical treatments with APF gels of varying viscosities, Pediatr Dent 7:175, 1985.

Ekstrand J, and Koch G: Systemic fluoride absorption following fluoride gel application, J Dent Res 59:1067, 1980.

Ekstrand J, Koch G, and Petersson LG: Plasma fluoride concentrations in pre-school children after ingestion of fluoride tablets and toothpaste, Caries Res 17:379, 1983.

Ekstrand J, et al: Pharmacokinetics of fluoride gels in children and adults, Caries Res 15:213, 1981.

Ellingsen JE, and Ekstrand J: Plasma fluoride levels in man following intake of SnF_2 in solution or toothpaste, J Dent Res 64:1250, 1985.

Fehr FR von der, Loe H, and Theilade E: Experimental caries in man, Caries Res 4:131, 1970.

Fejerskov O, Thylstrup A, and Larsen MJ: Rational use of fluorides in caries prevention, Acta Odontol Scand 39:241, 1981.

Granath L, and McHugh WD: Basic prevention for the individual. In Granath L and McHugh WD, eds: Systematized prevention of oral disease: theory and practice. Boca Raton, 1986, CRC Press Inc.

Hagan PP, Rozier RG, and Baseden JW: The caries-preventive effects of full- and half-strength topical acidulated phosphate fluoride, Pediatric Dent 7:185, 1985.

Harper DS, and Loesche WJ: Inhibition of acid production from oral bacteria by fluorapatite derived fluoride, J Dent Res 65:30, 1986.

Hattab FN: Diffusion of fluorides in human dental enamel in vitro, Arch Oral Biol 31:811, 1986.

Heifetz SB, et al: Prevalence of dental caries and fluorosis in four acres of Illinois: a 5-year follow-up survey, J Dent Res 66(special issue, abst 460):164, 1987.

Heifetz SB, and Horowitz HS: The amounts of fluoride in current fluoride therapies: safety considerations for children, ASDC J Dent Children 51:257, 1984.

Hock J, and Tinanoff N: Resolution of gingivitis in dogs following topical applications of a 0.40% stannous fluoride and toothbrushing, J Dent Res 58:1652, 1979.

Holloway PJ, et al: The value of self-applied fluorides at home, Int Dent J 31:232, 1981.

Horowitz HS: Abuse use of fluoride, J Pub Hlth Dent 37:106, 1977.

Horowitz HS, and Heifetz SB: Topically applied fluorides. In Newbrun E, editor: Fluorides and dental caries, Springfield, Ill, 1986, CC Thomas Publisher.

Horowitz HS, et al: Combined fluoride, school-based program in a fluoride-deficient area: results of an 11-year study, JADA 112:621, 1986.

Houpt M, Koenigsberg S, and Shey Z: The effect of prior toothcleaning on the efficacy of topical fluoride treatment, Clin Prevent Dent 5(4):8, 1983.

Iijima Y, and Katayama T: Fluoride concentrations in deciduous enamel in high- and low-fluoride areas, Caries Res 19:262, 1985.

Isman R: Knowledge and attitudes of dentists about fluoridation, JADA 109:924, 1984.

Katz S, et al: Preventive dentistry in action, ed 3, Upper Montclair, NJ, 1979, DCP Publishing.

Keltjens HMAM, et al: Microflora of plaque from sound and carious root surfaces, Caries Res 21:193, 1987.

Klimek J, Hellwig E, and Ahrens G: Fluoride taken up by plaque, by the underlying enamel and by clean enamel from three fluoride compounds in vitro, Caries Res 16:156, 1982.

Klimek J, et al: Movement of plaque fluoride under cariogenic conditions, Caries Res 17:315, 1983.

Lagerlof F, et al: Effects of inorganic orthophosphate and pyrophosphate on dissolution of calcium fluoride in water, J Dent Res 67:447, 1988.

Larsen MJ, and Jensen SJ: On the properties of fluoride solutions used for topical treatment and mouth rinse, Caries Res 20:56, 1986.

LeCompte EJ: Clinical application of topical fluoride products—risks, benefits, and recommendations, J Dent Res 66:1066, 1987.

LeCompte EJ, and Doyle TE: Oral fluoride retention following various topical application techniques in children, J Dent Res 61:1397, 1982.

LeCompte EJ, and Doyle TE: Effects of suctioning devices on oral fluoride retention, JADA 11:357, 1985.

LeCompte EJ, and Whitford, GM: The biologic availability of fluoride from alginate impressions and APF gel in children, J Dent Res 60:776, 1981.

LeCompte EJ, and Whitford GM: Pharmacokinetics of fluoride from APF gel and fluoride tablets in children, J Dent Res 61:469, 1982.

Leske GS, Ripa LW, and Sposato A: Posttreatment benefits from participation in a school-based fluoride mouthrinsing demonstration program: results after 4 to 6 years of rinsing, Clin Prev Dent 6(1):16, 1984.

Leske GS, et al: Posttreatment benefits from participation in a school-based fluoride mouthrinsing program: results after up to 7 years of rinsing, Caries Res 19:371, 1985.

Leverett DH, and Curzon MEJ: Effect of flossing and brushing immediately prior to weekly fluoride mouthrinsing, Pediatr Dent 5:187, 1983.

Levy SM: Expansion of the proper use of systemic fluoride supplements, JADA 112:30, 1986.

Levy SM: Compliance by health care providers with recommended systemic fluoride supplementation protocol, Clin Prev Dent 9(5):19, 1987.

Lyon TC: Topical fluorides: How much are you using? Dent Hyg 59:58, 1985.

Margolis HD, Moreno EC, and Murphy BJ: Effect of low levels of fluoride in solution on enamel demineralization in vitro, J Dent Res 65:23, 1986.

Mazza JE, Newman MG, and Sims TN: Clinical and antimicrobial effect of stannous fluoride on periodontitis, J Clin Periodontol 8:203, 1981.

McCall DR, et al: Fluoride ingestion following APF gel application, Br Dent J 155:333, 1983.

McClure FJ: Water fluoridation: the search and victory, Bethesda, Md, 1970, National Institutes of Health.

McDonald JL, Schemehorn BR, and Stookey GK: Influence of fluoride upon plaque and gingivitis in the beagle dog, J Dent Res 57:889, 1978.

Mellberg JR, and Mallon DE: Acceleration of remineralization in vitro by sodium monofluorophosphate and sodium fluoride, J Dent Res 63:1130, 1984.

Mellberg JR, et al: The relationship between dental caries and tooth enamel fluoride, Caries Res 19:385, 1985.

Mirth, DB et al: Comparison of the cariostatic effect of topically and systemically administered controlled-release fluoride in the rat, Caries Res 19:466, 1985.

More F, et al: Ingestion of fluoride during a topical application, J Dent Res 62:262 Abstr no 837, 1983.

Nakagaki H, et al: Distribution of fluoride across human dental enamel, dentine and cementum, Arch Oral Biol 32:651, 1987.

Narendran S, et al: Fluorosis in fluoridated and nonfluoridated communities, J Dent Res 66(special issue, abst 461):164, 1987.

Newbrun E: Mechanism of fluoride action in caries prevention. In Newbrun E, editor: Fluorides and dental caries, ed 3, Springfield, Ill, 1986, CC Thomas, Publisher.

Newbrun E: Topical fluoride therapy: discussion of some aspects of toxicology, safety, and efficacy, J Dent Res 66:1084, 1987.

Owen D, et al: Monitoring ingestion and urinary excretion of topical fluoride. IADR prog and abst 57(1256):405, 1979.

Ramsay DS, et al: Problematic gagging: principles of treatment, JADA 114:178, 1987.

Reintsema H, Schuthof J, and Arends J: An in vivo investigation of the fluoride uptake in partially demineralized human enamel from several different dentifrices, J Dent Res 64:19, 1985.

Retief DH, Harris BE, and Bradley EL: Relationship between enamel fluoride concentration and dental caries experience, Caries Res 21:68, 1987.

Ripa LW: Professionally (operator) applied topical fluoride therapy: a critique, Clin Prevent Dent 4(3):3, 1982.

Ripa LW: Need for prior toothcleaning when performing a professional topical fluoride application: review and recommendations for change, JADA 109:281, 1984.

Ripa LW: The roles of prophylaxes and dental prophylaxis pastes in caries prevention. In Wei Sh, editor: Clinical uses of fluoride, Philadelphia, 1985, Lea & Febiger.

Ripa LW: Topical fluorides: a discussion of risks and benefits, J Dent Res 66:1079, 1987.

Ripa LW, et al: Effect of prior toothcleaning on biannual professional APF topical fluoride gel-tray treatments: results after two years, Clin Prevent Dent 5(4):3, 1983(a).

Ripa LW, et al: Supervised weekly rinsing with a 0.2% neutral NaF solution: results after 5 years, Comm Dent Oral Epidemiol 11:1, 1983(b).

Ripa LW, et al: Supervised weekly rinsing with a 0.2% neutral NaF solution: results of a demonstration program after six school years, J Pub Health Dent 43:52, 1983(c).

Ripa LW, et al: Clinical comparison of the caries inhibition of two mixed $NaF-Na_2PO_3F$ dentifrices containing 1000 ppm F: results after two years, Caries Res 21:149, 1987.

Schamschula RG, et al: Interrelations between the fluoride concentrations in dental plaque and enamel and exposure to fluoride, Aust Dent J 27:360, 1982.

Seppa L: Effect of dental plaque on fluoride uptake by enamel from a sodium fluoride varnish in vivo, Caries Res 17:71, 1983.

Seppa L, and Pollanen L: Caries preventive effect of two fluoride varnishes and a fluoride mouthrinse, Caries Res 21:375, 1987.

Shannon IL, Edmonds EJ, and Madsen KO: Single, double, and sequential methods for fluoride applications, ASDC J Dent Children 41:115, 1974(a).

Shannon IL, Paoloski SB, and Wescott WB: Dental hygiene students in the fluoride laboratory, Dent Hyg 48:87, 1974(b).

Stallard RE, editor: Proceedings, international conference on fluorides and dental health, Nairobi, Kenya, New Brunswick, NJ, 1983, S & S Printing Services, Inc.

Steele RC, et al: The effect of tooth cleaning procedures on fluoride uptake in enamel, Pediatr Dent 4:228, 1982.

Stephan KW, et al: J Dent Res 66 (special issue, abst 459):164, 1987.

Stephan KW, McCall DR, and Tullis JI: Caries prevalence in northern Scotland before and after 5 years water defluoridation, Br Dent J 163:324, 1987b.

Stookey GK, et al: The effect of rinsing with water immediately after a professional fluoride gel application on fluoride uptake in demineralized enamel: an in vivo study, Pediatr Dent 8:153, 1986.

Teranaka T, and Koulourides T: Effect of a 100-ppm fluoride mouthrinse on experimental root caries in humans, Caries Res 21:326, 1987.

Tinanoff N, et al: Effect of a pumice prophylaxis on fluoride uptake in tooth enamel, JADA 88:384, 1974.

Tyler JE, and Andlaw RJ: Oral retention of fluoride after application of acidulated phosphate fluoride gel in air-cushion trays, Br Dent J 162:422, 1987.

U.S. Public Health Service, National Institute of Dental Research: The prevalence of dental caries in United States children, 1979-1980, NIH publication 82-2245, Washington, DC, 1981, Government Printing Office.

Vrbic V, and Brudevold F: Fluoride uptake from treatment with different fluoride prophylaxis pastes and from the use of pastes containing a soluble aluminum salt followed by topical application, Caries Res 4:158, 1970.

Vrbic V, Brudevold F, and McCann HG: Acquisition of fluoride by enamel from fluoride pumice pastes, Helv Odontol Acta 11:21, 1967.

Wefel JS: Critical assessment of professional application of topical fluorides. In Wei Sh, editor: Clinical uses of fluoride, Philadelphia, 1985, Lea & Febiger.

Wei SH: The potential benefits to be derived from topical fluorides in fluoridated communities. In Forester DJ, and Schulz EM, editors: International workshop on fluorides and dental caries reduction, Baltimore, 1974, University of Maryland School of Dentistry.

Wei SH, and Kanelis MJ: Fluoride retention after sodium fluoride mouthrinsing by preschool children, JADA 106:626, 1983.

White DJ, and Faller RV: Fluoride uptake from anticalculus dentifrices in vitro, Caries Res 21:40, 1987.

Whitford GM: Fluoride in dental products: safety considerations, J Dent Res 66:1056, 1987.

Whitford GM, et al: Topical fluorides: effects on physiological and biochemical process, J Dent Res 66:1072, 1987.

29 PIT AND FISSURE SEALANTS

OBJECTIVES: *The reader will be able to*

1. List three methods that have been used to prevent pit and fissure caries.
2. Discuss the role of sealants in a total preventive program.
3. Discuss research findings regarding sealant retention and caries reduction.
4. Describe the mechanism by which the sealant attaches to the tooth.
5. Discuss the effect that the shape of a pit or fissure has on the penetration of a sealant.
6. Discuss the factors to be considered when selecting teeth for the sealant application.
7. Describe three types of sealant material.
8. List the sequence of steps most commonly used when applying pit and fissure sealants.
9. Discuss possible reasons for under-utilization of sealant techniques in community and private practice settings, given their success as a preventive therapy.

One advance in the prevention of caries has been the development of occlusal sealants. These materials protect the pits and fissures from bacterial activity that creates carious lesions. It is interesting to note that although the occlusal surfaces account for only about 12.5% of the total surfaces at risk to caries, occlusal decay makes up almost 50% of the decay in children's teeth (Ripa, 1973).

In 1980, the National Dental Caries Prevalence survey reported that 16% of the caries experience of 5- to 17-year-old children occurred on the smooth surfaces of the teeth, while 84% involved surfaces with pits and fissures (NIH, 1983).

Methods other than sealants have attempted to lower the rate of pit and fissure caries. One approach was eradication of the occlusal anatomy by reshaping the occlusal grooves or by placing conservative occlusal restorations before decay actually occurs (Craig, O'Brien and Powers, 1983). As both of these methods eliminate sound tooth structure, it is unclear what is actually being prevented.

Obturation or closing the occlusal anatomy with materials such as silver nitrate, zinc chloride, potassium ferrocyanide, or red copper cement has also been tried. Such procedures have been unsuccessful primarily because of the material's physical or chemical properties.

Fluoride seemed an obvious answer to the problem of occlusal decay, as it would have a systemic effect on the actual quality of the enamel. Indeed, fluorides do reduce the absolute number of caries, but studies indicate that the proximal and smooth surfaces, not the occlusal surfaces, enjoy the most benefit from systemic or topical fluoride therapy (Ripa, 1973).

Reducing the retentive nature of the occlusal anatomy is the key to a significant reduction in pit and fissure caries. A fissure that is less likely to harbor debris and/or bacteria is less likely to decay. The sealants used today are materials that coat the occlusal surface. In this way the sealant acts as a physical barrier to prevent oral bacteria and nutrients from developing the acidic conditions necessary to destroy tooth structure. The factor that has made today's sealants more successful than other coverage techniques is an acid-conditioning process that alters or enlarges the naturally occurring enamel pores. With the increase in surface area due to this technique, the sealant is able to penetrate the enamel better and achieve a reliable mechanical bond (Gwinnett, 1973). The following studies indicate the significance of sealant materials in the patient's total prevention program. In a study of a single application of sealant on 113 permanent tooth surfaces, 87% had retained full coverage after 2 years. In the untreated control teeth, 60% became carious during the 2 years. Ninety-nine percent protection was obtained in the experimental surfaces of the permanent teeth (Buonocore, 1971).

In a 4-year clinical evaluation of pit and fissure sealants, 50% of the teeth had fully retained their single application of sealant. When sealant remained intact, the effectiveness in caries reduction was 84% (Going, 1977).

Retention and effectiveness of a single application of adhesive sealant after 5 years showed that 42% of the initially sealed sites retained their covering. When sealant was only partially lost, 93% of the sites remained caries-free. When sealant was fully retained, less than 1% became carious as compared with 18% of the untreated paired controls. When sealant was partially lost, 7% became decayed, missing, or filled as compared with 41% of the untreated pairs. Regardless of retention status, after 5 years of a single application of sealant a 39% effectiveness in preventing decay was attained (Horowitz, Heifetz, and Poulsen, 1977).

Even 10 years after a single application of a white-colored pit and fissure sealant to permanent first molars, 84% of the surfaces were sound. In a matched pair analysis of 12 pairs of teeth, 68% of the surfaces in the unsealed group became carious or were restored, compared with only 22% of the sealed group (Simonsen, 1987).

When fluorides and sealants are combined, the preventive benefits are enhanced. After 2 years a control group who participated in a weekly mouthrinsing program with 0.2% neutral NaF solution were 78.4% caries-free. The group that received sealants in addition to the weekly mouthrinsing remained 96.4% caries-free (Ripa, 1987).

THE BONDING MECHANISM

Buonocore (1975) suggested that the occlusal surface of a tooth is similar to an iceberg: much of what exists cannot be seen. In fact, with conventional explorer examination much cannot be determined with tactile sense. The explorer may "catch" in the tooth because of anatomy alone. Three principal types of pit and fissure configurations have been described: V types, U types, and I types (Figs. 29-1 to 29-3). In addition, miscellaneous shapes exist as small round openings, fis-

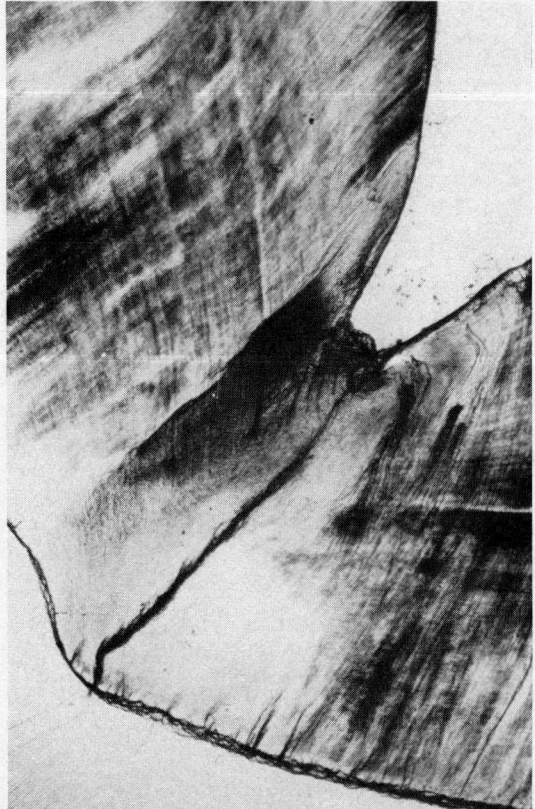

Fig. 29-1. Photomicrograph showing wide V-type fissure. (From Gwinnett AJ: J Am Soc Prevent Dent **3:**21, 1973.)

sures that have pits associated with their bases or walls, or continuous grooves that separate cusps (Fig. 29-4). To protect these anatomic defects from the inevitably high percentage of carious lesions, acid-etch resin sealants are useful. Success is dependent on a highly effective bonding technique and a leakage resistant material.

Mechanical bonding refers to a physical entrapment of material within pores or cavities occurring naturally or artificially created (Gwinnett, 1973). The etching process, also called conditioning, involves applying an acidic gel or a 30% to 40% acidic solution to the occlusal surface. The acid (usually 30% unbuffered phosphoric acid) removes inorganic material and creates tiny crevices or micro-pores. This rough and reactive porous surface provides a great amount of surface area, as well as tiny pits to which the sealant

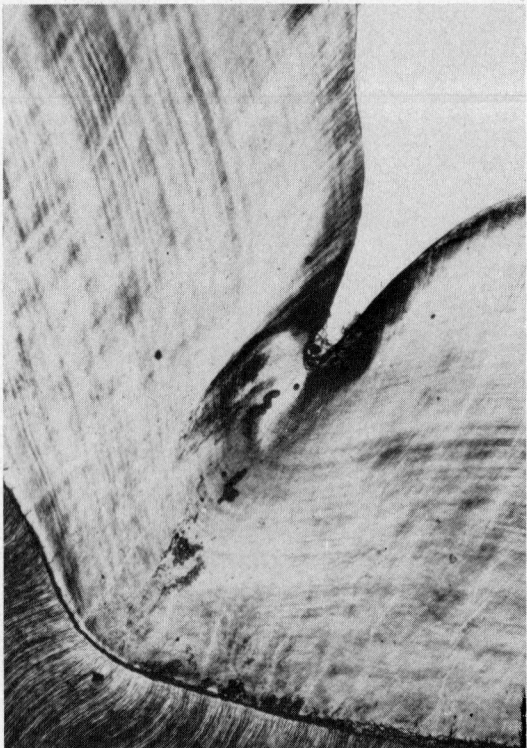

Fig. 29-2. Photomicrograph showing narrow V-type fissure. (From Gwinnett AJ: J Am Soc Prevent Dent **3:**21, 1973.)

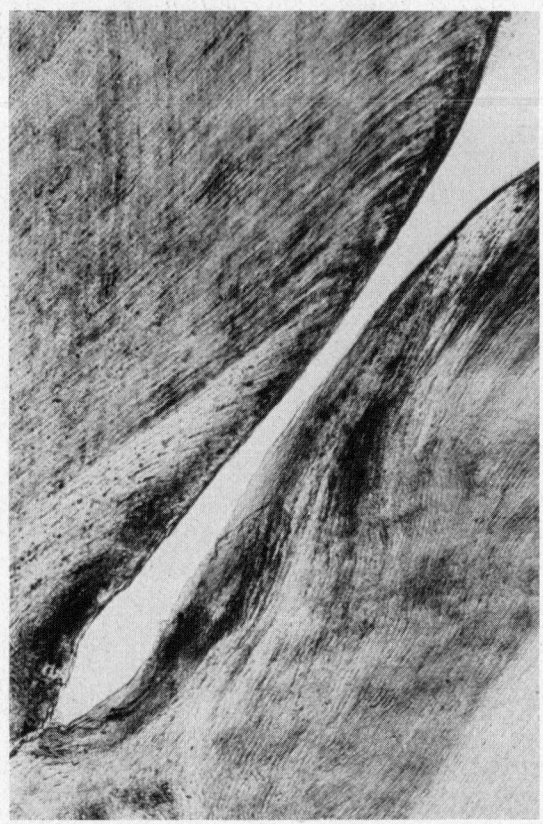

Fig. 29-3. Photomicrograph showing I-type fissure, a narrow constrictive configuration that is somewhat bulbous toward its base. (From Gwinnett AJ: J Am Soc Prevent Dent **3:**21, 1973.)

resin can adapt, forming a strong mechanical bond.

Three basic etching patterns can be observed by scanning electron micrograph. The conditioned enamel surface shows enamel rods that have lost material from the rod cores (Fig. 29-5). The surface may show a preferential loss of rod peripheries, or the enamel surface may show no specific pattern, but be etched satisfactorily. All three types of etching patterns can be observed on a single tooth. Irrespective of the etching pattern, satisfactory bonding occurs between the resin and enamel (Silverstone, 1987).

The studies mentioned previously indicate the degree of retention that is possible even after several years with only one application of sealant. In practice, sealants are examined regularly at recall intervals (3 to 6 months) and reapplied when necessary.

As conditioning does remove enamel structure,

does it harm the tooth? Generally, conditioning is confined to the cuspal planes of the occlusal surfaces that are to be covered with the sealant material. If conditioned enamel is left exposed, minerals in the saliva replenish the surface (Silverstone, 1987).

Researchers have reported that decay inadvertently sealed in a tooth does not appear to progress when the sealant is firmly bonded to the tooth (Mertz-Fairhurst, 1979; Handelman, 1983). The margins of sealed surfaces have been shown to resist leakage of dye and radioisotopes even after being boiled in water. A study of residual carious material under sealed lesions suggested a complete cessation of the carious process. No clinical or radiographic signs were seen to suggest that

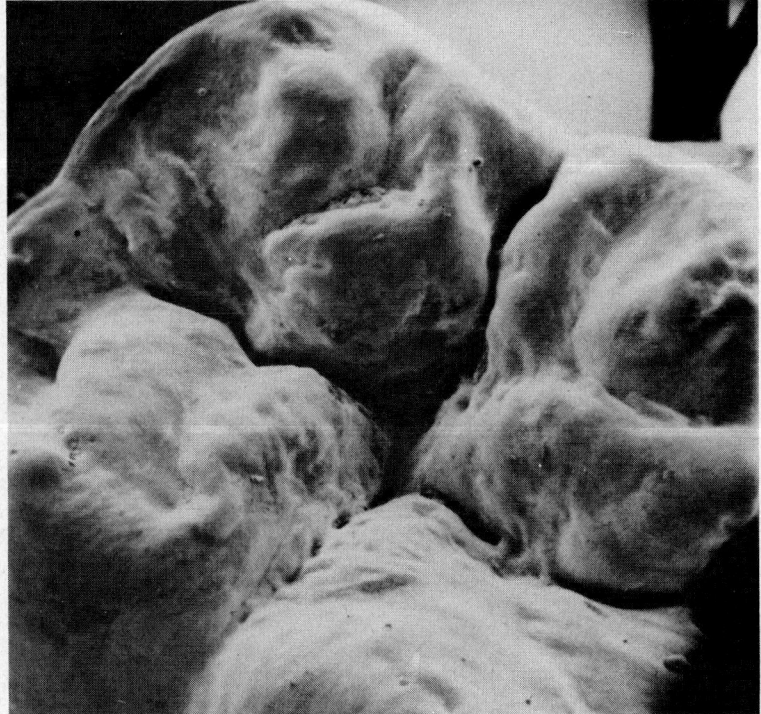

Fig. 29-4. Scanning electron micrograph showing random distribution of pits and fissures on occlusal surface. (From Gwinnett AJ: J Am Soc Prevent Dent **3:**21, 1973.)

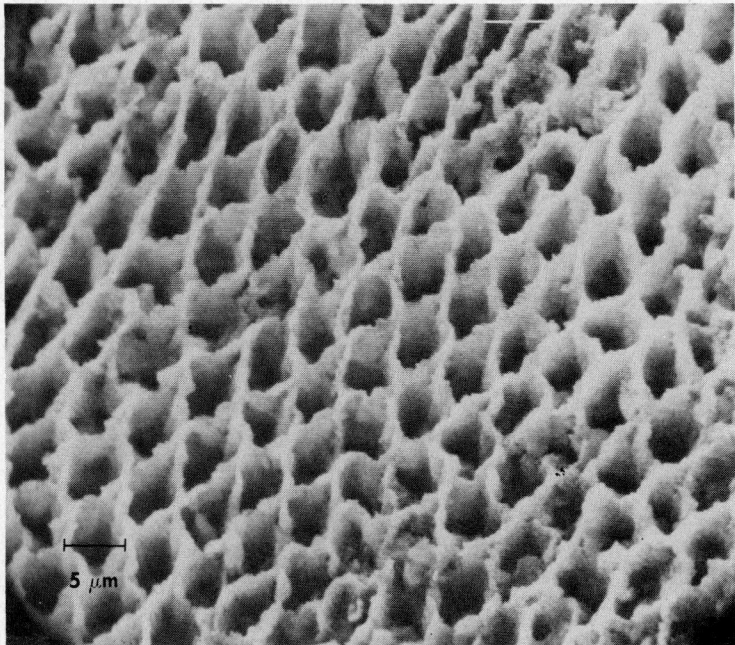

5 μm

Fig. 29-5. Scanning electron migrograph of enamel surface that has been etched (conditioned) with phosphoric acid for 60 seconds. Note loss of enamel prism core, which will encourage sealant retention. (From Silverstone LM: Preventive dentistry, Fort Lee, NJ, 1978, Update Publishing International, Inc.)

the health of the sealed tooth had been compromised (Mertz-Fairhurst, 1986). When carious surfaces or sound surfaces were sealed for the first time, the retention rates for the sealant materials were the same after a 2-year period (Handelman, 1987).

The results of these studies support the safety of sealing small, incipient caries. The nature of the sealant margin compares favorably with other current restorative material margins that, despite microscopic leakage, arrest the decay process and resist recurrence of caries to a high degree. Dennison and colleagues (1980) compared the margins of amalgam restorations with sealants retained after 18 months. Margin deterioration occurred in 50% of the amalgam restorations. Sealant margins remained undetectable in 55% of the cases. Sealants have proven themselves as effective materials for protecting the occlusal surfaces from the caries process.

SEALANT MATERIALS

Most sealants are bisphenol A-glycidyl methacrylate (BIS-GMA) materials, which are polymerized by an organic amine or ultraviolet or visible light (Craig, O'Brien, and Powers, 1983). Amine-accelerated materials are supplied as two-component systems and require mixing. Ultraviolet and visible light–polymerized materials require no mixing.

To ensure success with these materials, careful handling is necessary. It is especially important that the sealant material not be exposed to air during storage. This may cause evaporation, which would make the material less fluid and reduce penetration into the pits and fissures. Fresh sealant material should be used, and other sealant equipment such as brushes and light sources should be well maintained.

Mertz-Fairhurst and others (1982) reported a comparative clinical study of two pit and fissure sealants in which 49% of the teeth remained sealed with one product and 78% remained intact with the other product 6 years after a single application.

In a study comparing auto-polymerized versus light-polymerized fissure sealant, Houp and co-workers (1987) found no significant difference in the clinical performance and retention of these sealants after 31 months. Other studies compared

Acceptable

Concise Brand White Sealant, Minnesota Mining and Manufacturing Co.
Delton, Johnson and Johnson Dental Products Co.
Delton (tinted), Johnson and Johnson Dental Products Co.
Nuva-Seal P.A., LD Caulk Co, Division of Dentsply International, Inc.
Oralin Pit and Fissure Sealant, SS White Dental Products
Prisma-Shield, LD Caulk Co., Division of Dentsply International, Inc.
Prisma-Shield (tinted), LD Caulk Co., Division of Dentsply International, Inc.
Visio-Seal, ESPE

Provisionally Acceptable

Helioseal, Viadent USA
Delton Light Cure, Johnson and Johnson Dental Products Co.

Fig. 29-6. Pit and fissure sealant products approved by the Council on Dental Materials, Instruments, and Equipment. (From JADA **114**(5):671, 1987.)

products for their microhardness, bone strength, and abrasion loss (Strang, 1986).

New, improved sealant materials are being developed. A material that incorporates a slow-release fluoride is promising. A methacryloyl fluoride–methyl methacrylate (MF–MMA) copolymer resin showed after testing that 70% to 80% of the fluoride was tightly bound to the enamel, suggesting that such a sealant could protect the enamel from caries attack even after detachment (Tanaka, 1987).

Research shows that most sealant materials are comparable and effective. New product improvements are being made. There appear to be no health-related risks to either the patient or dental professionals. No systemic toxicity from the chemical use of sealants has been reported. Wearing protective glasses is recommended when using the light-cured materials (Dental Consensus Conference, 1983).

Materials approved by the Council on Dental Instruments and Equipment can be found in Fig. 29-6. The Council encourages manufacturers to submit their products for evaluation. Evaluations are based on lab test results of mechanical and physical properties and biological acceptability as well as clinical data on biocompatibility and effectiveness as a caries-preventive material. Clinical studies on retention may also be included. Participation by a manufacturer is voluntary.

INDICATIONS FOR SEALANT APPLICATION

In selecting teeth to be protected by sealant, the patient's caries susceptibility is important. This is reflected by the number of restorations and/or caries present and the patient's attitude about preventive dentistry. Occlusal sealants are not likely to be successful for reducing caries when adequate home care and dietary measures are lacking. Sealant protection is intended to be used as part of a total preventive program. Regular professional care, fluoride application (systemic and topical), and individual home care are the components of the preventive plan.

The patient's tooth anatomy is also a consideration. Deep, narrow pits and fissures tend to be more retentive of oral bacteria than teeth with shallow grooves, which retain less plaque and are more accessible to cleaning methods. In the permanent dentition, molars are more susceptible to caries than premolars. In the primary dentition, the second molars are more susceptible than the first molars (Ripa, 1973).

The pattern of dental caries differs greatly from tooth to tooth and surface to surface. At least 70% of occlusal surfaces in permanent molars eventually become decayed or filled. The peak in caries of this group is reached about 10 years after eruption between the ages of 16 and 22 years. Occlusal decay of premolars is less prevalent, with only 30% to 45% becoming carious. The peak for premolars is reached between the ages of 30 and 40 years. Sealants have the potential for preventing the need for occlusal fillings in 50% of molar teeth. Because the overall caries rate is less in premolars, sealants will do no better than saving 10% of the need for occlusal restorations in these teeth (Eklund, 1986). In general, when a patient is identified as being caries-susceptible, despite other preventive measures, the teeth should be protected as soon after eruption as possible.

In 1983, the consensus panel on sealants suggested these priorities for sealant application:

General population

Priority
1. Permanent first molars (ages 6 to 8)
2. Permanent second molars (ages 11 to 13)

High caries-susceptible children

Priority
1. Permanent first molars
2. Permanent second molars
3. Permanent premolars
4. Primary molars

Teeth should be selected as candidates for sealants after a careful evaluation with explorer and compressed air. A radiographic examination is also necessary. Occlusal sealing is contradicted where proximal surfaces are carious, as the restorative procedure will include a portion of the occlusal table. Occasionally there is a question about a "sticky" fissure. On explorer examination the instrument tip is retained or sticks for a brief instant in the pit or fissure. Usually the patient has no discomfort associated with this. If there is

---

1. Sealants are indicated for previously unrestored, deep, narrow pits and fissures that show no evidence of caries.
2. Presence of interproximal caries should be ruled out before sealant placement.
3. Sealants should be placed as soon as possible after eruption, when the tooth is free of gingival contact and when there is no tissue flap to interfere with application procedures.
4. Consider overall caries status. Seal newly erupted teeth promptly when there is evidence of current carious lesions and/or previous restorations on other teeth, malpositioned teeth, and any other condition promoting decay.
5. Only use sealant products accepted by the Council on Dental Materials, Instruments, and Equipment of the American Dental Association.
6. Sealants should be applied according to the manufacturer's instructions.
7. Fluoride treatment should be applied after sealant application.
8. If needed, one application per tooth may be allowed every 3 to 5 years with one repair allowed (lesser fee) in the intervening time.

Fig. 29-7. Sealant application guidelines for third-party payers.
(From DiLeone CM: Dental Hygiene **61**(1):18, 1987.)

no evidence of pathology with a bite-wing radiograph, placing a sealant is preferable to leaving the tooth in a vulnerable state or cutting a cavity for a prophylactic amalgam restoration (Ball, 1986). This practice may be controversial, but the rationale comes from the fact that sealed incipient caries do not progress, and it represents the most conservative treatment for preventing caries while preserving the most natural tooth structure.

Fig. 29-7 describes sealant application guidelines suggested for Medicaid and other insurance carriers and may be used as a summary of general considerations.

SEALANT APPLICATION

Although manufacturers' products differ, the basic steps in sealant application are similar. It is essential to note that the quality of the end product is determined to a great extent by the clinician's attention to (1) strict clinical dryness, (2) accurate timing for conditioning, (3) fresh sealant material, and (4) adherence to recommended setting (polymerization) procedures.

Application technique

1. Prepare the tooth surface, cleaning it of hard and soft deposits. Using a bristle brush, polish with a pumice and water. A polishing paste with fluoride or a fluoride treatment prior to the sealant application is contraindicated; the fluoride will interfere with the etching/conditioning technique (Silverstone, 1978). Rinse the teeth thoroughly with water.
2. Isolate the teeth with a rubber dam or a Garmer clamp with cotton rolls (Figs. 29-8 and 29-9). It is extremely important to keep the working area dry. The rubber dam procedure is recommended when the sealant is to be applied to several teeth in the quadrant. Satisfactory results can be obtained with frequent changing of cotton rolls. A study comparing rubber dam versus cotton roll isolation found the average 6-month retention rate was 95% regardless of the method of isolation used (Straffon, 1985). Once the teeth are isolated, dry the area with clean, dry compressed air (Fig. 29-10).
3. Apply the conditioner for the enamel-etching process. Following the manufacturer's directions for acid concentration and conditioning

time. A brush for painting the conditioner on the occlusal surface is recommended, although a cotton pellet can be used (Fig. 29-11). A fine brush is more accurate in placing the acid than a cotton pellet, which may absorb too much of the solution or cause air to be trapped in the fissure (Silverstone, 1983).
4. After the appropriate conditioning time (usually 60 seconds), rinse the area with water to thoroughly remove the conditioning solution. Immediately dry the teeth. Take care not to let saliva contact the conditioned surface, as this will interfere with the bonding of the sealant. *This is the most critical period in the sealant application.* Study results show that after any exposure of saliva of one second or greater, a

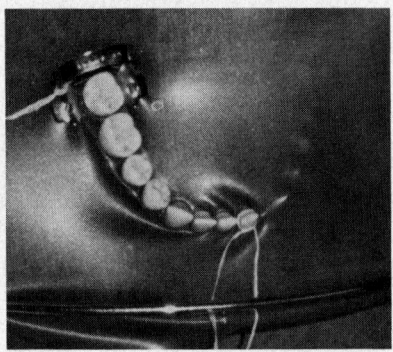

Fig. 29-8. One technique to maintain a dry working field during sealant procedure is to isolate teeth with a rubber dam.

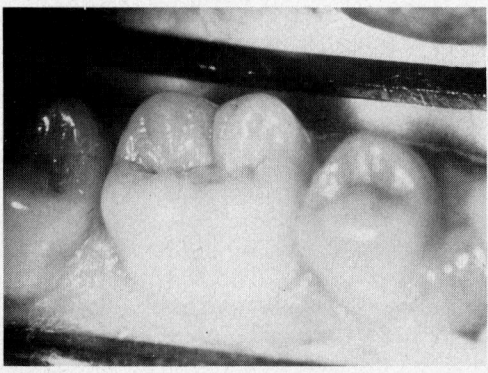

Fig. 29-9. Teeth are isolated with Garmer clamp and cotton rolls.
(Courtesy LD Caulk Co., Milford, Del.)

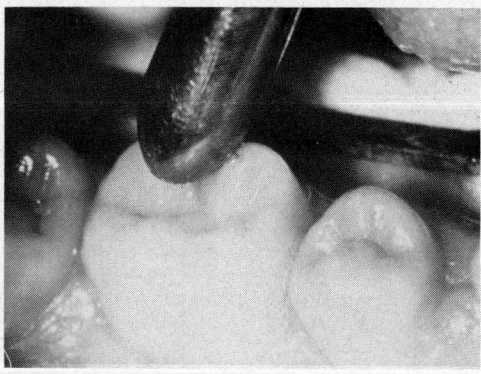

Fig. 29-10. Teeth are dried with compressed air.
(Courtesy LD Caulk Co., Milford, Del.)

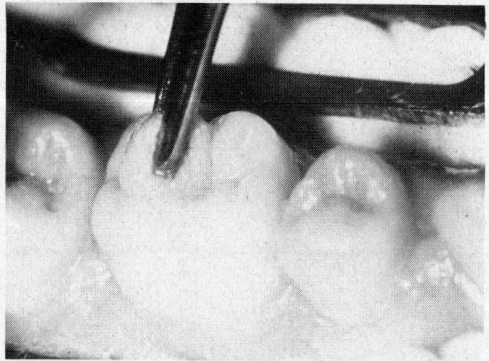

Fig. 29-11. Conditioner is applied according to manufacturer's directions.
(Courtesy LD Caulk Co., Milford, Del.)

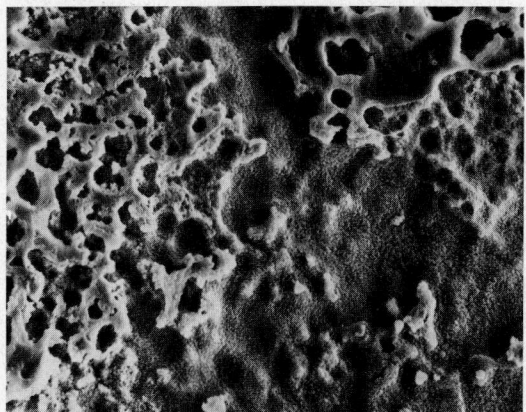

Fig. 29-12. Scanning electron micrograph showing human enamel that was etched for 60 seconds, then contaminated with human saliva for 5 seconds. Shown after rinse with water, the etched surface is completely obscured. Magnification × 1000.
(Courtesy LM Silverstone, Aurora, Colo.)

tenacious surface coating that cannot be removed by washing forms on the etched enamel surface (Fig. 29-12) (Silverstone, 1987). Inspect the teeth for a dull, chalky surface (Spohn and Berry, 1979) (Fig. 29-13). If the entire surface to be sealed does not appear chalky or if the teeth have been contaminated with saliva, repeat the conditioning procedure.

5. Apply the sealant by brushing the liquid on the conditioned tooth surface (Fig. 29-14). Concentrate the sealant in the central pits and fissures (Fig. 29-15). Apply the sealant to the cuspal planes to complete the coverage (Fig. 29-16). Trace the fissures with an explorer to enable air bubbles to rise and sealant to penetrate.

Sealants with a high coefficient of penetration (low viscosity) appear to penetrate the fissures by capillary action, reducing the likelihood of air entrapment. More viscous materials may allow more air to be trapped (Ball, 1987). It is especially difficult to get even coverage on maxillary molars because the sealant tends to flow from the mesial to the distal due to patient positioning. Take care not to apply an excess of sealant or to let the sealant flow into the contact area.

6. If polymerization is to occur chemically, follow the manufacturer's directions for the appropriate period of time (usually 1 minute). If ultraviolet light or visible light is needed for polymerization, follow directions for placement of the light wand and for correct exposure time. Not only do current ultraviolet machines vary in their output, but they also become less effective in time because of deposits on the ultraviolet lamp (Silverstone, 1983). Maintain the light source according to the manufacturer's specifications (Fig. 29-17). Observe the recommended warm-up time for the light source (2 to 5 minutes). Determine the efficiency of the light source by testing a

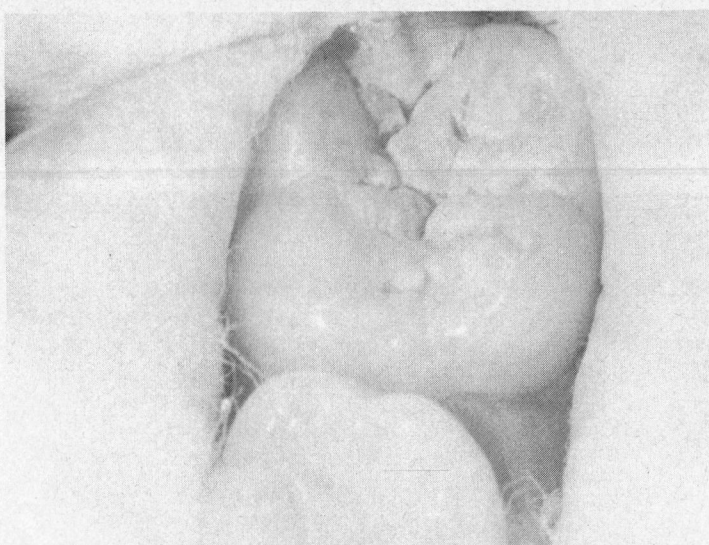

Fig. 29-13. Conditioner is rinsed off, and teeth are dried. Note dull, chalky appearance.
(From Spohn EE and Berry TG: Pit and fissure sealants. In Boundy SS and Reynolds NJ, editors: Current concepts in dental hygiene, vol 2. St. Louis, 1979, The CV Mosby Co.)

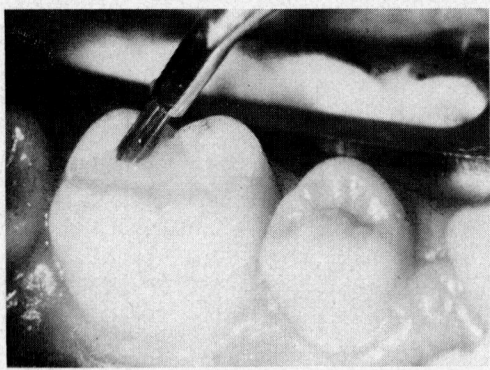

Fig. 29-14. Sealant is brushed on conditioned surface.
(Courtesy LD Caulk Co., Milford, Del.)

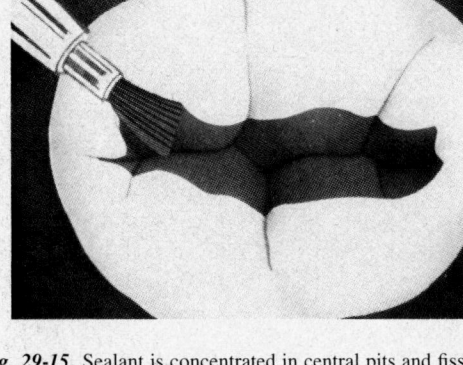

Fig. 29-15. Sealant is concentrated in central pits and fissures.
(Courtesy LD Caulk Co., Milford Del.)

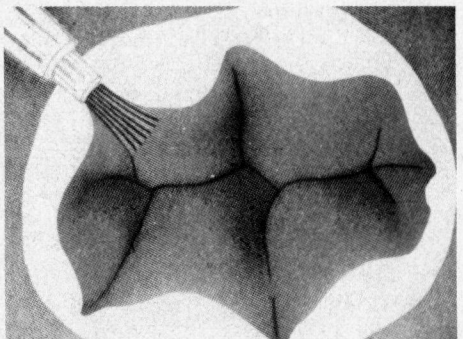

Fig. 29-16. Inclined planes of cusps are covered to complete coverage of occlusal surface.
(Courtesy LD Caulk Co., Milford, Del.)

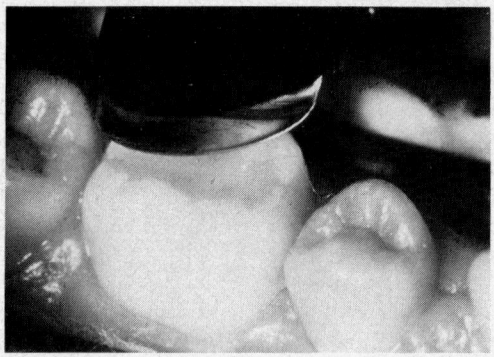

Fig. 29-17. Liquid sealant is polymerized with ultraviolet light according to manufacturer's directions.
(Courtesy LD Caulk Co., Milford, Del.)

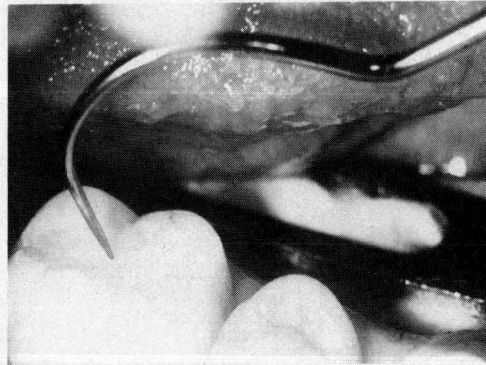

Fig. 29-18. Surface is evaluated with an explorer or probe to check total coverage.
(Courtesy LD Caulk Co., Milford, Del.)

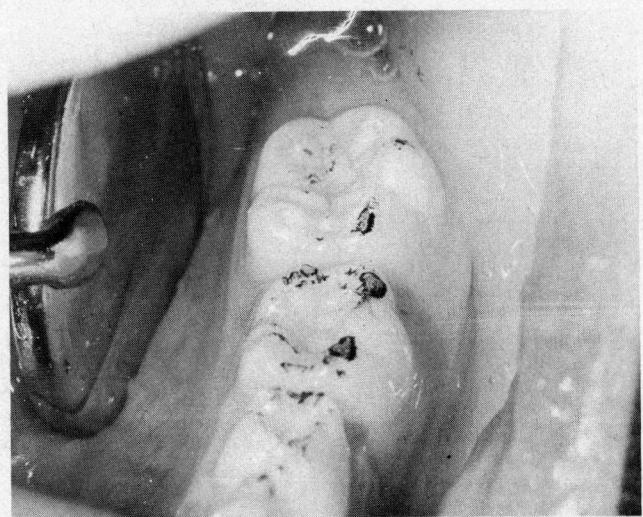

Fig. 29-19. Occlusal relationship is checked. In this case minimal occlusal contact occurs on sealant.
(From Spohn EE and Berry TG: Pit and fissure sealants. In Boundy SS and Reynolds NJ, editors: Current concepts in dental hygiene, Vol 2. St. Louis, 1979, The CV Mosby Co.)

drop of sealant on a glass slab with a 20-second exposure (Craig, 1983).

7. After polymerization occurs, rinse and wipe the occlusal surface. A small cotton pellet can be used to remove sealant that has failed to polymerize. Evaluate the surface carefully with a probe or an explorer to ensure that a smooth, hard surface has been achieved (Fig. 29-18). Check for incomplete coverage and voids. Repeat the entire procedure for defective areas.

8. Check the occlusal relationship with articulating paper (Fig. 29-19). Check the contact between the teeth with floss.

9. A fluoride treatment may be given after the entire sealant application is complete.

Alternative methods for preparing the teeth for sealants have been suggested by several authors. Mechanical preparation of the tooth can be beneficial. In a study where a #1 round steel bur was run at low speed over the fissure to remove plaque, organic debris, and surface enamel, the retention rate of the sealant was 88% as compared to 65% for the control group after 6 years (Shapira, 1986).

Some operators advocate going a step further, by using a dentin bonding agent after opening the fissure with a bur. In some fissures, enamel may be so thin that preparation of the tooth, even scraping with an explorer, may expose parts of the dentin. A very conservative composite restoration, or a glass ionomer cement, could be placed, then the entire surface sealed. There is minimal leakage because the restoration bonds with the cavity wall (Simonsen, 1978; Henderson, 1985). Houpt studied the concept of sealing for prevention rather than cavity extension for prevention. After 4 years, 156 out of 205 occlusal composite restorations showed complete retention of the sealant. Caries appeared in only 13 teeth. Conservative cavity preparation with sealant is successful and preserves valuable tooth structure (Houpt, 1985).

Another preparation technique involved using an air-polishing device (Prophy Jet). The study was done on extracted teeth. The mean sealant bond strength was higher for the teeth prepared with the air polisher than for the teeth prepared with a traditional pumice and water polishing technique. Further investigation is suggested (Scott, 1987).

The results of more invasive preparation techniques are being studied, but further consensus needs to be reached before new application recommendations are made.

Follow-up evaluation

Dental sealants should be followed clinically and radiographically. Close visual examination to assess wear, air bubble voids, and partial or complete loss should be completed every 6 months. Tinted sealants may be easier to examine visually than clear ones. At yearly intervals, a bite-wing radiograph can be taken to determine the status of the tooth underneath the sealant. The failure rate of sealants ranges from 5% to 10% the first year (Mertz-Fairhurst, 1984). During a 36-month study, 31% of the treatment teeth required at least one retreatment (Straffon, 1985).

Assessment of sealants can be complicated. Sealant products differ in appearance, and the patient may have more than one type of sealant if previous replacements have been made. The clinician needs to review the chart notations and complete a careful visual and explorer examination of all teeth. A decision about the status of each tooth with sealant should be made and recorded.

A recent investigation attempted to identify the evaluation instrument that would provide the

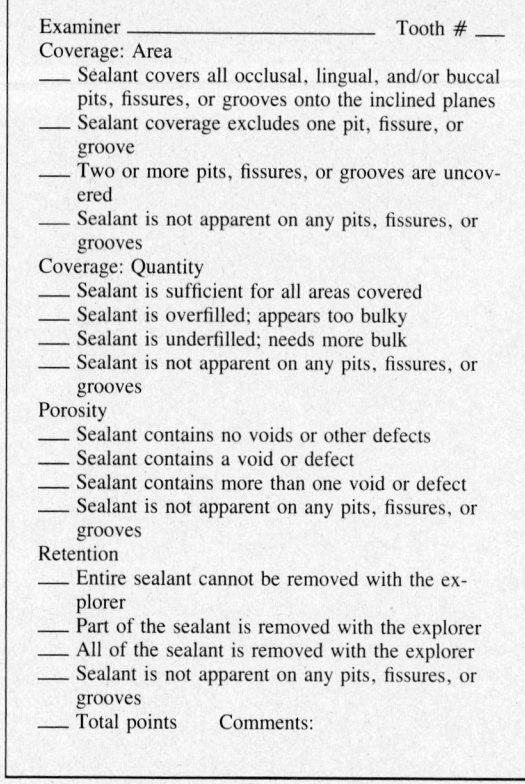

Fig. 29-20. Sealant evaluation form—criterion referenced. (From Daniel ST and Scruggs RR: J Dent Educ **51:**4, 1987.)

highest level of reliability for examiners. Global, checklist, and criterion-referenced instruments were compared. Experienced examiners achieved a higher reliability regardless of the evaluation instrument as compared to inexperienced examiners, but results suggest that written criteria encourage interexaminer reliability (Daniel, 1987). A sample evaluation instrument is found in Fig. 29-20.

The use of an evaluation instrument will provide some standardization in the way sealants are reviewed. Notes about the condition of the sealant will aid in deciding to watch or redo specific tooth surfaces at follow-up visits and will enhance record keeping about sealants.

Replacement procedure

When a sealant is identified as defective and in need of replacement, the tooth should be prepared by cleaning the surfaces as described in the Application section, step 1.

Following this, the sealant should be roughened up a bit with an explorer or small bur. This prepares the surface for the acid-etching process. Proceed with the customary application steps according to the manufacturer's instructions.

TRENDS IN SEALANT USE

Acceptance of the use of dental sealants in the general practice of dentistry has been slow. A 1985 National Health Interview Survey revealed that whereas the public is generally aware of the importance of a number of factors in the prevention of tooth decay, only 18% had heard of and knew the purpose of dental sealants (Corbin, 1987). It is possible that such a good educational campaign has been done with fluorides and oral hygiene that patients don't understand the added value of sealants for the prevention of occlusal decay (Gift, 1986).

Sealant usage has increased since 1983, when a Consensus Development Conference of the National Institutes of Health focused on dental sealants in the prevention of decay. In 1983, a survey of hygienists practicing in Minnesota and Wisconsin indicated that sealants were being used in only 54% of the offices in which they worked (Duffy, 1987). More recent studies showed that between 70% and 81% of general dentists used sealants to some degree (Bander, 1986; Faine, 1986; Rubenstein, 1986). Bander noted the dentist profile for sealant use suggests that younger dentists who practice with hygienists tend to have increased use of sealants. Factors that could influence this include recent exposure to sealants during professional school, the fact that younger dentists tend to have younger patients who may require the service more often, and the fact that the procedure is often delegated to hygienists. Rubenstein found that nearly 100% of pediatric dentists are applying pit and fissure sealants.

The consensus panel recommended that certain populations, including low-income, immigrant, disabled, and institutionalized children, have an urgent need for preventive measures including sealants (NIH, 1983). Several community-based sealant programs have published results that support the benefits sealants provide. In Iowa, a study found that for low socioeconomic status children who display more episodic than regular preventive dental care behavior, sealants were of greater importance than the usual prophylaxis-fluoride regimen (Jones, 1986).

A school-based study in New Mexico comparing children who received sealants on their first permanent molars with classmates who did not showed that after 6 years the sealed group had developed 6% occlusal decayed, missing, or filled teeth, whereas the unsealed group had 27% of the same surfaces decayed, missing, or filled (Calderone, 1987).

A Head Start program in Tennessee found that sealants are retained in primary molars after 1 year at a rate comparable to permanent molars. The program involved 3- to 4-year-olds and suggests the potential benefits of a sealant program with high caries–susceptible children (Hardison, 1987).

After 7 years of a fluoride mouth-rinsing program in an elementary school, there was a 50% reduction in tooth decay. The majority of carious surfaces involved pits and fissures. Ripa followed this study by combining sealants and the mouth rinsing program. After 2 years, the children remained 96% caries-free (Ripa, 1985, 1987).

Success with pit and fissure sealants is well documented, but there are other issues, related to the low use of sealant techniques. Concern over cost-effectiveness and the reluctance of insurance providers to cover sealants has affected the rate at which sealants are used. Because sealants can be applied by hygienists, state practice acts and the attitudes of employers have also determined the extent to which sealants have been used. There is a natural lag between validation of a technique in the academic world and widespread application or appreciation of it in the practical world.

Looking at costs, Ripa found that, assuming the cost of a single surface restoration to be twice the cost of a sealant, the cost for treating the unsealed group in the study was 1.64 times the cost of treating the sealed group (Ripa, 1985).

Eklund studied a variety of factors to assess the cost to an insurer of amalgam restorations versus that of sealants. Cost is tied to the level of dental caries in a population. If the potential caries rate is low, the cost of a preventive procedure is less likely to represent a true savings in the long run. Caries is likely to occur on the majority of permanent molars. Sealants as a covered benefit for molars may not increase insurance premiums if fees and copayments are properly balanced. A substantial decline in caries prevalence could diminish the economic argument for sealants (Eklund, 1986).

Related to cost effectiveness is the fact that hygienists can place sealants at a reduced cost compared with the cost of a dentist's time. The prophylaxis recall appointment provides an opportunity to check sealant status, making follow-up and reapplication a logical part of the hygienist's routine. In many cases, the dentist's willingness to delegate this function and the hygienist's desire to provide this service have determined how often sealants are used in practice. Most hygienists have received instruction about sealant application either during their training or through approved continuing education courses. The long-term effects of a 1-day course show a significant increase in the number of auxiliaries applying sealant and in the frequency of application (Tilliss, 1986).

Use of the sealant procedures varies according to the state dental practice act. A state sealant program in New Mexico focused attention on the hygienist's role in the program and brought eventual revision of the practice act to allow general supervision of hygienists (Siegal, 1986).

The issues of delegation and cost will continue to be debated. Several state Medicaid programs now offer sealants as a covered benefit, and the trend to do so will undoubtedly grow. For many years patients have been willing to pay for sealants regardless of insurance coverage because they desire comprehensive preventive dental care.

The dental profession needs to be involved in educating the public about sealants: their effectiveness, safety, and the rationale for their use. Encouraging adoption of guidelines for third-party payers in all states and seeking support for federally funded programs are worthwhile activities to be undertaken to increase the public's access to sealants.

Sealant techniques and materials are part of a new era of conservative restorations and caries prevention. Continued research, the development of new products, and increased use of these methods will assure that sealants will make an important contribution in the practice of dentistry.

ACTIVITIES

1. Practice sealant technique on a typodont or on extracted teeth using various manufacturer's products.
2. Practice techniques for isolation with rubber dam application or a clamp and cotton roll.
3. Practice a four-handed technique for sealant application.
4. Identify an appropriate patient, and apply a pit and fissure sealant.
5. Put together an informative brochure or poster about sealants for the patient waiting area.

REVIEW QUESTIONS

1. Describe the acid-etching process. What is the significance of this step in the sealant technique?
2. How might the following list of factors be considered in determining whether the sealant application is appropriate for this particular patient?

Patient age : 12 years old
New resident; moved from nonfluoride area
Teeth No. 3, No. 14, No. 19 and No. 30 restored
Teeth No. 18 and No. 31 erupted recently
No current interproximal caries radiographically
Home care and plaque control: good
Parents concerned about diet and regular dental care

3. List the steps to be followed in the sealant application procedure.
4. Sealants have been adopted slowly by dentistry over the past 20 years despite documentation regarding their success as a safe preventive measure. List possible reasons for this.

REFERENCES

Ball IA: An update on fissure sealants, I, Dent Update 13(8):380, 1986.
Ball IA: An update on sealants, II, Dent Update 13(9):419, 1986.
Bander VM: Dentist use patterns for pit and fissure sealants and topical fluorides, J Dent Educ 50(11):656, 1986.
Buonocore MG: Caries prevention in pits and fissures sealed with an adhesive resin polymerized by ultra-violet light: a two-year study of a single application, JADA 82:1090, 1971.
Buonocore MG: The use of adhesives in dentistry, Springfield, Ill, 1975, Charles C Thomas, Publisher.
Calderone JJ: The New Mexico sealant program: a progress report, J Pub Health Dent 47(3):145, 1987.
Corbin SB: 1895 NHIS findings on public knowledge about oral diseases and preventive measures, Pub Health Rep 102(1):53, 1987.
Craig RG, O'Brien WJ and Powers JM: Dental materials: properties and manipulation, ed 3, St Louis, 1983, The CV Mosby Company.
Daniel SJ, and Scruggs RR: The reliability of three methods for evaluation dental sealants, J Dent Educ 51(4):182, 1987.

Dennison JB, et al: A clinical comparison of sealant and amalgam in the treatment of pit and fissures, I: clinical performance after 18 months, Pediatr Dent 2:167, 1980.

Dennison JB, et al: A clinical comparison of sealant and amalgam in the treatment of pits and fissures, II: clinical application and maintenance during an 18-month period, Pediatr Dent 2:176, 1980.

DiLeone CM: Dental sealants: information and guidelines for insurance carriers, Dent Hyg 61(1):18, 1987.

Duffy MB, et al: Dental hygienists' knowledge, opinions, and use of pit and fissure sealants: a comparison of two states, J Pub Health Dent 47(3):121, 1986.

Eklund SA, and Ismail AI: Time development of occlusal and proximal lesions: implications for fissure sealants, J Pub Health Dent 46(2):114, 1986.

Eklund SA: Factors affecting the cost of fissure sealants: a dental insurer's perspective, J Pub Health Dent 46(3):133, 1986.

Faine RC, and Dennen T: A survey of private dental practitioner's utilization of dental sealants in Washington state, J Dent Child 53(5):337, 1986.

Gift HC, and Frew RA: Sealants: changing patterns, JADA 112(3):391, 1986.

Going RE, et al: Four year clinical evaluation of a pit and fissure sealant, JADA 95:972, 1977.

Going RE: The viability of microorganisms in carious lesions five years after covering with a fissure sealant, JADA 97:455, 1978.

Gwinnett AJ: The bonding of sealants to enamel, J Am Soc Prev Dent 3:21, 1973.

Handelman SL: Effect of sealant placement on occlusal caries progression, Clin Prev Dent 4(5):11, 1983.

Handelman SL: Clinical radiographic evaluation of sealed carious and sound tooth surfaces, JADA 113(5):751, 1987.

Hardison JR, et al: Retention of pit and fissure sealant on the primary molars of 3–4 year old children after one year, JADA 114(5):613, 1987.

Henderson HZ: The sealed composite resin restoration, J Dent Child 52(4):300, 1985.

Horowitz HS, et al: Retention and effectiveness of a single application of an adhesive sealant in preventing occlusal caries: final report after 5 years study in Kalispell, Montana, JADA 95:1133, 1977.

Houpt M, et al: Occlusal composite restorations: 4-year results, JADA 110(3):351, 1985.

Houpt M, et al: Autopolymerized versus light-polymerized fissure sealant, JADA 115(1):55, 1987.

Jones RB: The effects for recall patients of a comprehensive sealant program in a clinical dental public health setting, J Pub Health Dent 46(3):152, 1986.

Mertz-Fairhurst EJ, et al: Clinical progress of sealed and unsealed caries, I: depth changes and bacterial counts, J Prosthet Dent 42:633, 1979(a).

Mertz-Fairhurst EJ, et al: Clinical progress of unsealed caries, II: standardized radiographs and clinical observation, J Prosthet Dent 42:633, 1979(b).

Mertz-Fairhurst EJ, et al: Arresting caries by sealant: results of a clinical study, JADA 112(2):194, 1986.

National Institutes of Health: Consensus development conference on dental sealants and the prevention of tooth decay, JADA 108(2):233, 1984.

Ripa LW: Occlusal sealing: rationale of the technique and historical review, J Am Soc Prev Dent 3:32, 1973.

Ripa LW: The surface-specific caries pattern of participants in a school based fluoride mouthrinsing program with implications for the use of sealants, J Pub Health Dent 45(2):90, 1985.

Ripa LW: Caries prevention in children: the use of fluoride mouthrinses and pit and fissure sealants, NY State Dent J 53(2):16, 1987.

Rock WP, et al: A comparative study between a chemically polymerized fissure sealant resin and a light-cured resin, Br Dent J 152(7):232, 1982.

Rubenstein LK, and Dinius A: Dental sealant usage in Virginia, J Pub Health Dent 46(3):147, 1986.

Scott L, and Greer D: The effect of an air polishing device on sealant bond strength, J Prosthet Dent 58(3):384, 1987.

Shapira J, and Eidelman E: Six-year clinical evaluation of fissure sealant placed after mechanical preparation: a matched pair study, Pediatr Dent 8(3):204, 1986.

Siegal MD, and Calderone JJ: Controversy over the supervision of dental hygienists: impact on a community-based sealant program, J Pub Health Dent 46(3):156, 1986.

Silverstone LM: The current status of adhesive sealants, Dent Hyg 57(5):44, 1983.

Silverstone LM: The current state of sealant research, J Mass Dent Soc 36(1):15, 1987.

Simonsen, RJ: Potential uses of pit and fissure sealant in innovative ways: a review, J Pub Health Dent 42:305, 1982.

Simonsen RJ: Retention and effectiveness of a single application of white sealant after 10 years, JADA 115(1):31, 1987.

Spohn E, and Berry T: Pit and fissure sealants. In Boundy SS and Reynolds NJ, editors: Current concepts in dental hygiene, vol 2, St Louis, 1979, The CV Mosby Co.

Straffon LH, et al: Three year evaluation of sealant: effect of isolation on efficacy, JADA 110(5):714, 1985.

Strang R et al: Further abrasion resistance and bond strength studies of fissure sealants, J Oral Rehab 13(3):257, 1986.

Strang R, et al: Laboratory studies of visible-light cured fissure sealants: setting times and depth of polymerization, J Oral Rehab 13(4):305, 1986.

Tanaka M, et al: Incorporation into human enamel of fluoride slowly released from a sealant in vivo, J Dent Res 66(10):1591, 1987.

Tilliss TS: Application of pit and fissure sealant: long-term effects of a one-day continuing education course, Dent Hyg 60(7):300, 1986.

30 CONTROL OF TOOTH HYPERSENSITIVITY

OBJECTIVES: *The reader will be able to*

1. Discuss the interrelationships of dentin, cementum, enamel, the dentoenamel junction, and Tomes' fibers as they relate to hypersensitivity.
2. Describe the three general categories of stimuli that elicit pain response and give examples of each.
3. Explain the rationale behind the hydrodynamic theory.
4. Discuss the importance of plaque in the prognosis of treating hypersensitivity.
5. Describe antihypersensitive products available for home care.
6. Select and justify in-office procedures for treating sensitivity.
7. Comment on the current American Dental Association and Food and Drug Administration positions for desensitizing products.

Dentinal hypersensitivity can be described as an adverse reaction or pain in one or more teeth resulting from a thermal, chemical, or mechanical stimulus (Clark, 1985). Microscopic examination of clinically hypersensitive surfaces has shown them to be areas of dentin exposed by gingival recession, abrasion, erosion, periodontal therapy, defective restorations, or caries. The tubules in these areas are also shown microscopically to be wider and more numerous than in nonsensitive areas (Absi, Adam, and Addy, 1986). Hypersensitive dentin is found almost exclusively on the vestibular surfaces at the cervical margins (Graf and Galasse, 1977). The teeth most likely to be affected are the incisors, canines, and premolars.

It has been reported that approximately 40 million adults in the United States have dentinal hypersensitivity at one time or another and more than 10 million have long-term or chronic hypersensitivity (Kanapka, 1982). Hypersensitive dentin is most common among patients aged 20 to 30 years, and the condition is reported to occur equally often in males and females (Graf and Galasse, 1977).

Much research has been conducted on hypersensitivity in recent years. However, the exact mechanism of transmission of pain from the den-

tin to the terminal nerve endings has only been hypothesized. This chapter will summarize the factors currently thought to be responsible for dentinal pain and will review and critique the various treatment modalities commonly used.

ETIOLOGY OF HYPERSENSITIVITY

There are many possible causes of hypersensitivity. Dental procedures can contribute to or initiate the onset or progression of hypersensitivity. Periodontal therapy techniques may create or increase exposure of root surfaces, and it is recommended that concepts of hypersensitivity be explained to the patient when such procedures as root planing and other scaling procedures in the gingival margin area are to be performed. The root surface is covered with cementum, which is softer than calculus and often is removed by hand or ultrasonic instruments exposing the dentinal surface.

Caries or crown preparations by the dentist may also elicit sensitivity. For example, sensitivity may result if temporary filling materials are in contact with the dentin for too long a time after a cavity preparation has been performed. Temporary or permanent crowns on prepared teeth may create sensitivity problems around the exposed root surfaces. This postoperative sensitivity can be avoided if the dentist places a base material beneath restorations and crown preparations (Brannstrom, 1986).

Stimuli that may elicit hypersensitivity have been classified in three primary areas (Grant, Stern, and Everett, 1979). A direct *mechanical* stimulation can occur during dental instrumentation (e.g., during exploratory procedures or scaling).

Mechanical trauma can result from brushing, especially when toothbrushes with firm-textured bristles are used. It has been reported that incorrect brushing can cause gingival recession and root surface abrasion, and this may account for the high incidence of hypersensitive dentin on vestibular surfaces, particularly in teeth at the corners of the arch, in a region that is perhaps most susceptible to toothbrush trauma (Orchardson and Collins, 1987).

Patients who chronically clench and grind their teeth often complain of tooth sensitivity. Enamel loss through occlusal wear caused by bruxing can expose dentinal tubules and cause pain (Tachibana, 1985).

In addition, some highly acidic foods (e.g., lemons) can chemically strip the enamel, exposing the underlying dentin. Hypersensitivity also has been reported in cases of bulimic individuals due to the repeated exposure of the enamel to highly acidic gastric juices (Miles, 1985).

The second type of stimulus that elicits tooth sensation is *thermal*. Responses can occur when hot and cold foods or liquids are consumed or when cold air reaches the exposed dentinal areas.

Chemical stimuli can also cause pain, especially with sweet, sour, or highly acidic foods. Plaque also is associated with chemically induced pain.

MECHANISMS OF PAIN SENSITIVITY

The exact mechanism of the transmission of the pain response from dentin to terminal nerve endings is only hypothesized, although it is well established that the pulp is richly innervated and that the sensory nerves are present near the dentin between the odontoblast cells (Krauser, 1986).

Several theories have attempted to explain the mechanisms of dentin hypersensitivity. Two of these theories, the Transducer Theory and the Direct Nerve Endings Theory, are based on the premise that there is a direct nerve connection be-

tween the nerve endings in the pulp and the dentin-enamel junction. The Transducer Theory suggests that the odontoblast receives stimuli through processes within the dentinal tubules and transfers stimuli to the nerve endings in the pulp through a "synaptic-like" junction (Krauser, 1986). The Direct Nerve Endings Theory suggests the existence of nerve endings in the dentin that stem from the pulp and can be directly stimulated (Krauser, 1986).

It has been shown by scanning electron microscopy that nerves entering the tubules in the circumpulpal region only extend to the inner one third of mineralized dentin. Physiological studies also indicate that there are nerves in the most pulpal portion of the dentin and none near the periphery (Fran, Sauvage, and Frank, 1972). These findings invalidate the premises behind the two theories.

Currently, the most widely accepted theory about the transmission of dental sensation is the Hydrodynamic Theory.

Hydrodynamic theory

In the late 1950s, Martin Brannstrom conducted a series of experiments to explain the peculiar nature of dentinal sensitivity. How could an area of tooth that has no obvious signs of decay sometimes be so sensitive to the slightest stimulus? Why would exposure to a mere blast of air elicit a pain response? Why would exposure to sugar or salty foods cause pain when many chemical agents known to stimulate nerve fibers do not produce a response when applied to exposed dentin?

Brannstrom's theory is based on the observation that fluid within the dentinal tubules can flow in either an outward or an inward direction depending on the pressure variations in the surrounding tissues. This fluid movement is the basis of the Hydrodynamic Theory: Dentinalgia, or dentin pain, results from a stimulus causing minute changes in the fluid movement within the hollow, open tubules. This may subsequently deform the odontoblast or its process and hence cause an elicitation of pain via the intimately associated "mechanico-receptor-like" nerve endings (Brannstrom and Astrom, 1964). Simply stated, this means that pain-producing stimuli cause rapid movement of fluids within the dentinal tubules. This, in turn, stimulates the nerve processes in the pulpal dentin and the pulp. Based on this assumption, the Hydrodynamic Theory explains how so many different types of stimuli can elicit the same pain response.

The clearest example of this is dehydration of dentin (i.e., by air blast). The air causes dehydration, which cause the dentinal fluid to move in an outward direction, by capillary action. This would pull the odontoblastic process farther into the tubule, stimulating sensory pulpal nerves (Brannstrom and Astrom, 1964).

Heat applied to the dentin results in an expansion of the fluid, putting pressure on the odontoblast, which again stimulates a pain response (Brannstrom and Astrom, 1964).

Pain produced when sugar or salted solutions are placed in contact with exposed dentin can also be explained by tubule fluid movements. Fluids of a low osmolarity (i.e., the dentinal tubule fluid) will have a tendency to flow towards solutions of a higher osmolarity (i.e., salty or sugar solutions) (Berman, 1984). This outward flow of fluid elicits a pain response.

NATURAL DEFENSE MECHANISMS

The pulp has several natural defenses to protect itself from irritating stimuli.

Calcification

The tooth can naturally respond to sensitivity by causing calcification in the pulp chamber and the formation of secondary dentin to occlude the open canals (Krauser, 1986).

Bacterial plaque

Plaque can form in the acquired pellicle on the exposed dentin and, along with salivary occlusion, decrease sensitivity (Krauser, 1986). Obviously, this is not an ideal situation, because of the increased susceptibility to cervical decay.

Sclerosis

Peritubular dentin mineralization can partially or completely block the patent tubule, preventing the passage of painful impulses (Berman, 1984).

The majority of treatments for dentinal hypersensitivity attempt in some way to block fluid flow in the tubules. The following section describes some of the common agents as well as the difficulty of assessing their effects.

TREATMENT OF HYPERSENSITIVITY

Although many products are available for use either by the patient or in a professional office, no one accepted modality gives maximum or consistent benefit (Chasens, 1974; Everett, Hall, and Phatak, 1966; Goldman, 1982; Grant, Stern, and Everett, 1979; Peden, 1977; Yankell, 1982; Wycoff, 1982).

Since early in dental research, many agents have been tested for treating hypersensitive teeth. The essential criteria used to select agents to be tested have not changed since they were developed by Grossmann (1935). They are as follows:

1. Easy to use and apply
2. Nonirritating
3. Minimum number of dental appointments required (applications)
4. Painless
5. Minimum application time
6. Will not discolor teeth
7. No danger to teeth or soft tissues
8. Minimum expense

These criteria apply to both professional and over-the-counter (OTC) products.

Clinical studies to determine the effectiveness of agents or products for desensitization have been difficult to conduct because of the following factors:

1. Sole use of subjective evaluations
2. Lack of proper controls
3. Lack of objective measurements
4. Placebo effect in control group is strong

Many evaluations have been based on subjective reactions. In these studies, the person's reaction to the products being tested has been based on his or her impressions of whether there was poor, fair, good, or excellent improvement. In addition, several studies have been based on the patient's evaluation under unsupervised use and without using a placebo or control product (i.e., a product containing no known effective agent).

In 1984, the Council of Dental Therapeutics requested guidelines be established for evaluating the efficacy of agents used to reduce hypersensitivity:

1. The test data should be quantifiable and reproducible
2. A critical evaluation must be made of all subjective responses; the threshold of response should be established, preferably

quantified, and correlated to a clinically definable intensity; it is also recognized that the threshold is a range and not a point

3. The relationship between the experimental stimulus and the defined area of hypersensitivity must be established by controlled clinical research

4. There should be no commitment to a specific form of stimulus; if more than one stimulus is used, then these stimuli should be reproducible and interference between them must be minimized

5. Appropriate statistics should be used, and these should be justified according to the experimental design

To measure pain accurately, the investigations must assess the subjective pain as well as the characteristics of the stimulus producing the pain. Pain associated with dentin hypersensitivity has been difficult to assess. Research has not identified a physiological index that unequivocally relates to changes in pain sensation and is not simply related to stimulus intensity.

The criteria for accurate objective pain measurement are as follows (Ad Hoc Advisory Committee on Dentinal Hypersensitivity, 1986):

1. Reliability. The procedure yields consistent results with time; reliability across subjects and between test sessions should be determined

2. Validity. The procedure measures unequivocally a specific dimension of pain

3. Bias-free. The procedure is independent of method bias or patient or investigator response bias

4. Versatility. The procedure is applicable for both laboratory and clinical uses

Even the use of simple scales for assessing pain requires that the inducing stimulus be measurable and reproducible and that the measurements be expressed in physical terms (such as amperes, millimeters, degrees, centigrade). The stimulus must be (1) measurable; (2) reproducible; and (3) behavior predictable. Without quantification of the stimulus it is difficult, if not impossible, to compare the findings of the different investigators (Ash, 1986).

Two types of instrumentation have been developed that can be applied to the tooth surface to produce specified temperatures at the probe site

(Kanapka, 1982; Smith and Ash, 1964a, 1964b; Tarbet et al, 1982). This equipment has been used to evaluate agents with desensitizing potential and has recently resulted in acceptance of two products by the American Dental Association (Chasens, 1974; Kanapka, 1982).

A major problem with testing desensitizing agents or products can be the high degree of reduction in sensitivity that occurs in groups treated with control products. This may be due to a general decline over a period of time (often observed with sensitivity problems) or to improved cleaning by patients who become aware of being seen routinely by the dental professional.

Home care procedures should be emphasized as a primary factor when initiating treatment of sensitivity. It is important to have adequate plaque control procedures well developed by the patient before professional treatments are started (Chasens, 1974; Grant, Stern, and Everett, 1979; Green, Green, and McFall, 1977; Peden, 1977) and for long-term benefits (Wycoff, 1982). In addition to proper brushing and flossing procedures, the use of other topical and interdental aids to achieve cleaning and/or burnishing should be initiated. It is also important to discuss diet with the patient and, if necessary, to eliminate foods that are acidic or sour, as well as those that are fermentable carbohydrates, which can produce acids in plaque. It is also important to evaluate the patient's toothbrush and dentifrice product. It is suggested that soft or ultrasoft toothbrushes be used with dentifrices with minimum abrasive properties. There is no uniformity among toothbrush manufacturers as to the texture of the toothbrush bristles, and one manufacturer's soft bristles may be firmer than another manufacturer's medium bristles (Yankell and Emling, 1978). Toothpaste abrasiveness is difficult to monitor clinically, and it is up to the dental professional to individualize the dentifrice used by each patient. Regardless of treatment, it has been indicated that tooth sensitivity can improve with a change in oral hygiene procedures (Gedalia et al, 1978; Hiatt and Johansen, 1972).

COMMERCIALLY AVAILABLE PRODUCTS

Desensitizing toothpastes are widely promoted to both the dental profession and the public. Three of these toothpastes, Denquil (Richardson-Vicks, Inc.), Promise (Block Drug Co. Inc.), and Sensodyne (Block Drug Co. Inc.), contain potassium nitrate as the active ingredient and have been found to be an effective agent in clinical studies. The exact mechanism of action is not known. All these products have been "accepted" or "provisionally" accepted by the ADA and the Council on Dental Therapeutics (Council on Dental Therapeutics, 1986).

Thermodent's (Chas. Pfizer and Co.) active ingredient is strontium chloride. It works by occluding dentinal tubules with abrasive filler. The efficacy studies done on this product have produced mixed results (Berman, 1984).

A fifth product, Protect (J.O.Butler), contains dibasic sodium citrate in a pluronic gel. The action of this product is thought to be derived from the polyglycoid's ability to precipitate dentinal or salivary proteins. The studies on this product also have not shown significant improvements in desensitization (Clark, 1987).

PROFESSIONAL PRODUCTS

Most products used by dental professionals have not changed significantly in content or method(s) of application since they were comprehensively reviewed by Everett, Hall, and Phatak in 1966, and as described in many textbooks and review articles since then (Chasens, 1974; Grant, Stern, and Everett, 1979; Peden, 1977). None of these products has been classified as effective by the ADA Council on Dental Therapeutics (ADA Council, 1982) or the Food and Drug Administration.

Initial preparation of the teeth must be done before any desensitizing agent is professionally applied. Teeth must be free of all hard and soft deposits as assured by scaling, root planing, and polishing with a porte polisher if the teeth are very sensitive. In addition, 3% hydrogen peroxide can be applied to the teeth with a cotton pellet for further cleansing. Teeth are rinsed with warm water, dried, and isolated prior to treatment. Care should be taken to use air lightly or to dry the sensitive areas with cotton rolls. Rather than refer to specific products, only the active claimed ingredient(s) of products are indicated here.

It is claimed that *formalin,* in a concentration of 40%, precipitates albumin or denatures Tomes' fibers. A small amount of the solution is placed on a cotton pellet and rubbed into the sensitive area. A porte polisher is used to continue rubbing for a defined period. This agent should not contact the mucosa, as a reaction (precipitation of protein) with the tissues will occur, resulting in soft tissue irritation.

A solution of basic or ammoniated *silver nitrate* is alleged to precipitate albumin and denature Tomes' fibers. This solution is applied directly to the sensitive area and then is precipitated with a reducing agent such as eugenol. This preparation may be irritating to soft dental tissue and cause tooth discoloration.

Solutions of 40% *zinc chloride* and 20% *potassium ferrocyanide* are used in a two-step process. The clinical result of this combination is protein precipitation and denaturization of Tomes' fibers. The solution of zinc chloride is applied with a moist cotton pellet or porte polisher. With unwaxed floss or tape, the zinc chloride is rubbed vigorously on the interproximal surfaces and allowed to remain on the tooth for 1 minute. Excess solution is removed from the gingival margin. While the teeth are still moist, the second solution of potassium ferrocyanide is applied. This solution is rubbed vigorously until a white precipitate forms. Again, dental floss is worked interproximally. One minute is allowed for the reaction to occur, and then the excess is removed from the gingival margin.

Professional *fluoride gels and solutions* for caries treatment are used to treat hypersensitivity. As with caries prophylaxis, the teeth should be scaled and stain removed prior to fluoride treatment. With generalized sensitivity or many areas of gingival recession, tray or painting procedures are used. If specific teeth are sensitive, fluoride can be burnished into the area with a porte polisher. Also available are fluoride products with claimed desensitization properties. The first contains equal amounts of sodium fluoride, kaolin, and glycerin. This product is rubbed into the dried isolated sensitive area with a porte polisher for 1 to 5 minutes. The mechanism of action is attributed to the deposition of insoluble salts. Two products are available that contain *sodium silicofluoride.* The first of these is a saturated solution containing 0.7% in cold water or 0.9% in hot water. This preparation is rubbed into sensitive areas for 5 minutes. A calcium gel forms, which is stated to be an improved insulating barrier. Sodium silicofluoride is also combined with calcium hydroxide in a two-step procedure. Initially, the sodium silicofluoride is applied and allowed to react for 1 to 2 minutes. Then the area is painted with 5% calcium hydroxide and allowed to stand for 1 minute. This combination treatment is claimed to aid in a more rapid and complete precipitation and a more effective desensitization.

A *stannous fluoride* paste containing 8.9% stannous ion is being promoted for use in the treatment of sensitivity. During prophylaxis this paste should be rubbed into sensitive areas, preferably with a porte polisher.

In all of the aforementioned fluoride treatments, the suggested regimen is to apply the material at weekly intervals at least three times to obtain optimum results.

A promising product called *cyanoacrylate* has been shown in clinical studies to have an immediate and long-lasting effect on hypersensitive dentin. Data indicate that it is 33% more effective than sodium fluoride (Bahram, 1987).

Corticosteroid products also are available for dentin hypersensitivity. These products are used primarily for sensitivity due to cavity preparations but are also used for dentin hypersensitivity. Usually the agent is administered by being rubbed into the sensitive site. The mode of action is considered to be that of decreasing pulp hyperemia.

Great success has been found using *fluoride varnishes* and *unfilled resins* to cover the outside of the patent tubules (Clark, 1985).

Another proposed method of treating dental hypersensitivity is *iontophoresis*. The purpose of this procedure is to enhance movement of ions by electric currents. With this system, a negative ion such as fluoride would be pushed away from the toothbrush surface and encouraged to penetrate dental enamel. Another mechanism of action attributed to iontophoresis is the formation of secondary dentin. Several clinical studies have been reported on the use of iontophoresis alone or coupled with the use of fluoride material or a strontium chloride preparation. In general, iontophoresis alone has been claimed to be effective against hypersensitivity; when this procedure has been coupled with an active agent, an enhanced benefit has been reported.

There are several professional iontophoresis units available. Two are discussed here. The first of these is the Chayes-Siemon apparatus. This contains a 9-volt battery and an ammeter that must register 20, or about 0.4 milliampere, to ensure ion transfer. The patient holds the grip, or positive charge, of the equipment. The dental professional then applies the negatively charged end of the equipment, a sable brush dipped into a 1% sodium fluoride solution, in contact with the sensitive area for 1 minute. Because of a fairly high current, the patient may experience slight pain on initial contact with this equipment.

The second apparatus is the barrel-shaped Lemonstron apparatus with a sable brush at one end. The clinician moistens the brush with a 2% sodium fluoride solution and applies this to the sensitive tooth area. The circuit is completed by the clinician touching the patient. The brush is allowed to contact the sensitive area for 1 minute. Because this unit operates with two penlite batteries and there is no ammeter, the clinician is unsure of the quantity of current being dispensed.

As the research continues on the treatments for dentinal hypersensitivity, more efficient and effective products will be introduced to both the general public and dental professionals.

ACTIVITIES

1. Determine whether members of the class have areas of gingival recession and/or tooth sensitivity. Test both areas with the following: ice, a blast of air, cold water, hot water, and a sharp probe. What is the most severe reaction in terms of speed of reaction and pain? Do areas of recession and sensitivity differ? Why? What parameters do you think would be best for testing a new antihypersensitive agent?
2. Review two publications on desensitizing products, pre- and post-1980. Comment on the occurrence of placebo effect and on the measurements used.

REVIEW QUESTIONS

1. What are the primary areas where tooth sensitivity occurs?
2. What professional procedures contribute to tooth sensitivity?
3. What are the three stimuli that elicit hypersensitivity?
4. Classify the mechanisms of action of desensitizing agents.
5. True or false:
   a. The tooth area closest to the DEJ is the most sensitive.
   b. The placebo effect often occurs in treating sensitivity.

c. Regardless of treatment, improved oral hygiene can reduce sensitivity.
6. Describe how the fluoride treatment for caries is:
    a. Different from the fluoride treatment for sensitivity.
    b. Similar to the fluoride treatment for sensitivity.
7. Explain how fluid movement in dentinal tubules can cause a pain response.

REFERENCES

Absi EG, Adam D, and Addy M: The patency of dentinal tubules in hypersensitive and non sensitive dentine, Br Soc Dent Res (abst 89), 1986.

ADA Council on Dental Therapeutics: Dental therapeutics. ed 39, Chicago, 1982, American Dental Association.

Ad Hoc Advisory Committee on Dentinal Hypersensitivity, Council on Dental Therapeutics: Recommendations for evaluating agents for the reduction of dentinal hypersensitivity, JADA 112 (May):709, 1986.

Ash MM: Quantification of stimuli, Endod Dent Traumatol 2(4):153, 1986.

Avery JK: Anatomic considerations in the mechanisms of pain and sensitivity in the teeth and supporting tissues. In Chasens AI and Kaslick RS, editors: Mechanisms of pain and sensitivity in the teeth and supporting tissues, Rutherford, NJ, 1974, Fairleigh Dickinson University.

Bahram J; Cyanoacrylate—a new treatment for hypersensitive dentin and cementum, JADA 114 (Apr):216, 1987.

Berman Louis: Dentinal sensation and hypersensitivity, J Periodontol 56(4):216, 1984.

Brannstrom M: The hydrodynamic theory of dentinal pain: sensation in the preparations, caries, and the dentinal crack syndrome, J Endodont 12(10):453, 1986.

Brannstrom M, and Astrom A: A study of the mechanism of pain elicited from the dentine. J Dent Res 43:619, 1964.

Chasens AI: The management of tooth pain and sensitivity. In Chasens AI and Kaslick RS, editors: Mechanisms of pain and sensitivity in the teeth and supporting tissues, Rutherford, NJ, 1974, Fairleigh Dickinson University.

Clark DC: The effectiveness of a fluoride varnish and a desensitizing toothpaste in treating dentinal hypersensitivity, J Periodont Res 20:212, 1985.

Clark DC: The efficacy of a new dentifrice in treating dentin sensitivity: effects of sodium citrate and sodium fluoride as active ingredients, J Periodont Res 22(2):89, 1987.

Council on Dental Therapeutics: Acceptance of Promise with fluoride and Sensodyne—toothpastes for sensitive teeth, JADA 113:673, 1986.

Everett FG, Hall WB, and Phatak NM: Treatment of hypersensitive dentin, J Oral Ther Pharmacol 2:300, 1966.

Frank RM, Sauvage C, and Frank P: Morphological basis of dental sensitivity, Int Dent J 22:1, 1972.

Gedalia I, et al: The effect of fluoride and strontium application on dentin: in vivo and in vitro studies, J Periodontol 49:269, 1978.

Goldman HM: Dental sensitivity: a periodontist's perspective, Compend Contin Educ Dent (suppl)3:S110, 1982.

Graf H,, Galasse R: Morbidity, prevalence, and intraoral distribution of the hypersensitive teeth, J Dent Res 56(special issue A):A162, abst 479, 1977.

Grant DA, Stern IB, and Everett FG: Periodontics: in the tradition of Orban and Gottlieb. ed 5, St Louis, 1979, The CV Mosby Co.

Green BL, Green ML, and McFall WT Jr: Calcium hydroxide and potassium nitrate as desensitizing agents for hypersensitive root surfaces, J Periodontol 48:667, 1977.

Grossman LI: A systematic method for the treatment of hypersensitive dentin, JADA 22:592, 1935.

Hiatt WH, and Johansen E: Root preparation, I: obturation of dentinal tubules in treatment of root hypersensitivity, J Periodontol 43:373, 1972.

Kanapka JA: A new agent, Compend Contin Educ Dent (suppl)3:S118, 1982.

Kanapka JA: Clinical evaluation of dentinal hypersensitivity: a comparison of methods, 2(4):157, 1986.

Krauser JT: Hypersensitive teeth, 1: etiology, J Prosthet Dent, 2:153, 1956.

Levin MP, Yearwood LL, and Carpenter WN: The desensitizing effect of calcium hydroxide and magnesium hydroxide on hypersensitive dentin, Oral Surg 35:741, 1973.

Miles DA: Dental management and reported cases of bulimic erosion, Canada Dent Assoc J 51(10):757, 1985.

Orchardson R, and Collins WJN: Clinical features of hypersensitive teeth, Br Dent J (Apr):253, 1987.

Peden JW: Dental hypersensitivity, J West Soc Periodontol 25:75, 1977.

Smith BA, and Ash MM Jr: Evaluation of a desensitizing dentrifice, JADA 68:639, 1964 (a).

Smith BA, and Ash MM Jr: A study of a desensitizing dentifrice and cervical hypersensitivity, J Periodontol 35:222, 1964 (b).

Stanley HR: Dentin permeability and sensitivity. In Chasens AL and Kaslick RS, editors; Mechanisms of pain and sensitivity in the teeth and supporting tissues, Rutherford, NJ, 1974, Fairleigh Dickinson University.

Susi FR: Sensory receptor morphology in the teeth and their supporting tissues, Dent Clin North Am 22(1):3, 1978.

Tachibana Y: Dentin hypersensitivity following grinding of vital teeth, (Aug; spec no):153, 1985.

Tarbet WJ, et al: Home treatment for dentinal hypersensitivity: a comparative study, JADA 105:227, 1982.

Tronstad L: The anatomic and physiologic basis for dentinal sensitivity, Compend Contin Educ Dent (suppl)3:S99, 1982.

Yankell SL: At home treatment, Compend Contin Educ Dent (suppl)3:S115, 1982.

Yankell S, and Emling RC: Understanding dental products: what you should know and what your patient should know, Contin Dent Educ 1:(7), 1978.

Wycoff SJ: Current treatment for dentinal hypersensitivity: in-office treatment, Compend Contin Educ Dent (suppl)3:S113, 1982.

31 PAIN AND PAIN CONTROL: TOPICAL AND LOCAL ANESTHESIA

OBJECTIVES: *The reader will be able to*

1. Explain the relevance of psychosomatic, topical, and local anesthesia to dental hygiene practice.
2. Define pain, pain perception, and pain reaction; discuss the influences on pain reaction.
3. Develop an approach to be used to assist patients in coping with the pain that may be associated with dental treatment.
4. Explain why a thorough knowledge of the pharmacology, chemistry, and modes of action of anesthetic agents and vasoconstrictors and the possible medical complications is necessary for any dental personnel who apply topical anesthestic or administer local anesthesia.
5. Draw and label the nerve anatomy supplying the maxilla and the mandible.
6. Identify the tissues innervated by each of the nerves associated with dental local anesthesia.
7. Identify the tissues anesthetized by topical and local anesthesia.
8. Given several dental procedures, select the appropriate injections to be administered to achieve the desired anesthesia and identify the injection site.
9. Describe preliminary procedures to be performed prior to the administration of an injection.
10. When indicated, properly apply a topical anesthetic.

Pain and dental care go hand in hand for many people as is shown by the many cartoons and comedy routines centered around dental pain. This fear of being hurt or feeling pain prevents some people from seeking routine dental care. Dental personnel have used various methods to alleviate patients' pain, such as verbal reassurance, topical anesthetics, local anesthetics, conscious sedation, acupuncture, sedative premedication, general anesthesia, and hypnosis. As hygienists' responsibilities have increased to include various expanded duties, pain control procedures such as application of topical anesthesia, administration of local anesthetics, and nitrous oxide and oxygen conscious sedation have been added to hygienists' duties. Some states' laws have been modified to permit dental hygienists to perform these procedures. Currently hygienists are allowed to perform local anesthesia in the following states: Alaska, Arizona, California, Colorado, Hawaii, Idaho, Missouri, Montana, Nevada, New Mexico, Oklahoma, Oregon, Utah, and Washington (ADHA, 1988).

PAIN

Pain is a universal condition that everyone has experienced at some time. There are two aspects to pain, namely pain perception and pain reaction. *Pain perception* is the physical aspect, the process by which the pain is received and transmitted via the nervous system. The nerve end organs, pain perceptors, sense the painful stimulus, and it is transmitted through the peripheral nervous system to the central nervous system. Pain perception is the same for most healthy persons, unless the nervous system has been damaged by injury or disease (Bennett, 1984). *Pain reaction,* the other aspect of pain, is a person's expression of or reaction to the perceived pain. Pain reaction varies from person to person, being influenced by conscious and unconscious thinking as well as emotional, cultural, and ethnic factors (Burstein et al, 1979; Christensen, 1980; Foreman, 1979; Spear, 1977). Persons having minimal reactions to pain are said to have low pain reaction and high *pain reaction thresholds;* the pain reaction threshold is inversely related to pain reaction (Bennett, 1984).

PAIN CONTROL

Within dentistry, various methods are used to alleviate the patient's pain—both perception and reaction. These methods are referred to as *pain control;* some of the methods are listed at the beginning of the chapter. As described by Bennett (1984), there are essentially five methods of pain control. The first is *removal of the cause,* which is not always possible. If the cause of gingival pain during a scaling procedure is the clinician's use of a curette at too open an angle, the cause of the pain can be removed by closing the angulation. If, however, the cause of the pain is edematous tender tissue, the use of a topical or local anesthetic may be needed, because the cause (swollen gingiva) cannot be removed. A second method of pain control is the use of *psychosomatic methods,* such as verbal instruction or suggestion, hypnosis, relaxation techniques, and distraction methods. Psychosomatic methods alleviate the patient's pain by lessening his or her pain reaction. A third method of pain control is the use of a drug to *block the pathway of the painful impulse.* Topical and local anesthestic agents are used in this method to block the impulse before it is carried to the central nervous system. Blocking the impulse interferes with pain perception, thus lessening or eliminating pain. A fourth method of pain control is to *raise the pain reaction threshold* with drugs that have analgesic properties; this method is referred to as conscious sedation. One method of conscious sedation—nitrous oxide and oxygen analgesia—is discussed in Chapter 32. Many drugs have analgesic properties. Narcotics such as codeine or meperidine hydrochloride (Demerol), as well as other types of drugs including barbiturates and psychosedatives, have analgesic properties and are used in dentistry. These drugs can be used alone or in combination to achieve conscious sedation. The fifth method of pain con-

trol is achieved through *depression of the central nervous system* with general anesthetic agents. The general anesthesia prevents the patient's reaction to pain.

An introduction to psychosomatic methods and the use of topical and local anesthetic agents are presented in this chapter. After reading this chapter, the reader should be able to use some of the psychosomatic methods and topical anesthestic agents for pain control. Although the educational background of dental hygienists provides the prerequisite knowledge (i.e., chemistry, pharmacology, medical evaluation, anatomy, and emergency detection and procedures), any dental personnel—dentist or dental hygienist—should participate in an in-depth local anesthesia course before administering local anesthetics. The course should provide information about anesthetic agents, including the effects, contraindications, complications, reactions, patient evaluation, management, and injection technique. The administration of local anesthetics is a serious responsibility; a foreign substance is being placed into a person's body, and a drug is being administered that will probably produce the desired effect but that may also produce undesired effects. The practitioner must be able to differentiate among the desired and undesired effects of local anesthetics and initiate the appropriate care. A properly educated dental hygienist is capable of assuming the added responsibilities associated with the administration of local anesthetics, but *proper formal education is essential* (American Association of Dental Schools, 1980). Results from Lobene (1979) and a recent study by Sisty-LePeau (1986) describe the success of dental hygiene students in administering local anesthesia. After a specific expanded function course, the overall adequacy of anesthesia achieved for all procedures was 95%, indicating that dental hygienists can provide local anesthesia with a high degree of accuracy.

This chapter provides only a general overview of local anesthesia and emphasizes determining when a local anesthetic is needed and which injections will provide the desired anesthesia. The technique of administering an injection is not presented. The ability to determine which injection is needed, even if the hygienist does not perform the injection, allows the hygienist to request the proper injection; prepare the necessary armamentarium; and prepare the patient, including the application of the topical anesthetic. In addition, an understanding of the uses and limitations of topical anesthesia and local anesthesia will provide the dental hygienist with a realistic understanding of the capabilities of each agent for pain control.

INFLUENCES ON PAIN REACTION

As previously mentioned, pain reaction varies from person to person and may even vary for the same person depending on his or her mental and physical condition. Factors that influence a person's interpretation of an event as being painful can be divided into three categories: cognitive, emotional, and symbolic (Wepman, 1978).

Cognitive factors are those that influence how persons think about pain or when they interpret a sensation as being painful. There is evidence that what the clinician says can modify how patients think and react to painful stimuli. For example, Steblay and Beaman (1982) showed that telling patients that some of their physiologic sensations, such as temporarily increased heart rates, were due to the local anesthetic allowed the patients to properly associate the feelings with the anesthetic. This in turn seemed to allow the patients to be less fearful and experience less pain.

Wepman (1978) has reported an experiment in which patients were told that they would experience less pain if they listened to music through earphones during treatment (Melzack, 1973). The patients seemed to develop ways to cope with the pain, or to distract themselves from it, by tapping a foot, fingers, or humming. The patients reported less pain.

The above example helps illustrate the concept that people are less susceptible to pain, fear, or anxiety when they feel they have some control over the situation. Developing a way to cope with pain, as above, indicates having some control. When patients feel helpless or not in control, they are likely to experience greater pain. Thus it is important to allow the patient to have some control in managing the pain whenever possible (Wepman, 1978).

Emotional factors such as anxiety greatly influence patients' tolerance for pain. In general, increased anxiety is associated with decreased tolerance for pain, a high pain reaction, and a low pain reaction threshold (Bennett, 1984). For ex-

ample, a patient, nervous about a scaling procedure, who jumps when the clinician establishes a fulcrum has a high pain reaction and a low pain reaction threshold. Increased anxiety is many times exacerbated by patients' feelings of helplessness. Certainly, dental treatment is a situation in which patients have a limited amount of control. To help relieve anxiety, the clinician should strive to create an atmosphere in which the patient will feel accepted and able to express his or her concerns, thus giving the patient the feeling of shared control over dental experiences.

Events in patients' lives such as marriage, the birth of a child, change in a job, loss of a job, divorce, or the death of a loved one may also affect their ability to cope with pain. Because such events create stress and its associated anxiety, it is likely that patients may have a decreased pain reaction threshold. Careful listening, as described in Chapter 7, will help the clinician discern if life events are affecting a particular patient and perhaps his or her pain reaction.

The *symbolic factors* affecting pain are unique to each person, but universally pain symbolizes an attack, damage, or a threat. All persons have unconscious symbols and feelings of which they are unaware and which they usually are unable to explain. These unconscious feelings and symbols regarding pain affect patients' pain reactions (Wepman, 1978). The dental health professional can recognize that all persons react to pain and are affected by their unconscious feelings. It is not the role of the dental health professional to analyze why a patient reacts to pain in a certain manner. Rather, the role of the professional is to listen and observe so as to discern when patients are in pain and to take steps to alleviate the pain associated with dental treatment.

A variety of other factors such as fatigue, sex, race, and ethnicity may affect persons' pain reactions. When people are tired or fatigued, their pain reaction thresholds are decreased (Bennett, 1984). Various authors have indicated that pain reaction may be influenced by sex and race or ethnicity (Bennett, 1984; Christensen, 1980; Spear, 1977; Wepman, 1978). For example, men have a higher pain reaction threshold than women; Latin Americans and Southern Europeans have a lower pain reaction threshold than North Americans or Northern Europeans. As different groups have different cultures that regard expression of emotions and pain in a variety of ways, it is not surprising that pain reactions may vary. Yet these are generalizations that may be true for the majority of persons from a particular ethnic group; certainly there are many exceptions. Thus these generalizations may be helpful to the clinician, but every patient must be treated as an individual with particular reactions to pain (Wepman, 1978).

PSYCHOSOMATIC METHODS OF PAIN CONTROL

In order to provide dental treatment as painlessly as possible, the health care provider must incorporate knowledge about pain reaction and psychosomatic methods into a general approach to pain control.

Perhaps the most important element of an approach is to develop helping relationships with patients (see Chapter 7) in which they can trust the health care provider. This is more than establishing rapport, such as asking the obligatory "How are you?" (Wepman, 1978). Rather, it is offering a relationship in which the provider genuinely cares about patients' well-being, especially their dental health. The health care provider must be truthful and honest with patients about procedures that are painful. It is highly inappropriate for the health care provider to tell patients that procedures will not hurt or will only hurt a second if the health care provider knows otherwise. The health care provider should take seriously patients' reports of pain and use methods to alleviate the pain. Patients' complaints of pain may sometimes be verbal, but many times they are nonverbal communications such as knitted eyebrows, rolling eyes, or white knuckles clinging to the chair arms. The astute clinician will be attuned to such communications and question the patient to determine the source of the pain.

In addition to developing a helping relationship and being honest with the patient regarding pain associated with treatment, the health care provider must develop skills to alleviate pain. Some psychosomatic approaches include telling the patient about sensations associated with medication or treatment. Use of a soothing, not singsong, voice can help to relax or soothe the patient. The patient can be instructed to take a few deep breaths to help relax and ease tension. If the clinician is familiar with relaxation techniques such as tensing and relaxing muscle groups, these may be helpful for some patients (Atterbury, 1978; Foreman, 1979). Use of these techniques in a trusting, helping relationship may help the patient feel at ease with the clinician and more in control, thus increasing the patient's pain reaction threshold. Other methods that require further training, such as hypnosis, biofeedback, or progressive relaxation, also can be used.

The use of psychosomatic methods has been presented because these pain control methods are many times overlooked, as is the importance of the quality of the relationship between patients and the health care provider. These methods can potentiate other pain control measures such as topical or local anesthesia, nitrous oxide and oxygen conscious sedation, and general anesthesia. Psychosomatic methods alone are rarely successful in controlling the pain associated with dental treatment. The health care provider should use other pain control measures as necessary to alleviate the patient's pain.

LOCAL ANESTHESIA

An overview of local anesthetic agents, their use, and sites of injection is here presented before a description of topical anesthetics. An understanding of local anesthetics will enable the reader to better understand topical anesthetic agents and their use.

Local anesthetic agents

Local anesthetics are chemical agents that produce transient and completely reversible loss of sensation in a specific area. Other properties that are desirable for local anesthetic agents include the following (Bennett, 1978; Malamed, 1986):

1. The agent is sterile
2. It is stable in solution, but will readily undergo biotransformation in the body
3. It is nonirritating to the tissues
4. It will not cause permanent damage to nerve structure
5. It has a low systemic toxicity
6. It has a low potential for producing allergic reactions
7. It has adequate potency without use of harmful concentrations

8. Onset of anesthesia takes place within a short time
9. Duration of anesthesia is long enough to permit completion of the dental procedure, yet not so long as to require an extended recovery

The local anesthetic agents are water-soluble hydrochloride salt solutions. The chemical structure is made up of three portions, the lipophilic portion, the intermediate chain portion, and the hydrophilic portion (Fig. 31-1). The agent is classified by the intermediate chain linkage, which is either an ester or an amide. The hydrophilic portion is responsible for the water solubility of the agent. This ensures solubility within the dental cartridge and carries the solution through the interstitial fluid in the tissue to the nerve. The lipophilic group, composed of the aromatic ring structure, enables the agent to penetrate the lipid-rich nerve sheath and membrane where impulse conduction can be blocked (Hersh, 1987).

To understand how anesthetic agents work, a brief explanation of how a stimulus travels along the nerve to the brain is necessary. Impulse conduction relies on a permeable nerve membrane. An inactive nerve has a stable balance (polarization) between positive sodium ions on the outside of the nerve membrane and negative potassium ions on the inside of the membrane. This state of polarization is called the nerve's resting potential. When a stimulus such as pain, called an action potential, produces activity of the nerve fiber, the ion balance changes. This phase is called depolarization. The positive sodium ions (Na^+) move across the nerve membrane to the inside, and the negative potassium ions (K^-) move from the inside to the outside of the nerve membrane. To create equilibrium again, repolarization occurs, with the Na^+ ions moving back to the outside of the nerve membrane. This entire exchange process takes place in 1 millisecond. In this way, an impulse wave is transmitted along the nerve fiber.

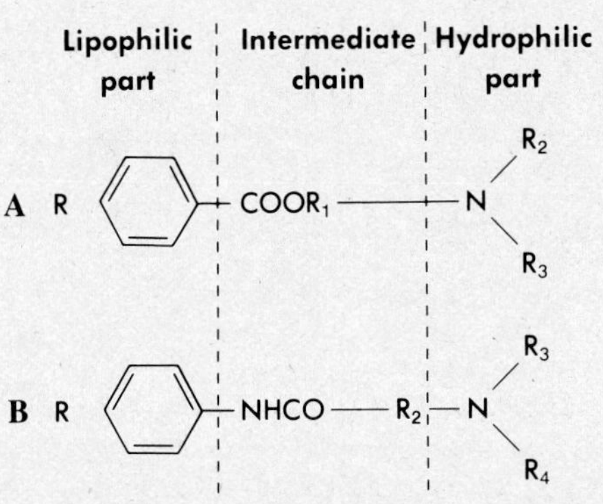

When a local anesthetic is injected in the area of a nerve fiber, the membrane becomes stabilized. Transfer of ions across the membrane is prevented and the resultant blockage of conduction prevents the patient from feeling any sensation.

The ester type of local anesthetic was the first type of anesthetic agent used successfully in dentistry. The best known ester is procaine (Novocain). Other types of esters are tetracaine (Pontocaine) and propoxycaine (Ravocaine) (ADA-CDT, 1982; Bennett, 1984). Additional types of anesthetic agents (nonesters) were developed because the esters produce allergic reactions in some patients. The esters are broken down primarily in the plasma and in the liver. Para-aminobenzoic acid is one of the metabolites formed from hydrolysis of the ester-type compounds. This substance is capable of inducing allergic-type reactions in a small percentage of the population (Blackmore, 1987).

The amides were developed after the esters had been used for a period of time. The most commonly used amides include lidocaine (Xylocaine), mepivacaine (Carbocaine), and prilocaine (Citanest). The amides are broken down in the liver, and there have not been any documented cases of allergic reactions to any of the *pure* amides (Bennett, 1984; Giovannitti and Bennett, 1979; Larson, 1977). Some allergic reactions have been reported as a result of amides that contain the preservative methylparaben (Bennett, 1984; Larson, 1977). Methylparaben is chemically similar to an ester, and it is thought that some patients have allergic reactions to this agent rather than to the amide anesthetic. Some amides are available without methylparaben.

Vasoconstrictors are added to some local anesthetics to increase their effectiveness and duration and to permit administration of smaller amounts.

Fig. 31-1. Typical chemical structure for a local anesthetic agent. **A,** Ester type. **B,** Amide type.
(From Malamed SF: Handbook of local anesthesia, ed 2. St. Louis, 1986, The CV Mosby Co.)

The vasoconstrictor constricts the blood vessels in the area, so that the anesthetic is carried away from the nerve at a slower rate. Commonly used vasoconstrictors include epinephrine, norepinephrine, levonordefrin, and others (ADA-CDT, 1982; Bennett, 1984).

Potency, toxicity, concentration, and maximum safe dose. The *potency* of a local anesthetic agent is the amount necessary to produce the desired effect. *Toxicity* refers to the amount of local anesthetic or vasoconstrictor necessary to produce a toxic overdose. Usually, the greater the potency of an agent, the greater the chance of a toxic overdose (Bennett, 1984). A toxic overdose occurs when the level of drug present in the blood or plasma is too high (Malamed, 1986). The signs, symptoms, and treatment of a local anesthetic or vasoconstrictor toxic overdose are discussed in Chapter 8. The blood plasma level of a local anesthetic or vasoconstrictive agent can become too high if (1) too much is given, (2) it is injected intravascularly, (3) it is rapidly absorbed, (4) it is metabolized slowly, or (5) it is unable to be excreted. Thus a toxic overdose can occur if the clinician's technique is faulty (1 and 2) or if the patient is medically compromised (3, 4, and 5). It is essential that the clinician review the patient's medical history and use proper injection technique. To prevent an intravascular injection, the technique includes aspirating, or putting negative pressure on the anesthetic cartridge, to test if the needle is in a blood vessel. If it is, blood will be drawn back into the cartridge. The needle should be withdrawn, and a fresh cartridge placed in the syringe. The needle is then reinserted and aspiration is completed again before depositing the solution.

Local anesthetic and vasoconstrictive agents are available in various *concentrations* (Table 31-1) according to their potency. A weakly potent agent would be produced in a higher concentration in order to achieve the desired anesthetic or vasoconstrictive effect.

Each local anesthetic and vasoconstrictive agent has a *maximum safe dose (MSD);* that is, the estimated greatest amount that can safely be given to a healthy 150-pound person (Bennett, 1984; Dafoe, 1982; Malamed, 1979; Rogo, 1982). Table 31-1 lists the MSDs for some local anesthetic and vasoconstrictive agents.

It should be noted that the MSDs are expressed in milligrams and that the anesthetic and vasoconstrictive agents are expressed in milligrams per milliliters. Whenever local anesthetic or vasoconstrictive agents are administered, the clinician should calculate the amount of each agent given to ensure that the MSD is not exceeded and record the amount in the patient's record. A standard cartridge contains 1.8 ml. A 1.0% solution contains 10 mg/ml, so a cartridge of 1% solution is equivalent to 18 mg of anesthetic agent. One cartridge of 2.0% solution is equivalent to 36 mg of anesthetic agent. Thus if a patient were given two cartridges of a 2.0% local anesthetic agent, the patient would have received 72 mg of the agent (Bennett, 1984; Dafoe, 1982).

The amount of vasoconstrictor administered should also be calculated and the MSDs observed. Epinephrine, the most commonly used vasoconstrictor, has an MSD of 0.2 mg for a healthy person and .04 mg for a person with a cardiac condition (Malamed, 1986). Again, the concentration of the agent must be considered in order to calculate the amount of drug administered. If one cartridge of solution containing epinephrine 1:100,000 is given, the patient will receive 0.018 mg of epinephrine. Table 31-2 presents the formulas and information necessary to calculate the amounts of local anesthetic and vasoconstrictive agents administered.

When local anesthetic and vasoconstrictive agents are used in conjunction, one of the two agents will determine the MSD. For example, the MSD for epinephrine may be reached before the MSD for the local anesthetic, and no more can be given.

The health care provider must adjust the MSD for patients with compromised medical histories. Patients with heart conditions, such as cardiac arrhythmias or hypertension, should have reduced amounts, or no vasoconstrictors. The MSD should also be adjusted downward for persons weighing less than 150 pounds (Bennett, 1984; Malamed, 1986). By weight, the MSD for Citanest (prilocaine) is 2.7 mg per pound up to a maximum of 400 mg. Therefore, a healthy person weighing 120 pounds can be given 324 mg, or 4 1/2 cartridges of prilocaine. A 60-pound child could receive 162 mg of prilocaine or 2 1/4 cartridges of the anesthetic agent. Calculating the

Table 31-1. Duration and maximal safe doses

Local anesthetic solution	Duration (min)		Anesthetic dose per cartridge (mg)	Vasoconstrictor dose per cartridge (mg)	Maximal safe dose of anesthetic		Maximal safe dose of vasoconstrictor (mg)	
	Pulpal	Soft tissue			mg/lb of body weight	Maximum (mg)	Healthy individual	Medically compromised individual
2% procaine	0-5	60-90	36		2.7/lb	400		
2% lidocaine	5-10	60-120	36		2.0/lb	300		
4% prilocaine	10-60	90-240	72		2.7/lb	400		
3% mepivacaine	20-40	120-180	54		2.0/lb	300		
0.4% propoxycaine, 2% procaine, and 1:20,000 levonordefrin	30-60	120-180	43.2	0.09	3.0/lb	400	0.5	0.50
2% mepivacaine and 1:200,000 epinephrine	45-60	120-240	36	0.0090	2.0/lb	300	0.2	0.04
2% lidocaine and 1:100,000 epinephrine	60-90	180-240	36	0.018	2.0/lb	300	0.2	0.04
2% lidocaine and 1:50,000 epinephrine	60-90	180-240	36	0.036	2.0/lb	300	0.2	0.04
2% mepivacaine and 1:20,000 levonordefrin	60-90	180-240	36	0.09	2.0/lb	300	0.5	0.50
4% prilocaine and 1:200,000 epinephrine	60-90	120-240	72	0.0090	2.7/lb	400	0.2	0.04
1.5% etidocaine and 1:200,000 epinephrine	90-180	240-540	27	0.0090	3.6/lb	400	0.2	0.04
0.5% bupivacaine and 1:200,000 epinephrine	90-180	240-540	9	0.0090	.9/lb	200	0.2	0.04

(Adapted from Malamed SF: Handbook of Local Anesthesia, ed 2, St Louis, 1986, The CV Mosby Co.; Hersh EV: Compend Contin Educ 8(**5**):374, 1987.)

Table 31-2. Computation of amounts of agents administered

Local anesthetic agents

FORMULA:

1.8 ml per cartridge × Number of cartridges × Concentration of solution = mg administered

1% = 10 ml
2% = 20 ml
3% = 30 ml
4% = 40 ml

EXAMPLE: 2 cartridges of lidocaine 2%
1.8 × 2 × 20 = 72 mg

Vasoconstrictive agents

FORMULA:

1.8 ml per cartridge × Number of cartridges × Concentration of agent = mg administered

Epinephrine
1:50,000 = 0.02 mg
1:100,000 = 0.01 mg
1:200,000 = 0.005 mg
Norepinephrine
1:30,000 = 0.03 mg
Nordefrin
1:10,000 = 0.1 mg
Levonordefrin
1:20,000 = 0.05 mg

EXAMPLE: 2 cartridges containing epinephrine 1:100,000
1.8 × 2 × 0.01 = 0.036 mg

MSD according to the patient's weight appears to be becoming the preferred method, particularly for children (Bennett, 1984; Malamed, 1986; Rood, 1981).

The MSDs given in Table 31-1 are helpful guidelines when working with healthy patients. The practitioner must keep in mind that the amounts are to be adjusted for medically compromised individuals and those with body weights of less than 150 pounds. The package insert accompanying the local anesthetic agent will assist the practitioner in determining the appropriate dosage in light of the calculated MSD.

Medical considerations

A complete and thorough review of the patient's medical history and vital signs is essential prior to the administration of a local anesthetic. Some patient's conditions may contraindicate a local anesthetic agent and/or vasoconstrictor. For example, patients with liver dysfunction should not be given an amide, because the liver's ability to break down the amide is compromised.

The use of effective local anesthetic formulations without vasoconstrictors (3% mepivacaine, 4% prilocaine) is advised in patients with severe and poorly controlled ischemic heart disease, with labile cardiac rhythms and potentially life-threatening arrhythmias, or with symptoms of uncontrolled hyperthyroidism (Jastak, 1983). These examples of medical complications emphasize the importance of reviewing patients' medical histories before the administration of local anesthetics and vasoconstrictors. If the clinician is unsure of the effect of these agents on a particular medical condition, the dentist or the patient's physician should be consulted. It is also important to be aware of other medications the patient may be taking. For example, if a patient were taking a sulfonamide, procaine would be contraindicated because it interferes with the action of the sulfonamide (Bennett, 1984).

The aging of the general population indicates that more elderly people will be requiring routine dental care. Bomberg (1986) pointed out that about 85% of the population over age 65 have one or more chronic disease conditions and that these patients often take between 3 and 12 medications simultaneously. It is important to establish the current physical state and medication regimen. Age-related changes in the liver, decreased liver mass and blood flow, and decreased renal function suggest that local anesthetic dosage must be revised downward for the medically compromised or frail elderly patient.

Allergic reactions to local anesthetics are mentioned in Chapter 8. Once the agent has been administered, the patient should be observed for at least 3 to 5 minutes, as most reactions occur within that time. If any untoward reaction occurs, the dentist should be informed, proper treatment provided, and the incident recorded in the patient's chart.

Armamentarium

The armamentarium necessary for an injection is illustrated in Fig. 31-2. The syringe is an aspirating syringe; the clinician can pull back the plunger by pulling back the ring. The tray also includes a topical anesthetic; an antiseptic; cotton-tipped applicators; gauze to retract, dry, and hold

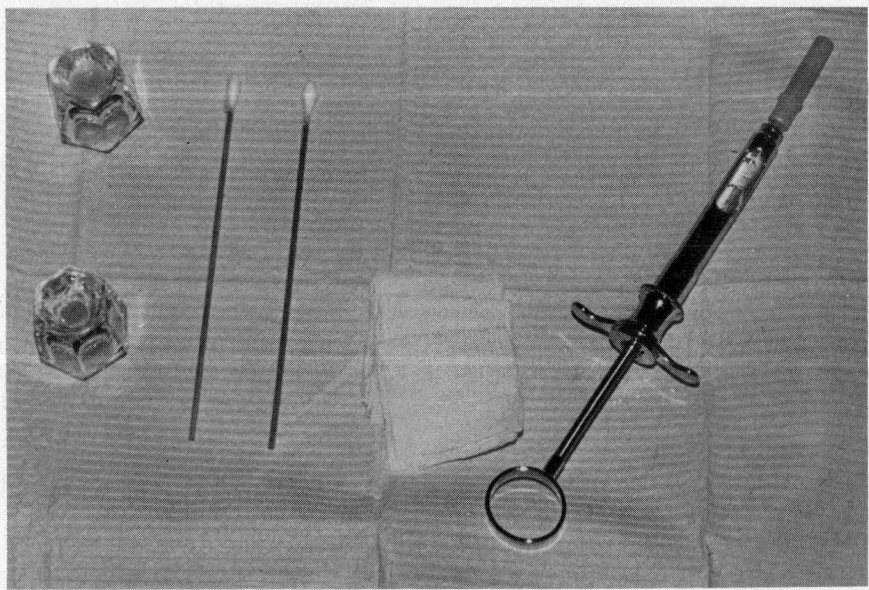

Fig. 31-2. Tray setup for administration of local anesthesia: topical anesthetic, antiseptic, cotton-tipped applicators, gauze, and assembled syringe.

movable tissues; and the assembled syringe. Fig. 31-3 shows the proper assembly of the syringe, cartridge, and needle. Needles are available in short or long lengths and a variety of gauges. The short needle is used for infiltration anesthesia, and the long needle is used for block anesthesia, including the posterior superior alveolar, mental, and inferior alveolar blocks.

The gauge of the needle refers to the diameter of the lumen; the most common gauges used in dentistry are 25, 27, and 30. Of the group, the 25-gauge needle has the largest lumen and is recommended for most dental injections that pose a risk of positive aspiration, such as the inferior alveolar, posterior superior alveolar, mental and incisive nerve blocks. Aspiration is easier through a larger needle lumen. The 27-gauge needles are useful for supraperiosteal and local infiltrations, and the 30-gauge needle for infiltration hemostasis (Malamed, 1986). The small lumen size of the 30-gauge needle does not permit adequate aspiration, so its use is limited to papillary injections.

Another form of armamentarium for anesthesia is the jet injector. This instrument is capable of delivering 0.05 to 0.2 ml of anesthetic solution at a pressure of 2000 pounds per square inch.

This technique is used primarily to produce topical anesthesia (Bennett, 1978; Malamed, 1986). The actual force of the injection may be disturbing to the patient. Although no needles are required, this type of injection does not produce adequate pulpal anesthesia, which limits its usefulness.

ADMINISTRATION

A knowledge and understanding of the anatomy of the nervous, vascular, osseous, and muscular structures of the head and oral area is necessary to determine which injections should be given and the technique for administration. Fig. 31-4 illustrates the innervation of the teeth and associated structures that are of interest to local anesthesia. The nerves supplying the oral structures pictured in Fig. 31-4 are branches of the fifth cranial nerve, the trigeminal nerve. Specific injections and injection techniques have been developed to anesthetize the nerve trunks and nerve branches. A nerve can be anesthetized along the nerve trunk before it branches; this is called *block anesthesia*. A branch of a nerve trunk can be anesthetized by depositing solution in the area of the nerve branch so that the solution filters through the underlying

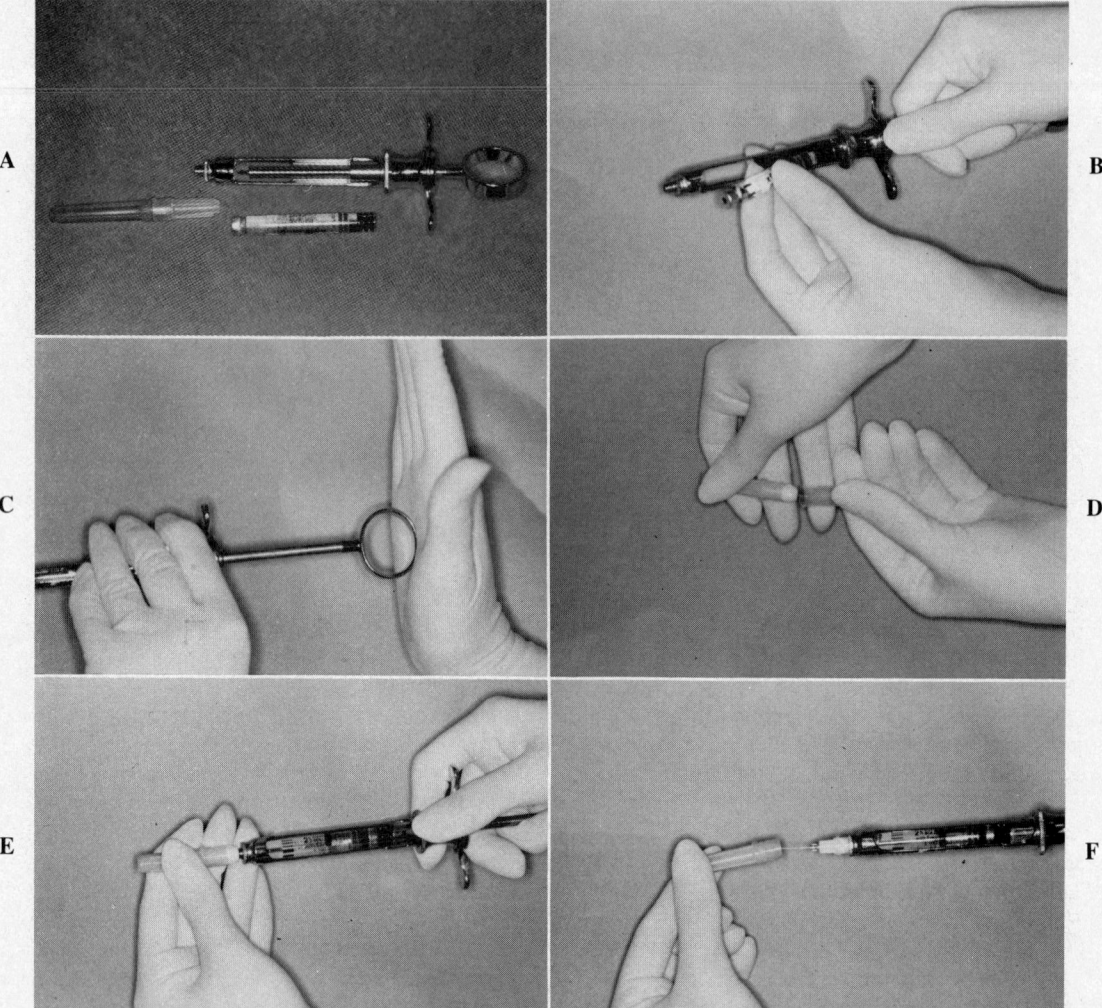

Fig. 31-3. Syringe, cartridge, and needle. Aspirator assembly is drawn back, and cartridge is inserted. Aspirating tip is engaged into plunger with several firm taps against ring. End of needle to be inserted into cartridge is uncovered. Needle penetrates diaphragm of cartridge and is screwed into syringe. Needle is exposed.

bone to reach the nerve; this is called *infiltration* or *field anesthesia* (Haglund and Evers, 1972; Sicher and DeBrul, 1975). Infiltration anesthesia depends on the solution filtering through the tissues and bone to reach the nerve; its effectiveness is dependent, in large part, on the thickness of the bone.

Table 31-3 lists the various injections along with the nerves and tissues anesthetized by each injection. Figs. 31-5 to 31-15 illustrate the injec-tion sites. This can help the clinician determine which injections could be given to achieve anesthesia in a given area. It is important to determine if soft or hard tissue anesthesia is necessary, as not all of the injections provide both. For example, the long buccal injection anesthetizes only the soft tissues over the mandibular molars; if the molars must be anesthetized, an inferior alveolar block must also be given. In some instances more than one combination of injections may be admin-

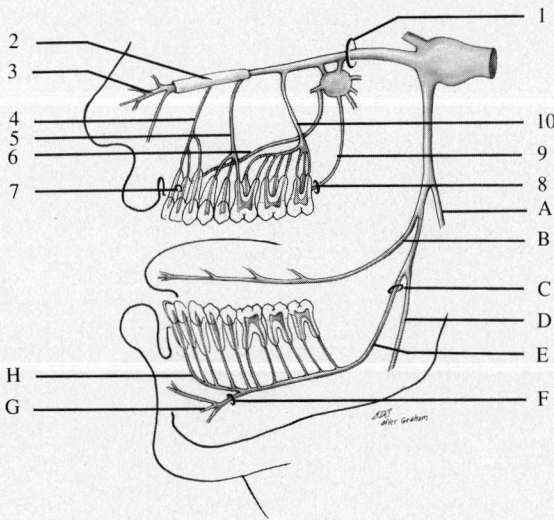

Fig. 31-4. Trigeminal nerve. Maxillary division: (1) foramen rotundum; (2) infraorbital canal; (3) infraorbital nerve; (4) anterior superior alveolar nerve; (5) middle superior alveolar nerve; (6) nasopalatine nerve; (7) incisive foramen (located on palate); (8) greater palatine foramen; (9) greater palatine nerve; (10) posterior superior alveolar nerve. Mandibular division: (A) auriculotemporal nerve; (B) lingual nerve; (C) mandibular foramen; (D) mylohyoid nerve; (E) inferior alveolar nerve; (F) mental foramen; (G) mental nerve; (H) incisive nerve. (After Graham KB: Local anesthesia and pain control: a modular approach, Kansas City, Mo, 1979, Biomedical Communication Services, University of Missouri—Kansas City School of Dentistry.)

istered to achieve the desired anesthesia. In those instances the clinician decides which injections to give based on such factors as which combination requires the fewest penetrations, which requires the least amount of solution, the desired duration, the patient's medical condition, and other relevant factors.

A local anesthetic may be required when the patient is experiencing pain in the gingiva and/or in the teeth. If verbal reassurance does not alleviate the pain, the clinician can consider nitrous oxide and oxygen conscious sedation and/or local anesthesia. Local anesthesia will provide complete anesthesia for a localized area from a single tooth to a quadrant or half of the mouth. It is rare that a patient is subjected to local anesthesia in all four quadrants at the same time; the maximum safe dose would be approached, and the patient may not appreciate a completely numb mouth. Most clinicians anesthetize a sextant or a quadrant to perform dental hygiene or periodontal procedures.

The clinician is concerned with the osseous, vascular, and muscular anatomy during the ad-

ministration of an injection (Bennett, 1984; Haglund and Evers, 1972; Reed and Sheppard, 1976). The osseous structures are the most reliable landmarks, as they are constant in shape and location. The musculature is important because penetration and trauma to the muscles must be kept to a minimum to avoid muscle trismus or soreness after the injection. A knowledge of the probable location of the blood vessels is important, since depositing solution intravascularly or rupturing a vessel can cause internal bleeding and the formation of a hematoma. The clinician must *always aspirate*—pull back the plunger—to create a negative pressure in the cartridge, which will draw blood into the cartridge if the tip of the needle is in a vessel. Blood vessels are associated with each of the nerves. Aspiration will help the clinician avoid injecting into the major blood vessels and decrease the chances of a hematoma or toxic overdose.

Steps for administration

1. Once the clinician has identified the injection to be given, he or she should palpate the an-

Table 31-3. Branches of the trigeminal nerve related to dental local anesthesia

Nerve	Tissues innervated/anesthetized	Injection
Maxillary division		
Greater palatine	Hard tissue: none Soft tissue: palatal tissue from teeth to midline from distal of third molar to cuspid	Greater palatine
Nasopalatine	Hard tissue: none Soft tissue: palatal tissues from left cuspid to right cuspid	Nasopalatine
Posterior superior alveolar (PSA)	Hard tissue: second and third molars; first molar excluding mesiobuccal root; associated supporting structures Soft tissue: overlying buccal tissues	Posterior superior alveolar (PSA)
Middle superior alveolar (MSA) branch of infraorbital	Hard tissue: first and second premolars, mesiobuccal root of first molar, and associated supporting structures Soft tissue: overlying buccal tissues and cheek or lip	Middle superior alveolar (MSA)
Anterior superior alveolar (ASA) branch of infraorbital	Hard tissue: cuspid and incisors and associated supporting structures Soft tissue: overlying facial tissues and lip	Anterior superior alveolar (ASA)
Infraorbital (includes both MSA and ASA)	Hard tissue: premolars, cuspid, incisors, and associated supporting structures Soft tissue: overlying facial tissue, cheek, and lip	Infraorbital
Individual terminal branches of MSA or ASA	Hard tissue: individual premolars, cuspid, incisors, and associated supporting structures Soft tissue: facial tissue and lip overlying individual teeth	Maxillary infiltration
Free nerve endings	Hard tissue: none Soft tissue: individual papillae	Interpapillary
Mandibular division		
Buccal (long buccal)	Hard tissue: none Soft tissue: buccal tissue of molars	Long buccal
Lingual	Hard tissue: none Soft tissue: lingual tissue from molar to midline, including anterior two-thirds of tongue	Lingual
Inferior alveolar (includes dental, mental, and incisive branches)	Hard tissue: molars, premolars, cuspid, and incisors to midline, as well as associated supporting structures Soft tissue: facial tissue anterior to mental foramen, including lip	Inferior alveolar or mandibular block
Mental branch of inferior alveolar	Hard tissue: none Soft tissue: facial tissue and lip anterior to mental foramen	Mental
Incisive and mental branches of inferior alveolar	Hard tissue: premolars, cuspid, incisors, and associated supporting structures Soft tissue: facial tissue and lip anterior to mental foramen	Incisive and mental
Individual terminal branches of mental and incisive	Hard tissue: individual cuspids, incisors, and sometimes premolars Soft tissue: facial tissue and lip overlying individual teeth	Mandibular facial infiltration
Anterior portion of lingual nerve	Hard tissue: none Soft tissue: lingual tissue in area of injection	Mandibular lingual infiltration
Third division nerve block (includes inferior alveolar, mental, incisive, lingual, mylohyoid, auriculotemporal, buccal nerves)	Hard tissue: mandibular teeth to midline; body of mandible; inferior portion of ramus Soft tissue: buccal and lingual tissue; anterior two-thirds of tongue and floor of mouth; skin over the zygoma; posterior portion of the cheek and temporal regions	Gow-Gates technique
Free nerve endings	Hard tissue: none Soft tissue: individual papillae	Interpapillary

(Data from Bennett, 1984; Reed and Sheppard, 1976; Sicher and DeBrul, 1975; and Malamed, 1986.)

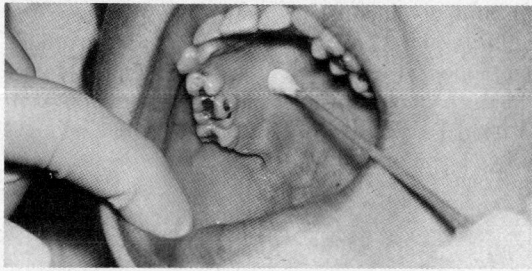

Fig. 31-5. Placement for greater palatine injection is at height of hard palate between first and second molars.

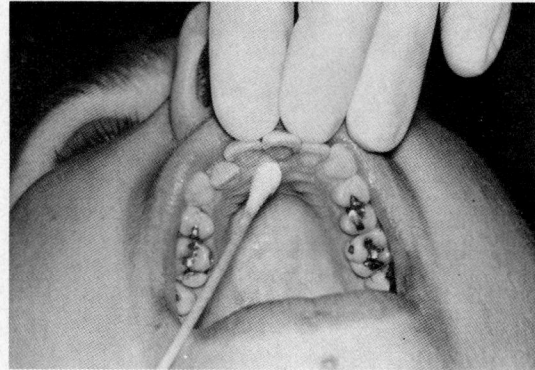

Fig. 31-6. Placement for nasopalatine injection is incisive papilla.

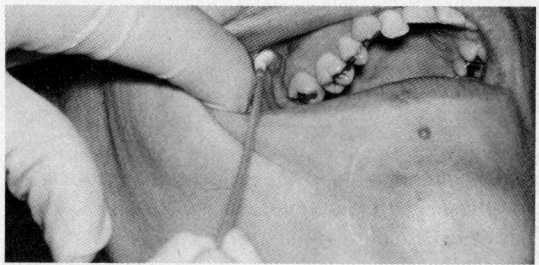

Fig. 31-7. Placement for posterior superior alveolar injection is at height of mucobuccal fold, distal to second molar.

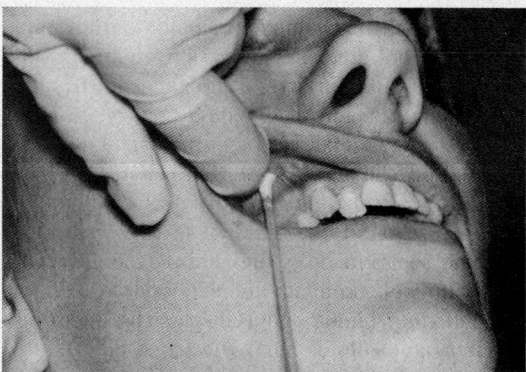

Fig. 31-8. Placement for middle superior alveolar injection is at height of mucobuccal fold between premolars.

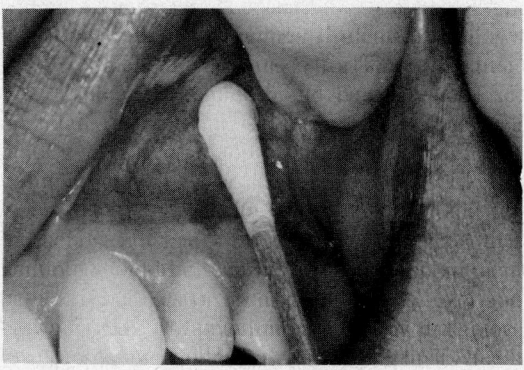

Fig. 31-9. Placement for maxillary infiltration is at height of mucobuccal fold over the desired tooth.

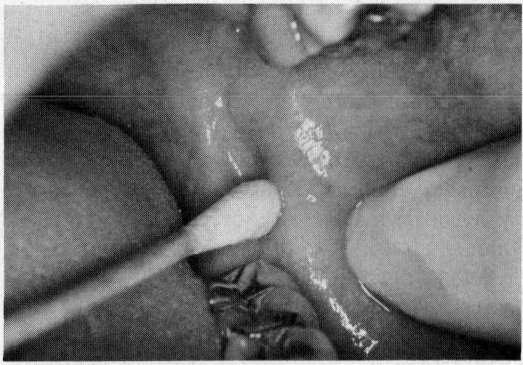

Fig. 31-10. Placement for inferior alveolar and lingual injection is distal to retromolar pad. Approach from across the arch.

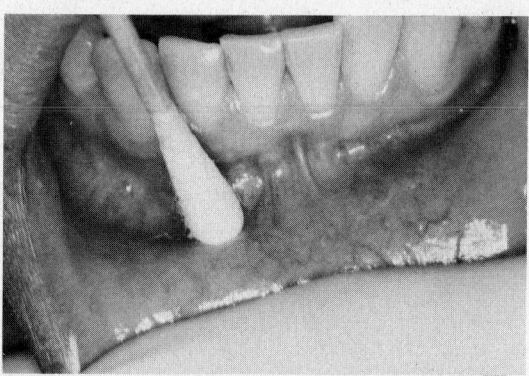

Fig. 31-13. Placement for mandibular facial infiltration is at depth of mucobuccal fold at desired tooth.

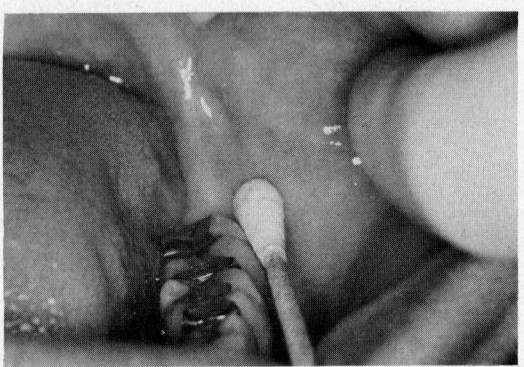

Fig. 31-11. Placement for long buccal injection is buccal to ramus and at height of molar.

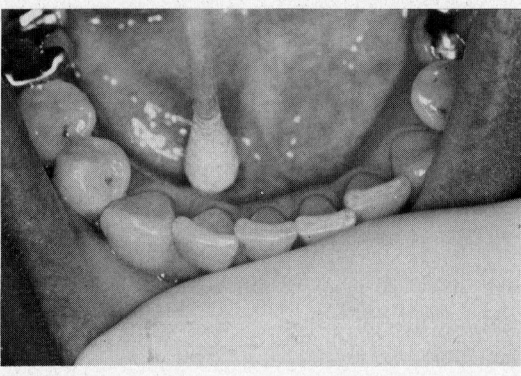

Fig. 31-14. Placement for mandibular lingual infiltration is at depth of mouth adjacent to tooth.

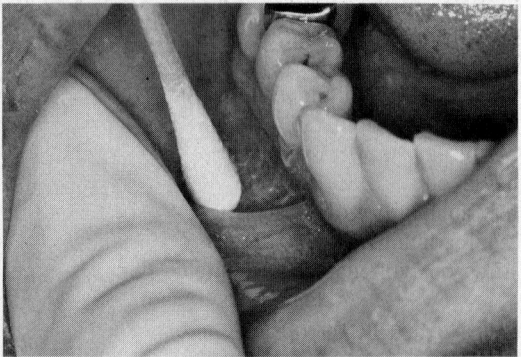

Fig. 31-12. Placement for mental infiltration is in mucobuccal fold, between premolars, approximating mental foramen.

atomical landmarks to locate the penetration site.

2. The penetration site is dried with a gauze square.
3. The topical anesthetic is applied to the area for the appropriate amount of time.
4. The topical anesthetic is rinsed and suctioned away, and the movable tissue is retracted so the clinician can see the penetration site. The area may be wiped with a gauze square to remove extraneous topical anesthetic.
5. The antiseptic solution is applied to the site just before the needle penetrates the tissue. Aseptic technique must be observed to protect the patient from a bacteremia or infec-

tion. The needle should touch nothing except the patient's tissues. The cap should remain on the needle unless the setup is being tested or the syringe is being used. Bennett (1984) has advocated the use of an antiseptic solution on the penetration site to lessen the chance of carrying bacteria and debris from the oral cavity into the tissue. Some clinicians do not use antiseptic solution before injection; others apply it before the topical anesthetic. These preferences in technique do not affect the result of the injection. The rationale used here is that the antiseptic should be the last agent on the tissue before the needle is inserted.

6. If possible, the clinician should establish a fulcrum against which to rest the syringe so it can be held steady during needle insertion, aspiration, and administration of the solution.
7. Before and during the injection the clinician should talk with the patient to provide reassurance.
8. The needle is inserted to the proper depth.
9. Aspiration technique is completed.
10. The solution should be injected slowly to increase the patient's comfort and reduce the chance of a toxic reaction.
11. When the desired amount of solution has been administered, the needle and syringe are removed.

Currently there is a controversy about recapping the needle at this point in the patient's treatment. The risk of needle stick injury is a serious concern because of the potential for disease transmission of hepatitis and AIDS. The latest ADA guidelines suggest that recapping a needle increases the risk of unintentional needle stick injury. Needles should not be recapped; rather, the unsheathed needle should be placed in a "sterile field" between injections (MMWR, 1986). Exposed needles may increase the likelihood of an accident, and inadvertent contamination of the needle may occur. Cardboard guards and wands that hold the cap so fingers may be kept away during recapping are possible alternatives. Another recapping technique involves placing the cap horizontally on the tray. The needle is aimed into the cap; once inside the cap, the syringe is tipped up vertically so the needle can be pushed in completely and the cap snapped into place at the hub (Blair, 1986). This is a procedure where judgment about the risks involved must be considered. At all times, handling a syringe with a used needle and disposing of needles requires extreme care.

The clinician or another properly trained person should remain with the patient for several minutes after the injection has been given, as an immediate reaction could occur.

Systemic reactions associated with local anesthetics and vasoconstrictors include syncope and allergic, toxic, and idiosyncratic reactions. An *idiosyncratic reaction* is an adverse reaction to a normal amount of local anesthetic that is unexplainable on a pharmacologic or biochemical basis. Treatment will vary according to symptoms and usually will be the same as for allergic or toxic reactions (Laskin, 1984). For more information, refer to the section on local anesthetic reactions in Chapter 8.

After several minutes, the clinician may tap the tissue and teeth to determine if anesthesia has been achieved. At the end of the appointment the patient should be reminded not to chew or bite the soft tissues that are numb. The patient should be instructed to call the office if any unusual sensations or rashes are experienced.

Some modifications in technique are necessary during the administration of local anesthesia to children. Malamed (1986) and Rood (1981) should be consulted if anesthesia is being given to children.

Assisting with administration of a local anesthetic

When assisting another person with the administration of a local anesthetic, these steps follow the review of the health history and the recording of the patient's vital signs:

1. Prepare the syringe with the appropriate anesthetic agent and a needle of the correct length (see Fig. 31-3). The setup may be tested by removing the cap and squeezing a few drops of solution onto a gauze square. This allows the assistant to examine the needle, position the bevel of the needle, and test the harpoon to make sure it is securely engaged in the plunger of the cartridge.
2. Apply the topical anesthetic for the appropriate time. Rinse the area (see page 601).

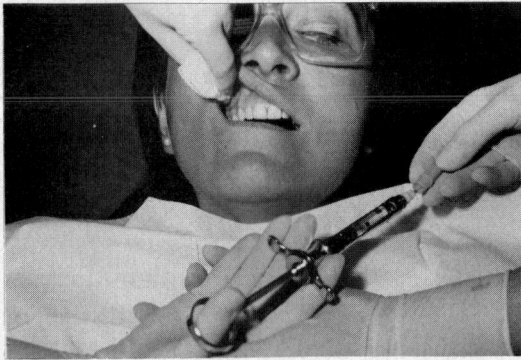

Fig. 31-15. Clinician grasps movable tissue with sterile gauze square and retracts tissue to achieve accessibility and visibility. Clinician is receiving syringe from assistant.

Date _____ Med History Update: Patient well, diabetes under good control, sees physician every 3 months, has taken insulin injection today and eaten within past 2 hours.
Vital signs: 129/84 R.A.S.
Treatment: Tooth #3—replace MO amalgam
            Tooth #4—MOD amalgam
Anesthesia: Lidocaine-topical, Betadine-antiseptic
            2% lidocaine-1:100,000 epinephrine
            One cartridge used for PSA, MSA, and
            greater
palatine injections: 36 mgs. lidocaine
                     .018 mgs. epinephrine
Remarks: Excellent anesthesia for 45 minutes, no adverse reactions.

Fig. 31-16. Sample chart entry after assisting with the administration of a local anesthetic.

3. When the clinician is ready, pass the antiseptic swab.
4. Pass the syringe to the clinician out of the patient's view. Each clinician has a preference for this transfer, but in general the assistant must hold the syringe in such a way that the operator can grasp it easily and securely. The assistant should not remove his or her hand until the clinician is in full control of the syringe (Fig. 31-15).
5. As the syringe is moved away from the assistant, the cap is removed and the needle should be positioned so the bevel of the needle is facing the tissue when the injection is performed.
6. Stand by to reassure the patient and to replace the cartridge if necessary.
7. Receive the syringe on a return transfer.
8. Rinse the patient's mouth.
9. Remain with the patient, unless the clinician is doing so.
10. Record the amount and type of anesthetic agents used in the patient's chart.

The treatment note in the patient's chart should identify the type and amount of local anesthetic used (Fig. 31-16).

Anesthetic complications

A few regional complications from local anesthesia will be mentioned.

Hematoma. Hematoma can occur upon injection into a highly vascular area or a region where a large blood vessel is located. During the injection the blood vessel is damaged or nicked, and bleeding occurs into the tissue. A small amount of blood can accumulate if a vein has been nicked, but a large hematoma can occur very rapidly if an artery has been affected. Usually the bleeding is self-limiting because of pressure that builds up in the tissues. When a hematoma is recognized, pressure should be applied to the area immediately. An ice pack may also be used. Only after 24 hours should moist heat be applied to the area. Swelling and discoloration will gradually disappear over 7 to 14 days. Aspiration is critical when administering local anesthesia and could prevent the vascular trauma just described.

Trismus. Trismus refers to difficulty opening the mouth due to spasm of the muscles of mastication or a motor disturbance of the trigeminal nerve. Needle insertion, especially multiple injections, can cause this. Usually the condition is much improved within 48 hours. Heat applications and gentle exercises are useful in managing this problem.

Tissue sloughing. The surface layers of epithelium are lost due to irritation; ulceration may result. This may occur as a reaction to a topical anesthetic. Following the recommendations for limiting the amount of agent will usually prevent this.

Lip and cheek biting. This occurs when the patient traumatizes the tissue while anesthesia is still present. It is seen most often in children, and the trauma can create a significant wound. The best prevention is to use an anesthetic agent that has a duration appropriate to the length of the dental appointment. Request that the patient does not eat, drink, or test the anesthetized area by biting until normal sensation has returned. For children, a sticker can be placed on the face or the shirt as a reminder to the patient and the parent to be careful.

Facial paralysis. The patient will sense a weakening of the muscles on the side of the face where the injection was given. The most notable findings are inability to close the eyelid, obliteration of the nasolabial fold, and drooping of the corner of the mouth (Laskin, 1987). This is the result of anesthetic solution being inadvertently deposited in the parotid gland, affecting the facial nerve, during an inferior alveolar nerve block. The condition is temporary, but the patient will require reassurance. It is probably a good idea to postpone the intended dental treatment until the patient is more comfortable. Recommend that the patient remove contact lenses and manually close the eye periodically to keep the cornea moist.

Most of these conditions can be prevented by proper injection technique, but occasionally they may occur due to differences in patient anatomy. Observe the patient very closely after an injection for anesthetic reactions and complications. Provide instruction for managing these uncomfortable conditions and always record the patient reaction in detail in the chart.

Other types of injections. Occasionally local infiltration or regional block anesthesia is inadequate. This may occur when infection is present in the site to be anesthetized. Teeth that require endodontic treatment often are in this category. The pH of normal tissue is around 7 (neutral) as compared to an area of infection, where the pH becomes more acidic, about 5. This lowered pH interferes with the ability of the anesthetic agent to effectively stabilize the nerve membrane and block impulse conduction. The result is decreased and delayed anesthesia in the area of infection. Infiltration into such an area is not recommended because of the risk of spreading the infection. Regional block anesthesia is more apt to be successful, but intrapulpal, intraosseous, or periodontal ligament injections may be useful additional techniques (Malamed, 1986).

For an intrapulpal injection, the pulp chamber is exposed and the needle is inserted in the pulp canal. The solution is deposited directly into the canal.

The intraosseous injection requires that a small incision be made in the apical region of the tooth. A bur hole is made through the cortical plate of bone. The needle is inserted and solution deposited into the cancellous bone.

The periodontal ligament injection requires that a needle be placed between the periodontal ligament and the tooth. The bevel of the needle is placed toward the tooth and a small amount of solution is deposited. This technique can be used on all four sides of the tooth to achieve anesthesia.

Care must be taken with intraosseous and periodontal ligament injections, especially if the solutions contain vasoconstrictors. The placement of the solution permits rapid absorption into the systemic circulation. Usually a vasoconstrictor is necessary to produce anesthesia of sufficient duration. Patients with severe cardiovascular disease and those with a history of anginal pain or arrhythmia should receive infiltration or regional block anesthesia rather than a periodontal ligament injection (Pashley, 1986).

TOPICAL ANESTHESIA

Topical anesthesia is achieved by direct application of an anesthetic agent onto the mucous membrane surface (Bennett, 1984). Once placed on the mucous membrane, the agent is absorbed by the free nerve endings in the area, creating an anesthetic effect. Only the free nerve endings are affected; as the topical anesthetic is not injected into the tissue, neither the nerve trunk nor its branches are affected. The topical anesthetic is absorbed by the blood vessels in the affected area, making a toxic reaction possible (Bennett, 1984; Rogo, 1982). In fact, a toxic reaction is even more likely to occur with a topical anesthetic than with a local anesthetic because topical anesthetics are supplied in much higher concentrations.

Topical anesthetic agents

Chemically, topical anesthetics are similar to local anesthetics. There are two groups of topical anesthetics: amides and esters. The amide used as a topical anesthetic is lidocaine (Xylocaine), and the main two esters used as topical anesthetics are tetracaine (Pontocaine) and ethyl aminobenzoate (benzocaine). Benzyl alcohol is also used as a topical anesthetic. In order for these agents to be effective, they are produced in greater concentrations than local anesthetics; for example, lidocaine is used in a 5% concentration; tetracaine is used in a 2% concentration; and benzocaine is available in 10%, 15%, and 20% concentrations (Bennett, 1984; Rogo, 1982). Because such high concentrations are placed in areas of the mouth where they are rapidly absorbed into the bloodstream, there is a danger of a toxic reaction.

Topical anesthetics are often liberally swabbed on the tissue. This technique can lead to overapplication and makes the dose difficult to quantify. Many practitioners regard topical anesthetics as relatively harmless agents. Nothing could be further from the truth; thus this emphasis on the chance of toxic overdose.

Topical anesthetics are available in three forms: gel, liquid, and spray. The gels and liquids are recommended for use prior to local anesthesia or during scaling procedures for superficial soft tissue anesthesia. Some practitioners also use topical anesthetics during radiographic series or impression taking to lessen patients' gag reflexes. Use of a topical anesthetic in these last two instances must be done judiciously to ensure that the patient maintains some of the necessary protective gag reflex. The use of topical anesthetic sprays is highly discouraged because their application and dose are difficult to control. The patient and clinician can inhale the agent, which is not recommended.

The precautions observed when selecting a local anesthetic, such as patient sensitivity to esters or methylparaben and compromised medical histories, also apply when selecting a topical anesthetic. If a patient has a history of allergy to ester anesthetics, then lidocaine topical anesthetic should be used. Methylparaben is used with some amide topical anesthetics so if a patient has a history of allergic reaction, the clinician should check the package insert accompanying the product to see if methylparaben is used. Patients with liver disease or dysfunction should not be given amide topical anesthetics, since they are broken down in the liver; rather, an ester should be used (Bennett, 1984; Rogo, 1982). Topical anesthetics do not contain vasoconstrictors, so the medical conditions affected by vasoconstrictors do not apply to topical anesthetics.

A complication of topical anesthetics, unlike local anesthetics, is tissue irritation. Because a topical anesthetic is applied directly to the mucous membrane, it has the potential to irritate or damage the tissue. This is of particular concern with benzocaine topical anesthetics because they are produced in very high concentrations. Benzocaine topical anesthetics can cause tissue sloughing if left in contact with the tissue too long.

Application

The use of a topical anesthetic before the injection of a local anesthetic and during a scaling procedure is presented in this section. Topical anesthetics are effective only on the soft tissue and are most effective on unkeratinized soft tissue, where they are more readily absorbed.

Before an injection, a topical anesthetic can be applied to the injection site. Figs. 31-5 to 31-15 illustrate the application of a topical anesthetic to some of the injection sites listed in Table 31-3. Before the topical anesthetic is applied, the area should be dried with either a gauze square or a stream of air (Fig. 31-17). A gauze square has the benefit of removing debris as well as moisture before the injection. Drying the tissue helps keep

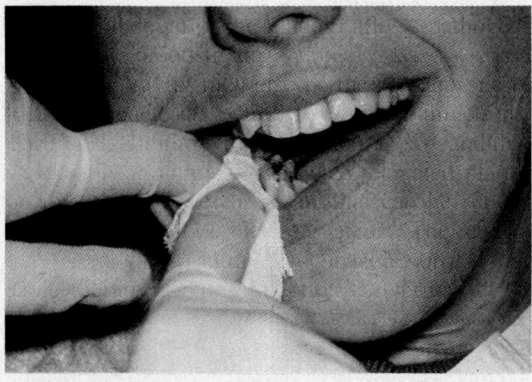

Fig. 31-17. Drying tissue with gauze prior to application of topical anesthetic.

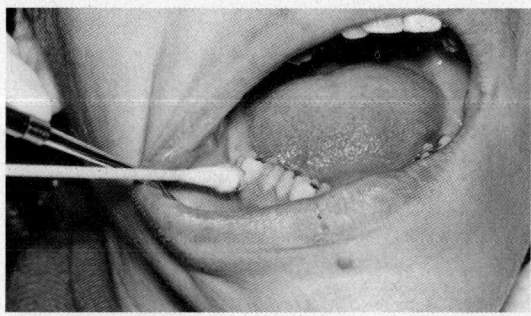

Fig. 31-18. Applying topical anesthetic for interpapillary injection with cotton-tipped applicator.

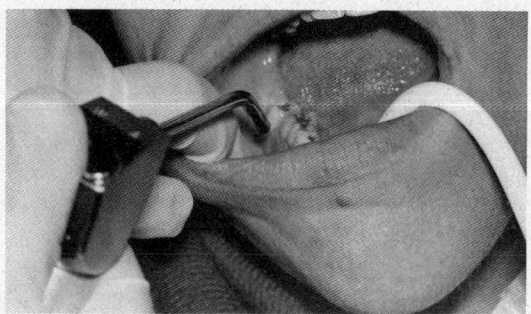

Fig. 31-19. Rinsing area at end of application time.

the agent in the desired area, and it also ensures that the desired amount is being applied. If there is saliva in the area, the topical anesthetic will be carried away, lessening the amount applied and producing undesired anesthesia in other areas of the mouth. The topical anesthetic should be applied with a cotton-tipped applicator that has been dipped into the agent. In order to maintain asepsis, the topical anesthetic should be removed from the container and placed into a dappen dish so that the container is not contaminated. The topical anesthetic on the cotton-tipped applicator (Fig. 31-18) is held in place for the appropriate amount of time. The length of application depends on the agent used and is determined by reading the manufacturer's directions accompanying the product. The highly concentrated benzocaine agents usually have very short application times of about 15 seconds; the less concentrated agents, such as lidocaine and tetracaine, may have longer application times of 30 to 120 seconds. The manufacturer's directions should be observed in order to obtain the desired effect and avoid tissue irritation.

Once the length of application is complete, the cotton-tipped applicator should be removed and the area should be thoroughly rinsed to remove the agent. Ideally, the area should be suctioned as it is rinsed. The patient should not swallow the rinse water. If a suction is not available, the patient should expectorate the rinse water and topical anesthetic. After the area is rinsed, an antiseptic, if one is used, is applied to the injection site and the injection is begun (Fig. 31-19).

The *application of a topical anesthetic during a scaling procedure* requires some modifications to the previous technique. It is still important to dry the area with either a stream of air or a gauze square, but the topical anesthetic can be applied in one of two ways. It can be applied with a cotton-tipped applicator or with a curette. Application with a cotton-tipped applicator will allow the topical anesthetic to reach the outer surface of the papilla and marginal gingiva but will not reach into the sulcus. Because the most sensitive tissue is likely to be the lining of the sulcus, it is recommended that one dip the curette into the topical anesthetic and carry it into the sulcus in this manner. Liquid topical anesthetic is most easily carried into the sulcus on a curette. The application time must still be observed and the area thoroughly rinsed.

During a scaling procedure the topical anesthetic of choice would provide a relatively long anesthetic effect and have a low toxicity. The MSDs of the agents must be observed. Benzocaine has a longer anesthetic effect and a lower toxicity than lidocaine or tetracaine. Benzocaine's longer effect and lower toxicity are due to its low water solubility; thus it is slowly absorbed. But also keep in mind that benzocaine is an ester and that tissue sloughing is more likely. If the patient is not allergic to ester drugs and the clinician observes the application time, benzocaine can provide adequate topical anesthesia. Lidocaine and tetracaine also provide adequate anesthesia and are less likely to produce an allergic reaction and tissue sloughing. As with many agents, the clinician should use several and develop his or her own preference, to be modified by the patient's medical history.

In general, the least amount possible of topical anesthetic necessary to produce the desired effect should be used. Also, the use of a topical anesthetic in highly vascular areas such as the floor of the mouth should be done with care. Observation of the application times and thorough rinsing are essential.

SUMMARY

Some psychosomatic, topical anesthetic, and local anesthetic approaches to pain control have been presented in this chapter. As the practitioner develops helping relationships with patients and uses the appropriate methods of pain control, his or her patients should have very little or no pain associated with dental treatment.

ACTIVITIES

1. Make up a sample of dental hygiene procedures that may require local anesthesia and decide which injections could be given. Refer to Table 31-3.
2. The innervation of the maxilla and mandible described in Table 31-3 is for the permanent dentition. Look up the innervation of the primary and mixed dentitions, and compare and contrast the innervations.
3. Obtain a copy of the laws that govern the practice of dental hygiene in the state. Is administration of local anesthesia permitted? If not, does the class think it should or should not be permitted? What can or cannot be done about the practice act in the state?
4. Participate in a formal local anesthesia course open to dental hygienists to learn how to administer local anesthetics.
5. Look at Table 31-1. Figure out the number of cartridges that could be given of each of the agents before reaching the maximum safe dose in healthy and medically compromised patients. Which agents are limited by the vasoconstrictor they contain?

REVIEW QUESTIONS

1. A dental hygienist graduated from a dental hygiene program that did not teach local anesthesia. The hygienist is now living in a state where he or she can administer local anesthesia. What additional education, if any, does the hygienist need? Why?
2. Draw and label the following nerves:
   a. Posterior, superior, middle superior, and anterior superior
   b. Lingual, buccal, and inferior alveolar

3. Name the tissues innervated by each of the following nerves:
   a. Posterior superior alveolar
   b. Greater palatine
   c. Buccal (long buccal)
   d. Infraorbital
4. Name the injections that should be given for each of the following procedures:
   a. Soft tissue curettage on the facial and lingual aspects of the mandibular right quadrant
   b. Class II mesioocclusal amalgam preparation on the maxillary left first molar; a rubber dam clamp will be placed on the second molar
   c. Root planing on the mandibular central incisor without soft tissue curettage

REFERENCES

ADA Council on Dental Materials, Instruments, and Equipment: Status report: the periodontal ligament injection, JADA 106:222, 1983.

ADA Council on Dental Therapeutics: Accepted dental therapeutics, ed 39. Chicago, 1982, American Dental Association.

Adriani J, and Campbell D: Fatalities following topical application of local anesthetics to mucous membranes, JAMA 162:1527, 1956.

Aldrete TA, and O'Higgins TW: Evaluation of patients with a history of allergy to local anesthetics, South Med J 64:115, 1971.

American Association of Dental Schools: Special report: curricular guidelines for comprehensive control of pain and anxiety in dentistry, J Dent Educ 44:279, 1980.

Atterbury R: Relaxation by vocal pre-sedation in dentistry, CAL 43:18, 1978.

Bateman PM: Multiple allergy to local anesthetic including prilocaine, Med J Aust 2:449, 1974.

Bennett RC: Monheim's local anesthesia and pain control in dental practice, ed 7. St. Louis, 1984, The CV Mosby Co.

Blair HW: Recapping needles (letter to editor), ADA News 18(23):4, 1987.

Blackmore JW: Local anesthetics: a review, Oral Health 77(2):11, 1987.

Bomberg TJ: Local anesthetics and the elderly patient, Gerodontics 2(5):157, 1986.

Burstein A, et al: Injection pain: memory, expectation, and experienced pain, NY J Dent 49:183, 1979.

Christensen LV: Cultural, clinical, and physiological aspects of pain: a review, J Oral Rehabil 7:413, 1980.

Dafoe BR: Providing pain control: local anesthesia, RDH 2(3):46, 1982.

Dietz ER: The dental assistant's role in preparing the anesthetic syringe, Dent Assist 56(3):26, 1987.

Dreyer R: Preparing the patients for anesthesia, Dent Assist 2(6):36, 1983.

Foreman PA: Behavioral considerations in patient management, Anesth Prog 26:161, 1979.

Fry BW, et al: Concentration of vasoconstrictors in local anesthesia change during storage in cartridge heaters, J Dent Res 59:1163, 1980.

Gangarosa LP. Sr: Newer local anesthetics and techniques for administration, J Dent Res 60:1471, 1981.

Gill GJ, and Orr DH: A double-blind crossover comparison of topical anesthetics, JADA 98:213, 1979.

Giovannitti JA, and Bennett RC: Assessment of allergy to local anesthetics, JADA 98:701, 1979.

Graham KB: Local anesthesia and pain control: a modular approach, Kansas City, Mo, 1979, Biomedical Communication Services, University of Missouri—Kansas City School of Dentistry.

Haglund J, and Evers H. 1972. Local anaesthesia in dentistry, London: Astra Läkemedel.

Hersh EV, et al: Local anesthetics: a review of their pharmacology and clinical use, Compendium, 8(5):374, 1987.

Jastak JT, et al: Vasoconstrictors and local anesthesia: a review and rationale for use, JADA 107(4):623, 1983.

Johnson WT, et al: Hypersensitivity to procaine, tetracaine, mepivacaine and methylparaben: a report of a case, JADA 106:53, 1983.

Kaufman E, et al: Difficulties in achieving local anesthesia, JADA 108(2):205, 1984.

Larson CE: Methylparaben—an overlooked cause of local anesthesia hypersensitivity, Anesth Prog 24:72, 1977.

Laskin DM: Diagnosis and treatment of complications associated with local anesthesia, Int Dent J 34(4):232, 1984.

Malamed SF: An update on pain and anxiety control in pediatric dentistry, II: inhalation sedation and local anesthesia, Alpha Omegan 72:29, 1979.

Malamed SF: Handbook of local anesthesia, St. Louis, 1986, The CV Mosby Co.

Malamed SF: The periodontal ligament (PDL) injection: an alternative to inferior alveolar nerve block, Oral Surg 53:117, 1982.

Melzack R: The puzzle of pain. New York, 1973, Basic Books.

Milgrom P, et al: Student differences in achieving local anesthesia, J Dent Ed 48(3):168, 1984.

Milgrom P, et al: Local anesthesia: adverse effects and other emergency problems, Int Dent J 36(2):71, 1986.

Miller S: Hypnosis—relaxation for you and your patient, NY State Dent J 45(5):221, 1979.

Mollen AJ, et al: Needles—25 gauge vs 27 gauge—can patients really tell? Gen Dent 29:417, 1981.

Morbidity and Mortality Weekly Report: Use and care of sharp instruments and needles, Mass Med Soc 35(15):238, 1986.

Mumma RD Jr, et al: Survey of administration of infiltration anesthesia, Dent Hyg 51:159, 1977.

Pashley DH: Systemic effects of intraligamental injections, J Endo 12(10):501, 1986.

Peterson DS, et al: Pain sensation related to local anesthetics injected at varying temperatures, Anesth Prog 25:164, 1981.

Prensky HD: Current concepts in pain control, Clin Prevent Dent 3(1):8, 1981.

Reed GM, and Sheppard VF: Basic structures of the head and neck, Philadelphia, 1976, WB Saunders Co.

Rogo ES: Providing safe comfortable pain control, RDH 1:12, 1982.

Rood JP: Notes on local anesthesia for the child patient, Dent Update 8:377, 1981.

Sharp J: Should dental hygiene students be taught to administer local anesthesia? NM Dent J 30:8, 1979.

Sheilds PW: Local anesthesia and applied anatomy, Aust Dent J 31(5):319, 1986.

Sicher H, and DeBrul EL: Oral anatomy, ed 6, St Louis, 1975, The CV Mosby Co.

Siskin L: Anaphylaxis due to local anesthesia hypersensitivity: report of case, JADA 96:841, 1978.

Sisty-LePeau N, et al: The administration of local anesthesia by dental hygiene students, Dent Hyg 60(1):28, 1986.

Spear FC: Cultural factors in clinical pain assessment, Int Dent J 27:284, 1977.

Steblay NM, and Beaman AL: Reduction of fear during dental treatment through reattribution technique, JADA 105:1006, 1982.

Walsh MM, et al: Mental imagery and local anesthesia, J Dent Ed 48(12):653, 1984.

Wepman BJ: Psychological components of pain perception, Dent Clin North Am 22:101, 1978.

Yaacob HB, et al: The pharmacological effect of Xylocaine topical anesthetics—a comparison with a placebo, Singapore Dent J 6:55, 1981.

Yoeman CM: Hypersensitivity to prilocaine, Br Dent J 153:69, 1982.

32 NITROUS OXIDE AND OXYGEN CONSCIOUS SEDATION

OBJECTIVES: *The reader will be able to*

1. State the indications for nitrous oxide and oxygen conscious sedation in dental hygiene practice.
2. Define the term *conscious* as used in the philosophy of conscious sedation.
3. Identify several methods of monitoring the patient's conscious state.
4. Describe the chemical nature of nitrous oxide.
5. Describe the pharmacologic mechanism that renders nitrous oxide effective.
6. Provide a list of representational examples of patient responses as the concentration of nitrous oxide is increased from 10% to 50%.
7. Complete a preoperative evaluation of a patient.
8. State the contraindications to nitrous oxide and oxygen conscious sedation.
9. Describe the safety features that a nitrous oxide and oxygen conscious sedation system should include.
10. Calculate the percentage of nitrous oxide delivered to a patient.
11. Prepare a patient for receiving nitrous oxide and oxygen conscious sedation.
12. Describe and demonstrate the technique for administering and monitoring nitrous oxide and oxygen conscious sedation.

For many patients, visiting the dental office is an anxiety-producing situation. Because of past experiences or current discomfort the patient worries that further discomfort is inevitable. Modern dentistry offers excellent pain control techniques. Local anesthetics are effective in blocking pain perception. Such techniques are necessary for most periodontal procedures and restorative dentistry. Before some patients are receptive to local anesthetic techniques, sedation techniques are helpful. Nitrous oxide and oxygen conscious sedation is a conscious inhalation sedation method that is used in many dental offices and clinics.

The hygienist performs procedures that may cause the patient discomfort. Patients who rely on nitrous oxide and oxgyen conscious sedation for other restorative dental procedures may require it for deep subgingival scaling, root planing, soft tissue curettage, and placement of temporary restorations or crowns.

Administration of nitrous oxide includes completing a health history, inducting the patient to the proper level of analgesia, monitoring the patient during analgesia (keeping track of the vital signs), and oxygenating the patient at the completion of treatment. The terms "assist" or "aid" in the administration of nitrous oxide are interpreted by state practice acts as the dentist inducting the patient to the proper level followed by the hygienist monitoring and oxygenating the patient following sedation. Currently 21 states allow hygienists to assist or administer nitrous oxide (Rogo, 1986).

Nitrous oxide has been used in dentistry for more than 100 years. Horace Wells, a dentist, first demonstrated its effectiveness during a surgical procedure in 1844 (Langa, 1976). Since that time, the properties and effects of nitrous oxide used with oxygen have been studied and documented.

Nitrous oxide and oxygen conscious sedation is most beneficial to dentistry because it comforts and relaxes the patient. Nitrous oxide alters pain reaction, which is a very individualized interpretation of actual pain perception. By raising the patient's pain reaction threshold, the patient is able better to relax and cooperate during dental procedures. A study designed to provide statistical estimates of the effects of nitrous oxide on pain and anxiety associated with tooth pulp shock demonstrated that nitrous oxide has a significant effect on raising levels of absolute sensation, pain threshold, and pain tolerance. Anxiety levels were reduced to a statistically significant degree (Dworkin, 1983). As an additional effect, nitrous oxide and oxygen conscious sedation alters the patient's perception of time, so dental appointments seem to pass more quickly. With a relaxed, conscious, and cooperative patient the appointment can be handled efficiently. Less stress results for both the patient and the clinician.

The basis of an understanding of nitrous oxide and oxygen conscious sedation is an appreciation of the conscious state. At no time during the administration of this form of inhalation sedation should the patient lose consciousness. The American Dental Society of Anesthesiology, Inc., defines *conscious* in this way: "A patient is said to be conscious if he/she is capable of rational response to command and has all protective reflexes intact, including the ability to clear and maintain his/her airway in a patent state" (Bennett, 1978). All parts of this definition must be observed. Rational response to command will be especially important in monitoring the patient's conscious state. Retaining the ability to breathe automatically and cough so that aspiration is avoided enables inhalation sedation to be administered without sophisticated technical support personnel and equipment. With nitrous oxide and oxygen inhalation sedation, vital signs and the function of cardiovascular and respiratory systems will remain within normal limits (Bennett, 1978; Roberts et al, 1982). Often there is a slight decrease in heart rate and cardiac output with a slight increase in total peripheral resistance, which is most likely due to breathing a high concentration of oxygen (Giovannitti, 1984).

Nitrous oxide affects the central nervous system by depressing the cerebral cortex, thalamus, hypothalamus, and reticular activating system. This results in nervous impulses either not being relayed to the cortex or being interpreted differently (Swepston, 1976). The patient will experience an alteration of mood, and the pain reaction threshold will increase. The patient will be in a relaxed and very suggestible state.

A 20% concentration of nitrous oxide has been compared to 15 mg of morphine administered subcutaneously (Chapman, 1943). In fact, a 35% concentration has been shown effectively to relieve the pain associated with myocardial infarction (Thompson, 1976). As an important note, this suggests that nitrous oxide sedation may be helpful in an emergency situation involving a myocardial infarction for providing supplemental oxygen and pain control for the patient until further emergency help arrives.

Nitrous oxide is a mildly potent anesthetic. *Potency* refers to the amount of medication necessary to achieve a desired effect. A clinical measure of relative potency has been experimentally determined. This is called the *mean alveolar concentration (MAC)*. MAC is defined as the concentration of anesthetic agent required to prevent movement (reflex reaction to pain) at the time of surgical incision in 50% of patients (DeMartina and Garber, 1979). A very potent medication such as halothane, a general anesthetic, has a MAC of 0.77%. Nitrous oxide has a MAC of 101% (Fordham, 1974). Since it is impossible to deliver a 101% concentration of pure nitrous oxide gas because of atmospheric conditions, relieving response to frank pain perception cannot be relied on. In a dental procedure where hard or soft tissue pain will be significant for the patient, nitrous oxide and oxygen conscious sedation must be accompanied by local anesthesia. Heft (1984) found that 33% nitrous oxide analgesia reduced the intensity but not the unpleasantness of painful tooth pulp sensations. Increasing the concentration of nitrous oxide will not significantly reduce true pain perception. A patient responding to pain while under nitrous oxide and oxygen conscious sedation will not be comfortable or cooperative for long.

Nitrous oxide is a colorless, nonexplosive, and sweet-smelling inorganic agent. It is prepared by heating ammonium nitrate crystals in an iron retort at 240° C (Bennett, 1978). This produces nitrous oxide and water. Commercially, nitrous oxide is supplied in pressurized cylinders as a liquid and a gas.

Nitrous oxide is nonallergenic and does not react with body tissues. It diffuses across tissue membranes much more rapidly than oxygen. When inhaled, nitrous oxide diffuses across the alveolar membrane in the alveoli of the lungs, entering the bloodstream. With a very low blood gas solubility (0.47) the nitrous oxide molecule travels unchanged in the blood. Nitrogen molecules are usually displaced in the bloodstream by the nitrous oxide. Nitrous oxide reaches equilibrium in the bloodstream rapidly and exerts its analgesic effect within minutes (Giovannitti, 1984). As long as the patient continues to breathe the flow of nitrous oxide and oxygen, a concentration of nitrous oxide that will affect the central nervous system will be maintained in the bloodstream. By controlling the external concentration of nitrous oxide and oxygen as it comes from the sedation equipment, the patient's alveolar concentration is controlled (DeMartina and Garber, 1979).

To calculate nitrous oxide concentration, a percentage is determined. The flow of nitrous oxide, expressed in liters per minute, is placed over the total flow of nitrous oxide and oxygen, creating a fraction that can then be converted to a percentage (Bennett, 1978):

$$Example\ 1: \frac{2 \text{ liters of N}_2\text{O}}{2 \text{ liters of N}_2\text{O} + 8 \text{ liters of O}_2} = \frac{2}{10} = 20\%$$

$$Example\ 2: \frac{3 \text{ liters of N}_2\text{O}}{3 \text{ liters of N}_2\text{O} + 6 \text{ liters of O}_2} = \frac{3}{9} = 33\ 1/3\%$$

The alveolar concentration, or percentage of nitrous oxide delivered, determines the sedative effect on the central nervous system that the patient will experience. Table 32-1 summarizes the range of responses possible at given concentrations (Bennett, 1978).

The sedation (depression) of the central nervous system resembles the state one experiences just before falling asleep. At concentrations higher than necessary for dental procedures sleep indeed occurs. To maintain the definition of consciousness, the patient must remain awake and responsive to verbal commands at all times. If the patient is unable to keep the mouth open or is falling asleep, the amount of nitrous oxide being delivered must be reduced.

In addition to being relaxed and having time perception altered, the patient may experience dissociation (DeMartina, 1979; Minnis, 1979). This refers to an effect on the patient's ability to

Table 32-1. Signs and symptoms in response to nitrous oxide and oxygen conscious sedation

Concentration N$_2$O	Response
10% to 20%	Body warmth
	Tingling of hands and feet
20% to 30%	Circumoral numbness
	Numbness of thighs
20% to 40%	Numbness of tongue
	Numbness of hands and feet
	Droning sounds present
	Hearing distinct but distant
	Dissociation begins and reaches peak
	Mild sleepiness
	Analgesia (maximum at 30%)
	Euphoria
	Feeling of heaviness or lightness of body
30% to 50%	Sweating
	Nausea
	Amnesia
	Increased sleepiness
40% to 60%	Dreaming, laughing, giddiness
	Further increased sleepiness, tending toward unconsciousness
	Increased nausea and vomiting
50% and over	Unconsciousness and light general anesthesia

From Bennett CR: Conscious sedation in dental practice, ed 2, St Louis, 1978, The CV Mosby Co.

maintain his or her spatial orientation. The patient may describe floating or sinking into the chair. The clinician's voice and sounds in the operatory may seem distant. Most people enjoy a slight bit of "escape" from the dentistry at hand. Other patients may interpret dissociation as a feeling of losing control of themselves or the situation. This in itself may be alarming to the patient, thereby reducing the comfort that the patient expects to feel.

Patient reactions vary a great deal at any given concentration of nitrous oxide. The clinician must be sensitive to the physiologic and psychologic personality of the patient. Observing the patient's responses constantly ensures that a comfortable level of sedation is maintained at all times.

A few parameters are noteworthy. When nitrous oxide is administered above a 40% concentration, the patient generally becomes increasingly sleepy and responds sluggishly to commands (Bennett, 1978; Hamburg, 1980). The patient may begin to perspire, look uncomfortable, move in an uncoordinated manner, and complain of nausea. Any of these signs indicates that the inhaled concentration is too high for the patient. Although vomiting is rare at recommended levels, it is potentially dangerous and unpleasant for everyone concerned.

A concentration of 30% to 35% is accepted as a range for maximum nitrous oxide and oxygen conscious sedation (Bennett, 1978). Many patients are comfortable at lower concentrations. An administration technique in which the concentration is preset is unacceptable. The patient is induced with small amounts of nitrous oxide and a constant flow of at least 6 liters of oxygen per minute. After a few minutes at each increment of nitrous oxide, the concentration is increased until a comfortable state is achieved.

As a general rule in dentistry, nitrous oxide sedation should never be administered in concentrations greater than 50%. If a patient requires more pain control, another anesthetic modality should be employed.

From one appointment to another the same patient may achieve desired sedation at different concentrations. The time of day, level of fatigue, general mood of the patient, and a variety of other factors influence this. In any case, delivering an excess of medication is, at worst, capable of producing a bad experience for the patient and, at best, unnecessary and wasteful.

PATIENT SELECTION

Before a patient experiences nitrous oxide and oxygen conscious sedation, a review of the medical status is necessary. Conditions that contraindicate this type of sedation include the following (DeMartina and Garber, 1979):

1. Recent myocardial infarction (within 6 months)
2. Chronic obstructive pulmonary disease (e.g., emphysema)
3. Pregnancy
4. Active asthmatic condition
5. Nasal obstruction resulting from current upper respiratory tract infection
6. Inability to communicate (very young children, severely retarded patients)

Patients with a history of recent myocardial infarction may be more likely to have a recurrent episode. Elective dental treatment is generally postponed until the patient is again medically stable.

Patients with emphysema, chronic bronchitis, or bronchial asthma in which the pulmonary system is chronically compromised may be prone to hypoxia. This refers to a lack of necessary oxygen in the bloodstream to adequately supply the patient's functional demand. If lack of oxygen is a problem for some, too much oxygen can also create a problem. Some patients, especially patients with emphysema, may rely on a lower level of oxygen circulating in the blood to stimulate the oxygen drive "reflex," which actually induces breathing. When abundant oxygen is delivered along with nitrous oxide, the drive to breathe is suppressed. Room air contains approximately 20% oxygen as compared with 70% to 80% delivered with inhalation sedation.

During pregnancy, the use of all medications is best avoided. Although studies do not confirm serious fetal effects, an unnecessary risk at this critical time in development is to be avoided.

The patient with active asthma is prone to breathing difficulty and may pose a serious problem should bronchospasm occur.

As nitrous oxide and oxygen conscious sedation relies on inhalation for its effectiveness, an upper respiratory tract infection and associated "stuffed" nose make the procedure useless. Because of the chance of cross-infection, elective dental care at this time is generally not advised.

The ability to communicate is essential, since this is a primary sign of the patient's consciousness. In patients with compromised ability, monitoring the patient is difficult.

The effects of nitrous oxide and oxygen conscious sedation are especially beneficial to the mild to moderately anxious and tense patient. Patients with more severe anxiety or less control of their emotions may not be helped with inhalation sedation of this type.

For patients with hypertension, the sedative effect of nitrous oxide is very beneficial because it keeps the blood pressure within the patient's normal limits.

Older patients who have Addison's disease or who have been taking corticosteroids should be carefully screened. If steroid therapy has been discontinued recently, the reaction to stress may be poor. The physician should be consulted about the possible need for steroids being reinstituted prior to treatment (Riklin, 1978).

For some medically compromised patients, the analgesia produced by nitrous oxide and oxygen may prove superior to other anesthetic/analgesic measures. Kaufman and others (1982) have reported the success of nitrous oxide and oxygen conscious sedation for the treatment of a hemophiliac, a patient with severe cerebral palsy, and a patient with severe disabilities caused by familial dysautonomia.

The clinician's discretion and the physician's consultation may be necessary for patients with epilepsy, multiple sclerosis, questionable emotional status, central nervous system disorders, and other medically compromised conditions. Patients with a history of previous substance abuse or dependency should be evaluated carefully before recommending nitrous oxide sedation. In general, no procedure should be performed for a patient unless the office personnel are able to support the patient should an emergency or life-threatening situation occur (DeMartina and Garber, 1979).

EQUIPMENT

Nitrous oxide and oxygen conscious sedation equipment is available as a portable or central system.

A portable unit is shown in Fig. 32-1. The small tanks of oxygen and nitrous oxide permit mobility of the unit throughout the office or clinic. If inhalation sedation is used often, frequent changing of the small tanks may create a problem. The "E" size cylinder of oxygen contains about 66 liters, while the "E" size nitrous oxide cylinder contains 1590 liters of compressed gas. These figures equate to a 2-hour duration for an oxygen cylinder (at 5 liters per minute flow) and a more than 5-hour duration for a nitrous oxide cylinder at the same flow rate (Dentist's Desk Reference, 1983).

Fig. 32-2 illustrates the regulators that attach to the portable unit tanks. These gauges indicate the pressure of the gas in the cylinder. Oxygen is

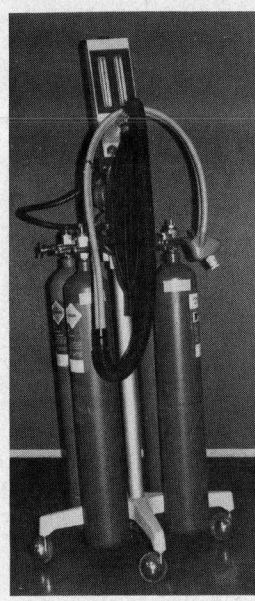

Fig. 32-1. Portable nitrous oxide and oxygen conscious sedation equipment.

supplied at a pressure of 2100 pounds per square inch (psi). As the oxygen is used, the pressure of the gas falls in direct proportion to this amount. Therefore if one half of the tank has been used, the regulator gauge will read 1050 psi.

Nitrous oxide is present as both a liquid and a gas and is supplied in cylinders at a pressure of 750 psi. The pressure remains the same in the tank until all the liquid is converted into gas. A nitrous oxide tank that is half empty will still read 750 psi; once all the liquid is converted, the pressure will drop until the tank is empty. A tag should be placed on the tank to keep track of the nitrous oxide used, with the date a full tank was opened and the dates and lengths of subsequent appointments when nitrous oxide was administered.

Central systems run from a bank of several large nitrous oxide and oxygen cylinders. These are called "H" and "G" tanks, respectively. With a central system, lines run to several wall hookups where the flow meter and mask unit are attached (Fig. 32-3). In addition to showing the pressure in the tanks, central systems usually include a wall- or desk-mounted alarm system that

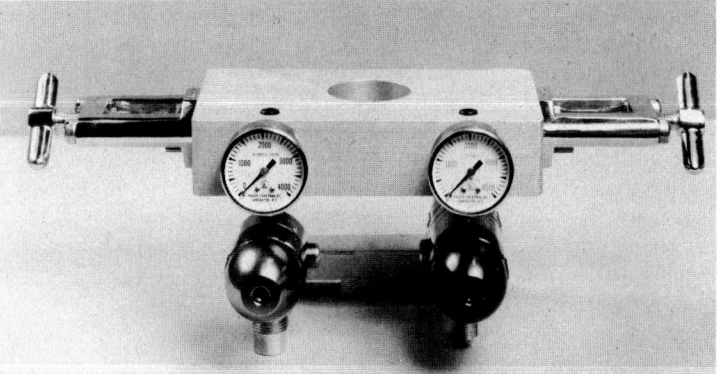

Fig. 32-2. Nitrous oxide and oxygen regulators that affix to portable analgesia machine. Pressure gauges indicate pressure of gas contained in cylinders.
(Courtesy Fraser Sweatman, Inc. From Bennett CR: Conscious sedation in dental practice, ed 2, St Louis, 1978, The CV Mosby Co.)

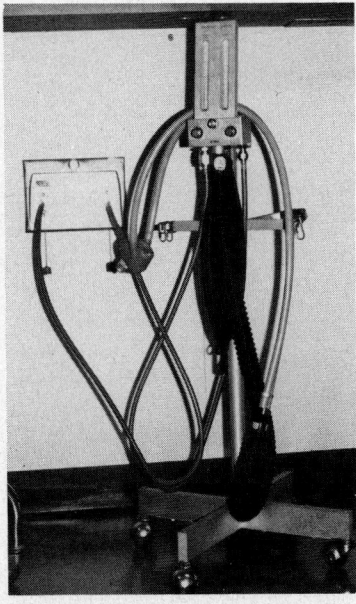

Fig. 32-3. Wall hookup for centralized nitrous oxide and oxygen conscious sedation system.

lights up or sounds if supplies are low (Fig. 32-4).

The following safety systems and devices have been developed to ensure proper use of inhalation sedation equipment (Bennett, 1978; DeMartina and Garber, 1979):

Universal color coding. The tanks and associated parts of the equipment (tubing, regulator gauge mount, flow controls) are colored *green* for oxygen and *blue* for nitrous oxide.

Pin index or diametric index system. The connection for the tanks and hoses for nitrous oxide will not adapt to the oxygen hookups. This prevents a person from mistakenly interchanging the gas systems.

Minimum oxygen flow. A preset flow of oxygen is provided at all times when the unit is on. This prevents the administration of pure nitrous oxide.

Fail-safe system. If for some reason the oxygen supply runs below the minimum level, the nitrous oxide automatically shuts off and begins to whistle.

Flow meter. This is a visual indication of liters per minute flow of both nitrous oxide and oxygen. The flow control valve (dial or lever) is color coded and labeled for each gas (Fig. 32-5). Automatic flow meters are available in which the concentration of nitrous oxide is dialed. The machine adjusts to higher or lower concentrations automatically when the dial is changed.

Nonrebreathing system. Expired gases are not recirculated.

Analgesia machine circuit. The analgesia machine circuit is a set of two tubes connected to the machine and to the nasal mask. The nasal mask has two valves—air dilution and exhalation. The air dilution valve would allow the patient to dilute the flow of nitrous oxide by inhaling room air. This is not desirable, because the clinician no longer can accurately estimate the alveolar concentration of nitrous oxide and oxygen being delivered by the

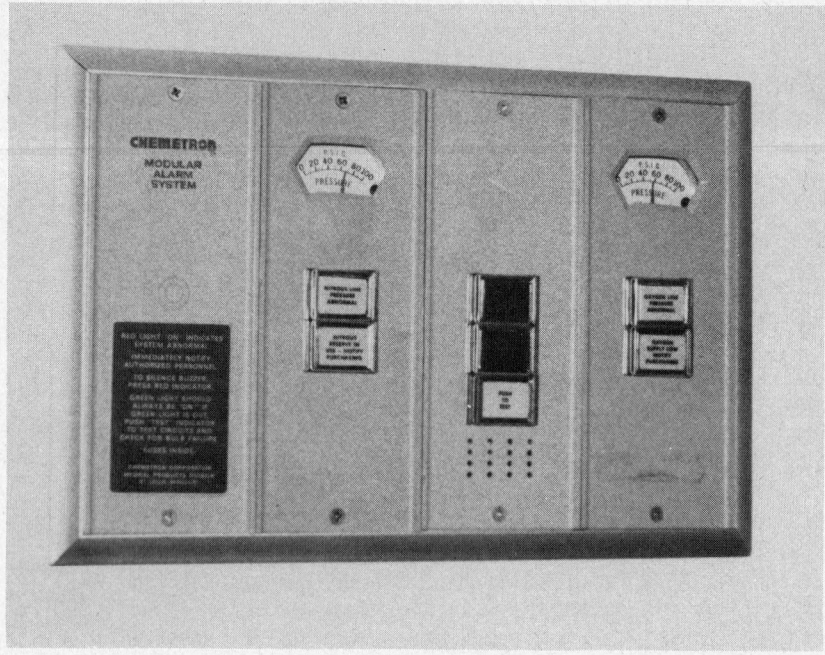

Fig. 32-4. Wall alarm system for centralized system.

Fig. 32-5. Fraser Sweatman analgesia machine with dials to regulate gas flow.

(Courtesy Fraser Sweatman, Inc. From Bennett CR: Conscious sedation in dental practice, ed 2, St Louis, 1978, The CV Mosby Co.)

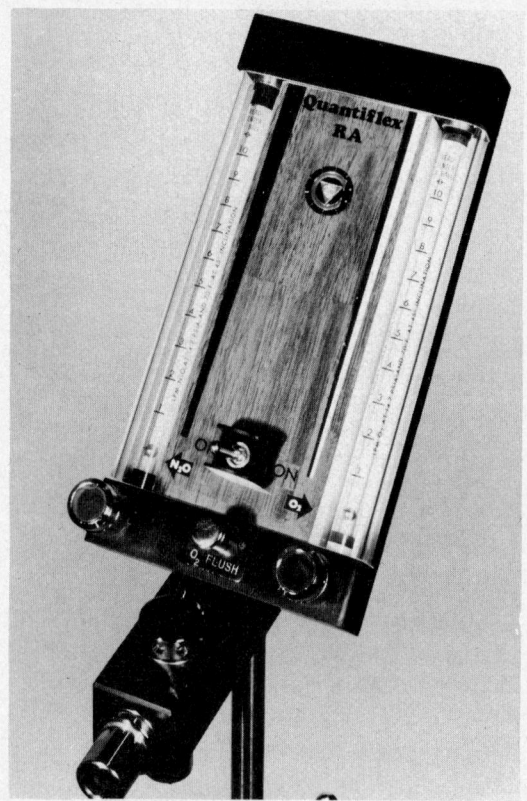

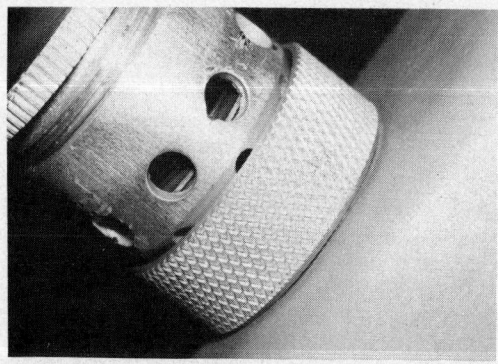

Fig. 32-6. Nasal mask with air dilution valve in *incorrect* position. Small holes indicate that air dilution valve is open.

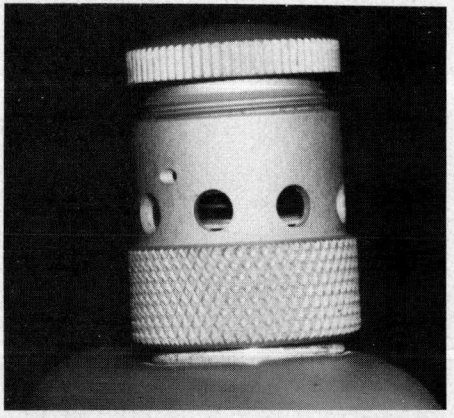

Fig. 32-7. Nasal mask with valves in *correct* position. Exhalation valve (large holes) open; air dilution valve (small holes) closed.

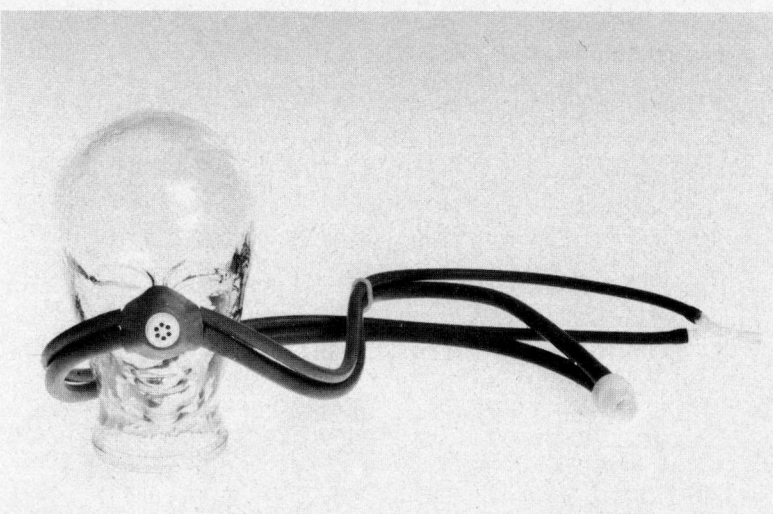

Fig. 32-8. Scavenging nasal mask.
(Courtesy Narco McKesson. From Bennett CR: Conscious sedation in dental practice, ed 2, St Louis, 1978, The CV Mosby Co.)

equipment. This valve, if present on the mask, is always in a closed position (Fig. 32-6). The exhalation valve allows the patient to exhale the previously circulated gases. This valve is always in the open position (Fig. 32-7). This is a nonscavenging system.

Scavenging system. This includes a mask or other device to remove expired gases from the operatory (Fig. 32-8). Studies on the effects of long-term exposure to small amounts of nitrous oxide and other anesthetic gases indicate that use of such a system is a recommended safety precaution.

Reservoir bag. The reservoir bag is filled by fresh gas and is large enough to accommodate the volume of the patient's greatest inspiration.

Flush valve. By activating this valve, the clinician is

able to deliver 100% oxygen at a high flow rate. This also enables the machine to be used in manual resuscitation.

Attention to nitrous oxide and oxygen conscious sedation eqiupment is essential. The installation of such equipment should be completed by qualified professionals. After installation, the equipment must be maintained and checked regularly to ensure proper functioning. The equipment must not be altered in any way, and guidelines from the manufacturer for safe handling must be followed.

CONCERN ABOUT ENVIRONMENTAL CONTAMINATION

In the last several years interest has been shown in the possible effects of chronic exposure to anesthetic gases. Although few studies have looked at nitrous oxide as a single agent, evidence does suggest that trace contamination of anesthetic gases may be a health hazard (Cohen et al, 1980; Jastak and Greenfield, 1977).

Major topics of study have included miscarriage, congenital malformation, cancer, and psychologic disorders. Knill-Jones and colleagues (1972) found that working female anesthesiologists reported spontaneous abortion rate of 18.2% as compared with 14.7% in nonanesthesiologists.

In a study sponsored by the Amercian Society of Anesthesiologists, female respondents reported a 1.25 rate of congenital abnormality per 100 live births as compared with a 0.21 rate reported by women responding from the American Academy of Pediatrics. The rates of the wives of men responding in the two associations were 1.56 and 0.9, respectively (Cohen et al, 1974).

In a 20-year study of the cause of death among anesthesiologists, Bruce and others (1968) found that the rate of lymphoid malignancy was significantly higher than normally expected.

In studies of psychologic effects, it has been found that traces of anesthetic gases may affect memory, reaction time, or temperament. Swepston (1976) has outlined a case presentation in which, after 3 months of daily misuse of nitrous oxide, a clinician experienced and was hospitalized for paranoid delusions.

When comparing individuals not exposed to inhalation anesthetics with those who were, Cohen and coworkers (1980) found that male dentists had a 1.7-fold increase in liver disease, a 1.2-fold increase in kidney disease, and a 1.9-fold increase in neurologic disease.

The morphology of the bone marrow of 21 dentists who habitually used nitrous oxide was investigated. The study provided direct evidence that occupational exposure to nitrous oxide may cause depression of vitamin B_{12} activity, resulting in measurable changes in bone marrow secondary to impaired synthesis of deoxyribonucleic acid (Sweeney, 1985). Studies conducted with laboratory rats subjected to prolonged nitrous oxide exposure show impaired bone marrow function, damaged spermatogenic cells with decreased testicular function, and an increase in fetal death in pregnant animals (Corbett, 1973; Kripke, 1976, 1977).

When humans have abused nitrous oxide for periods ranging from 3 months to 5 years, neurological symptoms appear. These include parasthesia of the extremities, loss of dexterity and balance, muscle weakness with gait ataxia, impotence, incontinence, and an electric shock sensation traveling upward from the feet to the neck after flexion of the neck. In most cases these symptoms are reversible after discontinuation of the drug abuse (Giovannitti, 1984).

Swenson (1976) studied the mean concentration of halothane and nitrous oxide, measured 15 inches in front of the nasal mask. In a nonrebreathing system in which partial recirculation of exhaust occurs, 1955 parts per million (ppm) of nitrous oxide were found. In a system in which no recirculation of exhaust occurs, 172 ppm of nitrous oxide were found. Scavenging devices and well-ventilated operatories are helpful in reducing the amount of exposure to nitrous oxide for dental personnel.

Investigators will continue to define the dangers and determine the safety standards for nitrous oxide use in dental practice. The National Institute for Occupational Safety and Health has recommended 50 parts per million as the maximum exposure to nitrous oxide waste gas in the breathing zone of the worker. In a study with pediatric patients, Badger and others (1982) noted that levels above the recommended persist in operatories in spite of scavenging equipment. Christiansen (1985) found that significant differences exist in the effectiveness of scavenging devices, and that neither rubber dam placement nor the patient's talking significantly affected levels of scavenged nitrous oxide. This suggests that better methods for eliminating waste gases and monitoring trace gases in the dental environment must be developed. Current guidelines for nitrous oxide scavenging and waste gas monitoring equipment are published by the American Dental Association Council on Dental Materials and Devices (Dentist's Desk Reference, 1983).

To reduce nitrous oxide levels in the dental operatory, the following recommendations can be implemented:

1. Use an approved nitrous oxide scavenging device
2. Fit the nasal mask to the patient as well as possible
3. Vent the exhaled gases and the patient suction machine to a safe disposal site outside the building
4. Use a fan to direct exhaled nitrous oxide away from the breathing zone of the operating personnel
5. Minimize patient conversation
6. Improve circulation of the operatory by opening a window or using a nonrecycling air conditioning system
7. Use a monitoring system; air sampling equipment is available and relatively inexpensive; a badge can be worn on the lapel to detect nitrous oxide levels in the operator's breathing zone
8. Maintain equipment; inspect the connectors and test for leakage at frequent regular intervals
9. Set conservative limits on the duration of nitrous oxide exposure for each patient
10. Shut off and secure the equipment after each day's use

There is no convincing evidence that trace concentrations found in dental operatories have any acute effect on the mental or motor functions of the dental personnel while the patient is sedated and treatment is under way. The threshold for psychomotor impairment is in the range of 10% to 20% concentration (Moore, 1983). This cannot be obtained through leakage in the breathing zone if the proper administration guidelines and safety practices are followed. The concern for dental professionals is from chronic low-dose exposure over a period of time.

Concerning professional liability, employers should be aware of the potential dangers of working with nitrous oxide and must inform their employees of the harmful effects. Besides providing information to employees, steps need to be taken that show the employer has followed the recommended and reasonable steps to eliminate danger in the workplace to both employees and patients (Troyer, 1983). If safe conditions do not exist, employees cannot be penalized for activities to preserve and pursue health and safety. If an employer refuses to acknowledge or correct potential nitrous oxide hazards, a formal complaint should be made to the regional Occupational Safety and Health Act office (Rogo, 1986).

ADMINISTRATION

Once the patient is identified as a candidate for nitrous oxide and oxygen conscious sedation, preparation for the experience is in order.

Often an initial experience is helpful for the patient. This is done at a time when no dentistry is to be performed. The patient is familiarized with the sedation equipment and experiences the relaxation effects. In this way the patient looks forward to a comfortable dental appointment. This step may in itself create an important change in the patient's attitude.

Dworkin (1984) found that providing information to people receiving a drug for pain relief yields higher sensation thresholds, pain thresholds, and tolerance of pain. This indicates that influencing thought processes in combination with analgesia can have the effect of increasing analgesia.

Occasionally the patient may have heard about nitrous oxide, or "laughing gas," and may be afraid he or she will do something embarrassing. The clinician should explain to the patient that this will not occur. The level of sedation will produce pleasant relaxation, but the patient will be aware of and in control of all actions. The patient is able to control the level of sedation by breathing deeply through the nose (increase effect) or by breathing through the mouth (decrease effect). These maneuvers affect the external concentration, thereby increasing or reducing alveolar concentration.

The clinician maintains a professional attitude. The patient's comments are listened to, and positive reassurance is offered. This encourages confidence in the clinician. During sedation, it will be important that the patient trust the clinician's suggestions.

Other suggestons before the dental appointment include attention to diet and dress. Before nitrous oxide and oxygen conscious sedation, the patient does not need to restrict diet altogether. A light meal 1 hour or so before the appointment is recommended. For patient comfort, neither an empty stomach nor a full stomach is suggested.

Comfortable, loose clothing is ideal. If desired, clothing at the neck can be loosened. If the patient is wearing contact lenses, they should be removed before inhalation sedation. Gas leaks around the bridge of the nose may produce drying of the eyes with potential irritation to the patient (Malamed, 1985).

Technique

Following are the steps for administering nitrous oxide and oxygen conscious sedation:

1. Review the patient's medical history. Take vital signs.
2. Discuss the procedure with the patient.
3. Prepare the sedation equipment by cleaning the nasal mask with disinfectant. Check to ensure that the supply of oxygen and nitrous oxide is sufficient to complete the procedure. Once the patient is seated in the operatory, the sedation equipment can be shown to the patient. Never force sedation on a patient. The patient should agree to try the experience. Reaffirm the comfortable feelings the patient will experience.
4. Turn the oxygen on to a flow of 6 to 8 liters per minute. This flow will be maintained throughout the procedure. The patient can hold the mask and feel the flow of oxygen. If the system does not include a scavenging mask, check the exhalation valve to be sure it is set at *open* and check the air dilution valve to be sure it is set at *closed*.
5. Fill the reservoir bag by activating the flush valve. The patient seats the nasal mask himself or herself and adjusts it to a comfortable position. A gauze square may be helpful if placed under the edges of the mask on sensitive areas of the face. This pads the mask against the face and closes any leaks around the mask if a perfect fit is not possible. It is especially important to have the oxygen flowing and the reservoir bag filled so that the patient may take a comfortable first breath of pure oxygen.
6. Allow the patient a few minutes to breathe the oxygen. Have the patient practice breathing through the mouth to show the patient how he or she has control of the inhalation technique.
7. Inform the patient that he/she may smell a sweet odor as the nitrous oxide is started at 0.5 to 1 liter per minute. Reassure the patient that the procedure is going well. Ask the patient to take a few deep breaths while relaxing arms, hands, and legs. Suggest that the patient rest back in the dental chair for a comfortable and enjoyable dental appointment. The patient may begin to show signs of less tension: relaxed facial expression, relaxed hands, and less movement of the eyes around the room. A patient who feels uncomfortable usually will say so or look distressed.

If a patient comments that nothing has changed, increase the nitrous oxide level another 1/2 or 1 liter per minute. Suggest the reactions that the patient will generally feel at that particular nitrous oxide concentration, such as, "You may be feeling warm or notice tingling in your hands and feet. Everyone responds a bit differently, but a feeling of floating comfortably or relaxing into the chair is common. These feelings are part of the relaxation technique."

A patient who is started on a sedation procedure should never be left alone. The operatory and supplies should be fully arranged before the sedation procedure is begun. Constant monitoring must be maintained (Fig. 32-9). One can arrange instruments, write notes, or begin examination procedures while observing the patient. Extremely close monitoring of the patient's every feeling may be anxiety producing if

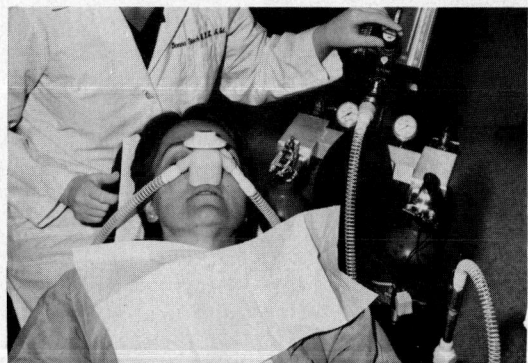

Fig. 32-9. Monitor patient at all times for consciousness, comfort, and cooperation.

the patient senses he or she is not feeling what has been suggested.

Careful observation of the patient will determine whether the nitrous oxide should be increased to the next step. When the patient is comfortable, he or she may sigh, readjust the body to a more relaxed position, become quiet, and smile slightly. Voices and other operatory noises may be exaggerated or muffled. The middle ear is an air space that is sensitive to pressure changes during nitrous oxide inhalation. Patients may report transient auditory changes (Duncan, 1984). Speak in a quiet voice, at a slower rate, and in a calming manner. Limit extraneous conversations with a third person in the operatory in order to create a more calm and quiet environment.

Minnis (1979) has noted that a person under nitrous oxide and oxygen conscious sedation is in a very suggestible state. The effect of the clinician's verbal and nonverbal communication is crucial; how things are said and done is very important. Experimental and control studies confirm the powerful role of mental processes in mediating pain experience (Dworkin, 1983). Be supportive and reinforce how well treatment is going. Comment on how comfortable the patient appears. Request that the patient let the clinician know if he or she feels otherwise. The softness and sincerity

of the clinician's voice may be one of the best instruments for relaxing and reassuring the patient. Weinstein (1986) found that the behavior of the clinician is a major influence on the fear-related behaviors of children, even when nitrous oxide is used. Certain verbal directions intended to distract the child's attention from the procedure at hand appear to be especially effective.

The comfort range for each patient varies with the individual. The optimum concentration of nitrous oxide should never exceed 35%. Use the formula mentioned earlier to compute the percentage.

8. Once a comfortable level of sedation has been achieved, a local anesthetic can be administered.
9. Proceed with the appointment plan.
10. Monitor the patient constantly for consciousness, comfort, and cooperation. If the patient is becoming very lethargic, closing his or her mouth often and tending toward sleep, reduce the percentage of nitrous oxide 1/2 to 1 liter per minute to lighten the level of sedation. Conversely, restlessness may also be a sign that the concentration of nitrous oxide is too high and the patient is no longer comfortable.
11. Near the end of the appointment, reduce the nitrous oxide concentration. The patient will usually maintain satisfactory relaxation if simple procedures are performed, such as polishing, flossing, carving amalgam, or checking occlusion. Place sensible limits on the duration of sedation in the individual case.

About 5 minutes before the end of the appointment, turn the nitrous oxide off completely.
12. Allow the patient to breathe 6 to 8 liters of pure oxygen per minute for at least 5 minutes. This step is necessary to avoid diffusion hypoxia, which may precipitate syncope.

Because nitrous oxide diffuses more rapidly than oxygen, the concentration of nitrous oxide in the bloodstream begins to diffuse into the alveolar spaces rapidly when the nitrous oxide is shut off. A temporary state of hypoxia (lack of oxygen) may occur if adequate oxygen is unable to diffuse from the lungs into the bloodstream during the phase of exhaling the nitrous oxide concentration. A lack of adequate oxygen or an increase in carbon dioxide levels in the bloodstream may produce syncope or other adverse cardiac and respiratory effects. By oxygenating the patient for several minutes following termination of the nitrous oxide flow, diffusion occurs gradually and a hypoxic state is avoided.

Generally, under short-term conditions such as are used in conjunction with outpatient dental treatment, the patient should be largely recovered after a 5-minute exposure to 100% oxygen at the conclusion of the appointment. However, further benefit is apparently gained from a somewhat longer recuperation before the patient engages in any activity requiring exacting psychomotor skills (McKercher et al, 1980).

13. Remove the nasal mask.
14. Slowly seat the patient is a semisupine position. Following the 5 minutes of breathing 100% oxygen, breathing room air for 10 to 15 minutes is appropriate. In most cases this much time is necessary to complete appointment procedures prior to dismissal. The patient remains in the chair until all sedation effects are gone. The patient should feel normal and be pleased with the dental appointment.
15. Disinfect the mask and equipment. Shut the entire system off after each administration if sedation is used infrequently or at the end of the day if the system is used frequently.

Because of the rapid euphoric effects nitrous oxide is capable of creating, there is potential for abuse of this medication. In fact, one or two deaths occur each year because of misuse of nitrous oxide (Swepston, 1976). Lock portable equipment and secure the central system to discourage any unfortunate occurrences.

16. Record the experience in the patient's chart. Note vital signs before nitrous oxide administration, concentrations of nitrous

oxide and oxygen administered, and length of time for inhalation sedation. Also record the length of time the patient received oxygen after the procedure and include any specific postoperative instructions given to the patient. A summary of the patient's reactions will be helpful for future reference.

Conditions during sedation

If a patient becomes uncomfortable or anxious and tries to remove the nasal mask, gently prevent this, as it predisposes the patient to diffusion hypoxia. Immediately flush the system with 100% oxygen while at the same time verbally reassuring the patient that you understand what is occurring and realize the patient feels uncomfortable (DeMartina and Garber, 1979). Ask the patient to breathe deeply as the pure oxygen is delivered. Within a few moments the patient will begin to feel better. Reassure the patient that everything is fine. He or she is safe and will be feeling better as each breath of oxygen is taken.

When a relaxed state is again achieved, complete the dental procedure. Do not let the patient have a bad experience with sedation. At the end of the appointment compliment the patient on his or her cooperation and the successful dental appointment.

An occasional patient may become nauseated and vomit. This usually does not happen when sedation is maintained with nitrous oxide and oxygen below a 35% concentration. If the patient felt well before the appointment and ate lightly before the dental appointment, this situation probably will not occur.

If vomiting does occur, help the patient to a position that will prevent aspiration from occurring. Hold the head over the cuspidor and use suction to assist evacuation (Swepston, 1976). Again, maintain the mask and flush the system so that the patient is breathing 100% oxygen. Supply the patient with a cool, wet towel to clean up. Refresh the operatory as quickly as possible. The patient probably will be embarrassed. Handle the situation promptly, comfort the patient, and finish the dental procedure. Prevention is possible by maintaining comfort at a lower level of nitrous oxide and observing the early signs of patient distress.

Although the most common side effects of nitrous oxide and oxygen sedation are nausea and vomiting, instances of dysphoria, claustrophobia, apprehension, and hallucination have also been described. Several cases of sexual phenomena have been reported that involved complaints to law enforcement agencies and required hearings before state dental boards. Usually these incidents have occurred when nitrous oxide was administered in concentrations greater than 50% and when the patient was sedated without an assistant in the room (Jastak, 1984). It is recommended that an additional person be present in the operatory when treating a patient of the opposite gender. In general, this seems a wise safety policy should an emergency occur for any of the individuals present in a clinical situation.

Conditions following sedation

In general, an episode of nitrous oxide sedation has no residual effects. The medication is inhaled, it influences the central nervous system while it circulates in the bloodstream, and it is exhaled unchanged. Depending on the nature of the patient and the length of sedation, the patient may retain a relaxed feeling. Often the dental procedure is itself tiring, and the patient may feel a bit fatigued. The age of the patient does not seem to be a significant factor in determining the response to nitrous oxide sedation (O'Reilly, 1983; Norton, 1984).

Normal functioning or driving is not contraindicated specifically because of nitrous oxide and oxygen conscious sedation, but the dentist or hygienist may recommend precautions according to the procedures performed or the patient's health status.

Patients returning to occupations that require operating heavy machinery, using highly skilled motor coordination, or making critical decisions may need to use discretion in returning to these functions. Conventional methods of assessing recovery from nitrous oxide may be inadequate. Somatosensory evoked potential tests may be useful in accurately describing recovery for specific tasks. Further studies are indicated, but early evidence shows recovery in some instances may be take longer than 25 to 30 minutes (Herwig, 1984). In general, recovery occurs within 15 minutes, with the patient feeling fine and able to perform as normal.

Care of the equipment

After the appointment, the inhalation equipment should be wiped with disinfectant. The nasal hood should be washed with soap and water, then placed in glutaraldehyde for 10 minutes. Rinse and dry the hood and wrap it for protection until the next appointment. Each week, all the tubing, reservoir bags, and nasal hoods should be placed in glutaraldehyde for 10 hours. They should be rinsed for 1 hour and dried (Yagiela, 1979).

CONCLUSION

Nitrous oxide and oxygen conscious sedation is a safe and effective means of providing comfortable dentistry to patients who require minor pain control and who are apprehensive about dental treatment. As the anxious patient gains confidence in the clinician and experiences several successful appointments, he or she may be weaned from nitrous oxide. One may find that increasing positive suggestion and decreasing nitrous oxide concentration produce the desired sedation. The patient is usually pleased with the realization of this new behavior. Seeing such a patient approach and accept dental care without fear is possibly the greatest benefit of nitrous oxide and oxygen conscious sedation.

ACTIVITIES

1. Given patient profiles, discuss the indication for nitrous oxide and oxygen conscious sedation.
2. Watch a demonstration of administration technique. Observe the experience of a clinic patient with nitrous oxide and oxygen conscious sedation.
3. Simulate administration of or actually administer nitrous oxide and oxygen conscious sedation to a lab partner. If actually administering sedation, share the variety of responses that were noted in the group.
4. Administer nitrous oxide and oxygen conscious sedation to an appropriate clinic patient.*

REVIEW QUESTIONS

1. Nitrous oxide and oxygen sedation is a form of conscious sedation. What does this mean (include a definition of conscious in your answer)?

*An instructor qualified to administer nitrous oxide and oxygen conscious sedation must supervise a student providing sedation to a clinic patient. Direct supervision during the induction phase and continued priority attention to this student and patient throughout the appointment are necessary.

2. Consider each of the following pairs. Check the characteristic that best describes nitrous oxide.
   a. Organic inhalation agent, odorless, and flammable
   a'. Inorganic inhalation agent, sweet smelling, and nonflammable
   b. Has a high blood gas solubility as compared with oxygen
   b'. Has a low blood gas solubility as compared with oxygen
   c. Eliminated unchanged by the lungs
   c'. Eliminated by the lungs as nitrogen
   d. An extremely potent anesthetic when administered with oxygen
   d'. A mildly potent anesthetic when administered with oxygen
   e. Affects the body's physiologic reaction to pain perception
   e'. Affects the person's psychologic reaction to pain perception
3. Explain why nitrous oxide and oxygen conscious sedation is contraindicated for persons with the following conditions:
   a. Emphysema
   b. Upper respiratory tract infection
4. Calculate the percentage of nitrous oxide being delivered to a patient at the flow of 4 liters per minute of nitrous oxide and 6 liters per minute of oxygen. How does this percentage relate to the level recommended for optimal sedation? If this patient were having a tooth extracted, would local anesthesia be indicated?
5. Identify three signs that indicate that the inhaled concentration of nitrous oxide is too great.

REFERENCES

ADA Council on Dental Materials and Devices: Expansion of the acceptable program, nitrous oxide scavenging equipment and nitrous oxide trace gas monitoring equipment. JADA 95:791, 1977.

ADA Council on Dental Therapeutics: Accepted dental therapeutics, ed 39, Chicago, 1982, American Dental Association.

Allen WA: Nitrous oxide in the surgery: pollution and scavenging. Some clinical experiences, Br Dent J 159(7):222, 1985.

Badger G, et al: Nitrous oxide waste gas in the pediatric operatory, JADA 104:480, 1982.

Bennett CR: Conscious sedation in dental practice, ed 2, St Louis, 1978, The CV Mosby Co.

Brown JP: Efficiency of three nitrous oxide relative analgesia scavenging systems, Dent Anaesth Sedat 13(1):5, 1984.

Bruce DL, et al: Causes of death among anesthesiologists: a 20 year survey, Anesthesiology 29:565, 1968.

Bruce DL, et al: Trace anesthetic effects on perceptual, cognitive and motor skills, Anesthesiology 40:453, 1974.

Chapman WR, et al: The analgetic effects of low concentration nitrous oxide compared in man with morphine sulfate, J Clinical Invest 22:871, 1943.

Christiansen JR, et al: Measurement of scavenged nitrous oxide in the dental operatory, Pediatr Dent 7(3):192, 1985.

Cohen EN, et al: Occupational disease among operating room personnel: a national study, Anesthesiology 41:321, 1974.

Cohen EN, et al: A survey of anesthetic health hazards among dentists, JADA 90:1291, 1975.

Cohen EN, et al: Occupational disease in dentistry and chronic exposure to trace anesthetic gases, JADA 101:21, 1980.

Control of occupational exposure to N_2O in the dental operatory. HEW Pub. (NIOSH) 77-171. Cincinnati, 1977, US Dept. of Health, Education and Welfare, Public Health Service Center for Disease Control. National Institute for Occupational Safety and Health.

Corbett TH, et al: Effects of low concentrations of nitrous oxide in rat pregnancy, Anest 39:299, 1973.

DeMartina BK, and Garber JG: Analgesia in dental practice, Contin Dent Educ 2:5, 1979.

Dentist's Desk Reference: Materials, Instruments, and Equipment, ed 2, Chicago, 1983, American Dental Association.

Dionne RA: The pharmacological basis of pain control in dental practice: N_2O_2, Compend Contin Educ Dent 2:271, 1981.

Duncan GH, et al: Nitrous oxide and the dental patient: a review of adverse reactions, JADA 108(2):213, 1984.

Dworkin SF, et al: Analgesic effects of nitrous oxide with controlled painful stimuli, JADA 107(4):581, 1983.

Dworkin SF, et al: Cognitive reversal of expected nitrous oxide analgesia for acute pain, Anesth Analg 62(12):1073, 1983.

Dworkin SF, et al: Cognitive modification of pain: information in combination with nitrous oxide, Pain 19(4):339, 1984.

Dworkin SF, et al: Psychological preparation influences nitrous oxide analgesia, replication of laboratory findings in a clinical setting, Oral Surg, Oral Med, Oral Pathol 61(1):108, 1986.

Fordham KC: Analgesia (medicated air). Booklet accepted for course credit by the Academy of General Dentistry, Radnor, Pa.

Getter L: Review and current status of scavenging and monitoring devices: report of ad hoc committee on trace anesthetics as a potential health hazard in dentistry, JADA 95:788, 1977.

Giovannitti JA: Nitrous oxide and oral premedication, Anesth Prog 31(2):56, 1984.

Hamburg HL: Establishing a standard technique for nitrous oxide/oxygen sedation, Dent Surv 56(3):28, 1980.

Hammond NI: Nitrous oxide and children's perception of pain, Pediatr Dent 6(4):238, 1984.

Heft MW, et al: Nitrous oxide analgesia: a psychological evaluation using verbal descriptor scaling, J Dent Res 63(2):129, 1984.

Herwig LD, et al: Time course of recovery following nitrous oxide administration, Anesth Prog 31(3):133, 1984.

Jastak JT, and Greenfield W: Trace contamination of anesthetic gases: a brief review, JADA 95:758, 1977.

Jastak JT, et al: Nitrous oxide and sexual phenomena, Dent Anaesth Sedat 13(2):56, 1984.

Kaufman E, et al: Nitrous oxide analgesia in selected dental patients, Anesth Prog 29:78, 1982.

Knill-Jones RP, et al: Controlled survey of women anesthetists in the United Kingdom, Lancet 1:1326, 1972.

Kripke BJ, et al: Testicular reaction to prolonged exposure to nitrous oxide, Anest 44:104, 1976.

Kripke BJ, et al: Hematological reaction to prolonged exposure to nitrous oxide, Anest 47:342, 1977.

Kucey SP: Nitrous oxide contamination in dentistry, Ont Dent 61(7):21, 1984.

Langa H: Relative analgesia in dental practice, inhalation analgesia and sedation with nitrous oxide, ed 2, Philadelphia, 1976, WB Saunders Co.

Littner MM, et al: Occupational hazards in the dental office and their control, IV: measures for controlling contamination of anesthetic gas, nitrous oxide, Quintessence Int 14:461, 1983.

Malamed SF: Sedation: a guide to patient management, ed 2, St Louis, 1989, The CV Mosby Co.

McKercher TC, et al: Recovery and enhancement of reflex reaction time after nitrous oxide analgesia, JADA 101:785, 1980.

Minnis R: Psychological effects of conscious sedation, Anesth Prog 26:150, 1979.

Moore PA: Psychomotor impairment due to nitrous oxide exposure, Anesth Prog 30(3):72, 1983.

Norton JC, et al: The effect of nitrous oxide and age on psychological and psychomotor performance, Anesth Prog 31(2):64, 1984.

O'Reilly JE, et al: The effects of nitrous oxide in the healthy elderly: nitrous oxide elimination and alveolar carbon dioxide, Anesth Prog 30(6):187, 1983.

Riklin BM: Nitrous oxide—oxygen sedation for the geriatric patient, J Am Soc Geriatr Dent 13(2):8, 1978.

Roberts GJ, et al: Physiological changes during relative analgesia—a clinical study, J Dent 10:55, 1978.

Rogo EJ, et al: Nitrous oxide: an occupational hazard for dental professionals, Dent Hyg 60(11):508, 1985.

Sweeney B, et al: Toxicity of bone marrow in dentists exposed to nitrous oxide, Br Med J 291(6495):567, 1985.

Sweeney B: Nitrous oxide: panacea or poison?, SAAD Dig 6(4):82, 1985.

Swenson RD: 1976. Scavenging of dental anesthetic gases, J Oral Surg 34:207, 1976.

Swepston BA: The practical use of oxygen—nitrous oxide conscious sedation in dental practice. Plano, Tex, 1976, Happiness Seminars.

Swepston B: Dental phobia becomes euphoria: advances of nitrous oxide, parts 1 and 2, Dent Pract 1(5):60, 1(6):42, 1980.

Thompson PL: Nitrous oxide as an analgesic in acute myocardial infarction, JAMA 235:924, 1976.

Troyer GT: Liability: important issue regarding nitrous oxide exposure, Dent Stud, 62(3):16, 1983.

Wald C: Nitrous oxide—are there any real contraindications? Quintessence Int 14:213, 1983.

Weinstein P, et al: The use of nitrous oxide in the treatment of children: results of a controlled study, JADA 112(3):325, 1986.

Yagiela JA, et al: Disinfection of nitrous oxide inhalation equipment, JADA 98:191, 1979.

33 MODIFICATION OF DENTAL HYGIENE CARE FOR PATIENTS WITH SPECIAL NEEDS

OBJECTIVES   *The reader will be able to*

1. Identify patients with special needs for whom dental hygiene care should be modified.
2. Modify dental hygiene care for patients with special needs in the following areas:
   a. Communication
   b. Appointment planning
   c. Environmental considerations such as equipment positioning and patient positioning
   d. Instruction for individualized home care
   e. Safety precautions in treatment
3. Identify the reasons for seeking specific resources to gain additional information regarding patients with sensory and physical limitations
4. Define the following:
   a. Dental phobia
   b. Shaping
5. Describe the oral side effects associated with different types of cancer therapy and discuss measures to prevent them or reduce their severity in oral cancer patients.
6. Describe major physiological and psychological changes associated with aging and suggest ways to accommodate these changes during dental hygiene treatment.
7. Discuss factors affecting the utilization of dental care by the elderly and suggest ways in which access barriers can be eliminated.
8. Discuss the role of the dental hygienist in alternative practice settings such as a nursing home, hospital, home care program, or other institutional setting.

Every patient needs to be treated as an individual with a unique personality, set of senses, and physical self. In fact, modifications in dental care are made regularly for patients with special needs. These patients include those who are very tall, very short, pregnant, or very young, as well as overweight and extremely fearful patients, patients with busy schedules, older patients, and patients who live far from the office.

In general, the professional team deals with these patients by modifying communication, appointment planning, chair and equipment considerations, and individualized instruction for home care. This same attention applies to patients who are handicapped in a mental, physical, or sensory way.

COMMUNICATION

Communication differs with each person. For patients who can see, looking at pictures, reading information, looking at and handling equipment, and observing other patients during dental procedures does much to acquaint them with care. Patients without sight can use hearing, touch, smell, and taste to explore dentistry. Depending on the sensory limitation, communication by way of the remaining senses helps the patient experience dentistry without fear. The clinician who takes time to reach out to these patients and to create a good dental experience will no doubt make friends as well as ensure the patients' cooperation.

Careful introductory procedures are useful for

patients who are deaf or blind. These patients lack essential sensory cues for determining what procedures are about to occur. A deaf person may be able to lipread. If so, the dental professional should speak to the patient only when the patient can see the professional's lips. It is usually annoying and embarrassing for the lipreading patient if the dental professional accentuates mouth movements in speaking or shouts. Speaking slowly but normally is usually most acceptable. A helpful tool for communication is to know sign language for the deaf or to write out a series of descriptions and questions for the patient.

For the blind patient, it is possible to describe procedures and allow the patient to feel the components of the dental operatory. For obvious reasons, sharp instruments should be felt only with caution and careful direction or not at all. Disinfection should follow the guided tour of equipment, and sterile instruments should replace those handled by the patient. This process should be explained to the patient to avoid arousing concern over why changes are being made.

Patients who may not understand the visual or verbal introduction to dentistry will need to take one step at a time. Every patient does better when surprises are minimized in a new and potentially frightening situation. Human qualities of friendliness, a calm manner, light touch, and gentle tone indicate in a universal language that the professional cares.

HOSPITALIZED, BEDRIDDEN, AND NURSING HOME PATIENTS

The oral health care of patients who are being cared for by others in the home, a hospital, nursing home, or other institution is all too often neglected because of the magnitude of other health problems, the inability to perform self-care, or the lack of time, knowledge, or motivation on the part of the individuals responsible for providing daily care. The dental hygienist can assist in the delivery of improved oral health care to patients who are bedridden and/or institutionalized by providing direct dental hygiene services to them and by teaching family members or institutional staff members how to provide effective, daily oral hygiene. Although the hygienist's role will be discussed in the context of a nursing home, much of the information in this section is applicable to

other settings as well, including care of the homebound, hospitalized, or any individuals who must depend on others for their care.

The federal government has specified certain requirements related to dental care that must be met by nursing homes in order to receive Medicare funding. All skilled nursing facilities must retain the services of an advisory dentist who is responsible for performing annual oral examinations, arranging for dental inservice training, establishing written policies regarding dental care, and providing emergency dental care. In some cases the advisory dentist may be the provider of routine dental care, or the facility may make arrangements for obtaining routine care with other dental services in the community. Intermediate care facilities are not required to retain an advisory dentist, although facilities that provide both skilled and intermediate care must follow the regulations that apply to skilled nursing facilities. State regulations governing dental care delivery in nursing homes vary from state to state, as does the degree of compliance of individual nursing homes to federal regulations. Dental hygienists who wish to work in nursing homes should familiarize themselves with the regulations which govern the provision of dental care in institutional settings.

Depending on the requirements of state dental practice acts, the hygienist may be permitted to perform some or all clinical procedures associated with dental hygiene treatment, including oral screenings, complete dental examinations, periodontal assessments, prophylaxis, taking radiographs, and oral hygiene instructions. Requirements for dental supervision of the hygienist within institutional settings vary from one state to another.

The delivery of care may occur in several different ways. Individuals who are mentally and physically capable of leaving the institutional facility may be transported to private dental practices or public dental clinics. Some larger health care facilities may be equipped with a dental operatory for on-site dental care. When patients who are homebound or in long-term care facilities cannot be transported to a dental office, dental treatment can be provided on-site with the help of portable dental equipment or in mobile vans equipped for dental procedures.

The dental hygienist also may assume an administrative function. Dental hygienists are well trained to serve as liaisons between the facility, the advisory dentist, and the professional dental community to coordinate the provision of dental care to residents. Tasks include assessing the needs of residents and staff members; planning for the treatment needs of residents and the educational needs of both staff and residents; establishing dental protocols, records, and schedules; securing necessary resources; coordinating treatment and examination procedures; and evaluating the success of the dental program in improving the oral health of the patient population. Knowledge of dentistry, communication skills, and skills related to assessment, planning, implementation, and evaluation of dental health programs are necessary prerequisites for this role.

The dental hygienist can provide oral health education to residents and inservice training to staff members. Residents who are capable of performing their own oral hygiene procedures should be taught proper plaque control and preventive skills and their importance for overall health and well-being. The nursing home responsible for their care must also ensure that these individuals have access to regular oral screenings or dental examinations to ensure prompt diagnosis of dental problems.

Planning for the needs of residents who cannot perform oral hygiene care independently requires a different focus for the dental hygienist. Unless the dental hygienist is a full-time employee of the institution, educational efforts are more effective if they are aimed at the care-providers rather than at the actual residents themselves. Time and resources should be directed toward teaching those staff members who are responsible for assisting residents with their oral hygiene care the importance of that task and how to perform it effectively.

Inservice programs provided by the dentist and/or hygienist should attempt to teach care providers, usually nurses' aides, the importance of maintaining their own personal oral hygiene and effective plaque control and preventive methods. Once they are informed and motivated to meet these needs for themselves, they will be more likely to understand the importance of providing daily oral hygiene care for others. Topics that may be covered during inservice programs include oral cancer screening, periodontal disease, dental caries (especially root caries), care of dental appliances, identification methods for dental appliances, and daily oral hygiene care.

The majoriy of oral hygiene care for residents of a nursing home is provided or monitored by nurses' aides. For these individuals, providing oral hygiene care is just one item in a long list of duties that they are assigned to perform or to assist the patient with daily. Time is a limiting factor in their ability to perform and/or monitor daily oral hygiene care. In addition, their understanding of the importance of oral health care and their motivation to maintain optimal oral hygiene may be limited. Many people, including other health care providers, may find it distasteful and unpleasant to clean someone else's mouth.

Therefore, the challenge that faces the dental hygienist is to share with these individuals how important it is for the overall well-being of their patients or residents to perform and/or monitor these tasks. Staff members also will be more interested and attentive when they understand how the information presented is relevant to their job performance and that they will find it helpful in solving day-to-day problems. They should be told why daily mouth care is important in terms of eating, speaking, sociability, and esthetics as well as for health reasons. Planning educational experiences that will help them understand how they would feel if they traded places with the patient or resident may help motivate them to perform these tasks.

Information presented should be useful, simple, and interesting. Adult learners tend to prefer activities, such as problem-solving sessions, demonstrations, and hands-on practice, rather than lecture presentations. Effective use of visual aids will also enhance audience attention and understanding of the information presented. The American Dental Association and the American Dental Hygienists' Association are excellent resources for both written and audiovisual materials that can be used to plan and deliver effective inservice presentations.

Oral hygiene care

Before determining the appropriate oral hygiene care for a resident or patient, the hygienist must have a clear idea of the dental and medical status of the individual. Close consultation among the dental hygienist, supervising dentist, nursing staff, and physician is necessary to ensure that there are no medical contraindications to the prescribed dental hygiene treatment or to the oral hygiene procedures. Based on this information, the hygienist can tailor dental hygiene procedures to meet individual patient needs. The following suggestions for daily oral hygiene care may be helpful for these patients.

Care for dependent patients. Dependent patients include individuals who are bedridden or those who must rely on nursing staff for daily oral care. They may be dependent because of mental incapacity, physical disability, or loss of consciousness. Oral hygiene care for these patients must be provided at least once and preferably twice daily.

If the patient is confined to an adjustable bed, position the bed at a 30- to 45-degree angle before performing oral hygiene procedures. The patient can also be elevated by propping several firm pillows behind the back. A towel should be placed over the patient's chest. Patients who can expectorate should have an emesis basin placed under their chin in which to empty the mouth. If the patient is unconscious or unable to expectorate, it is important that oral hygiene procedures do not introduce quantities of fluids that could be aspirated. Bedridden patients will also benefit from the use of portable oral evacuators to remove excess fluids during oral hygiene procedures. The patient's face should be turned toward the operator.

Patients who are not bedridden can be positioned for oral hygiene procedures in a chair or wheelchair located near a sink. The hygienist should stand behind the patient and lean the head back so that the oral cavity can be seen. Head support may be provided by the hygienist's arm or body or by a portable headrest attached to the chair. One hand is used to open the mouth and retract soft tissues while the other hand is used to clean the teeth and soft tissues. Use of disposable gloves is required when providing any type of intraoral care.

The lips should be lubricated prior to beginning oral hygiene procedures to prevent discomfort and cracking. If the patient cannot cooperate in open-

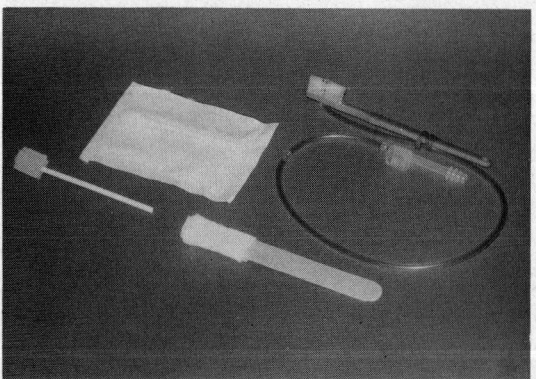

Fig. 33-1. Special aids for controlling plaque for hospitalized, institutionalized, bedridden patients. Top left: premoistened swabs; top right: tongue blade wrapped with gauze; bottom left: disposable foam "brush."

ing the mouth, the mouth may be propped open by a commercial mouth prop, a rolled washcloth or a mouth prop made by wrapping several tongue blades together.

If the patient has natural teeth, they should be brushed and flossed thoroughly. If the patient is unconscious or bedridden, do not use a regular foaming-type dentifrice due to the risk of aspiration of fluids. Instead, clean the teeth with a brush which has been moistened in water, mouthwash, or sodium bicarbonate solution. If use of a regular toothbrush is contraindicated due to bleeding problems or danger of bacteremia, a disposable foam toothbrush (e.g., toothette) or a gauze square wrapped around a finger may be substituted for more gentle cleaning. Patients who are conscious but bedridden may benefit from the use of a suction toothbrush, which is attached to oral evacuation equipment so that all excess fluids used during the brushing procedure are removed from the mouth through the head of the toothbrush (Fig. 33-1). A nonfoaming, ingestible dentifrice (e.g, NASAdent) may also be helpful for those patients. Teeth should be flossed by hand or with the help of a floss holder unless interproximal cleaning procedures are contraindicated by the patient's medical status.

The tongue should be lightly brushed or wiped clean. Other soft tissues in the mouth should be cleaned with moistened gauze squares, disposable sponge applicators, or anti-plaque rinse saturated swabs. Use of a brush-on fluoride gel is recommended for prevention of dental caries in long-term care patients who can tolerate that procedure. Following cleaning, patients who can rinse may do so with lukewarm water or a mouthwash. Water for rinsing may be delivered through a straw or by a syringe and then emptied into the emesis basin or evacuated with a suction device if one is available. For patients who cannot rinse, the mouth can be wiped with gauze squares or a clean damp washcloth. Soft tissues may be lubricated with mineral oil or artificial saliva preparations. Massaging the gums with the fingers may help stimulate circulation in those tissues.

Patients who wear dentures should have them cleaned daily and removed from the mouth at night. Denture care should follow the guidelines discussed in Chapter 27. Patients who do not require their dentures for eating or talking (e.g., unconscious patients) should have all removable appliances removed from the mouth.

Dentures should also be marked with the name of the individual or an identifying number so that they can be returned to the proper individual if they are misplaced. As this is a common problem in nursing homes, nursing home staff and dental consultants should be responsible for checking all dentures to make sure they are clearly labelled. Ways in which this can be accomplished are discussed in Chapter 27. These techniques should be discussed with nursing home staff so that they are able to perform this service themselves.

Care for those needing partial assistance. Patients who are capable of performing their own oral hygiene care should have access to the supplies necessary for daily home care. Oral hygiene kits can be organized and distributed according to the patient's dental needs. Items that might be supplied include the following:

1. *For patients with natural teeth:* Toothbrush, floss, mouthwash, disclosing tablets
2. *For patients with dentures:* Denture brush, denture cleaning tablets, denture cup, mouth swabs
3. *For patients with both teeth and dentures:* A combination of the items listed above
4. *For completely edentulous patients:* Mouthwash, mouth swabs

These residents may need individualized oral hygiene instructions provided either by the dental hygienist or trained nursing staff members. Special adaptations of oral hygiene aids should be recommended to those with physical handicaps (see Chapter 19).

The interest of the nursing staff is a critical factor in ensuring that these individuals are maintaining adequate oral hygiene and receiving positive reinforcement for their efforts. Oral hygiene care is one function that many patients can provide independently, and they should be encouraged to do so not only because it relieves the workload of the staff but especially because it reinforces the patient's self-esteem through the exercise of some independence and control. Because of the day-to-day contact that nursing staff have with institutionalized patients, they often are aware of factors likely to motivate individuals to maintain their oral hygiene, and they can be more successful in encouraging behavior change than dental professionals who are not known by the patients.

Residents of long-term care facilities should receive regular screening exams by nursing staff and complete oral examinations by dental professionals to detect problems that need treatment, including periodontal disease, caries, mobile teeth, soft tissue abnormalities, broken restorations or appliances, and poorly fitting dentures. Nursing staff who supervise and provide oral hygiene care should also be trained to recognize common oral problems and report them to a dental professional so that prompt diagnosis can be made.

Access to dental care must be provided for all individuals, including those who reside in institutions or those who are homebound. The dental hygienist can play an important role in providing access through the delivery of dental hygiene treatment and the provision of oral health education to care providers. Health promotion efforts to organize preventive programs where none exist and to involve other dental professionals in finding alternative ways to provide care for these individuals also are necessary. Dental hygienists' skills are needed in a variety of settings other than traditional private practice. Health promotion efforts should be focused on educating community leaders, other health care providers, and legislators regarding the skills which dental hygienists possess so that more of the access barriers that separate dental consumers with special needs from professional dental hygiene care can be eliminated.

DENTAL CARE FOR PREGNANT PATIENTS

A few modifications in care are necessary for *pregnant patients*. Women of childbearing age should be questioned about pregnancy through the medical history or recall history update before treatment. During the first trimester of pregnancy, the fetus is undergoing critical development of all organs and tissues. At this stage, called organogenesis, the unborn child is most susceptible to substances or events that could disturb normal growth. Exposure to certain medications and radiation could adversely affect the well-being of the mother and developing fetus. If there is a possibility that the patient may be pregnant, the taking of diagnostic radiographs should be delayed. Routine prophylaxis and examination can be performed if the patient is feeling well. Otherwise, all elective dental work can be postponed until the second trimester of pregnancy or until after the child is delivered.

It is best to provide treatment for the pregnant patient in the last half of the second trimester (fifth or sixth month). At this point, organogenesis is completed. The patient may be feeling quite well, and the weight and size of the fetus will generally not cause the patient discomfort when she is in the supine position. In later stages of pregnancy, the enlarged fetus puts pressure on major abdominal veins, causing blockage of venous return from the legs when the patient is supine. Hypotension and syncope can result if the patient is reclined for too long.

In general, all medications should be avoided throughout pregnancy. However, routine restorative dentistry can be provided with local anesthesia during the second and third trimesters. Additional vasoconstrictors are not necessary in anesthetic solutions. Nitrous oxide analgesia and general anesthesia are contraindicated. In emergency situations, many medications can be administered safely during pregnancy. The clinician should have the full support of the patient's obstetrician before prescribing or administering any type of analgesic, sedative, or antibiotic.

If radiographic diagnosis is essential, radiographs may be taken late in the second trimester or in the early part of the third trimester. To limit radiation to the patient, only a single film of the area in question should be exposed. The x-ray unit should have proper collimation and shielding. High-speed film and a long-cone/high-voltage technique are recommended. The patient is also protected by the lead shield drape as usual (Gier and Janes, 1983).

Patient education is important for the pregnant patient. This is an ideal time for the clinician to lay to rest the myths about decalcification of the mother's teeth and loss of teeth due to pregnancy. It is an especially good time to review the need for good home care habits and plaque control. In 1965 Löe studied 121 prenatal and postnatal women for signs of clinical inflammation. Gingival changes occurred in 100% of the subjects. Changes were noted as early as 8 weeks' gestation and were most severe by 8 months' gestation. The accumulation of plaque paralleled the gingival changes. When complete removal of plaque was accomplished, resolution of gingivitis usually occurred. Other factors contribute to gingivitis and oral problems during pregnancy. For example, preexisting periodontal conditions may be aggravated by hormonal changes. Home care habits may change as a result of general fatigue. Nausea and vomiting associated with "morning sickness' may make oral hygiene difficult. If the gag reflex is easily stimulated, the patient may avoid brushing and flossing. Vomiting will produce a temporary acidic state in the oral cavity, leaving the teeth more susceptible to attack. Providing understanding and support for the pregnant patient is as important as encouraging good oral hygiene habits and a noncariogenic diet.

The clinician should ask whether the patient is receiving nutritional information in conjunction with prenatal classes at the medical clinic or hospital. If not, this is something the dental staff should provide. The pregnant patient has increased demands for protein, calories, calcium, iron, and vitamins A, B-complex, C, and D (Williams, 1982). The function of these nutrients during gestation and the types of food or supplements they may be found in is important information to cover. (See Chapter 20 for more nutritional information.) The teeth begin to develop in the fetus at 6 weeks. Substances consumed during pregnancy can affect the development of the teeth. Overconsumption of fluoride during gestation can cause fluorosis of the deciduous teeth. Some antibiotics taken during pregnancy may stain developing teeth (Cheney and DePaola, 1979). A discussion of the importance of supplemental fluoride after the birth of the child to prevent decay can be mentioned at this time also. Ideally, the mother and child can be seen at a future appointment to review fluorides, eruption dates, and the beginnings of home care for the infant.

While the patient is pregnant is a good time to review the role of plaque and the frequency of sugar consumption as related to tooth decay. This will be beneficial to the patient and will be useful information in feeding the child later. Baby bottle syndrome is a condition that fits in nicely with such a discussion of sugar and decay. The patient may not be aware of the danger to the teeth when a child is put to bed with a bottle of milk or juice to nurse through the night. Characteristic rampant decay on the facial surfaces of the teeth can result from such a practice.

Usually the pregnant patient is very receptive to any information concerning the well-being of the expected child in addition to being interested in having a safe and healthy pregnancy. The clinician should be ready to act as a resource for any questions the patient may have throughout this time. If gingival problems occur, an appointment to remove irritating calculus and review plaque control may be appreciated. A parent who is informed and motivated about dental health will be an excellent model for the child. Seemingly routine information provided to the pregnant patient may be more meaningful than ever before.

MANAGEMENT OF PATIENTS ENCOUNTERING DENTISTRY FOR THE FIRST TIME

Occasionally a dental professional sees an *adult who is encountering dentistry for the first time or who is frightened because of previous negative dental experiences*. If fear of pain was the primary reason the patient avoided dental care, the "day of reckoning" when the patient does appear may be the zenith of anxiety for the patient. The very reason for the visit may be to alleviate the pain of a toothache or badly inflamed oral tissues. Thus the patient is in pain and is fearing further pain; a situation such as this requires careful handling. Even if the patient's long delay in seeking dental care is not directly related to fear, the messages about dentistry that people see on television, in cartoons, in comic routines, and in other media frequently connote pain and discomfort for the dental patient.

The patient may be expecting that dental care will be close to the stereotypes shown in the movies *Little Shop of Horrors, Marathon Man,* or *The Inlaws* or to the comic routines of Bill Cosby and others. The object of the first and subsequent encounters is to disprove those negative images.

The process begins with the phone call to the office, which may be a difficult, tenuous step for the patient. When accepting calls from new patients, the hygienist must listen for signs of distress and follow up with reflective listening that clarifies the source of the patient's anxiety. The patient should hear comfort and concern and encouragement. The patient could be reacting to anticipated pain and to cinematic or comedic stereotypes. Or the patient may be recalling a horrendous experience with dentistry, usually one in which the clinician would not stop treatment despite repeated complaints of pain.

The patient may have had a negative encounter with dentistry that has resulted in a high level of anxiety and avoidance; this is called *dental phobia,* which is a fear of dentistry that "has ballooned all out of proportion." The office staff should move into a *shaping* mode, in which the patient is incrementally reintroduced to dentistry through a series of nonthreatening encounters with staff, environment, equipment, and finally dental procedures. This often includes a preliminary appointment at which the patient is guided through sequential muscle relaxation and breathing exercises and may listen to audio tapes designed to soothe and distract him or her from anxiety. Relatively noninvasive procedures such as oral hygiene instructions and a head and neck examination may be introduced early, followed by a dental and periodontal charting at a subsequent visit. For some patients, shaping must be broken down into even smaller steps, including time to examine and hold a dental mirror, followed by the patient placing it in his or her own mouth and then the clinician holding it in the patient's mouth with no other instruments in sight. Each instrument and procedure is gradually introduced, with the clinician emphasizing by words and actions that the procedures will not be uncomfortable and that the patient can stop the clinician at any time. The patient should be given a hand signal to use to stop the clinician if discomfort is experienced (Kroeger, 1987).

Early steps in working with dental phobics may occur away from the dental office or in the consultation room away from the dental chair and other equipment. For some people, getting into the dental chair will be the seventh or eighth shaping step. Remember to explain to the patient that the chair will be placed in a supine position; moving into the flat-on-the-back position can trigger a sense of vulnerability. Gradually, patients can be reintroduced to dental procedures, including local anesthesia ("the needle") and "the drill," two of the most dreaded procedures. The patient should be reassured that these procedures can and will be performed so that there is little or no discomfort. Pain management techniques such as those suggested in Chapters 31 and 32 should be followed so that the implied promises of comfort are kept. When discomfort can be expected, the patient should be forewarned and the type of sensation described. Discomfort should never come as a surprise (Kroeger, 1987).

Similarly, if the patient has never had dental treatment, the emphasis is on introducing the patient to each item, describing its use and then moving ahead with procedures that are least threatening. The patient may be terrified of the anticipated evils that can be inflicted with an innocent tri-syringe; such terror can be avoided if the patient feels free to ask, "What is that?" The sequence for the first-time adult patient will typically move more quickly than that for the dental phobic.

Often the first-time adult patient or the dental phobic will call for an appointment because he or she is in pain. The pain should be relieved promptly. This situation may require the use of a sedative, analgesia, or some other method that makes dental care possible and as pleasant as pos-sible under the circumstances. Today's dentistry is unlikely to live up to the expectations of those who have avoided it because of fear, so even an uncomfortable procedure may be a pleasant experience in contrast to what the patient's mind has created or remembered.

A baffling experience for a clinician is the patient who complains of pain when the procedure typically does not create discomfort. A natural and typical reaction is one of disbelief. How could the patient complain about discomfort during a simple charting or polishing? An anxious patient has tense muscles. A person who has significant muscle tension is more likely to experience pain. Also, a person who believes a procedure will be painful will probably feel pain regardless of how benign the procedure may be. The memory bank of sights, sounds, smells, and feelings can be so vivid and so closely associated with pain that the patient reacts with pain as a conditioned response to those stimuli. If the patient can be relaxed and distracted from worry and negative stimuli, the psychological/physiological transmission of pain can be minimized. Any procedure that creates perceived pain should be halted and steps taken to distract, relax, or otherwise reduce the sensations. This may require anesthesia, analgesia, or other steps (Kroeger, 1987).

Introducing a *child patient* to dentistry follows many of the guidelines used for fearful or first-time adults. The child should be introduced sequentially to pleasant, simple procedures using a guided, experiential approach.

Infants who have a developmental disorder or whose parents have poor dental health should see the dentist not later than 6 months of age. Other children should be seen for their first appointment between the ages of 18 and 24 months (Wei and Nowak, 1982). Many clinicians follow the guideline of seeing children as soon as primary teeth appear. They use this appointment to introduce the parent to the day-to-day attention that should be given to the child's oral health so that the child grows up with good habits and an awareness of dental health.

The infant or toddler should be escorted into the operatory with the parent. The parent should sit in the dental chair and hold the child. The child's head should be placed in the crook of the parent's arm, with the other arm holding the child's body. This will help control the movements of the child and prevent accidents (Wright, Starkey, and Gardner, 1983). The clinician should focus on examining the oral structures for normal eruption patterns and overall proper growth and development. Counseling regarding diet, the use of pacifiers, the effects of finger- or thumb-sucking, and what to expect in the coming months with regard to eruption of teeth can occur during these early-age appointments. The parent can be shown how to wipe plaque from the gum pads and to brush the newly erupted teeth.

Once the child is old enough to aim a toothbrush into the mouth, dental appointments shift toward a shared parent/child responsibility for deplaquing the teeth. The child and parent are shown the evidence of plaque with disclosing solution, and a toothbrush and a pea-size portion of fluoride toothpaste are used to remove the plaque. The parent and the child are instructed in the proper use of the brush. The parent should be shown how to support the child's head while brushing his or her teeth, but the child should be given the opportunity to use the brush to imitate the proper motions. The goal is to remove all the plaque during the appointment and for the parent to ensure that it is removed daily, with both brush and floss, in order to minimize caries and gingival inflammation (Wei and Nowak, 1982).

It is vital that the parents minimize the child's exposure to fluoride toothpaste. Children tend to like the sweet-tasting paste and can be found eating it or loading it onto the toothbrush. The fluoride levels in toothpaste, particularly in the higher-concentration formulas, can contribute to fluorosis (permanent spotting of the developing enamel) and even to a toxic reaction when they are used in combination with fluoridated water and other dietary sources of fluoride. Children should either brush under supervision with only a minuscule portion of fluoride paste or be given nonfluoride toothpaste to use. Most clinicians will recommend the former of those two alternatives, opting for the benefits of frequent low doses of fluoride to remineralize enamel.

Dietary evaluation is an important part of early dental care. Patterns of snacking and foods typically eaten during mealtime should be examined for cariogenicity and for a good balance of essen-

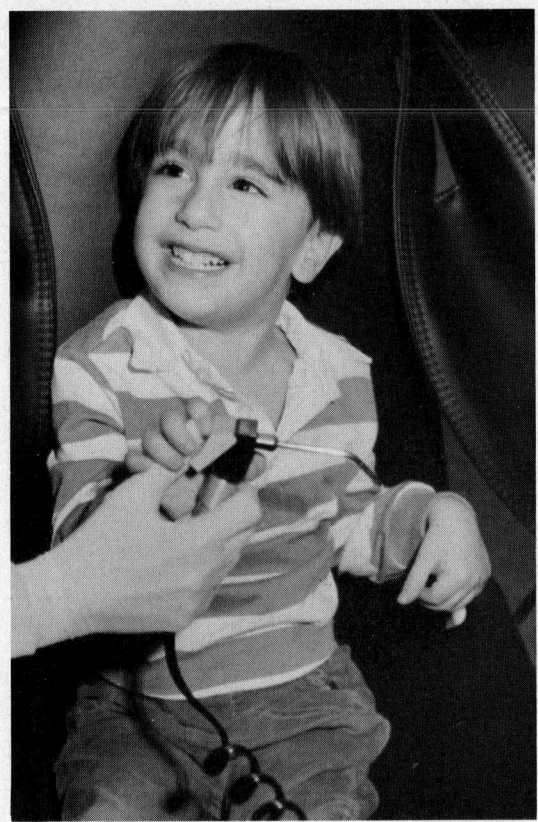

Fig. 33-2. A child's introduction to the dental environment should be experiential. Child may be given an opportunity to push buttons that cause the "spaceship chair" to rise and descend and to use the "squirt gun."

tial nutrients. Fluoride supplements should be prescribed if the water supply is not fluoridated. (See Chapter 28).

If a child of 2 or 3 years of age (or older) has never visited a dental office, time will need to be spent introducing the child to the dental equipment and procedures. The child may be encouraged to push the buttons once or twice or to make the "spaceship chair" rise and descend. The brave health care provider may even let the child operate the air and water "squirt gun" as long as the target is well-defined, such as a cup or sink (Figs. 33-2 and 33-3).

The mouth mirror and explorer may be the only two instruments needed for the first visit. The mirror is usually easily understood as a magic way to see the backs of the teeth and to shine

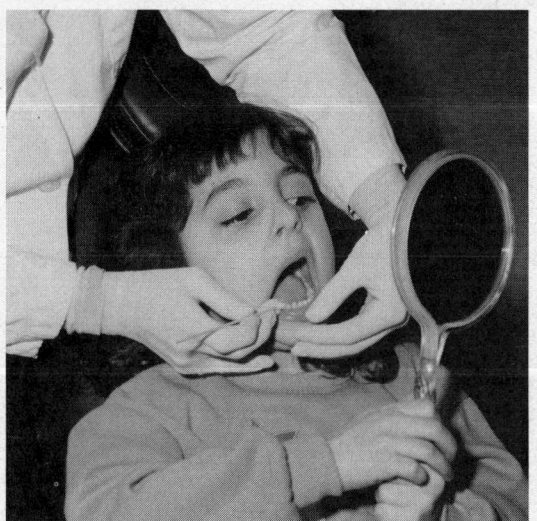

Fig. 33-3. Counting teeth with child observing in mirror involves child in beginning stages of care and familiarizes child with having a metal instrument and mouth mirror in mouth.

light into the dark corners. The explorer is a magic wand that counts sparkles on the teeth and checks to see if the teeth are strong. The child can hold a hand mirror while the clinician checks for caries and counts sparkles. For a preliminary procedure, it can be used to count teeth. Most children are amazed to learn that they have 20 or more teeth. While counting molars, it is possible to point out the large teeth that are nestled way in the back that need extra brushing. The clinician should always place a fingertip next to the sharp point of the explorer when moving in or out of the mouth or when moving from one tooth to another, in order to prevent sticking the child.

Occasionally, small pieces of calculus may be found on the lingual surfaces of the mandibular anterior teeth and on the facial surfaces of the maxillary molars; these can be removed with a scaler or curette. If the child is comfortable with the explorer feeling the teeth, the scaler should be easily accepted also. It may be necessary to gently caution the child to sit very still during the critical moments of adaptation. Asking the child to open wide, "like an alligator," helps keep a space available for getting hands and instruments inside the mouth. If the child has a tendency to inadvertently close slowly, the first and second fingers of the hand holding the mirror can be placed between the maxillary and mandibular arches to ensure at least a two-finger width space for access to the teeth. For the child whose jaws gently drift closed, this technique is quite useful and is tolerated well by the child. This technique becomes highly undesirable if the child closes forcibly. The resultant pain experienced by the clinician can be considerable. A rubber mouth prop is a better choice for this patient.

If stains are present on the teeth, it may be necessary to polish selected teeth with an abrasive. If a motor-driven handpiece is to be used, it can be described as an electric toothbrush. An unattached rubber cup can be handed to the child to squeeze to see how soft it is. The unattached cup can then be rubbed first on the child's fingernail to prove its harmlessness and then on the front of a central incisor. Explaining that toothpaste goes in the rubber cup helps the child figure out why the electric toothbrush has no brush.

It helps to show how the cup attaches to the prophylaxis angle and then to the handpiece. With all the parts assembled, the cup should again be rubbed on the tooth to show that it feels the same. A critical point is when the handpiece is activated and begins to hum or whistle. To prepare for that, it can be explained that the cup could be rubbed by hand on the teeth but that it would take a long time to do it. Most children have plans for some pleasant activity following a dental appointment, which they do not wish to delay. The electric toothbrush helps make sure the child will not be late. The rotating cup should be applied with *light intermittent pressure* on the fingernail and then on an incisor. Then polishing paste ("toothpaste") is added, and stains are polished off.

The saliva ejector attachment (a "straw") for the high-volume suction should be used to evacuate saliva and the abrasive, as small children cannot easily control swallowing and expectoration.

In many cases neither calculus nor stain will be evident on the teeth. Both scaling and polishing are in these cases unnecessary. More appropriate is the use of a disclosant with the child locating the calculus and brushing (and flossing with assistance) to remove it.

After plaque is removed, a topical fluoride treatment may be appropriate. (See Chapter 28). Care must be taken that the child does not swallow the fluoride. Ingesting the fluoride gel can cause nausea, vomiting, and illness. Large quantities can cause death.

Dental hygiene care procedures do not cause great discomfort; in many instances, there is none at all. Therefore the dental hygiene appointment can be an important opportunity to build a trusting relationship, free from fear, which can focus on preventing maladies that could require less pleasant dental appointments.

The following general guidelines are helpful in preparing for a child patient (Bailey, 1979; Goose and Kurer, 1973; Huggins, 1973; McDonald and Avery, 1983; Roche, 1975; Wei and Nowak, 1982; and Wright, Starkey, and Gardner, 1983; Andlaw and Rock, 1987; Pinkham, 1988):

1. Do not keep the child waiting.
2. Call the child by name, touch him or her gently, and give the child a big smile. Project that you are happy to see the child.
3. Gently guiding the child to the operatory or to the sink and plaque-counting area while holding the child's hand helps the child feel confidence in the clinician. For first visits it may be wise to start with plaque counting and finish with exploring and any necessary scaling, polishing, and fluoride treatment.
4. If the child is crying, it may help to whisper in the child's ear, "I can't understand you when you cry," or "You can't hear me when you cry." The whispering may do the trick; it is a shocking contrast to most people's response to crying. Another phrase that may help is, "Why are you crying?" whispered in the ear. After hearing the child's answer (usually "I want to go home"), point out all the assets of the day: "How many teeth do you think you have? We were going to count them! And we were going to make sure that your teeth are bright and shiny! If you go home, we're going to miss all that. Besides, I've been waiting all day to meet you. I'd really like to spend a little time with you."
5. Be *truthful*.
6. A voice intonation that reflects calm, firm, gentle control and understanding is often more important than the content of what is said.
7. "Attention must be obtained for communication to take place, and communication *must* occur before behavior shaping commences" (Wright, Starkey, and Gardner, 1983).
8. *Do not use baby talk.* Use a gentle adult-to-adult tone with simple words.
9. Use the "tell, show, do" method before every procedure.
10. Praise the child; take a genuine interest in the child's life, ideas, activities; help the child feel important.
11. If the child will not open his or her mouth, it can be useful to teasingly say, "I bet you don't have any teeth in there. Do you have teeth in there? Give me just a peek." As soon as the teeth peek out, praise them and exclaim, "I guess you *do* have teeth. How many?" The child will probably suggest a number such as 6, 7, or 58. Counting them answers the question and permits some preliminary inspection and caries detection.
12. Usually the parent of a child over 3 years of age remains in the reception area during treatment. However, if the parent must be in the room, it is wise to suggest that the conversation be limited to hygienist and child. A three-way discussion is confusing for the child, overly directive or distracting, and counterproductive. The parent should be fully involved during dental health education.
13. When working with a chairside assistant, be certain conversation is directed toward the child. The child should be the center of attention.

The child's first encounter with dentistry and all subsequent visits should be positive and rewarding for both patient and clinician and should contribute to lifelong oral hygiene and prevention. They should form a bond of professional friendship that makes dental care a pleasure.

DENTAL MANAGEMENT OF CANCER PATIENTS

In 1987 approximately 965,000 Americans were diagnosed as having cancer; of that number, 30,000 had some type of oral cancer (Silverberg, and Lubera, 1987). Advances in medical technology and increased awareness of the importance of early detection of cancer have resulted in increased survival rates among cancer patients. Therefore, it is important for the hygienist to educate and motivate all dental consumers to perform regular oral cancer self-assessments to improve the chances that abnormal conditions will be recognized and diagnosed at early stages. It is also important to stress the need for regular dental examinations for all patients, especially those in high risk categories for contracting oral cancer.

It is likely that dental hygienists will encounter patients in clinical practice settings who are preparing for cancer therapy or who have undergone cancer therapy. The dental hygienist can perform a critical role in helping patients preserve their dentition and prevent oral complications which can arise as a result of cancer therapy. The purpose of this section is to inform the dental hygienist of the general physical and oral side effects associated with cancer and its therapy and to discuss measures which can be used to prevent or manage oral complications of cancer therapy.

Types of cancer therapy

Cancer treatment may involve one or a combination of the following methods: surgery, radiation treatment, or chemotherapy. Therapy for types of head and neck cancer involves surgical removal of the tumor, which is most successful for localized, accessible tumors. Since a margin of healthy tissue surrounding the tumor must also be excised to ensure removal of all abnormal tumor cells, this treatment may involve loss of a significant amount of healthy tissue.

The oral complications of surgery may include facial disfigurement, speech impairment, the need for a special prosthesis to restore function, or the loss of function of muscles of facial expression or mastication. Consider the extent of these complications for each individual and be prepared to adapt regular treatment procedures and home care instructions so that they accommodate any loss of function that the patient may have experienced as a result of surgery. If the patient has been fitted with a special intraoral prosthetic device, consult with the maxillofacial specialist who designed the device regarding recommendations for its care so that instructions regarding the care of the appli-ances or prosthesis can be reinforced during regular dental visits.

A second approach is radiation treatment. Radiation can be delivered to the cancer site in one of four ways: (1) external irradiation, in which the source of radiation is outside the body; (2) perioral irradiation, in which the radiation beam is directed through a cone into the oral cavity directly to the surface of the tumor; (3) interstitial irradiation, in which radioactive material is implanted directly into the tissues to be treated; or (4) surface irradiation, in which an applicator containing radioactive material is applied to the surface being treated (e.g., lip) and the patient wears the applicator until the desired dose is delivered (Chen, 1986). Tumor size determines the dose. To improve the effectiveness of radiation therapy and to minimize the damage to normal tissues, the total dosage is delivered in equal daily doses over several weeks. For instance, a common dose of 6000 to 7000 rads is delivered in doses of 200 rads per day, five days a week, for six to seven weeks (Chen, 1986).

Radiation treatment can cause mucositis, taste alteration, limited mouth opening, xerostomia, rampant caries, and osteoradionecrosis. The occurrence, severity, and duration of these side effects vary among individuals according to the areas being treated, the type of radiation used, dosage, and duration of treatment.

Chemotherapeutic drugs have the capacity to destroy rapidly growing and reproducing cancer cells. Unfortunately, these drugs are not selective in their effects and also destroy actively producing normal cells, including hair follicles, bone marrow cells, and oral mucosa.

Oral side effects of chemotherapy include mucositis, dental neuropathy, xerostomia, dental caries, oral bleeding, and oral infections. Sonis and others (1978) found that 40% of all chemotherapy patients develop oral complications of treatment. The severity varies among individuals depending on the type, dosage, and duration of therapy (McClure et al, 1987a).

There are a number of other physical symptoms and problems that may affect cancer patients. These conditions may be due to the effects of the cancer itself, responses to cancer therapy, or psychological reactions to the diagnosis of cancer or to its treatment. They include: anemia, bleeding from skin or mucous membranes, constipation, diarrhea, fatigue, hair loss, itchy skin, loss of appetite, nausea and vomiting, pain, respiratory problems, sexual and reproductive problems, and urinary tract problems. Awareness of these potential problems helps the dental hygienist be more effective in treating cancer patients.

Pretherapy management

A dental consultation should be scheduled for all cancer patients before therapy begins. The chances of maintaining a healthy dentition and minimizing side effects of cancer treatment are closely related to the health of the oral tissues before treatment and the patient's ability to maintain a strict oral hygiene and preventive regimen during and after cancer therapy.

All dental treatment performed for patients who are about to begin cancer therapy should be discussed among the health professionals who will be providing treatment, including the surgeon, radiotherapist, and/or chemotherapist. Dental professionals must be advised regarding the immediacy of cancer therapy and the type of therapy planned. The need for cancer therapy may be immediate; if so, the dentist, in consultation with the medical team, must address the most critical dental needs without compromising the cancer therapy schedule.

Ideal preparation of the patient includes procedures that will eliminate or reduce oral infections. A complete oral examination is required to determine all treatment needs and their priorities. Sources of infection in the mouth can compound the potential for complications related to the cancer therapy. Therefore, whenever possible, all dental decay, dental abscesses, and periodontal infections should be treated before beginning cancer therapy. This includes thorough scaling, root planing, and polishing as needed in addition to a complete periodontal assessment. In addition, any surfaces within the mouth that could irritate oral tissues, such as sharp or broken tooth surfaces, broken or poorly contoured restorations or fixed prostheses, calculus, or poorly fitting dentures should be eliminated. Teeth with nonrestorable caries, periapical pathology, or serious periodontal involvement should be extracted before therapy because of their potential to cause infections that could become life-threatening or result in serious oral complications.

Before therapy, take impressions for custom-fitted trays for fluoride application or as mucosal guards. Show patients how to perform home fluoride applications, and stress the importance of daily fluoride therapy.

Stress the importance of frequent and effective plaque control and oral rinsing both during and after treatment to reduce the potential for infection and other oral complications. Home care instructions should be adapted to each individual's needs, depending on dental conditions, medical status, treatment side effects, patient ability, and compliance levels. Specific recommendations for management of oral side effects of cancer therapy will be discussed to assist the hygienist in designing an appropriate preventive treatment plan.

Oral problems related to cancer therapy and their management

Control of infection is the primary concern for patients being treated with chemotherapy. Infections are responsible for nearly half of the deaths in the general cancer population (McElroy, 1984). A combination of factors makes these patients especially susceptible to infection. The cancer may have left them in a weakened state or with few resources to fight off infections. Drug therapy suppresses bone marrow function, resulting in reduction of white blood cells, which are necessary for the body's defense against microbial infection. The oral mucosa, which normally acts as a physical barrier against the passage of pathogenic microorganisms into the bloodstream, is also affected by the drug therapy, and mucositis occurs with associated thinning and ulceration of the mucosa. Breakdown of the mucosa allows pathogens to enter the bloodstream.

The oral cavity may also be the primary site of localized bacterial, viral, or fungal infections. The most common fungal infection is Candidiasis. It appears clinically as white elevated plaque on mucosa, tongue, or palate that can be rubbed off, exposing raw, bleeding areas. The dentist may prescribe nystatin, ketoconazole, or clotrimazole therapy for this infection (Silverman et al, 1984).

Herpes simplex is a commonly occurring viral infection in these patients, usually beginning as small vesicles on the lips, which can spread to include gingival erosion and ulceration. They may eventually involve large areas of the oral cavity or surrounding tissues (Vuolo, 1987). Montgomery et al. (1986) found that 48% of immunocompromised patients contracted herpetic infections during chemotherapy.

Both gram-positive and gram-negative bacterial infections can occur in immunosuppressed patients as a result of increased virulence of normal oral strains, shifts in bacterial flora towards more pathogenic microorganisms, and lack of host defense mechanisms. Any of these oral infections can become life-threatening if they spread as a result of bacteremia.

Control of oral infections is a major responsibility. Perform a thorough scaling and polishing of teeth before therapy so that periodontal tissues are healthy and not sources of infection. During therapy, patients may benefit from more frequent supragingival polishing with a rubber cup as a means of plaque control, unless this procedure is contraindicated because of the patient's medical status. Patients with abnormally low white blood cell counts may need antibiotic coverage before any type of dental treatment. Consultation with the physician should always precede dental treatment.

Patients must know the importance of keeping the oral and dental tissues clean and free of bacterial plaque as a means of preventing infections, which could become life-threatening.

Another complication of chemotherapy is a decrease in the number of circulating platelets (thrombocytes) in the blood, resulting in a tendency to increased bleeding. In myelosuppressed patients, platelet counts may fall below 50,000/mm^3. Normal platelet counts range between 150,000 and 350,000/mm^3. Platelet counts of 50,000 to 100,000/mm^3 can result in excessive bleeding in response to injury. Spontaneous bleeding and prolonged bleeding are associated with platelet counts below 20,000/mm^3 (Fischbach, 1980). Depending on the platelet count, these patients may experience spontaneous bleeding of gingival tissues or increased bleeding in response to mechanical plaque removal. Oral factors that can predispose these patients to bleeding include trauma, gingival plaque and calculus, mobile teeth, restorations, and decayed or fractured teeth (Vuolo, 1987).

Prevention of oral bleeding requires removal of all rough surfaces in the mouth that might irritate or injure soft tissues before chemotherapy. Cus-

tom-fitted vinyl mouth guards should be constructed from impressions of the patient's teeth, for later use for both home fluoride therapy and for delivery of hemostatic agents to control bleeding. Patients who wear dentures may be advised not to wear them during chemotherapy or to wear them only when necessary, always removing them at night to prevent denture-related irritation of soft tissues (King & Martin, 1983; DePaola et al, 1983). For patients currently undergoing chemotherapy, medical consultation to assess blood cell counts is recommended before any dental treatment, even prophylaxis or home care instructions.

Treatment of oral bleeding may include pressure against localized bleeding sites with premoistened, sterile gauze sponges containing topical hemostatic agents such as Gelfoam, Surgicel, or Thrombostat until bleeding subsides. Hemostatic agents can also be placed in custom-fitted vinyl trays like those used for fluoride application and held in the mouth until localized bleeding has stopped. Bleeding may also be controlled by placement of a periodontal surgical dressing (McClure et al, 1987a).

Mucositis is an inflammation of the oral mucosa that is a common occurrence during both radiation and chemotherapy. Mild forms are characterized by erythema, leukoplakia or yellow patches, and mild discomfort. Symptoms of more severe forms include tissue thinning, ulceration and sloughing of necrotic tissue, and pain that interferes with normal oral functions (Vuolo, 1987). Damaged mucosa becomes a target for secondary infection of the many pathogens present in the oral cavity. The severity of this condition depends on the location of treatment and the type, duration, and dosage of radiation or chemotherapy given. Following irradiation, mucositis usually begins during the second week of treatment (Silverman and Greenspan, 1985). It is a reversible and temporary condition that is usually resolved by 1 to 2 weeks after end of therapy (McClure et al, 1987; Ritchie et al, 1985).

Plaque control procedures may have to be modified to reduce oral discomfort. The patient should be instructed to avoid extremely hot, spicy, acidic, coarse, or dry foods, tobacco, and alcohol. Commercial mouthwashes with alcohol, phenol, or astringents should be avoided (Wescott, 1985).

Rinsing with a mixture of salt, sodium bicarbonate and warm water ($\frac{1}{2}$ to 1 tsp of each in 1 qt of warm water) may provide some relief (Ritchie et al, 1985; Sullivan and Fleming, 1986; McClure et al, 1987a). This mixture should be used shortly after it is prepared, because the effervescence of the sodium bicarbonate lasts only about 20 minutes (McClure et al, 1987a). A solution of 0.5% hydrogen peroxide has also been suggested for cleaning oral tissues, although it is not recommended for continuous use because of the potential for irritation of soft tissues and potential carcinogenesis (Lowe, 1986; McClure et al, 1987a).

A 50% mixture by volume of Kaopectate and Benylin cough syrup may also soothe and reduce inflammation (Toth & Fleming, 1983; Toth & Frame, 1983; McClure et al, 1987a). Remedies to make eating and oral hygiene procedures more comfortable include the following:

1. A solution made from dyclonine hydrochloride 0.5% and diphenhydramine hydrochloride 0.5% in normal saline, applied topically to localized lesions with a cotton-tipped applicator or used as an oral rinse and expectorated (Wright, 1985);
2. Equal measures of 2% viscous lidocaine diphenhydramine elixir (12.5 mg/5 cc) and magnesia and alumina oral suspension (Maalox) (Wright, 1985);
3. A rinse prepared with unflavored Xylocaine HCl 2% Viscous in a 1:2 dilution with saline solution (Toth & Fleming, 1983; Toth & Frame, 1983; Lowe, 1986);
4. Dyclone Solution 0.5%

Topical anesthetic preparations should be used in moderation. The irritating chemical qualities of many of these agents can actually intensify and prolong mucositis if used frequently or over a long period (Toth & Fleming, 1983; Toth & Frame, 1983; McClure et al, 1987a).

Radiation therapy for head and neck cancer frequently involves the major and minor salivary glands, resulting in partial or total loss of salivary flow (known as xerostomia) including changes in the quality and the quantity of saliva. Saliva may become thick and ropey, or the flow is altered.

These changes usually begin 7 to 10 days after treatment begins and may become worse as treatment continues. These changes are usually irreversible (Sullivan and Fleming, 1986; Yasko &

Green, 1987). Some individuals may experience limited return of function within 6 to 12 months after treatment (Reynolds et al, 1980; Fay and O'Neal, 1984). Treatment of symptoms may need to continue indefinitely.

Xerostomia may also be experienced by patients treated with chemotherapy. However, it is a temporary condition, with normal function returning after the cessation of therapy (Vuolo, 1987). Treatment for drug-induced xerostomia and fluoride therapy to prevent xerostomia-related dental decay should be continued throughout chemotherapy and be discontinued after normal salivary flow has returned and normal home care can be resumed.

Salivary changes can create problems for patients, the most serious of which is rampant dental caries. Other problems include inadequate digestion of starches, irritation of mucous membranes, difficulties with talking, tasting, eating and swallowing food, and problems with denture retention.

Suggested remedies for relief of xerostomia include use of artificial saliva preparations (e.g., Moi-Stir, Orex, Salivart, Xerolube) and frequent rinsing with water or saline solution. Individuals can make their own saliva substitute by mixing 8 oz. of water with 4 or 5 drops of glycerine in a bottle equipped with a spray nozzle (Barker et al, 1982). Patients may have dentures modified to contain a reservoir that dispenses artificial saliva slowly into the mouth ('s-Gravenmade et al, 1984; Toljanic and Zucuskie, 1984; Vissink et al, 1986). Use of sugarless mints, candy, or gum may also help stimulate salivary flow.

Patients can use a water-based lubricant to prevent drying and chapping (e.g., Surgilube, K-Y jelly, or hydrous lanolin), cocoa butter, or a lip balm (McClure et al, 1987a; Yasko and Greene, 1987). Vaseline or petroleum jelly is anhydrous and will aggravate dryness (Barker, 1982; Debiase and Komives, 1983; Toth and Fleming, 1983; Toth and Frame, 1983). A cool mist vaporizer to increase room humidity and air filters to eliminate smoke may also help (Barker, 1982; Toth and Fleming, 1983; McClure et al, 1987a).

A special diet should be suggested of foods from each of the food groups that are already moistened, thereby making chewing and swallowing easier. Patients should drink up to 8 to 10 glasses of water daily (Yasko and Greene, 1987). Resources are available to assist the patient with planning and preparing foods that are easy to eat and nutritious (Goldberg, 1980; Rosenthal, 1980; Daly, 1985; Wilson, 1985). Pamphlets containing additional suggestions are available from the American Cancer Society and the National Institutes of Health.

Many factors related to radiation therapy combine to favor development of rampant caries in patients. "Radiation caries" may appear as any combination of the following: (1) dark brown to black discolorations with no apparent demineralization, (2) cervical decay, which may encircle the entire tooth, or (3) decay that begins on the incisal or cuspal surfaces of the tooth (Reynolds et al, 1980). This type of caries progresses rapidly and can occur at any time after the completion of therapy throughout the patient's lifetime. It can occur even in persons who have no history of decay if preventive methods are not employed both during and following radiation treatment.

Xerostomia is a primary factor in the initiation of rampant decay. Changes in the quantity and viscosity of saliva decrease its lubrication and cleansing abilities. There is also a loss in the buffering effects of the saliva (its ability to neutralize acids), and a reduction in output of the protective substances contained in saliva, and a decrease in remineralizing effect.

Radiation treatment also initiates a shift in the bacterial flora of the mouth that favors the growth of cariogenic bacteria such as *Streptococcus mutans*. Increase in bacterial acids reduce the pH of the saliva considerably. The patient's diet will likely contain less fiber and roughage because of the difficulty and pain of chewing these foods. Instead, high carbohydrate foods that are softer, easier to chew, and more adherent to teeth are eaten.

Prevention of rampant caries requires a rigorous program of strict oral hygiene and daily applications of fluoride. Patients should be taught proper and thorough means of mechanical plaque removal through use of a soft toothbrush, floss, and other appropriate plaque removal aids. It should be impressed on patients that no amount of professional help can compensate for a lack of strict compliance in their own daily home care. Patients who cannot or will not exercise strict

home care practices must be informed of the consequences. Development of rampant decay can destroy the existing teeth, and the resulting infections or treatment (e.g., extractions) can precipitate even more destruction due to osteoradionecrosis. The dentist may consider extraction of the teeth before therapy for patients with poor oral hygiene to eliminate the risks of further deleterious effects as a result of the cancer therapy.

A second critical step in the prevention of radiation caries is daily use of a topical fluoride gel. Tested products of either 1% sodium fluoride, 1.23% acidulated phosphate fluoride gel, or 0.4% stannous fluoride gel have been recommended for this purpose (Ritchie et al, 1985; Wescott, 1985; Wright, 1985; Schweiger and Salcetti, 1986; Sullivan and Fleming, 1986; McClure et al, 1987; Rothwell, 1987). Selection of the product may be based on the pH that the patient can tolerate comfortably. Sodium fluoride gels have the highest pH compared to the other two types and are less likely to irritate inflamed tissues. The lower pH of the acidulated gels, although tolerated well by some patients (Reynolds et al, 1980), may be irritating to the mucosa of others. If patients complain of irritation from an acidulated phosphate gel, its use should be discontinued and fluoride therapy should continue with either a neutral pH sodium fluoride gel or a stannous fluoride gel.

Place the fluoride in a custom-made vinyl tray. This ensures maximum adaptation of the gel to the tooth surfaces and minimizes leakage of the fluoride gel during the treatment. Trays should be applied once daily, preferably after the teeth have been cleaned, and left in place for a minimum of 5 to 10 minutes. After removing the trays, rinse them in cool water. The patient should expectorate excess fluoride and should refrain from eating, rinsing, or drinking for at least 30 minutes to receive maximum benefit from the treatment. This method is recommended for patients with poor oral hygiene or those who suffer from moderate to severe xerostomia (Sullivan and Fleming, 1986). Depending on oral conditions, some patients may need to use topical fluorides more frequently than once a day, especially if decay is detected or if severe xerostomia exists. Use of a toothbrush or disposable sponge brush may also be indicated for fluoride application if the fluoride trays cannot be tolerated.

Sullivan and Fleming (1986) suggest an alternate method of fluoride therapy for patients who have excellent oral hygiene and minimal mouth dryness. Using a toothbrush, the patient should apply 0.4% stannous fluoride gel to all teeth for 1 minute. The solution should then be swished vigorously around the teeth, held in the mouth for 1 minute, and then expectorated. The patient should not eat, drink, or rinse for 30 minutes afterwards. Since this method of application may not allow the gel to contact the tooth surfaces directly for the recommended treatment time, it is not the method of choice for patients who show signs of beginning decay or for those with less than optimal oral hygiene (McClure et al, 1987).

Daily fluoride treatments must be continued indefinitely by individuals suffering from radiation-induced xerostomia. The conditions that render these patients susceptible to rampant caries are likely to be present for the rest of their lives.

Osteoradionecrosis is the most serious complication of radiation therapy. When large doses of radiation are directed at bone, a number of changes occur. The blood supply to the bone is impaired, and the cells responsible for remodelling and repairing bone tissue are destroyed. Therefore, irradiated bone tissue is much more susceptible to infections and has a reduced ability to repair and remodel itself after trauma. According to Ritchie and coworkers (1985), osteoradionecrosis is a consequence of defective wound healing in which the tissue demands for oxygen, energy and nutrients exceed the available supply.

After radiation therapy, this bone defect can occur spontaneously, although commonly it occurs as a result of trauma to the bone. It is characterized by acute inflammation and destruction. Bone may be exposed to the oral cavity causing severe pain. This condition occurs more frequently in the mandible than the maxilla (Wescott, 1985), and represents permanent damage. Some cases of osteoradionecrosis have been reported as long as 25 years after the actual radiation treatment (McClure et al, 1987).

Osteoradionecrosis can have seemingly minor causes. Overzealous use of a toothbrush (Ritchie et al, 1985), or poorly fitting dentures could irritate the soft tissues to the extent that infection can occur in the underlying bone. Destruction can also be precipitated by periodontal infections (Fat-

tore et al, 1987). Because of the possibility of introducing infection and the reduced healing capacity of irradiated bone, invasive dental procedures, including extractions, periodontal surgery, apicoectomies, or deep scaling and curettage, are strictly contraindicated for patients at risk for osteoradionecrosis.

Prevention begins prior to radiation therapy. Existing infections must be eliminated, and all conditions which could precipitate future infection of either soft or hard tissues must be controlled. The patient must be educated about the potential for development of osteoradionecrosis, the seriousness of this side effect, and the importance of strict compliance with the recommended home care regimen to prevent dental infections. Patients who wear dental prostheses may be advised to wear them as little as possible during treatment and should be closely monitored to ensure that the prostheses do not cause any oral irritation.

If osteoradionecrosis does occur, it should be managed as conservatively as possible, because any surgical manipulation can make the situation worse. In addition to antibiotic therapy, good oral hygiene must be maintained; affected tissues can be irrigated with sterile saline solution and gently debrided to aid healing. Hyperbaric oxygen therapy has also been found to be useful for treatment of this condition (Ritchie et al, 1985). If conservative treatment fails to control the bone infection, jaw resection (surgical removal of large sections of the jaw) may be necessary to stop the destructive process (Wescott, 1985; McClure et al, 1987).

Loss of taste perception is a common side effect of radiation therapy. It usually begins during the second week of treatment. Damage to the taste buds and the microvilli of the tongue results in a loss of acuteness of the tastes of sweet, salty, bitter, and acidic substances. In many cases, this alteration is temporary, and varying degrees of taste perception return within a few months after the completion of therapy (Rothwell, 1987). Individuals who receive doses in excess of 6000 rads may have a permanent problem (McClure et al, 1987). This side effect contributes to a diminished appetite and thus poor nutrition. Individuals may also compensate for the loss of taste through overuse of salt and sugar and other spices, which could compound other medical or dental problems (e.g., hypertension, dental caries, mucositis). Since proper nutrition is critical to the overall health and recovery of these patients, nutritional counselling is indicated. Zinc sulfate (220-mg tablets) twice daily with meals has been reported to improve taste sensation for some patients (Mossman and Henken, 1978; Silverman and Thompson, 1984).

Irradiation of the temporomandibular joint or the muscles of mastication can cause muscle fibrosis and muscle spasms (trismus), which result in limitation of the patient's ability to open the mouth. This problem can prevent the patient from performing necessary oral hygiene and preventive procedures, and it interferes with eating. It can be treated by instructing the patient to perform a variety of exercises prescribed by the dental professional or by a physical therapist.

Before treatment, the maximal mouth opening should be measured and recorded. This measurement can then be used as a standard to identify a limitation of motion. Simple exercises to improve movement can be recommended such as opening the mouth to its maximum and then closing it 20 times in succession. This exercise should be repeated three times a day during and after radiation therapy (Peterson, 1983; Ritchie et al, 1985; McClure et al, 1987). Another exercise is to insert a mouth prop (formed by putting several tongue blades together) between the teeth and then rotate the blades to gradually force the teeth further apart. This exercise should be repeated two to three times a day with more tongue blades added as needed (Rubin and Doku, 1976).

Sullivan and Fleming (1986) suggested two others: placing the heel of both hands under the jaw and pushing up against the lower jaw while stretching the mouth open as wide as possible, and placing the middle and index fingers on the mandibular teeth and the thumb on the maxillary teeth and twisting the fingers to force the teeth apart for 2 seconds. This exercise should be performed ten times in succession with the right hand, then ten times with the left hand, and should be repeated four times daily.

An oral side effect of chemotherapy is **neuropathy.** Certain drugs used in cancer therapy may affect nerve function in various parts of the body, including the oral cavity, causing symptoms of pain or numbness. Toxic effects of these drugs on the nerve tissues may result in the patient complaining of pain in the teeth, periodontium, or jaw for which no apparent cause is detected (McClure et al, 1987a). Awareness of this complication and consultation with the oncologist will assist the dentist in diagnosing the source of the problem. Drug-induced neuropathy should cease after discontinuation of the drug (Vuolo, 1987).

Educating the cancer patient

The most important role of the dental hygienist in helping patients who are about to undergo cancer therapy is that of educator and motivator. The hygienist should inform patients (or those responsible for their care) of the possible oral side effects of their treatment while emphasizing that not all individuals will experience the same side effects or to the same degree.

The patient or the care provider must also be taught how to prevent or alleviate these side effects effectively, and they must be motivated to comply with instructions. Cancer patients must understand the importance of their role in preventing or reducing oral complications and in preserving their general and oral health (Engelmeier, 1987).

Due to the emotional nature of their medical problem, these patients are likely to be distracted, confused, and fearful during consultation for dental treatment. Therefore, it is wise to provide complete instructions to them verbally in front of another family member or companion and to provide written instructions for later reference.

Before therapy, patients should be instructed in a rigorous plaque control program to reduce inflammation. Patients should be shown sulcular brushing (the Bass method) using a soft-bristled nylon brush. Bristles can be softened further by rinsing or soaking them in hot water prior to use. After use, toothbrushes should be thoroughly rinsed and stored in a cool, dry area to reduce microbial contamination.

An approved fluoride dentifrice should be recommended. During treatment, if tissue irritation is a problem, a less irritating preparation such as a baking soda paste or solution may be substituted.

Proper use of dental floss and other interdental cleaning aids, as recommended by the hygienist, will help reduce bacterial plaque and control infection. Use of finger massage or rubber tip massage of gingival tissues may improve circulation following plaque removal. Oral irrigators may also be useful for cleansing and rinsing the mouth; these should be used on a low power setting (Yasko and Greene, 1987; Rothwell, 1987).

Adaptations in home care procedures must be made for patients with compromised ability to fight infection, abnormal bleeding tendencies, or extreme oral discomfort. It has been recommended that a normally aggressive home care regimen is appropriate as long as white blood cell counts are greater than $2,000/mm^3$ (20% polymorphonuclear leukocytes) and platelet counts are greater than $20,000/mm^3$ (Sonis et al, 1978; Wright et al, 1985). Modifications in home care, however, are necessary if severe mucositis, low white blood cell counts, or spontaneous bleeding occur.

Discontinue use of a toothbrush at the first sign of spontaneous bleeding. Teeth can be cleaned using a 4″ x 4″ gauze sponge moistened with a sodium bicarbonate and water solution and wrapped around the finger. Disposable sponges (toothettes) may also be used. These measures are also appropriate for individuals who are unable to tolerate the abrasiveness of a toothbrush. It has been suggested that lemon-glycerine swabs should not be used because they are anhydrous and can irritate friable tissues (Debiase and Komives, 1983). Flossing and use of any other sharp implement for plaque removal (e.g., toothpicks) should be discontinued until platelet counts return to normal.

Dentures should be cleaned thoroughly every night with a stiff brush and soaked in a denture cleaning solution overnight. Dentures should be thoroughly rinsed with water before being returned to the mouth to remove colonized microorganisms. The container used for soaking should be cleaned daily and solution replaced so that it does not serve as a bacterial reservoir.

Patients must also be educated regarding the need for frequent and regular recall appointments during and after their treatment to answer questions, provide additional remedies, and reinforce and monitor home care. Reinforcement is essential. Since many side effects of treatment are likely to be problems even after treatment for the cancer has been completed, continuous monitoring of the patient's oral health and prompt treatment of dental problems is important.

DENTAL CARE FOR THE ELDERLY

The percentage of elderly persons (65 years and older) in the United States population has been increasing steadily since 1900 and will undergo even more dramatic increases in the years to come. In 1900 the elderly comprised about 4% of the total population (Clark et al, 1982). Since that time, birth rates and life expectancies have increased due to advances in science and medicine, improvements in health, economic factors, and environmental factors. In 1985 elderly persons comprised about 12% of the population (Warren and Blandford, 1985).

The percentage of elderly is predicted to rise to 13.1% by the year 2000 and then to increase to 19.5% by the year 2025. Individuals born in the late forties and early fifties, known as the "baby boom" generation, will be reaching their seniority at that time. The growth of this segment of the population indicates the need for society to redirect its focus toward the concerns and needs of the elderly. Health care providers must be aware of the needs of this population group and be prepared to meet the challenges of serving it.

It is a mistake to attempt to categorize or to stereotype all elderly persons as homogeneous in terms of their physical or mental capabilities. Elderly persons are unique as individuals and perhaps more heterogeneous as a group than any other age group. Aging is a great diversifier (Warren and Blandford, 1985). There is no such thing as a "typical" elderly person, any more than there is a "typical" 18-year-old person.

An important objective of this chapter is to impress the dental care professional with the understanding that all people, regardless of their special needs relative to age, physical condition or mental status, must be treated as unique persons rather than stereotyped because of one condition or situation which affects their lives. Although special needs can fall neatly into categories, people do not. The challenge to dental care professionals and to all health care providers is to meet the individual needs of each patient.

Physiological changes related to aging

Warren and Blandford (1985) described aging as "a slow progressive decline in physiologic reserve during which the body loses some of its ability to adapt." Aging involves a complex interaction between the physiological changes that occur as part of the aging process and age-related diseases. Multiple chronic diseases in the elderly make them more vulnerable to stresses that would be considered minor to younger, healthier individuals.

Deterioration or debilitation often is attributed to physiological changes when it is really caused by disease. For example, only recently was it discovered that most senile dementia is not a normal consequence of aging, but is due to Alzheimer's disease. Xerostomia (lack of salivary gland function) is another example of a condition that is often present in the elderly, but it is usually caused by pathological changes or drug therapy rather than physiologic aging.

A genuine biological outcome of aging can be distinguished from disease through the following criteria: (1) it must be detectable in all human beings; (2) it occurs independent of outside influences; (3) it is progressive and irreversible in nature; (4) it is harmful to survival (Viidik, 1986). When measured against these criteria many conditions that were assumed to be part of normal aging are seen to be disease entities with a higher prevalence and incidence in the elderly.

Common diseases among the elderly

The dental hygienist should expect that most of the elderly patients who seek dental care will be functioning at physical and mental levels comparable to other adult age groups. Dental care providers should assume that most elderly dental care consumers will be healthy and active but that occasionally a patient will manifest significant changes in function or medical status that require modifications in the delivery of dental care.

A number of diseases occurring in the general population are more prevalent in the elderly. Common cardiopulmonary disorders, including valvular heart disease, may be present in more than 70% of the elderly population (Burch, 1975). The hygienist should be alert to those conditions that require medical consultation and prophylactic antibiotic premedication before dental treatment.

If the patient reports use of anticoagulant medications for treatment of cardiovascular problems, consultation with the patient's physician is necessary before performing any treatment that could induce bleeding, including periodontal probing and dental prophylaxis. Laboratory tests to determine bleeding time may also be indicated.

One of the most frequent diseases of the elderly is hypertension. Elderly individuals with a systolic blood pressure greater than 160 and diastolic blood pressure greater than 95 to 100 should be referred to their physician for further examination. In cases of severe hypertension, dental treatment should be postponed until the condition is under control. Drugs used to treat hypertension may also produce side effects, including xerostomia and postural hypotension.

Common nervous system disorders include cerebral vascular disease or stroke, development of tremors (Parkinson's disease) and dementias (Alzheimer's disease). Patients who have had a stroke may experience paralysis that affects their ability to move and walk. This disease may also affect their ability to understand others and to communicate their own thoughts. Appropriate modifications in home care instructions should be made so that they or those who care for them are able to perform effective oral hygiene procedures. Stroke patients may also be receiving anticoagulant therapy that requires special attention before dental treatment, as discussed previously. Persons with tremor disorders may have difficulty eating, which affects their overall nutritional status, and they may also experience difficulty with performing daily oral hygiene procedures for themselves. While in the dental chair, these patients may have difficulty remaining still, swallowing, and keeping their mouths open.

A number of rheumatologic disorders are also prevalent in the elderly, including arthritis and osteoporosis. Arthritis affects the ability of the individual to perform normal oral hygiene procedures and may require modifications of oral hygiene aides to facilitate their use by these patients. Some patients with severe osteoarthritis may have had joint replacement. These patients should receive antibiotic premedication before dental treatment to prevent infection of those joints. Consultation with the patient's physician is recommended.

Osteoporosis is most common in postmenopausal women and leads to fractures of the long bones, the hip joint, and the vertebral bodies of the spine. Individuals suffering from osteoporosis need extra time for positioning, and they may have difficulty remaining seated for long periods of time or may require extra cushioning while in the dental chair.

Hearing impairment, another common age-related problem, can occur as a result of both physiological and pathological changes. About 30% of the population aged 65 and over who live in the community and 99% of the elderly in nursing homes suffer from some level of hearing impairment (Dept. of HEW, 1979). Hearing disorders are probably the most common sensory disorder in the elderly and require extra attention to communication skills by the dental professional.

For many of these patients, the hearing loss involves the frequency of different sounds rather than a loss of volume. High-pitched consonant sounds such as "k," "sh," "ch," "t," "p," "th," and "f" are difficult for these persons to distinguish. Raising one's voice may be helpful in some situations, but shouting is not. Instructing these individuals while seated in operating position at the side or rear of the dental chair or talking with a face mask in place makes it more difficult for them to understand the message. Reducing background noises, such as office music, ultrasonic scalers, dental drills, or suction devices while speaking with the patient may improve communication. Patients who wear hearing aids may appreciate being advised when noisy equipment will be used so that they can adjust or remove their hearing aid rather than experience sound amplification.

Instructions should be written in large print for the patient whose vision is impaired. Vision problems including cataracts and glaucoma are common in the elderly population. Individuals with slight impairment may need more light in order to read or see demonstrations. Many also cannot distinguish certain colors, especially blues and greens. Some may have difficulty perceiving distances and depths, especially in low light environments. Adjusting the eyes from high to low light intensities may require a longer length of time (Brock, 1985).

Drug usage in the elderly

The elderly are the biggest consumers of both prescription and nonprescription drugs within the population. Drug usage increases with advancing age, with the average elderly person taking 3 or more drugs on a daily basis (Shapiro, 1986).

There are many problems associated with this high drug use rate. Elderly individuals are more susceptible to adverse drug interactions. Factors such as multiple drug use, age-related changes in bodily functions, and multiple illnesses all have the potential to interfere with the predicted action of a given drug in an elderly person. Depending on the specific medical and drug history of the individual, the absorption, distribution, effects, metabolism, and excretion of drugs can be altered in elderly individuals. Therefore, a complete medical and drug history is required (see Chapter 5).

If the dentist determines that drugs should be prescribed relative to dental treatment, the patient should be completely informed regarding the purpose of the drug, how it should be used, and possible side effects. For the elderly, instructions for use should also be communicated in writing and sent home with the patient. Since many elderly patients have difficulty managing containers with child-proof caps, that type of container should not be used.

Psychological aspects of aging

Erik Erikson (1959, 1963) believed that every human being works through certain psychosocial stages during a lifetime of development from child to adult, and he categorized these eight stages using terms that represent opposite ends of a continuum of development of the following life attitudes: (1) trust versus mistrust; (2) autonomy versus shame; (3) initiative versus guilt; (4) industry versus inferiority; (5) identity versus identity confusion; (6) intimacy versus isolation; (7) generativity versus self-absorption; and (8) integrity versus despair.

By the time adults reach old age, they have spent a lifetime developing their social and personal identities, but old age often brings a series of losses or limitations in their lives, including loss of health, spouse, family, friends, work and career, income, and sometimes even loss of the independence to direct their own lives. These losses can contribute to an individual's perception that many of the accomplishments and developments of a lifetime are now being slowly taken away, resulting in loss of identity and feelings ranging from anxiety, frustration, and confusion to depression, withdrawal, and anger. If the individual cannot adapt to these changes and resolve them so that a sense of identity and worth is maintained, the resulting conflict may cause a slipping away from the psychological goals achieved in adulthood and a return to a more childlike psychological outlook on life.

Of course, not all elderly individuals will have difficulty in all areas, but the unique situations of each person's life combined with the individual's personality will affect how these changes are handled psychologically. Erikson's descriptions of developmental stage in terms of these bipolar attitudes of psychological and social identity provide a useful framework for understanding how the individual may be affected by the losses and limitations that often accompany aging.

Trust versus mistrust. Elderly adults may have learned through a lifetime of experiences that there are some people who should not be trusted. As a result, they may "test" people before being able to trust them. Health care workers must demonstrate their trustworthiness in order to gain the cooperation and respect of these individuals.

Autonomy versus shame and doubt. Most adults have developed a valued sense of control over themselves and their lives. With aging, they may experience a loss of control in their lives. Losses extend to their lifestyle, income, health, family, friends, and a sense of being able to control their own fate. Instead of making their own choices, choices are made for them. This loss of independence can result in any number of negative feelings in the elderly adult. Elderly adults need to feel that they have control over the decisions and the events that surround their dental treatment.

Initiative versus guilt. As the child matures, he develops a sense of initiative towards behaviors and establishes a conscience about his actions. If he perceives that his behaviors are "bad," feelings of guilt emerge. When initiative is blocked in elderly persons, feelings of apathy or frustration are likely to occur. They now must learn to conform to the expectations of others who are assisting them with their care and may feel "bad" or guilty if they attempt to exercise their own initiatives and, as a result, displease those whose expectations were not met. Elderly

individuals should be encouraged to try new things and to exercise initiative within their lives without fear of reprisal or remediation.

Industry versus inferiority. As the child becomes a worker he becomes involved in producing rather than just consuming, and gains recognition for work and learns to work cooperatively and productively with other people. When an elderly adult is no longer employed or finds that he can no longer perform many of the tasks that made him feel productive, he may develop feelings of uselessness or of being a "burden" to others around him. Every adult needs to feel worthwhile and needs to experience recognition for his efforts, yet these needs are often overlooked in the elderly. As a result, elderly individuals may develop feelings of inferiority.

Identity versus identity confusion. A central task for any adult is to move through the process of acquiring a sense of identity that defines who he is and his place in society. The elderly may experience a loss of identity as a result of their isolation from social contacts, their loss of control over their lives, and their loss of privacy. In the dental office, the staff should not converse with a family member about the elderly individual's care or refer to him or her using third-person pronouns (he, she) as if the person were not present. Use of first names or pet names may represent a lack of respect for the person's seniority.

Intimacy versus isolation. Once a person has established her own identity she can begin to invest time and energy in the development of intimate relationships and commitments to others. The elderly person may become isolated from those with whom he has established intimate relationships, including family, friends, and coworkers. If new relationships and friendships are not formed the result is isolation, self-absorbtion, and loss of ego. Many elderly persons enjoy the dental visit because it provides a source of social contact. Dental professionals should understand this need for contact and be interested and willing listeners.

Generativity versus self-absorption. Generativity involves a person's concern for participation in the process of establishing and guiding the next generation. This process includes teaching their own children or other young persons about the lessons of life and therefore contributing to their understanding and ability to deal with life situations. When elderly individuals perceive that no one is interested in them, their knowledge, or their expertise, they can become bored, introverted, or withdrawn. They need opportunities to share their memories and experiences and to feel that something valuable can be learned from them.

Integrity versus despair. Integrity refers to a person's ability to accept that one has only one lifetime and that the events of the past were significant and meaningful. The person who has developed integrity feels satisfied with her life and she can look back on life and feel no regrets, while the person who is despairing feels like saying, "If only I could start all over." As an adult ages, she has more and more time for introspection: for examining her life, putting it into perspective, and coming to conclusions about how she has spent her time. These individuals need support as they work through this task, and they may need to talk and have someone listen as they attempt to sort out these issues.

An understanding of the relationship between a person's psychological needs and development and the aging process is important for understanding the implications of our behaviors and attitudes as health care providers toward the elderly. The dental hygienist should analyze each of the above concepts in terms of how they may affect the approach to providing dental hygiene treatment and patient education to elderly adults in a manner that will maximize their positive psychological perceptions of themselves.

Dental needs of the elderly

The elderly have a higher level of unmet dental needs than any other age group (Tyron, 1981). One encouraging trend is that edentulism rates are decreasing, meaning that people are retaining more of their teeth later in life. Recent data confirm that the prevalence of edentulism in the United States has continued to decline since the 1950s and that this trend can be expected to continue (Douglas and Gammon, 1985; Ismail et al, 1987). This trend is primarily due to increased exposure to preventive measures and dental treatment. It also indicates, however, that significantly more teeth will be at risk for dental diseases in elderly populations.

Although the rate of edentulism is declining, the treatment needs and education needs of the edentulous population are still significant problems. Currently, 90% of those over 65 are partially edentulous (Warren and Blandford, 1985) and approximately 34% are completely edentulous (Ismail et al, 1987). These individuals require regular dental examinations to evaluate whether partial and complete dentures fit properly, to examine soft tissues for the presence of disease, and to reinforce instructions for appliance care and oral hygiene.

Periodontal disease is estimated to affect 90% of the elderly who have natural teeth (Ettinger and Beck, 1982). Holm-Pedersen et al (1975) demonstrated that the periodontal tissues of the elderly are more susceptible to microbial-related inflammation than those of younger individuals. They also found that elderly persons tend to accumulate more plaque and to develop gingivitis more rapidly and more severely. These findings, along with recognition of the high prevalence of periodontitis among the elderly, have led to the idea that the prevalence and severity of active periodontal disease is higher in elderly population groups than in younger adult groups.

Page (1984), however, cautioned that in spite of the fact that the elderly do manifest more clinical evidence of periodontal destruction, these conditions may be a result of the cumulative effect of periodontal disease progression rather than a result of enhanced susceptibility to the disease due to aging. Furthermore, it is still not certain that this increased susceptibility actually results in higher prevalence and severity of active periodontitis in the elderly (Page, 1984).

Although examination of disease trends indicates that the prevalence of gingivitis is declining among the elderly, the prevalence of periodontitis has been reported to be stable for all elderly with the exception of women from 65 to 74 years of age. In this population group the prevalence of periodontitis showed an increase between studies done in 1960 through 1962 and 1971 through 1974 (National Center for Health Statistics, 1965, 1979; Douglas et al, 1983; Douglas and Gammon, 1985). Because the proportion of adults without periodontal disease has increased significantly since the 1960 through 1962 National Health Survey, a related decrease in the prevalence and severity of periodontal disease among the upcoming generations of elderly adults could be expected to follow (Bawden and Defriese, 1981; Hughes et al, 1982; Douglass et al, 1983; Page, 1984).

However, it is generally more difficult for the elderly to practice effective self-care measures because of functional limitations such as those resulting from arthritis or a stroke, or other debilitating disease. The preventive actions of the elderly may also be hindered by lack of understanding of the importance of preventive care or lack of knowledge regarding available preventive measures.

Dental caries continues into old age (Banting, 1984). However, coronal caries in the elderly is manifested primarily as secondary decay rather than primary decay (Hansen, 1977; Goldberg et al, 1981; Bergman et al, 1982, Banting, 1984).

Adults who have exposed root surfaces as a result of loss of periodontal attachment are also at increased risk of root caries. This is most commonly found on molar teeth, especially mandibular molars (Banting, 1984). It is generally agreed that prevalence rates increase with age, making this type of caries more common in the elderly (Banting, 1984; Beck, 1984).

The exact etiology of root caries has not yet been established. Research findings on the role of oral hygiene, gender, diet, and specific microbial factors as causative agents of root caries have been contradictory. There have been no conclusive studies regarding the nature of this disease using population groups considered representative of the general population (Seichter, 1987). It is generally agreed, however, that unique interactions of diet and bacterial plaque are important factors in its cause.

Currently recommended measures for prevention of root caries include mechanical plaque removal. Fluoride has been effective in the prevention of root caries as well as coronal caries (Seichter, 1987). Root caries has been less prevalent in populations that benefit from fluoridated water supplies in comparison to those who have lived in nonfluoridated areas (Stamm and Banting, 1980). Topical fluoride application in conjunction with recontouring and smoothing of shallow areas of root caries has been proposed as an acceptable alternative to restorative treatment in some cases. Additional studies are needed concerning the optimal concentration of fluoride and the most effective method for application of fluoride for the prevention of root caries. Prevention of periodontal disease is the best means of preventing root caries.

Oral cancer is also prevalent in the elderly. Cancer is the second leading cause of death in individuals aged 55 and above, with heart disease being the number one cause of death in these individuals. Silverman (1985) reported that about 95% of all oral cancers occur in persons over 40 years old and that the average age at the time of diagnosis is about 60. The elderly account for nearly 50% of all oral cancer cases reported annually in the U.S. (Baranovsky and Myers, 1986).

Oral cancer occurs more frequently in men than in women at a ratio of about 2:1. The tongue is the most frequent site of oral cancer, followed by the lip, oropharynx, and the floor of the mouth. About 95% of all oral cancers are squamous cell carcinomas (Silverman, 1985).

Hygienists can perform a valuable function by educating elderly patients of the need for regular oral examinations. This must occur not only in the private dental office, but also through community-wide efforts. Hygienists and dentists must promote preventive dental care for the elderly through educational in-services at retirement homes, nursing homes, and other institutions that serve the needs of the elderly. Educational programs should be presented in community centers that provide social activities and/or nutritional services to the elderly. Oral cancer screenings can also be scheduled at these sites or at community health fairs through the combined efforts of dentists and hygienists. Effective use of mass media (newspaper, radio, and television) is another excellent way to promote the message that preventive oral care can help preserve the health and well-being of dental consumers of all ages.

Use of dental care by the elderly

In spite of the tremendous need for dental care, use patterns for the elderly reflect fewer regular dental visits than other segments of the population. Data from the National Health Interview Survey indicated that in 1983 only 37.8% of adults aged 65 years and over who visited senior centers had visited a dentist within 1 year, compared to 51.8% of the total population. These dental care use rates were the lowest for any age group with the exception of children under age 6.

However, the demand for dental care among the socially active elderly may be increasing. Edentulous persons are less likely to have regular dental visits than those who have teeth. Dentate individuals are four times more likely to have visited a dentist yearly than those who are edentulous (Ismail et al, 1987).

A number of reasons explain why elderly do not utilize regular dental care, including: the cost of dental care, the priority of dental care as compared to other needs, lack of accessibility or availability of dental services, lack of perceived need on the part of consumers, negative attitudes on the part of both consumers and providers, and medical and psychological problems of the elderly.

The issues of the perceived need for dental care, the perceived accessibility of dental care, and the priority which is assigned to dental care compared to other basic needs are all closely related to the cost of dental care. Dental care is expensive for those elderly persons on a fixed income, and it must usually be paid for from out-of-pocket funds. Most elderly who may have previously enjoyed dental coverage from private insurance plans when they were employed are no longer covered by these plans. Of the two primary public assistance programs, Medicare offers no coverage for routine dental care, and coverage of dental services under Medicaid programs is extremely limited. The end result of these factors is that many elderly perceive that the cost of routine dental care makes it less accessible than other types of medical care and assign a lower priority status to their dental needs when compared to other basic needs of living (Marinelli et al, 1982; Blau, 1982; Antczak and Branch, 1985; Bomberg and Ernst, 1986; Gooch and Berkey, 1987).

Some may not seek dental care because they perceive a lack of respect and consideration for their needs on the part of dental professionals. Studies have shown that medical, dental, and nursing students believe the erroneous and stereotypical myths (Bomberg and Ernst, 1986). Solomon and Vickers (1979) noted that these stereotypes are held by persons regardless of socioeconomic or occupational status, or age, despite the increasing amount of factual information available regarding the elderly. These myths include: most elderly people are senile, frail and dependent; aging is a "second childhood"; most old people live below the poverty level; people become less intelligent as they age; most elderly are institutionalized; "you can't teach an old dog new tricks"; the elderly can no longer be creative, productive, and self-sufficient members of society.

Many elderly persons do not seek dental care because they do not feel that they have dental problems, that dental problems are an unavoidable consequence of aging, or because they do not believe their dental problems can be corrected.

Ettinger and Beck (1982) noted that the social, cultural, and historical experiences of the "old elderly" (75 years and over) resulted in ideas that dentistry is a luxury and that loss of teeth is an expected and inevitable part of growing old. The concept of prevention of oral diseases was unknown to these individuals.

In contrast, the "new elderly" (aged 60 to 64) grew up in an environment that allowed them to be better informed, resulting in greater demand for prevention. The economic prosperity of the fifties and improvements in dental technology also helped.

Ettinger and Beck went on to predict that the more positive attitudes of the "new elderly" toward dental care, coupled with the fact that more of them have retained more of their natural teeth, will result in an increase in the demand for dental services from this group.

Dental hygiene treatment planning for the elderly

Appointment scheduling. When scheduling appointments for elderly patients, consider their health status and stamina. Whenever possible, schedule appointments for midmorning, when the patient's energy reserves are highest. Patients who are physically debilitated, those with serious medical problems, or those with short attention spans or who exhibit restlessness should be scheduled for several short appointments rather than longer ones. Appointments should not interfere with eating schedules of diabetic patients or those whose meals are provided only at certain times. Patients with arthritis may need late-morning appointments to limber up before the dental appointment. Some patients may not want to drive or take public transportation during busy traffic periods or after dusk. Schedules may also need to be coordinated with individuals who drive the patient to the office.

Medical history. Obtaining and discussing the medical history is often the dental professional's first opportunity to establish an effective rapport with the elderly patient. Bomberg and others (1985) noted that a professional's clinical success with an elderly patient is more dependent on the professional's ability to communicate empathy for the patient through a positive attitude of caring and concern than on either clinical competence or technical skills.

A careful medical and drug history is imperative when treating elderly patients. Because some patients may not remember the exact names and dosages of their medications, suggest they bring the containers with them to the initial appointment or write down the information. Questions regarding the health history that the patient does not recall or cannot answer may be referred to family or friends or the patient's physician. Conditions that may contraindicate dental treatment should be discussed with the physician.

Oral examination. An examination should be performed in the same way as it would for any individual but with particular care for the fragility of oral tissues and alertness to oral conditions that are more prevalent in the elderly population.

The patient should be taught how to examine his or her own oral structures properly. (See Chapter 10). The importance of regular professional examinations of hard and soft tissues of the mouth should also be stressed, especially for those patients who are edentulous and may think they need not seek dental care.

Patient education. Preventive education is especially important for people in this age group, because they may not have grown up with preventive attitudes. Because more and more of the elderly will be retaining their natural teeth, preventive strategies should be designed to reduce the risk of dental caries and periodontal disease. Awareness includes recognition of the signs of dental disease in one's own mouth as well as an understanding of what has caused it. Explanations should avoid complicated terminology.

Emphasizing the positive aspects of preventive behaviors has a much better chance of creating patients' interest in themselves than does emphasis of negative possibilities. Therefore, motivating techniques should stress the positive outcomes of healthy behavior rather than focus on the consequences of disease and the patient's own fears.

Elderly people should be approached with the expectation that they are intelligent, responsible, and capable. It is also important for the elderly to believe in their own abilities to be self-sufficient and to provide care for themselves, rather than to be encouraged to depend on others for care, which decreases their self-esteem and sense of independence. Ignoring these abilities in the elderly and treating them or communicating with them as if they were dependent children, a process known as "infantilization," can lead to a loss of perceived ability on the part of the individual and can actually result in a vicious cycle in which individuals become less competent and self-sufficient because that is the perceived expectation of those around them (Dolinsky and Dolinsky, 1984).

Techniques should be demonstrated in the patient's mouth and then by the patient under the hygienist's supervision. Techniques should be observed and reinforced to ensure that they are being performed properly. If the elderly individual is being assisted with oral health care, follow the same procedures with that person.

Replacing old habits with new ones is difficult for an individual of any age. It requires patience and reinforcement. The hygienist must constantly evaluate the progress the patient is making and assess reasons for lack of improvement in oral health. Failure to improve oral health through the use of self-care methods may be attributed to lack of motivation, lack of understanding or improper technique.

Physically debilitating conditions may not permit use of normal oral hygiene aids. The hygienist should suggest appropriate modifications of the devices or a novel method of use that will compensate for the patient's problem. Manual toothbrushes may need to be modified to improve the access of the brush to all areas of the mouth. Floss holders may be helpful for patients with arthritis and limited dexterity. Electric toothbrushes may also be helpful for these persons. Use of a pulsating oral irrigator may also help in the control of supragingival and loosely attached subgingival plaque. Plaque control can be further enhanced through the supplemental use of tested antiplaque agents such as chlorhexidine, sanguinarine, essential oils, and stannous fluoride. These products can be used as a mouthrinse or diluted in oral irrigators as additional measures of plaque control (see Chapter 19).

Treatment planning. Gordon and Sullivan (1986) proposed that each of the following factors be evaluated when formulating treatment plans for elderly and/or compromised patients:

1. How the current dental situation affects the patient's quality of life
2. Whether the current situation is likely to get better, worse, or remain the same without treatment
3. The patient's desire for dental treatment
4. The potential for additional medical or dental problems that might occur as a result of treatment
5. The amount of time required to complete treatment and the length of time the treatment is expected to last
6. The limitations of the dentist in terms of technique, equipment, and access to the patient

After evaluation of each of these factors, the care provider presents as many viable treatment alternatives as possible to the patient or the patient's guardian and explains the benefits as well as the limitations or risks of each alternative so that the responsible party can give informed consent for the selected treatment plan.

Dental prophylaxis. Thorough scaling and selective polishing is an important part of the preventive dental treatment and maintenance for the elderly. Removal of supra- and subgingival deposits and extrinsic stain is important in controlling and maintaining health. History of periodontal disease may result in oral conditions that challenge the hygienist, including gingival recession, pocket formation, root sensitivity, furcation involvement, tooth mobility, and other conditions associated with this disease. The esthetics of a dental prophylaxis are as important to an elderly patient as they are to a younger one.

There is no conclusive evidence that older persons have either a greater or lesser sensitivity to pain than their younger counterparts (Chapman, 1984). Therefore, the hygienist should not assume

that elderly patients are likely to be more or less sensitive to the pain of treatment than anyone else simply because of their age. The need for careful manipulation of soft tissues during scaling, root planing, and polishing is as important in these patients as in any others.

Nonsurgical periodontal treatment may be the treatment of choice in elderly patients who either cannot withstand surgical treatment or who are poor medical risks for such treatment. Since many reports indicate that periodontal disease can often be treated as successfully by nonsurgical means as by surgical interventions, thorough scaling and root planing can be an important part of periodontal therapy for elderly patients.

Individual assessments should be made as to the amount and length of treatment which should be rendered at any one sitting. The comfort of the patient and ability to tolerate treatment procedures should be carefully considered when determining the treatment plan for each appointment.

Use of fluorides. The use of professional and home fluoride therapy should be based on the same criteria for elderly patients as for other patients. Presence of primary, secondary, or root caries, and reports of root sensitivity are all indications for active fluoride therapy. Selection of the type of fluoride to use should be based on the individual's unique dental needs.

Fluoride is an important part of the preventive regimen for dental caries in adults as well as in children. Both topical and systemic delivery of fluoride to susceptible tooth surfaces are effective means of preventing dental decay. Although the effect of topical fluorides on root caries has not been thoroughly documented, it has been shown that fluoride uptake is greater in root surfaces than in enamel and that high levels of fluoride are found in the cementum even after exposure to low concentrations of fluoride through topical or systemic applications (Brudevold et al, 1960; Singer and Varmstrong, 1962; Yardeni et al, 1963; Gedelia et al, 1965; Furseth, 1970; Stepnick et al, 1975).

Determination of recall intervals. Regular dental recalls are as important to members of this population group as to any other age group. Decisions about the amount of time between preventive visits should be based on the current periodontal status, the patient's ability to control plaque through chemical and mechanical measures, and the patient's ability to gain access to dental treatment (e.g., transportation, mobility, financial considerations). Research has shown that the most beneficial recall interval for patients with periodontal disease activity is no longer than 3 months. Patients who have difficulty maintaining satisfactory plaque control may need to return for more frequent professional maintenance than those whose plaque control is optimal.

ACTIVITIES

1. Invite a panel of pedodontists and dental hygienists who work with children to discuss management of behavior problems associated with fear or resistance to care.
2. Prepare a report of the causes and characteristics of pregnancy gingivitis.
3. Invite a clinician who works with handicapped patients in private practice or in an institutional setting to discuss practical modifications in care.
4. Experience sensory deprivation during a clinic or classroom session by dimming the lights, wearing waxed paper over lenses of prescription or safety glasses, wearing gloves, and putting cotton in your ears. After being a patient or a student under these conditions, discuss what frustrations you experienced as a result of the sensory deprivations. Relate these frustrations to those that an elderly or disabled patient might experience during treatment or patient education.
5. Review the "gate control theory," which describes the psychological/physiological transmission of pain, in Melzack R and Wall PD: The challenge of pain. New York, 1982, Basic Books, Inc.
6. Design a detailed shaping procedure for a dental phobic who needs a complete examination and a dental prophylaxis. Specify each step and the criteria that will be followed in deciding to introduce the patient to each subsequent step. Use your knowledge of behavior modification in designing the procedure.
7. Prepare a report describing the types of sedatives or analgesics that can be used to help control fear, pain, or lack of cooperation among special patients. Identify risk factors and advantages of each. Detail precautions that must be taken when working with patients who have been medicated with each agent.
8. Make arrangements to visit a nursing home. During your visit you may participate as a volunteer in assisting patients or interacting with them during social activities. Observe the atmosphere of a nursing home. Talk to staff members about different daily or weekly activities. If possible, discuss dental care with the dental consultant or members of the nursing staff.
9. Ask to accompany a home health nurse or public health nurse on home visits in your community for the purpose of consulting with clients about their dental health needs and with the nurses regarding their assessment of oral health needs of their clients.
10. Invite a radiation therapist, maxillofacial specialist, or oncologist to discuss procedures for management of complications arising from cancer therapy.
11. Increase your awareness of the achievements of elderly members of our society by looking for examples of individuals over the age of 65 who are still active contributors in the fields of politics, education, business, the arts, religion, or science. Get examples from newspapers, magazines, books, television, and movies.
12. Before class discussion, write down your answers to Palmor's Facts of Aging Quiz. Use the answers to discuss the myths and stereotypes that society associates with aging. Discuss possible reasons for some of these attitudes and how they may affect the delivery of dental care to the elderly.
13. The ADHA curriculum guide "Dental Hygiene Care for the Geriatric Patient" provides ideas for class activities that can be planned to help dental hygienists develop skills related to caring for elderly persons.

REVIEW QUESTIONS

1. True or false: If a child patient is reluctant to cooperate in receiving care, it is best to send the child home and suggest that he or she return when older.
2. In working with a patient who is new to dentistry (whether an adult or a child), it is wise to _____.
3. Describe several modifications in communication that are appropriate when treating a patient who is visually handicapped.
4. List four (or more) implements that can be used to ensure safe delivery of care for a mobile patient.
5. Identify several different modifications of treatment that should be assessed before treating the elderly patient.
6. At what age should a child first see a dentist or hygienist?
7. Should a child's teeth be polished as part of a dental hygiene appointment?
8. What type of brushing tool modification would be appropriate for a patient with limited arm movement?
9. List three areas of patient education to cover with a pregnant patient.
10. Which side effects of radiation cancer therapy are

permanent problems that require lifelong preventive measures?

11. What remedies can be suggested for patients who suffer from the effects of xerostomia?
12. Describe the recommendations for topical fluoride therapy for patients undergoing radiation therapy.
13. State reasons why a complete drug history is an important part of the assessment of elderly dental patients.
14. What dental problems are more prevalent in elderly populations than in their younger counterparts?
15. What three roles can a dental hygienist perform in a nursing home or other institutional setting?
16. Describe modifications in oral hygiene procedures for unconscious or bedridden patients.

REFERENCES

Andlaw RJ, and Rock WP: A manual of paedodontics, New York, 1987, Churchill Livingstone.

Antczak AA, and Branch AA: Perceived barriers to the use of dental services by the elderly, Gerodontics 1:194, 1985.

Bailey BE: Psychological management of the pedodontic patient. In Boundy SS, and Reynolds NJ, editors: Current concepts in dental hygiene, Vol 2, St Louis, 1979, The CV Mosby Co.

Bamberg TJ, et al: Developing the health history of the elderly patient, Gerodontics 1:165, 1985.

Banting DW: Dental caries in the elderly, Gerodontology 3:55, 1984.

Baranovsky A, and Myers MH: Cancer incidence and survival in patients 65 years of age and older, Ca 36:26, 1986.

Barker B, Barker G, and Gier R: Oral management of the cancer patient, Kansas City, Mo, 1982, University of Kansas City-Missouri.

Baum BJ: Salivary gland function during aging, Gerodontics 2:61, 1986.

Beck JD: The epidemiology of dental diseases in the elderly, Gerodontology 3:5, 1984.

Bernhoft C, and Skaug N: Oral findings in irradiated edentulous patients, Int J Oral Surg 14:416, 1985.

Blau ZS: Socioeconomic variations in dental status and behavior of today's elderly, Spec Care Dent 2:244, 1982.

Bomberg TJ, and Ernst NS: Improving utlization of dental care services by the elderly, Gerodontics 2:57, 1986.

Brock AM: Communicating with the elderly patient, Spec Care Dent 5:157, 1985.

Brudevold F, et al: Inorganic and organic components of tooth structure, Ann NY Acad Sci 85:110, 1960.

Burch GE: Fundamentals of clinical cardiology: interesting aspects of geriatric cardiology, Am Heart J 89:99, 1975.

Chapman CR: Pain perception in the elderly patient: an overview of the issues, Gerodontology 3:71, 1984.

Chen TY: Radiation, In Carl W and Sako K, editors: Cancer and the oral cavity, Chicago, Quintessence Publishing Co.

Cheney HG, and DePaola DP: Preventive dentistry. Post-graduate dental handbook series, Littleton, Mass, 1979, PSG/Wright, Inc. Publishing Co.

Clark J, et al: Care document of the geriatric area health education center, Baltimore, 1982, University of Maryland.

Daly KM, and Boyne PJ: Nutrition and eating problems of oral and head-neck surgeries. A guide to soft and liquid meals, Springfield, Ill, 1985, Charles C Thomas.

Debiase, CB, and Komives, BK: An oral care protocol for leukemic patients with chemotherapy-induced oral complications. Spec Care Dentist 3:207, 1983.

DePaola LG, et al: Dental care for patients receiving chemotherapy, JADA 112:198, 1986.

DePaola LG, et al: Prosthodontic considerations for patients undergoing cancer chemotherapy, JADA 107:48, 1983.

Dolinsky EH, and Dolinsky HB: Infantilization of elderly patients by health care providers, Spec Care Dent 4:150, 1984.

Douglass CW, and Gammon MD: Implications of oral disease trends for the treatment needs of older adults, Gerodontics 1:51, 1985.

Engelmeier RL: A dental protocol for patients receiving radiation therapy for cancer of the head and neck, Spec Care Dent 7:54, 1987.

Ernst, et al: Pharmacological considerations for the elderly patient, J Oral Med 39:131, 1984.

Ettinger RL, and Beck JD: The new elderly: what can the dental profession expect? Spec Care Dent 2:62, 1982.

Fattore LD, Strauss R, and Bruno J: The management of periodontal disease in patients who have received radiation therapy for head and neck cancer, Spec Care Dent 7:120, 1987.

Fay JT, and O'Neal R: Dental responsibility for the medically compromised patient, J Oral Med 39:218, 1984.

Fischbach FT: A manual of laboratory diagnostic tests, Philadelphia, 1980, JB Lippincott Co.

Fleming TJ: Use of topical fluoride by patients receiving cancer therapy, Curr Prob in Cancer 7:37, 1983.

Furseth R: A study of experimentally exposed and fluoride treated dental cementum in pigs, Acta Odontol Scand 28:833, 1970.

Gambert SR: Aging—an overview, Spec Care Dent 3:147, 1983.

Gambert SR: Drugs and the elderly, Spec Care Dent 4:102, 1984.

Gamboa GC: The dentist's role in oral cancer prevention and patient behavior modification, CDA J 13:50, 1985.

Gambucci JR, et al: Dental care utilization: patterns of older adults, Gerodontics 2:11, 1986.

Gedalia I, et al: Fluoride content of surface enamel, cementum, lamina dura and subperiosteal bone from mandibular angle of Hebrews, J Dent Res 44:452, 1965.

Gier RE, and Janes DR: Dental management of the pregnant patient: symposium on the patient with increased medical risks, Dent Clin North Am 27:419, 1983.

Goldberg PZ: So what if you can't chew, eat hearty! Springfield, Ill, 1980, Charles C Thomas.

Gooch BF, and Berkey DB: Subjective factors affecting the utilization of dental services by the elderly, Gerodontics 3:65, 1987.

Goose, DH, and Kurer J: A guide to children's dentistry, London, 1973, Henry Kimpton.

Gordon SR, and Sullivan TM: Dental treatment planning for compromised or elderly patients, Gerodontics 2:217, 1986.

's-Gravenmade EJ, et al: Artificial saliva in the management of patients suffering from xerostomia, Gerodontology 3:243, 1984.

Huggins B: Practical paedodontics, Edinburgh, 1973, Churchill Livingstone.

Ismail AI, et al: Findings from the dental care supplement of the national health interview survey, 1983, JADA 114:617, 1987.

Jacobsen PL: Advances in therapy for oral cancer, CDA J 13:25, 1985.

Keene HJ, et al: Dental caries and Streptococcus mutans prevalence in cancer patients with irradiation-induced xerostomia: 1-13 years after radiotherapy, Caries Res 15:416, 1981.

King GE, and Martin JW: Prosthodontic care of patients receiving chemotherapy and irradiation to the head and neck, Curr Prob in Cancer 7:43, 1983.

Kroeger RE: Managing the apprehensive dental patient, Cincinnati, 1987, Heritage Communications.

Lowe O: Pretreatment dental assessment and management of patients undergoing head and neck irradiation, Clin Prev Dent 8:24, 1986.

McClure D, et al: Oral management of the cancer patient, I: oral complications of chemotherapy, Compend Contin Educ Dent 8:41, 1987.

McClure D, et al: Oral management of the cancer patient, II: oral complications of radiation therapy, Compend Contin Educ Dent 8:88, 1987.

McDonald RE, and Avery BS: Dentistry for the child and adolescent, ed 4, St Louis, 1983, The CV Mosby Co.

McElroy TH: Infection in the patient receiving chemotherapy for cancer: oral considerations, JADA 109:454, 1984.

Marinelli RD, et al: Perception of dental needs of the well elderly, Spec Care Dent 2:161, 1982.

Melrose RJ: Etiology of oral cancer, CDA J 13:19, 1985.

Montgomery MT, et al: The incidence of oral herpes simplex virus infection in patients undergoing cancer chemotherapy, Oral Surg 61:238, 1986.

Mossman KL, and Henkin RI: Radiation-induced changes in taste acuity in cancer patients, Int J Radiat Oncol Biol Phys 4:663, 1978.

National Center for Health Statistics: Data from the national health interview survey, Health, United States, 1985. DHHS Pub 86-1232, Washington, 1985, US Government Printing Office.

Nethery WJ, and Fortman K: Prosthetic rehabilitation of patients with oral cancer, CDA J 13:35, 1985.

Peterson DE: Dental care of the cancer patient. Compend Contin Educ Dent 4:115, 1983.

Peterson D, and Sonis S: Oral complications of cancer chemotherapy, The Hague, Netherlands, 1983, Martinus Nijhoff Publishers.

Pinkham JR: Pediatric dentistry: infancy through adolescence, Philadelphia, 1988, WB Saunders Co.

Reynolds WR, et al: Dental management of the cancer patient receiving radiation therapy, Clin Prev Dent 2(5):5, 1980.

Ritchie JR, et al: Dental care for the irradiated cancer patient, Quintessence Int 12:837, 1985.

Roche JR: Preventive pedodontics. In Vernier JL, and Muhler JC: Improving dental practice through preventive measures, ed 3, St Louis, 1975, The CV Mosby Co.

Rosenthal G: Smooth food for all with dental problems . . . and everyone else, Washington, DC, 1980, Library of Congress.

Rothwell BR: Prevention and treatment of orofacial complications of radiotherapy, JADA 114:316, 1987.

Rubin RJ, and Kruger B: Hearing loss in the elderly. In Katzman R and Terry R, editors: The neurology of aging, Philadelphia, 1983, FA Davis Co.

Rubin RL, and Doku HC: Therapeutic radiology: the modalities and their effects on oral tissues, JADA 92:731, 1976.

Schachtele CF, et al: Diet and aging: current concerns related to oral health, Gerodontics 1:117, 1985.

Schweiger JW, and Salcetti MA: Dental management of the geriatric head and neck cancer patient, Gerodontology 5:119, 1986.

Seichter U: Root surface caries: a critical literature review, JADA 115:305, 1987.

Shapiro S, et al: Drug utilization by a non-institutionalized ambulatory elderly population, Gerodontics 2:99, 1986.

Silverberg E, and Lubera J: Cancer statistics, 1987, CA 37:2, 1987.

Silverman S, and Greenspan D: Early detection and diagnosis of oral cancer, CDA J 13:29, 1985.

Silverman S, et al: Occurrence of oral candida in irradiated head and neck cancer patients, J Oral Med 39:194, 1984.

Silverman S Jr, and Thompson JS: Serum zinc and copper in oral/oropharyngeal carcinoma: a study of seventy-five patients, Oral Surg 57:34, 1984.

Singer L, and Varmstrong WD: Comparison of fluoride content of human dental and skeletal tissues, J Dent Res 41(1):154, 1962.

Solomon K, and Vickers R: Attitudes of health workers toward old people, J Am Geriatr Soc 27:187, 1979.

Sonis ST, et al: Oral complications in patients receiving treatment for malignancies other than of the head and neck, JADA 97:468, 1983.

Spiro RH: Squamous cancer of the tongue, Ca 35:252, 1985.

Sreebny L, and Swartz SS: A reference guide to drugs and dry mouth, Gerodontology 5:75, 1986.

Stamm JW, and Banting DW: Comparison of root caries prevalence in adults with life-long residence in fluoridated and non-fluoridated communities, J Dent Res 59(A):abst 552, 1980.

Stepnick RJ, et al: The effects of age and fluoride exposure on fluoride citrate and carbonate content of human cementum, J Periodontol 46:45, 1975.

Sullivan MD, and Fleming TJ: Oral care for the radiotherapy-treated head and neck cancer patient, Dent Hyg 60:112, 1986.

Toljanic JA, and Saunders VW: Radiation therapy and management of the irradiated patient, J Prosthet Dent 52:852, 1984.

Toljanic JA, and Zucuskie TG: Use of a palatal reservoir in denture patients with xerostomia, J Prosthet Dent 52:540, 1984.

Toth BS, and Fleming TJ: Oral/dental considerations for pediatric patients receiving anticancer treatment, MDA J 63(3):33, 1983.

Toth BB, and Frame RT: Dental oncology: the management of disease and treatment-related oral/dental complications associated with chemotherapy, Current Problems in Cancer 7:7, 1983.

Tyron AF: A model for integrating geriatrics into the dental school curriculum Spec Care Dent 1:114, 1981.

US Department of Health, Education, and Welfare: National health survey: prevalence of chronic conditions and impairments, PHS pub 10000, ser 12,8. Washington DC, 1979, US Government Printing Office.

Viidik A: The biological basis of aging. In Holm-Pedersen P and Loe H, editors: Geriatric dentistry: a textbook of oral gerontology, Copenhagen, 1986, Munksgaard.

Vissink A, Huisman MC, and 's-Gravenmade EJ: Construction of an artificial saliva reservoir in an existing maxillary denture, J Prosthet Dent 56:70, 1986.

Vuolo SJ: Oral complications of cancer chemotherapy and dental care for the cancer patient receiving antineoplastic drug therapy: a literature review, NY J Dent 57:50, 1987.

Waldman HB: Knowing more about the elderly can help if we want to provide needed services, Gerodontology 4:83, 1985.

Warren GB, and Blandford DH: Geriatrics and geriatric dental education in the United States, Spec Care Dent 5:150, 1985.

Warren KL: Increasing access to dental care for the older patient: a special challenge, Spec Care Dent 2:248, 1982.

Wei SHY, and Nowak AJ: Implementing a preventive pedodontics practice. In Stewart RE et al, editors: Pediatric dentistry: scientific foundations and clinical practice, St Louis, 1982, The CV Mosby Co.

Wescott WB: Dental management of patients being treated for oral cancer, CDA J 13:42, 1985.

Williams SR: Essentials of nutrition and diet therapy. ed 3, St Louis, 1982, The CV Mosby Co.

Williams TF: Patterns of health and disease in the elderly, Gerodontics 1:284, 1985.

Wilson JR: Non-chew cookbook, Glenwood Springs, Colo, 1985, Wilson Publishing, Inc.

Wright GZ, Starkey PE, and Gardner DE: Managing children's behavior in the dental office, St Louis, 1983, The CV Mosby Co.

Wright WE: Periodontium destruction associated with oncology therapy: five case reports, J Periodontol 58:559, 1987.

Wright WE, et al: An oral disease prevention program for patients receiving radiation and chemotherapy, JADA 110:43, 1985.

Yarden J, Gedalia I, and Kohn M: Fluuoride concentration of dental calculus, surface enamel and cementum, Arch Oral Biol 8:697, 1963.

Yasko JM, and Greene P: Coping with problems related to cancer and cancer treatment, CA 37:106, 1987.

Zack L: The oral cavity. In Rossman I: Clinical geriatrics, ed 2, Philadelphia, 1979, JB Lippincott.

34 RESTORATIVE PROCEDURES

OBJECTIVES: *The reader will be able to*

A. Classification and nomenclature of cavity preparation
   1. Identify, spell, and describe the walls, cavosurfaces, line angles, and point angles of class I, II, III, IV, and V cavity preparations.
B. Isolation of the teeth
   1. Explain the advantages, disadvantages, and rationale of rubber dam isolation.
   2. List the armamentarium needed to place and remove a rubber dam.
   3. Given a specific tooth, identify the clamps that can be used.
   4. Explain the procedure to a patient.
   5. Place and remove a rubber dam.
   6. Evaluate a placed rubber dam and determine if the dam is clinically acceptable.
   7. Explain the importance of ensuring that all fragments of the rubber dam are removed.
C. Bases and liners
   1. Define bases and liners.
   2. Explain the purposes of bases and/or liners under amalgam and composite resin restorations.
   3. Describe the rationale for use and the clinical situations that require calcium hydroxide or varnish.
   4. Discuss the contraindications for using specific bases and liners under composite resin restorations.
   5. Place bases and liners in cavity preparations for amalgam and composite resin restorations.
D. Principles and general procedures for amalgam placement in class V and class I amalgam restorations
   1. List the ingredients of dental amalgam and explain the purpose of each.
   2. Discuss the indications for placement of an amalgam restoration.
   3. Discuss and follow accepted mercury hygiene precautions for both office personnel and patients.
   4. Explain the general procedure for placing an amalgam restoration, with special emphasis on physical properties.
   5. List and discuss the criteria for the placement of a successful class I, class II, and class V amalgam restoration—both the process and product.
   6. Place and carve class I, class II, and a class V amalgam restorations on typodonts or extracted teeth.
   7. After laboratory proficiency has been achieved, perform an amalgam placement procedure as dictated by the patient's needs.
E. Matrix for the conservative class II amalgam restoration
   1. Describe the functions of a matrix band, retainer, and wedge.
   2. Select correct matrix retainer, matrix band, and wedge for a given clinical situation.
   3. Assemble matrix band and retainer.
   4. Place assembled retainer, matrix band, and wedge on prepared tooth on a typodont.
   5. Evaluate the placed retainer, matrix band, and wedge according to criteria provided.
F. Restoration of the conservative class II amalgam preparation
   1. Place, condense, and carve amalgam in a conservative class II cavity preparation.

2. Remove Tofflemire retainer and matrix band without damage to the restoration.
3. Burnish accessible surfaces with apppropriate instrument.
4. Evaluate and adjust occlusal contacts on the restoration.
5. Evaluate the surface, anatomical form, marginal integrity, occlusal contacts, and proximal contours and contact using criteria provided.

G. Recontouring, finishing, and polishing amalgam restorations
1. Explain the rationale for recontouring, finishing, and polishing.
2. Differentiate between and describe the indications and contraindications for recontouring, finishing, and polishing procedures.
3. Identify the armamentarium necessary for amalgam recontouring, finishing, and polishing.
4. Explain how overhang removal is a part of the recontouring procedure and how hand instruments are used to achieve it.
5. List in order the instruments used to polish an amalgam.
6. Recontour, finish, and polish an amalgam.
7. Evaluate polished amalgam restorations to determine if they are acceptable according to the process and product criteria.

H. Properties of composite resin, acid-etching enamel: the class V and class III composite resin restoration
1. Explain the basic formulation of resin and its filler particles; explain the purposes of each.
2. Discuss the indications for placement of a composite resin restoration.
3. Discuss the basic rationale for acid conditioning of enamel, the procedure involved, and the precautions necessary.
4. Describe the difference between light-activated and chemically-activated composite resins; list the advantages of each.
5. Explain the general procedure for placing a composite resin.
6. List and discuss the criteria for a successful class III and class V restoration—both the process and the product.
7. Place and contour a class III, and class V composite resin restoration on a typodont or extracted tooth.
8. After laboratory proficiency has been achieved, perform a composite resin placement procedure as dictated by the patient's needs.

CLASSIFICATION AND NOMENCLATURE OF CAVITY PREPARATIONS

The pattern of carious destruction has many variations, and each preparation is therefore unique (see Chapter 11, Fig. 11-6). However, the basic principles of cavity design produce a similarity of cavity outline within each class of preparation.

The following basic components are common to all classes of cavity preparations:

Wall. A vertical or horizontal surface within the cavity preparation named in accordance with the closest external tooth surface (e.g., the facial, mesial, and lingual walls), or named for a structure it approximates

(e.g., the pulpal wall), or for its relationship to the long axis of the tooth (e.g., axial wall).

Cavosurface. The uncut tooth tissue adjacent to the cavity preparation.

Line angle. A line formed along the junction of two walls or of one wall and the cavosurface (referred to as the cavosurface margin) and named according to the walls and surfaces involved.

Point angle. A point formed by the junction of three walls within a cavity preparation and named according to the walls involved.

Class I cavity preparations

Because the class I preparation provides the foundation for developing terminology for cavity prep-

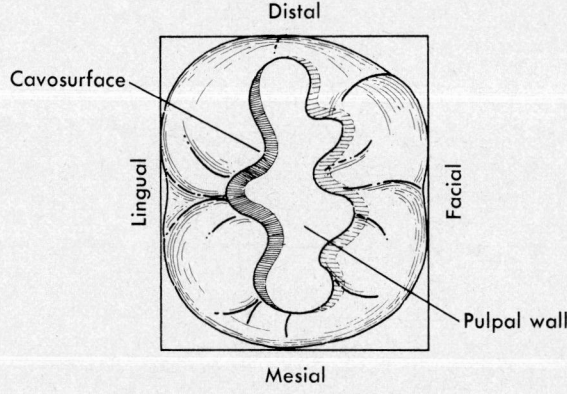

Distal

Cavosurface

Lingual

Facial

Pulpal wall

Mesial

Fig. 34-1. Outline of a class I cavity preparation. The outer surfaces of the tooth are designated mesial, lingual, distal, and facial. The wall at the bottom of the cavity is the pulpal wall. The unprepared external surface of the tooth adjacent to the preparation is the cavosurface.

(From Spohn EE, Halowski WA, and Berry TG: Operative dentistry procedures for dental auxiliaries, St Louis, 1981, The CV Mosby Co.)

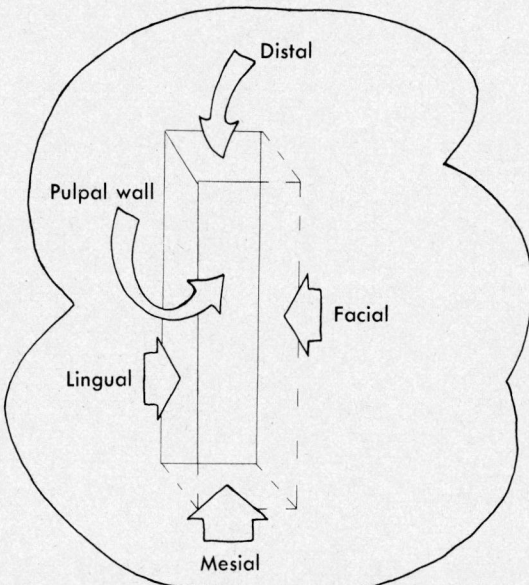

Distal

Pulpal wall

Facial

Lingual

Mesial

Fig. 34-2. Compare with Fig. 34-1. Preparation is a box with four walls and a bottom. The walls of the preparation are named for the external surfaces that they are adjacent to; the bottom is named pulpal wall because of its proximity to the pulp.

(From Spohn EE, Halowski WA, and Berry TG: Operative dentistry procedures for dental auxiliaries, St Louis, 1981, The CV Mosby Co.)

arations, it will be described in greater detail than any of the other classes. A class I preparation on a molar is used to illustrate the derivation of the nomenclature (Fig. 34-1).

Walls. This preparation normally has curving walls along the facial and lingual sides that blend with the mesial and distal walls. These vertical

walls end at a horizontal wall, called the pulpal wall. To simplify naming all the parts of the preparation, it is illustrated (Fig. 34-2) as a "box" within the tooth with the walls named.

Line angles. The three sets of line angles in the occlusal class I preparation are named according to the walls involved (Figs. 34-3, 34-4, and 34-5).

Rule number 1: When developing the name of a line angle or a point angle, drop the "al" and substitute "o" at the end of all words in the terms except the last one. For example, the line angle formed by the facial wall intersecting with the pulpal wall is termed the faciopulpal line angle. The term pulpofacial line angle is equally correct. The remaining line angles formed by the pulpal wall are shown in Fig. 34-3. In the actual cavity preparation, these line angles are not straight but follow the outline form of the preparation. The line angles formed by the intersection of one vertical wall with another are illustrated in Fig. 34-4. In the actual cavity preparation, these are not sharp corners but curves, and the names represent hypothetical places along the curves. Fig. 34-5 illustrates the four line angles formed by the intersection of the vertical walls with the cavosurface, or unprepared tooth structure.

Rule number 2: When cavosurface is one of the words used in developing a term, place it last in developing the name of a line angle. Therefore, the intersection of the facial wall with the cavosurface is named the faciocavosurface line angle. The other three cavosurface line angles are named in a similar manner.

Point angles. The four internal point angles of a class I occlusal preparation are illustrated in Fig. 34-6. The name of each is derived by combining the names of the involved walls using Rule number 1.

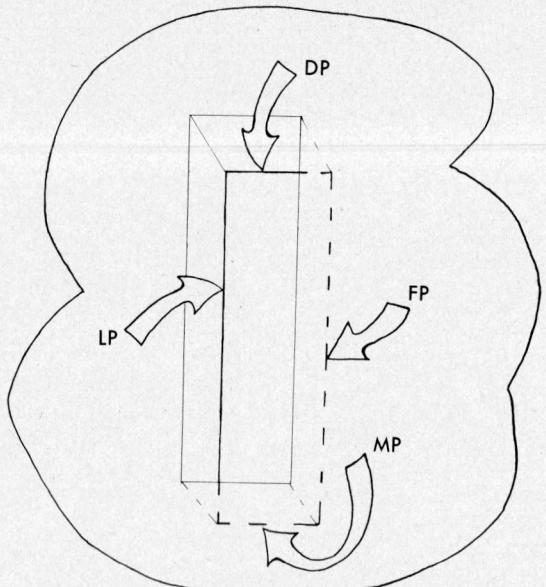

Fig. 34-3. The four line angles formed at the intersections of the vertical walls with the pulpal wall: the mesiopulpal *(MP)*, linguopulpal *(LP)*, distopulpal *(DP)*, and faciopulpal *(FP)* line angles.

(From Spohn EE, Halowski WA, and Berry TG: Operative dentistry procedures for dental auxiliaries, St Louis, 1981, The CV Mosby Co.)

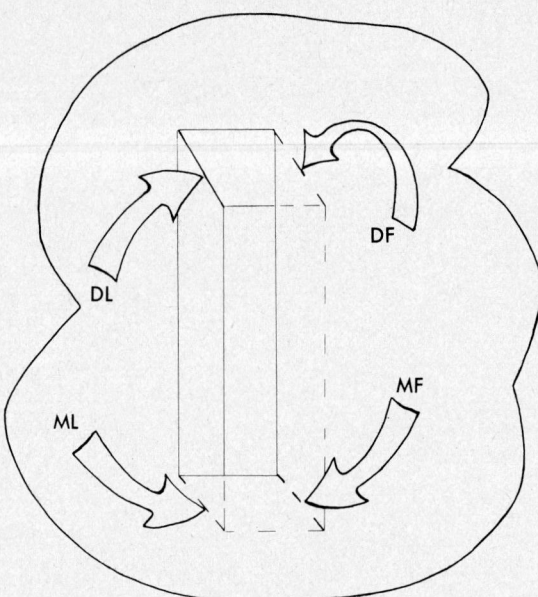

Fig. 34-4. The four line angles formed where the vertical walls intersect one another: the mesiolingual *(ML)*, distolingual *(DL)*, distofacial *(DF)*, and mesiofacial *(MF)* line angles.

(From Spohn EE, Halowski, WA, and Berry TG: Operative dentistry procedures for dental auxiliaries, St Louis, 1981, The CV Mosby Co.)

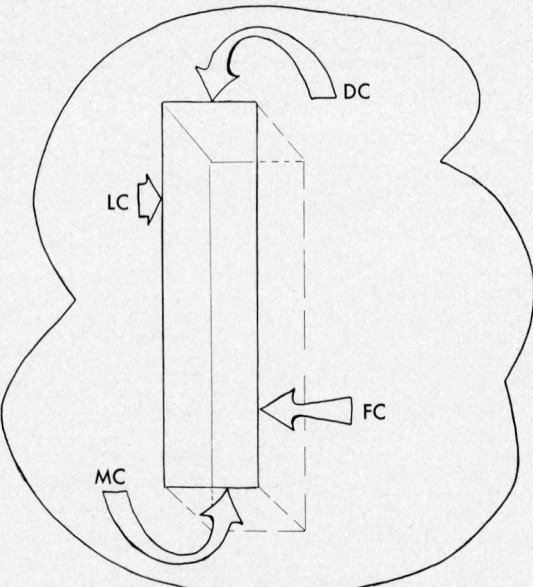

Fig. 34-5. The four line angles formed where the vertical walls intersect the uncut tooth surface (cavosurface): the mesial *(MC)*, lingual *(LC)*, distal *(DC)*, and facial *(FC)* cavosurface line angles.

(From Spohn EE, Halowski WA, and Berry TG: Operative dentistry procedures for dental auxiliaries, St Louis, 1981, The CV Mosby Co.)

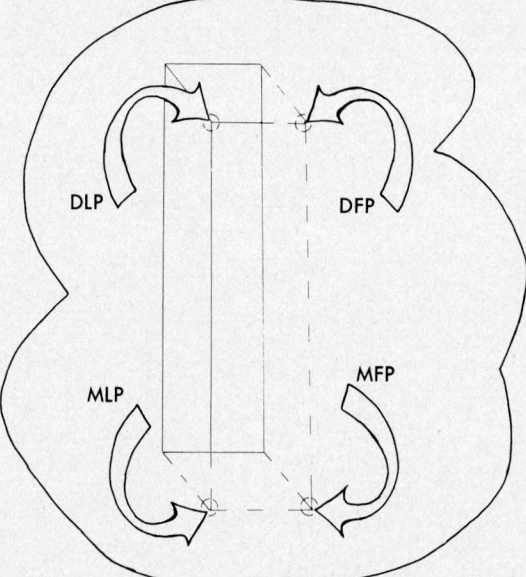

Fig. 34-6. The four point angles formed at the intersection of three internal walls. For example, the intersection of the three walls in the lower left is the mesiolinguopulpal *(MLP)* point angle.

(From Spohn EE, Halowski WA, and Berry TG: Operative dentistry procedures for dental auxiliaries, St Louis, 1981, The CV Mosby Co.)

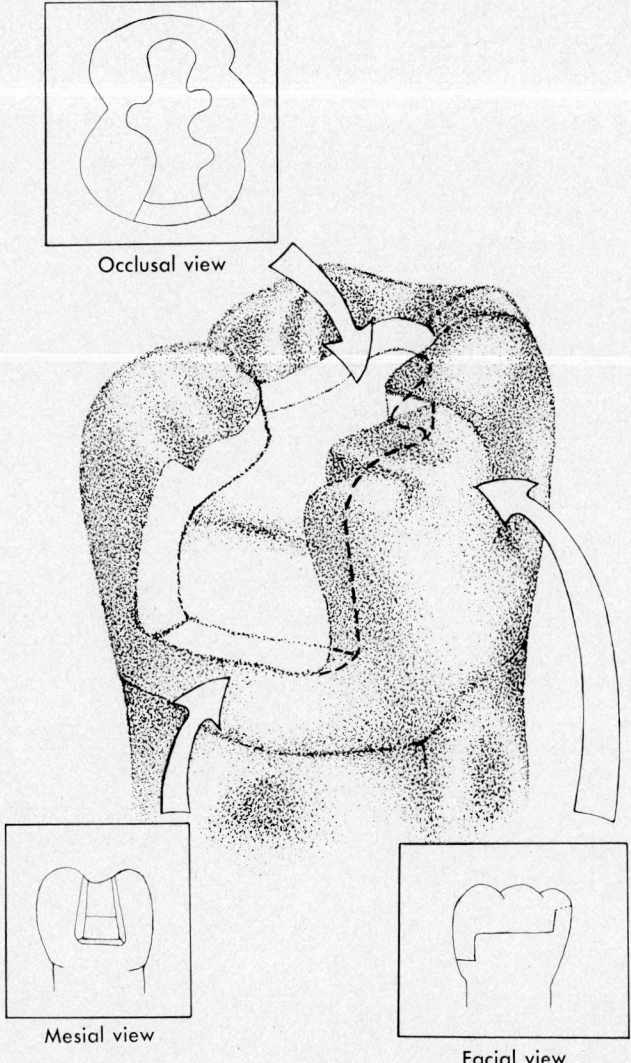

Occlusal view

Mesial view

Facial view

Fig. 34-7. Class II mesio-occlusal cavity preparation on tooth No. 19. Compare with the occlusal view in Fig. 34-1.

(From Spohn EE, Halowski WA, and Berry TG: Operative dentistry procedures for dental auxiliaries, St Louis, 1981, The CV Mosby Co.)

Class II cavity preparations

The class II cavity preparation is designed to remove the proximal surface. Because removal of proximal tooth tissue requires an occlusal approach, the marginal ridge is involved in the preparation (Fig. 34-7). The occlusal portion is prepared like a class I preparation. Therefore, a class II preparation is an extension of the class I preparation into the proximal area (34-7).

Walls and cavosurface. For the occlusal portion, the walls are identical to the class I preparation. The walls of the proximal portion, illustrated in Fig. 34-8, include an axial wall, which is parallel to the long axis of the tooth, and a gingival

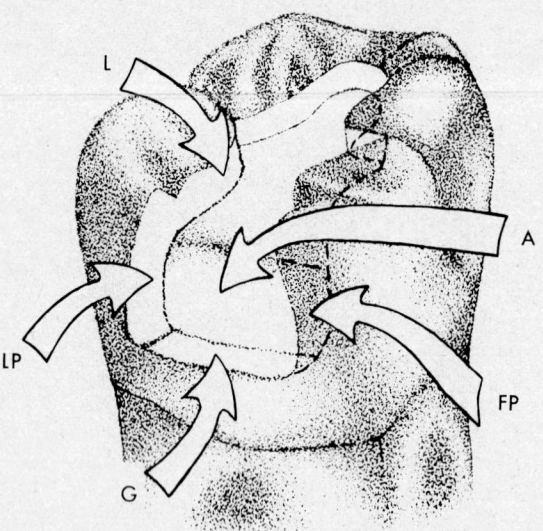

Fig. 34-8. The walls of the proximal portion of this preparation are the gingival *(G)*, linguoproximal *(LP)*, axial *(A)*, and facioproximal *(FP)* walls.
(From Spohn EE, Halowski WA, and Berry TG: Operative dentistry procedures for dental auxiliaries, St Louis, 1981, The CV Mosby Co.)

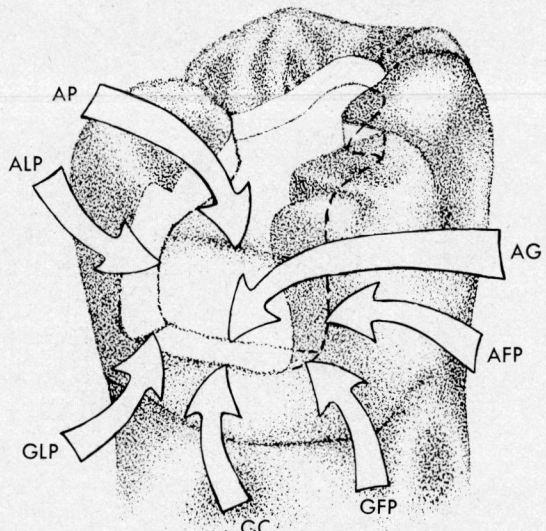

Fig. 34-9. The line angles of the proximal portion of a class II mesio-occlusal preparation: the gingivolinguoproximal *(GLP)*, axiolinguoproximal *(ALP)*, axiopulpal *(AP)*, axiogingival *(AG)*, axiofacioproximal *(AFP)*, and gingivofacioproximal *(GFP)* line angles.
(From Spohn EE, Halowski WA, and Berry TG: Operative dentistry procedures for dental auxiliaries, St Louis, 1981, The CV Mosby Co.)

wall, which is adjacent to the gingival tissues. The lingual and facial walls that continue from the occlusal portion to the proximal portion are termed the linguoproximal wall and the facioproximal wall, respectively.

Line angles. In the proximal portion of this preparation, the following new line angles occur:

Internal line angles (Fig. 34-9)

1. Axiopulpal
2. Axiogingival
3. Axiolinguoproximal
4. Axiofacioproximal
5. Gingivolinguoproximal (retentive feature)
6. Gingivofacioproximal (retentive feature)

External line angles (Fig. 34-10)

1. Linguoproximal cavosurface
2. Facioproximal cavosurface
3. Gingival cavosurface

Point angles. The intersection of the gingival and axial walls with each of the proximal walls forms two point angles: the axiogingivolinguoproximal and the axiogingivofacioproximal point angles (Fig. 34-11).

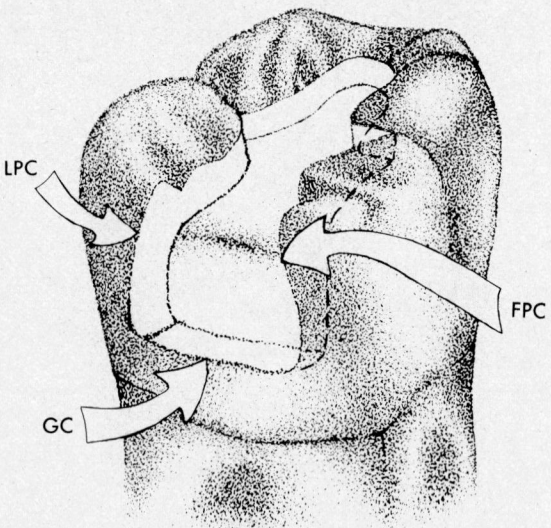

Fig. 34-10. The cavosurface line angles of the proximal portion of the class II preparation: the gingival *(GC)*, linguoproximal *(LPC)*, and facioproximal *(FPC)* cavosurface line angles.
(From Spohn EE, Halowski WA, and Berry TG: Operative dentistry procedures for dental auxiliaries, St Louis, 1981, The CV Mosby Co.)

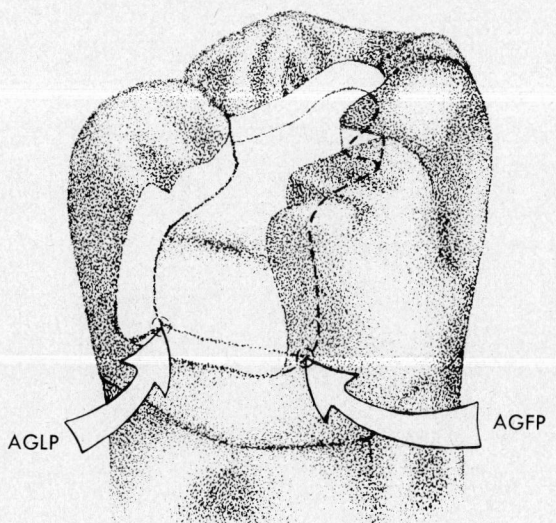

Fig. 34-11. The internal point angles of the mesioproximal portion of the class II mesio-occlusal preparation: the axiogingivolinguoproximal *(AGLP)* and axiogingivofacioproximal *(AGFP)* point angles.
(From Spohn EE, Halowski WA, and Berry TG: Operative dentistry procedures for dental auxiliaries, St Louis, 1981, The CV Mosby Co.)

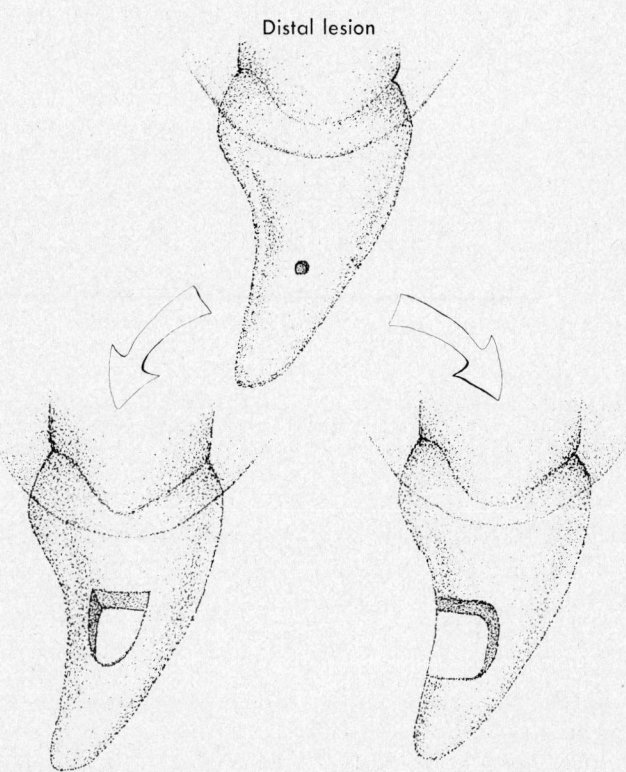

Fig. 34-12. Two variations (labial and lingual access) of the class III cavity preparation.
(From Spohn EE, Halowski WA, and Berry TG: Operative dentistry procedures for dental auxiliaries, St Louis, 1981, The CV Mosby Co.)

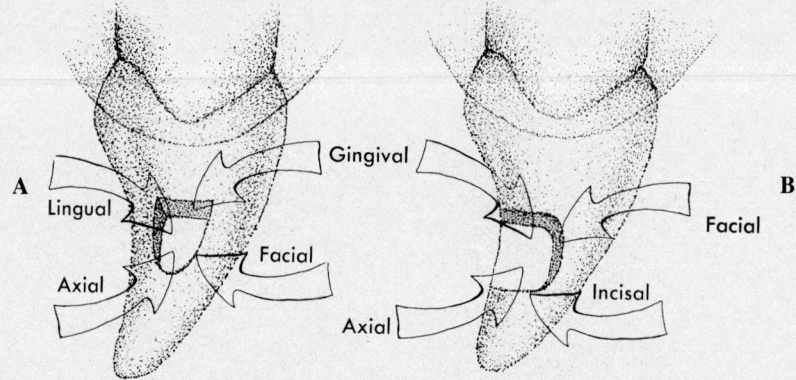

Fig. 34-13. Walls of the class III cavity preparation: **A,** labial access; **B,** lingual-slot access.
(From Spohn EE, Halowski WA, and Berry TG: Operative dentistry procedures for dental auxiliaries, St Louis, 1981, The CV Mosby Co.)

Class III cavity preparations

Dental caries on the proximal surface of anterior teeth may be removed by either a facial or lingual approach. Fig. 34-12 illustrates the cavity outlines resulting from each approach.

Walls and cavosurface. Fig. 34-13 illustrates the walls for the lingual-slot and the labial approach class III preparations. Using the rules and definitions previously stated, the reader can identify the line angles and point angles for each of the preparations.

Class IV cavity preparations

For the purposes of this chapter, illustrations are included for one form of a class IV restoration so that the student will have some basis on which to develop the nomenclature for this preparation. Fig. 34-14 is a proximal view of the class IV preparation.

Class V cavity preparations

This preparation is similar to a class I preparation except that its location is in the gingival one third of the facial or lingual surface. It also may be thought of as a "box" with four sides and a bottom. Fig. 34-15 illustrates the class V preparation on a posterior tooth. Note that on an anterior tooth, the occlusal wall is called the incisal wall.

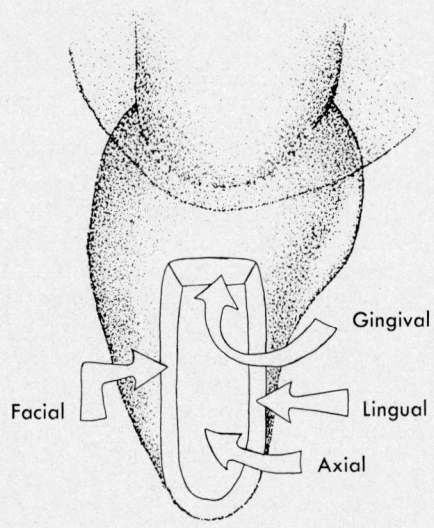

Fig. 34-14. Proximal view of the walls of the class IV cavity preparation.
(From Spohn EE, Halowski WA, and Berry TG: Operative dentistry procedures for dental auxiliaries, St Louis, 1981, The CV Mosby Co.)

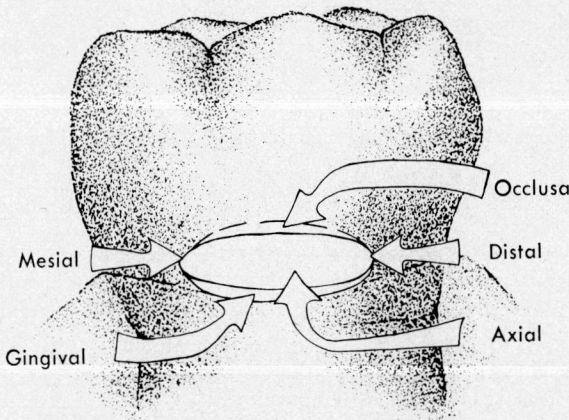

Fig. 34-15. Walls of the class V cavity preparation on a posterior tooth.

(From Spohn EE, Halowski WA, and Berry TG: Operative dentistry procedures for dental auxiliaries, St Louis, 1981, The CV Mosby Co.)

ISOLATION OF THE TEETH

Proper preparation of the operating field is necessary to perform operative dentistry procedures with optimal results. Isolating the operating field prevents moisture contamination, retracts and controls the soft tissues, protects the patient against aspiration of instruments and materials, and provides optimal visibility of the operating site. This should be accomplished without interfering with the operator's visual or mechanical access to the operating site, injuring soft or hard tissues, or causing discomfort.

The type of isolation required depends on the duration of the procedure and the degree of dryness necessary. For some procedures, cotton roll isolation can be used in conjunction with a saliva ejector and high-volume oral evacuation system. Mechanical cotton roll holders can be used in the mandibular arch. Absorbent triangles, placed over the parotid duct, can be used in conjunction with cotton rolls for increased moisture control. Cotton roll isolation offers ease and speed of application. However, there is risk of contamination of the operating field, limited retraction of soft tissues, and nothing to protect the patient from aspirating debris or small instruments.

The rubber dam meets the criteria for ideal isolation. Disadvantages are that the clamp can irritate the gingiva, placement of the dam can be time consuming for the beginning clinician, and some patients are sensitive to the rubber dam. Overall, however, the advantages of using a rubber dam outweigh the disadvantages.

Armamentarium

The necessary armamentarium for rubber dam placement is illustrated in Fig. 34-16. There are several types of rubber dam holders (Fig. 34-17). One of the most commonly used is the Young's frame. It is a metal U-shaped frame, which holds the dam away from the patient's face. The Woodbury holder is an elastic band that fits around the back of the patient's head and attached to the sides of the dam with three clips on each side. It provides excellent lip and cheek retraction.

The rubber dam clamp (Fig. 34-18) anchors the dam to the tooth. Therefore, this tooth is referred to as the anchor tooth. Clamps may be winged or wingless. The jaws of the winged clamp have small projections which allows the clamp to be mounted on the dam before placement on the teeth. The chart in Fig. 34-19 will be helpful in determining which clamps are most likely to fit particular teeth.

The dam material is available in several weights (light, medium, heavy, and extra heavy) and in four colors (green, blue, white, and gray). Medium or heavy material is usually used for restorative procedures because the heavier weight provides better retraction of the gingiva, lips, and cheeks and does not tear easily. Lightweight material is used more often during endodontic procedures because only one tooth is isolated, tearing is less of a problem, and the lighter material is easier to manipulate.

Preparing the patient

If the patient has never experienced a rubber dam, explain the benefits, such as eliminating debris in the mouth and the potential for a better restoration because of the isolation from oral fluids. Briefly explain the procedure to the patient so that the patient knows what to expect. As the patient will not be able to talk with the dam, suggest signals to be used in case the patient needs to communicate.

Examining the mouth

Examine the site where the dam is to be placed. Floss the teeth to determine if there will be difficulty in passing the dam between any of the teeth.

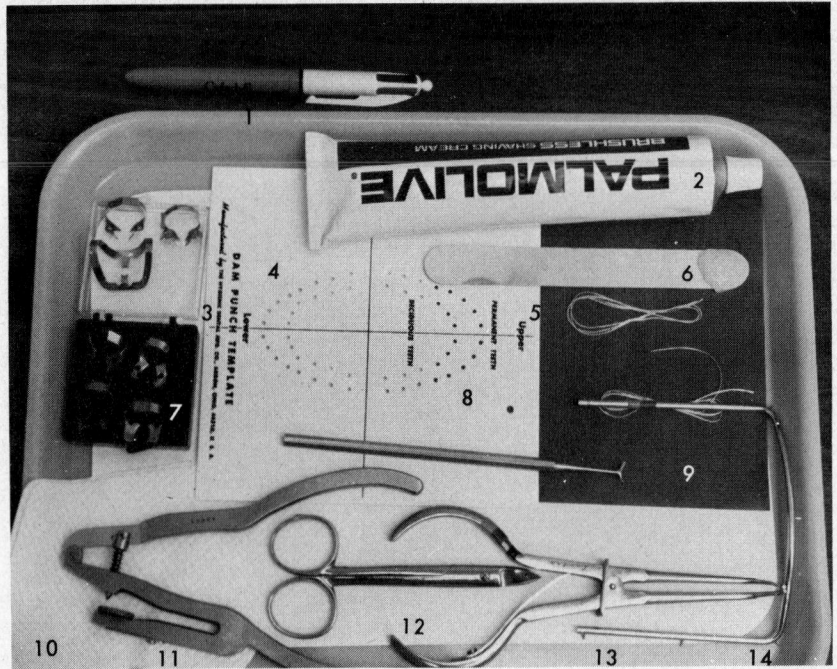

Fig. 34-16. Tray setup for rubber dam application includes: *1,* ball-point pen; *2,* lubricant for rubber dam; *3,* gingival retractors; *4,* rubber dam template; *5,* waxed dental floss; *6,* lubricant on tongue blade; *7,* assorted rubber dam clamps; *8,* T-ball burnisher; *9,* rubber dam material; *10,* rubber dam napkin; *11,* rubber dam punch; *12,* scissors; *13,* rubber dam clamp forceps; *14,* rubber dam holder.
(From Spohn EE, Halowski WA, and Berry TG: Operative dentistry procedures for dental auxiliaries, St Louis, 1981, The CV Mosby Co.)

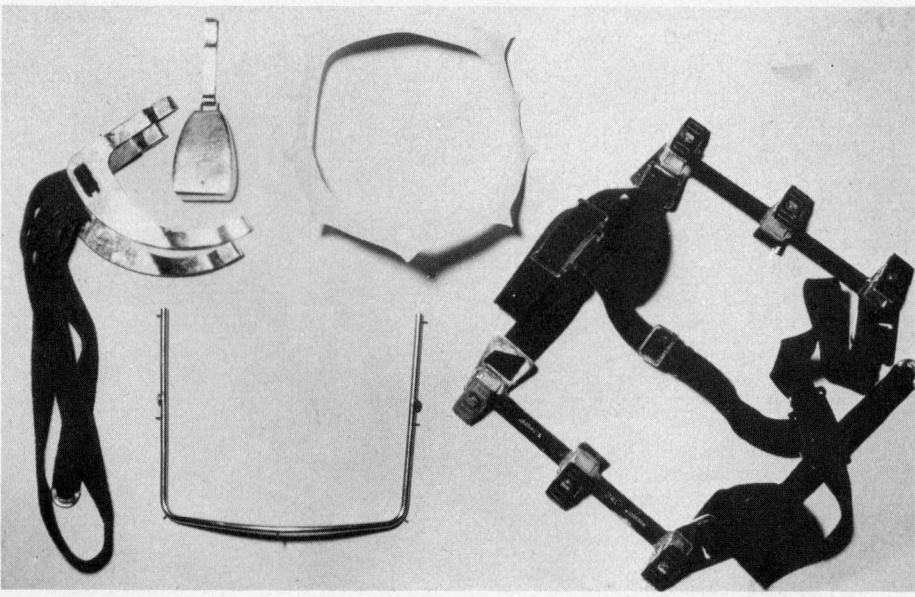

Fig. 34-17. Some examples of rubber dam holders. *Clockwise from upper left:* Wizard holder, weight, plastic frame, Woodbury holder, and Young's frame.
(From Gilmore WH, et al: Operative dentistry, ed 4, St Louis, 1982, The CV Mosby Co.).

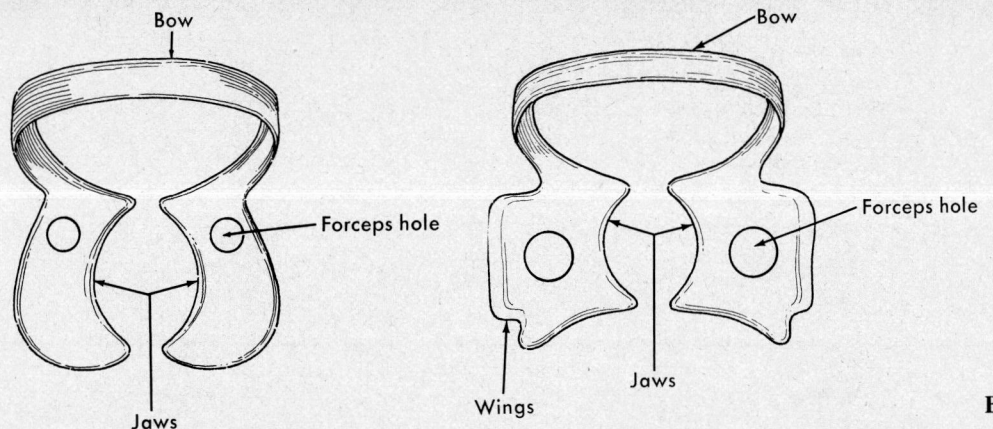

Bow
Forceps hole
Jaws
A
Bow
Forceps hole
Jaws
Wings
B

Fig. 34-18. Rubber dam clamps: **A,** wingless; **B,** winged.
(From Spohn EE, Halowski WA, and Berry TG: Operative dentistry procedures for dental auxiliaries, St Louis, 1981, The CV Mosby Co.)

SSW 212
Ivory S1
Maxillary premolars
SSW 27
Maxillary right molars
SSW 30
Ivory 11, 11A
Maxillary molars
Ivory 4, 8
Maxillary left molars
SSW 31
Ivory 10-10A
All molars
Ivory 7B, 14, 14A, 27
SSW 26
Mandibular right molars
Mandibular left molars
SSW 31
Ivory 10-10A
Mandibular molars
Ivory 7
SSW 30
Ivory 11, 11A
Mandibular premolars
and anteriors
Ivory 00, 0, 2
SSW 212
Ivory S1
Gingival retraction
SSW 212 Ivory S3
30 4(maxillary molars)
31 16 (molars)
Deciduous molars
SSW 1A Ivory 8A
2A

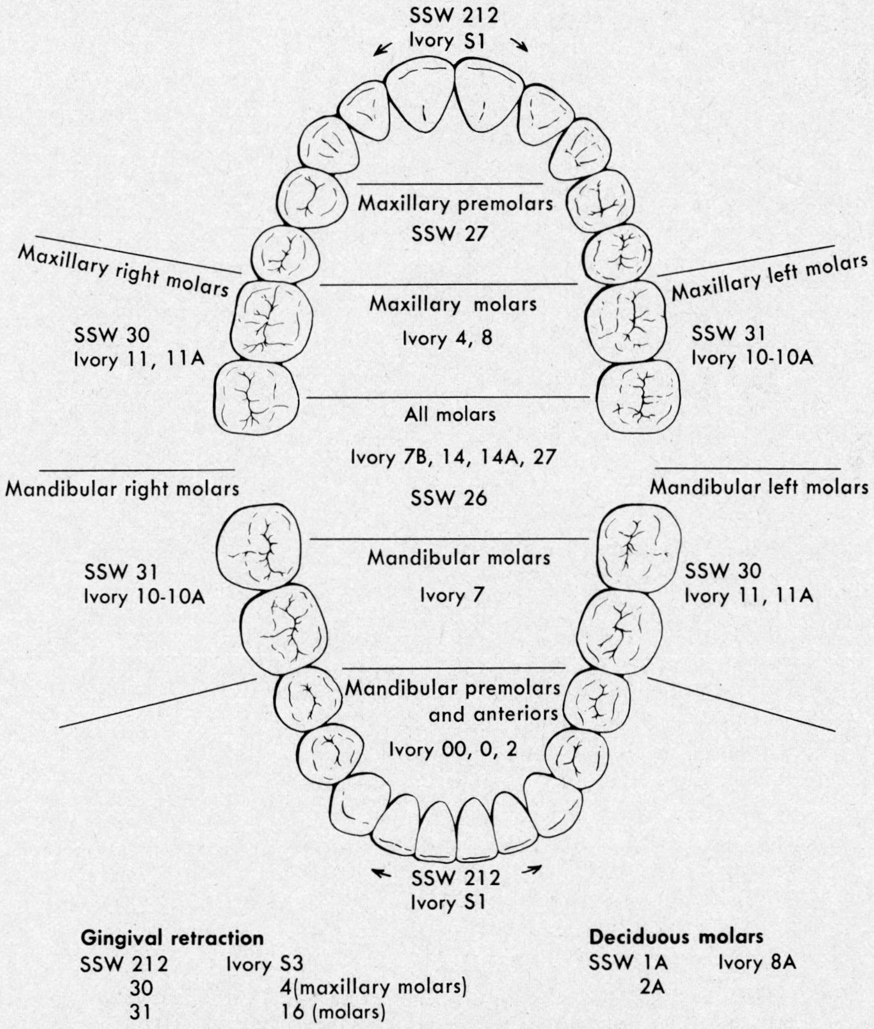

Fig. 34-19. Chart of suggested clamps to be used in various areas of mouth.
(From Howard WW, and Moller RC: Atlas of operative dentistry, ed 3, St Louis, 1981, The CV Mosby Co.)

If floss cannot be passed through any of the contacts, determine the cause. Calculus, restoration overhangs or rough proximal surfaces should be removed. Teeth with very tight contacts may need to be wedged apart before rubber dam placement. Place a wooden wedge into the involved proximal space for 1 to 2 minutes and then check the contact again with dental floss. Check the patient's occlusion to determine if any unusual anatomy may interfere with the restoration. Note the shape and size of the arch, position of the teeth, edentulous spaces, and fixed prostheses. This information will be needed to correctly punch the rubber dam.

Selecting the clamp

The rubber dam clamp is selected on the basis of the anatomy of the anchor tooth (see Fig. 34-19 for suggested clamps to be used in different areas of mouth). The location and number of the involved teeth will determine which teeth are to be isolated. Minimal access is obtained by isolating one tooth distal and two teeth mesial to the teeth being restored. For greater access, maximum retraction of the lips, cheeks, and tongue, and increased number of teeth available for a finger rest, the most distal tooth in the quadrant is clamped and isolation is extended to the opposite lateral incisor. When the operating site is exclusively the anterior teeth, the first premolar to the contralateral first premolar are isolated. In this situation, both premolars may be clamped or ligated with dental floss or the rubber dam wedged with a piece of rubber dam.

Determine the anchor tooth and select the appropriate clamp. Tie dental floss to the clamp to permit retrieval of the clamp if it slips off the tooth. Loop the floss around the bow of the clamp. Place the clamp in the forceps and squeeze the handles together to open the jaws of the clamp. With the tips of the forceps upward, the locking ring will slide toward the handle of the forceps and the jaws of the clamp will remain open (Fig. 34-20).

Position the clamp over the tooth, rotating it lingually to seat first the lingual jaw because vision is more restricted in this area. Rotate the clamp facially and seat the facial jaw. Be certain that the jaws do not drag across the tooth and scar the cementum. Squeeze the handles of the forceps

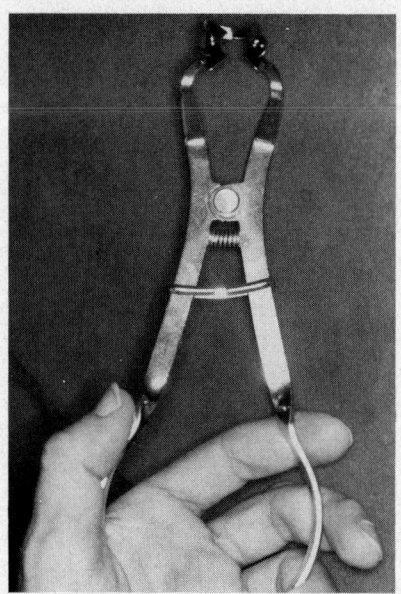

Fig. 34-20. Engage locking ring by pointing forceps upward, then squeeze and release.
(From Spohn EE, Halowski WA, and Berry TG: Operative dentistry procedures for dental auxiliaries, St Louis, 1981, The CV Mosby Co.)

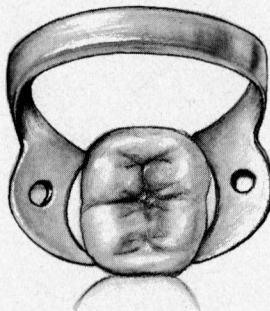

Fig. 34-21. All four prongs of clamp should be in contact with tooth.
(From Howard WW, and Moller RC: Atlas of operative dentistry, ed 3, St Louis, 1981, The CV Mosby Co.)

to release the locking ring and allow the jaws of the clamp to engage the tooth. When properly placed, all four prongs should contact the tooth cervical to the height of contour (Fig. 34-21). The clamp should be stable when rocked gently from side to side with light finger pressure and should not impinge on the soft tissue. If these criteria are not met, reposition the clamp or, if needed, select another clamp. If the clamp rotates on the tooth, slides off the tooth, or rests on the papilla, it is probably too big. If the clamp does not fit over the height of contour or tends to pop off the tooth, the clamp is probably too small. As the prongs are pointed and can cut the gingiva or gouge the root surface, forceps should always be used to disengage or adjust the clamp.

Preparing the rubber dam

The rubber dam is punched to suit each clinical situation. The factors to consider for determining the number, size, and location of the holes are the location of the teeth to be isolated, the size of the teeth, the shape and size of the arch, the position and spacing of the teeth, and the type of preparation. A template or rubber dam stamp can be used as a guide to mark the location of the teeth (Fig. 34-22). If these are not available, the dam can be punched according to Fig. 34-23. Mark the central incisors near the midline of the dam and allow 4 mm of rubber between anterior holes and 5 mm of rubber between posterior holes. Mark the holes for Class V restorations 1 mm to the facial side and allow an additional 1 mm of rubber between adjacent teeth for the gingival retraction needed for access to the Class V lesion.

The size of the tooth to be isolated determines the size of the hole to be punched. As a general guideline for a six-hole punch, use the smaller, size 2 hole for mandibular incisors and maxillary lateral incisors; the medium, size 3 hole for premolars, canines and maxillary central incisors; the size 5 hole for molars; and the size 6 hole for the anchor tooth and clamp. Fig. 34-24 *illustrates the use of a five-hole punch.* As the hole is punched, pull the dam up the punch spike to be certain the punch has cut completely through the dam.

Placing the rubber dam and frame

Before applying the rubber dam, lubricate the patient's lips with petroleum jelly to protect them against dryness and irritation from the dam. Place the powdered side of the dam facing the clinician to reduce glare from light reflection off the dam.

There are two alternative methods of placing the clamp and dam on the tooth. The decision which to use is based on the clinical situation, the operator's preference, and the availability of clamps. If a wingless clamp is used, place the clamp on the tooth and recheck its stability. Correctly orient the rubber dam and place the index finger of each hand on opposing sides of the hole that is to be placed over the clamped tooth.

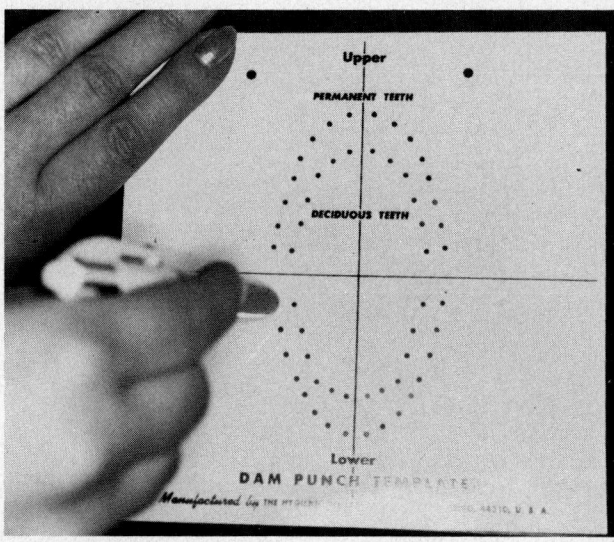

Fig. 34-22. Rubber dam template and a ball-point pen are used to mark the dam.
(From Spohn EE, Halowski WA, and Berry TG: Operative dentistry procedures for dental auxiliaries, St Louis, 1981, The CV Mosby Co.)

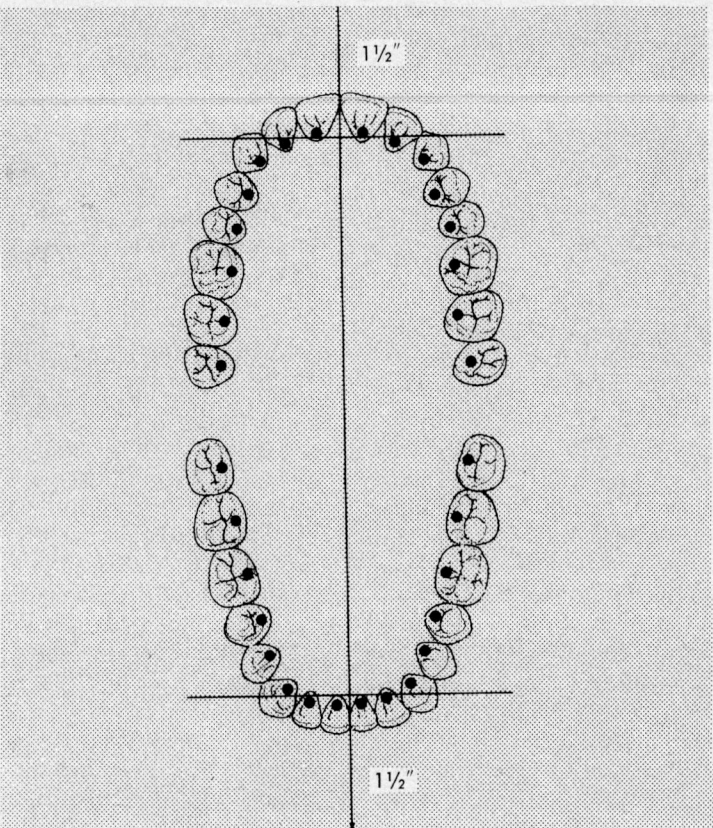

Fig. 34-23. For the average-sized arch, punch the central incisors approximately 1½ inches from the edge of the dam near the midline. Punch additional holes using guidelines in the text.
(From Spohn EE, Halowski WA, and Berry TG: Operative dentistry procedures for dental auxiliaries, St Louis, 1981, The CV Mosby Co.)

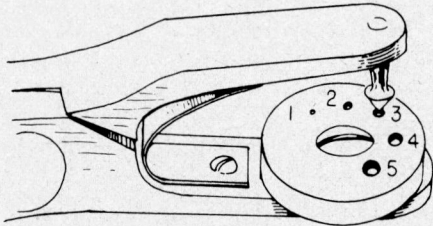

1. Smallest incisors
2. Incisors and cuspids
3. Cuspids and premolars
4. Premolars and molars
5. Molars and clamps

Fig. 34-24. Suggested sizes of holes to be punched in dam for various teeth.
(Modified from Howard WW, and Moller RC: Atlas of operative dentistry, ed 3, St Louis, 1981, The CV Mosby Co.)

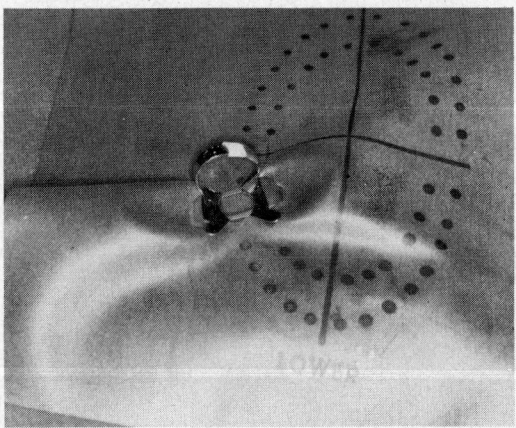

Fig. 34-25. Winged clamp being held by the dam before placement on the tooth.
(From Spohn EE, Halowski WA, and Berry TG: Operative dentistry procedures for dental auxiliaries, St Louis, 1981, The CV Mosby Co.)

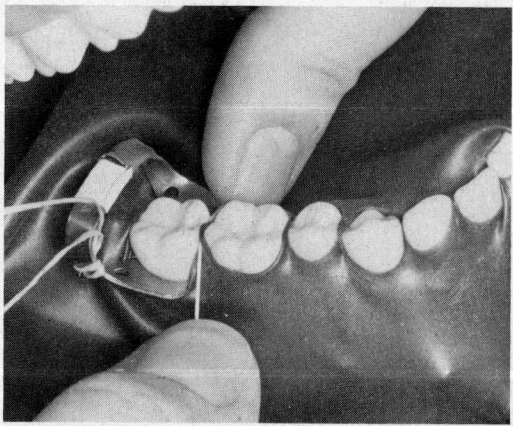

Fig. 34-26. When necessary, push the interseptal rubber through the contacts with dental floss.
(From Spohn EE, Halowski WA, and Berry TG: Operative dentistry procedures for dental auxiliaries, St Louis, 1981, The CV Mosby Co.)

Stretch the dam to enlarge the hole and slide it over the bow and under each of the jaws, one at a time. When the tooth and clamp are fully exposed and the rubber dam is against the gingiva, use the blade of the T-ball burnisher to pull the dental floss tied to the clamp through the hole.

The dam may also be placed on the bow of the wingless clamp before placement on the tooth. This method may be easier for the inexperienced operator because it allows for maximal access and visibility while applying the clamp. Care must be exercised, however, to avoid placing excess pressure on the clamp and traumatizing the tooth structure or surrounding gingiva as the rubber dam is seated.

To use a winged clamp, orient the clamp to the correct hole in the dam and engage the clamp onto the forceps. Slide one wing into the hole and then stretch the dam toward and over the opposite wing (Fig. 34-25). The dam may be placed on the frame at this stage if desired. Place the clamp on the anchor tooth as described previously, looking through the opening and under the dam to check the position of the clamp relative to the gingiva before releasing the forceps. Pull the rubber dam off the wings and under the clamp. Although vision is more limited when using this method, placement is faster because the clamp, dam, and frame are placed at the same time. After the dam is placed over the clamp, the most anterior tooth is isolated. The frame is placed next to hold the

dam away from the patient's face and to provide access to the working area. Position the base of the U-shaped frame downward, with the concave side of the frame toward the patient. Gently pull the rubber dam over the small metal protrusions on the frame to hold the dam in place.

Stretch the dam to open the holes and expose the remaining teeth one at a time. Next pass the rubber dam through the contact areas. This is more easily done with the help of an assistant. As the assistant stretches the dam over each contact area, push the rubber through the contact areas using waxed floss or tape (Fig. 34-26). Hold the floss against one proximal surface and then the other. Do not try to force the whole width of the septum through at once; this is difficult to accomplish and may result in tearing the dam. If the dam is not fully inserted into the interproximal areas, it will be difficult to tuck the dam into the facial and lingual sulci. Repeat the flossing procedure in any resistant interproximal areas.

After the dam is through each of the contact areas, the frame is readjusted to hold the dam more tightly. The frame should be as centered as possible and placed to avoid endangering the patient (i.e., the ends of the frame should be away from the patient's eyes). The floss attached to the clamp can be tied to the rubber dam frame so it is out of the operating field.

Tuck or invert the dam into the sulcus around each tooth to prevent seepage of sulcular fluid and

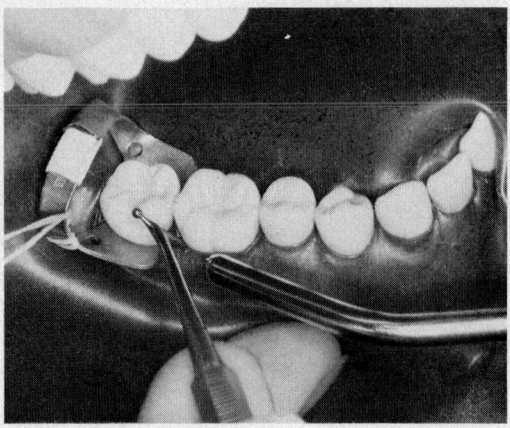

Fig. 34-27. Invert the dam into the sulcus using a thin (not sharp) blade. Air helps to dry the tooth and dam and creates a seal.
(From Spohn EE, Halowski WA, and Berry TG: Operative dentistry procedures for dental auxiliaries, St Louis, 1981, The CV Mosby Co.)

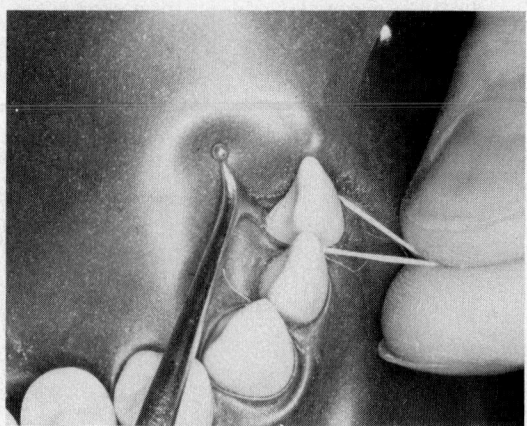

Fig. 34-28. Push the loop of ligature below the cingulum with the blade while pulling the ends in an apical direction.
(From Spohn EE, Halowski WA, and Berry TG: Operative dentistry procedures for dental auxiliaries, St Louis, 1981, The CV Mosby Co.)

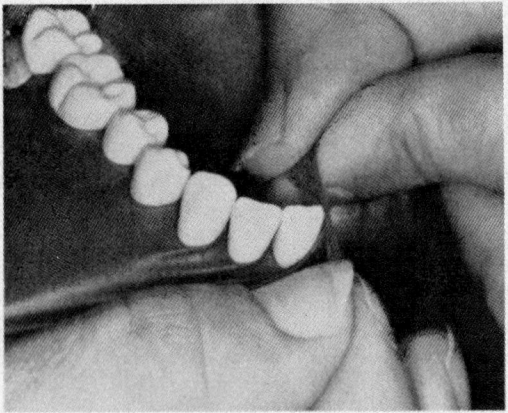

Fig. 34-29. Stretch the piece of rubber dam and push it into the contact area.
(From Spohn EE, Halowski WA, and Berry TG: Operative dentistry procedures for dental auxiliaries, St Louis, 1981, The CV Mosby Co.)

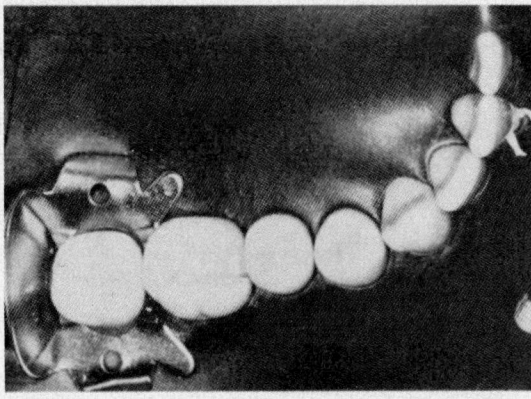

Fig. 34-30. Isolation achieved through a properly mounted rubber dam.
(From Spohn EE, Halowski WA, and Berry TG: Operative dentistry procedures for dental auxiliaries, St Louis, 1981, The CV Mosby Co.)

saliva from the oral cavity. Starting at the distal, position the blade of a plastic instrument or T-ball burnisher parallel to the distofacial line angle of the tooth, directed slightly into the sulcus, and slide it to the mesial line angle using the edge of the blade to push the rubber into the gingival sulcus (Fig. 34-27). Simultaneously, direct a stream of air into the sulcus to dry the tooth, rubber dam, and soft tissue to prevent the rubber dam from sliding back out of the sulcus. This step is re-

peated for each tooth on both the facial and lingual surfaces.

The rubber dam can be stabilized by ligating a piece of dental floss around the most anterior tooth (Fig. 34-28) or wedging a small piece of rubber dam into the embrasure between the last exposed tooth and the rubber dam (Fig. 34-29). For anterior rubber dam applications in which the teeth are isolated from first premolar to first premolar, the ligature or rubber dam wedge method of stabilization may be used instead of clamps. After the dam is correctly placed, a saliva ejector can be inserted under the rubber dam onto the floor of the mouth.

A properly applied rubber dam should (1) isolate the working area with no moisture present; (2) expose the teeth to be treated and provide sufficient visual access and sufficient finger rests for the clinician; (3) be stable and secure with no damage to the hard and soft tissues; (4) be inverted into the gingival sulcus; and (5) be comfortable (Fig. 34-30).

Applying the gingival retractor

The gingival retractor retracts or holds the gingival tissue and rubber dam material away from the site of the class V preparation. This retractor has two jaws, four prongs, two bows, and four

notches for the clamp forceps with specific lingual and facial sides (Fig. 34-31). When the gingival retractor is oriented to the tooth, the flat portion of the bow will be to the facial side of the tooth.

Insert the forceps into the notches and expand the jaws of the retractor. For greater access and visibility, seat the lingual jaw first. Position it by sliding it gently against the lingual surface until it is apical to the height of contour and flush with, but not impinging upon, the gingival tissue. Use the opposite hand to stabilize the lingual jaw while rotating the forceps to move the facial jaw along the facial surface in an apical direction until the facial jaw is apical to the height of contour and contacts the rubber dam overlying the gingiva. Using the jaws of the clamp, gently retract the gingiva and rubber dam to expose the gingival

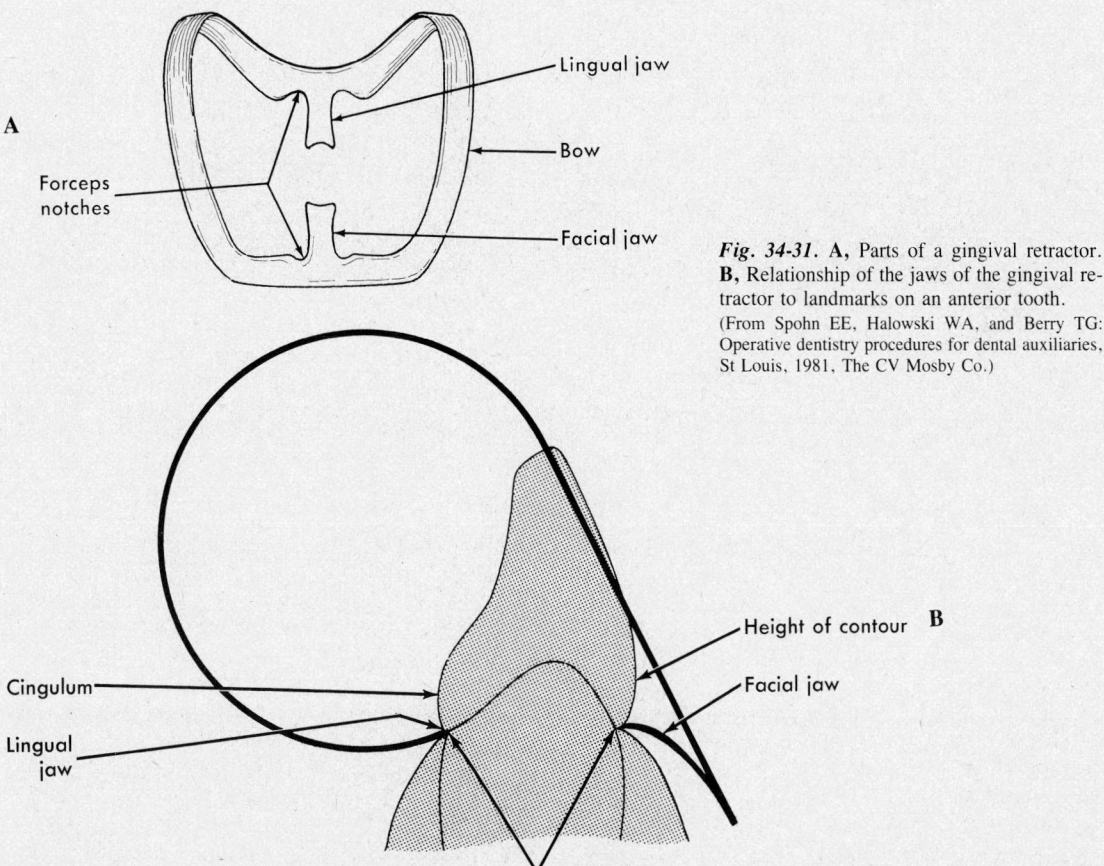

Fig. 34-31. **A,** Parts of a gingival retractor. **B,** Relationship of the jaws of the gingival retractor to landmarks on an anterior tooth. (From Spohn EE, Halowski WA, and Berry TG: Operative dentistry procedures for dental auxiliaries, St Louis, 1981, The CV Mosby Co.)

extent of the carious lesion. Make certain that the jaws are spread wide enough to avoid scraping against the tooth as the jaws are seated. This would scar the tooth, making it more susceptible to plaque accumulation and caries. If possible, retract the gingiva until it is at least 0.5 to 1.0 mm apical to the gingival extent of the lesion. The bows of the clamp should be parallel to the tooth's occlusal plane to ensure the even retraction of the gingiva in an apical direction. While removing the forceps from the retractor, continue to support the lingual and facial aspects of the retractor with the other hand until dental compound has been placed (Fig. 34-32).

Use dental compound to stabilize the gingival retractor to avoid slippage during the procedure. Trauma to the tooth structure and damage to the preparation or restorative material may occur if the clamp slips. Warm the compound over a flame until the end begins to sag, then temper it in warm water until the material is warm and malleable but not hot. The compound is applied to the top of one retractor bow and molded down onto the occlusal (incisal) surface, then broken off. Continue molding the soft compound onto the facial and lingual surfaces beneath and over the bow. This procedure is repeated for the other bow (Fig. 34-33).

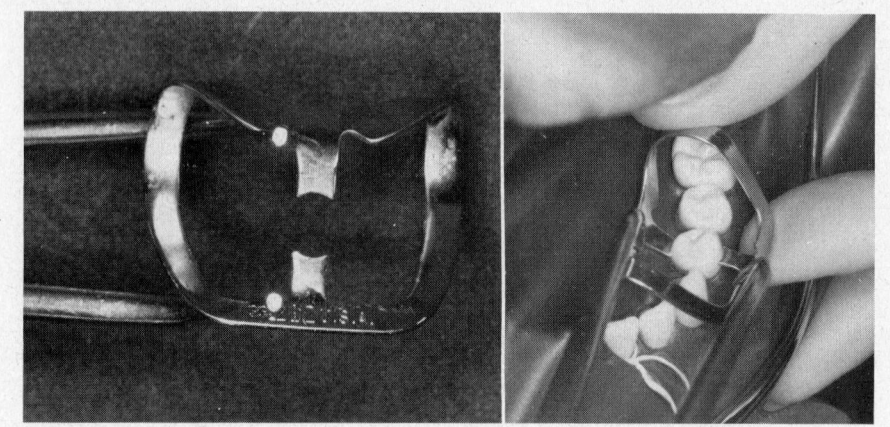

A   **B**

Fig. 34-32. Mounting gingival retractor. **A,** Position of gingival retractor in forceps for mounting in the maxillary left or mandibular right arches. **B,** Placement of retractor in mandibular left arch. (Notice that retractor is positioned in the other pair of notches and turned 180 degrees when compared with **A.**) Seat the lingual jaw first.
(From Spohn EE, Halowski WA, and Berry TG: Operative dentistry procedures for dental auxiliaries, St Louis, 1981, The CV Mosby Co.)

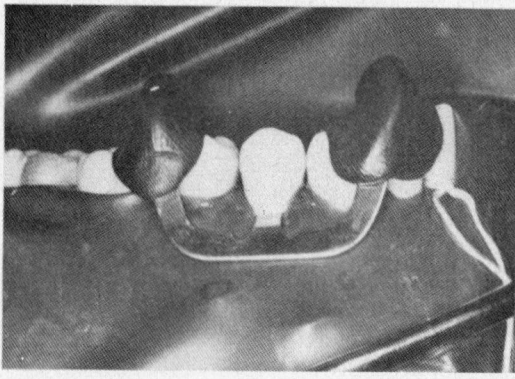

Fig. 34-33. Properly mounted gingival retractor with dental compound stabilizing it.
(From Spohn EE, Halowski WA, and Berry TG: Operative dentistry procedures for dental auxiliaries, St Louis, 1981, The CV Mosby Co.)

Check the retractor to make sure that it is stable, that is, it resists movement, and that it evenly retracts the gingiva and rubber dam. Check the stability with light finger pressure.

Removing the rubber dam

Before removing the dam, use high-volume evacuation to remove all debris from the operative field. If a gingival retractor has been used, it is removed first. Apply the forceps in an occlusolingual direction to break the compound off the teeth. The retractor is carefully removed in an occlusal direction without contacting the newly placed restoration or the tooth surface. Any remaining compound is removed with a sharp instrument. Remove the ligature or rubber dam wedge from the most anterior tooth. Stretch the dam to the facial away from the teeth and place one finger under the stretched dam (to protect the patient's lips and cheeks) while cutting the interdental areas of the dam (Fig. 34-34). The scissors should cut the entire septum with one stroke. Cut all the interproximal areas from the facial aspect, and pull the dam in a lingual direction.

Pulling the dam up through the contacts, or snipping the interproximal areas in stages may cause thin pieces of dam to tear or remain around the tooth. If a ring of the dam remained around the tooth, it would tend to migrate apically because the apex is the most constricted area of the tooth. As it progressed apically, it could cause severe bone destruction and possibly a gingival abscess or even loss of the tooth (Abrams, 1978).

The clamp, dam, and frame are removed at the same time. The rubber dam is laid on a light-coloured surface and checked to make sure that there are no small pieces of dam missing that could have remained in the patient's mouth. Except for the severed interdental pieces, the dam should appear as it did before placement (Fig. 34-35). Remove any piece left in the mouth with dental floss or an explorer.

The oral cavity should be rinsed and evacuated. The soft tissue should be examined for any trauma resulting from the clamp and the patient should be informed that he or she may experience some discomfort in this area after the anesthetic wears off.

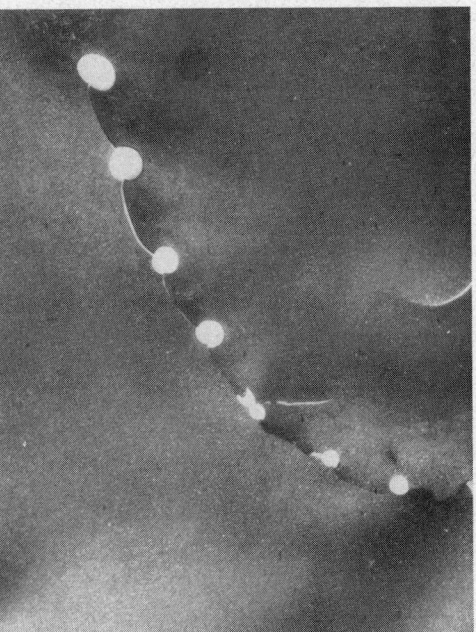

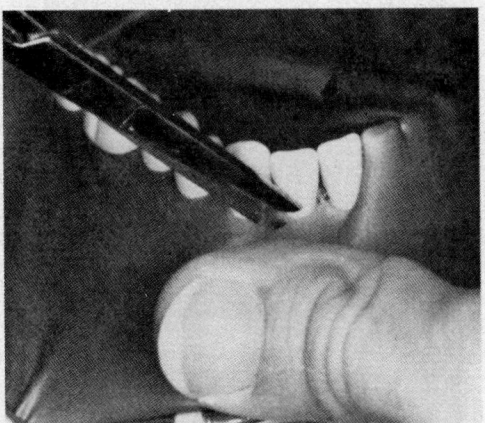

Fig. 34-34. Note that the tip of the lower scissors blade extends well beyond the rubber to ensure complete cutting of the septum each time.
(From Spohn EE, Halowski WA, and Berry TG: Operative dentistry procedures for dental auxiliaries, St Louis, 1981, The CV Mosby Co.)

Fig. 34-35. Note that a piece of rubber dam is missing next to the fourth hole from the bottom.
(From Spohn EE, Halowski WA, and Berry TG: Operative dentistry procedures for dental auxiliaries, St Louis, 1981, The CV Mosby Co.)

Evaluation criteria

Application of rubber dam

1. Isolated area is clean and dry
2. Number of teeth exposed provides visual access and finger rests
3. Clamp is stable and secure and does not impinge on gingiva
4. Ligature or wedges hold dam securely in place
5. Rubber dam is inverted into the gingival sulcus
6. Patient is comfortable
7. Gingival retractor (if used) is stable and evenly retracts the gingiva and dam

Removal of rubber dam

1. All rubber dam material, ligatures, and other debris have been removed
2. No significant soft tissue injury is present

PROBLEMS IN RESTORING TEETH

Pulpitis (inflammation of the pulp) is a concern before, during, and after operative dentistry procedures. Irritation of the pulp can occur from the cavity preparation and as a result of placing restorative materials. The physical cutting of enamel and dentin, heat generation from rotary instruments, and drying of the dentinal tubules by the use of air coolants during cavity preparation have all been shown to be potentially irritating to the pulp (Stanley 1961, 1971; Langeland, 1972). The most important factor in determining the response of the pulp is the thickness of dentin wall between the cavity preparation and the pulp chamber. Generally 2 mm of dentin thickness between the cavity preparation wall and the pulp provides an adequate insulating barrier against the operative techniques and the restorative materials (Cohen, 1980). A thickness of a 2.0 mm of dentin or more is adequate to protect the pulp from thermal, chemical, or bacterial irritation. However, the exact thickness of dentin is difficult to determine. Therefore, protection is often used to prevent the possibility of pulpal insult.

Some of the materials used in operative dentistry are potentially irritating to the pulp. Chemical irritation can occur when solutions from the materials seep through the dentinal tubules and contact the pulp.

The pulp is sensitive to temperature changes. Amalgam, a metal alloy, readily conducts heat and is, therefore, a potential conductor of thermal irritation to the pulp. Composite resin materials have a coefficient of thermal conductivity similar to that of enamel and dentin and do not pose a problem of thermal irritation (Harper, 1980).

Dimensional change due to thermal variations is another potential indirect contributor to pulpal irritation. Tooth structure and restorative materials are subjected to temperature changes in the oral cavity, resulting in expansion and contraction of restorative materials and the adjacent tooth tissues. The degree of expansion and contraction differs for amalgam, composite resin, enamel, and dentin allowing microscopic openings between restorations and adjacent tooth structure to be created. These openings permit the ingress and egress of oral fluids and debris along the interface. Browne and others (1983) have disclosed a strong positive correlation between the amount of pulpal inflammation and the extent of bacterial microleakage.

PROBLEM SOLVERS
Bases and Liners

Bases and liners are dental materials used to help the pulp recover from trauma that may have existed before the cutting of the cavity preparation and to help protect the pulp from trauma that may occur during or after the restorative procedures. Bases are materials applied to the pulpal floor or axial walls in relatively thick layers. Liners are materials applied as thin coatings to the walls and floor of the cavity preparation. These materials have specific indications for use depending on the health of the pulp, the amount of carious invasion, the depth of the preparation, and the restorative material being used.

The most common liner (or sealer) used is varnish. Varnishes are composed of natural or synthetic resins, such as copal or nitrated cellulose, dissolved in an organic volatile solvent, such as ether, acetone or chloroform. They are used under amalgam restorations to seal the cavity preparation in two ways. Varnishes seal the openings of the dentinal tubules, preventing chemical irritants from reaching the pulp. Free mercury from amalgam restorations is prevented from entering the tubules and causing discoloration of the tooth structure.

The sealer also seals the microscopic space between the tooth surface and restoration, thus reducing the leakage of fluids around the restoration (Murray, 1983; Yates, 1980). Because it is soluble in the oral cavity, the varnish near the cavosurface dissolves in time. However, the amalgam in this area is undergoing a corrosion process. The resultant corrosion products fill this crevice to some extent, sealing the interface between the amalgam and the tooth surface.

The copal-resin varnishes are contraindicated in composite resin restorations because varnish interferes with the setting reaction. If used, a layer of soft, semiset resin material remains along the interface of the restoration. This unset layer is rapidly lost at the cavosurface margin, leaving an opening for the ingress of fluids. Recently, new varnish-type dentin sealers have been introduced that are compatible with composite resins. The base of these varnishes is methylcellulose. Tjan and colleagues (1987) showed that these resin-compatible cavity varnishes are effective in reducing the dentin permeability to free monomer liquid, providing an effective barrier.

In recent years, the use of bases under amalgam restorations has undergone significant changes. Because bases are not as strong as amalgam, the thickness of the base affects the fracture strength of the amalgam. As the thickness of the base is increased, the fracture resistance of the amalgam is decreased (Hormati and Fuller, 1980; Farah et al, 1983). The most important factor of an insulator is the thickness of the base, not the type of material used. A thickness of 1 to 2 mm is sufficient to provide thermal insulation for the pulp.

An *obtundant* is a base placed to reduce the irritability of a pulp. Obtundants decrease the reaction of the pulp and reduce the pain. The most common obtundant used in dentistry is eugenol or oil of cloves and is found in zinc oxide–eugenol cement. In addition to its use as a base, this cement is recommended for use as an intermediary restoration when the prognosis of the tooth is questionable. Caution must be exercised when placing this material in patients who have exhibited a hypersensitivity to eugenol, exhibited as ulcers or sloughing of the gingival tissue. Eugenol interferes with the setting reaction of composite resin materials and is not used with them (Millstein, 1983).

Some bases are placed to stimulate the pulp to form reparative dentin in deep cavity preparations

where the remaining layer of dentin overlying the pulp is very thin. A pulp stimulator influences the pulp to form a layer of secondary dentin to protect itself from the irritation. Calcium hydroxide is a pulp stimulator when in direct contact with the pulpal tissue. It is commonly supplied as a two-paste system. Recently, light-activated calcium hydroxide has been introduced. It has the ability to seal and protect the pulp from chemical irritation. Peters and others (1981) found that a layer of calcium hydroxide provides short term thermal protection. It is radiopaque and clearly visible on radiographs.

PROCEDURES
Armamentarium

The armamentarium for the placement of varnishes and calcium hydroxide includes varnish, cotton pellets, cotton pliers, calcium hydroxide, and a mixing pad and placement instrument for the calcium hydroxide.

Procedural steps

The specific liner and/or base to be placed in a cavity preparation depends on the type of restorative material used, the depth of the cavity preparation, and the condition of the pulp.

Amalgam restorations

Minimal depth. Minimal-depth preparations extend from about 0.5 to 1.5 mm into the dentin. The remaining dentin is thick enough to provide both thermal insulation and protection during cavity preparation. However, a sealer is needed to seal the dentinal tubules and fill the space between the amalgam and tooth surface. Regardless of their depth, all cavity preparations that will be restored with amalgam require a sealer. Varnish is applied over the entire preparation, including both dentin and enamel, with a cotton pellet held with cotton pliers (Fig. 34-36). Two applications are needed to provide a complete coating of the tooth surface. The first layer of varnish is dried with a gentle stream of air before the second coat is applied. Strong blasts of air form ridges of varnish that may not dry before amalgam placement. Use a new cotton pellet to apply the second thin coat of varnish, allowing it to dry before placing the amalgam (Fig. 34-37). Some varnishes come with their own applicator. The solvent in the varnish is

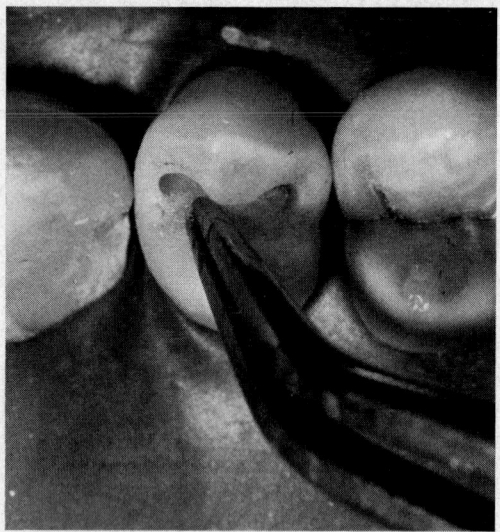

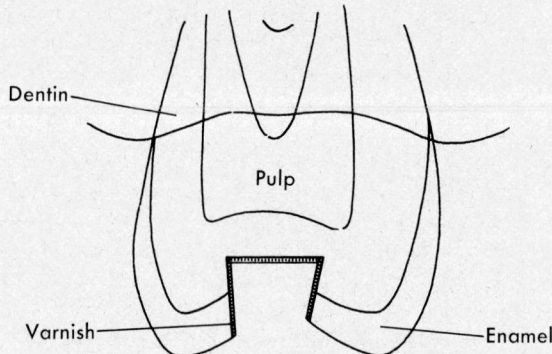

Fig. 34-37. Minimal-depth restorations have a sufficient bulk of dentin remaining to provide thermal insulation. Two coats of varnish are placed before placing the amalgam.
(From Spohn EE, Halowski WA, and Berry TG: Operative dentistry procedures for dental auxiliaries, St Louis, 1981, The CV Mosby Co.)

Fig. 34-36. Varnish is applied in all areas of the preparation, including over the cavosurface margin. A small cotton pellet helps control placement of the varnish.
(From Spohn EE, Halowski WA, and Berry TG: Operative dentistry procedures for dental auxiliaries, St Louis, 1981, The CV Mosby Co.)

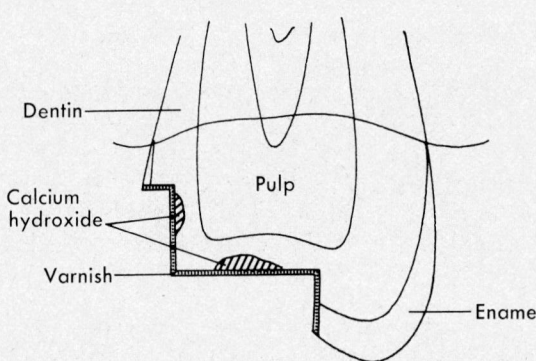

Fig. 34-38. Subaxial and subpulpal extensions in a class II preparation. Calcium hydroxide is placed in the extensions before the layer of varnish is applied.
(From Spohn EE, Halowski WA, and Berry TG: Operative dentistry procedures for dental auxiliaries, St Louis, 1981, The CV Mosby Co.)

highly volatile, so the bottle should be tightly capped immediately after use.

Subaxial or subpulpal extension. A subaxial or subpulpal extension is an area on the axial or pulpal wall extending deeper than the rest of the wall (Fig. 34-38). This places the amalgam closer to the pulp, leaving less dentin to protect the pulp. If there is a possibility that the pulpal tissue may be exposed microscopically or if there is concern that the pulp may need protection from thermal insult, calcium hydroxide should be applied in an even layer of 0.5 to 1.0 mm thick; otherwise apply varnish.

Near pulpal exposure. Cavity preparations that are very close to the pulp require special care (Fig. 34-39). The pulp is already irritated by the caries. Insult is added by the depth of the preparation. Knowledge of pulpal anatomy, history of the tooth's involvement, radiographic evidence, and experience will aid in determining the approximate location of the pulp. If the pink color of the pulp can be seen through the dentin, the dentin is very thin. In these situations, apply cal-

cium hydroxide over the deepest portion of the preparation (Fig. 34-40). Newer calcium hydroxide preparations are strong enough to be applied in layers thick enough to provide thermal protection as well as protection from chemical or bacterial irritation (Peters, 1981; Farah, 1981).

Dispense small, equal amounts of base and catalyst pastes on a mixing pad. The placement instrument can be used to mix the material to a homogeneous color. Wipe the instrument clean and pick up a small amount of material on the end of

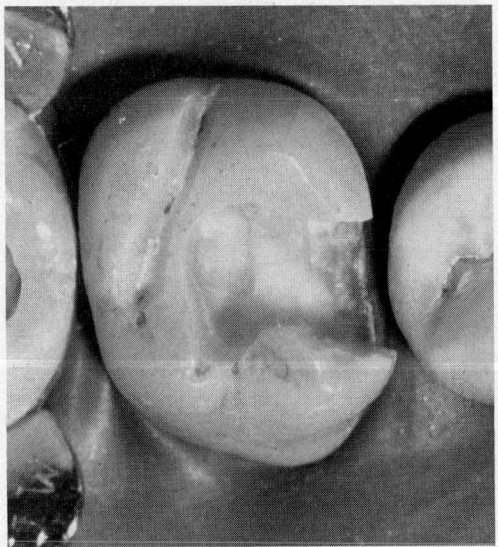

Fig. 34-39. Near pulpal exposures can occur on both the pulpal and axial walls.
(From Spohn EE, Halowski WA, and Berry TG: Operative dentistry procedures for dental auxiliaries, St Louis, 1981, The CV Mosby Co.)

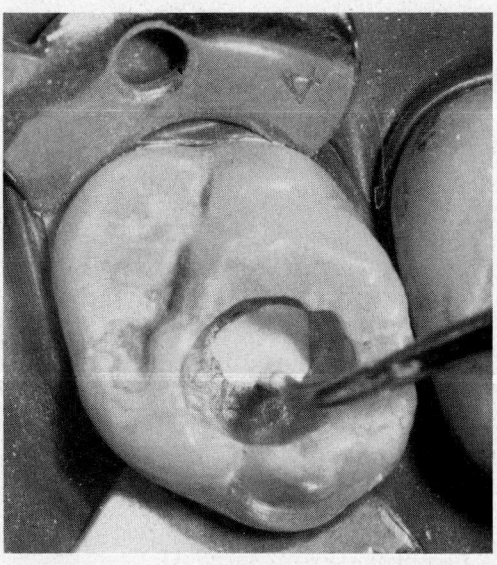

Fig. 34-40. Calcium hydroxide is placed in a thin, continuous layer on the deepest areas of the pulpal or axial wall.
(From Spohn EE, Halowski WA, and Berry TG: Operative dentistry procedures for dental auxiliaries, St Louis, 1981, The CV Mosby Co.)

the placement instrument. Place the material onto the desired area, spreading it over the dentin. An even layer of 0.5 to 1.0 mm is placed on dentin only. Calcium hydroxide placed on enamel must be removed. It is soluble in oral fluids and will quickly dissolve when exposed to oral fluids, leaving a space at the margin and making the restoration more susceptible to plaque accumulation and recurrent decay. To prevent interference with the retention of the restorative material, avoid placing the calcium hydroxide in any retentive grooves. Calcium hydroxide incorrectly placed can be removed using an explorer once the material has set. It tends to smear if removed before it sets. Two coats of varnish are applied over the entire preparation before continuing with the amalgam placement.

Pulpal exposure. Pulpal exposures can occur from either carious or mechanical causes. Depending on the severity and extent of the exposure, the decision may be made to treat the tooth endodontically. If, however, the decision is made to observe the tooth for a time to allow recovery, a temporary or intermediary restoration may be placed. Generally, zinc oxide–eugenol is used as a temporary restorative material because of its superior sealing qualities and its palliative effect on the pulp. Calcium hydroxide is placed over the exposure site and surrounding dentin to stimulate secondary dentin formation.

Composite resin restorations

Because thermal conductivity of composite resin material is similar to that of dentin, thermal irritation is not a potential problem. The major potential problem is chemical irritation from the monomer in the composite resin. The decision of which material to place is based on the depth of the preparation and the availability of the protective materials compatible with composite resin materials. Copal varnishes and zinc oxide–eugenol are contraindicated because they interfere with the setting of the material (Eliasson, 1979). When acid etching procedures are used with composite resins, the pulp must be protected from the phosphoric acid with calcium hydroxide placed on the pulpal floor or axial wall before conditioning the enamel. After the conditioning procedure is completed, it can be removed if not needed.

REVIEW OF PULPAL PROTECTION

Minimal depth

Minimal-depth preparations extend only 0.5 to 1.5 mm into the dentin so sufficient thickness of dentin remains to protect the pulp from potential chemical irritation. The composite resin is placed directly onto the cavity preparation.

Subaxial or subpulpal extension

A thin layer (0.5 mm) of calcium hydroxide is placed in the deepest portion of the cavity preparation. The calcium hydroxide should not be placed into the retentive grooves or along the enamel. Several applications of the material are easier to control than one large amount, particularily in preparations with minimal access.

Near pulpal exposure

Calcium hydroxide is placed in a thin layer (0.5 mm) over the deeper portions of the cavity preparation to provide protection from chemical irritation and stimulate secondary dentin.

Pulpal exposure

The exposure site, along with the surrounding dentin, is covered with a layer of calcium hydroxide, then a temporary zinc oxide–eugenol restoration is placed to allow time for observation of the tooth.

PRINCIPLES AND GENERAL PROCEDURES FOR AMALGAM PLACEMENT: THE CLASS V AND CLASS I RESTORATIONS

Dental amalgam is the most commonly used restorative material, accounting for almost three fourths of the restorations placed in dental practice (Gilmore et al, 1982). It is adaptable to many situations, offers good durability, and restores function to the tooth. It is easy to mix, place, and adapt into the preparation and to contour. Research on the long-term clinical performance of these alloys has indicated that they will last for decades, release less mercury than previous restorations, and not require resurfacing or replacement as would composite resins (Osborne et al,

1980; Lemmens et al, 1986; Osborne et al, 1987). Amalgam is a long-lasting, safe, inexpensive material that is tolerant of operator errors.

Amalgam is composed of several metals. Any combination of metals is refered to as an *alloy*. If an alloy is mixed with mercury, the result is an *amalgam*. The mixing process is known as *trituration*. Dental amalgam is often called silver amalgam because silver is its chief ingredient. Alloy composition varies among manufacturers; the ranges are shown below:

Percentage	Element	Function
40% to 69%	Silver	Combines easily with mercury
11% to 27%	Copper	Adds strength to the alloy, decreases corrosion and tarnish
15% to 30%	Tin	Aids in combining mercury with the alloy
0% to 1%	Zinc	Prevents alloy oxidation during the manufacturing process

All dental amalgams share the following physical properties:

1. *Dimensional change.* All amalgams undergo dimensional change, with the amount dependent upon many factors. Greater amounts of mercury cause greater expansion and a weaker restoration. Longer mixing time decreases expansion or increases contraction (although this is not a major factor within reasonable trituration times). Increased condensation pressure decreases expansion.

2. *Variance in strength.* Force applied directly to the thicker parts of the restoration is well tolerated. Amalgam exhibits good compressive strength. Force applied to a thin area such as an edge (margin) is not. Amalgam's tensile strength is only about one-fifth its compressive strength (Charbeneau et al, 1981).

3. Strength can be adversely affected by many factors. Inadequate trituration results in a drier mass, which in turn results in a mass containing voids (porosity). Excessive mercury produces a restoration that is weaker and more subject to corrosion and tarnish (Craig et al, 1980). The correct ratio of mercury to amalgam is specified by the manufacturer. It usually is approximately 1 to 1, although some alloys call for less than 50% mercury. Amalgam has relatively little strength early in its setting reaction and requires careful protection immediately after placement. It is subject to fracture if pressure is placed on an unsupported portion.

Other characteristics of the amalgam affect the procedures. These include the following:

1. Moisture can cause undesirable expansion of an amalgam restoration (Craig et al, 1980), as well as interfering with the blending of one carrier load of amalgam with the preceding one. It can increase the amount of corrosion and thus decrease the strength.
2. Amalgam begins the setting (hardening) process as soon as it is mixed. After 2½ to 3 minutes, the working stage of the material has passed. Although it can be loaded into an amalgam carrier and packed into the preparation with some difficulty, it will not become a part of the mass that has already condensed and will likely fracture or flake away. After 2½ to 3 minutes, mix a new batch of material that can be added to the already condensed amalgam.
3. When first placed, amalgam is relatively soft. Only the gross excess should be removed. Final carving should occur when the amalgam offers slight resistance to the instrument.
4. Because amalgam is initially very weak and can be fractured easily, carving strokes should not be directed toward unsupported amalgam; they should be directed from the tooth structure toward the amalgam. If this is not possible, use repeated, short, gentle carving strokes.

Product packaging

Alloy is packaged in powder or pellet form. The mercury may be packaged separately. The powder or pellets and the mercury may be loaded into separate dispensers so correct proportions can be dispensed into the mixing capsule. This method may cause mercury contamination through spills and aerosol production during trituration, and amalgam residue may contaminate future batches. For these reasons, only sealed prepackaged capsules containing correct proportions of the alloy and the mercury should be used.

The capsules are designed as "one-spill," "two-spill," or "three-spill" capsules. Small preparations may require only a one-spill capsule; large preparations will need one or more two- or three-spill capsules.

Dental mercury hygiene

All personnel who handle mercury should observe good mercury hygiene practices. Although cases are extremely rare, some individuals may develop a mercury sensitivity or allergy. The symptoms may vary from local dermatitis to a generalized erythema over the entire body. Symptoms of mercury toxicity can include tremor, which is observable in fine voluntary muscular movements (e.g., handwriting), eventually progressing to convulsions; loss of appetite; nausea and diarrhea; depression, fatigue, increased irritability, or moodiness; pneumonitis; nephritis; nervous excitability; insomnia; headache; swollen glands and tongue; ulceration of oral mucosa; and dark pigmentation of marginal gingiva and loosening of teeth. Excessive exposure to mercury or its vapor can cause toxicity.

The work area should be a well-ventilated space with fresh air exchange and outside air exhaust. The office should be monitored yearly for mercury contamination (more often if contamination is suspected). Periodic urinalysis for mercury should be done for all personnel. Follow the following additional precautions:

Use precapsulated alloy to minimize possible mercury spills.
Avoid direct contact with or handling of mercury, amalgam, or other mercury-containing materials.
Never heat mercury or amalgam.
Do not use mercury disinfecting solutions.
Prohibit eating, drinking, or smoking in the dental operatory.
Use recommended procedures for cleaning mercury spills and dispose of mercury-contaminated items properly.
Check clothing and shoes for mercury and amalgam before leaving the dental area, to avoid contamination of nondental areas.

Mixing the amalgam (trituration)

Trituration must wet all of the alloy particles with mercury within the appropriate time period. Mixing is done with a motor-driven mechanical device called an amalgamator, which shakes the capsule rapidly back and forth to break the barrier and allow the alloy and mercury to mix completely (Fig. 34-41). Some capsule designs require the barrier to be broken before the capsule is placed in the amalgamator. Refer to the manufacturer's directions.

Set the capsule firmly into the identations in the amalgamator arms. A capsule not held firmly in place may be flung loose. Set the timer to the number of seconds recommended by the alloy manufacturer for the amalgamator being used (this can vary from 2 to 25 seconds for a two-spill

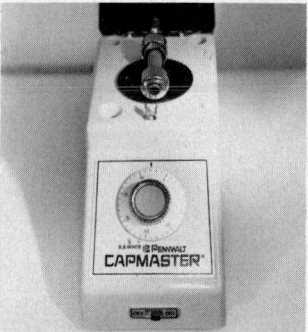

Fig. 34-41. Place the capsule securely in the rocker arms to prevent dislodgement. Close the cover before activating the amalgamator.

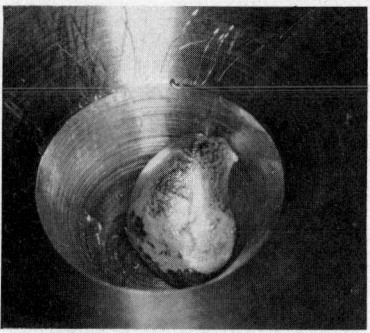

Fig. 34-42. The amalgam should be a single mass, not crumbly, and should have a dull shine.

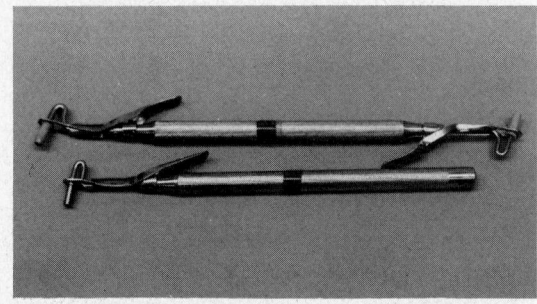

Fig. 34-43. Either the single- or double-ended amalgam carrier may be used. The double-ended carrier offers a choice of a large or small end to correspond to the size of the preparation.

capsule). The more alloy and mercury used, the greater the mixing time required. When the timer has been set, push the button to begin the mixing.

When trituration is completed, remove the capsule. Do not touch the amalgam directly with the fingers; this would cause moisture contamination and create a mercury hazard. Instead, drop the pellet directly from the capsule into an amalgam well or dappen dish. Immediately reassemble the parts to decrease the possibility of contamination.

The amalgam should be in a solid mass with a dull shine and no dry or grainy areas (Fig. 34-42). If the amalgam meets these criteria, it is ready to load into the amalgam carrier. If it appears dry and crumbles when pressure is applied, it cannot be well adapted to all the walls or into all the retentive features. It will not become one solid mass. Amalgam that is too wet with mercury will be very shiny and quite soft; it will set slowly, will be difficult to carve, and will have significantly less strength than a correctly proportioned mix (Craig et al, 1980).

Condensing amalgam

The amalgam carrier picks up the amalgam for transfer into the preparation. Although there are design variations, the carriers shown in Fig. 34-43 are most commonly selected. The end of the carrier is a hollow tube containing a plunger that extrudes the amalgam when the lever is depressed. The ends are two different sizes; select the one that fits the preparation. To load the carrier, place a finger under the lever and then insert the end of the carrier into the amalgam mass to

force amalgam into the tube. The finger under the lever holds the plunger in position, allowing the amalgam to enter the tube. After the carrier is loaded, wipe away the excess.

Place the first increment of amalgam into the most inaccessible portion of the preparation. This principle prevents the first increments of amalgam from hindering placement of the later segments. Place a partial load in a small or medium-sized preparation. If too much amalgam is deposited, it obscures the view, hinders the condensation strokes, and makes it difficult to determine if the amalgam is being well condensed. Only large preparations can accommodate placement of a full increment without risk of undercondensation.

Condensation forces the amalgam into all the areas of preparation and forces each particle of amalgam to attach or meld with previously placed particles to become one solid mass. This creates a tighter fit to decrease leakage of fluids between the amalgam and the tooth structure and also provides retention for the restoration, as amalgam does not bond or adhere to the tooth structure.

You must know the size and shape of the preparation and its retentive areas in order to condense a restoration properly. The retentive areas are usually located at or near the deepest portion of the preparation and consist of grooves cut into the walls that meet the axial or pulpal wall at the perpendicular angle. These grooves make the interior portion of the preparation larger than the external portion thus providing an "undercut" that locks the restorative material into the preparation. Amalgam is condensed into these areas first.

The condenser of choice should fit into all areas of the preparation. Before mixing the amalgam, insert the nib into the preparation to ensure that it will fit. A too-large nib will not force the amalgam into the retentive areas, while a too-small nib will simply push through the mass of amalgam without condensing it effectively.

Condensation pressure must be applied toward both the internal line angles of the cavity preparation and the walls themselves. A smaller condenser nib will aid in condensing into groove extensions and line angles. However, it may not be possible to insert even the smaller condenser into all areas. In such cases the side of the instrument can push the amalgam laterally into the area. Condensing strokes are primarily directed perpendicularly toward the axial or pulpal wall.

When condensing, each stroke must overlap the previous one. Well-condensed amalgam has two characteristics: (1) it shows overlapping indentations made by the condenser nib and (2) it is somewhat shiny because the condensing pressure has forced mercury from within the amalgam to the surface.

Each segment must be completely condensed. All loads are manipulated just as was the first segment. This makes the restoration a homogeneous mass rather than several "layers" that will not hold together.

When the preparation is filled, switch to the next larger condenser nib size. The large size will help adapt the amalgam to the cavosurface margins as the preparation is slightly overfilled by approximately 1 mm. Overfilling allows enough for removal of the mercury-rich layer on the top and ensures sufficient material to carve the original contours of the tooth. Direct the final condensation strokes toward the cavosurface margins at a 45-degree angle to ensure complete adaptation at the margins. A void at the margin could be fatal to the success of the restoration.

At this stage the amalgam should cover all margins, overfill the preparation, have a shiny surface without voids, and exhibit overlapping condensation strokes.

Burnishing amalgam

Initial. Burnishing rubs the surface, making it shiny or lustrous. Burnishing an amalgam restoration provides additional adaptation and compaction of the material over its surface and marginal areas, reducing marginal leakage and leaving a smoother surface that is easier to finish and polish (Kanai, 1966; Svare and Chan, 1972; Kato et al, 1968; Charbeneau, 1965).

After carving. With gentle pressure, move a smooth-ended instrument from the fresh amalgam toward and over the cavosurface margin to push the amalgam against the margin to improve adaptation. This action also wipes away excess amalgam. Care should be taken not to use too much pressure.

Burnish the amalgam immediately after condensation to smooth the surface and better adapt the amalgam. Burnish again after carving, when the amalgam has begun initial set.

Carving amalgam

Timing is important in carving. If started too late, the amalgam will be hard and difficult to carve. If started too soon, the amalgam may be too soft, resulting in overcarving as the instrument sinks into the surface. Test the hardness of the amalgam by pulling the carving instrument through an area of excess amalgam. Do not try definitive carving until the amalgam offers some resistance to the carving. However, do remove gross excess from the cavosurface margins early in the procedure.

Carving is a series of shaving strokes removing only the surface layer. Trying to remove too much at one time results in overcarving or fracturing the restoration. Control of the carving stroke is achieved by resting the instrument on tooth structure around the preparation. Adapting the instrument this way guides the instrument to shape the anatomy and prevents slippage and overcarving. The stroke should move the instrument from tooth onto the amalgam rather than

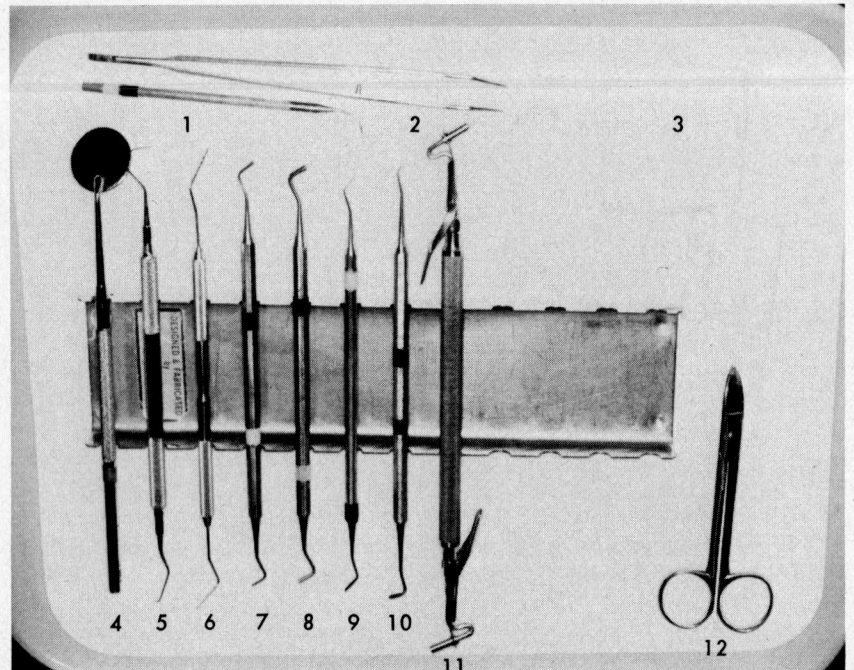

Fig. 34-44. Tray setup for Class V cavity restoration includes: *1,* calcium hydroxide placement instrument; *2,* cotton pliers; *3,* gauze and cotton pellets and rolls; *4,* mouth mirror; *5,* explorer; *6,* probe; *7 and 8,* amalgam condensers; *9,* No. ½ Hollenback carver; *10,* plastic placement instrument; *11,* amalgam carrier; and *12,* crown and bridge scissors.
(From Spohn EE, Halowski WA, and Berry TG: Operative dentistry procedures for dental auxiliaries, St Louis, 1981, The CV Mosby Co.)

from amalgam toward the cavosurface margins. This avoids removing too much amalgam at the margin ("ditching") leaving a ledge of enamel above the restoration.

Carving is much easier and better if the clinician has a good mental image of the anatomy of the tooth. The adjacent and contralateral teeth provide good reference for the anatomy of the tooth being restored. Grooves in the enamel surrounding the preparation must be carved into the adjacent amalgam. If this is not done, a ledge of amalgam will be left at the junction of the enamel groove and the amalgam. This ledge can be detected by drawing an explorer tip along the groove onto the amalgam surface. Amalgam extending out over the cavosurface margin is known as "flash" and must be removed. The restoration should not have a jagged outline (at the cavosurface margins) with abrupt changes in contour. Jagged contours usually indicate the presence of flash.

The restoration must reproduce the contours that were present before loss of the tooth structure. Resting the instrument on the surrounding enamel, with its blade angle corresponding with the angulation of the enamel surface, will reproduce the contours desired. No matter what the type or location of the restoration being carved, these principles remain the same.

The following sections will discuss the specific procedures involved in placement of the classes of restorations, each of which calls for unique variations and adaptations.

Armamentarium

The armamentarium suggested for amalgam restorations is shown in Fig. 34-44. Specific situations may require other instruments.

CLASS V AMALGAM RESTORATION

The class V occurs in the gingival one third of the facial or lingual surface of anterior and posterior

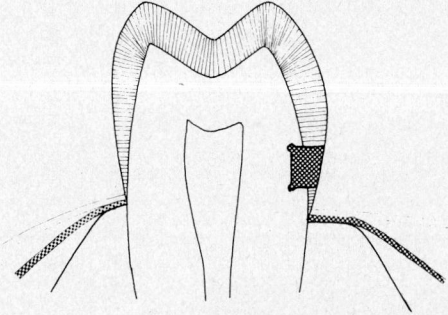

Fig. 34-45. Retentive grooves located in the gingivoaxial and occlusoaxial line angles.
(From Spohn EE, Halowski WA, and Berry TG: Operative dentistry procedures for dental auxiliaries, St Louis, 1981, The CV Mosby Co.)

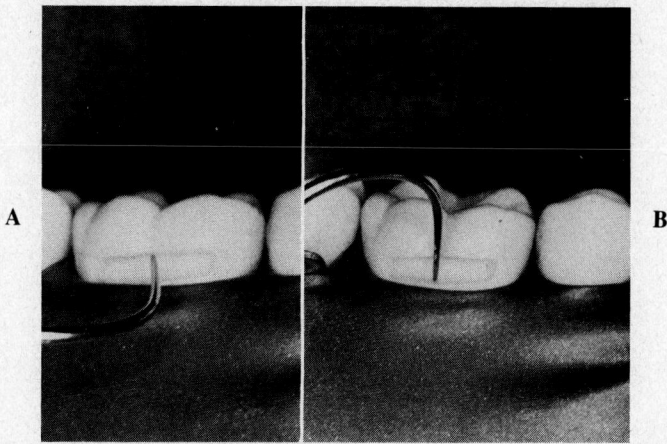

A   B

Fig. 34-46. Check retentive grooves with the tine of the explorer. A slight catch will be felt along the, **A,** occlusoaxial and, **B,** gingivoaxial line angles.
(From Spohn EE, Halowski WA, and Berry TG: Operative dentistry procedures for dental auxiliaries, St Louis, 1981, The CV Mosby Co.)

teeth (Fig. 34-45). Esthetic concerns contraindicate placement of an amalgam restoration in anterior teeth. The class V restoration is usually the least complex and easiest to place. Its basic shape is rectangular, although the walls are slightly curved. The axial wall meets the occlusal, gingival, mesial, and distal walls at nearly a right angle. Retention is provided by grooves placed at the occlusoaxial and gingivoaxial line angles. The preparation is essentially a "box" into which to condense the amalgam. The cavosurface margins of the preparation are usually smooth without undulations. Recognition of this outline aids in visualizing the preparation to determine the exact cavosurface margin to which to carve the restoration.

If indicated, place a base according to the criteria previously discussed. Before mixing the amalgam, check the retentive grooves with the explorer tip (Fig. 34-46, *A, B*) to remove any base material. Material left in the grooves prevents amalgam from being condensed into the area, reducing or eliminating retention of the restoration.

After the base is set, cover the entire cavity preparation with two coats of varnish.

Placement and condensation

Place one half of the first carrier load of amalgam against the axial wall (Fig. 34-47). Direct the first strokes at a 45-degree angle toward the gingivoaxial line angle to adapt the amalgam against the walls and along the whole length of the retentive

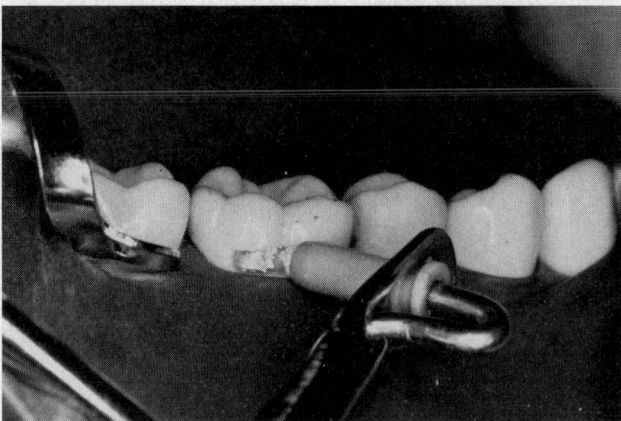

Fig. 34-47. First increment of amalgam being spread along the axial wall.
(From Spohn EE, Halowski WA, and Berry TG: Operative dentistry procedures for dental auxiliaries, St Louis, 1981, The CV Mosby Co.)

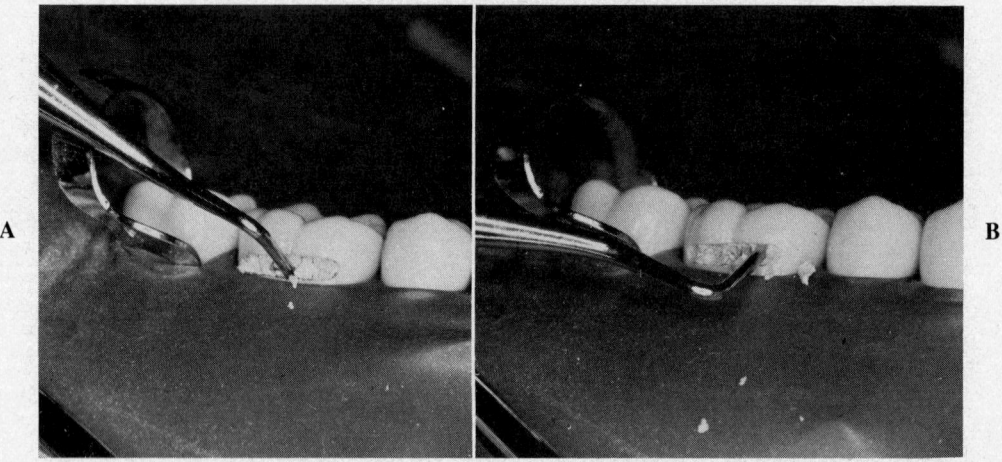

A   B

Fig. 34-48. A, Angle of condenser nib when condensing into the gingivoaxial retentive groove. **B,** Angling nib of condenser toward the occlusoaxial retentive groove.
(From Spohn EE, Halowski WA, and Berry TG: Operative dentistry procedures for dental auxiliaries, St Louis, 1981, The CV Mosby Co.)

grooves (Fig. 34-48, *A*). Continue condensation across the occlusoaxial line angle to the mesioaxial line angle (Fig. 34-48, *B*). All condensation pressure should be applied at 45 degrees to ensure good condensation of material against these line angles and into the retentive grooves.

The remaining amalgam should be compacted against the axial wall. Use overlapping strokes with enough pressure to produce slight indenta-

tions in the amalgam and to make the surface slightly shiny (Fig. 34-49). When all of the first carrier load is thoroughly condensed, add the second increment. Continue to condense until the whole axial wall is covered. Most of the condensation strokes will be directed at a 90-degree angle toward the axial wall. Some, however, should be as nearly perpendicular as possible to the occlusal, gingival, mesial, and distal walls (Figs. 34-

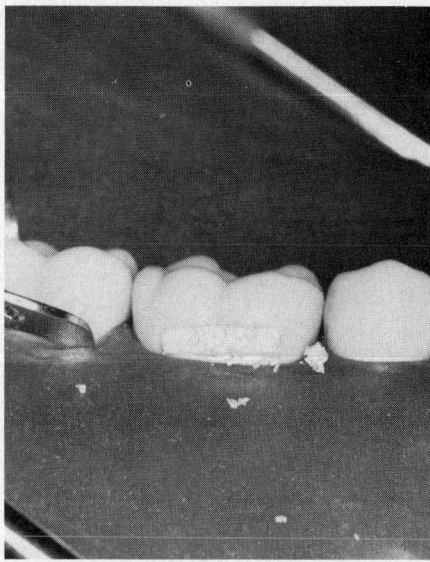

Fig. 34-49. Well-condensed amalgam has a slightly shiny surface with clearly visible overlapping condensing strokes.
(From Spohn EE, Halowski WA, and Berry TG: Operative dentistry procedures for dental auxiliaries, St Louis, 1981, The CV Mosby Co.)

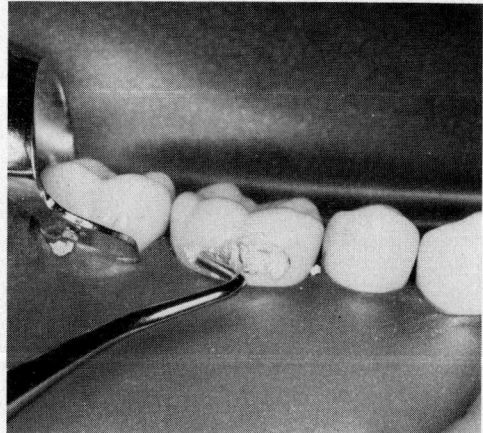

Fig. 34-50. Angle of condenser nib when directed toward the distal wall.
(From Spohn EE, Halowski WA, and Berry TG: Operative dentistry procedures for dental auxiliaries, St Louis, 1981, The CV Mosby Co.)

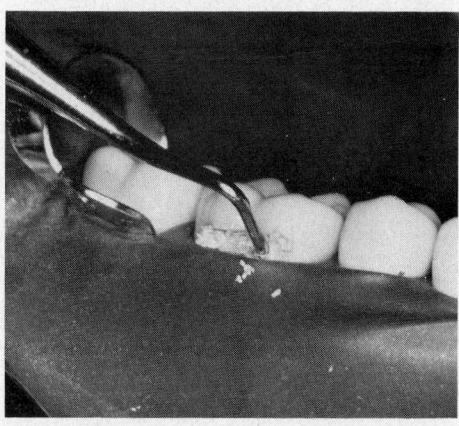

Fig. 34-51. Force of condensation directed toward the gingival wall.
(From Spohn EE, Halowski WA, and Berry TG: Operative dentistry procedures for dental auxiliaries, St Louis, 1981, The CV Mosby Co.)

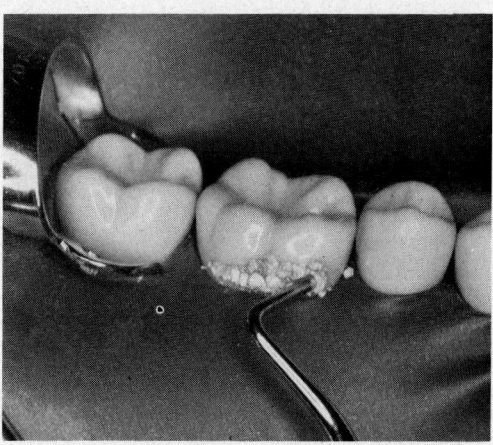

Fig. 34-52. Angle of condenser nib when directed toward the mesial wall.
(From Spohn EE, Halowski WA, and Berry TG: Operative dentistry procedures for dental auxiliaries, St Louis, 1981, The CV Mosby Co.)

50, 34-51, 34-52, 34-53). This helps to adapt the amalgam against those walls to increase retention and decrease leakage along the interface.

As the mass reaches the cavosurface, switch to the next larger condenser nib (Fig. 34-54) to make the final layer of amalgam easier to adapt over the margins.

Overfill the preparation by 0.5 to 1.0 mm (Fig. 34-55). The outer layer will be removed to eliminate mercury-rich amalgam. The last condensing strokes should be at approximately 45 degrees against the margins. Condense out over the margins slightly. Do not grossly overfill the prepara-

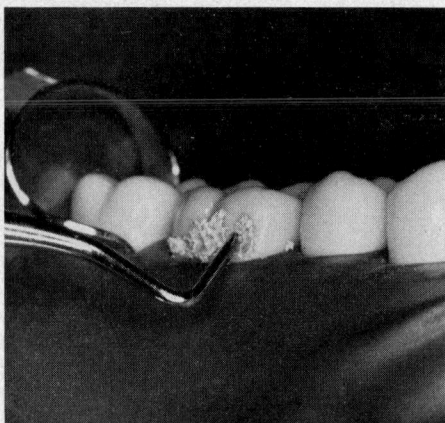

Fig. 34-53. The condenser nib is angled as nearly perpendicular to the occlusal wall as the preparation permits.
(From Spohn EE, Halowski WA, and Berry TG: Operative dentistry procedures for dental auxiliaries, St Louis, 1981, The CV Mosby Co.)

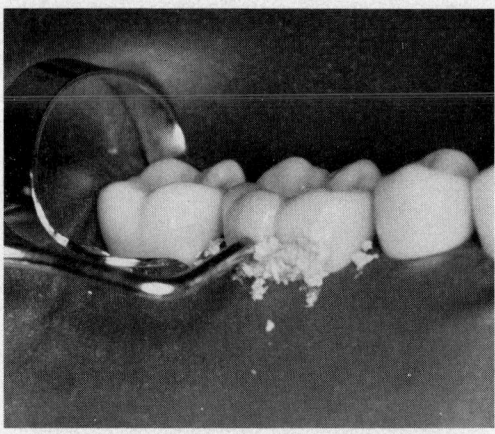

Fig. 34-54. The larger condenser nib is directed at and beyond the cavosurface margins.
(From Spohn EE, Halowski WA, and Berry TG: Operative dentistry procedures for dental auxiliaries, St Louis, 1981, The CV Mosby Co.)

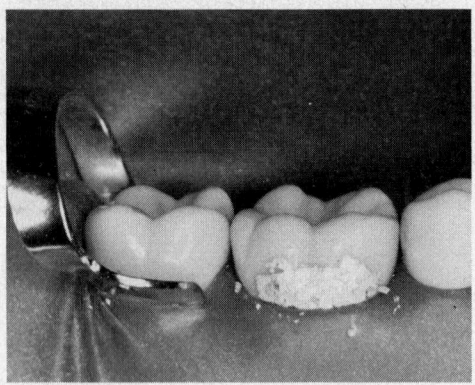

Fig. 34-55. The final increment of amalgam slightly overfills the preparation. Note the overlapping condensing strokes.
(From Spohn EE, Halowski WA, and Berry TG: Operative dentistry procedures for dental auxiliaries, St Louis, 1981, The CV Mosby Co.)

tion to avoid a more time-consuming and difficult carving process.

At this point, pause to evaluate the restoration carefully. It should meet the following criteria:

1. All margins are covered with amalgam
2. The preparation is overfilled by 0.5 to 1.0 mm of amalgam
3. The amalgam surface is shiny, without voids or grainy areas
4. Overlapping condensing strokes are clearly visible

If the restoration meets these criteria, the amalgam is ready to be burnished.

Initial burnishing

Choose a relatively flat-bladed instrument, such as a beavertail burnisher, for the rather flat class V restoration. Rest the tip of the instrument gingival to the margin with the side of the instrument contacting the gingival one-third of the restoration on its distal aspect. Pull the instrument along the gingival margin toward and over the mesial margin, then back along the gingival margin across the distal margin. This smoothes the material along the margins and better adapts it to the preparation wall (Fig. 34-56).

With the side of the instrument on the tooth occlusal to the restoration and the instrument tip on the amalgam, repeat the same steps done for the gingival margin. Take care not to allow the tip to dig into or gouge the amalgam.

The center portion of the restoration can be burnished by rubbing the instrument lightly over its entire surface from the distal cavosurface margin to the mesial cavosurface margin. Use only enough pressure to smooth the surface and better adapt amalgam to the margins. Excessive pressure on soft amalgam will gouge the amalgam, resulting in ditching or inadequate contours.

RESTORATIVE PROCEDURES

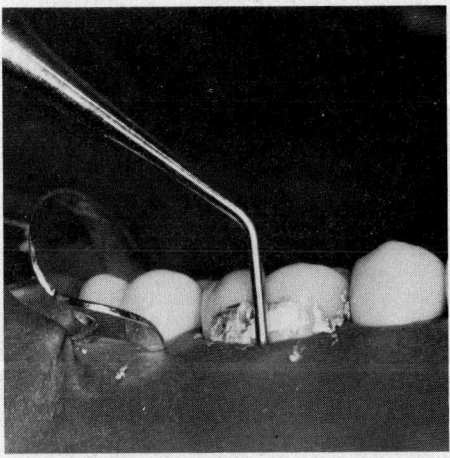

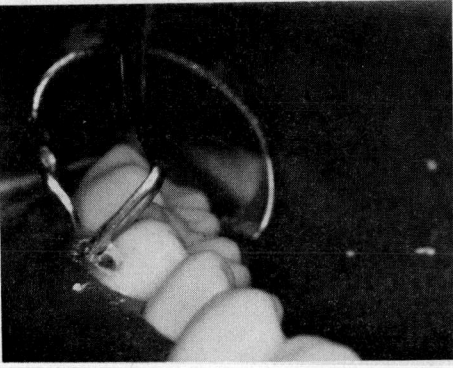

Fig. 34-57. Carving the occlusal margin. The tip of the instrument is not contacting the central portion of the restoration. (From Spohn EE, Halowski WA, and Berry TG: Operative dentistry procedures for dental auxiliaries, St Louis, 1981, The CV Mosby Co.)

Fig. 34-56. Burnish amalgam with the side of a condenser. A blade-shaped burnisher can also be used. (From Spohn EE, Halowski WA, and Berry TG: Operative dentistry procedures for dental auxiliaries, St Louis, 1981, The CV Mosby Co.)

The amalgam surface should be smooth, shiny, and tightly adapted to the margins. Some of the excess amalgam originally placed should have been pushed away from the cavosurface margins and eliminated. The class V restoration is ready for carving.

Carving the amalgam

Visualize the size and extension of the original preparation. Recall the mental image of the preparation developed before the amalgam was inserted.

Choose the ½ Hollenback carver to remove the excess material. Use the end with the blade that has a face perpendicular to the shank of the instrument so that the side of the instrument is adapted to the amalgam. With the blade resting on the tooth structure occlusal to the margin, pull the instrument through the excess amalgam (Fig. 34-57). Do not place the tip on the amalgam surface itself because it may gouge that surface. This procedure is quite similar to the one performed with the burnishing instrument except the blade edge will carve away amalgam.

Repeat the procedure along the gingival margin resting the tip of the instrument on the tooth gingival to the restoration and pulling it from the distal to the mesial and back (Fig. 34-58). The distal margin is carved with the carver tip resting on

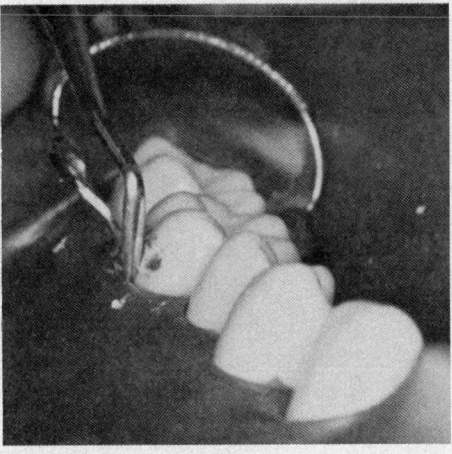

Fig. 34-58. The side of the bladed carver is adapted against both tooth structure and amalgam. The heel of the instrument is not contacting the central portion of the restoration. (From Spohn EE, Halowski WA, and Berry TG: Operative dentistry procedures for dental auxiliaries, St Louis, 1981, The CV Mosby Co.)

tooth structure distal to the restoration and moving occlusogingivally and then back again (Fig. 34-59). The same procedure is performed on the mesial margin.

In all these strokes, only the area immediately adjacent to the margin is being shaped. The intent is to remove obvious excess and begin to form the outer borders of the restoration.

Observe the occlusogingival contour from a mesial view (Fig. 34-60). Because the carving has

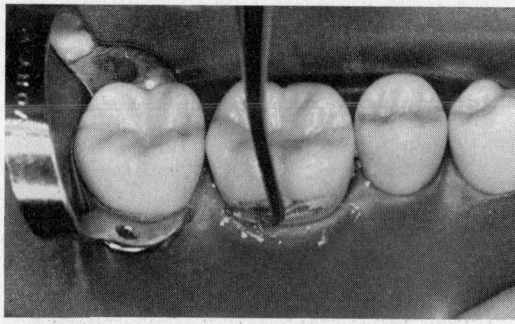

Fig. 34-59. Adaptation of the instrument when carving the distal margin.
(From Spohn EE, Halowski WA, and Berry TG: Operative dentistry procedures for dental auxiliaries, St Louis, 1981, The CV Mosby Co.)

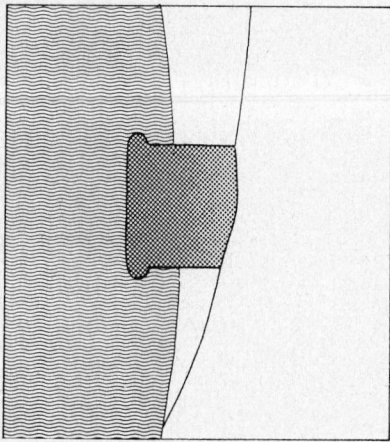

Fig. 34-60. Illustration of an overcontoured class V restoration. The margins are flush at the cavosurface; however, the center of the restoration is too bulky.
(From Spohn EE, Halowski WA, and Berry TG: Operative dentistry procedures for dental auxiliaries, St Louis, 1981, The CV Mosby Co.)

concentrated on the marginal areas, the middle third will be overcontoured.

Contour the middle of the restoration by positioning the instrument on the distal cavosurface margin and bringing it mesially past the mesial margin (Fig. 34-61). This is the first carving movement in which the blade of the instrument is not supported by tooth structure. Do not try to remove all the excess with the first stroke. Too aggressive removal may result in an undercontoured restoration. After the carving movement is made, reexamine the contours from the mesial to determine if additional reduction is needed. Remove amalgam until the contour is correct. The last carving strokes should blend all segments so the contour is smooth and continuous.

Using very light pressure and the side of an explorer, check all the margins carefully. If flash is detected, adapt the side of the ½ Hollenback carver along the marginal area as previously described. Shave away the excess amalgam and then reexamine. An *open margin* (a lack of amalgam or space between the body of the amalgam and the enamel wall), usually requires replacement of the amalgam (Fig. 34-62). A *submarginal area* (an area where the amalgam does not reach the level of the cavosurface margin) may be corrected if it is not too severe (Fig. 34-63). A difference of less than 0.2 mm (barely detectable with an explorer) is correctable by reducing the adjacent enamel during the finishing and polishing procedure. A difference of more than 0.2 mm usually requires replacement of the restoration.

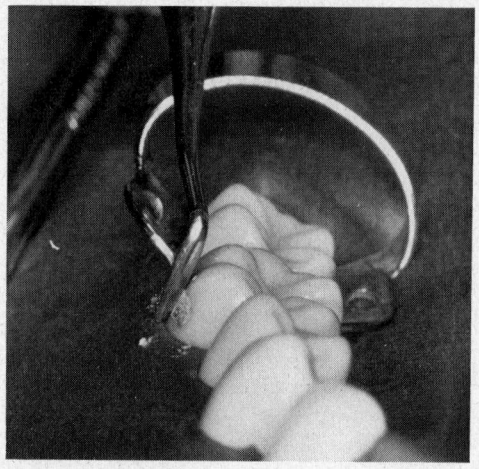

Fig. 34-61. Carving the central portion of the restoration "freehand." The side of the instrument is adapted to excess amalgam only.
(From Spohn EE, Halowski WA, and Berry TG: Operative dentistry procedures for dental auxiliaries, St Louis, 1981, The CV Mosby Co.)

Check the restoration for the following criteria:

1. Margins are flush with no open margins, submarginal areas, or flash
2. The anatomical contours are reproduced

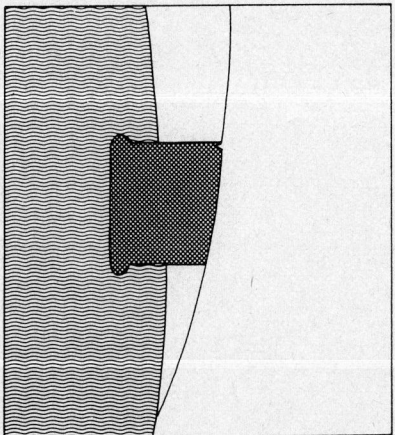

Fig. 34-62. An open margin may be the result of poor condensation at the cavosurface.
(From Spohn EE, Halowski WA, and Berry TG: Operative dentistry procedures for dental auxiliaries, St Louis, 1981, The CV Mosby Co.)

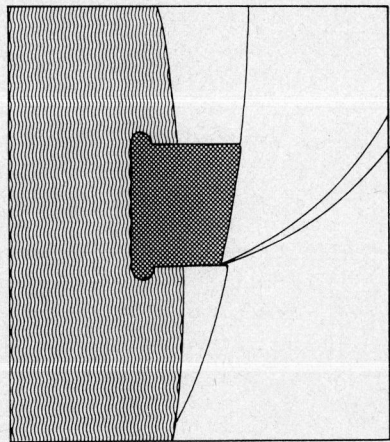

Fig. 34-63. Submarginal areas are detected as the explorer is moved from the restoration to the tooth surface.
(From Spohn EE, Halowski WA, and Berry TG: Operative dentistry procedures for dental auxiliaries, St Louis, 1981, The CV Mosby Co.)

3. The surface has been wiped with a damp cotton roll to help smooth the surface and wipe away debris

Final burnishing

If the amalgam has reached its initial set and is hard enough to resist alteration of contour, it may be burnished. Adapt the beavertail burnisher as described previously. Use a back-and-forth motion with enough pressure to produce a smooth shiny surface. Move the instrument over the whole restoration including the margins. Pressure must be applied to produce a shiny, smooth surface on the hardening amalgam. Reexamine the restoration to ensure that it meets all of the evaluation criteria listed in the check-off sheet at the end of the chapter.

CLASS I AMALGAM RESTORATIONS

The class I restoration is more difficult because it involves the grooves and pits of the occlusal surface and the ridges surrounding them. Anatomical features must be reproduced. Carefully examine the preparation's size and extensions into the grooves (Fig. 34-64). The outline form follows the extension of the carious lesion and the original anatomy of the tooth, but the cavosurface margins should be smoothly rounded with no sharp corners. The walls are parallel or slightly

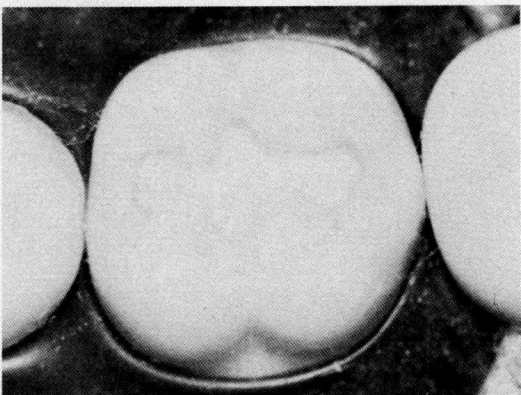

Fig. 34-64. Outline of a class I cavity preparation.
(From Spohn EE, Halowski WA, and Berry TG: Operative dentistry procedures for dental auxiliaries, St Louis, 1981, The CV Mosby Co.)

converging toward the occlusal. Apply base if it is indicated and two coats of cavity varnish.

Condensation

Deposit only one half carrier load into the distal portion of the preparation (Fig. 34-65). Push the carrier toward the pulpal wall and move it mesially as the amalgam is extruded, wedging the mass into the preparation.

Direct the first condensing strokes toward the

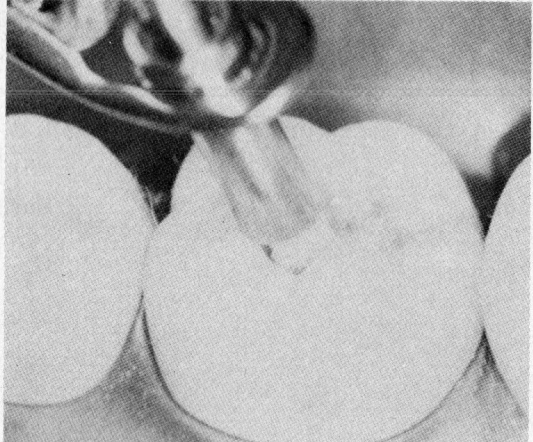

Fig. 34-65. Placement of the first increment of amalgam. (From Spohn EE, Halowski WA, and Berry TG: Operative dentistry procedures for dental auxiliaries, St Louis, 1981, The CV Mosby Co.)

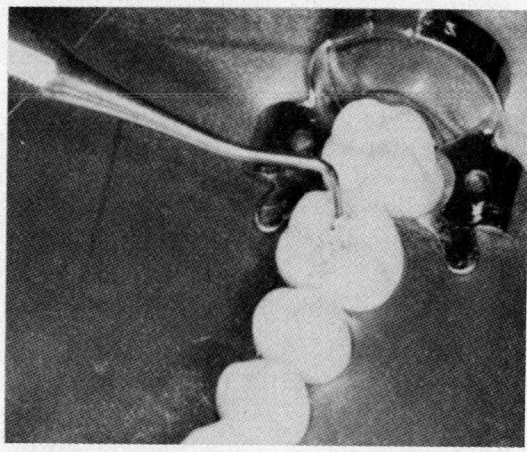

Fig. 34-66. Force of condensation directed perpendicular to pulpal wall. (From Spohn EE, Halowski WA, and Berry TG: Operative dentistry procedures for dental auxiliaries, St Louis, 1981, The CV Mosby Co.)

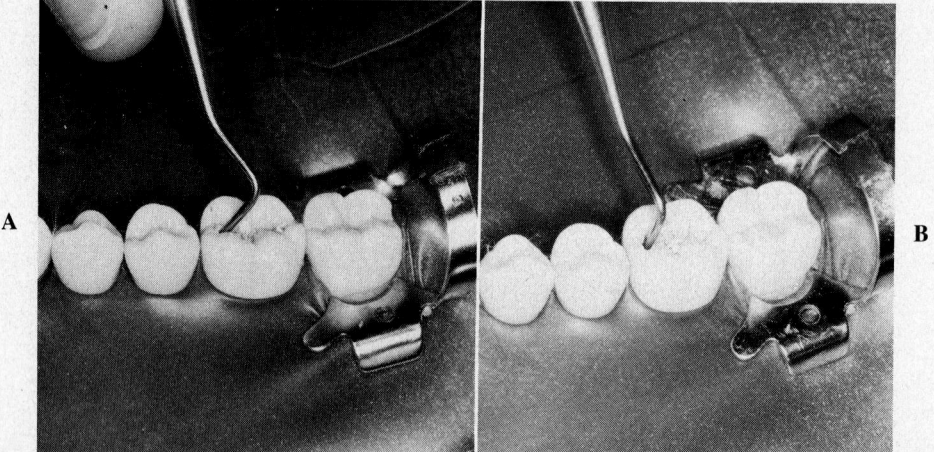

Fig. 34-67. A, Angle of condenser when directed toward the mesial wall and internal line angles. **B,** Angle of condenser when directed toward the lingual wall. (From Spohn EE, Halowski WA, and Berry TG: Operative dentistry procedures for dental auxiliaries, St Louis, 1981, The CV Mosby Co.)

distal and pulpal walls, using light pressure to further wedge the mass (Fig. 34-66) and begin condensing at the distal aspect and across the pulpal wall to the mesial wall. Direct the nib toward the internal line angles (Fig. 34-67). Begin with the distopulpal line angle and move the nib to include the facio-, mesio-, and linguopulpal line angles.

Add the next amalgam increment and condense it into the smaller grooves. Although most of the condensing will be accomplished with the nib end moving perpendicular to the pulpal floor, the side of the nib may be used to push amalgam sideways into groove extensions (Fig. 34-68).

Add and condense the amalgam until the prep-

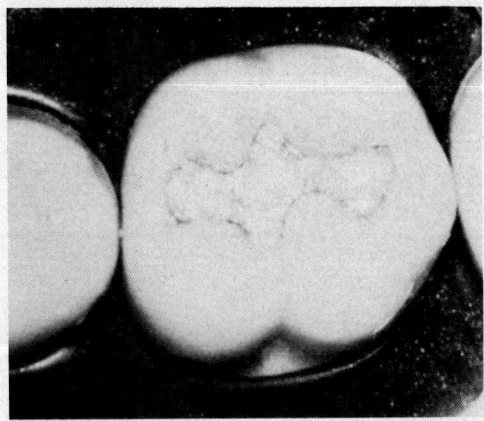

Fig. 34-68. Thoroughly condensed first increment of amalgam.
(From Spohn EE, Halowski WA, and Berry TG: Operative dentistry procedures for dental auxiliaries, St Louis, 1981, The CV Mosby Co.)

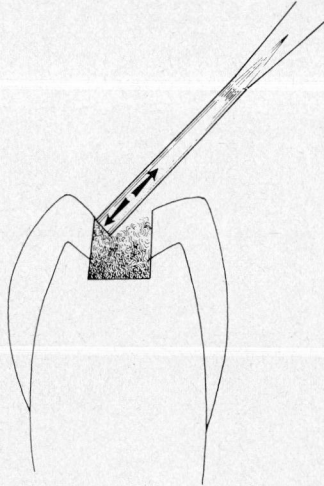

Fig. 34-69. Angle of condenser nib directed toward the internal walls during condensing of the second increment of amalgam.
(From Spohn EE, Halowski WA, and Berry TG: Operative dentistry procedures for dental auxiliaries, St Louis, 1981, The CV Mosby Co.)

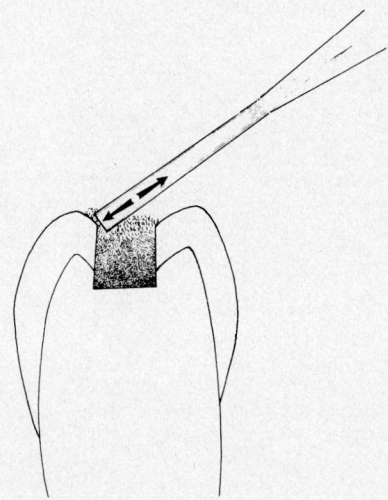

Fig. 34-70. Condensing the amalgam at the cavosurface margin. The nib is approximately perpendicular to the margin.
(From Spohn EE, Halowski WA, and Berry TG: Operative dentistry procedures for dental auxiliaries, St Louis, 1981, The CV Mosby Co.)

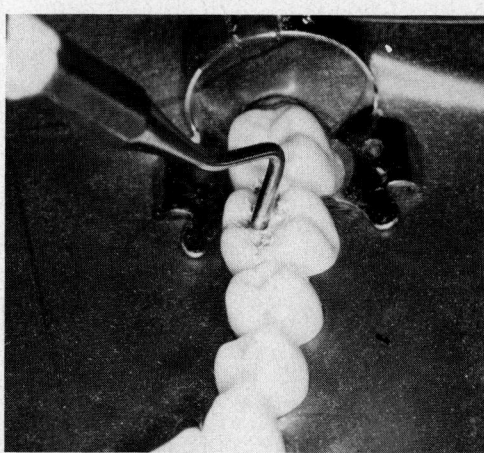

Fig. 34-71. Large condenser nib directed at an angle to the cavosurface margin.
(From Spohn EE, Halowski WA, and Berry TG: Operative dentistry procedures for dental auxiliaries, St Louis, 1981, The CV Mosby Co.)

aration is slightly overfilled (Figs. 34-69 and 34-70). Change to a larger condenser nib and direct the final condensing strokes at a 45-degree angle against the cavosurface margins to adapt the amalgam in these critical areas (Fig. 34-71). Evaluate the restoration after condensation is completed. It should exhibit the previously listed criteria for newly condensed amalgam.

Initial burnishing

The grooves and fossae or pits of a class I restoration require a football-shaped, egg-shaped, or ball

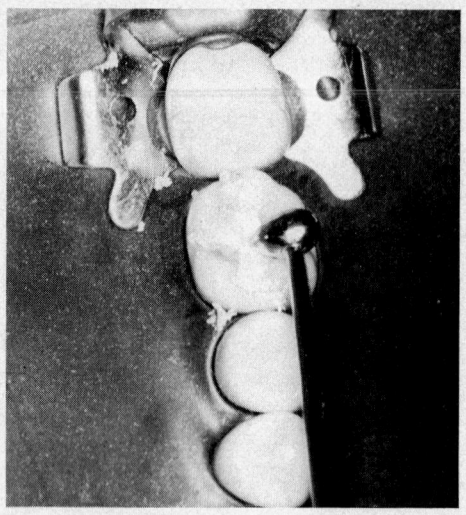

Fig. 34-72. Adapting the football-shaped burnisher along facial margin.
(From Spohn EE, Halowski WA, and Berry TG: Operative dentistry procedures for dental auxiliaries, St Louis, 1981, The CV Mosby Co.)

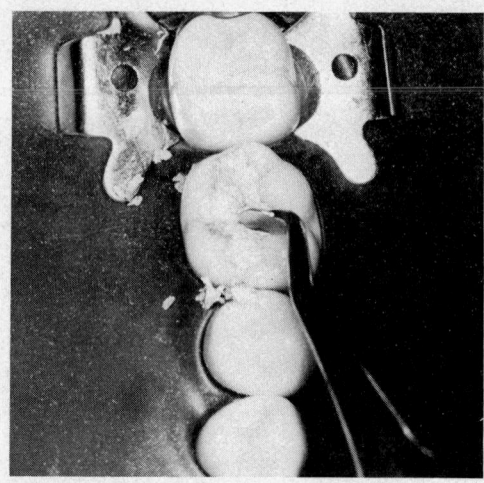

Fig. 34-73. Large discoid carver adapted on tooth surface and amalgam along the facial margin. The face of the blade is perpendicular to the tooth surface.
(From Spohn EE, Halowski WA, and Berry TG: Operative dentistry procedures for dental auxiliaries, St Louis, 1981, The CV Mosby Co.)

burnisher (Fig. 34-72). Place the more pointed end in the center of the tooth with the side resting on both tooth and amalgam. Beginning at the most distal aspect of the facial margin, move the burnisher to the mesial using relatively light strokes. Repeat the procedure along the lingual, mesial, and distal margins to complete the burnishing.

Carving the restoration

The instrument commonly used for carving the occlusal surface is the cleoid-discoid carver. Position the rounded or discoid end at the distal aspect of the facial surface with the side resting on both tooth and amalgam. Place the face of the blade perpendicular to the tooth surface. Move the instrument parallel to the faciocavosurface margin (Fig. 34-73) using short shaving strokes to remove the excess amalgam from the margin. Reposition the instrument and repeat the strokes along the linguocavosurface margin (Fig. 34-74). The instrument should be guided by the contours of the tooth to produce similar contours in the amalgam. Incorrect angulation will result in problems (Fig. 34-75).

Turn the instrument sideways to rest on the mesial marginal ridge (Fig. 34-76). Starting at the

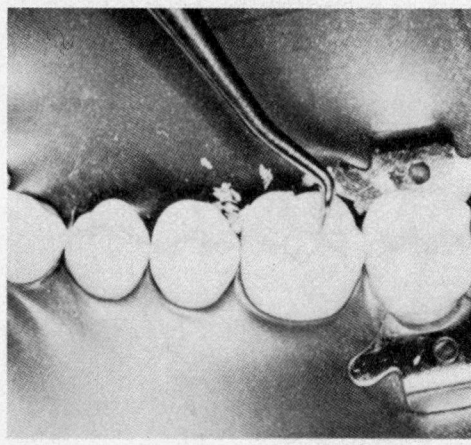

Fig. 34-74. Adaptation of large discoid carver along the lingual cavosurface margin. Amalgam is shaved away in thin layers.
(From Spohn EE, Halowski WA, and Berry TG: Operative dentistry procedures for dental auxiliaries, St Louis, 1981, The CV Mosby Co.)

mesiolingual line angle, move the instrument toward the mesiofacial line angle. The instrument will follow the contour of the mesial marginal ridge and produce a concavity just inside the marginal ridge. This is the beginning of the mesial

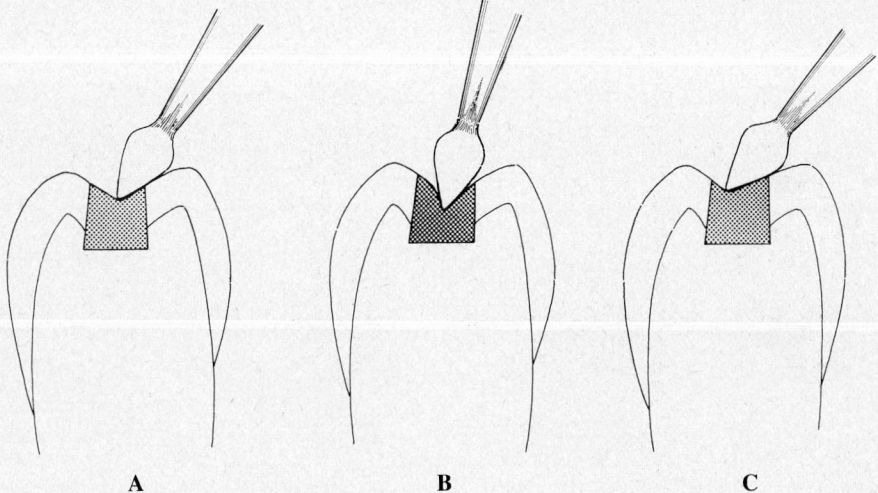

A   B   C

Fig. 34-75. **A,** Correct vertical angulation of the cleoid carver. The side of the blade is contacting tooth structure and amalgam. The tip is located in the central groove. **B,** Vertical angulation of the cleoid carver is too steep. **C,** Vertical angulation of the cleoid carver is too flat, and the tip is displaced too far toward the opposite cavosurface margin.

(From Spohn EE, Halowski WA, and Berry TG: Operative dentistry procedures for dental auxiliaries, St Louis, 1981, The CV Mosby Co.)

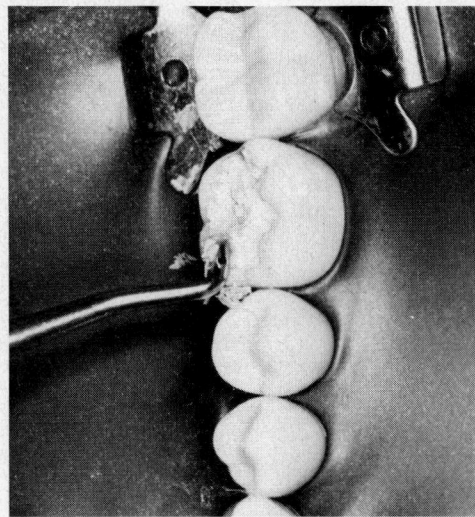

Fig. 34-76. Removing excess amalgam at the mesio-cavosurface margin.

(From Spohn EE, Halowski WA, and Berry TG: Operative dentistry procedures for dental auxiliaries, St Louis, 1981, The CV Mosby Co.)

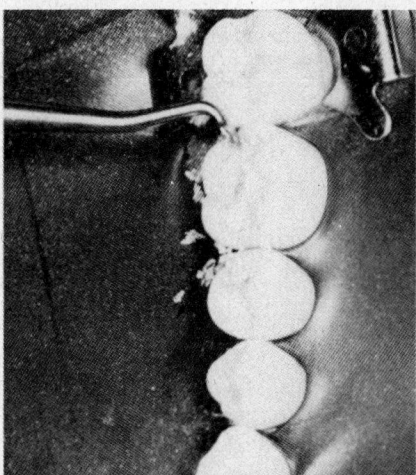

Fig. 34-77. The large discoid carver is adapted against the existing marginal ridge to aid in defining the distal margin and fossa.

(From Spohn EE, Halowski WA, and Berry TG: Operative dentistry procedures for dental auxiliaries, St Louis, 1981, The CV Mosby Co.)

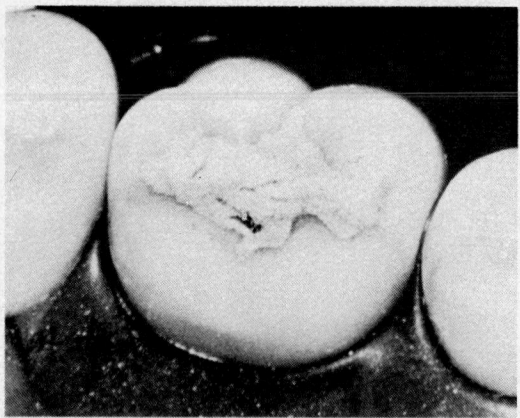

Fig. 34-78. The central groove is lightly defined in the surface of the amalgam. This serves as a reference point for placement of the tip of the cleoid carver.
(From Spohn EE, Halowski WA, and Berry TG: Operative dentistry procedures for dental auxiliaries, St Louis, 1981, The CV Mosby Co.)

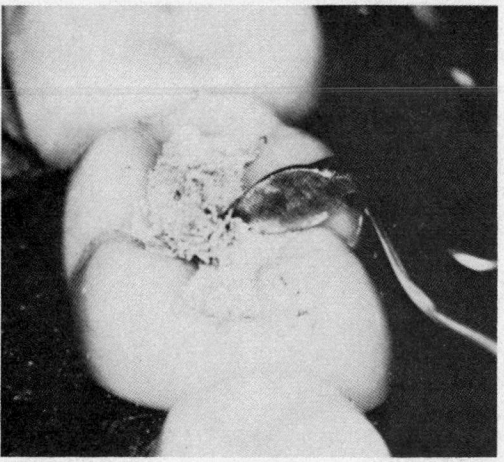

Fig. 34-79. The tip of the cleoid carver is maintained in the previously marked central groove as the excess amalgam is shaved away along the facial margin.
(From Spohn EE, Halowski WA, and Berry TG: Operative dentistry procedures for dental auxiliaries, St Louis, 1981, The CV Mosby Co.)

fossa. The same maneuver is repeated on the distal surface (Fig. 34-77). At this stage of carving, there should be little excess amalgam left on the occlusal surface.

Now concentrate on the details of the specific anatomy. Using the tip of the cleoid instrument, lightly mark the location of the central groove midway between the facial and lingual cusps tips. Starting approximately 1.5 mm from the disto-cavosurface margin, create a shallow central groove extending to within 1.5 mm of the mesio-cavosurface margin (Fig. 34-78).

Rest the cleoid carver on the most distal aspect of the facio-cavosurface margin with the tip extended to the central groove already marked. Pull the instrument mesially, allowing the blade to rise and fall as it is carried over triangular ridges and into fossae or grooves (Fig. 34-79). Repeat this movement along the linquocavosurface margin. The cusp ridges, central fossa, and central groove should be established.

Define the distocavosurface margin (Fig. 34-80). With the small discoid carver adapted against the distocavosurface enamel, move the instrument from the facial surface to the lingual on a line parallel to the distal marginal ridge. Reverse the face of the instrument and repeat the stroke back from the lingual to the facial margin. Do the same procedure to form the mesial fossa.

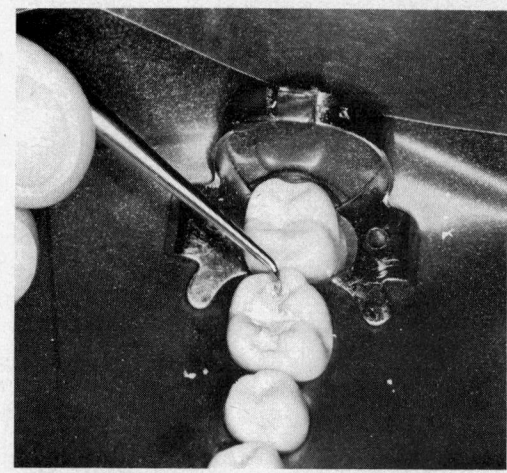

Fig. 34-80. The small discoid carver is used to define the distal fossa.
(From Spohn EE, Halowski WA, and Berry TG: Operative dentistry procedures for dental auxiliaries, St Louis, 1981, The CV Mosby Co.)

The remaining grooves and the central fossa are reproduced next. They need to be well defined but not deep. Place the small cleoid carver on the distofacial cusp ridge with the tip of the instrument touching the central groove. Pull the instrument mesially until it reaches the area halfway be-

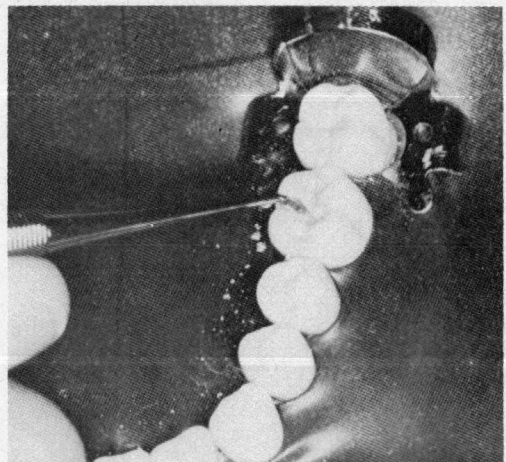

Fig. 34-81. Refining contours with the small cleoid carver adapted to the lingual margin. The tip is maintained in the central groove to avoid inadvertently creating grooves or scratches.
(From Spohn EE, Halowski WA, and Berry TG: Operative dentistry procedures for dental auxiliaries, St Louis, 1981, The CV Mosby Co.)

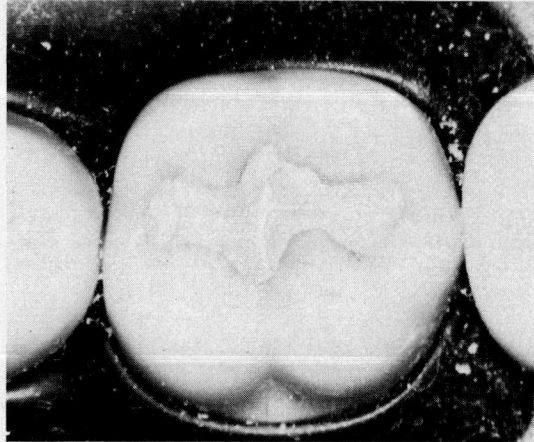

Fig. 34-82. Carving of the class I restoration is complete. The outline of the restoration is smooth with no jagged edges.
(From Spohn EE, Halowski WA, and Berry TG: Operative dentistry procedures for dental auxiliaries, St Louis, 1981, The CV Mosby Co.)

tween the distofacial and mesiofacial cusp tips. Keep the blade at the same angle to the surface of the tooth by rotating the handle of the instrument as it is moved from the height of the distal cusp ridge to the facial groove area. Reverse the steps just outlined, using the back of the cleoid carver as a push instrument to emphasize the contours as you move the instrument distally. Although the instrument does not carve as effectively when used as a push instrument, access and hand placement may be easier in this position. Next, place the instrument on the mesiofacial cusp ridge. Use the same technique to shape the distal incline of the mesiofacial cusp as was used for mesial incline of the distofacial cusp ridge. Then repeat the process on the lingual aspects of the restoration.

Final definition of the grooves may require use of the tip of the cleoid carver if the initial set of the amalgam has occurred (Fig. 34-81). If the amalgam offers resistance to removal, place the tip of the carver in the enamel groove and push the instrument from the enamel into the amalgam. Carry the stroke into the central groove or into a fossa. This same action is done for the lingual groove and any supplemental grooves present.

Check the restoration to ensure that the following criteria are met (Fig. 34-82):

1. Margins are flush with no open margins, submarginal areas, or flash
2. Major anatomical contours such as cusp ridges, fossae, and major grooves are present
3. All grooves and ridges present in the enamel are continued into the amalgam

Final burnishing

After initial set has occurred, burnish the contours using a small ball or football burnisher. Move the instrument back and forth from amalgam to tooth structure over the whole restoration with special emphasis on the margins. Use the tip to burnish in the fossae and down the grooves (Fig. 34-83). Use enough force to give the whole surface a shiny smooth appearance when finished (Fig. 34-84). Wipe the surface of the restoration with a damp cotton roll. Rinse the area using water spray and high volume suction to remove any debris. Remove the rubber dam.

Checking the occlusion

Check the patient's occlusion both visually and with the use of articulating paper. Before placing the articulating paper (or ribbon), dry both the maxillary and mandibular teeth. Use cotton pliers

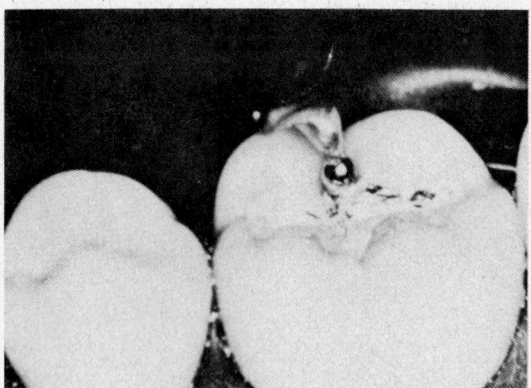

Fig. 34-83. Burnish the amalgam by moving the ball-shaped burnisher back and forth across the margins of the restoration.
(From Spohn EE, Halowski WA, and Berry TG: Operative dentistry procedures for dental auxiliaries, St Louis, 1981, The CV Mosby Co.)

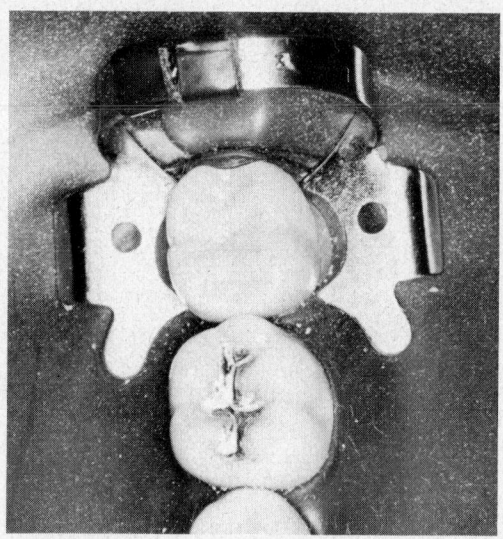

Fig. 34-84. The burnished restoration has a smooth, shiny appearance.
(From Spohn EE, Halowski WA, and Berry TG: Operative dentistry procedures for dental auxiliaries, St Louis, 1981, The CV Mosby Co.)

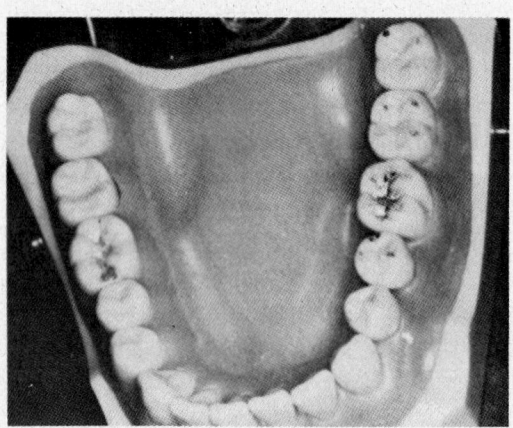

Fig. 34-85. Articulating-paper markings on the restoration must be of density equal to those on the surrounding tooth surface and adjacent teeth.
(From Spohn EE, Halowski WA, and Berry TG: Operative dentistry procedures for dental auxiliaries, St Louis, 1981, The CV Mosby Co.)

or Miller's holding forceps to insert the paper over the quadrant. Have the patient *gently* tap his or her teeth together to check contacts. Remove the paper. The marks on the restoration should be of the same density as those on the surrounding tooth structure and the adjacent teeth (Fig. 34-85). Use a cleoid or discoid instrument to remove any area where markings indicate extra heavy contact. Have the patient close again on the marking ribbon or paper and then move the mandible from side to side and forward to check for premature contacts in lateral and protrusive movements. Again, remove areas indicating excessive contact. Have the patient close and do the movements without the articulating paper in place. Prematurities may show as burnished or flattened spots on the amalgam surface (Fig. 34-86). Ask the patient how the new restoration feels when he or she closes gently. If the patient notices any difference in the way it feels compared with before the restoration was placed, recheck for prematurities. After any prematurities have been eliminated, recheck that the restoration meets all of the criteria listed in the check-off sheet at the end of the chapter.

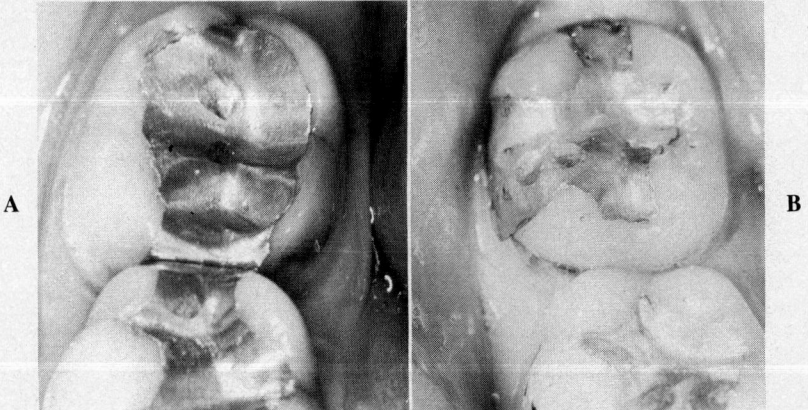

Fig. 34-86. Burnished spots on the amalgam surface.
(From Spohn EE, Halowski WA, and Berry TG: Operative dentistry procedures for dental auxiliaries, St Louis, 1981, The CV Mosby Co.)

MATRIX FOR CONSERVATIVE CLASS II AMALGAM RESTORATIONS

The class II cavity preparation removes the proximal surface of the tooth in addition to the occlusal grooves and fossae (Fig. 34-87). To create a "container" into which the amalgam is condensed, a temporary wall is established (Fig. 34-88). The matrix forms this temporary wall and creates a smooth external surface against which the restorative material can be condensed.

The matrix is a thin metal band that must be supported or stabilized, usually with a mechanical retainer, such as the Tofflemire matrix retainer. A wedge is used to adapt the band to the cervical region of the tooth and to separate the teeth to ensure proper proximal contact in the completed amalgam restoration. Variations in class II preparations will affect the width of the band selected and the positioning of the matrix retainer (facial or lingual).

The most common material used for the matrix is a thin stainless steel band contoured to approximate the shape of the missing proximal tooth structure. Precut stainless steel matrix bands of various sizes are manufactured for use with a Tofflemire retainer to accommodate variations in the location and size of the cavity preparation. The two most commonly used bands are the universal and the extension or MOD band (Fig. 34-89).

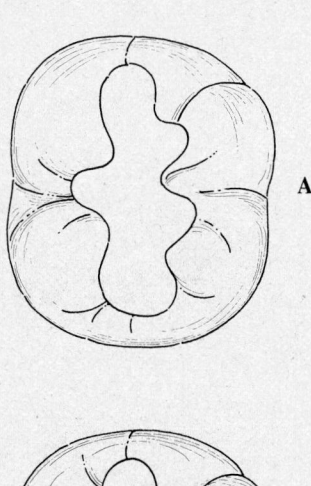

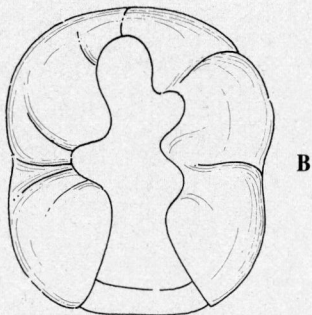

Fig. 34-87. Occlusal view of a class I, **A**; and a class II cavity preparation, **B**. A class II cavity is the extension of a class I cavity onto the proximal surface.
(From Spohn EE, Halowski WA, and Berry TG: Operative dentistry procedures for dental auxiliaries, St Louis, 1981, The CV Mosby Co.)

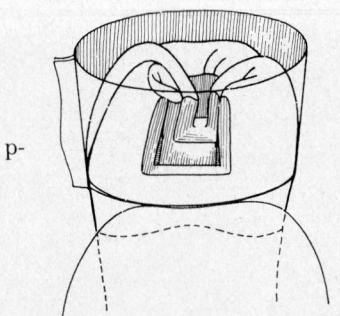

p-

Fig. 34-88. Proximal view of the class II cavity preparation with a matrix in place.
(From Spohn EE, Halowski WA, and Berry TG: Operative dentistry procedures for dental auxiliaries, St Louis, 1981, The CV Mosby Co.)

The universal band is used for routine extension class II preparations. The extension band, which is elongated in the proximogingival areas, is designed for use when the occlusogingival dimension of the preparation exceeds the height of the universal band. Other types of matrices are available for special applications (Fig. 34-90). The Automatrix® is a mechanical matrix device that tightens a band around the tooth and locks it into place.

Trimming the band may be necessary to fit variations in preparation design and size. In general, the principles for placement, wedging, and removal of the Tofflemire matrix will apply to all matrix systems.

The Tofflemire retainer is available in two forms: the straight and contra-angle versions (Fig. 34-91). The straight retainer is generally placed on the facial aspect, and the contra-angle retainer is positioned to the lingual (Fig. 34-92). Sizes are available for both adult and deciduous dentitions.

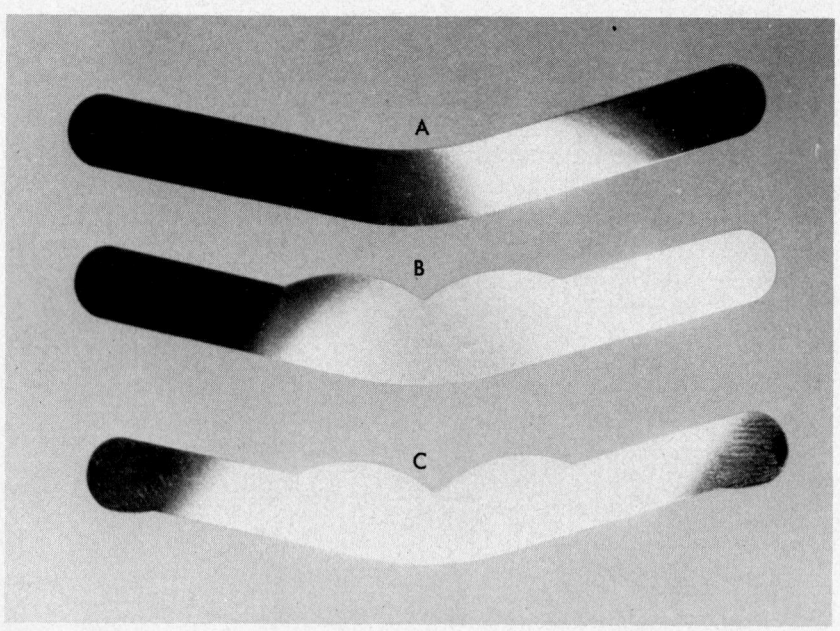

Fig. 34-89. Tofflemire matrix bands; **A,** universal band; **B** and **C,** variations of the extension band.
(From Spohn EE, Halowski WA, and Berry TG: Operative dentistry procedures for dental auxiliaries, St Louis, 1981, The CV Mosby Co.)

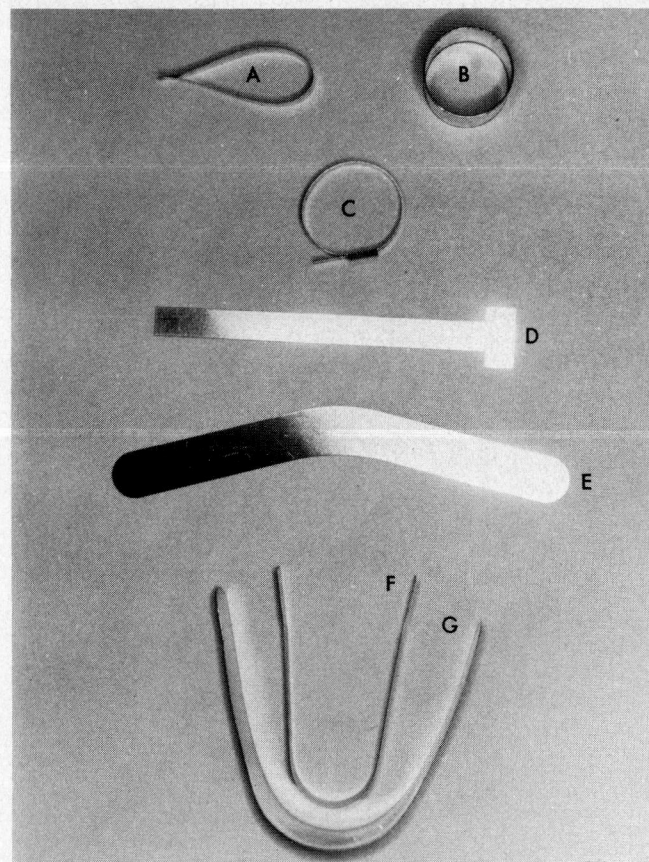

Fig. 34-90. Various forms of matrices: **A,** welded stainless steel; **B,** copper tube; **C,** T-band (assembled); **D,** T-band (unassembled); **E,** universal Tofflemire; **F** and **G,** precontoured stainless steel.
(From Spohn EE, Halowski WA, and Berry TG: Operative dentistry procedures for dental auxiliaries, St Louis, 1981, The CV Mosby Co.)

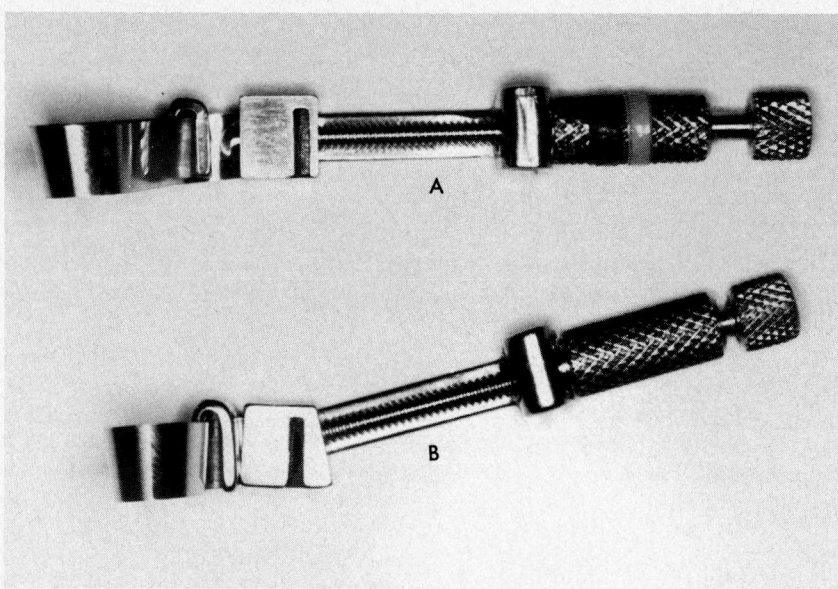

Fig. 34-91. Tofflemire matrix retainer and band assembled: **A,** straight; and **B,** contra-angle.
(From Spohn EE, Halowski WA, and Berry TG: Operative dentistry procedures for dental auxiliaries, St Louis, 1981, The CV Mosby Co.)

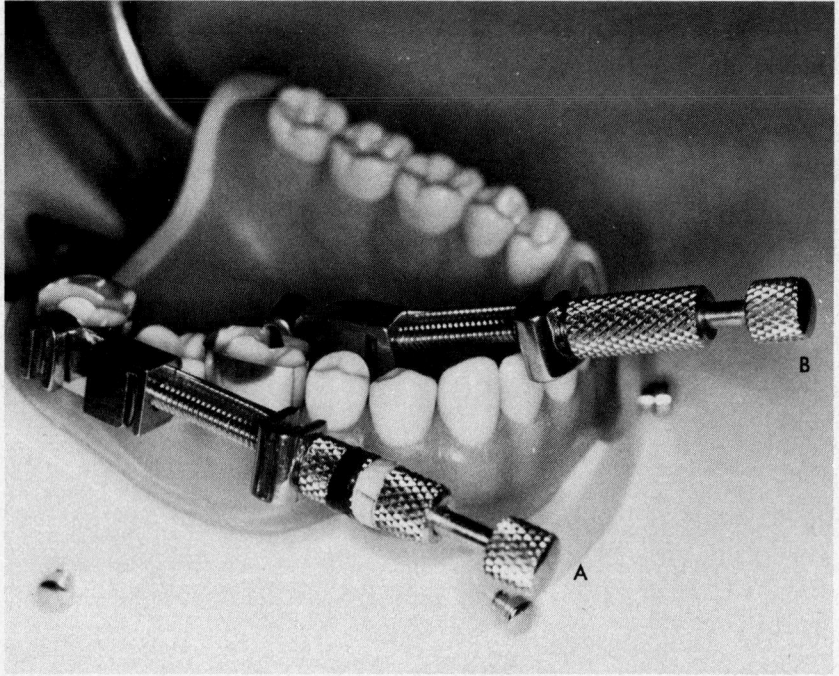

Fig. 34-92. Placement of the Tofflemire retainer and matrix band: **A,** straight retainer positioned from the facial aspect; and **B,** contra-angle retainer positioned from the lingual aspect.
(From Spohn EE, Halowski WA, and Berry TG: Operative dentistry procedures for dental auxiliaries, St Louis, 1981, The CV Mosby Co.)

Armamentarium

The armamentarium suggested for the placement of the Tofflemire matrix is shown in Fig. 34-93. Cleanse and dry the preparation. Bases and liners are applied before the matrix band is placed. Examine the occluso-gingival dimension to determine if the universal band may be used. The band should extend 1 mm apical to the gingival wall(s) and 1 mm occlusal to the future marginal ridge(s). If it does not, select an extension band. A band that extends too far occlusally obstructs the operator's mechanical and visual access to the preparation. A large facial extension of the preparation may require a contra-angle retainer that can be positioned from the lingual aspect. Large lingual extensions call for a straight retainer applied from the facial aspect.

Assembly of the retainer and band

Hold the retainer with the sliding body portion to the left and the slots opening toward the operator

as shown in Fig. 34-94. The outer knob is twisted counterclockwise to disengage the threaded set screw from the sliding body. The function of the outer knob is to turn the set screw in the sliding body and hold the matrix band in the slot. The inner knob moves the sliding body along the track towards or away from the head. Turn the inner knob counterclockwise until the sliding body resets against the head of the retainer (Fig. 34-94). The retainer is now ready to receive the matrix band.

The matrix band is shaped like a shallow V with the base of the V downward. Place the ends together to create a loop. A smaller opening is now toward the operator. Place the ends into the slot of the sliding body guiding the band through the first slot in the head. Then direct the band into the bottom slot (Fig. 34-95). Be certain that both ends of the bands have passed through the slots and have not been separated one from another. Lock the band in place by turning the outer knob

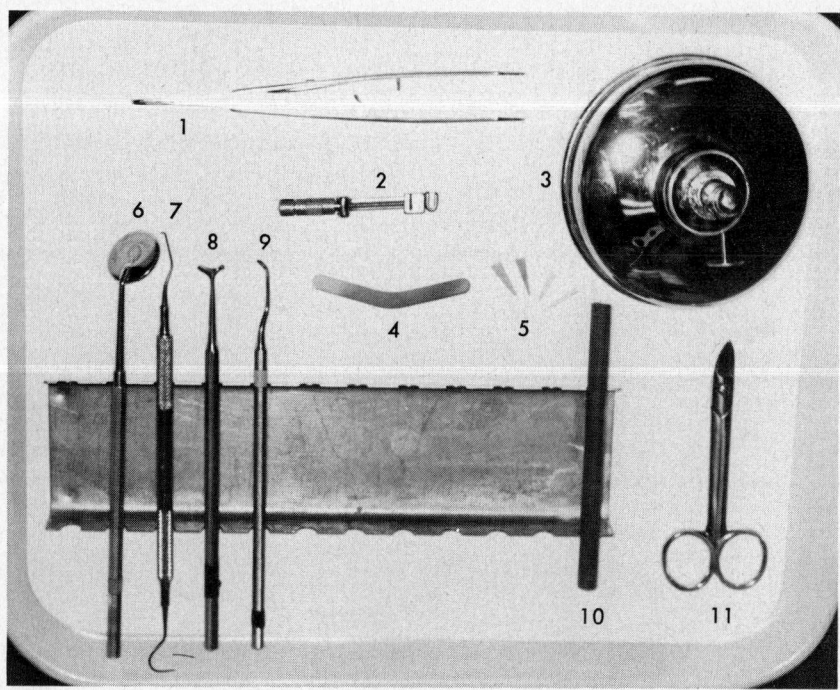

Fig. 34-93. The tray setup for placement of the Tofflemire matrix includes: *1,* locking cotton forceps; *2,* matrix retainer; *3,* alcohol lamp; *4,* matrix band; *5,* wooden wedges; *6,* mouth mirror; *7,* shepherd's hook explorer; *8,* T-ball burnisher; *9,* gold knife; *10,* low-fusing dental compound stick; and *11,* crown and bridge scissors.
(From Spohn EE, Halowski WA, and Berry TG: Operative dentistry procedures for dental auxiliaries, St Louis, 1981, The CV Mosby Co.)

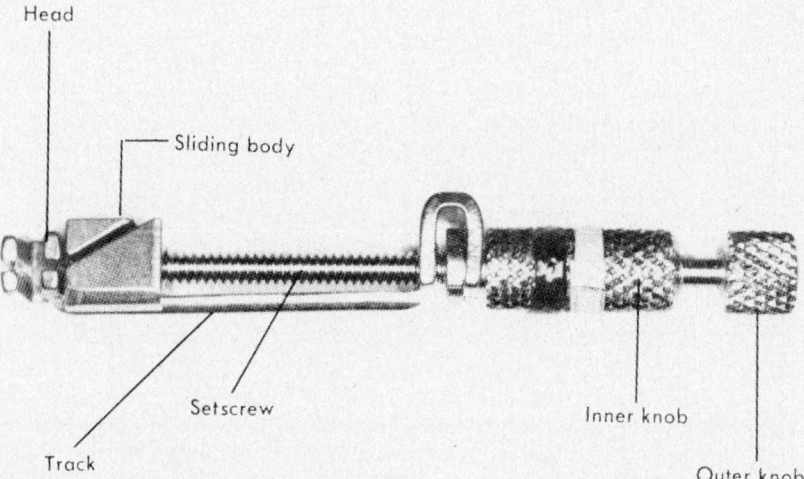

Fig. 34-94. The parts of the Tofflemire matrix retainer.
(From Spohn EE, Halowski WA, and Berry TG: Operative dentistry procedures for dental auxiliaries, St Louis, 1981, The CV Mosby Co.)

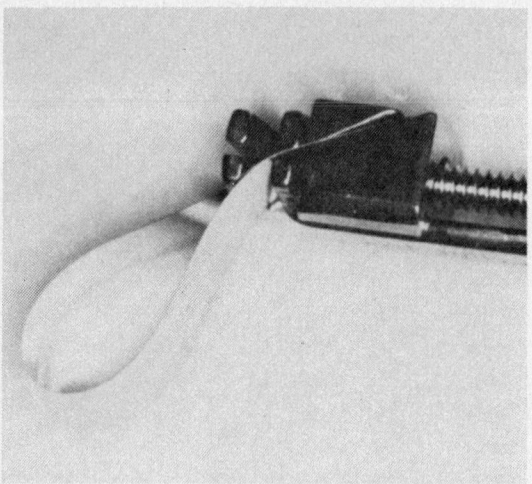

Fig. 34-95. The loop of the matrix band is then passed through the bottom slot in the head. The band is positioned for application in the mandibular right or maxillary left quadrant. (From Spohn EE, Halowski WA, and Berry TG: Operative dentistry procedures for dental auxiliaries, St Louis, 1981, The CV Mosby Co.)

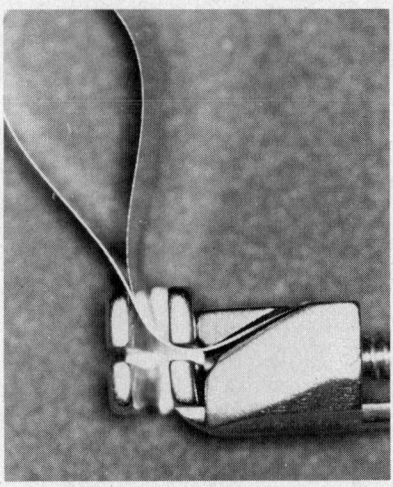

Fig. 34-96. The band is positioned for application in the mandibular left or maxillary right quadrant. (From Spohn EE, Halowski WA, and Berry TG: Operative dentistry procedures for dental auxiliaries, St Louis, 1981, The CV Mosby Co.)

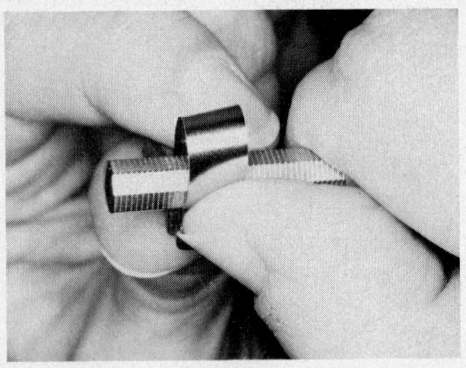

Fig. 34-97. Use an instrument handle to remove any creases in the band. (From Spohn EE, Halowski WA, and Berry TG: Operative dentistry procedures for dental auxiliaries, St Louis, 1981, The CV Mosby Co.)

clockwise until the set screw is tight against the band. Placed in this arrangement, the band can be used for class II preparations in the mandibular right or maxillary left quadrants. The band is directed through the upper slot in the head for mandibular left or maxillary right quadrants (Fig. 34-96). Note that the smaller opening of the loop of the matrix band is facing in the same direction as the slots of the head and body portions.

This is important for the removal of the matrix retainer.

After the band has been assembled on the retainer use a mouth mirror handle to contour the band (Fig. 34-97). Press your thumb against the band and mirror handle, and flatten any wrinkles or creases in the band. Avoid cutting your thumb on the sharp edge of the band.

Placement of the retainer and band on the prepared tooth

Position the retainer on the facial aspect of the tooth with the small opening towards the gingiva. This positioning allows the band to adapt to the conical shape of the crown. Use your thumb or index finger to apply pressure to the occlusal edge of the band, gently pushing the band gingivally through the proximal contact areas. Seat the band until it extends approximately 1 mm beyond the gingival wall of the cavity preparation. Avoid lacerating the gingival tissue with the edge of the band. Position the retainer parallel to the facial surfaces of the teeth (Fig. 34-98). While holding the band in position, twist the inner knob in a clockwise direction. This reduces the size of the loop and tightens the band around the tooth. Tighten the knob until it offers moderate resis-

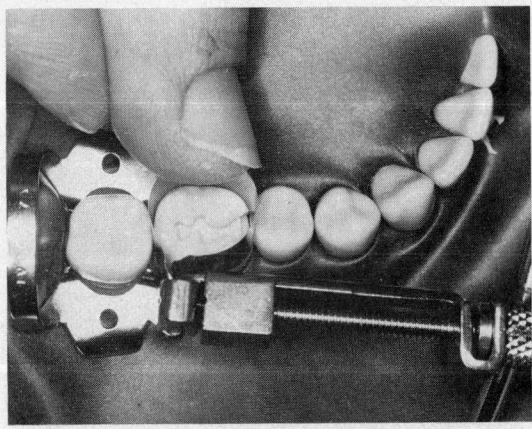

Fig. 34-98. Position the small opening of the band around the tooth.
(From Spohn EE, Halowski WA, and Berry TG: Operative dentistry procedures for dental auxiliaries, St Louis, 1981, The CV Mosby Co.)

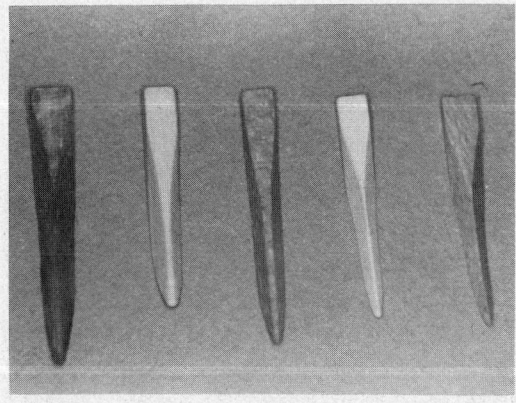

Fig. 34-99. Various sizes, shapes, and colors of precontoured wedges.

tance. Turning the knob too tightly may flatten the proximal portion of the band, resulting in an undercontoured restoration. Insufficient tightening may result in an overcontoured restoration and poor adaptation along the margins.

Placement of the wedge

The wedge holds the band against the proximal surface apical to the gingivocavosurface margin of the preparation. This minimizes the possibility of amalgam being forced beyond the cavosurface margin creating an overhang. The wedge also functions to separate the adjacent teeth slightly to compensate for the thickness of the matrix band. This movement of the teeth, made possible by the compressibility of the periodontal ligament, ensures contact between the teeth after the matrix band is removed and the teeth return to their normal position. Wedges are manufactured in various sizes and forms (precontoured and uncontoured) (Fig. 34-99). Precontoured wedges may be used with little or no modifications for many conservative class II preparations.

A description of the modification of uncontoured wedges is included because they are still in common use. Observe the height and width of the gingival embrasure, noting the level of the gingival margin and its relationship to the papilla. Evaluate the faciolingual contour of the prepared tooth. Note whether it is broad and flat (most mo-

lars) or cylindrical (most premolars). Select the correct wedge and alter it to the degree necessary to apply pressure to the band apical to the gingival margin.

The uncontoured wedges have two longer sides of equal length. The base of the triangle (shorter side) is placed against the gingival tissue. Grasp the wedge with a pair of locking forceps and insert it into the proximal embrasure from the lingual. Angle the tip of the wedge to avoid injury to the papilla. Release the wedge from the locking forceps. Using moderate force with the handle, push the wedge into the embrasure until it resists further movement (Fig. 34-100).

Evaluate the matrix and wedge. The band should be tightly adapted to the entire width at the gingival margin. To check this, place an explorer tip against the inside of the matrix at the gingival wall. If gentle force on the explorer tip creates an opening, the wedge is not holding the band against the tooth (Fig. 34-101). Either the wedge is too narrow, it has not been positioned far enough into the embrasure, or it is too wide.

If the contour of the proximal portion is relatively flat, then little or no contouring of the wedge is necessary. If the tooth contour is cylindrical in shape, it frequently is necessary to contour the wedge.

The wedge should be positioned slightly apical to the gingival wall of the preparation. If it extends too far occlusally, remove it and trim with a gold knife or scalpel (Fig. 34-102). Replace the

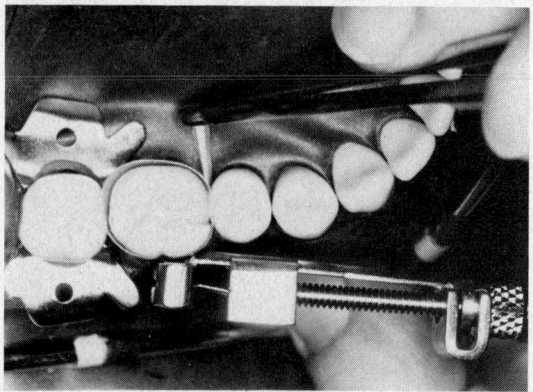

Fig. 34-100. Final positioning of the wedge with the handle of the forceps.

(From Spohn EE, Halowski WA, and Berry TG: Operative dentistry procedures for dental auxiliaries, St Louis, 1981, The CV Mosby Co.)

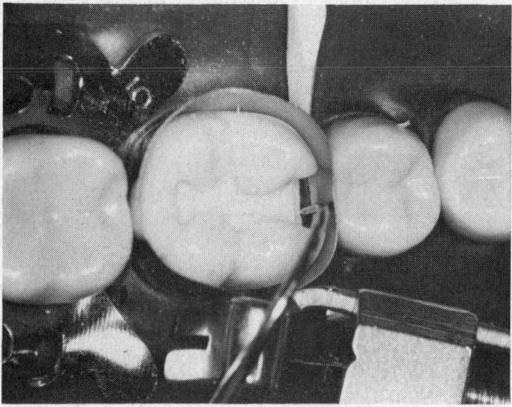

Fig. 34-101. Improper wedge selection or placement may result in the matrix band not being held against the tooth properly.

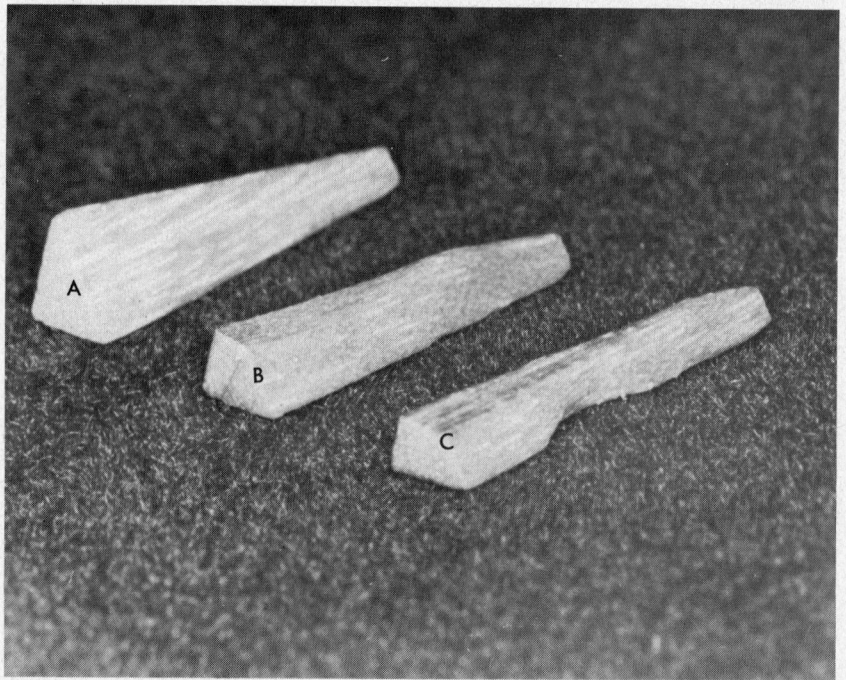

Fig. 34-102. The wedge trimmed for premolar application: **A,** untrimmed; **B,** occlusal height reduced; and **C,** proximal contour trimmed.

(From Spohn EE, Halowski WA, and Berry TG: Operative dentistry procedures for dental auxiliaries, St Louis, 1981, The CV Mosby Co.)

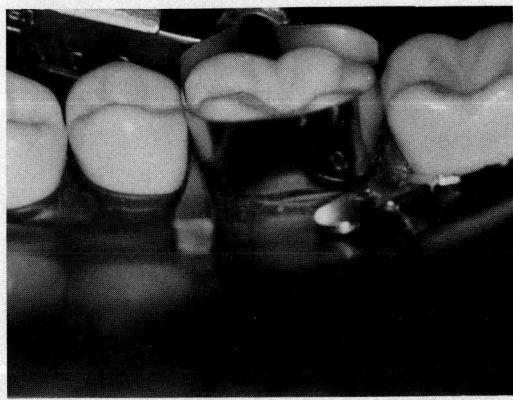

Fig. 34-103. Lingual view of a properly trimmed and positioned wedge.

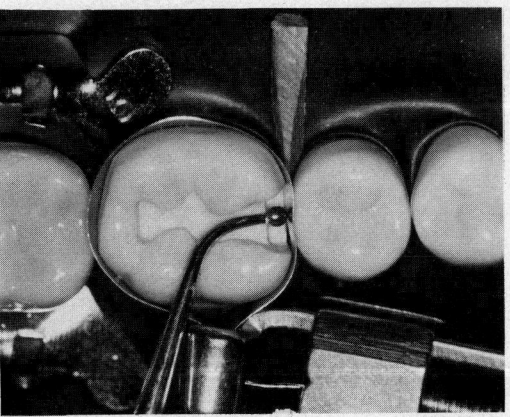

Fig. 34-104. Burnish the contact area before amalgam placement.

wedge and reevaluate it (Fig. 34-103). Burnish the matrix band in the area of the proximal contact using a small ball burnisher (Fig. 34-104). The contact area is at junction of the occlusal and middle thirds of the tooth. Burnishing slightly stretches and contours the matrix metal in the contact area to ensure that the contact with the adjacent tooth will be reestablished. Refer to the check-off sheet at the end of the chapter.

For complex amalgam restorations, a custom matrix is an alternative to the Tofflemire mechanical matrix in situations where the Tofflemire may not provide adequate extension and/or support for placement of the amalgam. The functions, principles of application, and evaluation criteria for the custom matrix are basically the same as those for the Tofflemire matrix. Clinical situations where a custom matrix may be indicated include cavity preparations that involve the following conditions:

1. Removal of one or more cusps
2. Teeth with unusually long clinical crowns
3. Teeth that have no contact with adjacent teeth
4. Interference with the placement of a Tofflemire retainer by the location of a rubber dam clamp
5. Adjacent class II preparations to be restored simultaneously

The Tofflemire matrix presents problems with large restorations. A gap occurs in the area where the band enters the slot in the retainer head. The band does not provide a proper contour if this portion of the tooth is involved in the preparation. The Tofflemire matrix may simply collapse when tightened because of insufficient support by the tooth. In general, the greater the extent of the cavity preparation, the less satisfactory is the mechanical matrix retainer.

The application of the matrix and wedges is influenced by the location of the margins of the cavity preparation. Extensions of the proximal walls facially or lingually or of the occlusal portion along the facial or lingual grooves or the removal of a cusp(s) will determine which matrix will be placed and the method by which it will be stabilized.

Fig. 34-105 illustrates a class II preparation of the mesial, occlusal, distal, and facial surfaces. The mesiofacial cusp has been removed, and a threaded pin has been placed in this area. The gingival wall now extends from the linguoproximal wall to the distal wall on the facial surface. Because there is no longer any tooth tissue to support the matrix band in this area, dental compound will be used to provide support for the band.

Several types of matrices are available, such as copper bands or tubes, brass T-bands, and stainless steel strips (bulk, roll, or precut) of various widths. The choice of the type of matrix is influenced by the clinical situation. Although these types of matrices are made of different materials and handle somewhat differently, the basic principles described for application apply to all types.

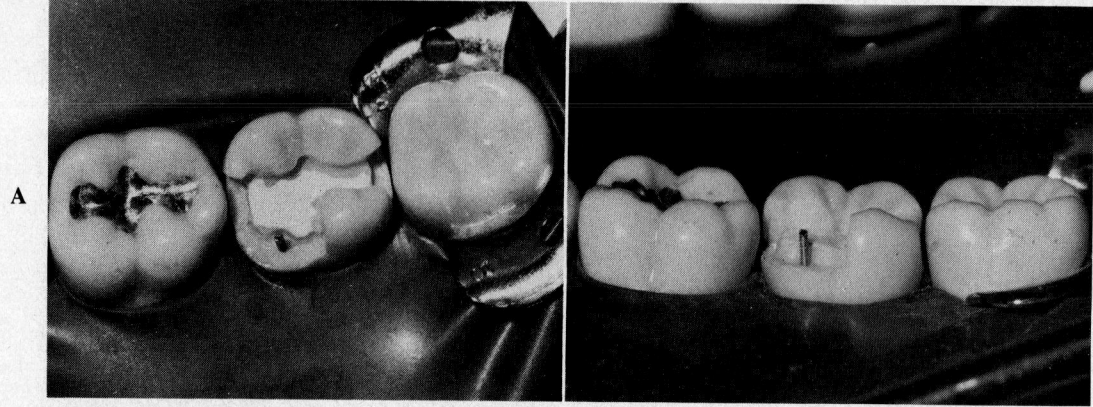

Fig. 34-105. A, Occlusal view of a complex class II amalgam preparation with the mesiofacial cusp removed. A retentive pin has been placed. **B,** Facial view of the preparation.
(From Spohn EE, Halowski WA, and Berry TG: Operative dentistry procedures for dental auxiliaries, St Louis, 1981, The CV Mosby Co.)

The copper band matrix is more rigid and tends to be more self-supporting than the stainless steel band; these are advantages for very extensive preparations. If the restoration is to serve as a temporary restoration and ultimately as a core over which a crown is to be placed, recreation of the anatomical form is less critical. In this situation, the copper band may be the matrix of choice because of the simplicity of selecting the band and adapting it to the cervical portion of the tooth, in addition to the advantages cited earlier.

The brass T-band matrix is available in both narrow and wide sizes. It is primarily used for the restoration of deciduous teeth but can be adapted and contoured for use on permanent teeth as well.

The welded stainless steel custom matrix is thinner than the copper tube, and therefore more desirable to use when contact with the adjacent teeth is to be reestablished. Consult a current textbook of operative dentistry for more information on this subject.

THE RESTORATION OF THE CONSERVATIVE CLASS II AMALGAM PREPARATION
Review the preparation

Access to the proximal surfaces is limited by the adjacent teeth, making it necessary to remove the marginal ridge of the affected tooth. The occlusal portion of the preparation is similar to that of the class I preparation (Fig. 34-106). The proximal

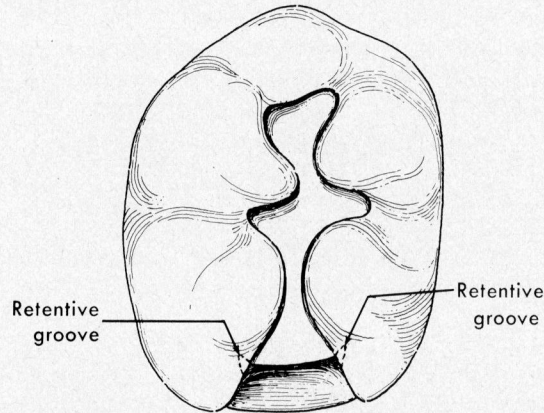

Fig. 34-106. The occlusal view of a class II preparation shows the outline and extension. The retentive grooves in the facioaxial and linguoaxial line angles are indicated by the arrows.
(From Spohn EE, Halowski WA, and Berry TG: Operative dentistry procedures for dental auxiliaries, St Louis, 1981, The CV Mosby Co.)

portion extends gingivally past the contact area to a depth near the gingival tissue. This preparation extends facially and lingually beyond the contact with the adjacent tooth (1 to 1.5 mm).

Retention of the restoration is provided by the parallel walls of the occlusal portion and the parallel or slightly convergent walls and retentive grooves of the proximal box (Fig. 34-107). The angulation of the walls resist an occlusal displacement of the restoration. The retentive grooves are located in the proximal facioaxial and linguoaxial

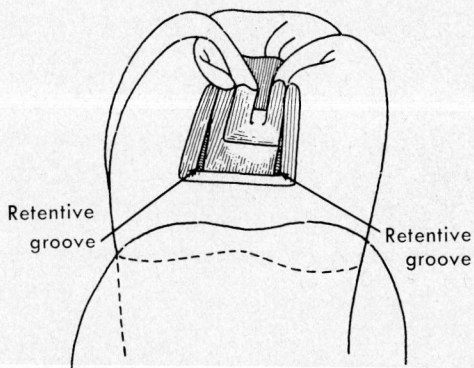

Retentive groove

Retentive groove

Fig. 34-107. The proximal view shows the proximal extension and the preparation's relationship to the gingival tissue. The retentive grooves are indicated by arrows.
(From Spohn EE, Halowski WA, and Berry TG: Operative dentistry procedures for dental auxiliaries, St Louis, 1981, The CV Mosby Co.)

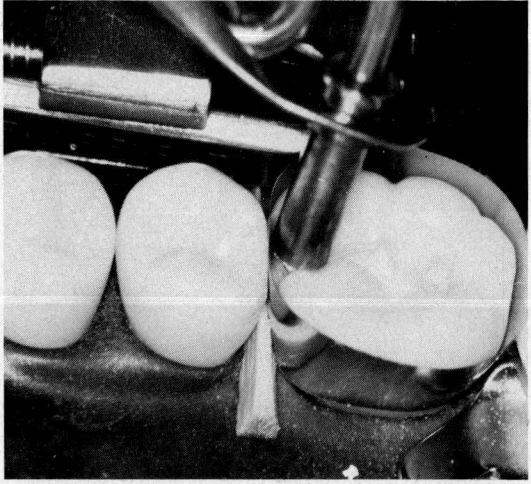

Fig. 34-108. Placing the first carrier load of amalgam into the proximal box enables the least accessible area to be condensed first.
(From Spohn EE, Halowski WA, and Berry TG: Operative dentistry procedures for dental auxiliaries, St Louis, 1981, The CV Mosby Co.)

line angles, extending occlusally from the gingival wall to the dentinoenamel junction.

The proximal contact is significant, in that if not correctly restored, the tooth may shift or drift, creating occlusion problems and upsetting the stability of other teeth in the arch. Inadequate contact and incorrect proximal contours may encourage food impaction and/or difficulty in maintaining adequate oral hygiene.

Before placing the rubber dam, observe the occlusal relationships of the involved tooth. If the tooth or teeth have long or sharp cusps, marginal ridge discrepancies, or other variations from normal, changes in the occlusal anatomy of the planned restoration may be necessary.

Condensing the amalgam

Mix the amalgam as previously described. Place the first increment into the least accessible area which is along the gingival wall of the proximal box (Fig. 34-108). Extrude only one-half of the amalgam carrier load. Select a condenser that will fit easily into the proximal box of the preparation.

Condense the amalgam against the gingival wall, holding the nib perpendicular to the gingival wall. Make overlapping strokes (Fig. 34-109). Condense the amalgam across the gingival wall from the facioproximal line angle to the linguoproximal line angle. Change the direction of the strokes to condense against the line angles. An

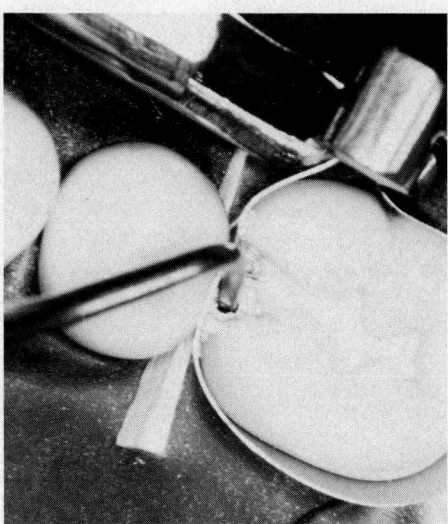

Fig. 34-109. The first condensing strokes are directed perpendicularly.
(From Spohn EE, Halowski WA, and Berry TG: Operative dentistry procedures for dental auxiliaries, St Louis, 1981, The CV Mosby Co.)

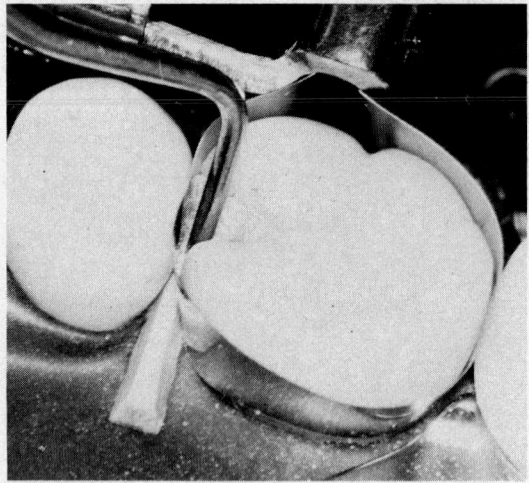

Fig. 34-110. The diamond-shaped nib can be used effectively to condense amalgam into the retentive grooves and the line angles formed by facial and lingual cavosurface margins and the matrix band.
(From Spohn EE, Halowski WA, and Berry TG: Operative dentistry procedures for dental auxiliaries, St Louis, 1981, The CV Mosby Co.)

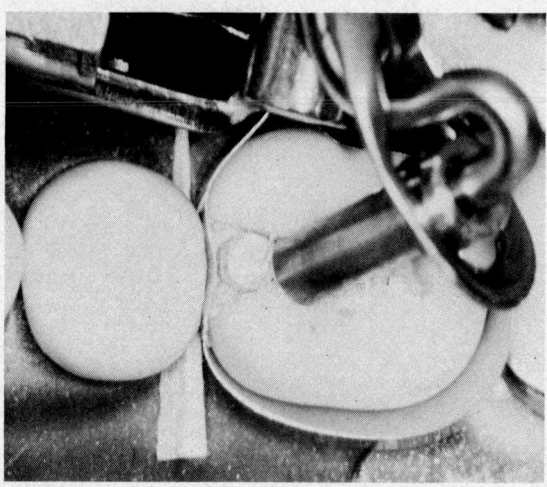

Fig. 34-111. The amalgam is placed onto the pulpal wall only after the proximal amalgam is condensed to the level of the pulpoaxial lline angle.
(From Spohn EE, Halowski WA, and Berry TG: Operative dentistry procedures for dental auxiliaries, St Louis, 1981, The CV Mosby Co.)

angle of approximately 30 to 45 degrees will insure thorough condensation in these corners. Condense the amalgam into the retentive grooves by using the end and sides of the condenser. Push with the side of the nib by moving the instrument laterally against the retentive grooves.

Condense the amalgam against the gingivocavosurface margin and the matrix band by directing the condenser against the side of the band and pushing it gingivally. This assures good condensation into the facial and lingual corners formed by the cavosurface margins and the matrix band.

Determine if the first increment of amalgam is adequately condensed. Place the second increment (one-half carrier load) into the proximal box. Make each condensing stroke quickly and firmly, overlapping it with the previous stroke. Direct the strokes toward the gingival wall, all the line angles, and the retentive grooves and against the axial walls. If both proximal surfaces have been prepared, repeat the condensation process for the other proximal box. Remember that 2½ to 3 minutes is the maximum time before a new batch of amalgam must be mixed.

When the amalgam reaches the level of the pulpoaxial line angle (Fig. 34-110), spread it onto the pulpal floor. Continue placing the amalgam in the same manner as for the class I. Focus attention on the marginal ridge area and along the matrix band to ensure adequate filling of the preparation. Be sure the amalgam is well condensed against the matrix band and has been carried to a height of approximately 1 mm occlusal to the height of the marginal ridge of the adjacent tooth (Fig. 34-111).

At this point the amalgam should overfill the occlusal surface of the preparation by approximately 1.0 mm and should spread to 0.5 to 1.0 mm beyond the cavosurface margins and exhibit no pits or voids.

Initial burnishing

Burnish as for the class I amalgam. Exercise caution when burnishing the area of the future marginal ridge to avoid elimination of too much material. Use an explorer or Hollenback carver to round the outer portion of the marginal ridge area. Place the instrument on the tooth structure slightly facial to the marginal ridge at the juncture of the marginal ridge and the facial cusp of the tooth. Hold the instrument at an angle of approximately 30 degrees to the long axis of the tooth. Move it lingually with the tip touching the matrix band to guide the stroke. End the stroke about halfway between the facial and lingual margins.

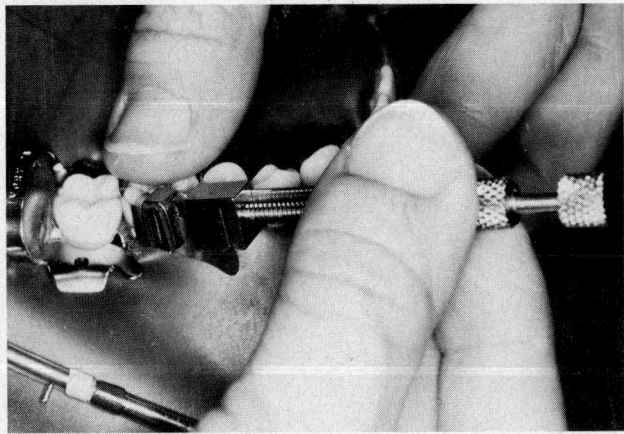

Fig. 34-112. Brace the matrix while turning the knob.
(From Spohn EE, Halowski WA, and Berry TG: Operative dentistry procedures for dental auxiliaries, St Louis, 1981, The CV Mosby Co.)

Determine if the marginal ridge is correctly rounded at a height equal to the adjacent marginal ridge. If it is too flat, increase the angulation of the explorer to approximately 45 degrees and repeat the stroke. This more vertical position will allow more rounding of the marginal ridge. Place the instrument at the same angle, slightly lingual to the lingual margin, and move it facially to blend this area.

Remove the gross excess from the rest of the occlusal surfaces as described for the class I restoration. Use the large discoid carver to initiate the carving of the mesial fossa. Because no marginal ridge serves as reference, take care not to form the fossa too near the proximal surface. Observe the marginal ridge on the opposite proximal surface and/or the adjacent tooth. The fossa should be located just proximal to the facial and lingual triangular ridges. Be careful not carve into the marginal ridge area.

Removal of the wedge, matrix band and retainer

Remove the wedge by pulling it lingually with the cotton pliers. To remove the retainer, place the thumb or index finger over the matrix band at the proximal surfaces to minimize pressure exerted on the amalgam (Fig. 34-112). Turn the inner knob one-half turn counterclockwise to increase the diameter of the loop. Release the set screw by turn-ing the outer knob counterclockwise. With a finger supporting the band, remove the retainer in an occlusal direction from the band. Then remove the band from the embrasure of the uninvolved proximal surface. Great care must be exercised when removing the band from the restored proximal to avoid fracturing the marginal ridge. Grasp the ends of the band a few millimeters from the tooth. If working with an assistant, have him or her place a large nibbed condenser on the marginal ridge area to counteract any forces exerted by pulling the band occlusally. Pull the band linguoocclusally until resistance is felt (Fig. 34-113). Change the direction of pull to a faciooclusal direction. Again, pull until resistance is felt (Fig. 34-114). Continue to pull and reverse direction when resistance is felt until the band is pulled free.

Carving of the proximal surface

Evaluate the gingival margin while the amalgam is still soft. Place the tip of the explorer into the gingival embrasure apical to the gingival margin. Gently pass the explorer past the gingival margin to check for an overhang. Pass the explorer from the amalgam to tooth surface to check for a submarginal defect (Fig. 34-115). Repeat this from both the lingual and facial embrasures. Use the side rather than the tip of the explorer to prevent scratching or gouging the surface.

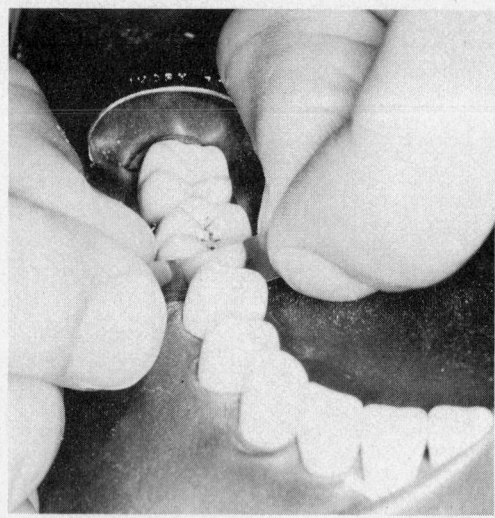

Fig. 34-113. The matrix band is pulled occlusolingually until resistance is felt.
(From Spohn EE, Halowski WA, and Berry TG: Operative dentistry procedures for dental auxiliaries, St Louis, 1981, The CV Mosby Co.)

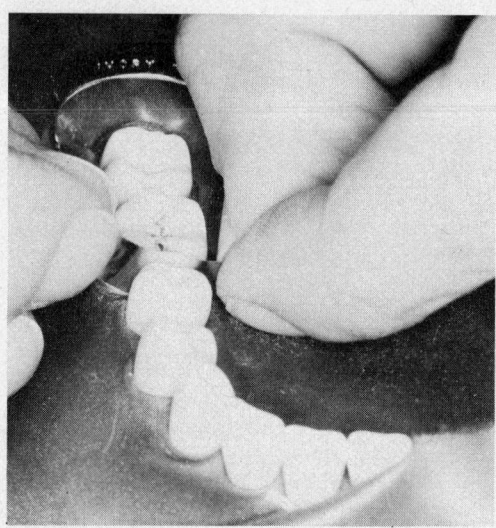

Fig. 34-114. The direction is changed to pull the band occlusofacially until resistance is felt.
(From Spohn EE, Halowski WA, and Berry TG: Operative dentistry procedures for dental auxiliaries, St Louis, 1981, The CV Mosby Co.)

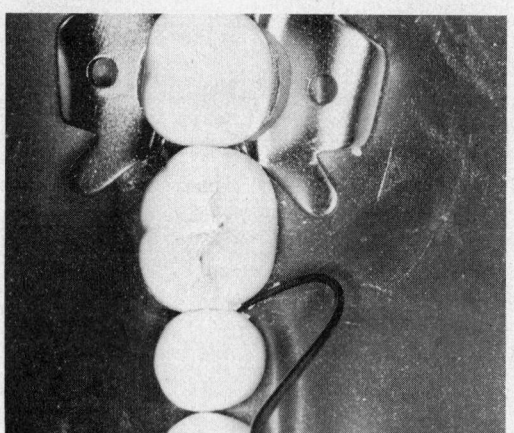

Fig. 34-115. Check for overextensions and submarginal areas with the explorer tip.
(From Spohn EE, Halowski WA, and Berry TG: Operative dentistry procedures for dental auxiliaries, St Louis, 1981, The CV Mosby Co.)

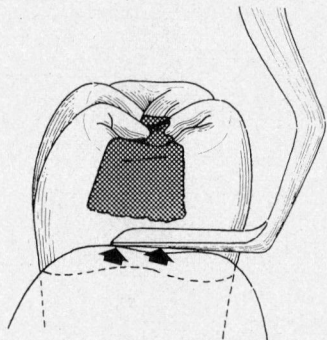

Fig. 34-116. The blade of the amalgam knife is inserted gingival to the gingival margin and is kept in contact with the tooth as it is moved occlusally past the margin. The amalgam is shaved away.
(From Spohn EE, Halowski WA, and Berry TG: Operative dentistry procedures for dental auxiliaries, St Louis, 1981, The CV Mosby Co.)

If an overhang exists, use the side of the explorer to burnish away the excess. Recheck to determine if the amalgam margin is flush with the enamel. If the amalgam has hardened somewhat, an amalgam knife is the instrument of choice. Insert the blade into the facial embrasure below the gingival margin and pull it in an occlusofacial direction in a smooth shaving stroke (Fig. 34-116). As the proximal contact area is reached, decrease the carving pressure and pull the instrument out into the facial embrasure to avoid removing the contact. Repeat the stroke from the

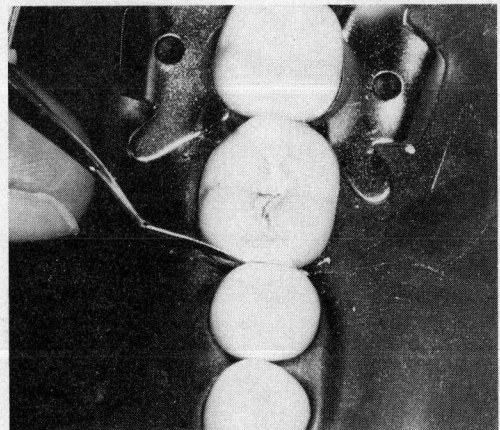

Fig. 34-117. Round the mesiofacial line angle with a ½ Hollenback carver. Use a shaving stroke to avoid the danger of fracturing the marginal ridge.
(From Spohn EE, Halowski WA, and Berry TG: Operative dentistry procedures for dental auxiliaries, St Louis, 1981, The CV Mosby Co.)

lingual aspect, overlapping the stroke made from the facial direction. Recheck the margin using an explorer.

Remove from the facial and lingual margins of the proximal surfaces any areas that are overcontoured or have flash. Hold the blade of the ½ Hollenback carver perpendicular to the facial margin of the preparation near the marginal ridge (Fig. 34-117). The blade is angled towards the adjacent tooth with the tip contacting it. The carving will be done with the edge rather than the tip of the instrument. Move the instrument in a gingival direction. This carving rounds the facioaxial line angle and opens the embrasure without danger of creating a ledge or corner on the proximal surface. Define the contour and the margin of the lingual portion in the same manner. Continue to make shaving strokes until the facial and lingual surfaces are rounded and the embrasures are sufficiently open.

Carving the final occlusal contours

Use a large discoid instrument to adjust the marginal ridge to approximately the same height as that of the adjacent tooth. Rest the instrument on the adjacent marginal ridge and move it from tooth to amalgam stopping short of the opposite cavosurface margin. If the teeth are malaligned,

supraerupted or not correctly restored, there may be a great discrepancy in marginal ridge height. The restored ridge height may be a compromise between matching the adjacent marginal ridge and restoring the original anatomy of the tooth. After the marginal ridge is adjusted, the adjacent fossa generally requires redefinition. Orient the small cleoid carver blade so the point of the instrument rests in the central groove area and the side of the blade rests on enamel. Move the instrument in a mesial or distal direction. The remaining tooth structure guides the pattern of the carving, reducing the possibility of overcarving. Do not carry the carving stroke into the marginal ridge; the marginal ridge may fracture. Continue to carve the occlusal portion as described during the Class I restoration. Evaluate the carving by the criteria previously listed.

Pass dental floss gently through the contact area to smooth the proximal surface, remove debris, and determine that the contact is tight enough. If the contact is adequate it will require pressure to pass the floss through the contact area. Remove the floss by pulling it in a facial or lingual direction.

Final burnishing

Burnish the occlusal surface as described for the class I restoration. Be particularly careful not to exert pressure on the marginal ridge to avoid fracture. If accessible, burnish the facioaxial and linguoaxial portions of the proximal area with the side rather than the cutting edge of the Hollenback carver. Adapt the carver with the tip against the adjacent tooth to avoid creating a defect.

Checking the occlusion

After removing the rubber dam, check the occlusion with articulating paper. Because the marginal ridge protion is not well supported and the amalgam has not reached final strength, have the patient close his or her teeth gently to avoid breaking the marginal ridge. Observe for burnish spots or dark blue spots especially on the marginal ridge (Fig. 34-118). Check the occlusal relationship of the unaffected teeth without the articulating ribbon in place. If prematurities are discovered, use the discoid carver to remove them. Instruct the patient to avoid chewing on the restored tooth for the next 24 hours and indicate that there may be some sensitivity to heat or cold.

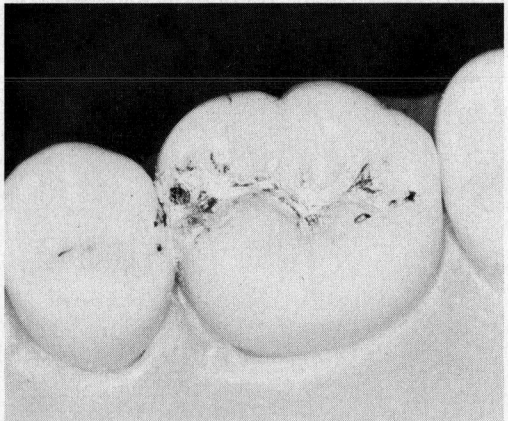

Fig. 34-118. The heavy mark on the marginal ridge indicates a prematurity that needs removing.
(From Spohn EE, Halowski WA, and Berry TG: Operative dentistry procedures for dental auxiliaries, St Louis, 1981, The CV Mosby Co.)

Evaluation criteria
Surface texture

1. The amalgam is smooth
2. No pits or voids are present
3. The amalgam has a dull luster; if the surface has been burnished, it is somewhat shiny

Anatomical form

1. The triangular ridges of the cusps extend to the central groove
2. The fossae are the correct size and depth and are in the correct location
3. The major grooves are distinct and correctly located
4. The supplemental grooves present in the adjacent enamel extend into the restoration

Marginal integrity

1. No open margins are present
2. No submarginal areas are present that cannot be smoothed during finishing and polishing
3. The amalgam does not extend beyond the cavosurface margin of the restoration

Occlusal contacts

1. The marks made by articulating paper or ribbon are of equal density on both the restoration and the surrounding tooth structure; contacts (as indicated by marks) occur in the fossae of the restoration if the relationship with the opposing tooth or teeth permits

2. The uninvolved teeth still occlude as they did before the procedure
3. The patient reports that the restoration does not feel "high"

Proximal contours and contact

1. The marginal ridge is rounded to form an occlusal embrasure
2. The proximal contour is primarily convex faciolingually
3. Occlusogingivally, the contact area is convex from the marginal ridge through the contact area
4. From the gingival border of the contact area to the cervical line, the contour is flat or slightly concave
5. The lingual embrasure is slightly larger than the facial embrasure
6. The proximal contact with the adjacent tooth occurs facial to the midline faciolingually and in the gingival portion of the occlusal one-third occlusogingivally

The procedures described above provide the basic techniques and approach to restoring a class II amalgam preparation with the loss of a minimum of tooth tissue. When more tooth structure is lost from the occlusal, proximal, facial, or lingual surfaces, the clinician must be more skilled and must use additional techniques, such as custom matrices to contain the amalgam and place it around pins that have been positioned to provide additional retention. For the restoration of complex amalgam preparations, consult current textbooks of operative dentistry.

RECONTOURING, FINISHING, AND POLISHING

It is important to recontour, finish, and polish both older and new restorations. However, the procedure should be performed only if the restoration is basically sound. If it is of questionable quality, it may need to be replaced. The decision to replace depends on factors such as marginal discrepancies of greater than 0.2 mm, open uncorrectable large overhangs, recurrent decay, and excessively deep occlusal anatomy.

Recontouring reduces or alters areas that are too bulky and/or overextended to blend with the normal contours of the tooth that has been restored. *Finishing* smooths the overall surface of the restoration and blends the specific details, such as margins, to the surrounding anatomy of the tooth. *Polishing* places a high shine or luster on the surface to give the best possible smoothness and resistance to corrosion and tarnish and to emphasize to the patient the quality and importance of the restoration. Recontouring, finishing, and polishing are not completely separate procedures but rather steps in a gradual removal of or reduction in the amalgam in decreasing amounts to produce the desired results.

Overhangs are overcontours on proximal surfaces. One radiographic survey study showed that 52% of class II restorations exhibit overhangs (Coxhead et al, 1978). These overhangs are associated with gingival and periodontal disease (Hakkarainen and Ainamo, 1980; Jeffcoat et al, 1980; Leon, 1977). Mechanical impingement may be a problem, but more important the overhang is a plaque retentive area, which complicates oral hygiene. Removal of overhangs and subsequent finishing and polishing of the area, in conjunction with plaque removal procedures by the patient, improve the health of the gingiva and supporting structures (Axelsson, 1981; Gorzo et al, 1979; Highfield and Powell, 1978; Rodriguez-Ferrer et al, 1980).

Armamentarium

A wide variety of instruments, including both hand and rotary instruments, is available for recontouring and finishing. Selection is based upon the accessibility of the area, the amount of reduction required, and the surface finish desired. Limiting the number of instruments will keep the technique simple and contribute to speed and efficiency. The rotary instruments most commonly used for recontouring and finishing are burs, abrasive stones, and finishing discs (Fig. 34-119).

The burs used for recontouring and finishing amalgam restorations are made of plain steel, rather than of carbide steel like those used for cavity preparation (Fig. 34-120). Finishing burs have more and smaller cutting edges (18 to 20) designed to leave a smoother surface. Various shapes and sizes are needed to gain access. The shapes recommended are a flame-shaped bur for narrow areas such as the embrasures, round or plug-shaped burs for fossae and grooves; and a pear-shaped or barrel-shaped bur for finishing cusp inclines. It is important to remember that the bigger the circumference of the rotary instrument, the greater the rotary speed of the external surface and the more surface of the tooth and restoration contacted. Greater circumference and greater surface contacted can be factors in heat generation.

Stones can be long and tapered for the occlusal or smooth surface restorations or rounded for use in fossae. Abrasiveness depends on the type of particles incorporated in the matrix of the stone. Particles in green stones are more abrasive than those in white stones. Green stones are used to remove amalgam bulk, and white stones are used for reducing small areas of enamel and/or amalgam around marginal discrepancies.

The thin, flat shape of disks can be adapted along broad, smooth surfaces. They are ideal for class V restorations or facial and lingual extensions of class II restorations. They are also used

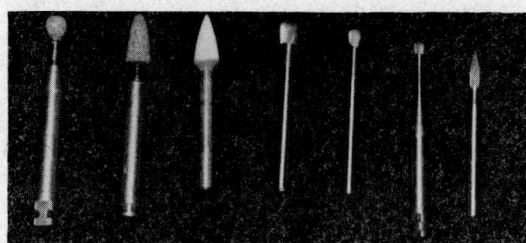

Fig. 34-119. Examples of burs and stones commonly used during finishing and polishing (left to right): round and tapered green stones, white stone, plug-shaped, round-shaped, and flame-shaped finishing burs. Available for both friction-grip and latch-type handpieces.

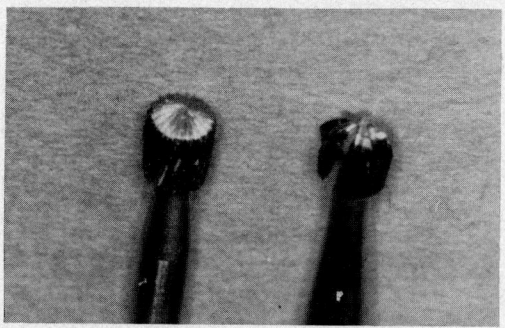

Fig. 34-120. The finishing bur on the left has more blades and produces a smoother surface than the cutting bur on the right.

to recontour the interproximal surface in the occlusal embrasure areas. Disks are available in different sizes and are attached to a mandrel inserted into a contra-angle. Both snap-on and screw-in mandrels with correspondingly designed discs are available in a variety of grits (Fig. 34-121). The most commonly used are garnet (coarse) and cuttle (fine). In most instances fine garnet is the most abrasive disc used and is followed by fine cuttle.

Hand instruments. Three types of hand instruments used to remove overhangs on the gingival cavosurface margin are the amalgam knife, files, and currettes. The amalgam knife is the instrument of choice. Files are used when the amalgam knife cannot be adapted. Universal curettes can remove small amalgam extensions and, when necessary, can smooth the amalgam after amalgam knives or files have been used.

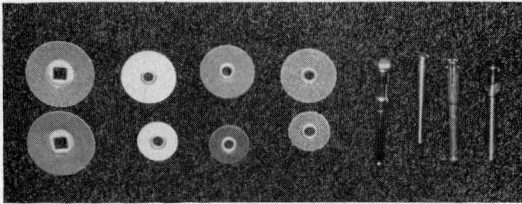

Fig. 34-121. Examples of the different types of mandrels and discs available.

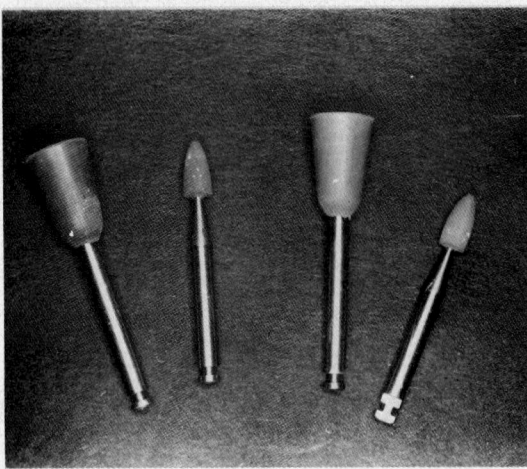

Fig. 34-122. Greenie and Brownie points and cups.

Polishing agents. Pumice is available in a variety of grits, or particle sizes. Finer grades, such as flour of pumice, are used in the first stage of polishing an amalgam restoration. Tin oxide has a much finer grit, so it is used as the final polishing agent to produce a high luster. Both are applied with flexible rubber cups or occlusal brushes.

Polishing can also be achieved with abrasive impregnated cups and points; Brownie, Greenie, and Supergreenie (Shofu Company). Both are convenient and less messy than pumice and tin oxide, but they are more expensive because they wear quickly. Results are equal to those obtained with pumice or tin oxide (Reavis-Scruggs, 1982) (Fig. 34-122). Coarser abrasive agents remove thin layers of amalgam and leave scratches. As finer abrasives are used, scratches become correspondingly finer. It is important to use abrasives in decreasing order of coarseness.

Heat from pressure and speed exerted by the rotary instruments is potentially detrimental to amalgam by bringing mercury to the surface, resulting in a dull appearance and more susceptibility to corrosion. This can be corrected only by removing the surface layer of amalgam, which could produce an undercontoured restoration. Heat production can be minimized by using moderate speed, intermittent moderate pressure, and wet abrasive agents.

Procedure

Because amalgam is not completely set until 24 hours after placement, recontouring, finishing, and polishing should not be initiated until then. Premature attempts interfere with the crystalline structure of the hardening amalgam, resulting in a weakened restoration. Although there have been experiments with polishing high copper amalgams within 10 minutes of placement (Corpron et al, 1982; Creaven et al, 1980; Schemlitzer et al, 1982; Nitkin, 1979) it is presently recommended that at least 24 hours pass (Creaven et al, 1980; Craig, 1980; Schemlitzer et al, 1982).

Recontouring and finishing the occlusal surface

Evaluate the occlusal contours of the restoration. Mark the occlusion with articulating paper in centric and excursive movements. If the markings indicate prematurities, the areas require reduction to

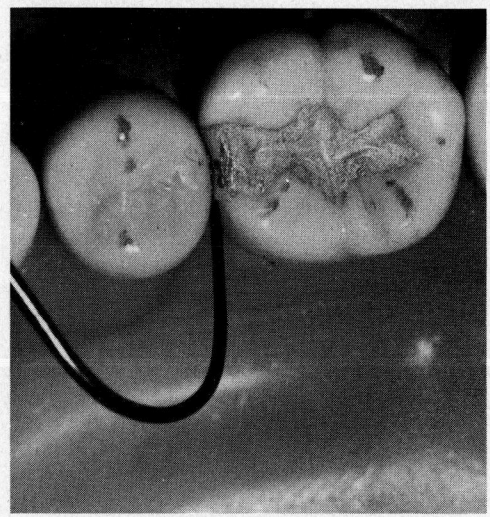

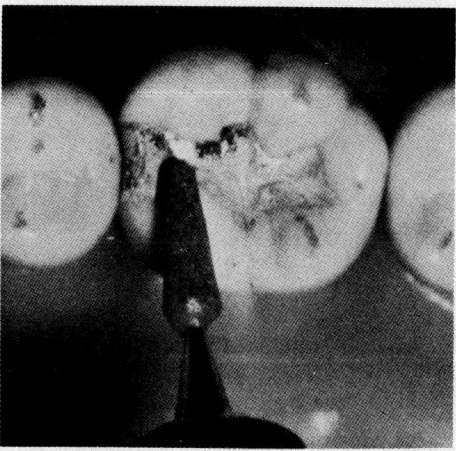

Fig. 34-124. The green stone removes excess amalgam rapidly. It is used only for recontouring because it leaves a rough finish.
(From Spohn EE, Halowski WA, and Berry TG: Operative dentistry procedures for dental auxiliaries, St Louis, 1981, The CV Mosby Co.)

Fig. 34-123. Heavy occlusal contacts are detected with articulating paper. Note the darker marking on the mesial marginal ridge. The explorer points to an overextension along the mesiolingual margin.
(From Spohn EE, Halowski WA, and Berry TG: Operative dentistry procedures for dental auxiliaries, St Louis, 1981, The CV Mosby Co.)

prevent occlusal trauma (Fig. 34-123). Place the side of the tapered green stone against the amalgam and move it back and forth with light intermittent pressure until the excess is removed (Fig. 34-124). Recheck the occlusion and continue until the prematurity is eliminated.

A pointed white stone is used to smooth a surface that is tarnished, corroded, and pitted and to eliminate any submarginal discrepancy less than 0.2 mm (Fig. 34-125). Place the side of the stone on the enamel, moving it back and forth at medium speed until the enamel is flush with the amalgam. To avoid excess heat and the possibility of removing too much enamel, do not leave the stone in one spot.

Finishing burs are used next to eliminate small excesses and to reshape and define the anatomy, producing smooth surface finish. Finishing burs are designed to cut when they are rotated either clockwise or counterclockwise. Smooth the occlusal margins with a round finishing bur by placing the side of the bur against both amalgam and tooth surface (Fig. 34-126). Light, short, intermittent strokes are used as the bur is moved along the entire occlusal margin. For larger restorations,

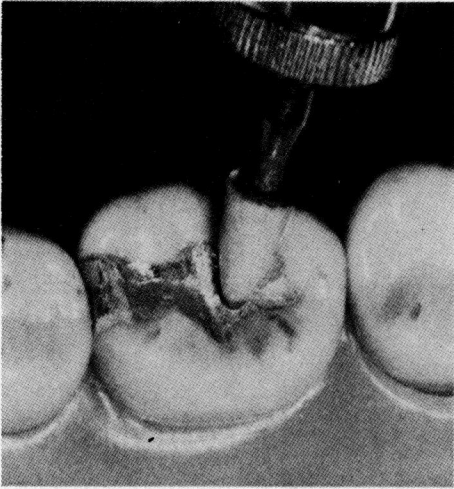

Fig. 34-125. The side of the stone is adapted to the enamel to correct marginal discrepancies of 0.2 mm or less.
(From Spohn EE, Halowski WA, and Berry TG: Operative dentistry procedures for dental auxiliaries, St Louis, 1981, The CV Mosby Co.)

a barrel- or pear-shaped finishing bur may be used.

The finishing burs also can improve the occlusal anatomy if the side of the round finishing bur is placed into the fossa (Fig. 34-127). The fossae should not be exaggerated but should ex-

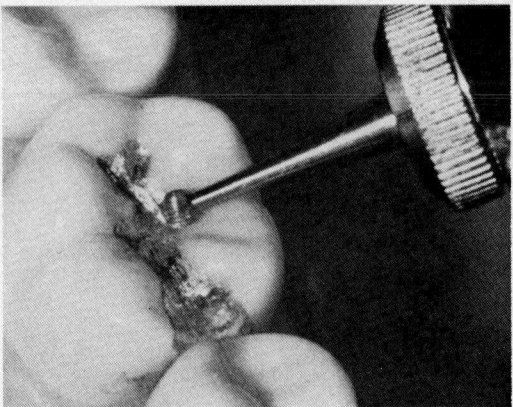

Fig. 34-126. The finishing bur is contacting both amalgam and tooth surface as it is moved along the entire cavosurface margin.
(From Spohn EE, Halowski WA, and Berry TG: Operative dentistry procedures for dental auxiliaries, St Louis, 1981, The CV Mosby Co.)

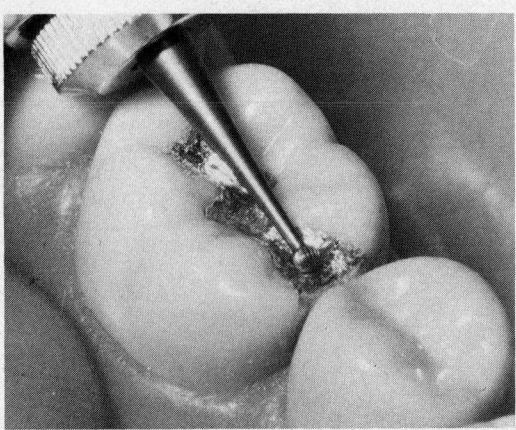

Fig. 34-127. Use the side of the plug-shaped finishing bur when defining mesial and distal fossae. Sweep the bur facio-lingually to create a convex area.
(From Spohn EE, Halowski WA, and Berry TG: Operative dentistry procedures for dental auxiliaries, St Louis, 1981, The CV Mosby Co.)

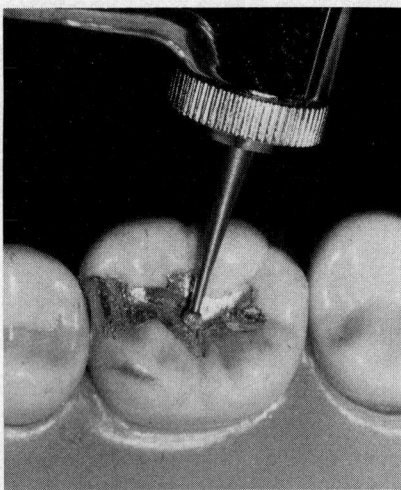

Fig. 34-128. A small finishing bur is used to define major developmental and supplemental grooves.
(From Spohn EE, Halowski WA, and Berry TG: Operative dentistry procedures for dental auxiliaries, St Louis, 1981, The CV Mosby Co.)

tend to a depth consistent with the rest of the occlusal anatomical contours. Define developmental grooves with a small No. 1 round or flame-shaped finishing bur. As the bur is not resting on tooth structure, control it carefully (Fig. 34-128). Use the bur in all the developmental and more promi-

nent supplemental grooves to make them distinct but not deep.

Recontouring and finishing facial and lingual surfaces

Use medium and fine finishing discs to recontour and smooth the facial and lingual surfaces. The edge of the disc (outer 1.0 mm) is adapted to each margin and light, sweeping strokes are used to move the disc from the margin towards the center of the restoration (Fig. 34-129). The clinician must take care not to overreduce the restoration. After recontouring, finish the surface of the restoration with a very fine disc.

A flame-shaped bur also can be used to recontour and smooth the surface (Fig. 34-130). The side of the bur is adapted along the margins, contacting both tooth and amalgam, and the same light, sweeping strokes are used over the entire margin. The clinician must use extreme caution along gingival margins, especially those extending onto the root surface. Rotary instruments can damage cementum and adjacent tissues. The side of the flame-shaped bur can be used along the gingival margin, minimizing contact with the adjacent cementum. A gingival retractor may be needed to increase access.

Developmental grooves of the facial and lingual surfaces are finished with round or flame-

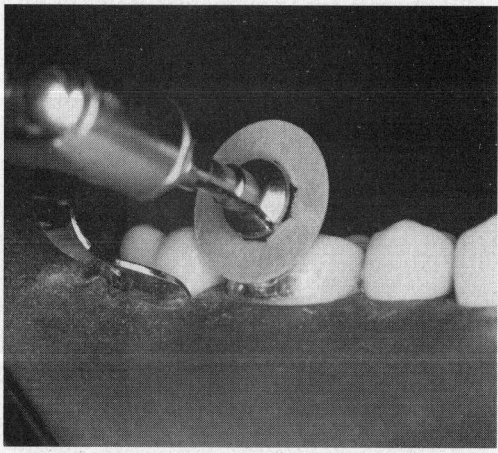

Fig. 34-129. The outer edge of the disc is adapted to the occlusal margin of a class V restoration.
(From Spohn EE, Halowski WA, and Berry TG: Operative dentistry procedures for dental auxiliaries, St Louis, 1981, The CV Mosby Co.)

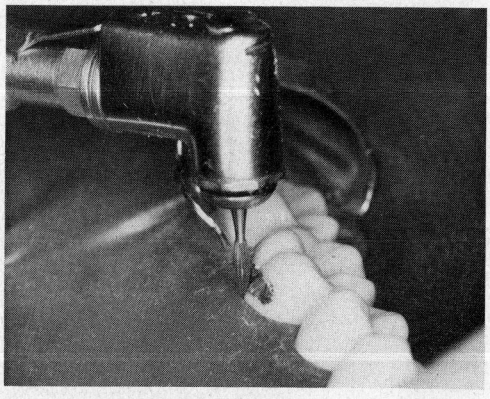

Fig. 34-130. The flame-shaped bur is adapted along the gingival margin of a class V restoration. Caution is needed to minimize contact of the tip with cementum.
(From Spohn EE, Halowski WA, and Berry TG: Operative dentistry procedures for dental auxiliaries, St Louis, 1981, The CV Mosby Co.)

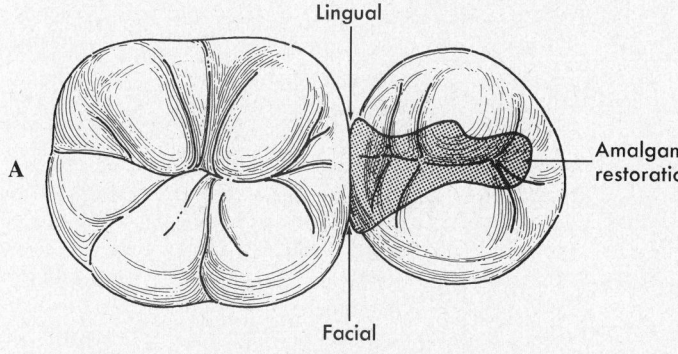

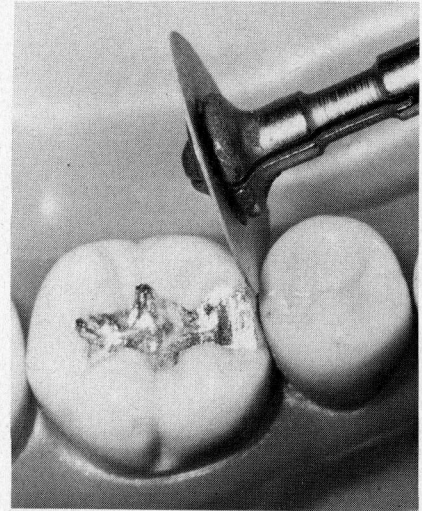

Fig. 34-131. A, This bulky, overcontoured occlusal embrasure may snag or tear dental floss. **B,** The finishing disk is adapted from the lingual aspect to contour the occlusal embrasure.
(From Spohn EE, Halowski WA, and Berry TG: Operative dentistry procedures for dental auxiliaries, St Louis, 1981, The CV Mosby Co.)

shaped burs. Select one that fits into the groove and use it in a manner similar to that used on the occlusal surface.

Recontouring and finishing the proximal surface

Small areas of excess amalgam located along the occlusal embrasure area are removed with a fine finishing disc. Rotate the disc to fit into the facial or lingual aspects of the occlusal embrasure and contact the excess amalgam (Fig. 34-131). Move the disc into the occlusal embrasure in a sweeping motion. Stop frequently and evaluate the results, as amalgam can be abraded quickly. This step is repeated on the opposite surface if indicated. A garnet disc may be used for gross excess. Follow this with a cuttle disc to remove flash from accessible facial and lingual margins. Adapt the edge

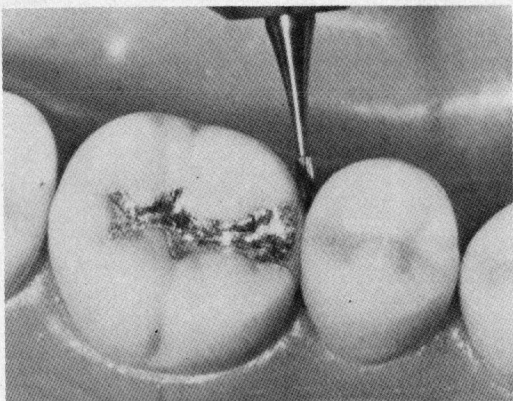

Fig. 34-132. The flame-shaped bur is held perpendicular to the lingual margin of the proximal box. Make sure the tip of the bur does not extend deep enough to affect the contact area. (From Spohn EE, Halowski WA, and Berry TG: Operative dentistry procedures for dental auxiliaries, St Louis, 1981, The CV Mosby Co.)

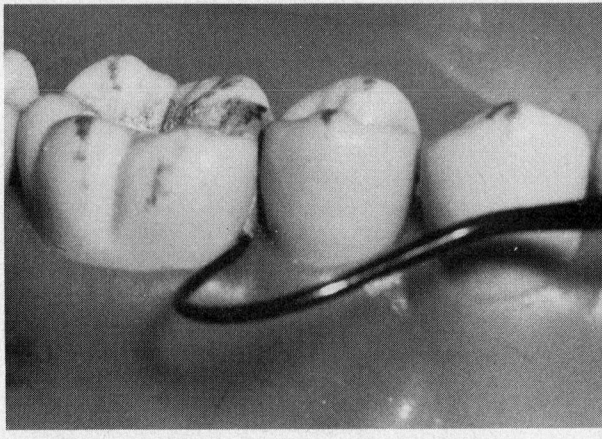

Fig. 34-133. An explorer can be used to detect an overhang, which is visible along the gingival margin. (From Spohn EE, Halowski WA, and Berry TG: Operative dentistry procedures for dental auxiliaries, St Louis, 1981, The CV Mosby Co.)

of the disc using the same light, sweeping strokes to move the disc along the amalgam surface. Do not push the rotating disc far enough into the proximal embrasure to damage the contact area or the papilla.

A flame-shaped bur also can be used to finish the facial and lingual margins of the proximal area. Place the bur perpendicular to the facial or lingual margin with the point extending into the embrasure and the side of the bur contacting both amalgam and tooth surface (Fig. 34-132). Move the bur parallel along the margin from the gingival margin to the marginal ridge. Avoid placing prressure on the tip of the bur to prevent creating a gouge or ledge in the contact area.

Removing gingival overhangs

The proximal area should be evaluated visually from both the facial and lingual aspects, tactilely by using floss and an explorer, and radiographically (Fig. 34-133). If an overhang is detected, the location, size, and shape must be determined, as with calculus deposits (Fig. 34-134).

Small overhangs often can be removed as part of scaling. Overhang removal is most successful with small to moderate overhangs.

In cross-section, the amalgam knife looks like an upside-down sickle scaler. The apex of the triangle is the cutting edge. The instrument must be

angled differently from a scaler (Fig. 34-135). The cutting edge of the amalgam knife is turned more toward the tooth than is the cutting edge of the sickle scaler. It is extremely sharp. Although some tissue displacement may be inevitable, no damage to the epithelial attachment and papilla should occur. Removing an overhang is different from removing calculus because the amalgam is shaved away. The instrument is *not* placed under the entire overhang and activated to remove the overhang in one stroke because the amalgam may fracture at the cavosurface margin necessitating placement of a new restoration.

Place the tip of the knife at the faciogingival aspect of the proximal box and insert it until the blade catches on a definite ledge (Fig. 34-136). Increase the pressure on the blade as it is moved from the gingival margin to the contact area to begin removing amalgam. Slowly move the blade farther into the proximal area while continuing the shaving strokes. On each stroke, the blade is inserted slightly deeper into the embrasure until the tip extends past the center of the proximal area. Avoid bringing the instrument too far occlusally and damaging the contact area. Make sure the blade does not cut into too much amalgam causing it to chip or fracture. Strokes are repeated until the excess is removed. Increased pressure may be needed on older restorations. Perform the same

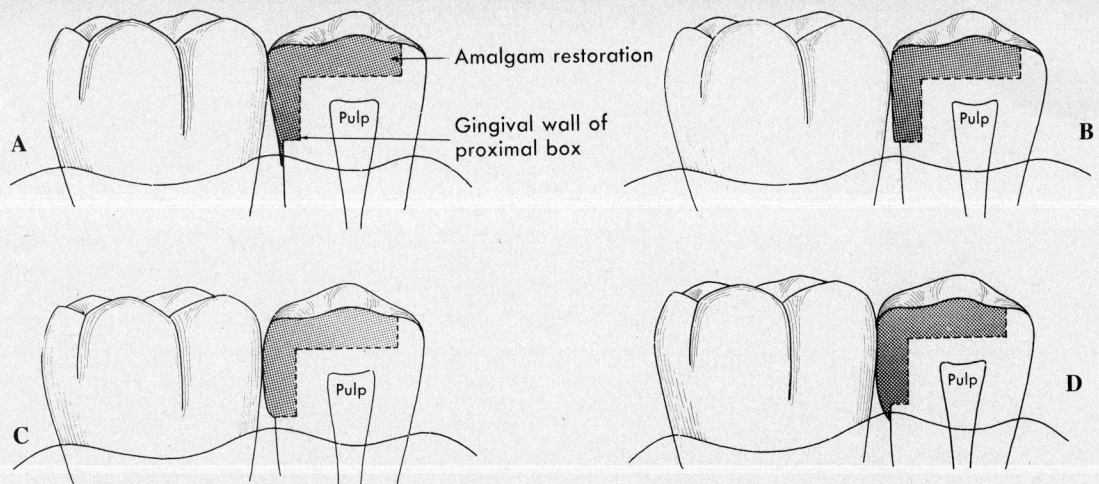

Amalgam restoration

Pulp

Gingival wall of proximal box

Pulp

Pulp

Pulp

A

B

C

D

Fig. 34-134. Excess amalgam in the proximal box can occur in a variety of ways. **A,** Excess amalgam can extend in a thin layer on the cavosurface apical to the gingival margin. **B,** Excess amalgam can extend as an overhanging ledge beyond the cavosurface margin. This ledge would be difficult to clean with floss. **C,** An overhang may be combined with an over-contoured proximal surface. **D,** An overhang and a severely over-contoured proximal surface reduce the gingival embrasure space and impinge upon the interdental papilla.
(From Spohn EE, Halowski WA, and Berry TG: Operative dentistry procedures for dental auxiliaries, St Louis, 1981, The CV Mosby Co.)

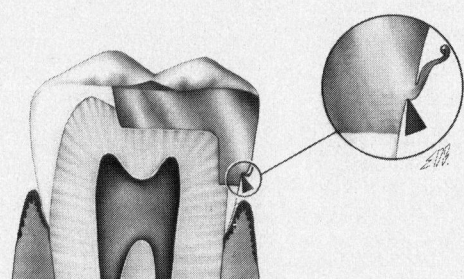

Fig. 34-135. Cross-section of amalgam knife being used to shave away an overhang.

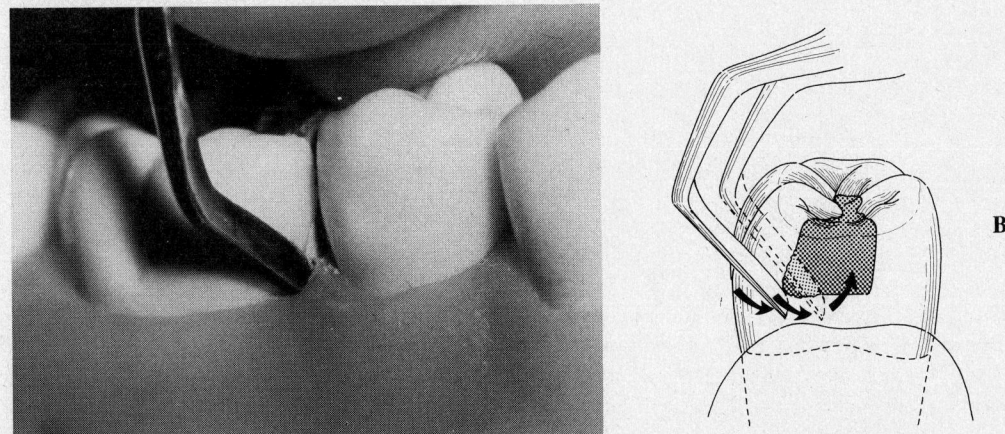

A

B

Fig. 34-136. **A,** Adaptation of the amalgam knife at the junction of the gingival and facioproximal cavosurface margins. **B,** Angle of the amalgam knife as it is inserted from the facial embrasure. The length of the stroke extends from the gingival margin to below the contact area.
(From Spohn EE, Halowski WA, and Berry TG: Operative dentistry procedures for dental auxiliaries, St Louis, 1981, The CV Mosby Co.)

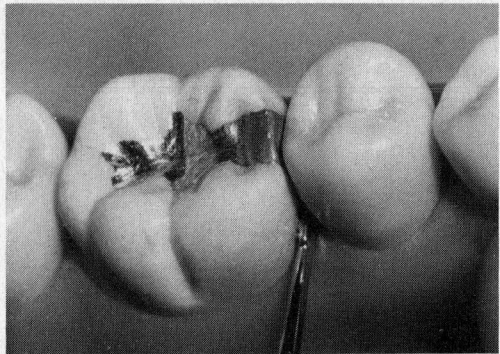

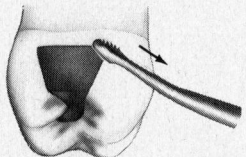

Fig. 34-137. The amalgam file is adapted flat against the gingival margin and adjacent tooth surface. The blades of the file shave the amalgam and produce a smoother margin.
(From Spohn EE, Halowski WA, and Berry TG: Operative dentistry procedures for dental auxiliaries, St Louis, 1981, The CV Mosby Co.)

Fig. 34-138. File is placed on tooth and amalgam and is used with a pull stroke directed obliquely or horizontally.

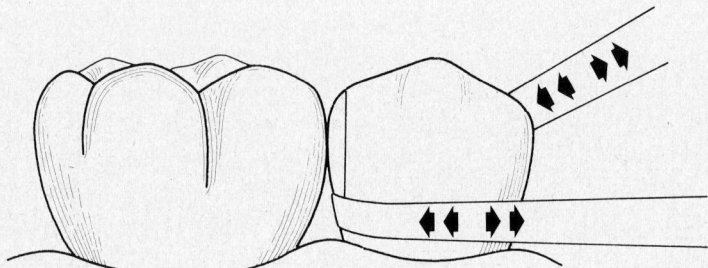

Fig. 34-139. The finishing strip is adapted against the gingival margin. As it is moved occlusally, avoid applying too much pressure, which may create an undercontoured surface.
(From Spohn EE, Halowski WA, and Berry TG: Operative dentistry procedures for dental auxiliaries, St Louis, 1981, The CV Mosby Co.)

steps from the lingual side, beginning at the linguogingival aspect of the proximal area.

The files are used when access to the gingival margin is very limited or to produce a smoother surface after the amalgam knife has been used. Three sets of files can be used: heavy, medium, and finishing files (Figs. 34-137 and 34-138). The files are used in order from heaviest to finest so that the deep striations are removed by each successively finer file.

After the files are used, a universal curette can be used to smooth the interproximal surface further. As the amalgam is being reduced, check the progress with an explorer. After the knife, file, and curette have been used, the amalgam should be flush with the tooth.

Another method of removing overhangs is with a reciprocating motor-driven diamond tip such as the Eva Prophylaxis System (Unitex Manufacturing Company). The tips, embedded with diamond particles, can remove the overhangs efficiently and effectively (Axelsson, 1981; Gelsky, 1982; Vale and Caffesse, 1979). The triangular tips are designed to be adapted to the proximal surface. Axelsson (1981) has recommended that the overhang removal be followed by finishing, polishing, complete plaque removal, and application of fluoridated paste with a plastic tip.

A finishing strip can be used to smooth the gingival margin of the restoration (Fig. 34-139). If gapped strips are used, the "safe" portion of the strip can be passed through the contact to avoid

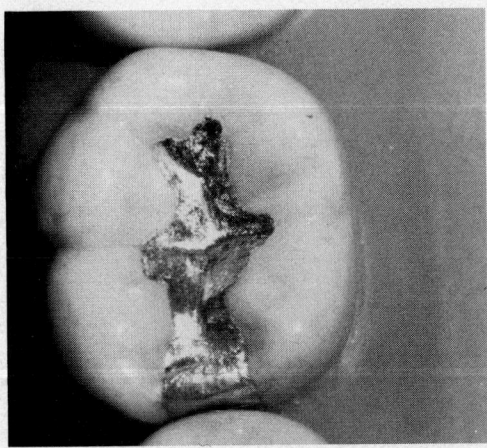

Fig. 34-140. The surface of the restoration after finishing and before polishing.
(From Spohn EE, Halowski WA, and Berry TG: Operative dentistry procedures for dental auxiliaries, St Louis, 1981, The CV Mosby Co.)

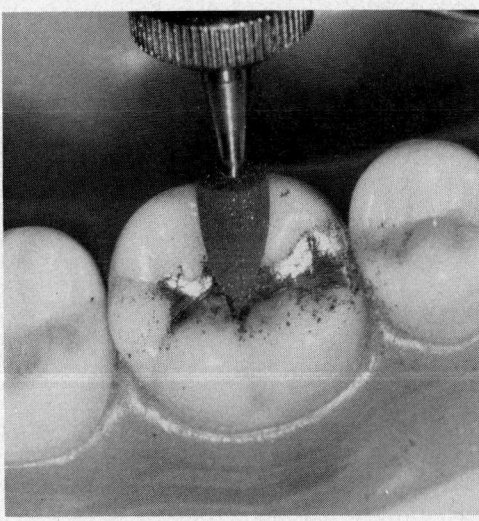

Fig. 34-141. Adaptation of a rubber point of the concave occlusal areas.
(From Spohn EE, Halowski WA, and Berry TG: Operative dentistry procedures for dental auxiliaries, St Louis, 1981, The CV Mosby Co.)

abrading the contact area of the amalgam. If ungapped strips are used, one end of the strip is cut into a point and threaded into the gingival embrasure. Position the strip so that half of it is on the tooth and half is on amalgam. A seesaw, back-and-forth motion is then used to remove any roughness. If the strip is on amalgam only, the edge of the strip could create deficient or open margin.

At this point, carefully evaluate the restoration (Fig. 34-140). The margins should be flush with the adjacent tooth surface, major anatomical contours should be consistent with surrounding tooth structure, and the surface should be smooth, with no major scratches present.

Polishing

Brown cups and points are more abrasive and are used first. The points are used in the concavities on the occlusal surface (Fig. 34-141). The end of the point is placed onto the fossae and grooves with the side contacting the facial or lingual inclined plane and then moved over the entire surface producing a slight luster. The cups are used on the more convex areas on the occlusal and proximal surfaces (Fig. 34-142). Watch for wear, and change the cups and points as needed to avoid marring the surface. The restoration should have a smooth, slight luster with no visible scratches from the bur (Fig. 34-143). Light, inter-

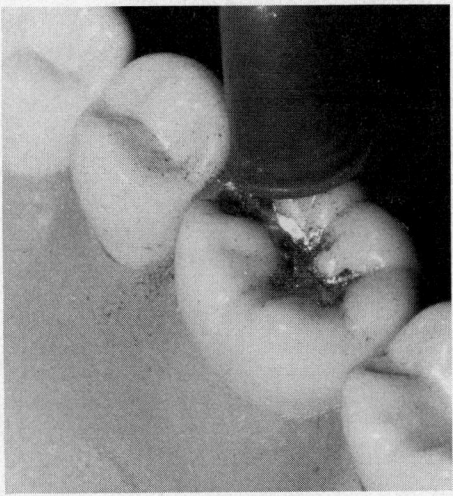

Fig. 34-142. Adaptation of a rubber cup on the more convex occlusal areas, such as the marginal ridge.
(From Spohn EE, Halowski WA, and Berry TG: Operative dentistry procedures for dental auxiliaries, St Louis, 1981, The CV Mosby Co.)

mittent pressure is needed to avoid creating excess heat. The green cups and points are used next in the same manner as the brown ones.

Powdered pumice and tin oxide may be used instead of the impregnated rubber cups and

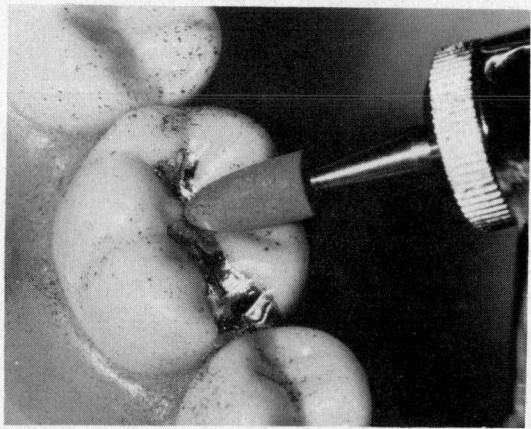

Fig. 34-143. A mirror-like finish is produced on the amalgam surface as finer abrasive agents are used.
(From Spohn EE, Halowski WA, and Berry TG: Operative dentistry procedures for dental auxiliaries, St Louis, 1981, The CV Mosby Co.)

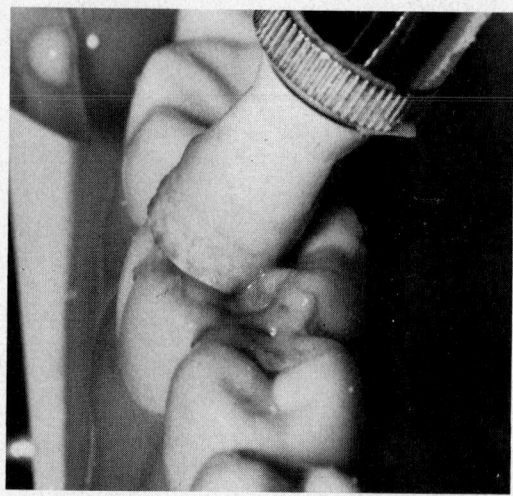

Fig. 34-144. A slurry of pumice can be applied with a rubber cup or occlusal brush.
(From Spohn EE, Halowski WA, and Berry TG: Operative dentistry procedures for dental auxiliaries, St Louis, 1981, The CV Mosby Co.)

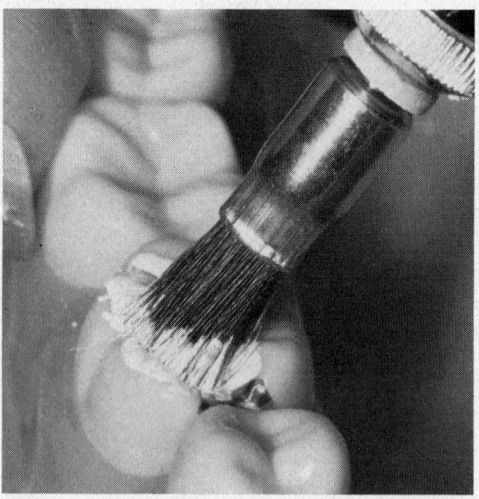

Fig. 34-145. Tin oxide is being applied with an occlusal brush.
(From Spohn EE, Halowski WA, and Berry TG: Operative dentistry procedures for dental auxiliaries, St Louis, 1981, The CV Mosby Co.)

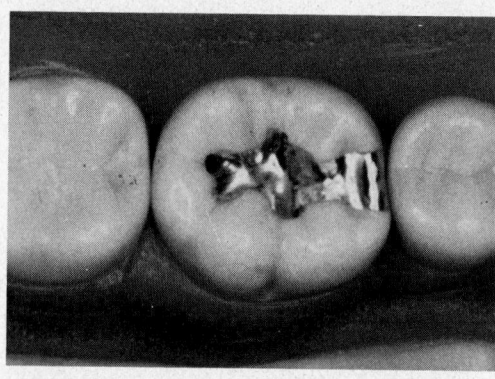

Fig. 34-146. Polished amalgam surface.
(From Spohn EE, Halowski WA, and Berry TG: Operative dentistry procedures for dental auxiliaries, St Louis, 1981, The CV Mosby Co.)

points. They are applied with a rubber cup or occlusal brush (Fig. 34-144). The flour of pumice is mixed with water to make a thin slurry and is applied using very light pressure and sweeping strokes to minimize heat. A slight luster appears and the scratches left from the bur are no longer visible. The proximal area gingival to the contact can be polished with dental tape covered with pumice. Contact areas should be flossed with care.

Apply tin oxide in a wet slurry using a rubber cup or occlusal brush (Fig. 34-145). A very light buffing motion is used with the cup to obtain a shiny, mirrorlike finish. The final step is to rinse thoroughly and floss the area to remove pumice and tin oxide. Provide thorough lavage of the area to remove all loose pieces of amalgam and other debris especially in the interproximal area.

The final restoration should be smooth with no visible scratches; it should have a shiny luster (Fig. 34-146). The adjacent tooth structure and soft tissue should be undamaged.

PROPERTIES OF COMPOSITE RESINS, ACID ETCHING OF ENAMEL, AND GENERAL PROCEDURES FOR PLACEMENT

Restoration of anterior teeth presents one significant consideration not as important for posterior teeth. Esthetic results are of paramount importance. Dental amalgam meets many of the criteria for the physical properties of the direct filling material, but it fails in its esthetic characteristics. Dental scientists have searched for a material that possesses good chemical and physical qualities, is relatively easy to handle, is biologically compatible, and yet has a pleasing esthetic appearance. No material yet developed meets all of these criteria completely, although the tooth-colored materials now available meet these criteria to an adequate degree. This section describes the chemical and physical characteristics of composite resin restorative materials. Acid etching of enamel to help retain composite resin materials is also discussed.

Resins contain inorganic filler particles in the resin matrix. These materials are commonly called "filled" or "composite" resins to distinguish them from the plain, or unfilled, resins. Four classes of composite resin have evolved (Table 34-1). The first-developed composite resins are now called "large-particle" or "conventional"

Table 34-1. Composite Resin Particle Size

Type of composite	Particle size
Conventional (large-particle)	Above 5 μM
Microfilled (fine-particle)	
Silica filler	.05 μM
Prepolymerized particles	10–70 μM
Small particle	0.5 μM – 5.0 μM
Blend (or hybrid): combination of microfilled and small particles	0.5 μM – 5.0 μM

composite resins. These were followed in the late 1970s by the "microfilled" and more recently by the "small-particle" and "hybrid" composite resins. These terms reflect the changes in filler particle size used in composite resin material.

Composition

Composite resins are made up of two major components: an organic polymer resin matrix and inorganic filler particles. The basic molecule (monomer) of the resin is chemically named bisphenol A-glycidyl methacrylate (BIS-GMA). The particles of the conventional filler component are composed of one of several inorganic materials, such as quartz, lithium aluminum silicate, barium aluminum silicate, and borosilicate glass. The filler particles of all resin systems are treated so that they will chemically bond with the resin during the setting reaction (Baum et al, 1985). In addition, small amounts of inorganic pigments are added to provide variations in shades.

The reaction that causes BIS-GMA molecules to be linked together, or polymerized, may be initiated chemically or by a special visible light source. The chemically activated products have two main components: a base (universal) portion and a catalyst (activator) portion supplied in paste form. When they are mixed together, the catalyst initiates the polymerization of the BIS-GMA molecules resulting in the formation of a solid mass. The light-activated materials have only one component containing both the resin monomer and the filler. When these are exposed to visible light, the polymerization is initiated and a solid mass is formed.

The polymerization reaction can take place between a material that has set and a newly activated material, resulting in a chemical bond. That property allows the repair of fractures and the correction of defects in either a restoration being placed or one placed at a previous appointment.

Due to the hardness and the relatively large size of the particles in conventional composite resins, the finishing process leaves a relatively smooth but yet slightly rough surface. The microfilled resin can be polished rather than just smoothed, resulting in a highly desirable surface finish. However, due to the small particle size and the low amount of filler material, these resins exhibit less desirable abrasion resistance. Therefore, the microfilled composites are reserved largely for areas not subject to heavy wear. Newer, small-particle and blend or hybrid composites have been developed to provide the smooth surface of the microfilled composite resins while possessing good wear resistance and strength. This is accomplished through higher proportions of filler particles; the undesirable characteristics of roughness and staining are minimized by using particles of smaller size.

Although the chemically cured material is satisfactory, several advantages of the light-cured have made it increasingly more popular. The light-activated material is supplied in one paste, which does not require mixing. This avoids the incorporation of air bubbles, which can occur when two components (pastes) are mixed together. In addition, the material can be added in layers and then shaped before curing with the light. In contrast, the clinician must wait until the chemically cured material is set before contouring. For these reasons, the light-activated material will be the one discussed here. The small-particle and hybrid composite resins are the materials most commonly used today. For certain clinical situations (e.g., class V), the microfilled resin often is selected because of its very smooth surface finish.

Manufacturers offer two different approaches to deal with the problem of surface finish. Some products include a glaze, which is the resin without the filler particles. This material is coated over the surface of the restoration to produce a very smooth finish chemically bonded to the restoration. The glaze is susceptible to abrasion, so the long-term benefits are limited. The other approach is the use of microfilled materials, which can be polished to a more lustrous finish. This reduces plaque retention particularly important for the class V restoration.

The composite resins may have adverse effects on the pulpal tissue due to free monomer molecules. A calcium hydroxide base is usually recommended under composite resin restorations in deep preparations.

Product packaging

The materials described apply to the light activated composite resin systems. The materials

used for acid etching are usually supplied as a kit containing the acid, the instrument for application, and the bonding agent. The acid (etchant) is usually supplied in gel form; it may be supplied in a syringe with disposable applicator tips for direct placement on the enamel (Fig. 34-147). A small disposable brush is supplied for application by some manufacturers.

The bonding agent is generally supplied in a squeeze bottle. One or two drops are dispensed onto a coated pad and picked up with a small brush or endodontic paper point for placement on the etched surfaces.

The composite resin comes in various shades of paste. It may be supplied in larger, multiple appli-

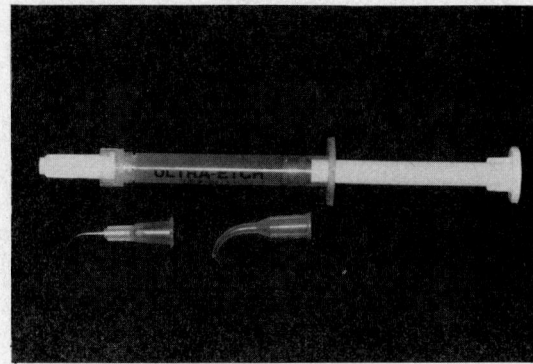

Fig. 34-147. Acid dispenser syringe and disposable applicator tips.

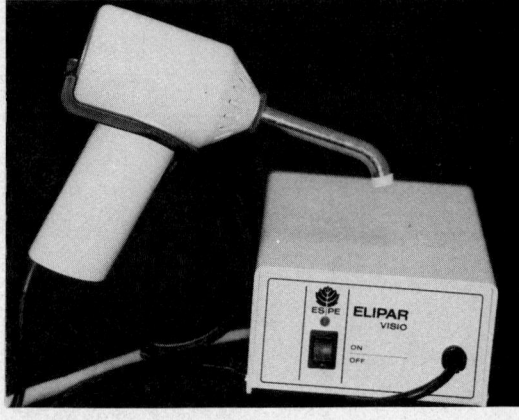

Fig. 34-148. An example of a visible light–projecting device.

cation syringes from which the material is dispensed for later insertion into the tooth. Alternatively, it may be supplied in single application carpules, which load into a syringe for injection into the preparation. These carpules are color-coded for easy identification.

The visible light–projecting devices used to cure the materials are available in several designs (Fig. 34-148). They all have the same objective. They initiate the setting process in the bonding agent and composite resin by projecting a bright light in the blue spectrum for a specified period of time.

Armamentarium

The armamentarium suggested for composite resin restorations is shown in Figs. 34-149. Specific situations may require other instruments.

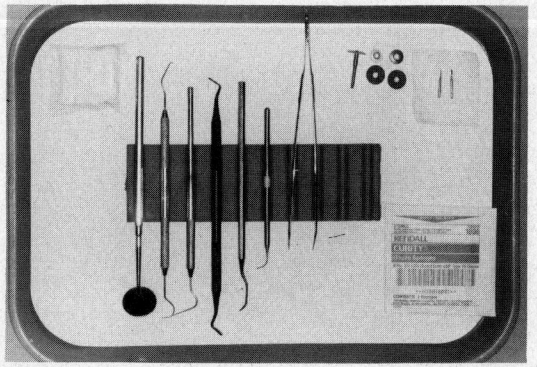

Fig. 34-149. Armamentarium for placement and finishing of a composite resin restoration includes: *1,* cotton rolls; *2,* mouth mirror; *3,* explorer; *4,* periodontal probe; *5,* placement instrument; *6,* gold knife; *7,* calcium hydroxide placement instrument; *8,* cotton pliers; *9,* mandrel; *10,* finishing discs; *11,* carbide finishing burs; *12,* gauze squares.

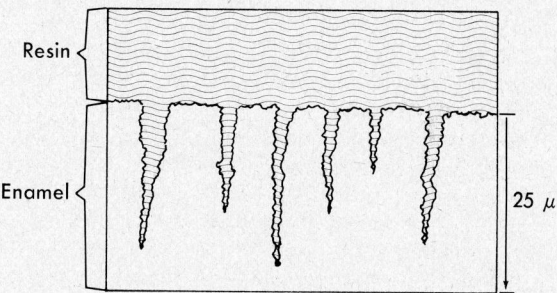

Fig. 34-150. The acid-etched enamel surface with resin applied. Note resin tags in the micropores.
(From Spohn EE, Halowski WA, and Berry TG: Operative dentistry procedures for dental auxiliaries, St Louis, 1981, The CV Mosby Co.)

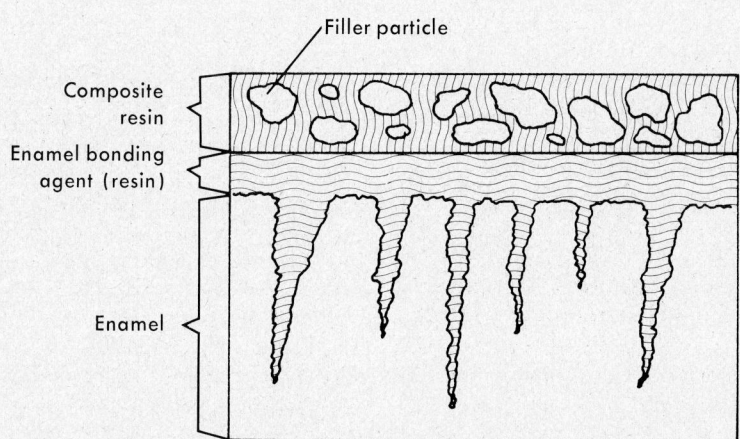

Fig. 34-151. The relationship of the acid-etched enamel, the enamel-bonding agent, and the composite resin.
(From Spohn EE, Halowski WA, and Berry TG: Operative dentistry procedures for dental auxiliaries, St Louis, 1981, The CV Mosby Co.)

Acid etching

Improvement in retention and significant decrease in marginal leakage can be achieved if the composite resin is placed over an enamel surface that has been etched with 30% to 40% phosphoric acid. This acid etching or acid conditioning selectively removes inorganic material from the enamel, leaving pits or micropores of up to approximately 25 µ in depth. Unfilled resin, referred to as a bonding agent, is then placed over the etched enamel. It flows easily into the countless micropores, forming tiny fingers or tags into the enamel surface (Fig. 34-150). When set, it locks onto the surface. Composite resin then is placed over the bonding agent to chemically bond with it (Fig. 34-151). The cavosurface margins may be prepared at an angle of approximately 30 to 45 degrees rather than at a 90-degree angle. This acute angle is referred to as a bevel. The bevel, because it is angled, provides a larger enamel surface to etch and to which to bond. Fig. 34-152 shows a class IV preparation with cavosurface margins that have been beveled and acid etched. The etched enamel appears chalky white in contrast to the unetched surface.

Two precautions about these retentive features are important. Additional retention may rely on undercuts in dentin in addition to micropores. The calcium hydroxide base must not be coated over the enamel or left in undercuts. After the acid etching process is completed, the etched enamel

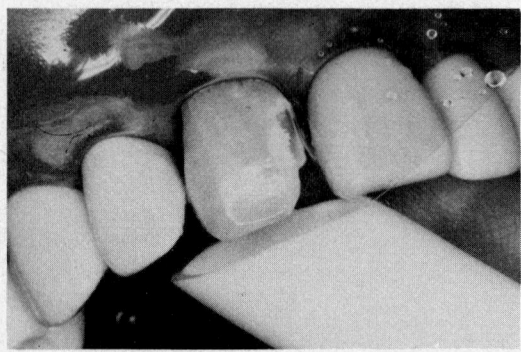

Fig. 34-152. The appearance of a class IV preparation following acid etching and rinsing of beveled margins. Note matrix strip placed to protect adjacent tooth during acid etching procedure.

cannot be contaminated with saliva or other fluids, as this will significantly decrease the retention.

Placing bonding agent

The bonding agent should be added carefully to avoid covering areas not conditioned. Use a matrix strip for preparations that involve the proximal surfaces to protect the adjacent tooth from the liquid resin. Bonding agent cured over unconditioned enamel will not bond to the tooth and will trap fluids between it and the enamel, thus allowing staining. It may fracture and leave jagged margins. Controlled placement of the bonding agent may best be achieved using a small brush or an endodontic paper point. Use a small cotton pellet to wipe away any agent on unetched enamel. Cure the agent by exposing it to the light for approximately 20 seconds. If it is a large preparation, it may be necessary to expose another area to the light for 20 seconds to ensure that all sections have been given adequate exposure time.

Placing and photocuring composite resin

Although manufacturers make a "universal shade" suitable for many situations, shade selection may be important. It must be done *before* the rubber dam is placed. For larger preparations, the darker shades generally are placed in the gingival section of the preparation with lighter and grayer ones placed towards the incisal edge of the restoration. Expose the composite resin to the light for a minimum of 20 seconds. Then add the next segment and repeat the curing process. Continue to add until the preparation is very slightly overfilled. Excess material is removed before curing.

Composite resin is not condensed but it does need careful adaptation into all areas of the preparation with special attention to the retentive areas and the cavosurface margins. For a small or medium-sized preparation, place only enough material to fill one half of the preparation to ensure that the material can be pushed into all areas at the depth of the preparation. A teflon-coated instrument with a blade on one end and a small nib on the other is a good choice for placement. The blade helps to pick up and carry material to the preparation. The nib is used to force the material into all areas of the preparation.

The material also may be placed using a syringe. The syringe technique may make it easier to make certain that the material completely fills all the areas of the preparation without undue entrapment of air bubbles. Special syringes that may be loaded with bulk material as well as prepackaged carpules with disposable syringe tips are available.

The materials generally are placed in the least accessible portion of the cavity preparation first. This usually will include any retentive features within the cavity preparation. In general, the materials need to be adapted to all walls with special attention to minimize the possibility of voids or defects at margins.

These materials are placed in layers no thicker than 2.5 mm (less for darker shades) so that photocuring will cause the resin to set to its full depth. If resin is placed in thicker increments, portions of uncured semisoft resin may be left in the body of the restoration. Hold the right rod as close as possible (1 to 2 mm) to the resin without touching it and make the exposure according to the manufacturer's recommendations (usually 20 seconds).

If the outer layer of the composite resin is not covered with a matrix strip, it will not cure completely because of the exposure to air. The resulting soft sticky surface *must* be removed to prevent such problems as excessive staining and premature wear. This surface can be finished easily to a very smooth texture.

Use of matrices

Matricing for composite resins follows the same principles as for amalgam restoration. The matrix is designed to confine the material to the preparation and to provide a smooth surface against which to adapt and cure the material. Class III or IV restorations require wedge placement to prevent flash along the gingival margin and to separate the teeth slightly to assure contact after the restoration is placed. Class V restorations may be placed without a matrix.

Finishing the composite resin restoration

The purpose of finishing composite resin restorations is to remove excess material in order to contour and smooth the surface of the restoration. Rotary instruments such as discs, white stones, and carbide finishing burs are used. Conventional coarse, medium, and fine discs may be used, as may the newer discs composed of silicone carbide or zirconium silicate (Shofu Company). Carbide finishing burs specifically designed for composite resins produce a relatively smooth surface and are available in a variety of shapes. Do not confuse these with regular finishing burs, which are not as effective in cutting the material. A gold knife is useful along the gingival cavosurface margin, particularly when the margin of the restoration extends onto the cementum in a limited access area on the proximal surface. Abrasive strips also are used to finish gingival and incisal proximal margins.

Start with the coarsest finishing materials and progress to the finest ones. Due to the hardness and the relatively large size of the particles in the resins, the finishing process results in a smooth surface but will not have the luster as a shining amalgam restoration.

THE CLASS V AND CLASS III COMPOSITE RESIN RESTORATIONS

This restoration must reproduce the form of the tooth, as did the class V amalgam restoration, and must be in harmony with the color of the tooth. The outline of the preparation is usually very similar to that of the class V amalgam preparation (Fig. 34-153). It may have beveled margins, and usually it has retentive grooves in the occlusoaxial and gingivoaxial line angles (Fig. 34-154). Al-

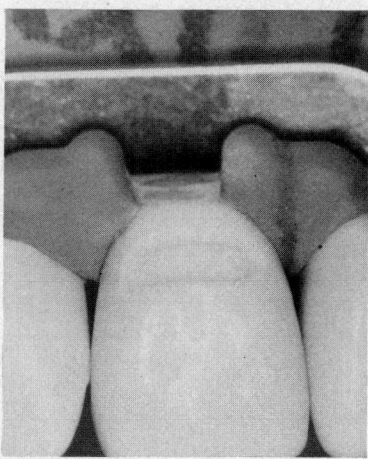

Fig. 34-153. Outline of class V cavity preparation for a composite resin restoration.

though most of the retention will depend upon enamel bonding, it is important to take advantage of additional retentive features if present.

The preparation must be clean and dry. Before placing a rubber dam, select a shade of material that will match the color of the tooth (Fig. 34-155). Ensure that the preparation is well isolated and the soft tissue is protected. A correctly placed rubber dam with a 212 clamp for gingival retraction is the best way to isolate the area.

Acid etching and bonding

The first step in the procedure is acid etching of the enamel to prepare it for the bonding agent. The etching solution is applied to all prepared enamel, including the bevel. In very conservative preparations with a thick layer of remaining dentin, calcium hydroxide may not be needed. However, deep preparations may call for placement of a calcium hydroxide layer to protect the pulp (Fig. 34-156). Apply acid to all areas of enamel to be covered by the restoration. The acid should

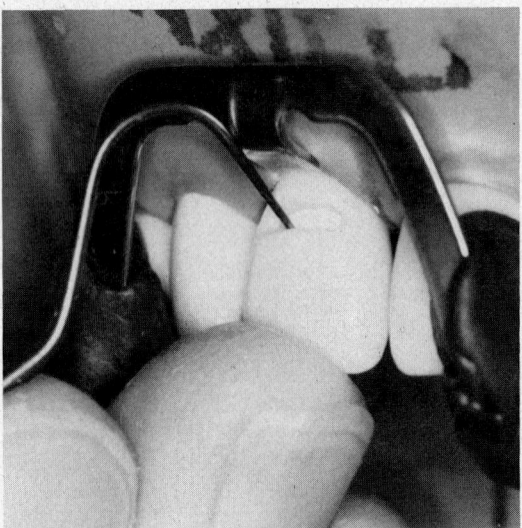

Fig. 34-154. Retention for the restoration may depend partly upon retentive grooves cut into the incisoaxial and gingivoaxial line angles.

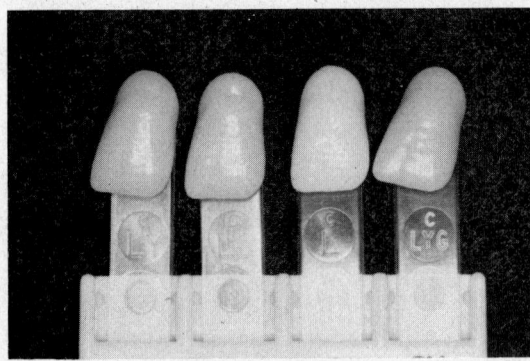

Fig. 34-155. The shade guide helps select the appropriate coloration of material.

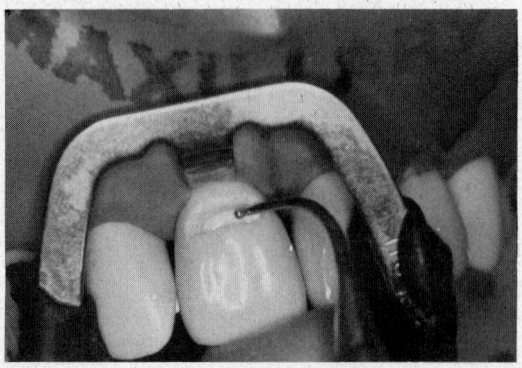

Fig. 34-156. Take care to place the calcium hydroxide on the dentin only. The dentin should be protected while the enamel is etched.

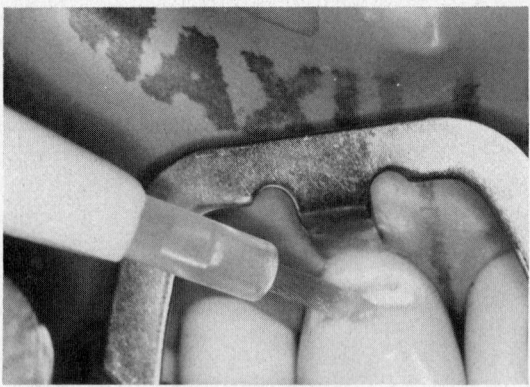

Fig. 34-157. The acid should be applied to the enamel walls and margins.

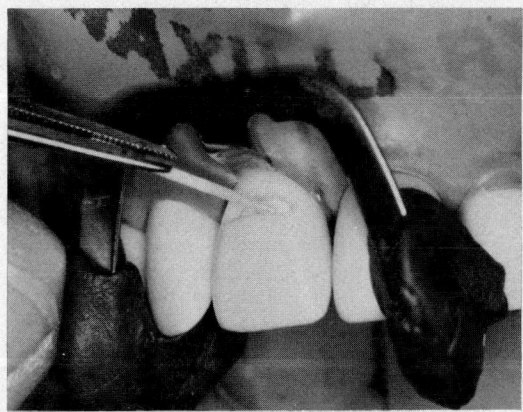

Fig. 34-158. The bonding agent is carefully applied to all of the etched surfaces but not onto the unetched enamel.

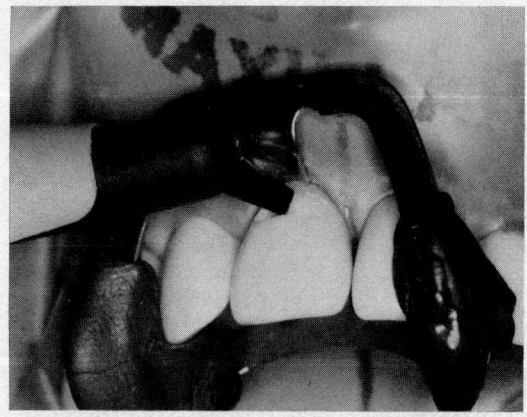

Fig. 34-159. Insert a layer of composite resin no thicker than 2 mm to ensure adequate curing.

be left on the enamel for 30 seconds for permanent teeth (Fig. 34-157). Saturation for less than 30 seconds may inadequately etch the surface; saturation for a longer time may overetch the surface, removing too much surface enamel. Either reduces the retentive characteristics of the surface. Note that deciduous teeth or teeth of patients in heavily fluoridated communities may require etching for longer periods. Rinse the surface thoroughly to stop the etching process and then dry it. Examine the etched enamel. A properly etched surface should have a chalky white appearance and a slightly rough texture. If it does not meet these criteria, repeat the etching procedure.

Dispense the bonding material and apply a thin, even layer over all etched enamel surfaces with the camel's hair brush or an endodontic paper point. It is important that the agent coat all etched surfaces to achieve maximum retention and marginal seal (Fig. 34-158). If this material is carried onto the calcium hydroxide base, it is of little consequence. To polymerize the material, direct the light source at the surface of the tooth from the recommended distance for 20 seconds. The surface is now ready for placement of the composite resin restoration.

Placement and photocuring

Using either the bladed instrument or a syringe, deposit the first increment of composite resin into the preparation (Fig. 34-159). Remember not to

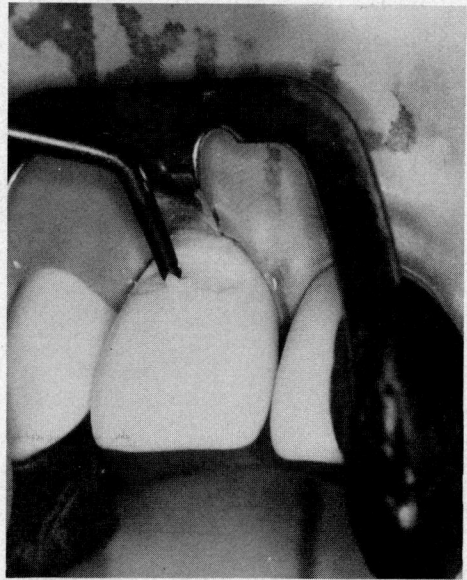

Fig. 34-160. Adapt the material into the incisoaxial line angle.

fill the preparation with the first increment. Using the nib, push the material into all the line angles and retentive areas to assure complete adaptation to the walls and to achieve maximum retention (Fig. 34-160). After the increment has been adapted, expose it to the light source for 20 seconds. Continue to add increments using the tech-

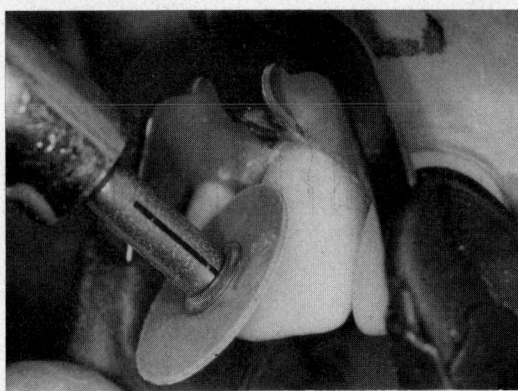

Fig. 34-161. Take care to adapt the disc carefully to the area to be reduced. Guard against abrading the enamel and overreducing the restoration.

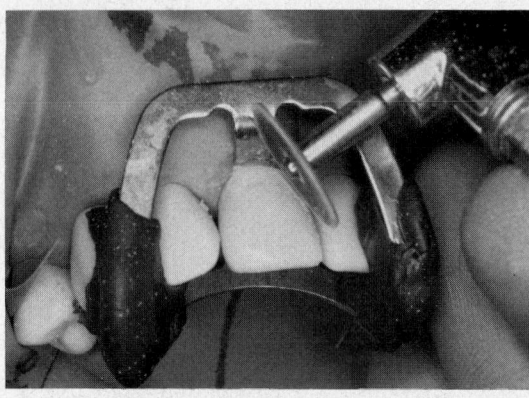

Fig. 34-162. The rest of the margins can be finished using the same careful adaptation of the disc.

nique described above. Completely cure the material in each new increment. Place increments no more than 2 mm thick before curing. This is especially important with darker shades, which do not allow light to penetrate as easily through the material.

After curing the material, evaluate the restoration visually and with an explorer. It should meet the following criteria:

1. Material extends 0.5 mm to 1.0 mm beyond the margins
2. Enough excess exists to allow removal of the outer layer
3. No voids, pits, or submarginal areas exist that are not correctable

If voids or ditching exist, add more material if the area has not been contaminated.

If gross excess is present, remove it from the incisal margin. Adapt the edge (outer 1 mm) of a medium disc to the area, using light sweeping strokes to contour the restoration (Fig. 34-161). Keep the disc adapted to the contours of the tooth by rotating it slightly as it is moved from the distal to the mesial side. Avoid excessive contact with the enamel.

The gingival margin is next to be corrected. Even greater care is needed to avoid contacting the tooth structure, because the cementum of the root surface is very susceptible to abrasion. Adapt the disc in a manner similar to that used on the

incisal margin (Fig. 34-162). Direct the sweeping strokes toward the center of the restoration. Avoid contact with the rubber dam. The gold knife may also be an effective instrument for removing flash from the gingival margin area. Use it to shave layers away pulling the blade incisally from tooth to restoration. Be careful not to break away larger amounts near the margins to avoid fracture of the margin itself.

Position the disc so only the outer edge is contacting first the mesial and then the distal margin. Use light sweeping strokes to contour these surfaces. Then contour the center of the restoration. To determine how much contouring is needed, examine the contour from the incisal and the mesial viewpoints. The middle of the restoration at this point may be bulky. Adapt the disc to reduce the bulk while blending the contours. Recheck the contour to assure they are blended correctly without overreduction.

Check the margins with an explorer, moving the tip from restoration to tooth and back to ensure that no flash, ditching, or submarginal areas are present. If flash or a bulk margin is noted on the gingival aspect, a flame-shaped carbide finishing bur may be helpful (Fig. 34-163). Its thin, tapered form lets it reach places not accessible to a bulkier instrument. Use sweeping motions with the bur to avoid creating a rippled effect.

Once the basic contours and bulk have been established, change to a fine grit finishing disc. Fol-

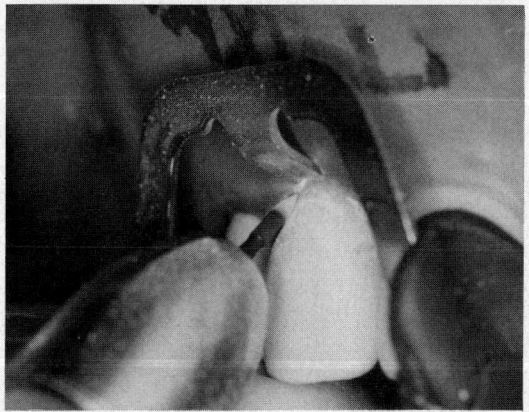

Fig. 34-163. The flame-shaped carbide finishing bur may be helpful to smooth the hard-to-reach areas along the gingival margin.

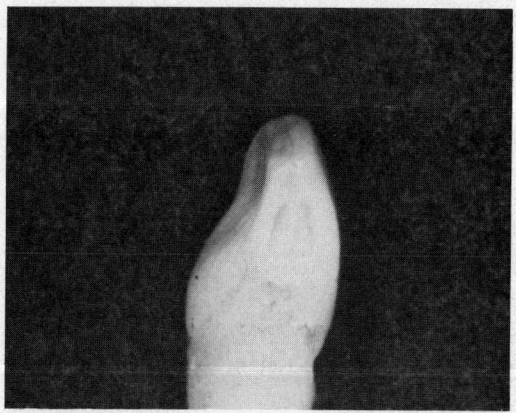

Fig. 34-164. Mesial view of a class III preparation showing the gothic-arch shape.

low the steps discussed for the medium grit disc. After you finish with the fine grit disc, evaluate the restoration according to the criteria listed at the end of this chapter for placement of composite resin restorations.

It is important to evaluate the restoration before removal of the rubber dam. If a problem is detected, it may be much easier to correct while the rubber dam still protects the operating field.

Remove the rubber dam. Reevaluate the esthetic results after the dam has been removed and the teeth are beginning to rehydrate. Inform the patient that the full esthetic results will not be realized until the tooth has regained all of its fluids.

The class III composite resin

Because the class III carious lesion occurs on the proximal surface, care must be paid to restore the functional and esthetic loss. Access to this preparation may be from the facial, the lingual, or from both directions. The preparation usually is shaped like an egg or a Gothic arch (Fig. 34-164) if the access is from the facial and slot-shaped if from the lingual. Retention is achieved by retentive areas cut into the incisoaxial and gingivoaxial line angles as well as by acid etching the enamel involved. The procedure that follows is for a preparation with facial access.

Visualize the outline to aid later in contouring and trimming the restoration. Determine whether

a bevel has been placed around the cavosurface margins. Apply calcium hydroxide base, taking care not to leave any on the enamel.

Acid etching and enamel bonding

Acid etch and rinse the enamel. Protect the adjacent tooth during the acid etching and bonding process by placing a Mylar strip between the teeth during these procedures (Fig. 34-165). Replace the calcium hydroxide if needed. Place bonding agent on the etched enamel surfaces and photocure.

A matrix and wedge are necessary for placement of a class III restoration to confine the material within the preparation, prevent an overhang at the gingival margin, and provide a very smooth surface against which to cure the composite resin. Slide the matrix strip between the teeth. The strip should do the following:

1. Extend gingivally past the gingival margin by 1.0 mm or more
2. Extend 1.0 mm to 1.5 mm incisally beyond the incisal margin
3. Extend far enough facially and lingually to be firmly grasped so the strip can be pulled tightly around the proximal surface

These extentions allow the matrix strip to cover the preparation area completely. To ensure that the strip can be pulled tightly around the

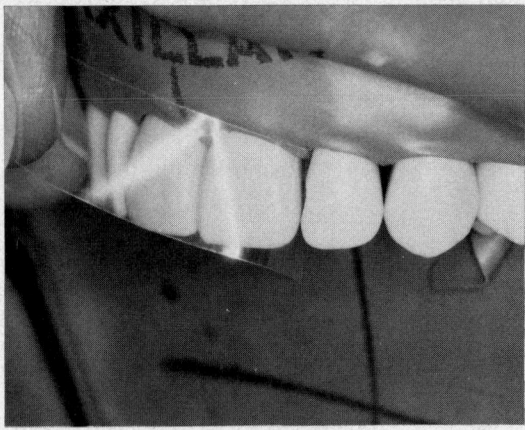

Fig. 34-165. A matrix strip will protect the adjacent teeth from the acid during the etching process.

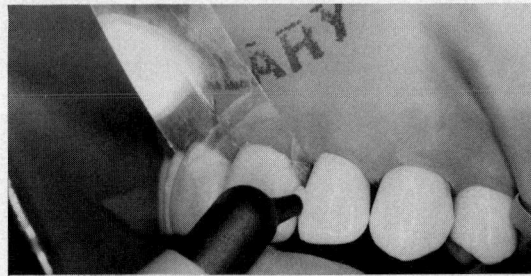

Fig. 34-166. Insert a limited amount to assure adequate curing depth. Do not try to fill the preparation.

tooth without wrinkling or slipping, test it by pulling it.

Select a wedge that will fit into the embrasure tightly enough to separate the teeth slightly and to press the strip against the tooth being restored. Direct the wedge into the lingual embrasure, as access to the preparation is from the facial. If the wedge extends through the interproximal far enough to hinder access to the preparation, shorten it. The incisal height of the wedge should be level with the gingival wall of the preparation.

Select the composite resin using the shade(s) chosen before rubber dam placement. Using either the bladed instrument or a syringe, insert the first segment into the preparation (Fig. 34-166). Use the nib end to press the material into all areas carefully. To keep the material from being pushed out the opposite side, support the strip on the lingual surface with your finger. Reflect the strip away from the preparation on the facial with your middle or first finger.

The strip is positioned to hold in the material on the lingual while allowing access from the facial. Expose the composite resin to the light for 20 seconds to cure the layer. Continue to add material until the preparation is very slightly overfilled. Check all areas facially and lingually to determine that all the contours are satisfactory and the margins are completely covered. If so, carefully adapt the strip against the tooth on the lingual surface holding it in place between the

thumb and index finger of one hand. Expose the lingual surface to the light. The finger should support the strip. Grasp the facial end of the strip between the thumb and index finger of your other hand. Slowly pull the strip across the facial surface toward the opposite proximal surface until the strip is tightly adapted. Pulling the strip slowly allows the excess composite resin to escape ahead of the strip as it closes. Once in place, use the thumb of the hand supporting the strip to hold the facial end in place. Expose the composite resin again to the light so that the outer surfaces and marginal areas are cured. During the time that the material is being cured, the matrix strip should be held tightly in place. The matrix will produce an extremely smooth, well-shaped surface, greatly reducing finishing time.

After the restoration has set, remove the wedge and matrix and evaluate the restoration. Decide how much contouring and finishing are necessary; this will determine which instruments are chosen. Remove thin layers of flash on the facial, lingual, and gingival surface using a gold knife. Position the tip of the blade gingival to the flash and pull incisally. Cut away material up to within approximately 1.0 mm of the cavosurface margins. Do not cut toward the gingiva to avoid damage to the underlying soft tissue.

Reduce the bulkier areas with rotary discs (Fig. 34-167). Place the slowly rotating disc into the facial embrasure contacting the restoration. Pull it in a facial direction, moving it in an arc over the proximal line angle past the facial margin. This movement produces a rounded line angle and opens the embrasure. Check the contours from a facial and incisal viewpoint. Make certain that the

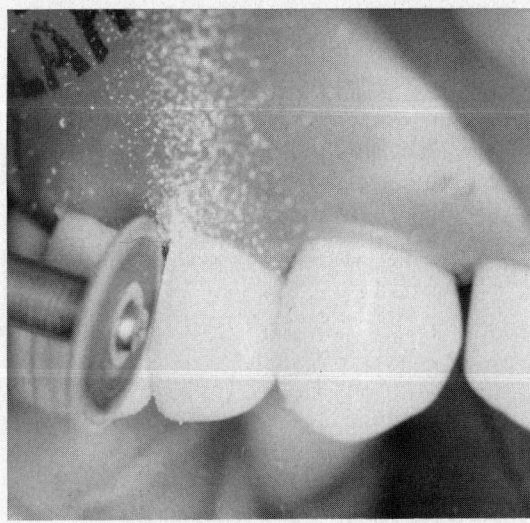

Fig. 34-167. Place the slowly rotating disc into the embrasure to shape and smooth the restoration.

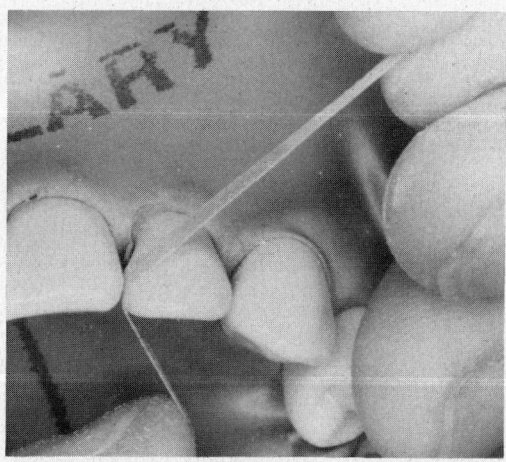

Fig. 34-168. A finishing strip, used with "shoeshine" motion, contours and smooths area that cannot be reached with a disc.

facioproximal contour is rounded and that a ledge is not being formed. A ledge is usually created when the disc is moved straight back into the embrasure against the contact area without the rounding motion. The key is to apply pressure only as the rotating disc is moved out of the embrasure and onto the facial surface.

The lingual margin should be finished in the same manner. If a large section of the lingual marginal ridge is involved, a white stone (cone-shaped or round) will be needed to form the concave surface. Move the stone mesiodistally from the marginal ridge to the lingual margin and back. The stone can also be pulled gingivoincisally to help form the incisogingival concavity found on the lingual surface. The marginal ridge should be the same height and contour as that of the adjacent tooth.

Once the contours are correct, use a fine grit disc to produce the final finish. Repeat the same procedures used with the medium grit disc. A finishing strip will contour areas such as the gingival margin that cannot be reached with the rotary disc.

The finishing strip has a coarse abrasive on one end and medium abrasive on the other. Use the coarse end first. Slide the safe zone of a finishing strip through the contact area. If tight contact pre-

vents the insertion of the finishing strip, place a wedge to separate the teeth slightly to allow insertion. Remove the wedge and slide the strip completely into place with its border located gingival to the gingival margin. Pull the strip back and forth in a shoeshine motion over the margin (Fig. 34-168).

Concentrate pressure on the area which most needs contouring. For instance, if the facial margin requires additional contouring, place the index finger of one hand lightly against the strip in the area of the margin and pull the strip mesiolingually with the thumb and forefinger of the other hand. This places the greatest pressure on the facial margin so that greatest reduction in roughness and/or contour occurs there. By concentrating on specific areas needing improvement, you can preserve the other contours already correctly established. The key is in using a finger to exert extra pressure in one area while drawing the strip through in a direction or at an angle which minimizes pressure in other area (Fig. 34-169). Use the fine abrasive strip to repeat the procedures used with the coarse strip.

Evaluate the margins and the contours to assure they are satisfactory (see checkoff sheet p. 735). Remove the rubber dam to check the occlusion. Have the patient close in centric occlusion and evaluate for premature occlusion on the restoration. Adjust prematurities if necessary, using the

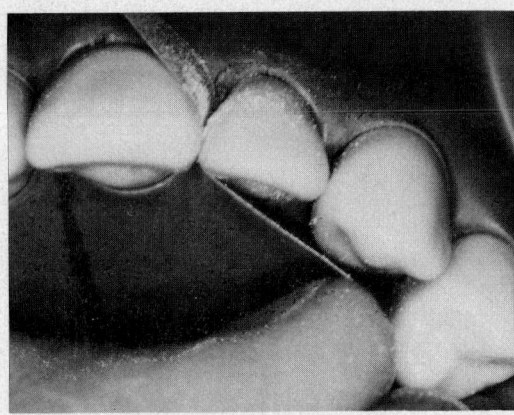

Fig. 34-169. When the strip is pulled in the direction shown, more pressure is applied to the lingual margins.

white stone. Have the patient perform excursive and protrusive movements. Reduce any prematurity with a white stone. Once the occlusion has been perfected, evaluate the restoration using criteria for placement of composite resin restorations (see checkoff sheet p. 735).

The class IV composite resin restoration involves replacement of the incisal angle of an anterior tooth. See current textbooks of operative dentistry to acquire additional information about the restoration of class IV cavity preparations.

ACTIVITIES

1. Investigate the laws to determine states where hygienists are permitted to perform restorative expanded duty procedures.
2. Conduct a panel discussion with dentists, hygienists, assistants, and technicians on the topic "Changing Roles of the Dental Auxiliary."
3. Conduct a panel discussion with hygienists who practice both traditional and expanded duties in restorative dentistry to learn about the challenge of doing both in dental hygiene practice.
4. Research the history of expanded duties in restorative dentistry in your province or state. Investigate the process of changing the laws that govern the practice of dental hygiene.
5. Research the practice of dental therapists in Britain, New Zealand, and Saskatchewan; determine how they provide dental care to the school children.
6. Evaluate a classmate's performance and final product when placing an amalgam or composite resin restoration using the criteria stated.

7. Given plaster three-dimensional models of teeth with class I, II, III, IV, and V cavity preparations, use an explorer to correctly identify the walls, cavosurface, line angles, and point angles.
8. Select correct matrix retainer and band and assemble for placement on a maxillary left first molar and a mandibular left first molar.
9. Acid etch the surface of a natural tooth and observe through a low-power microscope.
10. Practice placement of conservative class II amalgam restorations on maxillary and mandibular molars and premolar in a typodont. (A minimum of three acceptable restorations per quadrant is suggested.)
11. Conduct a survey among patients about their attitude toward auxiliary dental staff performing restorative procedures.

REVIEW QUESTIONS

1. List the walls and line angles of a class III (lingual slot) preparation on the mesial surface of a maxillary central incisor.
2. When applying the rubber dam, how do you determine which is the anchor tooth?
3. Describe three methods for placing the rubber dam clamp and rubber dam on the anchor tooth.
4. True or false: Varnish is placed under all amalgam restorations but only under very deep composite resin restorations.
5. True or false: When checking the occlusion of a class IV restoration, it is important to have occlusal contact in centric occlusion as well as in lateral and protrusive movements.
6. Describe the functions of the matrix band and wedge in the placement of a class II amalgam restoration.
7. True or false: Each of the following situations would indicate the necessity of placing a calcium hydroxide base.
   a. Minimal depth amalgam preparation
   b. Pulpal exposure
   c. Subaxial extension in a class III preparation
   d. Minimal depth composite resin preparation
8. Define an alloy.
9. Define an amalgam.
10. What is the chief ingredient of dental alloy?
11. Name the ingredients for most dental alloys.
12. What is trituration?
13. What are the characteristics of a correctly mixed amalgam?
14. Where should the first increment of amalgam be placed and condensed in a class V preparation on tooth #14? A class II preparation involving both the mesial and distal surfaces of tooth #30?
15. What problem(s) occurs if the operator continues

to add an amalgam after the approximately 2½ minutes of working time for that mix has elapsed?
16. What occurs when any instrument or container with amalgam is subject to heat?
17. What is submarginal area?
18. True or false: During finishing and polishing procedures, the rotary instruments are most effective when applied with constant, medium pressure at a high speed.
19. True or false: When finishing composite resin restorations, discs are used in order of decreasing coarseness to produce a smooth surface finish.

20. Describe the procedure of acid etching enamel and how this allows the bonding of a composite resin to the tooth.
21. Describe the two ways that polymerization of composite resins occurs and the advantages and disadvantages of each in the clinical situation.
22. List two situations in which a temporary rather than a permanent restoration would be placed.
23. Explain the difference between the strokes used to remove calculus and those used to remove excess amalgam on an overhang.

Rubber Dam Placement and Removal

Suggested check-off sheet
Mark **S** for satisfactory completion or **U** for unsatisfactory completion of each criterion in the appropriate space.

PERFORMANCE CRITERIA   FACULTY   STUDENT

1. Assemble the necessary armamentarium
2. Place the clamp properly
   a. Floss applied
   b. All four prongs contacting tooth
   c. Clamp stable
   d. Clamp centered on tooth
   e. Clamp does not impinge on gingiva
3. Properly punch the dam
   a. Correct number of holes
   b. Position of holes modified for patient
4. Place the dam properly
   a. Dam stretched over clamp first
   b. Most anterior tooth isolated and ligated
   c. Frame placed
   d. Dam carried through contact areas with tape
   e. Frame readjusted
   f. Clamp ligature pulled to outer surface
   g. Dam tucked into sulcus around each tooth
   h. Area rinsed and suctioned
5. Remove the dam properly
   a. Ligature on most anterior tooth cut
   b. Interdental areas of dam pulled buccally and cut
   c. Lingual portion of dam freed interdentally
   d. Buccal portion of dam freed interdentally
   e. Clamp ligature held and clamp, dam, and frame removed
   f. Patient's mouth rinsed and suctioned
   g. Dam and patient's mouth checked for rubber dam debris

Placement of Base and Varnish

Suggested check-off sheet

Mark **S** for satisfactory completion or **U** for unsatisfactory completion of each criterion in the appropriate space.

PERFORMANCE CRITERIA   FACULTY STUDENT

1. Select the correct base   _____
2. Mix base correctly.   _____
3. Place the calcium hydroxide properly   _____
   a. Cover all subpulpal and subaxial areas   _____
   b. Does not cover any enamel   _____
   c. Applied in layer approximately 0.5 to 1.0 mm thick   _____
   d. Does not fill retentive grooves   _____
4. Correctly place varnish for amalgam restorations   _____
   a. Place over all walls including cavosurface margins   _____
   b. No pooling or placement of varnish in thick layers   _____

Tofflemire Matrix Retainer and Band Placement and Removal

Suggested check-off sheet

Mark **S** for satisfactory completion or **U** for unsatisfactory completion of each criterion in the appropriate space.

PERFORMANCE CRITERIA   FACULTY STUDENT

1. Assemble the necessary armamentarium   _____
2. Place the band in the retainer properly   _____
   a. Occlusal opening of band faces curved portion of prongs   _____
   b. Band held securely in retainer   _____
3. Place the band on the tooth properly   _____
   a. Retainer on facial surface with knobs extending anteriorly   _____
   b. Gingival portion of band around cervical area of tooth   _____
   c. Retainer centered on buccal surface of tooth   _____
   d. Band 1 to 2 mm above occlusal surface   _____
   e. Band 1 to 2 mm below gingival margin   _____
   f. Contact area burnished into band   _____
4. Place the wedge properly   _____
   a. Inserted from lingual aspect   _____
   b. Base of wedge placed against gingiva   _____
   c. Wedge not extending into preparation   _____
   d. Band held against tooth tightly   _____
5. Remove the retainer, band, and wedge properly   _____
   a. Retainer removed   _____
   b. Wedge removed   _____
   c. Band removed from unrestored area   _____
   d. Band removed from restored area from lingual to buccal aspect   _____
   e. Restoration undamaged   _____

Amalgam Restoration Placement

Suggested check-off sheet

Mark **S** for satisfactory completion or **U** for unsatisfactory completion of each criterion in the appropriate space.

PERFORMANCE CRITERIA   FACULTY   STUDENT

1. Assemble the necessary armamentarium   _____
2. Correctly mix the amalgam   _____
3. Place the amalgam and condense adequately   _____
   a. Deposite first carrier load in least accessible area   _____
   b. Throughly condense amalgam   _____
   c. Condense into all areas of prep   _____
   d. Condense out over cavosurface margins   _____
   e. Slightly overfill preparation   _____
4. Burnish the restoration   _____
   a. Adapt amalgam to margins   _____
   b. Smooth surface   _____
5. Establish occlusal anatomy   _____
   a. Grooves, fossae, ridges and cusps in the proper location   _____
   b. Create stable occlusal contacts   _____
6. Establish proper proximal contours   _____
   a. Establish proximal contact in the desired location   _____
   b. Create the desired embrasure form and location   _____
   c. Eliminate any amalgam overhang   _____
7. Completely adapt all amalgam margins to the surrounding enamel   _____
8. Burnish and smooth the entire restoration surface   _____
9. Completely remove all amalgam particles and other debris   _____

Amalgam Finishing and Polishing

Suggested check-off sheet

Mark **S** for satisfactory completion or **U** for unsatisfactory completion of each criterion in the appropriate space.

PERFORMANCE CRITERIA   FACULTY   STUDENT

  1. Assemble the necessary armamentarium   _____
  2. Assess the amalgam   _____
  3. Check the occlusion and make necessary modifications   _____
  4. Isolate teeth   _____
  5. Observe the order of instrumentation   _____
     a. Discs   _____
     b. Finishing strips   _____
     c. Pear-shaped bur   _____
     d. Bud- or flame-shaped bur   _____
     e. Round bur   _____
     f. Pumice with brush   _____
     g. Pumice with rubber cup   _____
     h. Pumice with floss or tape   _____
     i. Wet tin oxide with rubber cup   _____
     j. Wet tin oxide with floss or tape   _____
     k. Dry tin oxide with rubber cup   _____
  6. Finish and polish the amalgam restoration   _____
     a. Lavage area after each abrasive   _____
     b. Reproduce original contours of tooth   _____
     c. All margins flush   _____
     d. Amalgam smooth and shiny   _____
     e. Remove dam and recheck occlusion   _____
     f. Adjacent hard and soft tissues undamaged   _____

Placement of Composite Resin Restorations

Suggested check-off sheet

Mark **S** for satisfactory completion or **U** for unsatisfactory completion of each criterion in the appropriate space.

PERFORMANCE CRITERIA   FACULTY   STUDENT

  1. Assemble the correct armamentarium   _____
  2. Select the desired shade(s) of material   _____
  3. Correctly acid condition enamel   _____
     a. Place acid on desired area only   _____
     b. Leave acid no more than 30 to 60 seconds   _____
     c. Completely rinse and dry the surface   _____
     d. Correctly evaluate the adequacy of the etching process _____
  4. Place bonding agent   _____
     a. Place on etched surfaces only   _____
     b. Place without pooling resin   _____
     c. Cure by exposing to the light source   _____
  5. Correctly insert material   _____
     a. Place first increment in least accessible area   _____
     b. Place increments in layer 2 mm or less in thickness   _____
  6. Expose all areas of material to light source for minimum of
     20 seconds   _____
  7. Slightly overfill prep   _____
  8. Contour the restoration before each exposure to the light
     source   _____
  9. Confine the material to the preparation with the matrix (if
     present)   _____
 10. Shape and smooth the restoration   _____
     a. Establish the contours compatible with the general tooth
        contours   _____
     b. Create proximal and/or occlusal contacts (when applica-
        ble)   _____
     c. Create correct embrasure form (when applicable)   _____
     d. Establish a margin that blends completely with surround-
        ing enamel   _____
     e. Produce a smooth, shiny surface free of pits and voids _____

Amalgam Overhang Removal (Margination)

Suggested check-off sheet

Mark **S** for satisfactory completion or **U** for unsatisfactory completion of each criterion in the appropriate space.

PERFORMANCE CRITERIA   FACULTY   STUDENT

1. Assemble the necessary armamentarium   _____
2. Assess the overhang   _____
3. Observe the order of instrumentation   _____
   a. Amalgam knife   _____
   b. Large files (e.g., Orban)   _____
   c. Medium files (e.g., Hirshfeld)   _____
   d. Fine file (e.g., Rhein 31/32)   _____
   e. Universal curette   _____
   f. Discs   _____
   g. Finishing strips   _____
   h. Dental tape with pumice   _____
   i. Dental tape   _____
4. Remove the overhang properly   _____
   a. Area thoroughly lavaged   _____
   b. Margins flush   _____
   c. Amalgam smooth   _____
   d. Contact present with adjacent tooth   _____
   e. Interproximal contour of tooth reproduced   _____
   f. Adjacent hard and soft tissues undamaged   _____

REFERENCES

Abrams H et al: Gingival sequela from a retained piece of rubber dam: report of a case, J Ky Dent Assn 30:21, 1978.

Axelsson P: Concept and practice of plaque control, Pediatr Dent (special issue) 3:101, 1981.

Baum L et al: The textbook of operative dentistry, ed 2, Philadelphia, 1985, WB Saunders.

Browne RM et al: Bacterial microleakage and pulpal inflammation in experimental cavities, Int Endo J 16:147, 1983.

Charbeneau GT et al: Principles and practice of operative dentistry, ed 2, Philadelphia, 1981, Lea and Febiger.

Charbeneau GT: Suggested technique for polishing amalgam restorations, J Mich Dent Assoc 47:420, 1965.

Cohen S and Burns RC: Pathways of the pulp, St Louis, 1980, The CV Mosby.

Corpron RE et al: A clinical evaluation of polishing amalgams immediately after insertion: 18 month results, Pediatr Dent 4:98, 1982.

Coxhead LJ et al: Amalgam overhangs — a radiographic study, NZ Dent J 74:145, 1978.

Craig RG, editor: Restorative dental materials, ed 6, St Louis, 1980, The CV Mosby Co.

Creaven PJ et al: Surface roughness of two dental amalgams after various polishing techniques, J Prosthet Dent 43:289, 1980.

Eliasson ST: Compatibility of composite resins with pulp insulating materials, J Dent Res 58:397, 1979.

Farah JW et al: Effect of cement base thickness on MOD amalgam restorations, J Dent Res 62(2):109, 1983.

Farah JW et al: Cement bases under amalgam restorations: effect of thickness, Oper Dent 6(3):82, 1981.

Gelsky SC: Overhanging amalgam restorations: their prevalence, ramifications, and irradication, Can Dent Dyg 16:19, 1982.

Gilmore W et al: Operative dentistry, ed 4, St Louis, 1982, The CV Mosby.

Gorzo I et al: Amalgam restorations, plaque removal, and periodontal health, J Clin Periodontol 6:98, 1979.

Hakkarainen K and Ainamo J: Influence of overhanging posterior tooth restorations on alveolar bone height in adults, J Clin Periodontol 7:114, 1980.

Harper RH et al: In vivo measurements of thermal difussion through restorations of various materials, J Pros Dent 43(2):180, 1980.

Highfield JE and Powell RN: Effects of removal of posterior overhanging metallic margins of restorations upon the periodontal tissues, J Clin Periodontol 5:169, 1978.

Hormati A and Fuller J: Fracture strength of amalgam overlying base materials, J Pros Dent 43(1):52, 1980.

Jeffcoat MK et al: Alveolar bone destruction due to overhanging amalgams in periodontal disease, J Periodontol 51:599, 1980.

Kanai S: Structural studies of amalgam, II: effect of burnishing on margins of occlusal amalgam fillings, Acta Odontol Scand 24:46, 1966.

Kato S et al: Effect of burnishing on marginal seal of an amalgam restoration, J Prosthet Dent 19:393, 1968.

Langeland K: Prevention of pulpal damage, Dent Clin North Am 16:709, 1972.

Lemmons PLM et al: Influence on the incidence of bulk fracture of amalgam restorations, J Dent Res 65 (special issue):Ab. 30, p. 729, 1986.

Leon AR: The periodontium and restorative procedures: a critical review, J Oral Rehabil 4:105, 1977.

Millstein PL and Nathanson D: Effect of eugenol and eugenol cements on cured composite resin, J Pros Dent 50:211, 1983.

Murray GA et al: Effect of four cavity varnishes and a fluoride solution on microleakage of dental amalgam restorations, Oper Dent 8:148.

Nitkin DA: Placing and polishing amalgam in one visit, Quintessence Int 10:23, 1979.

Osborne J et al: Dental amalgam: clinical behavior up to eight years, J Oper Dent 5(1):24, 1980.

Osborne J et al: Personal communication, unpublished data, 1988.

Peters DD and Augsberger RA: In vivo cold transference of bases and restorations, JADA 102(5):642, 1981.

Reavis-Scruggs R: Comparing amalgam finishing techniques by scanning electron microscopy, Dent Hyg 56(9):30, 1982.

Rodriguez-Ferrer HJ et al: Effect of gingival health of removing overhanging margins of interproximal subgingival amalgam restorations, J Clin Periodontol 7:457, 1980.

Schemlitzer LD et al: A six month clinical evaluation of polishing techniques on the marginal integrity of a high copper alloy, J Ind Dent Assoc 61:17, 1982.

Stanley HR: Traumatic capacity of high-speed and ultrasonic dental instrumentation, JADA 63:749, 1961.

Stanley HR: Pulpal response to dental techniques and materials, Dent Clin North Am 15(1):115, 1971.

Svare CW and Chan KC: Effect of surface treatment on the corrodibility of dental amalgam, J Prosthet Dent 19:393, 1972.

Tjan AH et al: The efficacy of resin-compatible cavity varnishes in reducing dentin permeability of free monomer, J Prosthet Dent 57:2, 1987.

Vale JD and Caffesse RG: Removal of amalgam overhangs, J Periodontol 50:245, 1979.

Yates JL et al: Cavity varnishes applied over insulation bases: effect on microleakage, Oper Dent 5:43, 1980.

PART FOUR

EVALUATION

Chapters 35 to 37 address the need to *evaluate* the success, or at least the outcomes, of practice. Success is defined as the success of therapy (in terms of both short- and long-term goals) for the individual patient and also as the relative success that the health care provider experiences as a result of his or her participation as a dental professional.

Evaluation is discussed as the final stage of the project development cycle, but because project development is a cycle and evaluation almost always prompts ideas for change, evaluation may blend in with a new phase of assessment and its subsequent phases. Evaluation then becomes not the end but the beginning.

35 CASE DOCUMENTATION

OBJECTIVES: *The reader will be able to*

1. Discuss the value of case documentation in relation to record keeping.
2. Identify several ways in which case documentation can be used as an educational resource.
3. List the components of a case documentation.
4. Present a case documentation, using either a written or verbal format.

Case documentation refers to a thorough record of the patient's dental therapy. This record is both visual and written. The visual record is composed of intraoral photographs, radiographs, and study models. The written information includes examination notes, diagnostic chartings, and recordings of treatment. A comprehensive documentation is composed of initial assessment data, the treatment outcome, and an evaluative summary of the therapy.

A lengthy record of each patient or each phase of care may not always be necessary. However, some patients with particular needs are well suited for case documentation. Patients who require extensive reconstruction therapy that includes home care instruction, initial hygiene periodontal preparation, and major restorative and periodontal procedures are candidates for documentation. With such cases, care is delivered in phases over an extended period of time. Thorough records of each phase that reflect the actual therapy are important for following care to completion. Occasionally a patient may expect an outcome that cannot be achieved. Records that document the steps of therapy may help the patient or other professionals evaluate the appropriateness of care.

Another patient may need to realize that even with impeccable home care procedures, fibrotic tissue from chronic inflammation will not change over several months. By documenting the condition, the decision for a minor surgical procedure can be made with the patient. A patient with a condition such as acute necrotizing ulcerative gingivitis, for which dental therapy will dramatically reduce the gingival conditions, is another type of case well suited for documentation.

Documentation of treatment enhances the accuracy of the patient's record. Too often, when records are reviewed, information on specific patient conditions and treatment procedures lack pertinent details.

In addition to improving record keeping, case documentation has several educational benefits.

For the clinician, the components of a documentation allow practice in almost all skill areas. Putting it all together in such a way is helpful for the clinician (especially a student) in appreciating and evaluating total care for the patient.

For the patient, involvement in the case documentation creates a particular commitment to the goals of treatment. The patient is motivated by participating in the data collection and seeing the results of therapy. At the completion of care, the patient takes pride in his or her role in the therapy and wants to maintain the successful outcome.

For colleagues and other patients, a documentation can be presented as an example from which to learn. Documentation of the success (or failure) of a particular treatment plan or mode of therapy is helpful to other clinicians. The comparison of actual cases is an excellent format for discussion and professional sharing.

For the lay person, the prospect of a significant amount of dentistry may be overwhelming. Examples of completed cases may be helpful in proposing or convincing a patient of the need for specific therapy. Seeing examples of the course of care may be reassuring to the patient.

Showing patients the successful results of prevention-oriented dental therapy is one of the best motivators for preventive home care methods (Figs. 35-1 to 35-4).

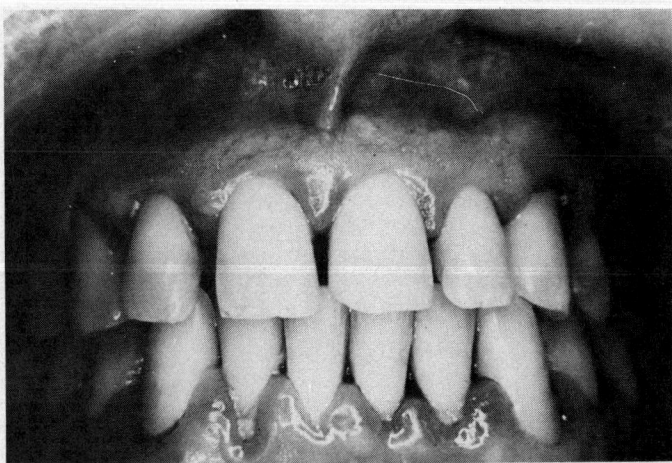

Fig. 35-1. Initial photograph. This 40-year-old man had multiple periodontal abscesses, one of which is clearly seen in mandibular right cuspid area. There are no systemic etiologic factors. Tissue bleeds readily and is swollen and edematous. Papillae are separated from lingual soft tissue. Maxillary and mandibular incisors are mobile, diastemas are present, and there is fremitus of anterior teeth in excursive movements.
(From Corn H, and Marks M: Contin Dent Educ **1:**10, 1978.)

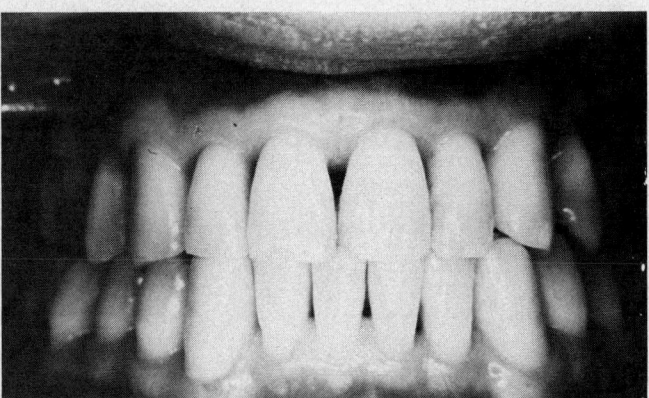

Fig. 35-2. This 12-year result clearly shows that reinforcement of plaque control procedures along with secondary preventive dentistry therapy has enabled patient to achieve this aesthetic result. Sequence of treatment was *1,* successful completion of plaque control program and its reinforcement, *2,* root scaling and root planing, *3,* soft tissue curettage, *4,* occlusal adjustment in centric relation, *5,* minor tooth movement to retract maxillary anterior teeth, and *6,* occlusal adjustment to gain group function in excursive movements and eliminate fremitus patterns. Result shows how stability of tooth position as well as a healthy gingival attachment can be achieved once dental disease has been arrested.
(From Corn H, and Marks M: Contin Dent Educ **1:**10, 1978.)

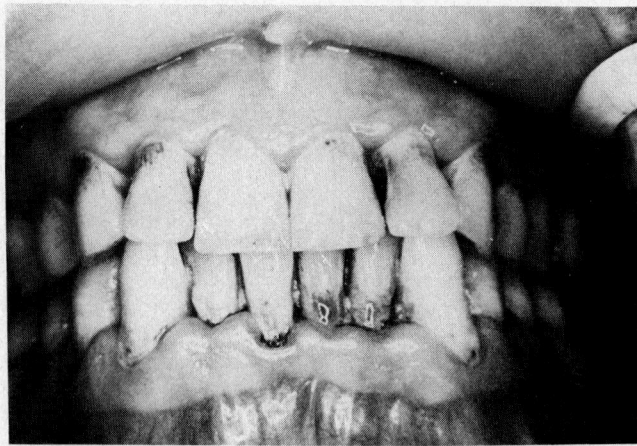

Fig. 35-3. This 50-year-old man had never been to a dentist and had no understanding of the benefits of preventive dentistry care. His treatment consisted of initial therapy and restoration of carious areas.
(From Corn H, and Marks M: Contin Dent Educ **1:**10, 1978.)

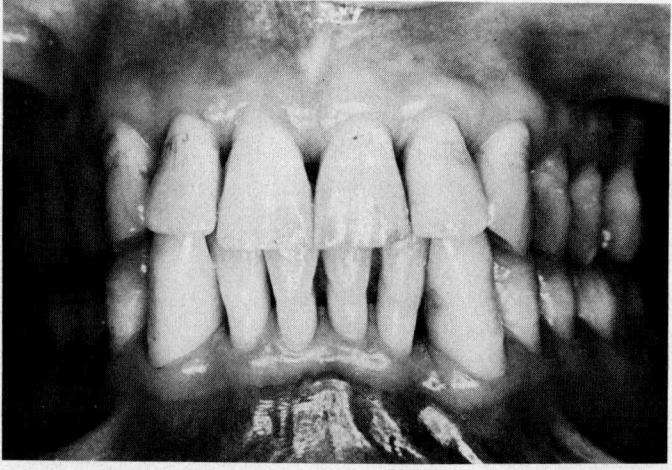

Fig. 35-4. Results of root scaling and root planing along with extensive soft tissue curettage have provided this 14-year postoperative result. It is important to ensure that patients not be discouraged at the initial examination, since it is likely that they are unaware of the benefits that preventive dentistry can provide. Secondary preventive procedures enabled this man to have renewed pride and enthusiasm for aesthetics that were achieved during periodontal therapy.
(From Corn H, and Marks M: Contin Dent Educ **1:**10, 1978.)

DOCUMENTATION PROCEDURES

There is no doubt that documentation of care is time consuming. As a clinician approaches case documentation, the key word is *organization*.

The components of a case documentation are as follows:

1. Review of the comprehensive health history
2. Initial clinical findings (intraoral and extraoral examination)
3. Chartings (periodontal survey, and indices—gingival, plaque, bleeding)
4. Radiographs
5. Diagnostic study casts
6. Photographs
7. Treatment considerations (goals, treatment plan)
8. Record of treatment
9. Posttreatment findings (review components 2 to 6)
10. Evaluation summary

The consistent quality of diagnostic aids is important. Periodontal records, radiographs, study models, and photographs are necessary to show changes in the patient's tissues as therapy progresses. Instruction for each of these procedures is given in earlier chapters.

Documentation involves making detailed notes of the dental appointment.

Sample chart note: 2/6/88—Prophylaxis with fluoride

A record entry this general tells us very little about what actually occurred. A record entry noting the plaque index, results of a periodontal screening, indications of trouble spots in the dentition, the preventive education, the patient's response to care, the care rendered, and plans for future therapy documents the content of the appointment more specifically. Three months from the date of the appointment, the detailed chart notes will facilitate patient follow-up.

Documentation procedures are completed throughout treatment. Planning, with particular attention to the time needed to complete necessary documentation procedures, is recommended to avoid frustration during each appointment or frustration with the results of poor documentation.

PRESENTATION OF CASE DOCUMENTATION

The format for a case documentation presentation can be either written or verbal. A verbal presentation of case documentation is most common. One format for presentation is described; however, many formats are acceptable. The prospective audience, the facilities for presentation, and the purpose for the presentation will play a large part in determining the most appropriate format.

Patient assessment

Introduce the patient profie. Provide a summary of the health history, stating the chief complaint and the history of the present condition. Summarize the clinical findings and present pertinent information from the intraoral and extraoral examination. Show the initial intraoral photographs (slides), study casts, periodontal charting, indices, and radiographs. Describe the dental health education assessment. Use an order of presentation that emphasizes the important aspects of the individual case.

When extensive information is to be presented, a handout is helpful to complement the verbal presentation. The audience is able to take notes during the presentation so that important aspects of the presentation can be reviewed at a later time.

Patient planning

At this point, general concerns about the patient and reasons for selecting the case for documentation may be presented. State the goals of the treatment, and outline the proposed treatment schedule.

Implementation phase

Describe the treatment actually rendered at each appointment. Provide photographs and other indicators of ongoing care, such as periodontal indices. These aids support the treatment being described and allow the audience to follow the healing and restorative process.

Detailed slides of particular instrumentation procedures are excellent for educational purposes. A series illustrating ultrasonic scaling or soft tissue curettage procedures may illustrate a particular technique. This allows the presenter to discuss instrument selection, the choice of materials, or the sequence of therapy.

In this phase, implementation of the preventive education plan is presented. In what area was home care instruction given? What motivational appeal was used? How was the patient involved in learning? What positive reactions or roadblocks were encountered?

Treatment plans often are changed. Revisions are easily pointed out as the implementation phase is presented.

Posttreatment evaluation

This portion of the presentation allows for comparison of initial assessment data and follow-up data. Present the follow-up series of intraoral photographs, periodontal charting, indices, study models, and radiographs (if appropriate). When facilities allow, showing before and after slides simultaneously on two screens is effective.

Discuss or summarize the outcome in relation to the stated goals. If the outcome was not as anticipated, present the factors that may have influenced this. Alternative approaches to care may be included in the discussion also.

With a written presentation, the main consideration is organizing and including all the pertinent information. Present the patient with objective comments. Use information as it was found in chartings and as reflected by photographs, models, and radiographs. Detail the posttreatment data to demonstrate the effectiveness of the clinical course.

Judgments and evaluations are appropriate after the objective data are presented. Provide the rationale for therapy, and summarize the treatment outcome in relation to expected goals.

Text continued on p. 753.

SAMPLE CASE
Case Documentation

PATIENT PROFILE: Ms. Smith is a 23-year old black woman. She lives in Philadelphia. She originally came to the dental school for pain in the maxillary left area. The patient presented with large occlusal caries in No. 16, which was eventually extracted.

CHIEF COMPLAINT: Ms. Smith came to the dental hygiene clinic because she felt her "gums were in bad shape."

PAST DENTAL HISTORY: The patient was seen by a private dentist about 4 years ago to have her teeth cleaned. She has not been to a dentist since except for the emergency care in which No. 16 was extracted.

MEDICAL HISTORY SUMMARY: Ms. Smith reports having had mumps and chickenpox when she was a child. No residual effects were reported. She had a cyst removed from her left cheek 2 years ago. This did not necessitate entering the hospital, as it was done on an outpatient basis. No complications were reported. The patient has broken her right leg and left arm in sports-related accidents. Both these accidents occurred more than 5 years ago, and the patient has recovered full function in both limbs.

The patient takes no prescribed medications at the current time. She does take a daily multivitamin. The patient does not take aspirin, because it upsets her stomach.

The patient's family history reveals that her father died of heart trouble when he was 52 years old. Her mother is alive and has high blood pressure. She has one sister who is alive and well. The patient is obese and follows a diet and exercise schedule prescribed by her physician. In the past 6 months she has lost 75 pounds.

SAMPLE CASE

Case Documentation—cont'd

REVIEW OF SYSTEMS:

HEENT: Wears glasses; recent sore throat

Skin, appendages: Reports her skin becomes dry when she diets

Bones, joints, muscles: Denies any related symptons

CV: Denies chest pains, palpitations, syncope; blood pressure 130/86

Resp: Reports having bronchial trouble now and then, usually related to sore throats; quit smoking 2 months ago; denies excessive coughing

GI: When patient was taking liquid protein, she experienced gastrointestinal discomfort; no symptoms currently reported

GU: Drinking a great deal of water with the diet; states that this causes more frequent urination

Hemo: Denies excessive bruising or bleeding during extraction

Endo: Denies symptoms related to diabetes, thyroid disorder, and hormone function

CNS: Denies dizziness, restlessness, and hallucinations

CLINICAL FINDINGS:

Extraoral examination: The patient's facial symmetry, lips, TMJ, and larynx were within normal limits. Submandibular and posterior cervical lymph nodes were palpable.

Radiographic findings: Horizontal and vertical bone loss present between all mandibular anterior teeth. Radiographic calculus is apparent, especially on mandibular anterior teeth. Caries was detected on the distal of No. 29.

Intraoral examination: The patient presented with generalized periodonitis, most severe in the mandibular anterior area. The posterior pharyngeal wall appeared inflamed. Tonsils were present and appeared enlarged. Bilateral mandibular tori were present. Calculus was generalized throughout the mouth with the heaviest deposits located on the lower anterior teeth. The gingiva was inflamed and edematous with some suppuration evident in the lower anterior area. Except for the lower anterior section, the tissue was generally scalloped with normal pigmentation. Tooth No. 9 has mesioincisal fracture, and occlusal caries was detected on Nos. 2, 20, and 29 by exploration.

Periodontal examination: To document reduction in periodontal pocket depth, only the chartings of the maxillary left buccal and of the mandibular anterior facial are noted.

Maxillary left

9	10	11	12	13	14	15	16
423	334	435	625	524	335	424	X

(tooth number)

Pocket depth in mm (mesial buccal distal)

Mandibular anterior

323	335	544	535	534	533
27	26	25	24	23	22

DENTAL-HEALTH EDUCATION:

1. The patient brushed her teeth once a day but did not floss. A random scrubbing method was used for cleaning the teeth and gingiva.
2. Initial bleeding index: 22
3. Initial plaque index: 30 (on a 30-point scale)

INITIAL ASSESSMENT: See Figs. 35-5 to 35-8 for initial assessment.

Continued.

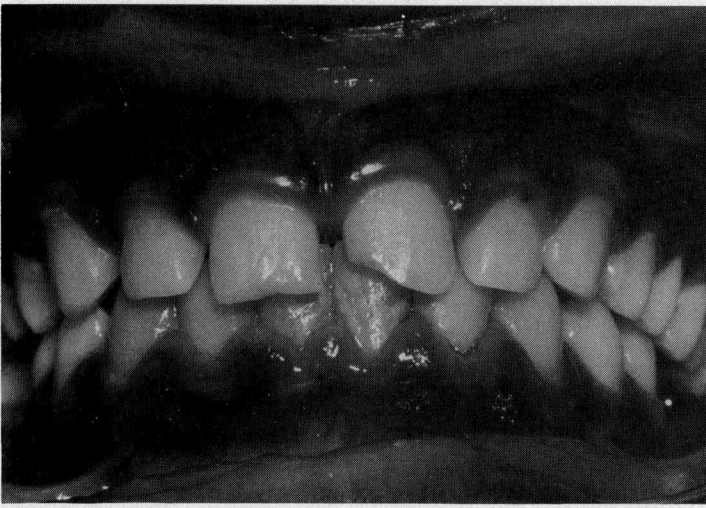

Fig. 35-5. Patient appeared for treatment with generalized periodontitis more severe in lower anterior area. Gingiva is edematous with suppuration evident.

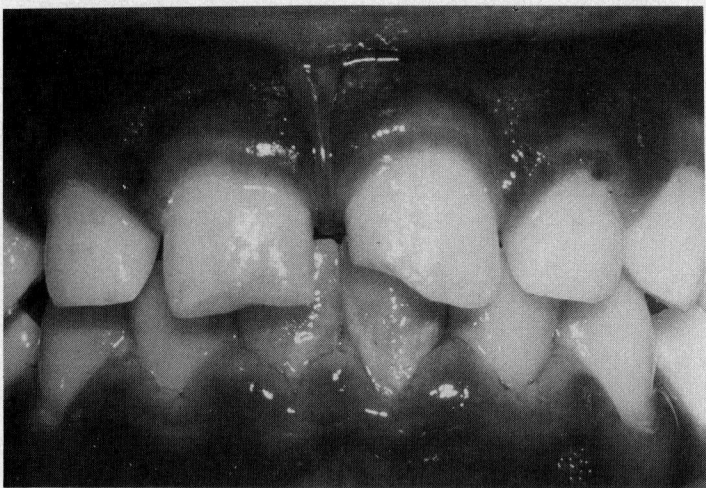

Fig. 35-6. Calculus is generalized but appears heaviest on facial and lingual aspects of mandibular anterior teeth. Several 4- to 5-mm pocket depths were noted on examination.

SAMPLE CASE
Case Documentation—cont'd

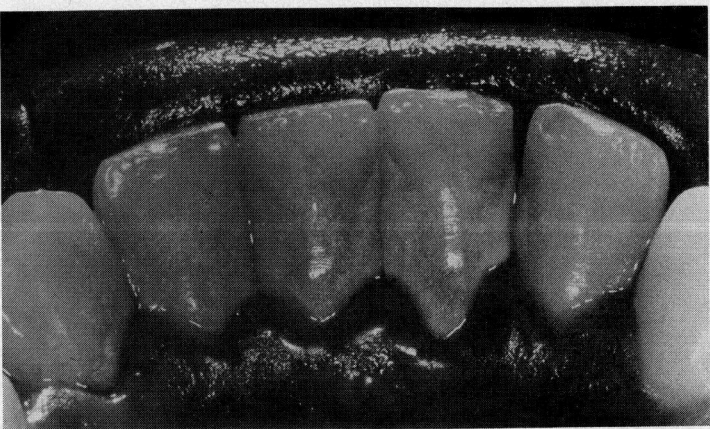

Fig. 35-7. Initial photograph of lingual tissue and heavy calculus deposits on lower anterior teeth. Note tissue contours due to inflammation.

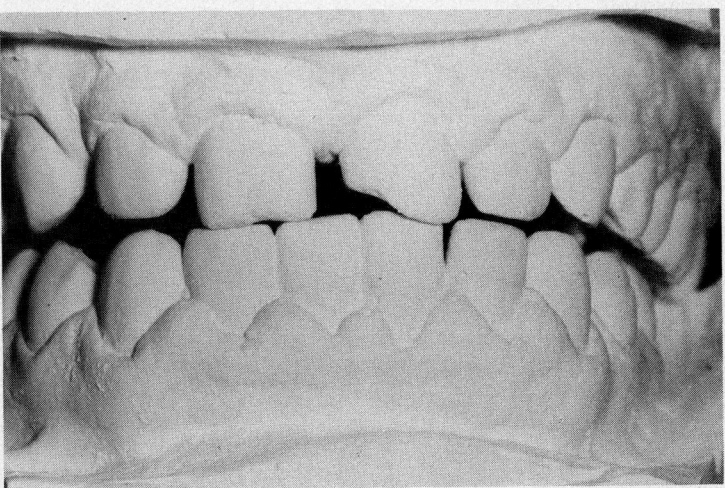

Fig. 35-8. Close-up of initial study models shows fractured maxillary central incisor and topography of gingival tissue.

Continued.

Case Documentation—cont'd

PLANNING:

Rationale for case selection: Due to the nature of the calculus deposits, the depth of the periodontal pockets, and the patient's willingness to improve her oral conditions, I feel this patient will benefit by participating in documentation procedures. I anticipate that with proper home care instruction and periodontal procedures including ultrasonic scaling, scaling and root planing, and soft tissue curettage, the patient's tissue will respond well.

Goals:

1. Improve the health status of the gingiva, teeth, and supporting ligaments, especially in the lower anterior area.
2. Remove all hard deposits so that the patient can effectively clean her own mouth.
3. Have the patient demonstrate how to correctly brush and floss to effectively remove plaque.
4. Reduce the depth of periodontal pockets.

Initial treatment plan:

Appointment 1. Medical history; intraoral, extraoral examination

Appointment 2: Complete series of radiographs; initial study casts

Appointment 3: Complete periodontal charting; initial series intraoral photographs

Appointment 4: Dental health education: emphasis on brushing technique; perform ultrasonic scaling for the entire mouth

Appointment 5: Dental health education: review brushing skills; emphasis on flossing techniques; complete mandibular scaling and root planing

Appointment 6: Dental health education: review flossing skills: assess for possible periodontal aids; complete maxillary scaling and root planing

Appointment 7: Dental health education: review all home care procedures; complete polishing and fluoride treatment; follow-up intraoral photographs

Appointment 8: Extension if necessary

IMPLEMENTATION: The treatment proceeded as planned. The patient was receptive to documentation procedures. No skill roadblocks were encountered with dental health education. The patient was able to demonstrate adequate skills with a modified sulcular brushing and loop flossing technique. The plaque index decreased steadily. Hygiene procedures were accomplished with a minimum of difficulty. Photographs were taken immediately after the ultrasonic scaling at appointment 4 (Figs. 35-9 and 35-10).

SAMPLE CASE
Case Documentation—cont'd

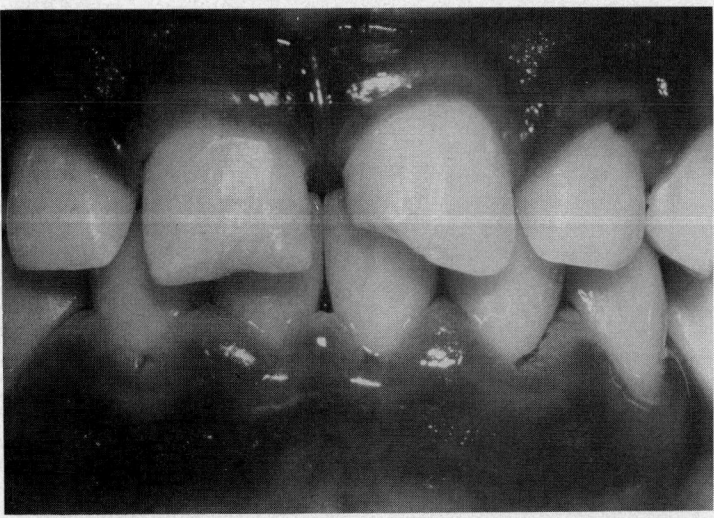

Fig. 35-9. Appointment 4. Following dental health education emphasizing brushing technique, entire mouth was ultrasonically scaled. Facial aspect of mandibular anterior teeth immediately following ultrasonic procedure.

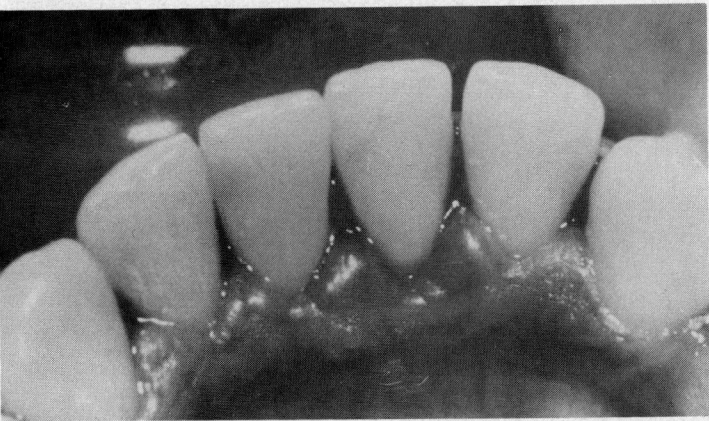

Fig. 35-10. Lingual aspect of mandibular anterior teeth following ultrasonic procedure. Compare with initial photograph, Fig. 35-7.

Continued.

SAMPLE CASE
Case Documentation—cont'd

Treatment revisions:

Appointment 7: Observed lower anterior tissues for possible curettage

Appointment 8: Reviewed dental health education and completed soft tissue curettage facial and lingual of Nos. 22 to 27; placed a periodontal pack

Appointment 9: Observed healing of lower anterior tissue; administered maxillary infiltration between Nos. 9 and 10, using approximately one-fourth Carpule (0.5 cc) or 14 mg mepivacaine (Carbocaine) 3% anesthetic solution; placed a composite resin on mesioincisal edge of No. 9

Appointment 10: Dental health education reinforcement; completed follow-up photographs and study models

Appointment 11: Follow-up periodontal charting; discussed recall and further restorative treatment needs

EVALUATION: Ms. Smith was treated in the dental hygiene clinic for a period of 2 months. The follow-up photographs and study models indicate that the tissue in the lower anterior area responded well to deposit removal and soft tissue curettage (Figs. 35-11 to 35-14). The patient can demonstrate an adequate technique for brushing and flossing. She effectively removes plaque and values her newly acquired skills and the appearance of her tissue. Continued home care has been reinforced to maintain this area. The final plaque index was 4, and the final bleeding index was 1. Following are the chartings of pocket depth after treatment in the areas originally noted.

Maxillary left

9	10	11	12	13	14	15	16	(tooth number)
323	333	323	413	313	325	323	X	

(Pocket depth in mm mesial buccal distal)

Mandibular anterior

323	323	223	322	223	332
27	26	25	24	23	22

The patient and I are pleased that our goals for this phase of treatment have been accomplished. Ms. Smith will continue with restorative treatment and will be seen for periodontal recall in 2 months.

Case Documentation—cont'd

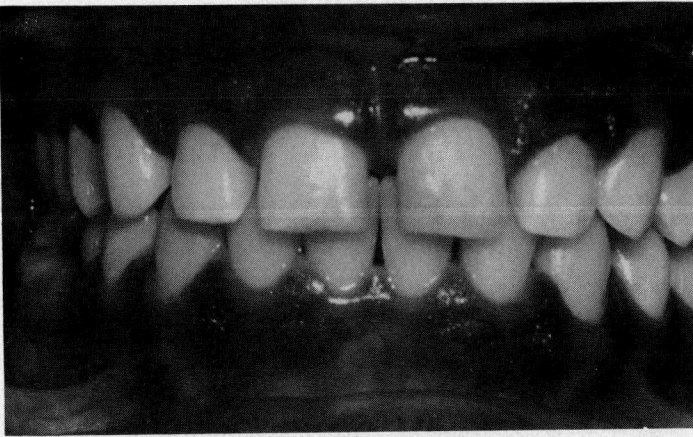

Fig. 35-11. Appointment 9. Composite resin was placed on maxillary left central incisor. Soft tissue curettage of lower anterior tissues had been completed at previous appointment.

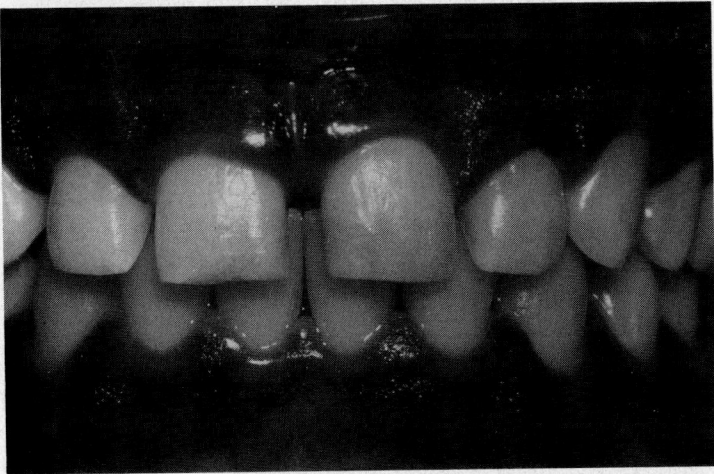

Fig. 35-12. Ten days after curettage, healing process in lower anterior area is evident. Deepest pocket depth noted in this area was 3 mm.

Continued.

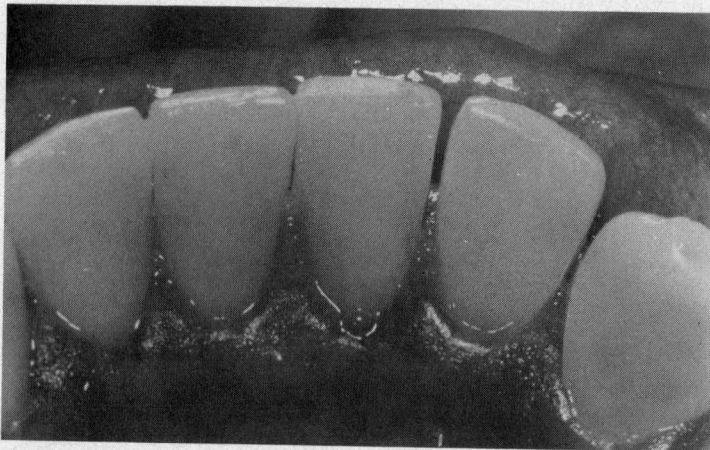

Fig. 35-13. Follow-up photograph of mandibular lingual anterior tissue reveals much improved gingival contour after deposit removal, root planing, and soft tissue curettage. Note papillae edge and stippled texture as compared with that in Fig. 35-7.

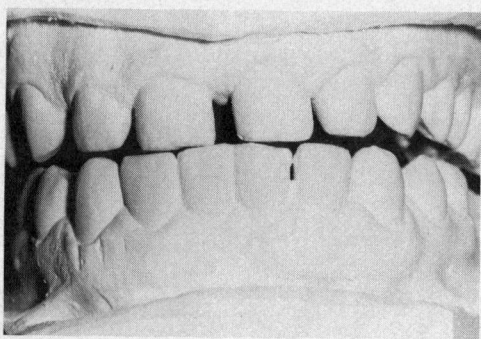

Fig. 35-14. Follow-up study models document healing process that occurred in mandibular anterior region and restoration of maxillary central incisor.

ORTHODONTIC CASE DOCUMENTATION

Orthodontic specialization for dental hygienists is an exciting career option. The skills a hygienist uses are varied and the influence of the hygienist on the patient during the course of treatment is tremendous.

The following case is presented to illustrate some of the ways a hygienist participates in orthodontic care. Although not every educational program for hygienists includes some of these skills, the basic foundation of anatomical sciences, traditional clinical preventive services, and patient management skills can be enhanced through special courses and on-the-job training. State laws that provide for delegation of duties and general supervision of hygienists have made it possible for hygienists to become very active in orthodontic care.

The hygienist's involvement begins with the pretreatment evaluation. This includes gathering information about the patient's medical and dental history and learning about the patient's oral habits and home care practices. Photographic records can be completed by the hygienist. These include extraoral photographs, radiographs, cephalometric, temporomandibular joint views, and intraoral views. The patient is examined clinically to determine the health of the teeth and the periodontal tissues. The hygienist is able to complete plaque scoring, and periodontal and restorative chartings. Following this, impressions and study models are completed. These initial records are used to prepare a treatment plan. Hygienists with an educational background in craniofacial growth and development may be involved in preparing parts of the treatment plan and presenting it to the patient.

The hygienist will be able to help the patient and his or her family understand the proposed treatment and to answer questions during treatment.

As treatment moves to the active phase requiring removable or fixed orthodontic appliances, the hygienist will be the one who sees the patient the most during the frequent checks at the dental office. During this phase of care, modifying home care techniques, cleaning the teeth, applying fluoride treatments, and adjusting appliances will become the hygienist's responsibility. The ability to communicate with the patient about personal oral care, attention to diet, compliance with recommended hours for wearing various appliances, and so forth will be important for keeping the treatment plan on target and supporting the patient through the changes.

The hygienist can participate in removing and replacing various appliances and in keeping the records current by repeating photographs and chartings if necessary during treatment. When the treatment is completed, new photos, radiographs, and models will be made to document the results of the care. As the patient is usually followed for a period of time, the hygienist will stay involved with a recall schedule to monitor the posttreatment care. The opportunity to be skilled in many clinical areas and an understanding friend throughout the years is a rewarding part of delivering primary care.

This orthodontic case documentation shows the value of written and photographic records. In actuality, many more records make up the patient's portfolio. This sample covers the essential aspects of the patient's care.

Text continued on p. 761.

Orthodontic Case Documentation

PATIENT PROFILE: A 10-year, 2-month-old caucasian male. Resident in a Cleveland suburb. Patient came to orthodontist from referral of neighbor.

CHIEF COMPLAINT: Crowded teeth.

PAST DENTAL HISTORY: Patient involved in regular recall with primary care dentist. Patient experienced trauma to upper anterior teeth, resulting in fracture of both upper central incisors.

MEDICAL HISTORY: Negative, other than usual childhood diseases; no complications or hospitalizations.

CLINICAL FINDINGS (Fig. 35-15): The patient appeared for treatment with a facial profile characterized by a slightly turned up nose with obtuse nasolabial angle, a long upper lip, retrognathic chin, and a sublabial crease which is indicative of a strong mentalis muscle. A slight mid-opening click of the left temporomandibular joint was noted. Several deciduous teeth were present; several were loose.

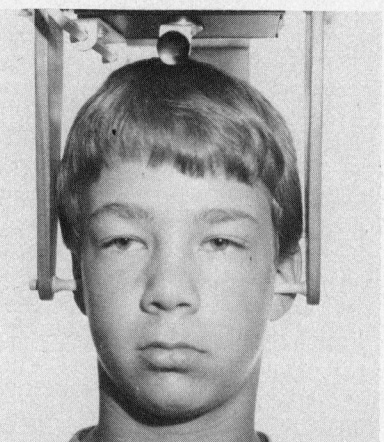

B

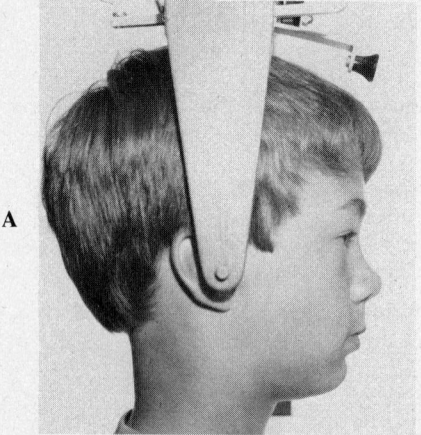

A

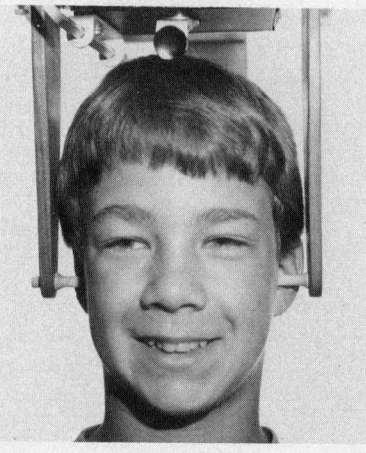

C

Fig. 35-15. Facial photographs before orthodontic treatment. **A,** Profile. **B,** Frontal. **C,** Smile.

SAMPLE CASE
Orthodontic Case Documentation—cont'd

INTRAORAL FINDINGS (Figs. 35-16 to 35-19): Patient exhibited excessive protrusion with a deep bite and crowded upper and lower teeth. Molars were in an approximate class I bilateral occlusion. Generalized gingivitis was noted.

INITIAL TREATMENT: A recommendation was made by the orthodontist to the parents requesting the patient have several deciduous teeth extracted. The patient was seen at 9-month intervals until the permanent teeth erupted.

After approximately 18 months of observation, the orthodontist requested the patient be evaluated for full orthodontic treatment. The parents consented. A complete series of diagnostic records was gathered and processed by the dental hygienist. The diagnostic series of records taken included the following: panographic x-ray; frontal x-ray; lateral cephalometric x-ray; hand-wrist x-ray; facial photographs, including frontal, lateral, and smile; a series of intraoral 35 mm slides; impressions for diagnostic casts; and a maxillary intercuspation bite registration. A request was made for a complete series of periapical x-rays, which was to be obtained from the primary care dentist and forwarded to the orthodontist.

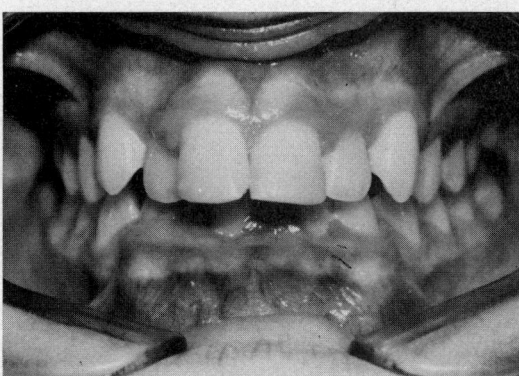

Fig. 35-16. Direct anterior view of teeth in occlusion before orthodontic treatment.

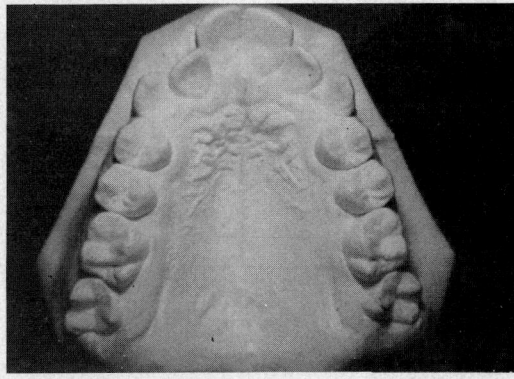

Fig. 35-17. Occlusal view of maxillary diagnostic cast before orthodontic treatment.

Continued.

SAMPLE CASE

Orthodontic Case Documentation—cont'd

REVIEW OF DIAGNOSTIC RECORDS AND TREATMENT PLAN: Confirmed the clinical observations and suggested the need for the removal of permanent teeth to relieve the crowding and advance the mandible to improve skeletal balance and the soft tissue profile. The treatment plan that would best accomplish these goals and work toward rehabilitation of the temporomandibular joint included the removal of all four permanent second molar teeth. This would create space for the relief of crowding and allow the full unhampered development of the third molars. Functional jaw orthodontics would accomplish mandibular advancement and improve the functional relationships in the temporomandibular joint.

TREATMENT CONSULTATION WITH PARENTS: Parents met with the dental hygienist for review of treatment recommendations made by the orthodontist. Parents consented to treatment.

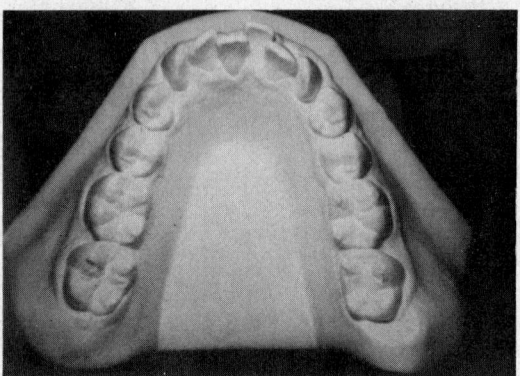

Fig. 35-18. Occlusal view of mandibular diagnostic cast before orthodontic treatment.

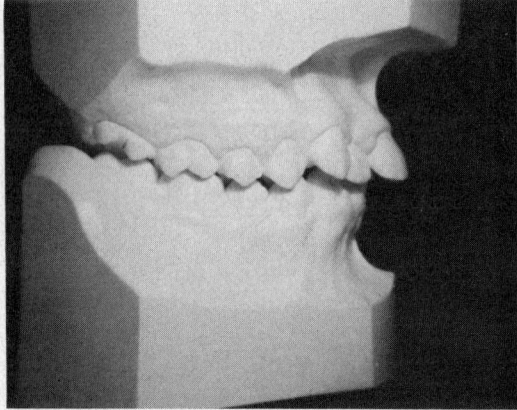

Fig. 35-19. Right lateral view of diagnostic casts in occlusion before orthodontic treatment.

Orthodontic Case Documentation—cont'd

TREATMENT: The patient met with the dental hygienist at a special patient orientation appointment for discussion and demonstration of proper oral hygiene and appliance care.

The four second molar teeth were removed by an oral surgeon. Removable functional appliances (Sagittal appliance followed by an orthopedic corrector) were worn by the patient for approximately 2 years (Figs. 35-20 and 35-21). The patient wore the appliances 24 hours daily. He had recall appointments at 3- to 6-week intervals for adjustments to the appliances and monitoring of treatment progress and oral hygiene evaluation. During this time, he was advised to see his primary care dentist for his routine dental health care.

Retainers were placed after the 2 years of removable appliance treatment. The patient was monitored for another 18 months while the third molars erupted.

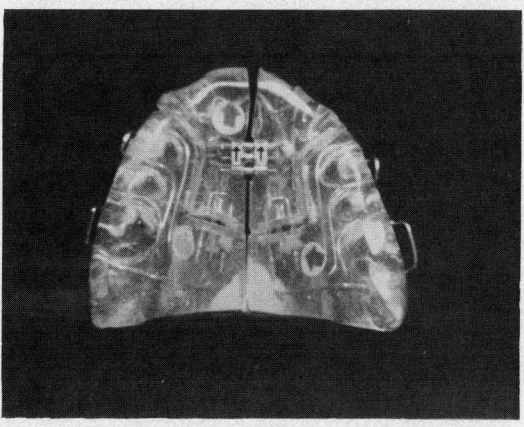

Fig. 35-20. Removable sagittal appliance.

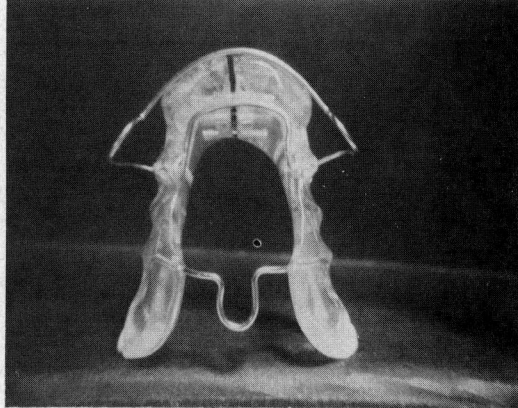

Fig. 35-21. Removable orthopedic corrector appliance.

Continued.

Orthodontic Case Documentation—cont'd

Final treatment records were gathered by the hygienist for review by the orthodontist (Figs. 35-22 to 35-26). The orthodontist dismissed the patient from treatment.

EVALUATION: Stable treatment results were obtained during the growth years. The third molars erupted without incident. The patient and parents were delighted that treatment results could be accomplished without fixed appliances.

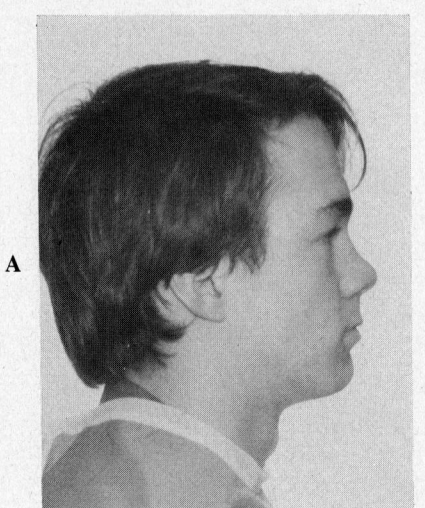
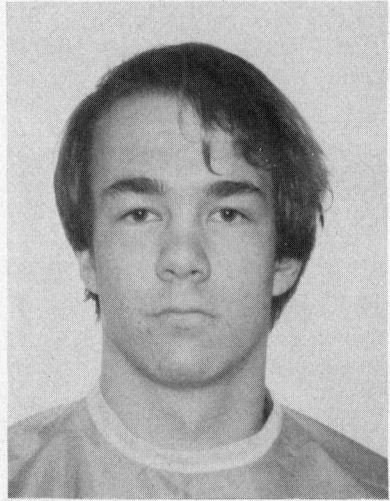

Fig. 35-22. Facial photographs following orthodontic treatment. **A**, Profile. **B**, Frontal. **C**, Smile.

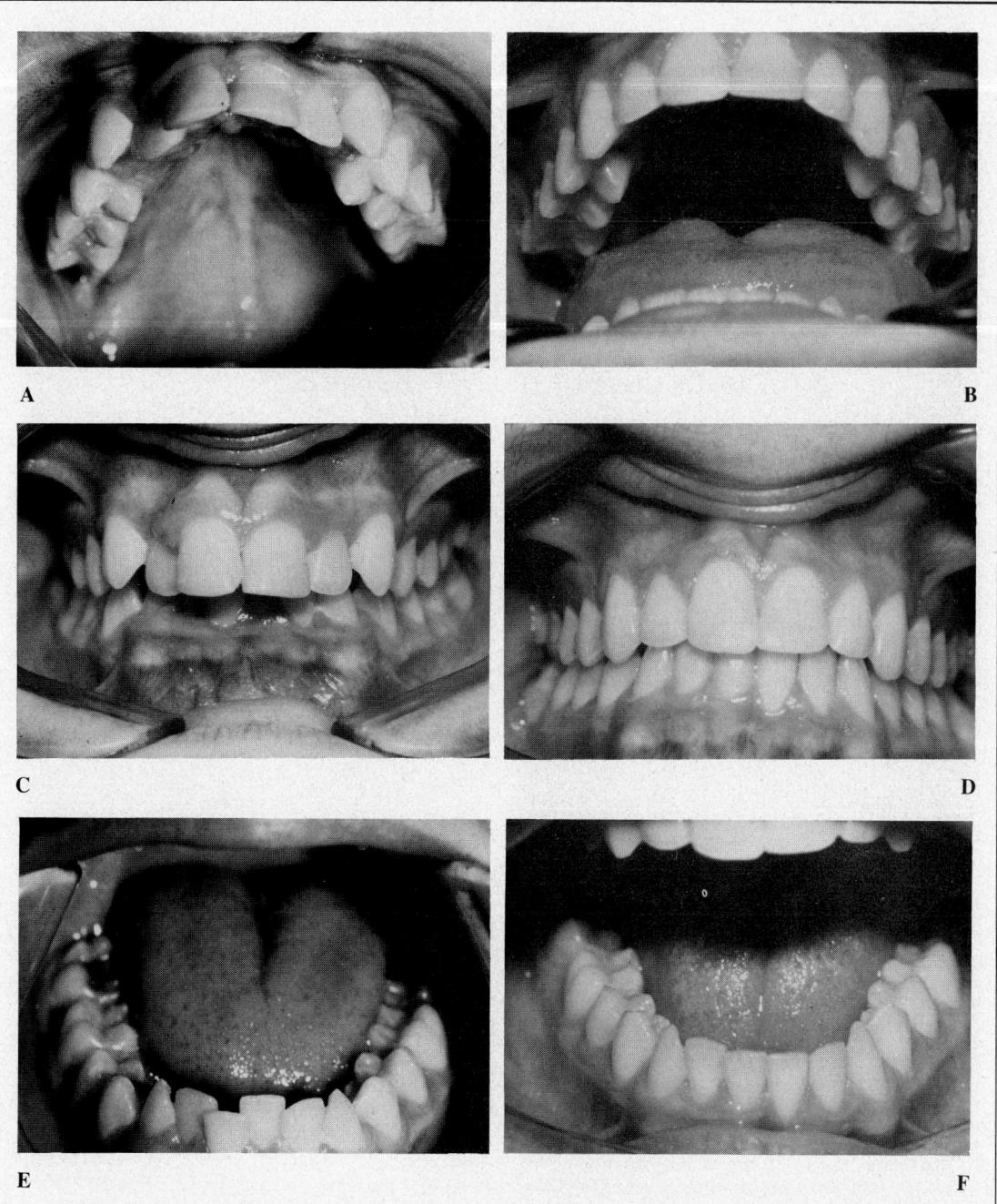

Fig. 35-23. Documentation of position of patient's teeth before and after orthodontic treatment. **A,** Initial maxillary occlusal view. **B,** Final maxillary occlusal view. **C,** Initial facial view of teeth in occlusion. **D,** Final direct anterior view of teeth in occlusion. **E,** Initial mandibular occlusal view. **F,** Final mandibular occlusal view.

Continued.

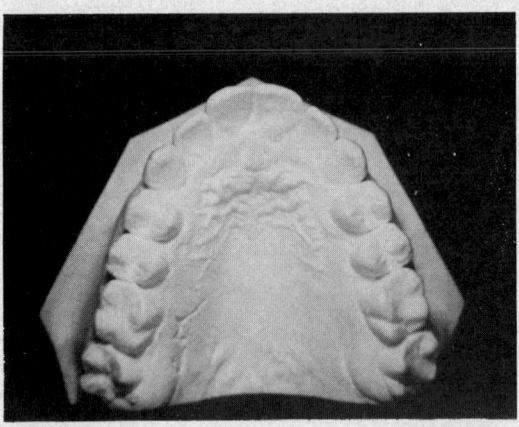

Fig. 35-24. Occlusal view of maxillary cast, following orthodontic treatment.

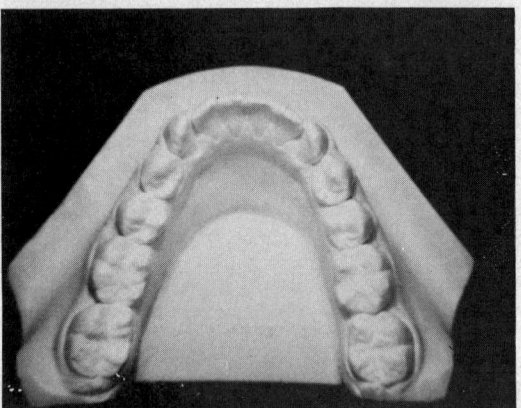

Fig. 35-25. Occlusal view of mandibular cast, following orthodontic treatment.

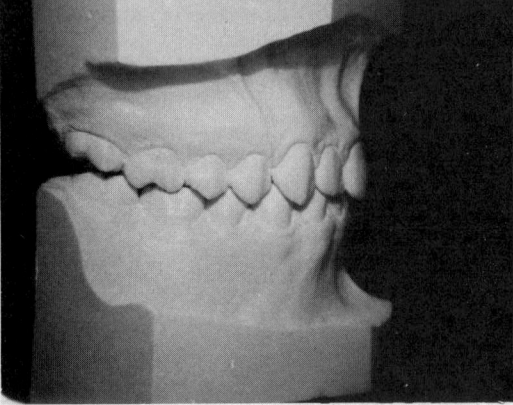

Fig. 35-26. Right lateral view of casts in occlusion following orthodontic treatment.

CONCLUSION

Student peers and professional colleagues enjoy learning from case documentations. This situation places the clinician/observer in a position to empathize with the care being delivered. Treatment options may be explored and discussed in an environment conducive to sharing past experiences and new ideas.

The clinician who presents a case documentation has the opportunity to display an aspect of his or her patient care. Fellow clinicians learn from observing the type and quality of care provided to the patient.

Practicing presenting a case documentation will be valuable experience as the student clinician enters the professional world. Maintaining standards for recording comprehensive quality care will become the responsibility of the clinician. Beyond this, sharing cases with others will be a primary area for professional contact and postgraduate education.

ACKNOWLEDGEMENTS

We wish to thank Deborah Drazek, R.D.H., for permission to publish the sample case documentation with original photographs and study models and to thank Michael R. Sabat, D.D.S., M.S., A.B.O., F.A.C.D., Lynda Sabat, R.D.H., and their patient for permission to publish the orthodontic case documentation with original photographs and study models.

ACTIVITIES

1. Listen to case documentations presented by faculty, visiting clinicians, or more advanced students.
2. Create a format for presentation to suit specific clinic needs if necessary.
3. Prepare and present a case documentation.*†
4. According to class size, present documentations in groups of five or six. Select one documentation to be presented to the entire class and/or junior class.*†

REVIEW QUESTIONS

1. List the components of a case documentation.
2. Describe how case documentation does the following:
   a. Enhances record keeping
   b. Can be used in patient education

*After the student has completed the necessary instruction on the components of a documentation, identify a patient (one or more) who presents conditions where observable tissue changes will occur. Because of the extent of procedures to be completed and the time required for follow-up, 10 weeks to a full semester may be necessary to complete the documentation.

†Evaluation. A case documentation presentation is designed primarily to demonstrate the effectiveness of performing a particular therapy. Although an aspect of the clinician's techniques and management skills will be demonstrated, a case documentation is not designed to measure the clinician's overall skills and abilities. Considering the scope of the documentation and the length of treatment, a variety of factors that may be out of the clinician's control may affect the outcome. In our experience, evaluation of the documentation presentation by providing feedback, suggestion, and support has been the most helpful and appropriate mechanism.

36 EVALUATING SUCCESS OF DENTAL HYGIENE CARE

OBJECTIVES: *The reader will be able to*

1. Explain how a philosophy of accountability for professional practice can affect a person's overall approach to providing care.
2. Identify several ways in which a dental hygienist can take account of the effectiveness of his or her professional practice, including the following:
   a. The degree to which prevention is emphasized in each day's routine
   b. The overall effect on health levels of the population group he or she serves
   c. The degree to which clinical protocols approximate nationally accepted standards
   d. Approach behaviors of patients to dental hygiene care
   e. Personal gratification and health
   f. Cost-effectiveness
   g. Participation in professional advancement
3. Integrate mechanisms for personally evaluating the quality and effectiveness of care that he or she provides as a student and as a graduate clinician.
4. Share personal convictions regarding the goals of professional practice, personal goals regarding professional life, and the future outcomes of an "accountable" approach to health care delivery.

After several years of being a student (and, typically, undergoing the concomitant financial burden), a recent graduate views the opportunity for employment as the chance to earn money, to develop a solid base for a career, and to realize many of the dreams long associated with being grown up and employed. The graduate probably feels a newfound freedom to purchase personal possessions, to travel, to start a family, and to be self-sufficient. These are understandable goals shared by most of us; the first step toward these goals is or was an exciting one for each of us.

When a clinician graduates and enters practice, the assumption is that the clinician will contribute to the well-being of patients and, in general, "make a difference" in the lives of the people who seek care from that person. The overall expectation is that care will be of the highest quality and that it will be delivered ethically. The graduate hygienist is expected to be an asset to society, certainly not a drain or detriment. In this age of consumerism, patients believe they have a right to expect competent, high-quality care. They also

believe they have the right to complain or even to sue if those expectations are not met.

Some people assume that the recent graduate not only will work hard to provide quality care but also will contribute to the well-being of the profession. The new dental hygienist is viewed as a valuable resource to help ensure that dental hygiene grows and remains a valuable career for new generations of students.

Health care professions in general have made several attempts to reconcile their individual and collective responsibilities to provide quality care with their personal goals. They may have to work long hours rather than living in relative leisure. They may have to purchase expensive equipment rather than a new house or car. Recently, they have struggled with professional obligations to listen to consumers and meet their needs. Those obligations often seem to conflict with the professional person's admitted needs for autonomy and authority. A dentist or hygienist might be thinking, "Now that I am a professional, I'm in charge. What I think and say are important." No sooner does a graduate leave the continuing recommendations and expectations of the faculty than he or she confronts the needs and expectations of patients. But if the professions once were viewed as omniscient, such is no longer the case. Dental hygiene, like the other professions, finds itself more accountable. The hygienist, whether a recent graduate or a long time member of the profession, needs to be able to identify how much he or she is contributing to the well-being of society, of the profession, and finally of himself or herself. Consumers, insurance companies, the government, family members, and the clinician's conscience will be asking the questions. Clinicians are advised to think about measures for evaluating their performance and contributions.

A sound system of accountability will include ways to answer these and other questions: (1) Why am I doing what I am doing? (2) Do I make life better for each patient who seeks care? (3) Is the care I recommend justified? (4) Do I charge reasonable, just fees for care? (5) Do I listen to the wants and needs of my patients? (6) Does the care I deliver meet up-to-date protocols? (7) Could another hygienist review my care and find it to be of impeccable quality? (8) How do I know the answers to these questions?

DEFINING GOALS

At the base of every system of accountability lies a series of goals, statements of what seems to matter in regard to achievement. These goals exist whether or not they are ever written down or expressed aloud. The process of defining and actually writing out these personal and professional goals or values can help clarify what needs to be evaluated to determine success or achievement. An exercise at the conclusion of this chapter provides one way in which these goals can be clarified and delineated for each individual.

Once a series of goals is defined, it is possible to project ways in which their achievement can be measured or at least examined. The following areas of evaluation are suggested for beginning a comprehensive program of self-evaluation.

PREVENTION ORIENTATION

Most of the literature that discusses the relative merits of prevention and treatment in erradicating disease supports prevention as the logical area of emphasis. Health care providers will be forever behind in keeping up with disease unless it can be prevented from occurring. Public health emphasizes prevention on a large scale. Clinical practice can emphasize it on a smaller scale.

If a clinician has established the value that preventing dental disease is a goal for professional practice, then the clinician may wish to document and evaluate the degree to which that orientation is apparent in daily practice. Some relatively simple measures can be recording and assessing the percentage of time spent in helping patients to care for themselves by plaque removal, routinely performing oral cancer self-examination, and adopting nutritional patterns that promote health. How many minutes per hour are spent educating the patient to prevent disease? Is time provided for measuring blood pressure to detect hypertension? Is the medical history updated at each visit? Are patients routinely evaluated for fluoride therapy and sealants?

If the vast percentage of the day is spent removing hard and soft deposits that reappear soon after the recall visit, has the clinician's goal of prevention been actualized or is it a value not yet integrated into behavior?

Effect on health levels

A more long-term measure of disease prevention is to evaluate the pattern of health needs each patient has had while receiving care. If prevention efforts are successful, disease prevalence should decrease in the clinician's patient population. If the primary etiologic factors in dental disease are avoided or controlled by the patient, the advanced incidence of dental caries, periodontal disease, and oral cancer should decrease.

It may be useful to gather and retain the assessment data relative to plaque, gingival, and bleeding indices; calculus formation; caries rate; and any other indicators of health status. A historic overview of the patient's progress in oral health each year will reveal whether the patient is developing little or no dental disease, is showing a steady recurrence of problems, or is on a rapid downhill course to tissue destruction and tooth loss.

This overview can be accomplished at a recall visit when new assessment data are gathered. Sharing the findings with the patient can provide evidence of the effectiveness of the health partnership of clinician and patient. Observing health levels (or at least the absence of signs of disease) rise and remain high over the years provides a long-term evaluation of the quality of a preventive program.

COMPARISONS WITH NATIONAL STANDARDS

Regardless of whether the daily clinical procedures are prevention oriented or directed toward treating active disease to restore health, the health care provider may find it particularly helpful to compare his or her approaches to practice and specific procedures with those published as national standards.

Standards regarding acceptable treatment practices are (1) sometimes published by professional associations, (2) discussed and reported in journals and other professional literature, and (3) presented at professional meetings and continuing education sessions.

A significant form of self-evaluation is to systematically compare clinical protocols used in practice with those that have gained general acceptance. Such an evaluation process challenges one's modes of operation, conceptual base for practice, and belief systems. It also permits the individual to challenge the national standards, and it can stimulate inquiry into improved clinical practice and involve the clinician in research efforts to validate the efficacy of any "accepted" procedure.

One method is to join a professional study club or a peer group whose function it is to investigate, test, and validate clinical protocols and assist peers in the group in integrating the agreed-on procedures into their daily practices.

Being recognized as an open, up-to-date, competent clinician among peers can carry great personal reward and satisfaction.

APPROACH BEHAVIORS OF PATIENTS

It is a simple fact that regardless of the strength of a preventive program and the degree to which national protocols are challenged or observed, little overall success can be claimed by a clinician if the patient does not continue to seek care. If patients appear and disappear, there is some indication that the health care provider needs to assess the way patients are viewed in the overall health process. Is the patient a means to an end, whether it be clinical requirements or a reasonable income? Is the patient an object of care? Does the patient feel that the health care provider respects, values, and looks forward to seeing him or her?

If the treatment files show large numbers of long-term patients who have continued to seek care over the years, a relationship has developed that the patients see as helpful and worth maintaining.

The other point of view might be examined also. What are the approach behaviors of the clinician to patients? Does the health care provider have a preconceived notion of what a patient ought to be? Does the health care provider reject patients who do not meet the expected standards of behavior, or does the health care provider see each person as valuable and worthy of care regardless of initial compliance or noncompliance with the criteria for the "ideal" patient?

PERSONAL GRATIFICATION AND HEALTH

An annual physical can be a way of measuring success. If the health professional's own health includes such elements as varicose veins; slumped shoulders; chronic headaches; regular use of drugs for indigestion, anxiety, insomnia, or "pep"; fatigue; and hostility, the "health" professional may need to carefully examine the relationship of clinical practice to these problems. Successful practice should allow time for relaxation, pleasure, exercise, and a broadening understanding of life and the surrounding world, and it should be a source of pleasure rather than a daily drudgery. Physical and mental health reflect the degree to which the day's focus and activities stimulate gratification or anxiety.

The very process of evaluating annually the success of the preventive program, short- and long-term health progress of patients, compliance with accepted standards of practice, and approach behaviors of patients can produce a picture of gratification or dissatisfaction. One bottom line question is: Do the process and outcome of what I am doing with my life bring me gratification? If the answer is yes, the self-evaluation can bring a renewed spirit for the continuation of practice. If the answer is no, the clinician may need to identify what kind of change is necessary.

COST EFFECTIVENESS

In an economy that is based on competition, one element that is not easily ignored is the evaluation of the cost-effectiveness of practice. Providing the highest quality health care services at a cost that is greater than the income generated from these services guarantees a short-lived practice. The basic costs of a health care facility (rent, insurance, utilities, supplies, salaries, etc.) must be covered by generated income. Therefore a complete evaluation of success should include an analysis of the ledger. A practice that does not break even or generate profit will need professional analysis of its operation and suggestions for change.

Cost-effectiveness implies more than generating sufficient income. Its primary connotation in terms of accountability to the profession and the public is the degree to which the expended health dollar actually improves health. Do patients pay money every 6 months for a slow immersion into advanced periodontal disease or eventual full mouth reconstruction, or does the money they pay ensure the restoration and maintenance of health over the years? The answer to this question brings the health care provider back to the evaluation of prevention effectiveness.

PARTICIPATION IN PROFESSIONAL ADVANCEMENT

Closely tied to monetary success is professional advancement. Many people see their profession as a career ladder. Over the years following graduation, they acquire experience and advanced education so that they can assume new responsibilities and meet new challenges, either in the same job setting or in a series of different jobs. Goals can be set and measured along a pathway for advancement and opportunities.

A second aspect of professional advancement is tied to ensuring that the profession of dental hygiene is nurtured and guided as it changes over the decades. This usually involves a commitment to association activities at the local, state, national, or international levels. It is easy to acquire a degree and use that degree for personal advancement. However, in a "loner" profession such as dental hygiene where interaction with other hygienists is frequently sparse, it also is easy to lose track of what is happening to the profession through educational, regulatory, political, and legal changes. Five or ten years after gradua-

tion, the profession can look quite different in terms of the security it provides, its attractiveness to new applicants, and its ability to provide quality care. An accountable dental hygienist should be able to point to specific contributions he or she has made to help guide and sustain the profession.

CONCLUSION

Each area of evaluation helps the dental hygienist assess his or her individual contribution to the quality of life—his or her own life, the profession's and of course that of each patient and thus of society.

A well-planned, thoughtful approach to this process may make dental hygiene a truly rewarding career and a source of lifelong fulfillment, or it may be a means for planning career changes and personal growth in new areas.

A format that can be used for generating personal and professional goals and for displaying evaluation findings from the year(s) is suggested on page 711.

ACTIVITIES

1. Using the evaluation of success format presented on page 766 define personal and professional practice goals that are, in your opinion, signs of success. Then form groups of three to share those goals. Note similarities and differences in goals and values among the members of the small groups. Suggest ways in which these goals could be evaluated in practice on a regular, periodic basis.
2. Analyze the degree to which prevention-oriented procedures make up the clinical efforts in your daily practice as a student.
3. As a student, conduct a year-long or a 1-semester system of accountability that measures the extent to which personal and professional goals are approximated or achieved.
4. Invite representatives of the local or state hygienists' association to discuss how members and leaders contribute to improving the profession.

REVIEW QUESTIONS

1. How can a philosophy of accountability of professional practice affect one's overall approach to providing care?
2. Identify seven ways in which a health professional can measure effectiveness or success in practice.
3. What can a health care provider do if he or she sees little evidence of success or gratification in professional or personal life?

Defining and Evaluating Personal and Profession Goals

Use the following format for recording your response to questions 1 to 7.

	1	2	3	Question 4	5	6	7
PROFESSIONAL GOALS:							
PERSONAL GOALS:							

1. List each goal that is important for your sense of success (short- and long-term).
2. Rank each goal you have listed according to its relative importance and significance in your determination of success.
3. Give the earliest date you will be able to evaluate your progress toward each goal.
4. How will you know progress has been achieved (what is your measure)?
5. How will you know when each goal has actually been achieved?
6. When do you expect that each goal will be achieved?
7. What roadblocks to achievement of each goal can you identify? How can you reduce them?

37 EXPECTATIONS, ACTUALITIES, AND STRATEGIES FOR CHANGE IN DENTAL HYGIENE PRACTICE

OBJECTIVES: *The reader will be able to*

1. Recognize the need to systematically apply the philosophy and procedures of dental hygiene care to a practice setting.
2. Identify strategies for integrating dental hygiene care into a practice setting in which:
   a. The practice has never had a dental hygienist on the team.
   b. The practice has had a hygienist for many years who has established well-accepted procedures for the practice.
   c. The practice has had a series of dental hygienists over the years who have integrated a variety of different approaches in varying degrees.
3. Set personal priorities for integrating various aspects of dental hygiene care into dental practice.
4. Describe the positive and negative aspects of developing a dental hygiene practice.

Many clinicians find their first employment in a private practice or group clinic. The recent graduate may encounter an ideal situation that makes the transition from school to work an easy one. Such a practice would ensure that the clinician can provide the broadest range of responsibilities, tapping to the fullest extent what he or she learned. Ideal protocols may be followed, helping the new clinician feel confident about how care is delivered and the practice is managed. The clinician may feel appreciated, welcome, involved, respected.

It is more likely that any employment situation will be less than ideal. Even a carefully selected site will have surprises and disappointments. How can a clinician/employee work well within a practice that could adopt more up-to-date protocols? How can he or she work with other employees who present interpersonal challenges? How can he or she relate well to the employer or office manager?

Some of the challenges or difficulties emerge the first day on the job. Others can occur after months, years, or even decades.

The purpose of this chapter is to help clinicians be aware of potential problems that can occur when he or she attempts to "fit in" or when an ideal employment site begins to go sour. A second purpose is to provide possible strategies that can be used to make the best of every situation. This chapter consists of four scenarios. They are stories of successes, of learning experiences, of disappointment, of resolution. Read them carefully. Discuss them with fellow students and faculty. Identify alternative responses that might improve the outcome or that could be fruitless.

After years in practice, the needs of a dental hygienist may change, bringing difficult decisions. A hygienist may decide to assume more responsibility for the business aspects of a practice and adopt a situation where he or she works with a dentist as an independent contractor. Or the hygienist may be placed in a situation where working unsupervised appears to be the best option. While the legality of each of these situations differs from state to state, it is important to assess the opportunities and problems associated with each.

"REAL LIFE" SCENARIOS

To offer suggestions for addressing these possibilities, four scenarios or monologues are provided for review and discussion.

Although each of the monologues is fictitious, together they represent the collective experiences and suggestions of dental hygienists who have returned to the educational environment to discuss their successes and their failures, their values, and their commitment. A helpful sequel to this chapter may be to invite recent graduates and dental hygienists who have had years of experience, preferably in a variety of practice settings, to discuss what they encountered in dental hygiene practice and to answer questions regarding the implementation of dental hygiene care in dental practice.

Scenario 1: I remember the first weeks of practicing in the office of Dr. J. It felt so good to be out of school and really working in a dental practice as a dental hygienist. Dr. J. had given me a great deal of freedom to schedule my patients so that I could build up speed and ensure that each patient received high-quality care. Quality was a very big item with Dr. J. I also had a great deal of freedom in selecting instruments, so one of my first official acts was to order eight new sets of scalers and curettes so that I could improve on the few instruments that were left from the previous dental hygienist. The bill for the instruments was quite a shock to both the employer and to me, but Dr. J. seemed more than willing to go along with my suggestions as long as clean teeth and smooth roots could be accomplished.

For the first month Dr. J. checked every tooth surface with an explorer and a probe to find any remaining deposits. It reminded me a great deal of the early days in school, and I found myself praying that my clinical skill had developed sufficiently so that little if anything would be found. There were, of course, a few remaining pieces of calculus or root roughness found now and then, but it soon appeared that I had met the dentist's standards of excellence. Soon the careful checks of each surface were reduced to spot checks and a friendly conversation with the patient about the progress of care. Occasionally the patient was asked directly for his or her opinion as to whether I had done a good job.

The message became clear that the highest priority for this dentist was the clean tooth at the end of the dental hygiene appointment. As my speed picked up, I decided that instead of reducing the time of the dental hygiene appointments, I would begin to integrate other kinds of dental hygiene procedures into this new free

time. I decided to polish all the amalgams over a series of recall visits so that eventually all the amalgams would be smooth and less likely to retain plaque and stain. I began to institute a much more thorough plaque control program, as the patients regularly returned with high plaque counts and seemed more willing to have me clean it off than to remove it themselves on a daily basis. I started teaching all the patients the oral cancer self-examination to round out the prevention program in the practice. I even dared to discuss the possibility of some heavy smokers reducing their use of tobacco to reverse some of the beginning signs of tissue change, such as nicotine stomatitis.

It never occurred to me that the dentist might not agree that this series of decisions was appropriate or desirable. I had wanted to integrate this new approach as a sort of surprise for the dentist that would make for an even better feeling about my performance. I think what triggered the negative reaction was the complaint of a long-standing patient that he did not have time to sit around and practice flossing in a mirror or feeling the inside of his own cheeks. The patient hadn't seemed hostile during the appointment; I noticed nervousness but thought that was just because it was a new procedure. Anyway, the patient complained to the dentist, who wasn't fully aware of what I was doing. The dentist seemed to join sides with the patient and basically told me to cut out all that frivolous stuff and get back to scaling teeth. The dentist wanted to know whether I was charging the patients for all this "prevention"; I had to tell the dentist I wasn't because I hadn't wanted anything to block the patient's acceptance of the procedure.

That decision and my decision to forego discussion of my plans with the dentist were grave errors in this case. The dentist decided I was giving away my time that could be used to clean and plane teeth, which generated income for the office. The dentist also, it turned out, really didn't have much faith in prevention as a reasonable approach to dental disease. The philosophy that emerged in the somewhat heated discussion of how I was spending my time was that dental disease was basically inevitable, that all the dental health education in the world wouldn't reverse that trend, and that the most efficient way to spend time was to clean those teeth every 6 months. The final comment was that the practice could not afford to lose patients such as the one who had complained and that I was to cease and desist from my fancy prevention techniques and get back to basics.

Back to basics it was. My appointment times were reduced to 45 minutes per appointment. I was allowed to bring patients back for additional scaling or other technical procedures, but not for extensive plaque control. There was a lot less agitation in the office with this edict, but somehow I felt as though I had missed an opportunity to integrate some prevention into an otherwise (in my opinion) fine clinical practice by having made some critical mistakes in integrating the changes. The two basic mistakes seemed to be the unilateral decision I made to include those procedures and ignoring the possibility that the patients' and the dentist's philosophies might be quite different from mine. The other contributing factor I had ignored was the financial implications of my decision.

Confronting this same kind of situation, what do you think could have been done differently to make the change more positive? What do you think one can do now to help improve the situation? Would you continue in this practice?

Scenario 2: My first position as a dental hygienist was in a practice in which there had been an entire string of dental hygienists, each of whom had stayed for 1 or 2 years and then left. The dentist seemed quite accepting of the fact that no dental hygienist would ever have the commitment to stay and really develop within the dental team. It must have appeared that dental hygienists were born vagabonds who came and left after a short period of time. The dentist just wanted to have a dental hygienist to make sure that the recall program continued. The busy restorative schedule in the practice left no time for the dentist to perform routine prophylaxes.

A highlight of the practice was that I was involved in the initial examination of the patient. The dentist was quite willing to delegate the complete head and neck examination and the preparation of all dental chartings and radiographic series. All new patients were given a full 30-minute initial visit for the preparation of these assessment findings, which did not seem like much at first. As I was able to pick up speed, I realized that the time was ample as long as I was fairly efficient in my procedures. After having talked with some of my classmates who were expected to fit it all into 10 minutes, I began to see how "generous" this time allotment was. I really enjoyed performing the initial procedures as well as completing the recall scaling and polishing.

I had noticed at my interview that there was an autoclave in the laboratory but that only surgical instruments seemed to be prepared for that sterilization method. The tray of blue solution in the dental hygiene operatory was filled with explorers, scalers, and mirrors—a certain indication of the standard protocol for "sterilizing" instruments. I also had failed to see any oxygen supply in the office, and there was no fire extinguisher in the laboratory or anywhere, for that matter. I made a mental note to address these concerns early in my employment.

I had the notion that either I could just start using the autoclave to make my point as to how I wanted to sterilize my instruments or I could discuss the situation with the employer and with the other members of the dental team, especially those who were in charge of operating it for surgical instruments. I suppose in some instances I could have chosen the former option and just gone ahead, but something told me that I should discuss it with the people involved. I think it was the sense of ownership of the laboratory equipment I saw in the eyes of the dental assistant who prepared the instrument trays. This person apparently had never had anything to do with "hygiene instruments," and it appeared that there was a set schedule for using the autoclave.

My decision to discuss it was wise. I swallowed hard and used the cold disinfectant solution for the first morning of my employment there. I kept telling myself that this is the procedure used in many practices, and that I could reduce the number of microorganisms if I used fresh solution, few instruments, and an adequate soak time. I knew I was compromising my principles to use this technique, but I felt in the long run I could avoid many more opportunities for cross-contamination if I was able to reach my goal of using the autoclave for all my patients without alienating the staff. At lunchtime the dental assistant placed a batch of instruments into the autoclave, and we went to lunch. I asked the assistant if the dental hygienists had ever used the autoclave for their instruments. The answer was no. I then asked whether it would cause any problems if I used the autoclave. There was a skeptical look, but the reply was that as long as it didn't interfere with the regular schedule of use for dental instruments, there would be no problem. We clarified what that schedule was. I made certain it was understood that I would be happy to autoclave my own instruments at other times, and the dental assistant agreed that there would be no major problem.

That afternoon, I continued to use the disinfecting solution, hoping it would be for the last time. At the end of the day, I asked to speak with my employer. Dr. P expressed confidence in my work, which I appreciated, and said half-heartedly that it would be nice if I decided to stay for a while in the practice. Dr. P was surprised when I said that I looked forward to a long working relationship. I felt the beginning of closure in our conversation and decided to ask the big question: "Would you see any problems in my using the autoclave for sterilizing my instruments?" Dr. P frowned a bit and said that she really had no other qualms about using the autoclave for dental hygiene but that she wasn't sure how the dental assistant would respond to having a whole new batch of instruments to run several times per day, and she felt the dental assistant wanted control over the autoclave, as other people using it had seemed to increase the frequency of malfunction. I explained to Dr. P that I had sensed that problem and had discussed it with the dental assistant. I shared with Dr. P the fact that the dental assistant and I had agreed on a schedule and the fact that I could autoclave my own instruments. The next day the new system began, and the tray of blue solution was no longer used. Everything in the dental hygiene operatory could either be autoclaved or was disposable.

Several months later I brought up the issue of the oxygen and the fire extinguisher to the dentist. I felt it was important to move slowly with my suggestions, or the team might feel I was out to criticize and improve rather than to join what was already a solid dental team. The dentist responded fairly well to my suggestion that when funds were available we ought to purchase some emergency equipment—at least an oxygen unit and a fire extinguisher. Action wasn't immediate, but a few weeks later a purchase order for one item was sent in by the dentist. The second item was purchased 2 months later. We even had a session on how to use the equipment and set down some procedures in anticipation of an emergency situation. It seemed to me that I had been quite successful in bringing about meaningful change in the practice.

What I hadn't noticed was that a change had occurred in me as well. When I told Dr. P that I might want to have a long-standing relationship with the practice, I wasn't sure if I was being entirely truthful. Now that I have become a part of the practice and feel comfortable with the people I work with, I have decided that I really do want to remain in clinical practice with this team of people. I guess the proof of this is that I started working in that position 10 years ago, and I'm still there.

What would you have done in this situation?

Scenario 3: I was really lucky to find a practice in which the dentist was young and interested in adding a dental hygienist as the practice grew. I had all kinds of ideas about integrating dental hygiene into a clinical practice and really did not want to have to follow in the footsteps of a dental hygienist who had established all kinds of patterns and expectations over the years that might conflict with my ideas. I was certain that because the dentist was young, there would be great opportunity for innovation, especially in performing expanded functions such as local anesthesia and placement of restorations. I wanted to add myofunctional therapy and conduct a mini-research study of the efficacy of using a behavioral approach to modification of the swallowing habit. Somehow I felt that such therapy often failed because the educational techniques failed, and that this

was true for dental health education in general. A small clinical study over many years could provide answers to those questions.

I remember having big plans and being excited about my new position. My first letdown was seeing the operatory in which I was to work. The equipment was ancient. There was an old belt-driven engine that squeaked relentlessly, an old cuspidor, and a bulb syringe and glass of water for irrigating the mouth. There was no high-speed evacuation and no stool to sit on. The comforting factor was that the dental chair had been partially converted from the old style to a lounge-type chair. However, I still had to pump it up with my foot and figure out all the levers for adjusting the back. My first reaction was one of grief and then of anger. The dentist had said he would equip an operatory for me, but I never thought it would be with this kind of equipment. I decided to confront Dr. W with the problem of my expectations versus his. At first, he was a bit defensive, saying he couldn't imagine how such equipment would be a problem. When I discussed how difficult it would be to work without evacuation, without a tri-syringe, and without a stool, he admitted that he simply could not go any deeper into debt to buy modern dental equipment. He wanted to add a dental hygienist to the team but couldn't add the luxury equipment that was necessary for ideal practice. What surprised me the most was how little he seemed to know about the needs of a dental hygienist in providing services for patients. The idea of a high-speed evacuation system for dental hygiene care was a new one to him. Also, he hadn't seemed to generalize what he had learned about sit-down dentistry to dental hygiene. It seemed as though all the guidelines for efficient, relatively comfortable practice were not applicable to a dental hygienist.

Overcoming that first shock took quite a while. Plus there was the need to set up a reasonable recall system, to order appropriate supplies (sparingly to help balance the budget), to develop a system for appointing patients, and to set down even basic protocols regarding when a dental hygienist becomes involved in dental treatment. The dentist and I spent long hours discussing whether a dental hygienist *could* record the medical history and then we discussed whether a dental hygienist *should* record the medical history, even if the skill was well developed.

Procedure by procedure, we worked out the protocols. I was glad that I had a solid rationale for each of the procedures I was to perform and that I had good skills in performing them. Step by step, we integrated dental hygiene into the practice. It required almost 1 year to accomplish this. The actual procedures were moved into place very slowly. The dentist did not wish to rush into anything, and he was very concerned about the patients' acceptance of a dental hygienist. He himself had never had dental care from a dental hygienist.

Through all of these slow developments, I could see progress, but I couldn't help remembering my dream to use the expanded functions I had learned and to begin my small clinical study of myofunctional therapy.

I first discussed my hopes with the dentist after I had been there for 18 months. He did seem to trust me now. I decided to inquire about beginning the myofunctional therapy study first, as that would be slow to start and he didn't seem to have much problem with detecting malocclusion and referring patients to orthodontists for care. I described what I wanted to do. The reply was a solid no. His rationale was basically that he didn't trust those kinds of efforts, that he had been taught in school that the only way to modify swallowing habits was with long-term orthodontic treatment, and then even then, the techniques seemed to fail. It became apparent that there was no point in discussing it as an appropriate project. Such an idea was ludicrous to Dr. W.

I returned to traditional practice for another few months and decided to approach the topic of giving my own anesthesia as needed prior to root planing and curettage. So far, the dentist had been performing the pain control procedures at the beginning of appointments where local anesthesia was indicated. I had learned and practiced local anesthesia in school and had received high praise from the dental hygiene faculty, the oral surgery faculty, and from periodontics faculty who had witnessed my technique and who had quizzed me on rationale, anatomy, pharmacology, and complications. I was careful to keep my skills up-to-date on all the expanded functions, including anesthesia, by taking every refresher course that was available at the local university and through my local dental hygiene component. I served as a clinical instructor 4 hours per week, working with the course director demonstrating and observing these procedures. I really knew my stuff.

Again I tried to approach the topic as a suggestion for modification of my functions in the practice and pointed out to Dr. W that my performing the anesthesia procedure would make scheduling for his patients a good deal easier. He commented that it was really essential that a person who was specially trained be ready to respond to an emergency if local anesthesia procedures should trigger such an event. I pointed out to him that he routinely left patients who had received an injection to be monitored by a dental assistant and that the first few moments following an injection are those during which an untoward response such as toxic or allergic reaction is most likely to occur. I told him about my background and my abilities and suggested that I would certainly be as able as the dental assistant to monitor signs and symptoms and that I had had a full course in emergency procedures, including CPR. My defense was offensive. There was no further discussion.

I retreated to traditional dental hygiene procedures. Fortunately, there was a great deal of diversity among the procedures I could perform, and I derived satisfaction from the manner in which I had been able to integrate so much into a practice, even if it had taken months and months to do so.

Based on the two previous reactions to my requests, I was, of course, hesitant to ask about restorative procedures. I wanted to be able to place the rubber dam and the matrix, place temporary restorations as needed, and place and carve amalgam and tooth-colored restorations. The dental practice was building, and the appointment book was filled for 3 weeks in advance. The practice was making a better income, and I was rewarded with new equipment for my operatory. I was asked to select the kind I wanted from three basic designs. Still, somehow I still wanted to be able to practice expanded functions. I kept thinking that if I could add restorative functions to my list of procedures, perhaps local anesthesia could be added eventually. When I inquired, I was informed that the dental assistant would be the one to perform those skills if the dentist ever decided to delegate them. Dr. W did not feel it was within the scope of practice of the dental hygienist to become involved with restorative procedures. He felt it was imperative that the dental hygienist perform preventive procedures, as was originally intended for the dental hygienist.

I am still practicing traditional dental hygiene in an efficient, well-designed, modern clinical practice in which dental hygiene procedures as they have been defined for decades are valued and fully integrated into daily routines. I know I will probably never have the freedom to do the things I had hoped to do in research projects and with anesthesia and restorative procedures. If that day ever does arrive, it will have been so long since I used those skills that I will probably not be able to prove my ability. I have to make a decision regarding whether I should stay or try to find a position in which I can do what I really want to do. I keep remembering what my boss said regarding the matter of local anesthesia: "If you really want to do all these things, why don't you go to dental school?"

Scenario 4: My choice was a difficult one. I was forced after 16 years of clinical practice in a dental office to look for alternatives. I had worked for the same dentist from the day I passed my licensure examinations. I knew every patient by name and watched babies grow up to be young adults. I went to patients' funerals and weddings. I knew those people, and I thought I knew the dentist.

Things were going more slowly in the practice. The

new children did not need extensive restorative care—something for which we were genuinely grateful. It looked as though we were winnning the prevention battle. But as the practice aged, Dr. S's appointment book was not booked as far ahead and his days were quite easy compared to the humming activity of the 1970s. It was a gradual change, but it happened. My salary was not increased for 5 years, and I was required to take my vacation when he took his—which became less frequent and of shorter duration. Then we dropped medical insurance. I kept hoping that Dr. S would try some new ideas to bring life to the practice. It seemed that his colleagues were fresher in their approaches to drawing patients to the practice. Finally he went to a practice management seminar that was coming to town. I breathed a sigh of relief and wished him well.

When he returned, he was full of ideas for the practice, including some clever ways to attract patients. He seemed incredibly happy, but something was different in the way he approached me and the office manager. One week after his return he left the office without saying goodbye. The next day was Saturday, and I was greeted by a special delivery letter. In it was a check for 2 weeks' pay and a brief typed note that thanked me for my years of service. It added that he could no longer afford to pay me my salary and that he had opted to hire a dental hygienist right out of school who was willing to work for $20 less per day. This apparently was one of the fine ideas learned at the seminar.

It was impossible then to find a job as a hygienist without working for peanuts. I tried to swallow my pride and say I could take a 30% cut in my salary. But the thought brought tears of rage to my eyes. How was I going to live? I filed for unemployment and collected it while I sorted out my anger and my plans. At least Dr. S did not contest the unemployment. But I still felt like a discarded piece of dental equipment. I missed my patients in that practice, and I resented that they would be receiving care from someone new. I hoped I would never lay eyes on the hygienist or ever again on Dr. S. I was betrayed. I seemed to have counted for nothing.

I took stock of my savings and visited a business management consultant. I told her I wanted to set up my own practice—a few blocks from Dr. S. There was a small office suite with two treatment rooms available there. With her help, I developed a business plan, and I was able to secure a sizable loan that helped me buy used dental equipment. I placed announcements in the local newspapers and used all of my connections in the community to ensure that people knew I was setting up my own business and would love to provide them with dental hygiene care. I used the idea of the "gentle first step" in seeking dental care to attract patients who have the financial means (usually through insurance) to obtain care but who are frightened of the prospect of visiting the dentist.

I lost money for 8 months. I watched my loan and my savings dwindle as I worked as hard as I could to draw in sufficient numbers of patients to pay the rent, utilities, a competent staff person, and the supply bill. It was very difficult to compete with the low fees dentists charge for dental hygiene care. The amount of time needed to provide complete dental hygiene care clearly is worth more than we were charging at Dr S's. In my practice, there is no "flexible fee" associated with restorative care to make up the difference in a practice that relies upon dental hygiene services for its income. For 2 months I broke even. I kept working to draw in patients, give them the best care possible with the most flexible appointment times, and develop reasonable relations with the local dental community.

Putting all my energy into building the practice actually helped me get over the anger of my dismissal. It also helped that so many of the patients I treated at Dr. S's felt as strongly about me as I did about them. They came to me for dental hygiene care, even though nearly all of them went to him for annual dental exams and whatever other dental care they needed. A few went to other dentists, saying that they just didn't feel the same way about him after what he had done. One even described it as unethical for him to fire me.

Relations with area dentists were not so easy. I can understand how they would want to be cohesive and protect the right of a dentist to fire an employee. They also wanted to help protect Dr. S's good reputation and, by extension, their own. At first, they tried just about everything to keep me from opening my practice, including putting pressure on the bank to turn down my loan and trying to influence the State Board to say I could not see any of Dr. S's patients; they even tried to say I could not legally expose radiographs or use fluoride (a prescription agent) in the care of my patients. Fortunately, another hygienist who footed most of the legal battle costs had won decisions regarding those issues within the past 6 months. My financial costs were relatively minor in fighting off the efforts. But the emotional costs were high, and it was a very hard time for me.

The way I overcame it was to meet with one dentist at a time, usually over lunch. I would take the dentist to a nice restaurant near my practice, introduce him or her to my philosophy of dental hygiene care, present the forms I would use for data gathering and for transmitting information to the dentist after each visit, and discuss what special information he or she would like from me when I referred a patient. I tried to be disarmingly charming and impeccably professional. I made certain that the care I would deliver would be "by the book," meeting all accepted standards based on current research. I tried to be confident and sincere in my request for suggestions. I ended up by asking how the dentist felt about my treating patients from his or her practice. I then asked if he or she would like to receive new patients from me.

I worked hard to draw in people who had been unwilling to visit the dentist, and I made certain that they were referred promptly for their dental care. I spread around the referrals among the dentists whose work I knew was good. I complimented dentists on the quality of dental work I saw when one of their patients visited me. I worked hard to develop a supportive relationship. That was what pushed me from losing money to eventually making money. I don't think I will ever really prosper financially in my practice, but I certainly have much higher job security than I did as an employee. I am not at another person's mercy. I do, however, have to work very hard and concentrate continually on building the practice and making it even better than it is. I "stick to the knitting," ensuring that it gets all the attention it needs.

I also am more aware of how I treat my staff. I am careful to remember to give them the same respect and consideration I had hoped for in my employment situation. I have a strong sense of pride in what I have accomplished. I'll probably finish my years in dental hygiene in this, my own practice. The irony is that I never intended to be an independent businessperson when I selected dental hygiene. I wanted to work with a dentist. But I also expected commitment from my employer and a sense of self-worth that is nurtured by people who respect me for what I do well. Probably the hard times of the early 1980s had more to do with Dr. S's decision to fire me, but there should have been more between us than financial considerations. If I ever am in a position to work "for" a dentist, I'm going to be mighty careful to find one who seems to value me as a person and as a contributor to the goodwill of the office. I'll still give my very best, I'll just be more cautious.

How do you feel about the hygienist's experience with her employer dentist? What would you have done in her situation? What risks did the hygienist take in setting up her own practice? What are the problems she continues to face? Would you feel comfortable in this situation?

ACTIVITIES

1. Discuss each of the scenarios, analyzing the choice of actions the dental hygienist had in each of the situations and the appropriateness of the action selected. Focus on the likely outcomes of alternative choices of action. Place yourself in the position of the dentist in each case, and project how the dentist may be seeing the actions and attitudes of the dental hygienist.
2. Were the dentists in the scenarios male or female? Is it confusing to picture a dentist as a woman? Did you picture the dental hygiensts to be women? Which one might have been a male hygienist? Why would you make that assumption? How does sex role bias affect the way we interpret and anticipate behavior, regardless of the professional role?
3. Set the personal priorities of what you hope to accomplish and what you expect to find in the "ideal" dental practice. Share those expectations with a small group of classmates. Explain how you will make a choice regarding whether to try to change or to agree to live with less than ideal conditions. Ask others in the group how they would feel if they had a dental practice and you were to implement the approaches to change that you feel would work best in solving the less than ideal conditions.
4. Role-play a variety of encounters with hypothetical employers and patients regarding attempts to change the following:
   a. Integration of preventive measures into a practice
   b. Integration of additional assessment procedures into the scope of practice of the dental hygienist
   c. Integration of expanded functions into the scope of practice of the dental hygienist
   d. Procedures regarding sterilization, instrument purchase, office cleanliness, and nonfunctional equipment
5. Invite hygienists from the area to discuss how they succeeded or struggled to integrate comprehensive dental hygiene care into their work settings.
6. Search back issues of *RDH* magazine for articles about independent contracting and independent practice and how hygienists breaking new ground in these areas felt they had succeeded or struggled.

SUGGESTED RESPONSES

CHAPTER 1

1. The patient is viewed as a partner in care, involved extensively in decision making and in the self-care components necessary for health.
2. A faculty member has had an opportunity to compare expectations with reality and to develop an educational approach that blends the ideal with the real. Individual faculty members differ according to their clinical, conceptual, and futuristic perceptions of practice.
3. a. Dental practice acts define the scope and limitations of dental practice and dental hygiene practice in each jurisdiction (usually defined by state boundaries). In many instances they differ widely from one another, resulting in significantly different roles and responsibilities for dental hygienists, depending on the jurisdictions in which they reside.
    b. The practice acts often limit programs within their jurisdiction to include only those skills that are legally allowable for practice in that jurisdiction. Thus programs differ widely in the functions and responsibilities they may legally include.
4. Legalization of independent dental hygiene practice would allow entrepreneurial hygienists to open their own practices and perform the full array of legal dental hygiene services learned in dental hygiene school. It would open practice opportunities for hygienists currently unable to find work as employees in solo dental practices, where only 42% of dentists use dental hygiene services. It could perhaps extend dental hygiene, and eventually dental care, to a population group that currently does not seek care because of fear.
5. *Professional culture* refers to those characteristics that are unique to a given profession. It refers to the attitudes, knowledge base, functions, demographics, and other features that make that profession distinct from others.

CHAPTER 2

1. Should; turning the light on and off wears out the switch and causes the lamp to burn out more quickly
2. a. Tilt chair back
    b. Lower back of chair to supine position
    c. Adjust headrest
    d. Raise chair as necessary to proper height
    e. Rotate chair if necessary
3. To direct a stream of water; to direct a stream of air; and to spray air and water in an area
4. Become unscrewed and fall off
5. Most traditional dental hygiene functions require slow-speed torque; high speed will be less effective and could be dangerous
6. The angle needs cleaning to remove abrasive and other foreign elements from the gears
7. The clinician's feet are flat on the floor and thighs are parallel to the floor; the abdominal rest should fit snugly below the rib cage as the clinician inclines forward
8. The assistant's eye level is approximately 5 inches above the clinician's eye level and thighs are parallel to the floor
9. An oil soap to clean and soften the material
10. Ultrasonic cleaner (for removing debris) and autoclave and dry heat oven (for sterilizing)

CHAPTER 3

1. Except for surgeons, few other health professionals come in closer contact with patients for longer periods of time than the dental clinician. The oral cavity is abundant in organisms that are potentially pathogenic. The close physical contact with the patient, the nature of the work performed, and the instruments used all contribute to the clinician's susceptibility to infectious disease. The air, saliva, blood, and aerosols from instrumentation or breathing are potentially dangerous. The clinician must be aware of sources of infection and take precautions to protect himself or herself, the operatory environment, and patients from the spread of infectious organisms.
2. a. *Mycobacterium tuberculosis:* tuberculosis; indirect transmission from inanimate sources or respiratory droplets
    b. *Treponema pallidum:* syphilis; indirect contact, break in skin, or contact with lesion
    c. *Clostridium tetani:* tetanus; airborne transmission by means of dust-carried spores
    d. Respiratory virus (e.g., adenovirus): respiratory tract infection; respiratory droplet, aerosol
    e. Hepatitis B virus: serum hepatitis; oral or fecal

route, saliva or respiratory droplets, or direct transmission by means of contact with contaminated blood

f. Rubeola virus: measles; respiratory secretions, saliva, blood

3. a. True f. True k. True
   b. False g. True
   c. True h. True
   d. False i. True
   e. True j. False

4. Sanitation: the mechanical and/or chemical cleaning of an object
   Disinfection: the destruction of bacteria and other microorganisms by means of chemicals or heat
   Sterilization: total destruction of all forms of microbial life

5. Start with an initial scrub that includes a thorough lathering of all surfaces using a brush, soap that may or may not contain an antiseptic, and copious amounts of running water; all jewelry should be removed; the initial scrub should be a series of three latherings, each followed by a thorough rinsing; the initial scrub should last 2 to 3 minutes

6. Steam under pressure, dry heat, ethylene oxide gas, chemical vapor sterilizer, and chemical solutions (glutaraldehyde only)

7. Steam under pressure: 121° C (250° F) at 15 to 20 psi for 15 to 20 minutes
   Dry heat: 160° C (320° F) for a minimum of 1 hour
   Ethylene oxide gas: 49° C (120° F) for 2 to 3 hours *or* room temperature for 12 hours
   Chemical vapor sterilizer: 127° C (260° F) at 20 to 25 psi for 30 minutes
   Chemical solution (glutaraldehyde): room temperature for 6 ¾ to 10 hours, assuming that the chemical concentration is optimal and the instruments have been properly prepared

8. Tri-syringe: Sterilize tips if possible; wipe the unsterilized portion twice with an effective tuberculocidal disinfectant, using two separate gauze sponges
   Handpiece: Sterilize if possible in the autoclave, chemical vapor sterilizer, or ethylene oxide sterilizer (depending on the manufacturer's instructions); if it cannot be sterilized by an approved method, it must be carefully scrubbed twice with a tuberculocidal disinfectant, using two separate gauze sponges

CHAPTER 4

1. The complete dental record is a medicolegal record that provides the information necessary to safely and knowledgeably treat a patient and provides protection for both the patient and the dental health care provider in a court of law

2. a. Demographic data (name, address, and so on): to include the patient's identifying and emergency information
   b. Medical and dental histories: to identify the patient's past and present needs
   c. Examination findings: to identify the patient's present health status
   d. Treatment performed: to promote continuity of care and to protect the patient and the health care provider in a legal proceeding
   e. Fees charged and paid: as part of legal financial records
   f. Dates of all treatments: to promote continuity of care and to protect the patient and the health care provider in a legal proceeding
   g. Results of treatment: to provide follow-up, especially if the result was unexpected or unusual
   h. Radiographs: to provide a diagnostic aid to chartings, examinations, and tests
   i. Correspondence: to protect the patient and the health care provider in a legal proceeding

3. The primary difference is that the problem-oriented approach includes a problem list that is not included in the treatment-oriented approach

4. The purpose of a chart audit is to ensure that the health care providers are maintaining complete, thorough, and accurate dental records

5. A complete format would include the date, subjective findings, objective findings, medications administered, treatment, results, the patient's reactions, whether treatment is complete or incomplete, treatment to be performed at the next appointment, the amount of time before the next appointment, and the signature of the health care provider

CHAPTER 5

1. An appropriate response would be: "I realize this is time consuming, but it is important for us to discuss your general health before I check your teeth. Certain medical conditions and medications a patient may be taking may affect their dental treatment. For example, some patients with specific types of heart problems actually need to take an antibiotic before we treat them to prevent serious complications. The health history is the foundation for your total care. All this information is kept confidential. If some of the questions puzzle you, I'll be happy to explain why they are significant. My concern is that you receive safe and proper treatment. The few minutes we take at this point to get to know you and complete a thorough record are necessary to ensure that 'checking your teeth' stays as simple as it sounds."

2. All of the above (e) is the correct answer
   a. Rheumatic heart disease: Consult the physician

to determine if damage to heart valves makes antibiotic premedication necessary

b. History of myocardial infarction: Consult the physician to obtain a history of the most recent heart attack and to determine the severity of disease; the physician may advise on the patient's tolerance to stress and on the advisability of vasoconstrictors in local anesthetics

c. Blood pressure reading of 160/100 (hypertension): Consult the physician to determine if medication is required for the patient

d. Hemophilia: Consult the physician to determine the extent of the bleeding disorder, the need for transfusion before treatment, and other possible contraindications to treatment

3. Antibiotic premedication is necessary for patients who report a history of (a) rheumatic heart fever with valve damage and/or (b) surgical replacement of a heart valve or a joint; depending on the physician's consultation, the following conditions may also require antibiotic prophylaxis: (a) congenital heart defect repair and (b) pacemaker implant

4. Communication principles:
Ask direct but open questions
Follow a logical order
Guide, but do not dominate the interview
Show support and empathy
Reflect the patient's response to clarify meaning
Avoid "yes" and "no" questions
Avoid "why" questions
Use nonverbal signs to encourage patient response
Ask probing questions concerning the topic at hand
Close the interview with a summary

5. As part of the review of a patient's health status, the dental hygienist must be aware of the medication a patient is taking; the *Physicians' Desk Reference* is helpful in identifying medication and providing information on drug composition, action, dosage, precautions, and side effects that may affect dental treatment

CHAPTER 6

1. To retract tissue, to reflect light, for indirect vision, and for transillumination

2. To detect root irregularities and hard deposits; to measure the depth of the gingival sulcus or periodontal pocket; to trace the topography of the soft tissue attachment to the tooth; and to measure recession, masticatory mucosa, and the size of lesions

3. To explore the teeth for caries; and to explore the teeth for irregularities such as calculus deposits, root roughness, anatomic defects, and margins of restorations

4. a. True
   b. False. If the first 1 to 2 mm is used, detection

can identify the specific location and less soft tissue trauma is likely to occur

c. True

d. False. The terminal shank should be parallel to the long axis of the tooth

5.

Clinician position	Patient's head position
Right handed	
a. 11 o'clock	Straight
b. 9 o'clock	Away from clinician
c. 9 o'clock	Away from clinician
d. 11 o'clock	Toward clinician
e. 11 o'clock	Toward clinician
f. 9 o'clock	Away from clinician
g. 9 o'clock	Away from clinician
Left-handed	
a. 1 o'clock	Straight
b. 3 o'clock	Toward clinician
c. 1 o'clock	Toward clinician
d. 3 o'clock	Away from clinician
e. 3 o'clock	Away from clinician
f. 1 o'clock	Toward clinician
g. 1 o'clock	Toward clinician

CHAPTER 7

1. If the hygienist ignores the patient's request to have her teeth polished, the patient will probably go elsewhere for the service or try it herself at home with a strong abrasive. If the hygienist is willing to simply polish at the first visit (after at least a medical history), there is a greater likelihood that the patient will return for further care (as explained by the hygienist) *after* the big event. The mother of the groom wants white teeth now, not sore gums. In some instances in which no harm can result, a patient can be satisfied in this manner, with long-term positive results for both the hygienist and the patient.

2. It is difficult to determine whether the patient is dependent on the dentist, believing that he will retain his teeth as long as he returns periodically for care, or if he does not really care if he keeps his teeth but does not want to experience pain either (thus the necessity of dental visits). The hygienist might do well to point out the string of appointments for restorations and simply ask the patient if he expects to retain his teeth. Mentioning rather objectively that soon the restorative material will hold his teeth together and that soon after that the teeth will begin to give up may make an impression on the patient. Often a follow-up of, "If you decide you really *do* want to keep them, let me know. I think there might be a couple of things you can to to prevent losing them over a period of time," will move the patient to ask for help. The hygienist can always resort to blatant fear tactics to awaken such a patient,

but usually they are less effective than a calm inquiry and suggestion. Different degrees of subtlety and different opening lines are appropriate for each person. There is no key phrase that works for all. In any case, the hygienist is unwise to proceed with a speech about flossing and diet. The patient will tune him or her out if possible.

3. Such a statement might imply a great deal of trust in the dental hygienist. It may also imply a dependency relationship in which the patient has transferred responsibility for oral health to the dental hygienist. Rarely do such patients have a thorough program of preventive self-care.

4. a. Excessive familiarity
   b. Professional closeness
   c. Professional closeness (but worthy of discussion)
   d. Professional aloofness

5. There are several possible actions, including refusing to provide care for the patient, having the patient sign a disclaimer for risks resulting from the omitted procedure, or working around the missing procedure until trust is increased and the need for the procedure becomes more apparent to the patient.

6. These are *possible* replies. The key to a *listening* response is that the *content* of the message is rephrased and the *affect* or emotion behind the statement is reflected.
   a. "It sounds like you're worried about what I'm going to see in there."
   b. "You don't feel as comfortable lying down for your dental work."
   c. "You sound a little disturbed that you can feel this more than you could with other hygienists."
   d. "You sound upset that the dentist has hired someone else to clean your teeth. You think the dentist is the person who should do it."

   Each listening response enables the patient to confirm or correct the understanding the hygienist has of the patient's statement. Even more important, it allows the patient to say more, to elaborate on the problem or feeling, and to express wants, needs, or expectations.

7. a. While reassuring, it cuts off a message the patient is trying to give: there is some reason the hygienist will be unhappy. It may be very important for the patient to say it before the hygienist looks in. It also sounds like the patient may feel guilty. The patient may feel he or she is reporting into the hygienist for judgment. A glib, nonlistening comment shuts off the patient's next statement and any exploration of what is behind the opening comment.
   b. This, too, shuts off communication, because the hygienist is presenting a logical argument in favor of reclining chairs. The patient and the hygienist are both right, but the hygienist is actually denying the validity of the patient's statement by presenting his or her own and thus arguing.
   c. Problem solving immediately after a comment closes off communication. The hygienist is closing out lots of information that the patient might have revealed if the hygienist had saved problem solving for later.
   d. No matter how tempting it may be to lecture, the patient should be listened to *first* so that accurate perceptions are clear. Information to enlighten the misinformed should follow the reflection and listening. The patient then knows the hygienist understands, and he or she is more likely to listen.

CHAPTER 8

1. Dental visits often are likely to create anxiety for patients. Patients who have a propensity for syncope (fainting) or other physical responses to anxiety are more likely to respond this way in the dental environment. Also, the drugs used in dentistry, including local anesthetics, may cause an emergency situation. The dental hygienist may be the first person to recognize and respond to the situation.

2. Primary drugs
   Noninjectable drugs
   Oxygen
   Nitroglycerin (spray preferably)
   Injectable drugs
   Epinephrine (allergy)
   Chlorphenexamine (antihistamine)
   Diazepam (anticonvulsant)
   Narcotic antagonist (Naloxone)
   Equipment
   Oxygen delivery system for portable oxygen
   Suction and suction tips
   Syringes for drug administration
   Tourniquets

3. All emergency equipment should be readily available and functioning. Drugs maintained in the kit should be up to date. All members of the team should be able to recognize signs of patient distress, and they should be prepared to respond appropriately. Rehearsing the proper procedures for any kind of an emergency can be critically important if quick, responsible action is to occur. Emergencies can be prevented by the use of medical histories and fire and accident prevention devices and by careful monitoring of the patient.

4. a. Move instruments and other dental equipment away from the patient, place the patient in a full supine position (a patient in the late stages of pregnancy should be turned on her side), place a

cool cloth on the patient's forehead, alert another team member, prepare an ammonia ampule for wafting under the patient's nose if he or she loses consciousness, and administer oxygen until the patient is recovered.

b. Place the patient is an upright position, send a team member to call for emergency assistance, administer oxygen, place a nitroglycerin tablet under the tongue, monitor vital signs, and begin CPR in the event of cardiac arrest. If the pain is associated with angina, the nitroglycerin will relieve the discomfort. If it is associated with heart failure or myocardial infarction, the pain will persist.

c. Place the patient in a supine position, and check for vital signs. Begin CPR if breathing and a heartbeat are absent, and have a team member send for emergency assistance. If the patient is breathing and has a heartbeat, waft an ammonia ampule under his or her nose and administer oxygen. Continue monitoring vital signs until the patient is fully recovered. An awareness of the patient's medical history should help determine if there are causes other than syncope that could account for the loss of consciousness, such as hypoglycemia, hyperglycemia, cardiovascular problems, or acute adrenal insufficiency.

5. The unconscious patient does not possess protective reflexes; therefore, a head tilt/chin lift maneuver must be maintained to prevent the tongue from causing an airway obstruction, thus producing respiratory arrest. The unconscious patient must be monitored in case respiratory arrest occurs. In this event, oxygen would be delivered by positive pressure on an ambu bag. The patent airway would be maintained by the head tilt/chin lift maneuver.

The conscious victim still possesses protective reflexes and, unless an obstruction occurs, is capable of inhaling and exhaling without assistance. The patient should be closely monitored in case the situation deteriorates.

CHAPTER 9

1. d. Use of the clinician's fingernail to test instrument sharpness is a violation of acceptable methods of contamination control when used during patient treatment. Any of the other three methods would be preferable to this method.

2. a. False. The Arkansas stone is a natural stone.
   b. True. Cutting edges of good-quality stainless steel instruments are not dulled by steam sterilization (Parkes and Kolstad, 1981—see references for Chapter 9)
   c. False. Only the lower cutting edge of Gracey

curettes is used for periodontal procedures. Therefore only that cutting edge should be sharpened.

3. The internal angle of 70 to 80 degrees forms a complementary angle with the sharpening stone, which is applied at 100 to 110 degrees.

4. Both the rounded toe and the rounded back of the curette design must be preserved during sharpening procedures.

5. a. Facial surface

6. b. Pressure is applied only to the downstroke to minimize formation of wire edges.

CHAPTER 10

1. To gather assessment data for diagnosis and treatment planning; to provide early detection of disease, thus improving the prognosis for recovery; to detect contraindications to dental treatment; to provide baseline and continuing data of the patient's health status; and to provide descriptions of the patient's health status for use as legal records

2. Pulse, respiration rate, temperature, and blood pressure

3. a. Adult pulse: 60 to 80 beats per minute
   b. Adult respiration rate: 14 to 20 breaths per minute
   c. Adult temperature: 98.6° F (37° C)
   d. Adult blood pressure: 120/80 mm Hg
   e. Borderline temperature for fever: 99.6° F
   f. Borderline blood pressure for hypertension: 160/95 mm Hg

4. a. Pulse rate: Rest the patient's arm in a comfortable position. Place the index and second fingers on the radial artery found on the thumb side of the wrist. Compress this area gently, and count the beats for 1 minute.
   b. Blood pressure: Rest the patient's arm in a comfortable position. Roll up the patient's sleeve. Place the sphygmomanometer on the patient's arm about 1 inch above the bend in the arm. Feel the radial pulse, and inflate the cuff until the pulse is no longer felt. This provides an estimate of the systolic pressure. Release the air in the cuff. Let the patient's circulation return to normal. Inflate the cuff 20 to 30 mm Hg higher than that previously noted. Slowly deflate the cuff. Note the point at which the first sound is heard and the point at which the sound completely disappears. Record the first sound as systolic pressure and the last sound as diastolic pressure. Confirm this recording a second time. Remove the cuff.

5. a. Inspection: a visual examination of each of the structures before they are palpated for signs of abnormal color, texture, or consistency

b. Palpation: feeling or pressing on structures of the body: used for examining most intraoral and some extraoral structures

c. Auscultation: listening for sounds produced within the body: used for examining the temporomandibular joint and larynx

d. Percussion: striking tissues with the fingers or with an instrument to hear the resulting sounds and patient response; not previously described as a method used during the intraoral examination, but often used as a means of assessing pulpal disease in individual teeth

6. a. Submandibular lymph nodes: Standing behind the patient, push the soft tissues from one side of the submandibular area over to the other side; grasp these tissues with the cupped fingers of the hand, and roll tissues over bone of the mandible. Repeat for the other side.

b. Floor of the mouth: Place the fingers of one hand intraorally on the floor of the mouth and the fingers of the other hand extraorally beneath the same area. Use bimanual palpation to examine the entire floor area.

c. Buccal mucosa: Place one hand or several fingers intraorally and the other hand extraorally. Use bimanual palpation to examine the entire area from the labial mucosa back to the retromolar area.

7. To prevent the clinician from touching lesions in the mouth that might be contagious, such as syphilis; to prevent the clinician from contracting diseases transmittable through the bloodstream, such as hepatitis; to identify conditions that would contraindicate dental treatment for the patient's well-being, such as strep throat; and to prevent discomfort of the patient due to palpation of painful lesions such as ulcers

8. a. Auricular chain
   b. Cervical chain
   c. Occipital chain
   d. Submandibular (posterior) and submental (anterior) chains

CHAPTER 11

1. Legal record of the patient's initial condition and changes in oral status over a period of time; helpful in preparing a treatment plan; useful in cross-checking financial records; and combines radiographic and clinical findings into a comprehensive record for diagnosis

2. a. Anatomic: most precise replica of tooth characteristic
   b. Geometric: stylized version of teeth and findings; usually makes charting neater and easier to read

c. Numerically coded: provides a complete time line of oral conditions and changes on a single piece of paper

		Universal	Palmer's notation	International	Description
3.	a.	3	6⌋	16	Maxillary right first permanent molar
	b.	29	5⌋	45	Mandibular right second premolar
	c.	16	⌊8	28	Maxillary left third molar
	d.	n	⌐b	72	Mandibular left primary lateral
	e.	13	⌊5	25	Maxillary left second premolar

4. a. Class II
   b. Class III
   c. Class V
   d. Class I
   e. Class VI
   f. Class IV

5. a. A, amalgam
   b. T, temporary
   c. TC, tooth-colored restoration
   d. FGC, full gold crown
   e. GF, gold foil
   f. C, caries
   g. SSC, stainless steel crown
   h. DGO, defective gold onlay
   i. RC, root canal
   j. PAP, periapical disease

6. a. Tooth anomaly: Mark with an asterisk, and describe the condition elsewhere on the page, preceded by the asterisk
   b. Pontic: Mark the root as missing, fill in the crown with the appropriate restoration, and draw horizontal bars to connect it to the adjacent pontic or abutment
   c. Drifting: Draw a horizontal arrow parallel with and above the occlusal table, pointing in the direction of the drift
   d. Rotation: Begin an arrow on the proximal side of the proximal surface of the tooth that is rotated facially, and arc the arrow across the facial as-

pect of the tooth to suggest the direction of rotation

e. Attrition: Draw a horizontal line through the facial view of the teeth to indicate the amount of tooth lost due to mastication
f. Unerupted teeth: Circle
g. Calculus: Draw in with a triangle, or include a written statement in the summary
h. Overhang: Place an *O* in the appropriate box
7. Retained root tip, unerupted teeth, bone loss, root canal restoration, widened periodontal ligament space; loss of continuity of lamina dura, unerupted supernumerary teeth, periapical disease, and other disturbances of the hard tissues

CHAPTER 12

1. A calculus charting procedure assists beginning clinicians in identifying and classifying calculus as tactile sense and dexterity with instruments increase. It assists in developing abilities in differentiating between normal anatomy and calculus deposits. It provides valuable baseline data regarding a patient's oral conditions and is a useful tool in designing a treatment plan for dental hygiene care.
2. a. Ledge: A ring or part of a ring that encircles the tooth, projecting from the tooth toward the gingiva, thus appearing like a ledge. Such deposits are usually located subgingivally, although they may be visible above the margin of the gingiva if the tissue has receded.
   b. Veneer: Veneer calculus, a thin sheet of burnished calculus that marks the location of a deposit incompletely removed by either an improperly adapted instrument or a dull instrument. The calculus is usually located subgingivally and is difficult to detect because it has been mechanically smoothed.
   c. Crustaceous: A chalky, white amorphous mass of calculus, usually appearing supragingivally on the lingual aspect of the mandibular anterior teeth and on the facial surfaces of the maxillary molars. It may be afforded some shape by the action of the tongue and the other musculature.
   d. Fingerlike projections: Projections of calculus that dip into the pockets formed during the advancement of periodontal disease. They tend to cover large surface areas of the roots and are found almost exclusively subgingivally.
3. Although research continues into the etiology of periodontal disease, it is the general consensus that calculus is a less important factor than plaque in the initiation and progression of periodontal disease.

Calculus is usually covered with masses of microorganisms (plaque) that continuously affect the tissues.
4. a. True
   b. True
   c. False; the outer portion is more porous
   d. False; there are two: one associated with microorganisms and one not
   e. True

CHAPTER 13

1. Acquired pellicle: a, f, h
   Materia alba: e, g
   Food debris: d, g
   Plaque: a, b, c, i
2. Calcification
3. Acid or low; decalcification of tooth structure or caries
4. a. Days 1 and 2: Microbial composition begins with gram-positive cocci
   b. Days 3 and 4: Filamentous forms of organisms start to occur and eventually grow into the coccal layer and replace these initial organisms
   c. Days 6 to 10: A more mixed bacterial flora begins to appear; plaque becomes more gram negative and contains anaerobic organisms
   d. Days 10 to 21: Inflammation of gingivae begins; plaque is composed of densely packed spirochetes and vibrios
5. a. black pig. Bacteroides; b. Fusobacterium; c. Treponema; d. Acidominococcus; e. Wolinella; f. Selenomonas; and g. Actinobacillus
6. a. erythrosin; b. sodium flouroscein; c. FD&C green No. 3; and d. FD&C red No. 30 and FD&C blue No. 1.
7. Visual signs of inflammation (size, shape, texture, consistency); bleeding (when probed or sprayed with compressed air)
8. The routine inclusion of indices in clinical practice provides baseline data for each patient, aids the health care provider in following a patient's progress or regression, and can generate valuable data regarding the overall success of the practice in minimizing or eradicating dental disease. If such data follow unchanging criteria and are performed by one clinician or by clinicians carefully following the same standardized procedures, valid epidemiologic information about the patient's population can be provided. Finally, the indices are valuable tools for patient motivation in assuming greater personal responsibility for lowering plaque levels and thus dental disease.

CHAPTER 14

1. Establish baseline data on the patient; aid in establishing a diagnosis; serve as a resource during treatment planning; aid in implementation of the treatment plan; as a reference for evaluating treatment success; as a source of legal evidence; and in forensic dentistry
2. The amount of masticatory mucosa on the buccal surface of the tooth minus the buccal pocket depth of the same tooth equals the amount of attached gingiva.
3. Overangulate. The consequence of overangulation in a given area is that the reading may be slightly higher than the actual pocket depth. This would alert the hygienist or dentist to a potential problem area before it existed to that degree. If the probe is underangulated, the clinician runs the risk of assuming that an area is healthier than it actually is, and it may be overlooked in the dentist's diagnosis and treatment plan. Which would be worse for the patient?
4. No. Pocket depths are essentially meaningless unless the height of the gingival margin is also known. The depth of the pocket must be viewed in the context of whether or not there has been abnormal enlargement of the tissues or apical migration of the junctional epithelium. Without this context, the clinician would not know whether a 3 mm pocket could be interpreted as normal, the result of gingival inflammation, or the result of periodontal destruction.
5. a. False. The probe should be adapted as close to parallel as possible as long as the clinician is certain that the tip is closely adapted to the tooth; the parallel relationship will exist for buccal and lingual adaptation, but the probe should be angled slightly for best assessment of the interproximal areas.
   b. False. In situations in which calculus prevents the clinician from adapting the probe to the base of the sulcus or pocket, it is often necessary to perform some scaling before accurate pocket depths can be determined.
   c. False. Although where pocket readings are taken in six prescribed areas, it is the deepest point within each area that is recorded. This may not necessarily occur at exactly the same point on every tooth; in fact, it is unlikely that that would be true. In addition, if two distinctly separate vertical defects are detected within the same area of the tooth, the clinician may choose to include an extra reading to further define the bony morphology around that tooth.

CHAPTER 15

1. a. Overbite: the vertical distance that the maxillary teeth overlap the mandibular teeth
   b. Occlusal trauma: forces that cause damage to the supporting structures
   c. Occlusal traumatism: Damage due to abnormally arranged forces
2. Tooth position, tooth-to-tooth habits, foreign object-to-teeth habits, oral musculature habits, and iatrogenic factors
3. Subjective: aching muscles, teeth that move, pain when biting, or pain with temperature changes. The patient may report grinding or clenching teeth or a habit of holding a pipe with the teeth or chewing or sucking a foreign object.
   Clinical: mobility; wear patterns; changes in tooth position; poorly contoured restorations; plunger cusps; severe overbite or overjet; overdevelopment of the muscles of mastication; clicking, pain, or improper movement of the temporomandibular joint; and tooth sensitivity
   Radiographic: widened periodontal ligament space, necrosis of the periodontal ligament, cemental tears, loss of the lamina dura, bone resorption, and root resorption.
4. a. False; there must be damage to the supporting structures caused by occlusal trauma for the condition to be considered occlusal traumatism
   b. False; occlusal trauma does not cause periodontal pockets. Periodontitis is an inflammatory disease that affects the supporting structure; occlusal traumatism is a *non*inflammatory disease that affects the supporting structure.
   c. True in most cases.

CHAPTER 16

1. Permanent records, diagnostic aid, educational aid, and fabrication of temporary appliances
2. Water-to-powder ratio, water temperature, and method of manipulation
3. The tray should be large enough to permit ¼ inch (6 mm) of alginate to flow between the tray and oral structures without impinging on the soft tissues and without causing pain.
4. Fill the tray to the level of the beading wax; smooth alginate with wet fingers; retract one cheek with the fingers; retract the other cheek with the side of the tray as it is being inserted; loosen the cheek and insert the other side of the tray; center the tray; place the posterior border of the tray first, and then the rest of the tray; muscle mold; and hold the tray gently.
5. Border molding is forming pliable materials (i.e., alginate) to conform to the muscle attachments of

the soft tissues to include the muscle attachments in the cast for diagnostic and fabrication purposes.

6. The clinician can try to divert the patient's attention, reassure the patient, and/or ask the patient to breathe through the nose. If the patient reports a history of a gagging problem, the clinician can ask the patient to hold an ice cube in the mouth before inserting the tray or rinse the mouth with an anesthetic mouthwash.

7. Distortion and/or ripping of the alginate

8. To permit the dental personnel to correctly relate the mandibular cast to the maxillary cast during the trimming procedure

9. Initially, the gypsum is flowed into the tray in small increments to coat the tooth surfaces, and the excess is allowed to run out of the impression tray. Gradually, larger increments are added and flowed around the impression.

10. Compare your drawing with Fig. 16-28.

CHAPTER 17

1. Any four of the following: diagnostic aid, treatment planning, case presentation, case documentation, education/motivation, and instruction/peer review

2. Single-lens–reflex camera body, 100 mm automatic short-mount lens or 100 mm macrolens, fully automatic bellows, electronic point-source flash attachment, rotating bracket for flash, proper color correction filters, and pistol grip and cable release

3. a. 9
   b. 10
   c. 5
   d. 2
   e. 1
   f. 8
   g. 7
   h. 6
   i. 4
   j. 3

4. a. Wet the cheek retractor.
   b. Ask the patient to relax the lips and open the mouth slightly.
   c. Place the rim of the retractor onto the edge of the lower lip.
   d. Rotate the handle of the retractor until it is parallel to the corner of the mouth.
   e. Instruct the patient to bite down. Pull the retractors out laterally and forward.

5. a. Mandibular anterior lingual: A lingual view of the mandibular anterior teeth and gingiva from the distal of the right cuspid to the distal of the left cuspid
   b. Buccal of right side: A direct buccal view of the right maxillary and mandibular teeth in occlusion

from the distal of the right cuspid to the retromolar or maxillary tuberosity area
   c. Anterior direct: A direct view of the maxillary and mandibular teeth in occlusion from the distal of the right cuspid to the distal of the left cuspid
   d. Maxillary occlusal: A view of the maxillary occlusal surfaces and palatal tissues

CHAPTER 18

1. The nature of the patient's condition; a suggested plan of treatment; discussion of likely outcomes of treatment; risks involved in treatment; the likely outcome of not proceeding with care; and alternative treatment approaches

2. Technical assault or technical battery

3. The final treatment plan is more likely to be acceptable to the patient, and it will reflect a blending of the needs as seen by the patient and the dental hygienist, which will facilitate a partnership relationship and will increase the probability of cooperation in care and the achievement of health goals.

4. Emergency

5. The dental hygienist should perform thorough, reliable assessments; draw preliminary conclusions from the data, including proposed treatment and scheduling; use the dentist as a resource and arbiter of decisions regarding the patient's status and proper treatment; and follow through with high-quality care, providing status reports as care progresses.

CHAPTER 19

1. Education of the public and of private patients in dental health has always been part of the profession of dental hygiene. Because of the nature of the work the clinician performs (monitoring the health of the oral tissues, cleaning the teeth, and providing periodontal or restorative therapy), he or she is in an excellent position to educate the patient as to the causes of dental disease and the steps necessary to avoid disease. Considering the number of patients with periodontal disease, preventive education is perhaps the hygienist's most important role.

2. Dental plaque has been identified as an important factor in inflammatory gingival disease. The relationship of oral hygiene and plaque has led scientists to conclude that controlling or disorganizing dental plaque is still a good way to prevent dental disease at the current time.

3. An individualized approach to preventive education is valuable because the patient easily sees his or her role. The patient is involved in decisions about goals and has an opportunity to feel commit-

ment to a plan designed particularly for him or her. By personalizing the dental health education plan, the hygienist finds that instruction is less likely to become routine from patient to patient.

4. a. Small step size allows the rate of instruction to not overwhelm the patient
   b. Active participation allows the patient to become involved and practice using the new concepts or skills.
   c. Immediate feedback provides the patient with cues and encouragement about performance so that corrections can be made or reinforcement can be given early in practice.
   d. Self-pacing gives the learner a significant role in determining what instruction will be given and when.

5. a. Skill does not seem to be the problem, so do not bore the patient.
   b. This is a bit extreme at this point in treatment.
   c. The best response. Most likely the patient is having a difficult time understanding or accepting the need for improved home care. Perhaps he/she is having difficulties adjusting to new routines, and a few words of encouragment or helpful suggestions are all that is needed.
   d. You've given up too soon if you consider yourself a preventive educator.

6. a. Short-term; security
   b. Long-term; social
   c. Short-term; security
   d. Long-term; esteem

7. Disagree. A specific technique is less important than the degree of thoroughness in cleaning. Many brushing techniques are adequate. Brushing can be performed several times a day, but unless the bacterial plaque is thoroughly and consistently disorganized, disease will continue. Also, regular interproximal cleaning must be performed in addition to following a brushing routine.

8. Keeping the tissue in tone is an important consideration. The patient may find an interdental stimulator such as the periodontal aid, wood wedge, rubber tip, or oral irrigator helpful. For the bridge, a floss threader will be necessary to clean under the bridge and to floss the abutment teeth. The oral irrigator can flush food debris and plaque from this area also. Yarn may be suggested for polishing the last tooth in the arch adjacent to the removable partial denture if regular floss is not cleaning thoroughly. Variable-diameter floss and an oral irrigator for flushing and stimulation may be the aids of choice. Selecting the aid the patient is most comfortable using is most important.

9. a. A disclosing agent is needed to identify the plaque and to evaluate areas missed in cleaning. It is probably the only way to ensure thoroughness in the initial preventive program.
   b. Brushing in a random or haphazard fashion rarely results in thoroughness. Establishing a habit of brushing in sequence is a mechanism for ensuring that all areas are attended to.
   c. Because of the anatomic limitations of this area, the usual application of the brush is difficult. The patient needs particular instruction in this area.
   d. The tongue and soft tissue collect bacterial plaque and decomposing food particles. Tissue regeneration accounts for sloughing of dead cell layers also. Although the saliva functions to rinse the oral cavity, brushing or scraping the tissues enhances the cleanliness of the mouth.

10. Plaque control, importance of fluoride in caries prevention, how to identify changes in the normal structures of the mouth, nutritional and diet education, and the need for specialized dental care for individual needs

11. a. False; it changes the quality of the plaque and reduces gingivitis
    b. True
    c. True
    d. False; it is a blunt needle used primarily by the clinician to deliver agents subgingivally
    e. True

12. a. Essential oils, over the counter
    b. Chlorhexidine, prescription
    c. Sanguinaria, over the counter
    d. Cetylpryidinium chloride, over the counter
    e. Uncertain, probably soaping agents, over the counter
    f. Stannous ion, prescription

CHAPTER 20

1. Carbohydrates, fats, and proteins
2. Any of the three nutrients consumed in excess can cause weight gain. Their total contribution to daily caloric intake determines fat deposition (if it is in excess of expended calories) or fat utilization (if it is less than expended calories).

3. a. 6   j. 4
   b. 7   k. 3
   c. 5   l. 12
   d. 9   m. 2
   e. 10
   f. 14
   g. 11
   h. 13
   i. 1

4. Often the patient is fully aware of what he or she *ought* to include in the daily diet. Information about what to do and what not to do may not be what is

needed. After the patient demonstrates his or her level of knowledge about diet and nutrition, it is easier to decide what kind of information still needs to be provided in the follow-up discussion. The self-assessment process itself may cause the patient to develop a need to know or a need to change.

5. The RDAs and the four food groups provide a guideline or standard for evaluating the appropriateness and healthfulness of a person's diet. If these guidelines are generally followed or met, all essential nutrients should be provided in the diet. With these guidelines, missing elements in a person's diet can be readily identified and suggestions for change can be made.

6. Plaque provides a matrix for absorbing fermentable carbohydrates, which are converted by bacteria into acid, which demineralizes the tooth structure. Plaque promotes smooth-surface caries, providing an attachment to the teeth that maintains acid contact.

7. Saturated and unsaturated fats; salt-cured, smoked, and salt-pickled foods; alcohol; and food contaminants, including additives; alcohol in combination with tobacco promotes oral cancer

8. Vegetables, especially raw vegetables (lettuce, celery) and cruciferous vegetables, in particular (cabbage, cauliflower, brussels sprouts, broccoli)

CHAPTER 21

1. When calculus is located with a cutting instrument, increased horizontal or lateral pressure against the tooth is used to engage the blade next to the deposit so that it is removed with a working stroke. For calculus removal, the blade must be angled to the tooth to ensure that the cutting edge can be engaged effectively and to reduce tissue damage by the unused blade.

2. a. True
   b. False; it is used with a push stroke on the proximal surfaces of anterior teeth with the shank perpendicular to the long axis of the tooth
   c. True
   d. True
   e. False; the size, shape, and length of the shank and blade dictate where the various universal curettes may be used
   f. False; the sickle scaler is best reserved for supragingival calculus and for calculus that is barely below the margin of the gingiva
   g. False; all plaque and endotoxin must be removed from the root surface, or the disease will continue to advance subclinically

3. Exploring; observing signs of continued inflammation in localized areas; and air directed on the teeth and into the sulcus

CHAPTER 22

1. a. While there are many other criteria used in patient selection for ultrasonics, the presence of large amounts of deposits is the primary factor.
2. Severe diabetes
3. No. Ultrasonic devices should not be used for children (young, growing tissues).
4. a. The clinician and the assistant should wear face masks and protective lenses. The patient should wear protective lenses.
   b. Immediately following the procedure, the area should be thoroughly wiped with a disinfectant
   c. A laminar air flow system should be used to reduce the numbers of airborne microorganisms.
   d. Patients known to have virulent pathogens such as hepatitis viruses or tuberculosis mycobacteria should not have ultrasonics used at all.
5. Ultrasonic instruments use high-frequency sound waves to fracture deposits from teeth and to cavitate the accompanying water supply to mechanically flush the area.
6. Decreased; increased
7. Chisel, beaver tail, universal curette style, and periodontal probe style
8. All of the statements are *true*.

CHAPTER 23

1. a. In scaling, a variety of instruments are used, including scalers, hoes, chisels, files, curettes, and ultrasonic instruments; root planing requires the use of fine curettes with small blades and shank designs that facilitate access to any area. Examples of these are the Gracey curettes.
   b. Root planing requires many more strokes over an area than scaling.
   c. Root planing is best accomplished when a variety of different stroke directions overlap onto the same area; hand scaling is usually accomplished with several strokes in a single optimal direction.
   d. Scaling often requires heavy lateral pressure during the working stroke; root planing starts with moderate, even pressure, which is decreased as the surface becomes harder and smoother.
2. a. Gracey curettes generally have a smaller blade size than universal curettes.
   b. Gracey curettes have offset cutting edges, with one located lower than the other; cutting edges are parallel on the universal curette blade. Both edges of a universal curette are used; only the lower edge of the Gracey curette is used.
   c. The universal curette has a simple shank design, facilitating its use throughout the mouth; Gracey shanks are designed so that each is optimally used in specific areas of the mouth.
3. Tactile sensations reveal that the root is regular,

smooth, and hard; audio clues reveal a high squeaky pitch or no sound at all during working strokes; visual clues reveal a homogeneous, shiny, tooth-colored surface; and tissue resolution reveals shrinkage of pocket depth, normal architecture, and no sulcular bleeding.

4. a. If these are the sole criteria, more tooth structure may be removed than is necessary. Hardness is deceptive because you can plane well into healthy dentin without detecting a significant change in hardness. Not all teeth will achieve glasslike smoothness, so these criteria may be misleading.

   b. The differences between diseased cementum, healthy cementum, and healthy dentin are not clinically apparent; even an experienced clinician cannot always detect the differences between them through tactile evaluation.

CHAPTER 24

1. a. Soft tissue curettage: The use of the sharp blade of a curette to remove diseased tissue from the soft tissue pocket wall, thus converting a chronic inflammatory wound into a surgical wound to promote healing of the area

   b. Coincidental curettage: The inadvertent scraping of the cutting edge of an instrument against the soft tissue wall of a pocket or sulcus while the working edge is engaged in scaling or root planing

2. Shrinkage is the only predictable result of this procedure.

3. False; if the procedure is done thoroughly and correctly, the underlying subsulcular connective tissue that is diseased and part or all of the junctional epithelium will also be removed

4. As it is stated that the lack of healing cannot be attributed to poor plaque control, then it may be because of incomplete removal of diseased tissue during the curettage, excessive trauma to the tissues during curettage, or incomplete root planing and submarginal plaque control causing reinfection.

5. a. Indication
   b. Contraindication
   c. Indication
   d. Contraindication
   e. Indication
   f. Contraindication
   g. Contraindication
   h. Contraindication

6. a, c, and d

CHAPTER 25

1. A periodontal dressing protects the area from irritants, protects newly exposed root surfaces, stabi-

lizes mobile teeth, protects sutures, maintains the position of repositioned tissue, and helps control bleeding.

2. Either one can be used, depending on clinician preference. The eugenol pack is believed by some practitioners to soothe the tissues; other practitioners believe that eugenol irritates the tissues. Other factors to be considered are storage time, mixing time, consistency of the pack, and ease of manipulation of each material.

3. Refer to Fig. 25-15 for the suggested response.

4. If the sutures were tied on the facial surface, then the lingual pack should be removed first. The sutures can be cut on the lingual portion, and then they can be removed from the buccal portion at the same time the pack is removed. The clinician must be sure *never* to pull the knot through the tissue.

5. Dressings may promote the accumulation of plaque and associated inflammation resulting in prolonged wound healing; dressings also may contribute to patient discomfort.

CHAPTER 26

1. a. Exogenous: stains that originate outside the tooth
   b. Endogenous: stains that develop within the tooth
   c. Extrinsic: exogenous stain on the exterior of the tooth; removable by the patient or professional
   d. Intrinsic: within the tooth structure, not removable by the patient or by basic polishing or scaling

2. It removes and prevents formation of stains and/or discolorants (pellicle).

3. Essentially the same abrasives are used in both; higher concentrations are present in professional products.

4. Abrasive hardness, particle size, shape, concentration, and the pressure and speed used.

5. Operate at a low speed (minimal speed at which the attachment can be applied to the tooth without stalling); use *moderate intermittent* pressure on the tooth; and use sufficient amounts of abrasive to minimize direct contact of rubber and brush with the tooth

6. Portability, provides gentle massage, can reach surfaces obscured by malposed teeth, generates minimal frictional heat, generates minimal noise, is easily cleaned and sterilized, and generates minimal aerosol

7. It is slow and tedious and requires considerable hand effort.

8. The presence of stains that cannot be readily removed by the patient

9. Air pressure and water force a slurry of sodium bicarbonate against the tooth structure, loosening stain and polishing the tooth.

CHAPTER 27

1. c and d
2. c
3. b
4. False
5. Candida albicans
6. Clean dentures regularly, soak in diluted vinegar overnight when calculus first forms; never scrape a denture surface—bring it in for professional cleaning instead
7. Wear mask, gloves, and glasses; isolate denture and solution in sealed plastic bag during cleaning; never reuse solution
8. Clean over a sink partially filled with water or with a rubber mat or towel placed in the bottom; hold denture firmly

CHAPTER 28

1. Streptococcus mutans
2. a. True
   b. True
   c. True
   d. True
   e. True
   f. False; the optimal concentration is 1 ppm
3. Dental fluorosis is a change in the color of the enamel that occurs during its formation prior to eruption due to ingesting too much fluoride. It ranges from a white, chalky appearance to brown discoloration.
4. After the teeth erupt, the fluoride and other minerals that are ingested or are in the saliva pass over the enamel, adding to its ability to resist caries.
5. a. Once-daily rinsing
   b. Twice daily rinsing
   c. Once-weekly rinsing
   Read the manufacturer's directions for amount and duration of rinsing. Typically, 10 ml of the rinse is swished for 60 seconds and then expectorated. The rinses are not to be given to persons who cannot control the swallow reflex or who cannot thoroughly expectorate.
6. No. Laboratory and clinical trials have demonstrated that it makes no difference whether the teeth are polished, brushed, flossed, or left without intervention prior to administering fluoride. However, dental hygiene procedures emphasize clean teeth; therefore, it is recommended that selective polishing, combined with the patient demonstrating proper plaque removal with a brush and floss, precede fluoride application. This procedure is intended to reinforce good at-home oral hygiene rather than to enhance fluoride uptake.
7. The Grand Rapids/Muskegon and Kingston/ Newburg trials were instituted to determine whether or not fluoride in the water creates measurable changes in dental caries. Two of the cities contained insignificant amounts of fluoride, two were fluoridated to optimal levels of 1 ppm. The decayed, missing, and filled surfaces were significantly fewer in the fluoridated communities than in the nonfluoridated communities at the evaluation points, paving the way for widespread communal fluoridation of water supplies.
8. See the check-off sheet (p. 524) for each step.
9. c. All teeth to be treated must be covered by the fluoride gel or solution before the 4-minute timing begins.
10. Adults: 5 to 10 g
    Children: 32 mg/kg body weight
    The amount of fluoride gel or solution applied is somewhere in the range of 125 to 200 mg.
11. d. All three are acceptable antidotes for acute fluoride poisoning. Seek immediate emergency care if symptoms persist or if the amount ingested is more than 3.5 mg/kg body weight, or is unknown.
12. The total fluoride dose would be about 192 to 195 mg.
13. This dosage would not be above the CLD (certainly lethal dose) for a 2-year-old child, which is estimated to be 320 mg.
14. Yes, hospitalization is indicated for this level of overdose. The total ingested dose of 192 to 195 mg is well beyond both the STD and the PTD estimates, and it is equivalent to a dose of more than 190 mg F/kg body weight (estimated body weight for a 2-year-old is 10 kg or 22 lb).

CHAPTER 29

1. The acid-etching process (conditioning) is the most critical part of the sealant technique. An acidic gel or solution is painted on the occlusal surface for 60 seconds. This removes inorganic material from the occlusal enamel and leaves a reactive porous surface. The increased surface area allows the sealant resin to penetrate the enamel and form a mechanical lock for the sealant. Due to the etching, a strong bond can be formed between the enamel and the sealant material that is highly resistant to bacterial leakage and occlusal wear.
2. This patient is at a caries-prone age and shows a history of restorations in commonly susceptible teeth. The patient's susceptibility may be exaggerated, as she previously lived in a nonfluoridated area. Clinically, the patient appears for treatment with good home care and a good preventive attitude reinforced by the parents. The newly erupted teeth are sound, and radiographic data reveal that there are no interproximal caries. These factors indicate

that the patient is a good candidate for sealant protection. In a consultation among the hygienist, dentist, patient, and family, information about the sealant procedure, the benefits, risks and responsibilities should be discussed and a decision made. (We would elect to seal teeth No. 18 and No. 31 and recommend that the patient return when teeth No. 2 and No. 15 erupt if this occurs prior to the next regularly scheduled visit.)

3. Steps in the sealant application procedure: (1) remove hard and soft deposits; (2) polish with pumice; (3) rinse thoroughly; (4) isolate and dry teeth; (5) condition the teeth; (6) rinse and examine (recondition if necessary); (7) reisolate and dry teeth; (8) apply sealant; (9) polymerize sealant; and (10) rinse and examine.

4. Possible reasons:
   a. New ideas are accepted slowly.
   b. The dental professions needed time to realize the benefits, practicality, and safety of sealant use.
   c. Dentists and auxiliaries needed to learn the sealant technique.
   d. The public was unaware of the benefits of sealants so did not demand the service.
   e. State laws have limited the hygienist's role in providing the service.
   f. Employer attitudes about new techniques and delegation of sealants have changed slowly.
   g. Insurance carriers have not recognized sealants as a service to be covered in their dental plans.

CHAPTER 30

1. Areas where the dentin is exposed, primarily as a result of enamel and/or cementum being eroded abraded or planed away

2. Root surface scaling, gingival surgery (causing gingival or root exposure recession), cavity preparation, and placement of crowns

3. Mechanical, thermal, and chemical

4. Depositing of precipitating insoluble materials at nerve endings (Tomes' fibers); denaturing nerve endings; stimulating secondary dentin formation; and reducing pulp hyperemia

5. a. True
   b. True
   c. True

6. a. Differences: Fluoride is applied more frequently; can be burnished on very sensitive areas
   b. Similarities: Teeth should be clean (scaled and polished) and dry prior to application. The same preparations can be used. If the entire mouth is treated, the same mode of application (tray, painted on dried teeth) can be used.

7. The Hydrodynamic Theory states that pain-producing stimuli cause a movement of the fluids in the tubules in either an outward or an inward direction, depending on the pressure variations in the surrounding tissue. This movement stimulates the nerve processes in the pulpal dentin and the pulp.

CHAPTER 31

1. The hygienist should participate in a formal local anesthesia course that provides in-depth information about nerve anatomy, the chemistry and pharmacology of local anesthetics, the modes of actions of each, medical complications, and treatment of the complications. The course should also include a laboratory portion that teaches the techniques of administering local anesthetics.

2. Refer to Fig. 31-4.

3. a. Hard tissue: Second and third molars and the first molar, excluding the mesiobuccal root and the associated supporting structures; soft tissue: overlying facial tissue
   b. Hard tissue: None; soft tissue: palatal tissue from the margin of the gingiva to the midline and from the distal aspect of the posterior-most molar to the cuspid
   c. Hard tissue: None; soft tissue: buccal tissue of mandibular molars
   d. Hard tissue: Premolars, cuspid, incisors, and associated supporting structures of the maxilla; soft tissue: tissue overlying facial tissues and the lip

4. a. Mental, long buccal, and lingual
   b. Posterior superior alveolar, infiltration over the mesiobuccal root of the first molar, or middle superior alveolar; a greater palatine if the patient's palate is sensitive to the clamp
   c. Mandibular facial infiltration in the area of the central incisor

CHAPTER 32

1. Conscious sedation refers to a state of relaxation or central nervous system depression in which the patient remains conscious at all times. A conscious patient is defined as one who is capable of rational response to command and has all protective reflexes, such as maintenance of an airway and the cough reflex, intact.

2. a'. Inorganic inhalation agent, sweet smelling, and nonflammable
   b'. Has a low blood gas solubility as compared with oxygen
   c. Eliminated unchanged by the lungs
   d'. A mildly potent anesthetic when administered with oxygen
   e'. Affects the person's psychologic reaction to pain perception

3. a. The patient with emphysema has a compromised

respiratory system. Various concentrations of oxygen may decrease this person's ability to function. Expiration is difficult and may affect elimination of nitrous oxide from the blood-stream.

  b. Generally the patient with an upper respiratory tract infection is experiencing difficulty in breathing through the nose. Since this is necessary to permit effective inhalation sedation, the patient will not benefit from the procedure.

4. $\dfrac{4}{4+6} = \dfrac{4}{10} = 40\%$

This is higher than the recommended optimal level for sedation (30% to 35%). Although patient responses vary, close observation is necessary to avoid an adverse response to too high a concentration. Although nitrous oxide and oxygen conscious sedation raises the pain threshold, the body perceives the pain and reacts to it. In the case of a tooth extraction, local or regional anesthesia is necessary.

5. Any three of the following: the patient appears lethargic, falls asleep, begins to perspire, complains of nausea, moves in an uncoordinated fashion, becomes uncooperative, and/or reports dreaming. See Table 32-1 for other responses.

CHAPTER 33

1. False. An attempt should be made to provide some service for the child, even if it is just counting teeth with a mouth mirror. The child may be more willing to cooperate if all procedures are carefully explained in simple terms that attract the patient rather than create fear.

2. Carefully explain each procedure, perhaps showing how pieces of equipment to be used function. Child patients may be allowed to manipulate some of the simpler pieces of equipment such as the air-water spray or the dental chair. A child may be allowed to feel the rubber cup. Encourage the patient to ask questions regarding the care he or she will receive so that he or she does not build up unnecessary fears.

3. For the patient who is visually handicapped, the hygienist can communicate by way of the other functioning senses. If the patient can hear, describe the procedures to be performed. Let the patient touch the equipment and hear it work before an intraoral procedure is attempted. Guide the patient with a gentle touch, and support his or her cooperation. Verbally introduce each step of care. Concerning home care techniques, allow the patient to feel the method for brush and floss manipulation, in addition to feeling it intraorally. Repeat each step of instruction as necessary. Emphasize the feel of clean, plaque-free teeth.

4. Implements for delivery of safe dental care: physical restraints, mouth props (bite blocks), steel mirrors, rubber dam application, instruments secured with floss, and thimbles modified for finger protection.

5. Assessments should be made to determine the patient's sensory abilities and ability to communicate before treatment begins so that appropriate modifications can be made. Manipulation of tissue should be kept to a minimum to avoid unnecessary trauma and resultant slower healing. Medical history assessments should be thorough, as complicated medical histories may be encountered when older patients are treated. Appropriate modification based on medical histories should be made.

6. At age 6 months if the child has a developmental disorder or if the parents have poor oral health; other children should be seen between the ages of 18 and 24 months.

7. Only if stains are present. Preferred practice is to have the child (or parent) deplaque the teeth with a brush and fluoride paste, practicing proper technique and checking results with a disclosant. Topical fluoride can then be applied.

8. Depending on the limitation and the patient's ability to use his or her hand, wrist, and fingers, a brush could be modified by heating the plastic handle to turn the brush head in a way that would be more useful. The brush handle could be enlarged or elongated by attaching the brush to an object such as a ball or a wooden dowel. If the patient has head and neck mobility, an electric toothbrush could be mounted on a surface so that the patient could place the mouth on the brush and move the head position. It is important to evaluate the patient's abilities before helping select or create a modified tool.

9. The answer should include at least three of the following responses:
  a. Inform the patient when dentistry should be provided and what to avoid (radiographs, medications, treatment in the first and third trimesters).
  b. Dispel any myths the patient may have about dentistry and pregnancy.
  c. Stress the need for plaque control to prevent gingival inflammation.
  d. Stress the need for a balanced diet and nutrient supplements.
  e. Explain the role of sugar and decay—baby bottle syndrome.
  f. Discuss fluorides, the development of teeth, and/or eruption dates.

10. Xerostomia, rampant caries, and osteoradionecrosis
11. Use of artificial saliva preparations; more frequent rinsing; preparation of foods that are easy to chew and swallow; use of sugarless mints, gum, or candies; use of lubricants on lips; or modifications in the living environment (e.g., vaporizer, air filter)
12. Patients should apply topical fluoride gel using customized fluoride trays once a day during treatment and continuing indefinitely. Choice of gel is dependent on patient's tolerance of an acidic pH; APF and SnF_2 gels have lower (more acidic) pHs than sodium fluoride gels. Brush-on application may be appropriate for patients with good oral hygiene and minimal mouth dryness.
13. Dental care providers can use a drug history to identify medical conditions which exist; it allows them to research oral side effects of prescribed drugs and potential interactions with drugs used for dental treatment; it also provides an opportunity for care providers to assess whether or not the individual is complying with prescribed drug therapy.
14. Periodontal disease, root caries, oral cancer, edentulism
15. Provider of direct patient treatment services, educator of patients and other care providers, dental coordinator or consultant
16. Treatment is provided in bed with the patient propped up slightly; use of fluids for rinsing or use of a foaming dentifrice may be contraindicated due to danger of aspiration of fluids into the lungs; use of portable suction devices is helpful; mouth props may be needed.

CHAPTER 34
1. Walls: Gingival, axial, facial, and incisal
   Line angles: Incisoaxial, facioaxial, gingivoaxial, faciogingival, facioincisal, linguoaxial
2. Generally, for posterior teeth, the anchor tooth is the most distal tooth in the quadrant to provide maximum visibility and access to the operating field. Minimal access is obtained by clamping one tooth distal to the teeth being restored.
3. The clamp and dam can be applied by placing the clamp on the tooth and stretching the dam over the clamp onto the tooth; the dam can be placed over the bow of the clamp, the clamp placed on the tooth, then stretching the dam over the tooth; or the dam can be stretched over the wings of the clamp and both the clamp and wings are placed together.
4. False; varnish is indeed placed under all amalgam restorations; however, it interferes with the setting reaction of composite resin material

5. False; it is important to have contact in centric occlusion but contact in lateral and protrusive movements should be eliminated because of the limited strength of the restoration
6. The matrix band forms the missing wall(s) to complete the "container" into which the amalgam can be condensed. It also restores the proximal anatomical contours and contact areas to the tooth. The wedge adapts the matrix band to the cervical region of the tooth. It also separates the teeth to ensure proximal contact for the restored tooth.
7. a. False; there is no indication for placing calcium hydroxide because calcium hydroxide is effective as a pulp stimulator only when in direct contact with the pulp
   b. True; calcium hydroxide would stimulate the pulp to form secondary dentin
   c. True; calcium hydroxide would protect the pulp from possible irritation from the monomer in the composite resin material
   d. False; there is sufficient thickness of remaining dentin to protect the pulp from potential chemical irritation from the monomer
8. An alloy is any combination of metals
9. An alloy of any metal(s) with mercury is referred to as an amalgam
10. It is silver—42% to 69%
11. They are silver, copper, tin, and zinc
12. It is the process of mixing mercury with an alloy
13. It should be in one pellet or mass that holds together without crumbling, has a slightly dull shine, and does not appear dry or grainy
14. In Class V preparation, the first increment should be placed and condensed along the axial wall at the distogingival line angle. In a Class II MOD preparation, the first increment is placed and condensed against the gingival wall of the distal box.
15. a. The amalgam is more difficult to load, place, and condense
    b. It will not adhere well with the previously placed loads and will be subject to fracture/flaking
16. Mercury vapor is released, resulting in potential mercury poisoning of those present
17. It is an area at the cavosurface where the amalgam is not at the same height as the cavosurface enamel; either too little amalgam was added originally or too much amalgam has been carved away
18. False; light intermittent pressure is used to avoid heat production, which would bring mercury to the surface of the amalgam
19. True; finishing with the least coarse disc leaves the smoothest finish on the surface of the restoration.
20. Phosphoric acid in concentrations of 30% to 40% is applied to the enamel for 30 seconds to 1

minute. The phosphoric acid selectively removes inorganic material from the enamel surface leaving micropores or pits in the surface. The resin component of the composite resin flows into these countless pits to form resin tags which hold tightly by mechanical means to the surface. The many, many tags provide great retention.

21. The setting reaction can be initiated chemically by mixing a reactor with the base material, or it can be activated by exposing the material to a visible light in the blue spectrum. The chemically cured composite resins require no special and expensive light and can be cured in a large mass. The light cured allow methodical shaping of the restoration before curing. It also comes in one paste, which requires no mixing and thus avoids incorporation of air bubbles.

22. A temporary restoration would be placed in situations where the vitality of the pulp is questionable, a tooth has been painful and is awaiting definitive diagnosis, there was insufficient time to place a permanent restoration, or the tooth is awaiting the placement of a cast intracoronal restoration.

23. When removing the calculus, the instrument is placed under the deposit and then activated to remove as much of the deposit as possible. When removing excess amalgam, the amalgam is shaved off in layers to avoid fracturing the amalgam and creating an open margin.

CHAPTER 35

1. Components of a case documentation: health history review, initial clinical findings, chartings, radiographs, study casts, photographs, treatment plan, record of actual treatment, posttreatment findings, and evaluation summary

2. a. Case documentation enhances record keeping by ensuring that accurate data are available for the clinician to follow the patient's care. Documentation of before-and-after treatment establishes the initial condition and treatment outcome. Such information may be useful and necessary for reference and comparison at a later date.

   c. Participating in case documentation procedures is motivating for the patient as he or she is able to realize the changes that have occurred throughout the course of treatment. Examples of other patient documentations demonstrate potential modes of therapy and may aid the patient in making a decision for personal treatment.

CHAPTER 36

1. A system of accountability defines goals that can provide a direction or a target for the daily activities of practice. Such a system can add meaning to a lifetime of clinical practice. Accountability can also develop a support system for encounters with malpractice or third-party payer investigations.

2. The degree to which prevention is emphasized in each day's routine (i.e., the amount of time or effort spent on prevention and preventive educational activities); the overall effect on health levels of the population (maintenance, improvement, or loss of health over time); the degree to which clinical protocols approximate nationally accepted standards, through comparison with published protocols, reviews of the literature, and participation in peer group study clubs; approach behaviors of patients to dental hygiene care through the development of a long-term patient population; personal gratification and health; cost effectiveness; and participation in professional advancement.

3. Decide to live with the dissatisfaction or develop a plan for change

INDEX

Page numbers in *italics* indicate boxes and illustrations. Page
numbers followed by *t* indicate tables.

791

Blood pressure—cont'd
  measurement of, technique for, 171-174
Boiling water for disinfection, 41
Bonding of composite resin restorations, 722
    class III, 727-728
    class V, 725
Bone levels, charting of, in periodontal examination, 255
Bony defects, charting of, in periodontal examination, 255
Boxing wax for pouring study model, 302, *304*
Brachial pulse, location of, 166
Brush, interproximal, in plaque control, 377, *379*
Brushite in calculus formation, 226
Buccal mucosa in intraoral examination, 188-189
Buccal pocket walls in soft tissue curettage, 478-479
Buccal views, posterior, photographic technique for, 331
Bulimia nervosa, identification of, 194
Bulla, definition of, 177

C

Cabinetry, storage, 19
Calcification as natural defense mechanism of pulp, 578
Calcium in general and oral health, 393-394
Calcium carbonate in toothpastes, 511
Calcium pyrophosphate in toothpastes, 511
Calculus
  burnished, 224
  charting of, 219, 227-229
  clinical significance of, 224-225
  deposits of
    crustaceous, 223
    fern-like, 224
    fine, removing, 443-466; *see also* Scaling, fine
    finger-like, 224
    heavy, removing, 409-441
      by hand scaling, 409-425; *see also* Scaling, hand
      by ultrasonic and sonic instruments, 426-441
    nodular, 224
    spicular, 224
    supragingival, 223-224
    supramarginal, 223-224
    types of, 223-224
  detection of, 223-230
  formation of, stages of, 225-227
  periodontal disease and, 445
  scoring of, 229-230
Camera system for intraoral photography
  bellows, 318-319, 320
  instant close-up, 317
  loading film in, 325
  macro-lens, 318, *319*
  making photograph with, 327-328
  removing film in, 327
  selecting, 316-321
    camera adjustments in, 320-321

Camera system for intraoral photography—cont'd
  selecting—cont'd
    camera body in, 318
    film selection in, 321
    lens in, 318-319
    lighting units in, 319-320
    viewing system in, 318
Cancer
  diet and, 396-397
  oral
    in elderly, 643
    self-examination for, 196-200
  patient with, dental management of, 630-638
    education in, 637-638
    oral problems specific to, 632-637
    pretherapy, 632
    therapy type and, 631-632
Carbohydrates
  dental caries and, 395-396
  in general and oral health, 391-392
Cardiac arrest
  emergency management of, 146
  signs, symptoms, and treatment for, 139*t*
Caries, 234
  charting of, 215
  diet and, 395-396
  fluoride and, 536-537
  rampant, complicating radiation therapy for cancer, 635
  recurrent, charting of, 215
  root, in elderly, 643
  tooth discoloration from, 510
Carotid pulse, location of, 166
Caruncle, sublingual, 189
Case documentation
  implementation phase in, 743-744
  orthodontic, 753, *754-760*
  patient assessment in, 743
  patient planning in, 743
  posttreatment evaluation in, 744
  presentation of, 743-744, *745-752*
  procedures for, 743
Case presentation, 343-351*t*
  designing, 340-341
Casts, diagnostic, 289-313; *see also* Study models
Cavity preparation(s)
  Class I, 652-653, *654*
  Class II, 655-656, *657*
  Class III, *657, 658*
  Class IV, 658
  Class V, 658, *659*
  classification and nomenclature of, 652
Centric occlusion, 279
Centric relation, 279-280
  in occlusal analysis, 283-284, *285*
Cepacol in daily plaque control, 385